T0226121

KGMU BOOK OF
CLINICAL CASES IN MEDICAL SCIENCES

KGMU BOOK OF
CLINICAL CASES IN MEDICAL SCIENCES

The Georgians

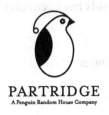

PARTRIDGE
A Penguin Random House Company

To order additional copies of this book, contact
Partridge India
000 800 10062 62
orders.india@partridgepublishing.com

www.partridgepublishing.com/india

KGMU BOOK OF
CLINICAL CASES IN MEDICAL SCIENCES

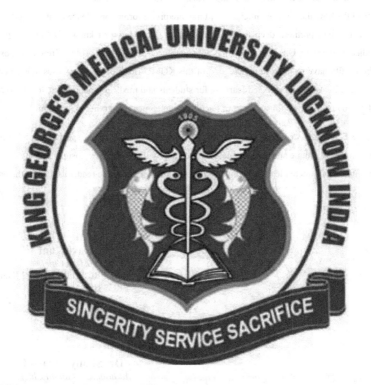

Editor In Chief
Dr. Ravi Kant
Vice Chancellor, KGMU, Lucknow
FRCS (England), FRCS (Ireland), FRCS(Edinburgh), FRCS (Glasgow), FAMS, MS, DNB, FACS, FAIS

Additional Editor-In Chief
Dr. Shally Awasthi
Head, Department of Medical Education & Prof. of Pediatrics, KGMU, Lucknow
MD, DNB, MMSc, FNAS, FIAS, FIAP, FAMS

Preface

It is an accepted fact that teaching and learning are driven by assessment. This could be formal assessment, as during the examinations, or informal self assessment. There are various tools for assessment of knowledge but the most reliable, valid and objective one is the use of multiple choice questions. The art of writing a multiple choice question testing the higher domains of learning requires an experienced writer with critical thinking skills. An ideal writer is a medical teacher. Teachers' close interaction with the students makes them understand the how the students interpret and misinterpret information. Hence clinical vignettes prepared by experienced teachers promote deep thinking and test the core imbibed knowledge of examinees. King George's Medical University, U.P., Lucknow, has an experienced faculty of 400 plus. Knowledge, expertise and wisdom of the faculty have resulted in the creation of this KGMU Book of Clinical Cases in Medical Sciences. This will serve as a book for self directed learning for students and medical practitioners. Institutions elsewhere will be benefitted by using this book as a part of Faculty Development Program for Assessment.

Medical Science is vast. We have compiled clinical vignettes from 31 specialties and sub-specialties and this makes the book unique and remarkable. Each reading will result in new insight into the subject. This in turn would promote self-directed learning which would result in benefit of the reader as well as the patients.

Dr. Ravi Kant
Editor –In Chief
FRCS (Engl). FRCS (Edin), FRCS (Glasg),
FRCS (IREL), MS, DNB
Vice Chancellor,
King George's Medical University,
Lucknow (UP) India

Dr. Shally Awasthi
Additional Editor-In Chief
MD (Pediatrics) DNB (Pediatrics) MMSc
(Clin Epid, USA)
Professor, Department of Pediatrics
Head, Department of Medical Education
King George's Medical University,
Lucknow

FOREWORD

I thank Professor Shally Awasthi for asking me to write Foreword of this book entitled, "KGMU Book of Clinical Cases." When I remember my days as an undergraduate (MB,BS – 1957-62), and post-graduate (MS, Surgery – 1962-65) student and examinee, we used to get a question paper (two question papers in each subject), one of external examiner and the other of internal examiner having 4 long descriptive questions and one "write short notes on 4-5 small topics". This system worked very well for many long years.

During subsequent years as the number of teaching institutions and teachers increased some people started questioning this system of examination and said that it is not the test of complete knowledge (extent of knowledge) of a candidate. It is a sort of a 'chance' examination. As a large number of students used to do selective study depending upon the "guess" of some members of faculty and also on the utterances of the Professor and Head of the concerned Department a few days or weeks before the examination when the papers were being set.

When I became a teacher in Surgery in 1966 and an examiner, I modified the paper on my own (without any objection from anybody) to increase the range of questioning in the following manner –

- First two long questions consisted of one about a disease (etiology, pathology, clinical features, investigations and treatment), and the other about the causes, differential diagnosis and treatment of a symptom or sign.
- Next two long questions consisted of one, "what are the causes or signs or complications of –
- Fifth question as usual short notes on 4-5 topics.

This system of examination paper examined the depth, descriptive power and extent of knowledge.

Present system of objective questioning

The present examination system is entirely based on a battery of short questions with 4-5 answers with one correct answer which has to be marked by the candidate. Hence, it tests a candidate extensively on that particular subject. But it has led to:

- Reduction of serious or deep study of textbooks as most of questions was superficial with 'spot the diagnosis' type of answers, not made by deep learning, thinking and planning.
- It increased the demand of objective question-answer books and reduced the demand of serious textbooks. The market is now flooded with objective question-answer type books.
- Additionally, the one-year period of internship lost its clinical learning and training appeal, and became a preparatory year for PGME.

KGMU book of clinical cases

This book is the result of deep thinking and planning questions on a clinical problem by a team of dedicated teachers on each subject. The answers to these questions can only be given by carefully understanding the problem. It is hoped that this system will stimulate or force students to do serious study not only to remember but assimilate the subject.

I congratulate Prof Ravi Kant, Professor Shally Awasthi and their team of learned teachers to bring out this excellent book.

Whatever is old is not all bad and whatever is new is not all good. Hence, I will suggest the examination paper should have 50% of old system and 50% of new system, when the candidates will be examined both in depth and extent.

Dr T. C. Goel
Professor Emeritus of Surgery
King George's Medical University, Lucknow

FOREWORD

The editor Hon'ble Vice Chancellor Dr. Ravi Kant must be congratulated for having initiated this book written by almost all faculty members of the King George's Medical University. The book has been compiled keeping the requirements of undergraduates, postgraduates and clinicians in an easy multiple choice format as is the requirement today in all International Medical Universities. To keep up with the continued and rapid evolution of internal medicine practices and advances in management is an arduous task. The subjects chosen include Anatomy, Physiology, Biochemistry, Pharmacology, Toxicology, Pathology, Community Medicine, Obstetrics & Gynaecology, Anesthesiology, Forensic Medicine, Internal Medicine, Radiology, Radiotherapy, Pediatrics, Respiratory Medicine, Translational Medicine, Neurology, Cardiology, Psychiatry, Nephrology, Endocrinology, Gastroenterology, Haematology, Medical emergencies along with Dermatology which cover the entire gamut of the MBBS course. The illustrations and photographs of cases, CT scans and MRI's are very well presented. However, I feel the undergraduates need a more detailed description of disease as was in vogue two decades ago as it is important that they write sentences correctly and as future medical teachers are able to convey in simple language (English) details of various medical conditions. I am happy to recommend the book to all clinicians, undergraduate and postgraduate students pursuing MD, DM and DNB. Practicing physicians will also find perusing this book a rewarding experience.

Devika Nag
Emeritus Professor
Department of Neurology
King George's Medical University U.P.
Lucknow

Dr. Surya Kant, *Professor & Head*
Dr. Ajay Kumar Verma, *Assistant Professor*

Section Editors:
1. **Otolaryngology**
   Dr. Anupam Mishra, *Professor*
2. **Forensic Medicine**
   Dr. Anoop Kumar Verma, *Professor & Head*
3. **Physiology**
   Dr. Sunita Tiwari, *Professor & Head*

Section Editors:
1. **Microbiology**
   Dr. Vimala Venkatesh, *Professor*
2. **Pathology**
   Dr. Ashutosh Kumar, *Professor*

Section Editors:
1. **Anesthesiology**
   Dr. Jaishri Bogra, *Professor & Head*
   Dr. Anita Malik, *Professor*
2. **Surgical Gastroenterology**
   Dr. Abhijeet Chandra, *Professor & Head*
3. **Surgery (Gen.)**
   Dr. Abhinav Sonkar, *Professor & Head*
4. **Physical Medicine & Rehabilitation**
   Dr. Anil Kumar Gupta, *Assistant Professor*

ACKNOWLEDGEMENT

We acknowledge the intellectual inputs and time devoted by the faculty of King George's Medical University Lucknow. We are grateful to the patients who formed the basis of case scenarios. We thank Mr. Nikhil Saxena for his tireless efforts in computing and formatting and other staff, Mr. Mohammad Faizan Siddiqui for facilitating the logistics and coordination.

I N D E X

Chapter-1

Anatomy

CEREBELLUM
Dr. A. K. Srivastava, Professor, Department of Anatomy

A 56 year old man who is a chronic alcoholic, visited a doctor when he noticed that he had a tremor in his right hand whenever he attempted to shave, button his shirt or when he tried to insert the key in the lock. He also noticed that he developed a tendency to fall on his right side during walking. On examination, the doctor found hypotonia of muscles of upper and lower limb of right side. When the patient was asked to walk heel to toe along a straight line, the patient swayed to the right side. Speech was normal and nystagmus was not present.

1. Which part of the brain is likely to be involved?
    (A) Cerebrum
    (B) Cerebellum
    (C) Basal ganglia
    (D) Brain stem
2. Majority of the efferent fibres from the cerebellum are carried via
    (A) Superior cerebellar peduncle
    (B) Middle cerebellar peduncle
    (C) Inferior cerebellar peduncle
    (D) All of the above
3. A medulloblastoma involving the vermis in children will mostly present in the form of
    (A) Truncal ataxia
    (B) Tremor
    (C) Disorder of speech
    (D) Disturbance of gait
4. The type of tremor seen in cerebellar disease is
    (A) Essential tremor
    (B) Resting tremor
    (C) Intention tremor
    (D) Postural tremor

Answers:
1. B
    Essential function of Cerebellum is to coordinate muscle activity, body posture and muscle tone.
2. A
    Fibres from the dentate, emboliform and globose nucleus leave through the superior peduncle whereas the fibres from fastigial nucleus leave through the inferior peduncle.
3. A
    Vermis controls the muscle coordination of the head and trunk.
4. C
    Voluntary muscles contract irregularly and weakly causing tremor, seen when movements like shaving, buttoning the shirt etc. are attempted.

Reference:

1. Snell RS. Clinical Neuroanatomy, 7th edition.New Delhi: Wolters Kluwer (India) Pvt. Ltd.; Chapter 6, The cerebellum and its connections. 2010, pp 233-245.

CEREBROSPINAL FLUID CIRCULATION
Dr. A. K. Srivastava, Professor, Department of Anatomy

A 2 year old child is brought to the hospital by his parents because of the large size of his head as compared to other children of his age. After a careful history and examination of the child he is diagnosed as a case of hydrocephalus.
1. The cerebrospinal fluid (CSF) is formed by the
    (A) Choroid fissure
    (B) Choroid plexus
    (C) Arachnoid villi
    (D) Arachnoid granulation

2. The CSF leaves the ventricles of the brain and enters the subarachnoid space through openings in the
    (A) Lateral ventricle
    (B) Third ventricle
    (C) Cerebral aqueduct
    (D) Fourth ventricle
3. A non communicating type of hydrocephalus may develop due to
    (A) Obstruction of internal jugular vein
    (B) Obstruction of foramen of Magendie
    (C) Obstruction of cerebral aqueduct
    (D) Sagittal sinus thrombosis

Answers:
    1. B
        The CSF is formed mainly in the choroid plexus of the lateral, 3rd & 4th ventricle. Some of it is also originates from ependymal cell lining the ventricles and from the brain substance through periventricular spaces.
    2. D
        From the 4th ventricle fluid passes through median aperture and lateral foramina of lateral recesses to the subarachnoid space.
    3. C
        In non communicating hydrocephalous, the raised CSF pressure is due to blockage at some point between its formation and exit.

Reference:
    1. Snell RS. Clinical Neuroanatomy, 7th edition.New Delhi: Wolters Kluwer (India) Pvt. Ltd.; Chapter 16, The ventricular system, the cerebrospinal fluid, and the blood brain and blood CSF barriers. 2010, pp 459 -467.

FUNCTIONAL AREAS OF CEREBRUM
Dr. P. K. Sharma, Professor, Department of Anatomy

A 64 year old woman suffered from a cerebrovascular lesion. Following recovery she was found to have a difficulty in speech. She was able to understand spoken speech but had difficulty in understanding written speech.
1. A defect in understanding written speech is called
    (A) Agnosia
    (B) Aphasia
    (C) Alexia
    (D) Agraphia
2. Motor speecharea of Broca is present in the
    (A) Inferior frontal gyrus
    (B) Inferior parietal gyrus
    (C) Precentral gyrus
    (D) Postcentral gyrus
3. Damage to the cerebral cortex posterior to primary auditory area would cause
    (A) Aphasia
    (B) Acalculia
    (C) Word blindness
    (D) Word deafness
4. The inability of a person to recognize a key placed in his hands when his eyes are closed (Astereognosis) would occur due to lesions involving
    (A) Superior Parietal lobule
    (B) Inferior Parietal lobule
    (C) Occipital lobe
    (D) Post central gyrus

Answers:
    1. C
        Damage to angular gyrus often leads to alexia meaning inability to read.

2. A

Motor speech area of Broca , Brodmann areas 44 and 45 are located in the inferior frontal gyrus of the dominant hemisphere.

3. D

Damage posterior to the primary auditory area damages the secondary auditory area which causes failure in interpretation of sounds(word deafness).

4. A

Lesions of superior parietal lobule damage the somesthetic association areas and the person is unable to appreciate texture, form and size with eyes closed.

Reference:

1. Snell RS. Clinical Neuroanatomy. 7th edition. New Delhi Wolters Kluwer/ Lippincott Williams & Wilkins; Chapter 8, The structure and functional localization of the cerebral cortex. 2010, pp 296-297.

FUNCTIONAL AREAS OF CEREBRUM

Dr. P. K. Sharma, Professor, Department of Anatomy

A 45 year old right handed man suffered with severe headache. A few minutes later he became unconscious and was taken to the emergency. Later he regained consciousness, but, continued to suffer from severe headache. He gave history of hypertension of long duration. There was weakness on the lower right side of face and his speech was slurred. On examination there was weakness and sensory loss in the right upper limb.

1. Which artery is most likely to be involved in the cerebro vascular accident in above case?
   (A) Middle meningeal artery
   (B) Posterior cerebral artery
   (C) Middle cerebral artery
   (D) Anterior cerebral artery
2. Why there is weakness in only lower half of right side of face?
   (A) Cortical area for upper part of face is supplied by anterior cerebral artery
   (B) Bilateral cortical representation of upper part of face
   (C) Involvement of facial nerve at the level of pons
   (D) Bilateral supply of upper part of face by facial nerve
3. Slurring of speech in above case is due to involvement of Brodman area number-
   (A) 4 of left side
   (B) 4 of right side
   (C) 44,45 of left side
   (D) 44,45 of right side

Answers:

1. C

Occlusion of the middle cerebral artery may produce contralateral hemiparesis and hemisensory loss involving mainly the face and arm(precentral and post central gyrus) and aphasia if the left hemisphere is affected.

2. B

The part of facial nerve nucleus that supplies the upper part of face receives corticonuclear fibers from both cerebral hemispheres so a unilateral damage will not manifest as paralysis in upper part of face.

3. D

Motor speech area of Broca (Brodmann areas 44 and 45), is located in the inferior frontal gyrus. This area is important on the left/ dominant hemisphere and ablation of this area will result in paralysis of speech.

References:

1. Snell RS. Clinical Neuroanatomy. 7th edition. New Delhi: Wolters Kluwer/ Lippincott Williams & Wilkins; Chapter 17, The blood supply of the brain and spinal cord. 2010, pp 483.
2. Snell RS. Clinical Neuroanatomy. 7th edition. New Delhi: Wolters Kluwer/ Lippincott Williams & Wilkins; Chapter 11, The cranial nerve nuclei and their central connections and distribution. 2010, pp 346.
3. Snell RS. Clinical Neuroanatomy.7th edition. New Delhi: Wolters Kluwer/ Lippincott Williams & Wilkins; Chapter 8, The structure and functional localization of the cerebral cortex. 2010, pp 290.

TRACHEO-OESOPHAGEAL FISTULA

Dr. Navneet Kumar, Professor, Department of Anatomy

Two days old infant was admitted in pediatrics ward with complaints of increase rate of breathing, cough and recurrent regurgitation of milk. On examination, respiratory rate was 50/ minute, child was cyanosed and bronchial breathing was present in right lung. DLC showed 20% lymphocytes and 80% neutrophils. Chest radiograph revealed consolidation of right lung and stomach full of air.

1. Which anomaly is present in this patient?
   - (A) Hiatus hernia
   - (B) Hirschsprung's disease
   - (C) Volvulus
   - (D) Tracheo esophageal fistula
2. Esophageal epithelium develops from
   - (A) Endoderm Foregut
   - (B) Ectoderm Mid gut
   - (C) Mesoderm Hind gut
3. Stomodeum 3. Lungs develop from
   - (A) Foregut
   - (B) Mid gut
   - (C) Hind gut
   - (D) Stomodeum

Answers:
1. D

   Newly born child with breathing problem and stomach full of air define the connection   between esophagus and trachea ie trachea- esophageal fistula.
2. A
3. A

Reference:
1. Gordon A Mackinlay. Surgical pediatrics. In: Neil McIntosh, Peter J. Helms, Rosalind L Smyth, Stuart Logan, Forfer & Arneil's editors. Text book of pediatrics. 7th edition. Edinburgh. Churchill Livingstone Elsevier 2008.

CHROMOSOMAL ANOMALY

Dr. Navneet Kumar, Professor, Department of Anatomy

A 6 month old child presented with complaints of growth retardation, low-set ears, protruded swelling in abdomen and bluish discoloration of skin. On examination severe developmental delay, strawberry-shaped head, club feet, omphalocoel and abnormal heart sounds were found. An investigation revealed Ventricular Septal Defect and after karyotyping diagnosis of Edward syndrome was made.

1. Which chromosomal anomaly is present in this patient?
   - (A) Trisomy 21
   - (B) Trisomy 18
   - (C) Fragile X chromosome
   - (D) Triple X chromosome
2. What is the sequence of Edward syndrome, Patau syndrome and Down syndrome?
   - (A) Trisomy 18, 15, 21
   - (B) Trisomy, 21, 13, 18
   - (C) Trisomy, 15, 18, 21
   - (D) Trisomy, 18, 13, 21
3. Omphalocoeal is
   - (A) Partial intestine outside abdominal wall
   - (B) Testis in inguinal canal
   - (C) Enlarge umbilicus due to intestinal loop
   - (D) Urinary bladder without anterior abdominal wall

Answers:
1. B

2. D
3. A

Reference:

1. Michael A. Patton. Genetics. In: Neil McIntosh, Peter J. Helms, Rosalind L Smyth, Stuart Logan, Forfer & Arneil's editors. Text book of pediatrics. 7th edition. Edinburgh. Churchill Livingstone Elsevier 2008.

BRAIN STEM LESION
Dr. Punita Manik, Professor, Department of Anatomy

A 60 years old woman was admitted to the hospital with the complaints of sudden onset of bouts of vomiting, hiccups and severe dizziness (vertigo). She also mentioned that she had hot and painful sensation in the skin of the left side of the face. On examination it was noticed that the soft palate moved to the right side when asked to say "ah". Drooping of the left upper eyelid, sunken left eyeball and a constricted pupil on the left side was also seen. Pain and temperature sensations were impaired in the trunk and extremities on the right side.

1. What is the diagnosis of the above mentioned case?
   (A) Lateral medullary syndrome
   (B) Medial medullary syndrome
   (C) Weber's Syndrome
   (D) Millard Gubler's syndrome
2. Which of the following arteries is involved in this syndrome?
   (A) Posterior inferior cerebellar
   (B) Anterior spinal
   (C) Posterior spinal
   (D) Basilar
3. Which of the following nucleus is involved in causing sudden onset of bouts of vomiting, hiccups and severe dizziness (vertigo) ?
   (A) Nucleus Ambiguous
   (B) Vestibular Nucleus
   (C) Medial Lemniscus
   (D) Spinal nucleus of trigeminal nerve
4. Impaired pain and temperature sensations on the right side of the trunk was due to the involvement of
   (A) Inferior cerebellar peduncle
   (B) Spinothalamic tract
   (C) Pyramidal tract
   (D) Spinal tract and nucleus
5. Drooping of the upper eyelid, sunken eyeball and constricted pupil on the left side were due to the involvement of
   (A) Spinothalamic tract
   (B) Spinal tract and nucleus
   (C) Descending sympathetic fibres
   (D) Inferior cerebellar peduncle

Answers:

1. A
   The diagnosis of the above mentioned case is Lateral medullary syndrome.

2. A
   The posterolateral region of medulla oblongata is supplied by medullary branches of posterior inferior cerebellar artery (PICA). It supplies nucleus ambiguus, nucleus of tractus solitarius, vestibular nucleus, spinal nucleus and tract of trigeminal nerve, spinothalamic tracts, inferior cerebellar peduncle and descending sympathetic fibres.

3. B
   The vestibular nucleus is present in the lateral part of grey matter of medulla oblongata near the inferior cerebellar peduncle.

4. B
   Spinothalamic tract is situated posterolateral to the inferior olivary nucleus and carries pain and temperature sensations from the contralateral half of the body.

5. C
   Involvement of the descending sympathetic fibres in the reticular formation leads to Horner's syndrome on the ipsilateral side.

Reference:
1. Snell RS. Clinical Neuroanatomy, 7th edition. New Delhi: Wolters Kluwer/ Lippincott Williams & Wilkins; Chapter 11, The Brainstem. 2010, pp 217 - 218.

SPINAL CORD LESION
Dr. Punita Manik, Professor, Department of Anatomy

A 40 year old man came to the hospital with the complaints of gradual onset of weakness in the legs, arms and trunk, tingling & numbness which had progressively worsened. On examination, there was bilateral spastic paresis. He also had bilateral loss of vibration, pressure and touch sense, exaggerated tendon reflexes and positive Babinski's sign.

1. What is the most probable diagnosis?
   (A) Tabes dorsalis
   (B) Syringomyelia
   (C) Subacute combined degeneration
   (D) Brown Sequard syndrome
2. Which level of spinal cord is commonly involved in above disease?
   (A) Cervical
   (B) Upper thoracic
   (C) Lower thoracic
   (D) Lumbosacral
3. Which of the following tracts are commonly involved?
   (A) Posterior column
   (B) Anterior spinothalamic
   (C) Lateral spinothalamic
   (D) Tectospinal
4. Bilateral exaggerated tendon reflexes and positive Babinski's sign is due to involvement of
   (A) Lateral corticospinal tract
   (B) Lateral spinothalamic tract
   (C) Dorsal column
   (D) Anterior spinothalamic tract

Answers:
   1. C
      Subacute combined degeneration of the spinal cord causes bilateral spastic paresis and loss of vibration, pressure and touch sense, exaggerated tendon reflexes and positive Babinski's sign.
   2. D
      Usually affects lumbosacral region of the cord.
   3. A
      Bilateral Posterior column and Lateral corticospinal tracts are involved in this disease.
   4. A
      Involvement of upper motor neuron fibres lead to spastic paralysis, exaggerated tendon reflexes and positive Babinski's sign which is also positive in new born and infants due to incomplete myelination of the corticospinal fibres.

Reference:
1. Snell RS. Clinical Neuroanatomy, 7th edition. New Delhi: Wolters Kluwer/ Lippincott Williams & Wilkins; Chapter 11, The Brainstem. 2010, pp 340-360.

CRANIAL NERVE INJURY
Dr. Jyoti Chopra, Professor, Department of Anatomy

A 25 year old football player came to an ophthalmologist with a complaint of double vision particularly when he goes down stairs for last two weeks. He told that three weeks ago he had a severe blow on his head following which he lost consciousness. After few minutes he was all right so he didn't consult any doctor. On examination, it was observed that his head was tilted towards right side. The doctor asked him to follow his finger with his head in straight position. When he asked him to look towards right and then downwards, his left eye was unable to move downwards. On looking vertically downwards his left eye was slightly deviated towards medial side.

1. In your opinion which nerve has been damaged?
   (A) Occulomotor

(B) Trochlear
(C) Trigeminal
(D) Abducens

2. This nerve emerges from which part of brainstem?
   (A) Right ventral pons
   (B) Left ventral pons
   (C) Right dorsal midbrain
   (D) Left dorsal midbrain

3. When the doctor asks to look towards right and then downwards which muscle of left eye is being tested?
   (A) Lateral rectus
   (B) Inferior rectus
   (C) Superior oblique
   (D) Inferior oblique

4. When doing the above maneuver which muscle of right eye is being tested?
   (A) Lateral rectus
   (B) Inferior rectus
   (C) Superior oblique
   (D) Inferior oblique

5. Which muscle is responsible for medial deviation of left eye on looking vertically downwards?
   (A) Lateral rectus
   (B) Inferior rectus
   (C) Superior oblique
   (D) Inferior oblique

Answers:

1. B

   Superior oblique is supplied by trochlear nerve.

2. C

   Trochlear nerve is the only cranial nerve that emerges from dorsal surface of brainstem (midbrain) and decussates immediately with the nerve of opposite side.

3. C

   The pulley of superior oblique muscle lies medial and anterior to its insertion. To test this muscle patient is asked to look medially, thus placing the muscle in optimum position and then is asked to look downward. If it is paralyzed patient fails to look downwards.

4. B

   The origin of inferior rectus muscle is situated medial to its insertion. To test this muscle patient is asked to look laterally (thus placing the muscle in optimum position to lower the eyeball) and then is asked to look downward.

5. B

   When patient is asked to look vertically downwards, both superior oblique and inferior rectus are tested, if superior oblique is paralyzed eye will be deviated slightly medially due to unopposed action of inferior rectus.

References:

1. Snell RS. Clinical Anatomy by Regions. 9th edition. New Delhi: Wolters Kluwer/ Lippincott Williams & Wilkins; Chapter 11, The Head and Neck. 2012 pp 551, 557-559.
2. Snell RS. Clinical Neuroanatomy. 7th edition. New Delhi Wolters Kluwer/ Lippincott Williams & Wilkins; Chapter 11, Cranial nerve nuclei and their central connections and distribution. 2010, pp 340, 360.

PARKINSON DISEASE

Dr. Jyoti Chopra, Professor, Department of Anatomy

A 50 year old man was brought to the neurologist by his son with complaints of difficulty in initiating and performing new movements, slow shuffling gait, slurred speech and tremors. The doctor observed that his facial expression was mask like, swinging movement of arm while walking was absent and tremors disappeared when he was asked to write. When he tried to flex his arm, he felt a series of jerks, similar to cogwheel. Superficial and deep reflexes were normal.

1. Damage to which structure may cause such problem?
    (A) Substantia gelatinosa
    (B) Substantia nigra
    (C) Cerebellum
    (D) Caudate nucleus
2. Deficiency of which neurotransmitter is responsible for these symptoms?
    (A) Dopamine
    (B) Glutamate
    (C) GABA
    (D) Serotonin
3. The motor symptoms are caused because of _____ output to motor cortex from basal nuclei
    (A) Decreased inhibitory
    (B) Decreased excitatory
    (C) Increased inhibitory
    (D) Increased excitatory

Answers:
    1. B
        Patient is suffering from Parkinson disease, a degenerative disease, involving substantia nigra.
    2. A
        There is degeneration of dopamine secreting cells of substantia nigra.
    3. C
        The basal ganglia normally exert a constant inhibitory influence on a wide range of motor systems, preventing them from becoming active at inappropriate times. When a decision is made to perform a particular action, inhibition is reduced for the required motor system, thereby releasing it for activation. Dopamine acts to facilitate this release of inhibition. When the dopamine level is low it causes increased inhibition of motor cortex.

Reference:
    1. Snell RS. Clinical Neuroanatomy. 7th edition. New Delhi: Wolters Kluwer/ Lippincott Williams & Wilkins; Chapter 10, Basal nuclei and their connections. 2010, pp 322-325.

INTRACRANIAL HEMORRHAGE
Dr. Anita Rani, Professor, Department of Anatomy

An 18 year old boy was brought to the trauma center in unconscious state by his friend following a hit by a cricket ball on his right temple region. His friend told the medical officer that immediately after the hit, the boy fall down and was unconscious for about 10 minutes. He gained consciousness for some time. On examination, his skull did not show any evidence of fracture. An urgent CT scan confirmed right sided extradural hemorrhage.

1. The term extradural refers to the potential space between
    (A) Inner table of skull bones and their periosteum
    (B) Inner periosteum of the skull bones and meningeal duramater
    (C) Duramater and arachnoid mater
    (D) Piamater and brain substance
2. Which of the following region of the lateral wall of skull is thinnest?
    (A) Parietal eminence
    (B) Pterion
    (C) Asterion
    (D) Zygomatic arch
3. Damage to which of the following structure may lead to extradural hemorrhage in this region?
    (A) Petrosquamous sinus
    (B) Middle meningeal vessels
    (C) Middle cerebral artery
    (D) Superficial temporal vessels

4. Which of the following area of the cerebral hemisphere is most vulnerable for compression by collected blood in this region?
   - (A) Area around central sulcus
   - (B) Visual area
   - (C) Premotor area
   - (D) Insula
5. Centre of Pterion can be marked on the temporal fossa by placing your fingers
   - (A) 4 cm above the midpoint of zygomatic arch
   - (B) Just behind the frontozygomatic suture
   - (C) Just infront of tragus
   - (D) On the pulsations of superficial temporal artery

Answers:

1. A
   Cerebral dura mater consists of two layers, outer endosteal layer is the one which forms the periosteum of skull bones and the inner menigeal layer actually protects the brain. The space between endosteal layer and inner table of bone is described as Epidural or Extradural space.

2. B
   Area of lateral skull where anteroinferior angle of parietal bone, greater wing of sphenoid,frontal and squamous part of temporal bone articulate with each other at a H shaped suture, is termed as pterion . This is the thinnest area and is most likely to injure when hit.

3. B
   Middle meningeal artery and vein runs deep to petrion in extradural space.

4. A
   Anterior branch of middle meningeal artery ascends upwards parallel to central sulcus.

5. A
   To drain the blood, burr hole is made through pterion.

Reference:

1. Snell RS. Clinical Anatomy By Regions. 9th edition. New Delhi: Wolters Kluwer/ Lippincott Williams & Wilkins; Chapter 11, The Head and Neck. 2012, pp 532, 543.

SWELLING IN THE POSTERIOR TRIANGLE OF NECK

Dr. Anita Rani, Professor, Department of Anatomy

A 7 year old boy, resident of Kanpur district, was brought to a pediatric OPD, with complaint of painless swelling in right side of his neck. His mother gave history of anorexia and weight loss for last four months and lethargy during evening hours. Physician suspected the swelling as an enlarged and matted lymph nodes. Swelling was located in the posterior triangle of neck in relation to sternocleidomastoid muscle. Thorough examination and lymph node biopsy confirmed the diagnosis of tubercular lymphadenitis.

1. Which of the following group of lymph nodes of head and neck is classified as deep cervical group?
   - (A) Submental, submandibular, retroauricular and occipital
   - (B) Pre-tracheal, prelaryngeal and retropharyngeal
   - (C) Jugulo-omohyoid, jugulo-digastric and supraclavicular
   - (D) Palatine, pharyngeal, lingual and tubal tonsils
2. What is the relationship of jugulo-omohyoid lymph nodes with the sternocleidomastoid muscle?
   - (A) Superficial to muscle along the external jugular vein
   - (B) Along the anterior border of muscle in digastric triangle
   - (C) Along the posterior border of muscle in posterior triangle
   - (D) Deep to muscle around internal jugular vein
3. If the swelling was suspected to arise from jugulo-omohyoid nodes then which of the following areas of head and neck should be examined by the physician to rule out any other primary site of infection in above case?
   - (A) Ear
   - (B) Tonsil
   - (C) Tongue
   - (D) Tooth
4. Which of the following maneuver would you like to perform to confirm the relationship of swelling with right sternocleidomastoid muscle?
   - (A) Extending the neck against resistance
   - (B) Flexing the neck against resistance

(C) Rotating the neck against resistance towards left

(D) Bending the neck towards right

5. While taking the biopsy of lymph node, which important structure has to be taken care of?

(A) Internal Jugular Vein

(B) Spinal Accessory Nerve

(C) Common Carotid Artery

(D) Long thoracic nerve

Answers:

1. C

The lymph nodes of the head and neck are arranged as a regional collar that extends from below the chin to the back of head and as a deep vertical terminal group.

2. D

Jugulo-omohyoid lymph nodes are embedded in the carotid sheath around internal jugular vein, which itself lies deep to sternocleidomastoid muscle.

3. C

Lymphatics from the tongue may directly drain into lower cervical deep lymph nodes (jugulo-omohyoid and supraclavicular group) without involving primary lymph nodes.

4. C

Sternocleidomastoid muscle, when acting on one side helps in turning the head to the opposite site.

5. B

Spinal accessory nerve emerges behind the posterior border of sternocleidomastoid, a little above the middle of it and then runs in a fascial tunnel towards trapezius muscle in the roof of posterior triangle.

Reference:

1. Snell RS. Clinical Anatomy By Regions. 9th edition. New Delhi: Wolters Kluwer/ Lippincott Williams & Wilkins; Chapter 11, The Head and Neck. 2012, pp 603-604.

VOCAL CORD PARALYSIS

Dr. Anita Rani, Professor, Department of Anatomy

A 45 year old female consulted her surgeon with the complaint of alteration in her voice quality after a surgery of thyroid gland , conducted a month back. On laryngoscopy, her right vocal cord was found in cadaveric position and the left cord was shifted towards its right fellow on saying " E".

1. Which one of the following nerves is most likely to be damaged during thyroid surgery leading to vocal cord paralysis?

(A) Superior laryngeal

(B) External laryngeal

(C) Internal laryngeal

(D) Recurrent laryngeal

2. During laryngoscopy, true vocal folds are recognized as

(A) Mobile and avascular

(B) Immobile and vascular

(C) Mobile and vascular

(D) Immobile and avascular

3. In 'Cadaveric Position' the vocal cords are

(A) Midway between abduction and adduction

(B) Adducted

(C) Abducted

(D) Immobile and relaxed

4. Which of the following muscle is responsible for abduction of vocal cord?

(A) Posterior cricoarytenoid

(B) Lateral Cricoarytenoid

(C) Thyroarytenoid

(D) Vocalis

5. In which of the following type of recurrent laryngeal nerve injury, tracheostomy is mandatory to save a person's life?

(A) Unilateral complete section

(B) Bilateral complete section

19

(C) Unilateral partial section

(D) Bilateral partial section

Answers:

1. D

All intrinsic muscles of larynx except cricothyroid are supplied by recurrent laryngeal nerve.

2. A

The vocal fold moves with respiration and its white colour is easily seen when viewed with a laryngoscope. The vestibular fold is fixed and pink in colour.

3. A

In unilateral complete injury of recurrent laryngeal nerve, vocal cord of that side assumes a position midway that of adduction and abduction and is commonly referred as cadaveric position.

4. A

Posterior cricoarytenoid muscle causes abduction of vocal cords.

5. D

In bilateral partial injury of recurrent laryngeal nerve abductors of both vocal cords are paralysed hence rima glottidis is closed and acute breathlessness and stidor results which necessitates immediate cricothyroidotomy or tracheostomy to save life of a person.

Reference:

1. Snell RS. Clinical Anatomy By Regions. 9th edition. New Delhi: Wolters Kluwer/ Lippincott Williams & Wilkins; Chapter 11, The Head and Neck. 2012, pp 644-651.

DIAPHRAGMATIC HERNIA

Dr. Archana Rani, Associate Professor, Department of Anatomy

While examining a one day old male infant who was born via a normal vaginal delivery, the pediatrician noticed that his respiratory rate was increased to 60 (normal=30). Auscultation revealed an absence of breath sounds on the left side but good breath sounds on the right side of the chest. The heart sounds were loudest in the right chest and the abdomen appeared to be scaphoid. The chest x-ray demonstrated bowel within the thorax. The child was diagnosed as a case of congenital postero-lateral diaphragmatic hernia and was ventilated through the endotracheal tube.

1. What are the sources for development of diaphragm?

(A) Septum transversum, pleuroperitoneal membrane, body wall

(B) Body wall, oesophageal mesentery, pericardio-peritoneal canal

(C) Oesophageal mesentery, pleuroperitoneal membrane, foregut

(D) Septum transversum, pleuro-pericardial membrane, liver bud

2. What is the cause of postero-lateral congenital diaphragmatic hernia?

(A) Defect in right crus of diaphragm

(B) Failure of closure of pericardio-peritoneal canal

(C) Congenitally small oesophagus

(D) Failure of development of muscular fibres of diaphragm

3. Above hernia is associated with

(A) Malrotation of midgut loop

(B) Displacement of lung and heart

(C) Disturbed relation of cardio-esophageal junction to diaphragm

(D) Defective development of foregut

Answers:

1. A

Diaphragm develops from the septum transversum, which forms the central tendon of diaphragm; two pleuro-peritoneal membranes; muscular components from somites at cervical segments three to five and the mesentery of oesophagus, in which the crura of the diaphragm develop.

2. B

The cause of postero-lateral congenital diaphragmatic hernia is failure of one or both pleuro-peritoneal membranes to close the pericardio-peritoneal canals.

3. B

The abdominal viscera in the chest push the heart anteriorly and compress the lungs, which are commonly hypoplastic.

Reference:
1. Sadler TW. Langman's Medical Embryology. 11th edition. New Delhi, Philadelphia: Wolters Kluwer Health/ Lippincott Williams & Wilkins; Chapter 11, Body Cavities. 2010, pp 159-162.

DESCENT OF TESTIS

Dr. Archana Rani, Associate Professor, Department of Anatomy

A twenty year old boy was found to have absence of testis on right side of scrotum as he was undergoing medical examination before joining the police force. On deep palpation, a small and firm structure was felt in front of the upper part of right thigh.

1. What is the diagnosis?
   (A) Undescended testis
   (B) Anorchism
   (C) Monorchism
   (D) Ectopic testis
2. The testis appears in scrotum usually between
   (A) 5th-6th month
   (B) 6th-7th month
   (C) 7th-8th month
   (D) 8th-9th month
3. Appendix of testis is a remnant of
   (A) Mesonephric tubules
   (B) Mesonephric duct
   (C) Paramesonephric duct
   (D) Sex cords
4. Sertoli cells are derived from
   (A) Coelomic epithelium
   (B) Mesenchyme of genital ridge
   (C) Primordial germ cells
   (D) Neural crest

Answers:
1. D
   Abnormal position of testis is known as ectopic testis. It may be under the skin of the lower part of abdomen, under the skin of the front of thigh, in the femoral canal, under the skin of the penis and in the perineum behind the scrotum.
2. D
   Testis develops in relation to the lumbar region on the posterior abdominal wall. It gradually descends and reaches the iliac fossa during 3rd month, rests at deep inguinal ring up to the 7th month, traverses the inguinal canal during 7th-8th month and in the scrotum at the end of 8th month of intrauterine life.
3. C
   It is a remnant of degenerated cephalic part of paramesonephric duct.
4. A
   Sertoli cells are derived from coelomic epithelium in the presence of testis determining factor.

Reference:
1. Sadler TW. Langman's Medical Embryology. 11th edition. New Delhi, Philadelphia: Wolters Kluwer Health/ Lippincott Williams & Wilkins; Chapter 15, Urogenital System. 2010, pp 247-248, 260-261.

ALLANTOIC DIVERTICULUM

Dr. Archana Rani, Associate Professor, Department of Anatomy

An eighty year old man complaint of urine discharge from the umbilicus. History revealed that he had difficulty in micturition. After examining him, the surgeon found that he had a benign enlargement of prostate gland.
1. What could be the probable cause of urine discharge from umbilicus?
   (A) Ectopia vesicae
   (B) Patent vitellointestinal duct

(C) Posterior urethral valve

(D) Patent urachus

2. The structure involved in the above case is the remnant of

    (A) Allantoic diverticulum

    (B) Cloaca

    (C) Primitive rectum

    (D) Primitive urogenital sinus

3. How would you explain such late presentation of this congenital anomaly?

    (A) Decreased tone of abdominal muscles

    (B) Decreased tone of detrusor muscle

    (C) Increased intravesical pressure

    (D) Decreased elasticity of periumbilical skin

Answers:

    1. D

    Patent urachus is the condition in which the interior of the urinary bladder communicates with the exterior at the umbilicus.

    2. A

    The structure involved is urachus, which is a remnant of allantoic diverticulum.

    3. C

    Enlargement of prostate gland in the later life causes urinary obstruction. This result inincreased intravesical pressure and urine takes the least pathway of resistance through the urachus to the umbilicus.

Reference:

    1.   Sadler TW. Langman's Medical Embryology. 11th edition. New Delhi, Philadelphia: Wolters Kluwer Health/ Lippincott Williams & Wilkins; Chapter 15, Urogenital System. 2010, pp 243-245.

RADIAL NERVE INJURY

Dr. R.K. Diwan, Assistant Professor, Department of Anatomy

A patient consulted a doctor because he was unable to extend his right wrist. History revealed that 2 days back, he fell down and a local doctor gave him tetanus injection in back of right upper arm. On examination, extension of right wrist and fingers was absent. Extension at right elbow was weaker as compared to left.

1. Which deformity is present in the patient?

    (A) Claw hand

    (B) Ape thumb deformity

    (C) Wrist drop

    (D) Dinner-fork deformity

2. Which nerve is injured in the above deformity?

    (A) Ulnar

    (B) Radial

    (C) Median

    (D) Musculo-cutaneous

3. What is the site of injury of above nerve in relation to humerus?

    (A) Anatomical neck

    (B) Surgical neck

    (C) Bicipital groove

    (D) Spiral groove

4. In which area doctor has to look for sensory loss?

    (A) Dorsal aspect of arm

    (B) Dorsal aspect of arm and forearm

    (C) Dorsal aspect of forearm and hand

    (D) Dorsal aspect of hand

Answers:

    1. C

    The patient is unable to extend the wrist and the fingers; this occurs as result of the weakness of extensors and unopposed action of flexor muscles of wrist.

    2. B

The extensors of wrist and fingers are supplied by radial nerve.
3. D

IM Injection in the upper posterior part of the arm can injure radial nerve in spiral groove.
4. C

In the spiral groove radial nerve gives lower lateral cutaneous nerve of arm and the posterior cutaneous nerve of the forearm .Cutaneous innervations of dorsum of hand androots of lateral 3 and ½ fingers is derived from terminal branches of superficial branch of radial nerve.

Reference:
1. Snell RS. Clinical Anatomy By Regions. 9th edition. Philadelphia: Walter Kluwer/ Lippincott Williams and Wilkins; Chapter 6, The upper limb. 2012, pp 377, 392,431.

FASCIAL SPACES OF HAND
Dr. R.K. Diwan, Assistant Professor, Department of Anatomy

A 55 years old painter cut his left ring finger by sharp edge of broken glass of window. After about 3 to 4 days he developed fever and his entire ring finger was semiflexed, swollen and painful. Any attempt to extend the finger was associated with extreme pain.

1. Infection of which of the following structure can give rise to above presentation?
   (A) Mid palmar space
   (B) Ulnar bursa
   (C) Digital synovial sheath
   (D) Pulp space
2. Infection of ring finger can infect
   (A) Ulnar bursa
   (B) Midpalmar space
   (C) Radial bursa
   (D) Thenar space
3. Which structure is surgically open to drain the pus from mid palmar space?
   (A) Thenar space
   (B) Lumbrical canal
   (C) Space of Parona
   (D) Digital synovial sheath

Answers:
1. C

Infection of a Digital Synovial sheath results in distention of pus, swollen and distended sheath is stretched results in pain.
2. B

Anatomically, the digital sheath of ring finger is related to the midpalmar space.
3. B

The lumbrical canal is a potential space surrounding the tendon of each lumbrical muscle and is normally filled with connective tissue. 2nd, 3[rd]and 4th canals communicates with midpalmar space.

Reference:
1. Snell RS. Clinical Anatomy By regions. 9th edition. Philadelphia: WalterKluwer/ Lippincott Williams and Wilkins; Chapter6: The upper limb. 2012, pp 398-404.

SHOULDER DISLOCATION
Dr. R.K. Diwan, Assistant Professor, Department of Anatomy

A 22 years old badminton player while delivering a shot suffered with severe pain in his right shoulder. He was brought to the casualty. He was holding his arm at the side of the body in external rotation. On examination, his right shoulder was found to be flattened and head of humerus was palpable in the infraclavicular fossa. Orthopedic surgeon tested for sensations on the upper part of arm. On passive abduction of arm contraction of deltoid was felt. An AP radiograph of the shoulder region confirmed the diagnosis of anterior dislocation of head of humerus.

1. Which nerve is injured in the anterior dislocation of shoulder joint?
   (A) Musculocutaneus

(B) Ulnar

(C) Axillary

(D) Median

2. Which of the following muscles cause external rotation at shoulder joint?

    (A) Teres minor and infraspinatus

    (B) Teres major and supraspinatus

    (C) Teres minor and supraspinatus

    (D) Teres major and infraspinatus

3. Which artery is liable to damage in above case?

    (A) Subclavian

    (B) Axillary

    (C) Brachial

    (D) Profunda brachii

Answers:

    1. C

    Anterior dislocation of shoulder joint lead to injury of axillary nerve.

    2. A

    Teres minor and infraspinatus muscle lead to lateral rotation and stabilization of shoulder joint.

    3. B

    Anterior dislocation of shoulder joint lead to injury of axillary artery.

Reference:

1. Kulkarni NV. Clinical Anatomy by the regions. 2nd edition. New Delhi: Jaypee Brother's publication; Chapter 5, The upper Limb. 2012, pp 118-119.

LYMPHATIC DRAINAGE OF BREAST

Dr. R.K.Diwan, Assistant Professor, Department of Anatomy

A 65 years old woman consulted a surgeon with complaint of hard painless lump in her left arm pit. Examination revealed a breast lump of approximately 2 cm in size in upper outer quadrant and loss of mobility of the breast. An enlarged axillary lymph node was palpable on left side. Mammography and FNAC confirmed a diagnosis of breast carcinoma. Chest radiograph did not reveal any abnormality.

1. Lymph from upper and outer quadrant of breast is primarily drained into which group of lymph nodes?

    (A) Supraclavicular

    (B) Anterior axillary

    (C) Central axillary

    (D) Paravertebral

2. Invasion of which of the following structure by cancer cells can lead to fixation of left breast in above case

    (A) Lactiferous duct

    (B) Lymphatics

    (C) Skin of breast

    (D) Ligaments of Cooper

3. Radiological examination of skeletal system is mandatory to rule out bony metastasis in carcinoma breast. What is the route of spread of cancer cells to bones?

    (A) Venous

    (B) Lymphatic

    (C) Arterial

    (D) Transcoelomic

Answers:

    1. B

    Approximately 60% of carcinomas of the breast occur in the upper outer quadrant.

    2. D

    The fibrosed ligaments of cooper, at the base of the breast cause fixation of the breast to the underlying pectoral fascia leading to loss of mobility of the breast.

    3. A

    The cancer cells spread to vertebral column, cranial bones, ribs and femur by entering the venous circulation. During rise in intra-thoracic pressure (in acts like coughing, straining, etc.) there is reversal of blood flow in the inter-vertebral vein, which facilitates the spreadinto the internal vertebral venous plexus, vertebral bodies and cranial bones.

Reference:
1. Kulkarni NV. Clinical Anatomy by the regions. 2nd edition. New Delhi: Jaypee Brother's publication; Chapter 5, The upper Limb. 2012, pp 90-92.

KNEE JOINT INJURY

Dr. Arvind Kumar Pankaj, Assistant Professor, Department of Anatomy

A patient came to an orthopedic OPD and told that while playing football he fell down and since then he is having severe pain at right knee. On examination doctor noticed that there was localized tenderness on the medial side of right knee joint line. Drawer test was negative.

1. On the basis of examination which structure do you think is most probably involved?
    (A) Medial collateral ligament
    (B) Medial Meniscus
    (C) Anterior cruciate ligament
    (D) Poterior cruciate ligament
2. Medial collateral ligament is detached part of which muscle?
    (A) Tibialis anterior
    (B) Extensor digitorum longus
    (C) Adductor magnus
    (D) Semitendinosus
3. Injury of medial meniscus is more common because it is-
    (A) Attached to the capsule of knee joint
    (B) Attached to popliteus muscle
    (C) Attached to medial collateral ligament
    (D) Bigger as compared to lateral meniscus

Answers:
    1. B
        Tenderness at knee joint line is typical of meniscal injury
    2. C
    3. C
        Strong attachment to medial collateral ligament restricts its mobility

Reference:
1. Snell RS. Clinical Anatomy by Regions. 9th edition. New Delhi: Wolters Kluwer/ Lippincott Williams & Wilkins; Chapter 10, Lower Limb. 2012, pp 500-503.

LYMPHATIC DRAINAGE OF LOWER LIMB

Dr. Arvind Kumar Pankaj, Assistant Professor, Department of Anatomy

A 35 years old farmer suffers a cut on the medial side of his right knee while climbing over a palm tree. He presented with an infected wound, high grade fever and painful swelling in the upper part of front of right thigh, in the emergency department five days later.

1. Which group of lymph nodes would be the first to receive drainage from infected area?
    (A) Medial horizontal group of superficial inguinal
    (B) Lateral horizontal group of superficial inguinal
    (C) Vertical group of superficial inguinal
    (D) Deep inguinal
2. Deep inguinal group of lymph nodes enlarge in which of the following condition?
    (A) Carcinoma of the glans penis
    (B) Infected wound of fifth toe
    (C) Abscess in superolateral quadrant of buttock
    (D) Cellulitis around umbilicus
3. Which of the following problem may cause enlargement of popliteal group of lymph nodes?
    (A) Melanoma in great toe

(B) Inflammation in little toe along lateral margin of foot
(C) Infected sebaceous cyst in scrotal region
(D) Gluteal abscess

Answers:
1. C
   The vertical group of superficial inguinal lymph nodes receives superficial lymph vessels from the territory drained by great saphenous vein (including medial aspectof the knee), and lies along its termination near the saphenous hiatus.
2. A
   The deep inguinal nodes receive lymph from the superficial inguinal lymph nodes (horizontal and vertical groups), popliteal lymph nodes, the glans and body of penis and clitoris.
3. B
   Popliteal group of lymph nodes receive superficial lymph vessels from lateral side of foot and leg. These accompany the small saphenous vein to the popliteal fossa.

Reference:
1. Snell RS. Clinical Anatomy by Regions. 9th edition. New Delhi: Wolters Kluwer/ Lippincott. Williams & Wilkins; Chapter 10, Lower Limb. 2012, pp 454, 478.

CONGENITAL DEFORMITY OF FOOT
Dr. A.K. Pankaj, Assistant Professor, Department of Anatomy

A 9 month old boy was brought to orthopedic OPD with the complaint of deformed feet since birth. Parent told that the child is reluctant in walking. His feet were pointing downwards and inwards, with both sole facing backwards.

1. What is the most probable diagnosis?
   (A) Congenital talipus equinovarus
   (B) Pes planus
   (C) Pes cavus
   (D) Talepus calcaneo valgus
2. What do you understand by the term "forefoot"?
   (A) Tarsals
   (B) Tarsals and metatarsals
   (C) Metatarsals
   (D) Metatarsals and Phalanges
3. Which of the following deformity is present in above case?
   (A) Adduction and planter flexion of foot
   (B) Abduction and planter flexion of foot
   (C) Adduction and dorsi flexion of foot
   (D) Abduction and dorsi flexion of foot

Answers:
1. A
   Congenital talipus equinovarus has three element- equinus, varus (i.e. inversion) and adduction. The talus point downward (equinus), the calcaneum faces inwards (varus) and the forefoot is adducted.
2. B
3. A
   In clubfoot, foot is planter flexed at the ankle joint and inverted at midtarsal joint.

Reference:
1. Snell RS. Clinical Anatomy by Regions. 9th edition. New Delhi: Wolters Kluwer/ Lippincott Williams & Wilkins; Chapter 10, Lower Limb. 2012, pp 512.

PLEURA
Dr. R. K. Verma, Assistant Professor, Department of Anatomy

A 30 year old patient consulted his physician with the complaint of high grade fever and severe pain in his right chest which exaggerates on respiration and coughing. The pain was also radiating down to the front of upper abdomen. On examination, patient was found febrile and respiratory rate was increased. On auscultation of chest, decreased breath sound was heard over lower part of right side of chest. Chest X-ray revealed obliterated costodiaphragmatic recess of right side.

1. Obliterated costodiaphragmatic recess in the radiograph suggests collection of fluid in which of the following spaces?
   (A) Pleural cavity
   (B) Mediastinum
   (C) Thoracic cavity
   (D) Pericardial cavity
2. Which site of intercostal space should be the safest for performing thoracocentesis in above case?
   (A) At midaxillary line along the lower border of 9th rib
   (B) At midclavicular line along the lower border of 9th rib
   (C) At midclavicular line along the upper border of 10th rib
   (D) At midaxillary line along the upper border of 10th rib
3. Which is the correct anatomical order of structures that are pierced during thoracocentesis (outside to inside)?
   (A) Skin, superficial & deep fascia, muscles, endothoracic fascia and parietal pleura
   (B) Skin, superficial & deep fascia, muscles, endothoracic fascia and visceral pleura
   (C) Skin, superficial & deep fascia, endothoracic fascia, muscles and parietal pleura
   (D) Skin, superficial & deep fascia, endothoracic fascia, muscles and visceral pleura
4. What is the anatomical basis of perception of pain in right upper abdomen, while the disease is affecting lung and its membrane?
   (A) Parietal pleura and anterior abdominal wall are innervated by lower intercostal nerves
   (B) Visceral pleura and viscera of upper abdomen have same autonomic nerve supply
   (C) Parietal pleura and viscera of upper abdomen have same autonomic nerve supply
   (D) Visceral pleura and anterior abdominal wall are innervated by lower intercostal nerves

Answers:
   1. A
      In pleurisy, fluid collects in most dependent part of pleural cavity, a potential space between visceral and parietal pleura, causing obliteration of costodiaphragmatic recess.
   2. D
      To avoid injury to the neurovascular structures in intercostal space, thoracocentesis is done along the upper border of lower rib of corresponding intercostal space in the midaxillary line.
   3. A
   4. A

Reference:
   1. Snell RS. Clinical Anatomy by Regions. 9th edition. New Delhi: Wolters Kluwer/ Lippincott Williams & Wilkins; Chapter 2, The Thorax:Part I-The Thoracic Wall & Chapter 3, The Thorax:Part II-The Thoracic Cavity. 2012, pp 46,61,64.

THORACIC DUCT
Dr. R.K. Verma, Assistant Professor, Department of Anatomy

A 55 year old patient was admitted in hospital with complaints of difficulty in swallowing food and severe weight loss for last one month. He was diagnosed as a case of carcinoma of lower third of esophagus. Resection and reconstruction of esophagus was planned. During surgery, the surgical field began to fill with a clear to milky fluid.

1. What is the cause of appearance of milky fluid in the surgical field?
   (A) Injury to the pleural cavity
   (B) Penetration in the pericardial cavity
   (C) Laceration of thoracic duct
   (D) Laceration of right auricle of heart
2. Which of the following is the correct relation of thoracic duct with oesophagus in superior mediastinum?
   (A) Runs along left edge of esophagus
   (B) Runs along right edge of esophagus
   (C) Lies posteriorly
   (D) Crosses in front and reaches the left border
3. Which one of the following is tributary of thoracic duct at the root of neck?

(A) Right jugular trunk
(B) Left jugular trunk
(C) Ascending trunk
(D) Descending trunk

Answers:
1. C
Thoracic duct is related to left margin of oesophagus in superior mediastinum,which may damage during surgery causing leakage of milky fluid in the surgical field.
2. A
3. B

References:
1. Standring S. Gray's Anatomy. 40th edition. Spain: Churchill Livingstone Elsevier; Chapter 55, Mediastinum. 2008, pp 943.
2. Snell RS. Clinical Anatomy by Regions. 9th edition. New Delhi: Wolters Kluwer/Lippincott Williams & Wilkins; Chapter 3, The Thorax: Part II-The Thoracic Cavity. 2012, pp 98 - 99.

BLOOD SUPPLY OF HEART
Dr. R.K.Verma, Assistant professor, Department of Anatomy

A 40 year old businessman of good health consulted his physician as recently he has started experiencing chest discomfort during his morning jogging hours. A thorough cardiac evaluation revealed 90% narrowing of the anterior interventricular artery, 60% narrowing of the circumflex artery and left coronary artery dominance. The cardiologist strongly recommended a cardiac bypass procedure plus stenting to relieve the blood flow condition.

1. The term "left coronary dominance" indicates
    (A) Both the arteries in above case are branches from right coronary artery
    (B) The circumflex artery give rise to right posterior interventricular artery
    (C) The narrowing of anterior interventricular artery is causing diminished flow to the SA node
    (D) The circumflex artery descends in the anterior interventricular groove passes around the apex of heart
2. The circumflex coronary artery
    (A) Arises from anterior aortic sinus
    (B) Branch of right coronary artery
    (C) Continues as left marginal artery
    (D) Give left diagonal artery
3. Which of the following are true about coronary bypass surgery EXCEPT:
    (A) It can only be done after a coronary angioplasty procedure
    (B) A segment of the saphenous vein is often used to bypass the obstructed segment of the affected coronary artery
    (C) The internal thoracic artery may be used to directly supply the distal segment of a coronary artery
    (D) It is done in cases of coronary artery stenosis

Answers:
1. B
In left coronary dominance, the posterior interventricular artery arises as a branch of   circumflex artery, which is a terminal branch of left coronary artery
2. C
3. A

Reference:
1. Snell RS. Clinical Anatomy by Regions. 9th edition. New Delhi: Wolters Kluwer/ Lippincott Williams & Wilkins; Chapter 3,The Thorax: Part II-The Thoracic Cavity. 2012, pp 87, 89.

BRONCHOPULMONARY SEGMENTS
Dr. R.K.Verma, Assistant Professor, Department of Anatomy

A 65 year old farmer presented in OPD with complaints of chronic cough and weight loss. After several investigations he was diagnosed as a case of benign neoplasm which was restricted to the apical bronchopulmonary segment in superior lobe of left lung. Patient is scheduled for a segmental resection of his left lung.
1. A bronchopulmonary segment is aerated by
    (A) Secondary bronchus

(B) Tertiary bronchus
(C) Respiratory bronchiole
(D) Terminal bronchiole

2. Which of the following are segments of superior lobe of left lung?
   (A) Apical, posterior and anterior
   (B) Medial and lateral
   (C) Apical, posterior, anterior, superior & inferior lingular
   (D) Apical medial, lateral and posterior basal

3. Area of the bronchopulmonary segment aerated by respiratory bronchiole is known as
   (A) Bronchopulmonary segment
   (B) Pulmonary unit
   (C) Lobe of lung
   (D) Alveolar sac

Answers:
1. B
2. C
3. B

Reference:
1. Snell RS. Clinical Anatomy by Regions. 9th edition. New Delhi: Wolters Kluwer/ Lippincott Williams & Wilkins; Chapter 3, The Thorax: Part II-The Thoracic Cavity. 2012, pp 71, 72.

ECTOPIC PREGNANCY
Dr. Garima Sehgal, Lecturer, Department of Anatomy

A 28 year old married woman was brought to the emergency department with severe cramping pain in the right lower abdomen for last 10 hours. She told that she was not having menstruation for last 2 months; previously, menses occurred at regular 28-days interval. She had mild intermittent vaginal bleeding, sometimes associated with lower abdominal pain, for past 3 days. Mild tenderness was present in the right lower quadrant. Bimanual pelvic examination revealed a tender walnut-sized mass in the right parametrium. She was diagnosed as a case of ectopic pregnancy.

1. The commonest site for implantation in uterus is
   (A) Upper part of anterior wall
   (B) Upper part of posterior wall
   (C) Lower part of anterior wall
   (D) Lower part of posterior wall

2. The uterus and the developing fetus are visualized most commonly by
   (A) X – ray
   (B) CT scan
   (C) MRI
   (D) Ultrasonography

3. Most common site of ectopic pregnancy is
   (A) Ampulla of uterine tube
   (B) Lower part of uterine cavity
   (C) Ovary
   (D) Rectouterine pouch

4. The term parametrium refers to
   (A) Outer most layer of uterus
   (B) Pelvic fascia on either side of uterus
   (C) Broad ligament
   (D) Uterovesical fold of peritoneum

Answers:
1. B
   Normal implantation takes place in the endometrium of the body of the uterus, most frequently on the upper part of the posterior wall near the midline.
2. D
   A sonogram of the female pelvis can be used to visualize the uterus and the developing fetus and the vagina.

3. A

Occasionally, implantation takes place outside the uterus, resulting in extrauterine or ectopic pregnancy. Ectopic pregnancies may occur at any place in the abdominal cavity, ovary, or uterine tube . However, 95% of ectopic pregnancies occur in the uterine tube, and most of these are in the ampulla.

4. B

The supravaginal part of the cervix is separated in front from the bladder by cellular connective tissue, the parametrium, which also passes to the sides of the cervix and laterally between the two layers of the broad ligaments.

References:

1. Snell RS. Clinical Anatomy by Regions, 9th edition. Philadelphia: Wolters Kluwer / Lippincott Williams & Wilkins; Chapter 7, The Pelvis: Part II – The Pelvic Cavity. 2012, pp 292.
2. Snell RS. Clinical Anatomy by Regions, 9th edition. Philadelphia: Wolters Kluwer / Lippincott Williams & Wilkins; Chapter 7, The Pelvis: Part II – The Pelvic Cavity. 2012, pp 289.
3. Sadler TW, editor. Langman's Medical Embryology, 11th edition. New Delhi: Wolters Kluwer (India) Pvt. Ltd.; Chapter 4, Second week of Development: Bilaminar Germ Disc. 2010, pp 52.
4. Standring S. Gray's anatomy- The anatomical basis of clinical practice, 39th edition.New York:Elsevier/Churchill Livingstone; Chapter 104, Female Reproductive System. 2005, pp 1332.

APPENDIX

Dr. Garima Sehgal, Lecturer, Department of Anatomy

A 25 year old lady, suffering from nausea, vomiting and pain in abdomen for last 2 days, was admitted in emergency. She gave history that pain was earlier periumbilical in location but later it shifted to the right lower quadrant (RLQ) of the abdomen. Her menstrual cycles were regular. She was lying down in the bed motionless with her hips and knees in a flexed position. Her body temperature was 101°F. On examination, tenderness was elicited in the right lower quadrant. A diagnosis of acute appendicitis was established and a standard medical treatment was started.

1. Which of the following features of appendix makes it a preferable site of infection?
    (A) Rich blood supply
    (B) Long, narrow, blind tube
    (C) Scarcity of lymphatic tissue
    (D) Close relation to caecum
2. Mc Burney's point, the point of maximum tenderness in cases of appendicitis is located at junction of
    (A) Lateral ⅓ rd and medial ⅔ rd of a line joining right anterior superior iliac spine to umbilicus
    (B) Lateral ⅔ rd and medial⅓ rd of a line joining right anterior superior iliac spine to umbilicus
    (C) Lateral ⅓ rd and medial ⅔ rd of a line joining right anterior superior iliac spine to pubic symphysis
    (D) Lateral ⅔ rd and medial⅓ rd of a line joining right anterior superior iliac spine to pubic symphysis
3. Gangrenous perforation is commonly seen in distal part of the appendix because
    (A) Distal part is devoid of arterial supply
    (B) Appendicular artery is an end artery beyond midpoint
    (C) Distal part of artery lies away from wall of appendix
    (D) Appendicular artery has no anastomosis
4. Intraoperatively, which of the following anatomical feature helps in locating appendix?
    (A) Base of caecum
    (B) Ileocaecal junction
    (C) Absence of appendices epiploicae
    (D) Convergence of taeniae coli

Answers:

1. B

It is a long, narrow, blind-ended tube, which encourages stasis of large-bowel contents. It has a large amount of lymphoid tissue in its wall. The lumen has a tendency to becomeobstructed by hardened intestinal contents (enteroliths), which leads to further stagnation of its contents.

2. A

The appendix lies in the right iliac fossa, and in relation to the anterior abdominal wall its base is situated one third of the way up the line joining the right anterior superior iliac spine to the umbilicus (McBurney's point).

3. B

Although the appendix is well supplied by arterial anastomoses at its base, the appendicular artery is an end artery from the midpoint upwards and its close proximity to the wall makes it susceptible to thrombosis during episodes of acute inflammation. This may render the distal appendix ischaemic and explains the frequency of gangrenous perforation seen in the disease.

4. D

The three taeniae coli on the ascending colon and caecum converge on the base of the appendix

References:

1. Snell RS. Clinical Anatomy by Regions, 9th edition. Philadelphia: Wolters Kluwer / Lippincott Williams & Wilkins; Chapter 5, The Abdomen: Part II – The Abdominal Cavity. 2012, pp 185.

2. Snell RS. Clinical Anatomy by Regions, 9th edition. Philadelphia: Wolters Kluwer / Lippincott Williams & Wilkins; Chapter 5,The Abdomen: Part II – The Abdominal Cavity. 2012, pp 182.

3. Standring S. Gray's anatomy- The anatomical basis of clinical practice, 39th edition. New York:Elsevier/Churchill Livingstone; Chapter78, Gastrointestinal Tract - Large Intestine. 2005, pp 1190.

4. Snell RS. Clinical Anatomy by Regions, 9th edition. Philadelphia: Wolters Kluwer / Lippincott Williams & Wilkins; Chapter 5,The Abdomen: Part II – The Abdominal Cavity. 2012, pp 182

URETER

Dr. Garima Sehgal, Lecturer, Department of Anatomy

A 38 year old male, visits the physician with complaints of severe pain in the left flank, nausea and vomiting. The patient narrates that the pain is travelling from loin to groin and his urine is red (haematuria). There is no accompanying history of any other urinary complaint. The plain radiograph of abdomen revealed a radio-opaque shadow in the line of left ureter.

1. Pain sensation from ureter reaches to which one of the following spinal segments?
   (A) T5 – T8
   (B) T7 – T10
   (C) T9 – T12
   (D) T11- L2

2. The line of projection of the ureter on a radiograph lies-
   (A) On the lateral margin of all lumbar vertebral bodies
   (B) In front of tips of transverse processes of all lumbar vertebrae
   (C) Lateral to tip of transverse processes of all lumbar vertebrae
   (D) Along the lateral border of psoas shadow

3: Both types of renal stones, radio-opaque or radiolucent, may be diagnosed with help of which of the following investigations
   (A) Pyelography
   (B) Cholecystography
   (C) Plain skiagram of KUB region
   (D) Barium meal

4. The most common site of impaction of renal stone in ureter is -
   (A) Renal pelvis
   (B) Pelviureteric junction
   (C) at the level of ischial spine
   (D) against the tip of transverse process of L4 vertebra

Answers:

1. D

The renal pelvis and the ureter send their afferent nerves into the spinal cord at segments T11 and 12 and L1 and 2.

2. B

The ureter runs down in front of the tips of the transverse processes of the lumbar vertebrae, crosses the region of the sacroiliac joint, swings out to the ischial spine, and then turns medially to the bladder.

3. A

Most stones, although radiopaque, are small enough to be impossible to see definitely along the course of the ureter on plain radiographic examination. An intravenous pyelogram is usually necessary.

4. B

There are three sites of anatomic narrowing of the ureter where stones may be arrested,namely, the pelviureteral junction, the pelvic brim, and where the ureter enters the bladder.

References:

1. Snell RS. Clinical Anatomy by Regions, 9th edition. Philadelphia: Wolters Kluwer/ Lippincott Williams & Wilkins; Chapter 5, The Abdomen: Part II – The Abdominal Cavity. 2012, pp 212.
2. Standring S. Gray's anatomy- The anatomical basis of clinical practice, 39th edition. New York:Elsevier/Churchill Livingstone; Chapter 91, Kidney and Ureter. 2005, pp 1274.

GALL BLADDER

Dr. Garima Sehgal, Lecturer, Department of Anatomy

A 42 year old obese female presents in the emergency with severe right upper quadrant pain associated with nausea and vomiting. On examination she is febrile and she has rebound tenderness and guarding in right upper quadrant. WBC counts – 14,000 (normal 4,000 – 11, 000), liver function tests are normal (LFTs) and C reactive protein is raised. She is diagnosed as a case of acute cholecystitis.

1. During clinical examination, the fundus of the gall bladder is mostly palpated deep to the tip of which costal cartilage?
   (A) 7th
   (B) 8th
   (C) 9th
   (D) 10th
2. Gall stones that perforate the gall bladder in the region of the neck, pass most commonly into which part of the duodenum
   (A) First
   (B) Second
   (C) Third
   (D) Fourth
3. Calot's triangle is bounded by
   (A) Cystic duct, Common Hepatic artery, Liver
   (B) Common hepatic duct, Common Hepatic artery, Liver
   (C) Cystic artery, Common bile duct, Liver
   (D) Cystic duct, Common hepatic duct, Liver

Answers:

1. C

   It often lies in contact with the anterior abdominal wall behind the ninth costal cartilage where the lateral edge of the right rectus abdominis crosses the costal margin.

2. B

   Neck lies anterior to the second part of the duodenum and the right end of the transverse colon.

3. D

   The near triangular space formed between the cystic duct, the common hepatic duct and the inferior surface of segment V of the liver, is commonly referred to as Calot's triangle.

Reference:

1. Standring S. Gray's anatomy- The anatomical basis of clinical practice, 39th edition. New York:Elsevier/Churchill Livingstone; Chapter 86, Hepatobiliary System. 2005, pp 1228- 1229.

SKIN

Dr. Archana Srivastava, Junior Resident III year, Department of Anatomy

A 70-year-old woman sustained burn injury over her upper limbs and chest. On admission to the hospital her BP was 100/60 mmHg and pulse rate was 64/min. The haemoglobin level was 11.0g/dl, total leukocyte count 14000/ml and platelet count 2,35000/ml. She was diagnosed to have first degree skin burn.

1. The layer of the skin which is **NOT** affected in first degree skin burn is
    (A) Stratum basale
    (B) Reticular layer
    (C) Stratum spinosum
    (D) Stratum corneum
2. All of the following cells of the skin are affected in first degree burns **EXCEPT**
    (A) Melanosomes
    (B) Keratinocytes
    (C) Langerhans cells
    (D) Fibroblasts
3. The percentage area of burn in this patient according to "Wallace Rule of Nine" is
    (A) 18%
    (B) 36%
    (C) 27%
    (D) 54%
4. All are functions of epidermis of skin **EXCEPT**
    (A) Protection from physical injury
    (B) Prevention of dehydration
    (C) Sensation of temperature
    (D) Production of antibodies
5. Pigment containing cells of the skin is
    (A) Pigmentoblasts
    (B) Keratinocytes
    (C) Melanocytes
    (D) Dendritic cells

Answers:
    1. B
        The epidermis is affected in first degree burn. The epidermis has following layers stratum basale, stratum spinosum, stratum granulosum, stratum lucidum and stratum corneum. The reticular layer is part of the dermis and is not affected in first degree burn.
    2. D
        Keratinocytes, melanosomes, langerhans cells are present in the epidermis. The fibroblasts are present in dermis they produce collagen fibres.
    3. B
        Rule of Nine is used to calculate the percentage area of burn in adults. The body is divided into anatomical regions that represent 9% (or multiples of 9).
    4. D
    5. C
        Melanocytes are the pigment containing cells of the skin.

Reference:
    1. Snell RS. Clinical Anatomy by Regions. 9th edition. Philadelphia: Wolters Kluwer; Chapter 1, Introduction. 2012, pp 1-33.

PALMAR APONEUROSIS
Dr. Archana Srivastava, Junior Resident III year, Department of Anatomy

A 50-year old male presents with complaints of pain in the right palm with bending of ring and little finger. He is unable to extend his affected fingers. There is no history of burn injury or soft tissue injury. The X-ray of the hand is normal. Thyroid function test showed normal hormone levels.
1. The anatomical structure affected in this clinical condition is
    (A) Flexor retinaculum
    (B) Palmar aponeurosis
    (C) Interosseous muscles
    (D) Ulnar nerve
2. Palmar aponeurosis is a modified form of
    (A) Superficial fascia
    (B) Deep fascia
    (C) Subcutaneous adipose tissue
    (D) Panniculus Carnosus

3. In Dupuytren's contracture the histological examination of skin will show
   (A) Increased elastic fibres
   (B) Increased collagen fibres
   (C) Increased adipose tissue
   (D) Deposition of calcium in the dermis
4. All of the following structures are modified deep fascia **EXCEPT**
   (A) Carotid sheath
   (B) Rectus sheath
   (C) Interosseous membrane
   (D) Retinacula
5. All of the following statements are correct about palmar aponeurosis **EXCEPT**
   (A) It is degenerated portion of palmaris longus tendon
   (B) It is thickest over thenar and hypothenar regions
   (C) It gives attachment to the skin of palm
   (D) It protects underlying tendons

Answers:

1. B
   Dupuytren's contracture occurs due to contracture of fibrous tissue of the palmar aponeurosis. The disease results in flexion deformity of ring and little finger. It is seen above the age of 40 years and is more common in males.

2. B
   Palmar aponeurosis is derived from deep fascia. It is thick in the middle and thin over the hypothenar and thenar regions thereby facilitating movements of the fingers.

3. B
   In Dupuytren's contracture, there is increased fibroblast activity and the normal type I collagen of skin is replaced by increase amounts of type III collagen in early stages. In advanced stage type I collagen is present in tendon like cords.

4. B
   Rectus sheath is aponeurosis of muscles of anterolateral abdominal wall.

5. B
   Palmaraponeurosis is thin over thenar and hypothenar eminence.

Reference:

1. Singh V. General Anatomy, 1st edition. India: Elsevier; Chapter 5, Skin, superficial fascia and deep fascia. 2008, pp 70-91.

Chapter-2

Anaesthesiology

TRACHEO- OESOPHAGEAL FISTULA
Dr. Anita Malik, Professor, Department of Anaesthesiology

A one day old, 2500 gm. newborn male is admitted in emergency with a history of inability to pass Ryle's tube in delivery room and choking on the first glucose water feed. The chest X ray reveals the tube curled in the proximal oesophageal pouch and the presence of a gastric air bubble.

1. The most probable diagnosis is
   (A) Achalasia cardia
   (B) Tracheooesophageal fistula
   (C) Pyloric stenosis
   (D) Congenital diaphragmatic hernia
2. Which type of Tracheooesophageal anomaly is the most common?
   (A) Type A
   (B) Type B
   (C) Type C
   (D) TypeD
3. VACTERL syndrome includes all of the following except
   (A) Tracheooesophageal fistula, anal anomalies
   (B) Vertebral,cardiac anomalies
   (C) Respiratory anomalies
   (D) Limb anomalies
4. Bag mask ventilation is contraindicated in which of the following situations
   (A) Anal atresia
   (B) Omphalocoel
   (C) Tracheooesophageal fistula
   (D) Gastroschisis
5. For repair of Tracheooesophageal fistula the distal end of endotracheal tube is placed
   (A) Proximal to fistula
   (B) At the level of fistula
   (C) Distal to fistula
   (D) Inside the fistula

Answer:
1. **B**
   Oesophageal pouch with inability to pass Ryle's tube and inability to feed suggests diagnosis of trachea-oesophageal fistula.
2. **C**
   The most common lesion (more than 90% of cases) is type C, in which a fistula exists between the trachea and the lower esophageal segment at a point slightly above the carina, and the upper esophageal segment ends blindly in the mediastinum at the level of the second or third thoracic vertebra.
3. **C**
   The term VACTERL (Vertebral, Anal, Cardiac, Tracheo Esophageal, Renal, Limb) association refers to these anomalies, because they commonly coexist in various combinations with Trachea-oesophageal fistula /Esophageal atresia.
4. **C**
   Positive pressure ventilation will force gas through the fistula into the stomach which may add to the respiratory compromise.
5. **C**
   Ideally, the stomach should not distend with inspired gases (i.e., ventilation does not enter the stomach via the fistula, or the fistula itself has not been intubated).

Reference:
1. Brett. C, Davis PJ: Anesthesia for general surgery in the neonate in Smith's Anesthesia for Infants and Children, 8th Edition, 2011, Elsevier; pg 574-578.

CONGENITAL DIAPHRAGMATIC HERNIA
Dr. Anita Malik, Professor, Department of Anaesthesiology

In a one day old newborn with respiratory distress, physical examination reveals a scaphoid abdomen, bulging chest, decreased breath sounds, distant or right-displaced heart sounds, and bowel sounds in the chest.

Radiographic examination of the chest shows a bowel gas pattern in the chest, mediastinal shift, and little lung tissue at the right costophrenic sulcus.

1. Most common occurrence of diaphragmatic hernia is
   (A) Left Posterolateral
   (B) Right Posterolateral
   (C) Paraesophageal
   (D) Anterior (Morgagni)
2. Which of the following should be avoided in anaesthetic management of congenital diaphragmatic hernia?
   (A) Nasogastric Tube
   (B) Mask ventilation
   (C) Patient may be needed to be kept intubated in postoperative period
   (D) Low pressure ventilation
3. The new lung-protective (gentle ventilator) strategy for congenital diaphragmatic hernia includes all except
   (A) A small tidal volume
   (B) A large tidal volume
   (C) An adequate positive end-expiratory pressure (PEEP) to keep the airways open
   (D) Permissive hypercapnea
4. In congenital diaphragmatic hernia with right-to-left Shunting, low concentrations of inhalation anesthetics (sevoflurane or isoflurane)
   (A) Decrease pulmonary vascular resistance
   (B) Increase pulmonary vascular resistance
   (C) Decrease systemic vascular resistance
   (D) Increase systemic vascular resistance
5. Improved oxygenation without causing pulmonary barotrauma in congenital diaphragmatic hernia in specialized units is provided with
   (A) High-frequency oscillatory ventilation(HFOV)
   (B) Inhaled nitric oxide (NO)
   (C) Extracorporeal membrane oxygenation (ECMO)
   (D) All of the above

Answer:

1. A
   The most common defect is posterolateral (Bochdalek'shernia), occurring in 90% of cases, of which 75% are left sided.
2. B
   Positive pressure ventilation by mask and bag has risks, because attempting to expand the noncompliant lungs may damage the hypoplastic lung by over distention, as well as distend the stomach and intestines (which are in the left hemi thorax), further decreasing chest compliance.
3. B
   Avoiding volutrauma includes a small tidal volume, appropriate PEEP (5 to 7 cm H2O) to avoid atelectasis and shear stress trauma (low volume injury), adequate oxygenation measured with pulse oximetry [SpO2] 90% to 95%) and permissive hypercapnea as needed, while maintaining adequate pH (>7.25).
4. A
   Decrease pulmonary vascular resistance may be advantageous in producing pulmonary vasodilatation, but if effects on SVR> PVR, right-to-left shunting may actually worsen.
5. D
   All of the above

Reference:

1. Brett. C, Davis PJ: Anesthesia for general surgery in the neonate in Smith`s Anesthesia for Infants and Children, 8th Edition, 2011, Elsevier; , pg 567-573

DAY CARE SURGERY

Dr. Jaishri Bogra, Professor & Head, Department of Anaesthesiology

A 25 year old female presented with complaints of amenorrhea for 2 months, pain in abdomen for 1 day and bleeding per vaginum for 1 day. Her urine pregnancy test was positive and Ultrasonography showed bulky uterus with undeveloped fetus. Her vitals were stable and she had mild pallor. A diagnosis of incomplete abortion was made. She was posted for dilatation and curettage under monitored anaesthesia care.

1. Contraindication to day care surgery are all except:

(A) No responsible adult in home to care for the patient after surgery.

(B) Infants less than 45 weeks post conceptual age.

(C) Potentially life threatening chronic illnesses.

(D) ASA physical status III and IV.

2. Which of the following statement is true about day care surgery:

(A) Preanaesthetic evaluation is not required for day care surgery.

(B) Routine preoperative testing is not recommended before ambulatory surgery.

(C) ASA minimum monitoring standards are not mandatory for day care surgery.

(D) No postoperative observation is required in day care surgery.

3. Which of the following drug is not preferred in day care surgery:

(A) Propofol

(B) Remifentanyl

(C) Pancuronium

(D) Bupivacaine

4. Fast tracking eligibility criteria for ambulatory surgery includes all except:

(A) Ability to drink fluids and pass urine.

(B) Postoperative pain assessment.

(C) Hemodynamic stability.

(D) Respiratory stability.

5. True about procedural sedation and monitored anaesthesia care:

(A) Both require presence of a trained anaesthesiologist.

(B) ASA preoperative fasting guidelines must be followed in both cases.

(C) Both require availability of resuscitation equipments and trained personnel to use them.

(D) They represent different level of sedation.

Answers:

1. D

Selected patients with ASA physical status III and IV can undergo day care surgery and it is not a contraindication for day care surgery.

2. B

There is no routine preoperative testing recommended before ambulatory surgery. And investigation should be done as indicated by clinical assessment.

3. C

Pancuronium is a long acting muscle relaxant which is not recommended for day care surgery.

4. A

Ability to drink fluids and pass urine is not considered mandatory before discharging patient after day care surgery.

5. C

Availability of resuscitation equipments and trained personnel is required before any procedure requiring sedation or use of anaesthetic agents..

References:

1. White PE, Eng MR. Ambulatory Anesthesia. In: Miller RD (Eds) Miller's Anesthesia, 7th edition. Elsevier, Philadelhia 2010,pp 2419-2460.

2. White PF, Song D. New criteria for fast tracking after outpatient anesthesia: A comparison with the modified Alderete's scoring system. AnesthAnalg 88:1069,1999.

ORAL CANCER

Dr. Jaishri Bogra, Prof. and Head, Dept. of anaesthesiology

A 55 year old female presented with complaint of an ulcerative growth on lower lip for 8 months. She was tobacco chewer for last 30 years. The biopsy of the lesion showed squamous cell carcinoma. Wide local excision of the lesion with modified radical neck dissection with reconstruction was planned. Her airway examination showed restricted mouth opening of 2 finger breath with Mallampati grade III. General and systemic examination was unremarkable.

1. Mallampati grading indicates:

(A) Mouth opening.

(B) Ease of ventilation.

(C) Space in oral cavity to accommodate laryngoscope and endotracheal tube.

(D) Anterior larynx.

2. In "cannot ventilate, cannot intubate" situation, following can be used except:
   (A) Supraglottic airway.
   (B) Fibreoptic laryngoscopy.
   (C) Cricothyroidotomy.
   (D) Jet ventilation.
3. Following types of endotracheal tubes can be used for lower lip surgery except:
   (A) Poly Vinyl Chloride oronasal endotracheal tube.
   (B) Red rubber nasal endotracheal tube.
   (C) South facing RAE endotracheal tube.
   (D) Flexometallicendotracheal tube.
4. Following nerve block can be used for lower lip surgery:
   (A) Infraorbital nerve
   (B) Mental nerve
   (C) Supratrochlear nerve
   (D) Lingual nerve
5. Contraindication for awake fibreoptic intubation is:
   (A) Facial trauma
   (B) Uncooperative patient
   (C) Cervical spine instability
   (D) Microagnathia

Answer:
1. C
   Mallampati grades indicate about the space available in oral cavity to accommodate laryngoscope and endotracheal tube.
2. B
   Fibreoptic laryngoscopy is not used during emergency situations as it requires preparation and time to perform.
3. C
   South facing RAE endotracheal tube is used in upper lip surgery.
4. B
   Mental nerve is not used for lower lip surgery
5. B
   Use of fibreoptic laryngoscope requires cooperative patient.

References:
1. Khan RM, Maroof M (Eds). Airway Management. 4th edition. Paras medical publisher. 2011.
2. Ban CH. Peripheral nerve blockade. In: Barash PG, Cullen BF (Eds). Clinical anesthesia. 6th edition, Lippincott Williams and Wilkins, Philadelphia, 2012: pp 960-963.

DECORTICATION
Dr. Shashi Bhushan, Professor, Department of Anesthesiology

A 30 year old male presented with complaints of cough for 3 months, exertionaldyspnoea for 1 month and right side chest pain for 1 week. He also reported weight loss in last 3 month. His examination revealed coarse crepts and rhonchi on right side. His x ray chest,and sputum examination was done and he was diagnosed to be suffering from pulmonary tuberculosis. ATT was started as per standard protocol. After 4 months of ATT, his symptom did not improve. Xray chest and CT thorax was done and a loculated right sided empyema thoracis was diagnosed. He was posted for right decortications.

1. Three legged stool of prethoracotomy respiratory assessment includes all except:
   (A) Respiratory mechanics
   (B) Cardiopulmonary reserve
   (C) Chest radiography
   (D) Lung parenchymal function
2. Most common arrhythmia after pulmonary resection is:
   (A) Atrial flutter
   (B) Atrial fibrillation
   (C) Ventricular tachycardia
   (D) Heart block

3. Arterial blood gas analysis is recommended during one lung ventilation because:
   (A) PaO2 provides indication of risk of desaturation before SpO2
   (B) ETCO2 is less reliable indicator of PaCO2 during one lung ventilation.
   (C) Accuracy of pulse oximeters differ significantly and needs to be verified intraoperatively with ABG.
   (D) All of the above
4. The options for lung isolation in adults include all except:
   (A) Double lumen tubes
   (B) Fogharty catheter
   (C) Bronchial blockers
   (D) Univent tubes
5. Specific indications for right sided Double Lumen Tubes are all except:
   (A) Left sided tracheobronchial tree disruption
   (B) Left sided empyema thoracis
   (C) Left sided sleeve resection
   (D) Descending thoracic aortic aneurysm

Answers:
   1. C
   Chest radiography is not a part of three legged assessment.
   2. B
   Atrial fibrillation is the most common arrhythmia after pulmonary resection.
   3. D
   Due to gross ventilation perfusion mismatch, the routine indicators of oxygenation and ventilation (SPO2 and EtCO2) are not very reliable during one lung ventilation.
   4. B
   Fogharty catheter is used in children for lung isolation.
   5. B
   Left sided empyema thoracis can be performed with right as well as left sided double lumen tubes.

References:
   1. Peter DS, Javier HC. Anesthesia for thoracic surgery. In: Miller RD (eds) Miller's anesthesia. 7th edition. Elseviier, Philadelphia,2010; pp 1819-1880.
   2. Slinger PD, Johnston MR: Preoperative assessment: An anesthesiologist's perspective. ThoracSurgClin 15:11,2005.

BRONCHOPLEURAL FISTULA
Dr. Shashi Bhushan, Professor, Department of Anesthesiology

A 15 year old male presented with complaints of fever for 1 month, cough with purulent expectoration for 1 months and exertionaldyspnoea for 10 days. He has taken irregular medication from local practioner. His examination revealed coarse crepts on left side. His x ray chest and sputum examination was done and he was diagnosed to be suffering from pneumonia with pleural effusion. Antibiotics were started as per culture report. An intercostal drain was placed and purulent pleural fluid was drained from the ICD. After 15 days, his symptom did not improve. Xray chest and CT thorax was done and an empyema thoracis with bronchopleural fistula was diagnosed. He was posted decortication with repair of bronchopleural fistula.

1. The preferred method of lung isolation in bronchopleural fistula involving left mainstem bronchus:
   (A) Bronchial blocker
   (B) Right double lumen tube
   (C) Left double lumen tube
   (D) Univent tube
2. Factors correlated with increased risk of desaturation during one lung ventilation are all except:
   (A) Supine position
   (B) High percentage of ventilation or perfusion to the operative lung on preoperative V/Q scan
   (C) Left side thoracotomy
   (D) Normal preoperative spirometry or restrictive lung disease
3. Monitoring mandatory during thoracotomy are all except:
   (A) ECG
   (B) Invasive blood pressure
   (C) Temperature
   (D) Capnography

4. The endobronchial cuffs of double lumen tubes are:
    (A) High volume, high pressure
    (B) High volume, low pressure
    (C) Low volume, high pressure
    (D) Low volume, low pressure
5. First step of management of sudden severe desaturation during one lung ventilation:
    (A) FiO2 increased to 1.0
    (B) Resume both lung ventilation
    (C) CPAP (continuous positive airway pressure) to nonventilated lung
    (D) PEEP (positive end expiratory pressure) to ventilated lung

Answers:
1. B
    Right double lumen tubes are preferred method for bronchopleural fistula as they provide better isolation and surgery does not interfere with surgical procedure.
2. C
    Right side thoracotomy is a risk factor for desaturation.
3. B
    Invasive blood pressure monitoring is not mandatory for all thoracotomies.
4. D
    Low volume, low pressure cuff are used in endobronchial cuffs.
5. B
    Termination of one lung ventilation should be done in case of sudden severe desaturation.

References:
1. Peter DS, Javier HC. Anesthesia for thoracic surgery. In: Miller RD (eds) Miller's anesthesia. 7th edition. Elseviier, Philadelphia,2010; pp 1819-1880.

INTESTINAL OBSTRUCTION
Dr. Ajay Chaudhary, Associate Professor, Department of Anesthesiology

A 37-years old female with distention of abdomen. She cannot pass flatus and stool since last 12 hours but otherwise is good general condition. Her past surgical history was significant for cholecystectomy 3 years ago, under general anesthesia, and cesarean delivery 1 year ago with spinal anesthesia. Both procedures were without complication. She weight 65 kg. In the preoperative holding area, her vital signs were heart rate, 97 beats per minute, blood pressure, 130/65 mm Hg, and respiratory rate, 18 breaths per minute. She was found to have acute abdominal tenderness, and she had a nasogastric tube in place. The tube was draining approximately 25mL per hour of bilious fluid. Her hematocrit was 39%.

1. What's your diagnosis?
    (A) Pregnancy
    (B) Bowel obstruction.
    (C) Worm infection.
    (D) Paralytic's ileus.
    (E) None of the above
2. What are the mechanisms a conscious person has to prevent regurgitation and pulmonary aspiration?
    (A) Lower esophageal sphincter
    (B) Gastro esophageal angle
    (C) Diaphragmatic crura
    (D) Upper esophageal sphincter
    (E) All of the above.
3. Discuss the risk factors for regurgitation and pulmonary aspiration during general anesthesia.
    (A) History of gastritis or ulcer
    (B) Esophageal disorders or previous esophageal surgery
    (C) Recent meal
    (D) Diabetes mellitus, if associated with gastro paresis
    (E) All of the above.
4. How should the nasogastric tube be managed before induction?
    (A) Nasogastric tube be suctioned before induction.
    (B) Nasogastric tube Both increase, les and upper esophageal sphincter tone.

(C) Application of cricoid pressure

(D) Increase the gastric pressure associated with induction.

(E) None of the above.

5. Describe the effects of commonly used anesthetic agents on lower esophageal sphincter tone decrease.

(A) Metoclopramide

(B) Metoprolol

(C) Neostigmine

(D) Pancuronium

(E) Inhalation agent.

Answers:

1. B

Respiratory rate, 18 breaths per minute. She was found to have acute abdominal tenderness, and she had a nasogastric tube draining approximately 25mL per hour of bilious fluid. Her hematocrit 39%.

2. E

Normal functioning of lower esophageal sphincter and preserved gastro esophageal peristalsis prevent the gastro esophageal reflux and regurgitation.

3. E

High-risk Patient for aspiration Like Full Stomach Patient, History of gastritis or ulcer Esophageal disorders or previous esophageal surgery,Recentmeal,Diabetes mellitus, with gastro paresis.

4. A

Nasogastric tube be suctioned before induction to prevent regurgitation and aspiration of patients.

5. E

Effect of Drugs Used in Anesthesia on Lower Esophageal Sphincter Tone Increase;

Metoclopramide, Domperidone, Prochlorperazine, Cyclizine, Edrophonium, Neostigmine, Succinylcholine, Pancuronium, Metoprolol, Antacids,

Effect of Drugs Used in Anesthesia on Lower Esophageal Sphincter Tone decrease; Halothane, Isoflurane, Enflurane.

References:

1. Boet S, Duttchen K, Chan J, 2011. Boet S, Duttchen K, Chan J, et. al.: Cricoid pressure provides incomplete esophageal occlusion associated with lateral deviation. J Emerg Med 2011; 5: pp. 1.

2. Cotton BR, Smith G, 1984. Cotton BR, Smith G: The lower oesophageal sphincter and anaesthesia. Br J Anaesth 1984; 56: pp. 37.

3. Ehrenfeld JM, Cassedy EA, Forbes VE, 2011. Ehrenfeld JM, Cassedy EA, Forbes VE, et. al.: Modified rapid sequence induction and intubation. AnesthAnalg 2011; 10: pp. 1.

4. El-Orbany M, Connolly LA, 2010. El-Orbany M, Connolly LA: Rapid sequence induction and intubation. AnesthAnalg 2010; 110: pp. 1318.

5. Nellipovitz DT, Crosby ET, 2007. Nellipovitz DT, Crosby ET: No evidence for decreased incidence of aspiration after rapid sequence induction. Can J Anesth 2007; 54: pp. 748.

6. Ng A, Smith G, 2001. Ng A, Smith G: Gastroesophageal reflux and aspiration of gastric contents in anesthetic practice. AnesthAnalg 2001; 93: pp. 494.

BLUNT INJURY ABDOMINAL

Dr. Ajay Chaudhary, Associate Professor, Department of Anesthesiology

A 18-year-old man flying kite from the roof of a two story apartment building slips and falls to the ground. On arrival to the emergency trauma centre KGMU lucknow30 minutes later, he is awake and alert and can accurately state his name. He is oriented to time place, and person, but he cannot recount actually what happened. He is complaining of pain. No ENT bleeding and vomiting. On physical examination, he is shivering, has a grossly deformed right proximal femur, and has a tender abdomen to palpation. His vital signs are heart rate 135 beats per minute, blood pressure 88/69 mm Hg, respirations 22 breaths per minute, and oxygen saturation by pulse oximetry (SpO$_2$) 99% on facemask oxygen.

1. What's your diagnosis:

(A) Head injury.

(B) Abdominal injury.

(C) Femur injury.

(D) Abdominal and femur injury.

(E) Head, abdominal and femur injury

2. What will you do if primary intubation attempts fail?
   (A) one person assigned to administer medications
   (B) To hold cricoid pressure
   (C) To maintain in-line cervical stabilization,
   (D) To manage the airway.
   (E) All of the above.
3. The fluid of choice for treating simple hypovolemia in a nonbleeding patient is
   (A) Isotonic crystalloid solution.
   (B) Normotonic crystalloid solution.
   (C) Hypertonic crystalloid solution.
   (D) Colloid solution.
   (E) None of the above.
4. What are the anesthesiologist's intraoperative priorities?
   (A) Provide immobility and amnesia
   (B) Monitor arterial blood pressure
   (C) Maintain normothermia.
   (D) Diagnose and treat medical issues and electrolyte abnormalities
   (E) All of the above.
5. What are the airway management options?
   (A) benefit to awake, nasal, blind, or fiberoptic intubation
   (B) asleep oral direct laryngoscopy
   (C) hold cricoid pressure
   (D) maintain in-line cervical stabilization
   (E) All of the above.

Answers:

1. D
   He is complaining of pain. No ENT bleeding and vomiting. On physical examination, he is shivering, and has a tender abdomen to palpation. His vital signs are heart rate 135 beats per minute, blood pressure 88/69 mm Hg, respirations 22 breaths per minute, and oxygen saturation by pulse oximetry (SpO$_2$) 99% on facemask oxygen.
2. E
   if primary intubation attempts fail than first to call for help and maintained the airway and oxygenate the patient.
3. A
   Isotonic solutions (physiological saline, Ringers lactate) are widely used as volume expanders. Their use inevitably results in an increase in the volume of interstitial fluid. The subsequent increase in lymphatic return is responsible for interstitial albumin being drawn into the plasma sector. Because of these effects, along with a lack of adverse effects, crystalloid solutions are the first choice for intravenous infusion solutions.
4. E
   He or she is continuously monitor your vital functions, including your pulse, blood pressure, oxygen level, ventilation (breathing) and level of anesthesia. On occasion anesthesiologist is form additional procedures to more closely monitor your blood pressure or your heart function depending on your medical condition and type of surgery. In addition, your anesthesiologist keeps a close eye on your fluid status and administers any necessary intravenous fluids or blood and blood products during your surgery. We will also administer any required pain medication and anti-nausea medication before you leave the operating room.
5. B
   Successful airway management ensure adequate tissue oxygenation. Most airway related deaths and morbidity result from a failure to ventilate and oxygenate rather than a failure to intubate. It is important for the anaesthetist to be skilled at airway management without tracheal intubation.

References:

1. Abdul Rahman YS, Al Den AS, Maull KI, 2010. Abdul Rahman YS, Al Den AS, and Maull KI: Prospective study of validity of neurologic signs in predicting positive cranial computed tomography following minor head trauma. Prehosp Disaster Med 2010; 25: pp. 59.
2. American College of Surgeons:, 2008. American College of Surgeons : ATLS Student Course Manual. Chicago: American College of Surgeons, 2008.
3. Diez C, Varon AJ, 2009. DiezC, and Varon AJ: Airway management and initial resuscitation of the trauma patient. CurrOpinCrit Care 2009; 15: pp. 542.

4. Healey MA, Samphire J, Hoyt DB, 2001. Healey MA, Samphire J, Hoyt DB, et al: Irreversible shock is not irreversible. J Trauma 2001; 50: pp. 826.
5. Herman NL, Carter B, Van Decar TK, 1996. Herman NL, Carter B, and Van Decar TK: Cricoid pressure. AnesthAnalg 1996; 83: pp. 859
6. Lieurance R, Benjamin JB, Rappaport WD, 1992. Lieurance R, Benjamin JB, and Rappaport WD: Blood loss and transfusion in patients with isolated femur fractures. J Orthop Trauma 1992; 6: pp. 175.

LABOUR ANALGESIA
Dr. Rita Wahal, Professor, Dept of Anaesthesiology

A 28 yrs old primigravida, otherwise healthy lady with 38 weeks pregnancy in labour pain is requesting for pain - relief

1. What are the adverse effects of labour pain apart from –
   (A) reduced uterine blood flow
   (B) reduced O2 delivery to the fetus
   (C) prolonged labour
   (D) maternal hypoventilation
2. Following agent cannot be used for pain relief in labour –
   (A) Entonox
   (B) Sevoflurane
   (C) I.V.Fentanyl
   (D) Epidural Ropivacaine
3. Epidural analgesia is not advised for the following reasons but one –
   (A) Maternal refusal
   (B) Allergy t LA
   (C) Bleeding tendency
   (D) Previous LSCS
4. Drug , which is not used for Epidural analgesia is -
   (A) Ropivacaine .1% 10ml + 2 mic/ml fentanyl
   (B) Levobupivacaine .1%
   (C) Bupivacaine .0625% + 2 mic/ml fentanyl
   (D) Lignocaine 2%
5. For Patient controlled epidural analgesia -
   (A) It Provides safe and effective technique
   (B) Provides no patient safety
   (C) Increases amount of LA used
   (D) Increases the incidence of motor block

Answers:
1. D
   Labour pain results in hyperventilation resulting in respiratory alkalosis and shifts the oxygen dissociation curve to left and reduced oxygen delivery to fetus.
2. C
   I.V. fenyanyl is not recommended as it causes respiratory depression.
3. D
   Previous LSCS is not a contra indication
4. D
   Epidural Lignocaine is short acting and causes motor blockade, there not recommended.
5. A
   It is a safe technique.

References:
1. Update on modern neuraxial analgesia in labour : a review of literature, C.Loubert et al, Feb.2011 onliinelibrary.wiley.com
2. Labour Analgesia , Miller's Anaesthesia pg. 2215

TMJ ANKYLOSIS - ANAESTHETIC MANAGEMENT

Dr. Rita Wahal, Professor, Department of Anaesthesiology

A 7 years old boy with bilateral TMJ Ankylosis is admitted in the Fascio-maxillary department. He fell from the mango tree at the age of 3yrs and thereafter his mouth opening is reducing gradually. Now, he is unable to open his mouth. His nutritional status is poor. He is small for his age. H/O snoring is present. On examination, TMJoint movements are not palpable, interincisor gap is zero and there is crowding of teeth. He is having retrognathia and prominent antigonial notch.

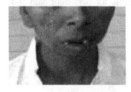

1. Preoperative assessment should include measurement of the following parameters except –
    (A) Mento-hyoid distance
    (B) Thyromental distance
    (C) Mallampatti grading
    (D) Patency of nostrils
2. Anaesthetic management to secure airway in this patient may include the following techniques apart from –
    (A) Blind nasal intubation
    (B) Fibreoptic guided intubation
    (C) Bougie with ILMA
    (D) Tracheostomy
3. Awake intubation in TMJ Ankylosis does not require –
    (A) Trans tracheal injection of LA
    (B) Superior laryngeal nerve block
    (C) Consent and LA sensivity test
    (D) Rocuronium
4. Inducion of anaesthesia in TMJ ankylosis patient should not include –
    (A) Atropine
    (B) Sevoflurane
    (C) Propofol
    (D) Suxamethonium
5. FibreopticBronchopycannot be performed if the following is present except –
    (A) Heavy secretions
    (B) Bleeding not relieved by suction
    (C) LA allergy
    (D) Hypercapnia

Answers:
1. C
    Patient is unable to open his mouth; therefore Mallampatti grading can not be performed.
2. C
    Bougie and ILMA can not be introduced, as mouth opening is nil
3. D
    Muscle relaxant should not be given
4. D
    Suxamethonium should not be used till the airway is secured in patients with difficult airway
5. D
    Hypercapnia creates no problem in fibreoptic intubation

References:
1. American Society of Anaesthesiologists Task Force on Management of the Difficult Airway. Practice Guidelines for management of difficult airway: an updated report by the American Society of Anaesthesiologists Task Force on Management of the Difficult Airway. Anaesthesiology. 2013;118:251-270
2. Airway management, Clinical Anaesthesia – Barash 6th edition (2009) pg. 751

PAIN MANAGEMENT: FOLLOW-THROUGH CASE OF CARCINOMA GALL BLADDER

Dr. Sarita Singh, Associate Professor, Department of Anaesthesiology

A 55 years old female patient referred from the gastro surgery department with persistent pain in right hypochondrium since 3 month duration, with history of off and on fever, itching and dark color urine. On examination she had jaundice and lump in right hypochondrium, with mild ascites. She was initially treated by physician for 1 month. When no response then investigation were done and referred to gastro surgeon for further treatment. After reviewing the case by surgeon she was referred to pain clinic for persistent pain and palliative care.

1. What could be most likely diagnosis:
   (A) Carcinoma stomach
   (B) Carcinoma head pancreas
   (C) Carcinoma gall bladder
   (D) Carcinoma Colon
2. What could be the most important investigation:
   (A) Ultrasound
   (B) CT scan
   (C) ERCP
   (D) X-ray Abdomen
3. What could be the cause of persistent pain in this patient:
   (A) Metastasis in liver
   (B) Distention and stretching of CBD and gall bladder
   (C) Infiltration to the retro peritoneum
   (D) All of the above
4. In this case which plexus are responsible for pain perception:
   (A) Celiac plexus
   (B) Splanchnic plexus
   (C) Hypogastric plexus
   (D) a+b
5. If patient is not responding with conventional analgesics then what will be options:
   (A) Celiac plexus block
   (B) Splanchnic block
   (C) Hypogastric block
   (D) Stellate ganglion block

Answers:
   1. B
   Carcinoma Head Pancrease.
   2. C
   CT scan
   3. D
   All of the above
   4. D – (a +b)
   5. A
   Celiac plexces block

Reference:
   1. Joshi Murlidhar –Text book of Pain Management 2nd edition Hyderabad India, Joshi Institute of pain 2009.

TRIGEMINAL NEURALGIA

Dr. Sarita Singh, Associate Professor, Department of Anaesthesiology

A young man of 25 years is presented with sudden onset of recurrent electric shock like pain over the right side of face for 6 month, aggravated by chewing, brushing and washing of the face.The was no H/O toothache in past, tooth carries &trauma. He was referred from dental OPD to pain clinic for further treatment.

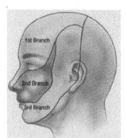

(Distribution of Trigeminal nerve)

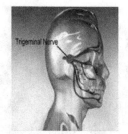

(Branches of Trigeminal Nerve)

1. What will be the most likely diagnosis:
   (A) Mandibular neuralgia
   (B) Horner syndrome
   (C) Trigeminal neuralgia
   (D) Glossopharngeal neuralgia
2. What could be most appropriate investigation:
   (A) CT
   (B) MRI
   (C) Angiography
   (D) X-ray
3. Most common branch involve in Trigeminal neuralgia:
   (A) Ophthalmic
   (B) Mandibular
   (C) Maxillary
   (D) Mandibular+ Maxillary
4. What are the interventional procedure in this disease:
   (A) Radiofrequency ablation of the nerve
   (B) Balloon decompression
   (C) Steroid phenol, glycerol injection
   (D) All of above.
5. Suicide disease – is the name of:
   (A) Trigeminal neuralgia
   (B) Migrane
   (C) Cancer
   (D) Glossopharyngeal neuralgia

Answers:

    1. C
       Trigeminal Neuralgia
    2. B
       MRI
    3. D
       Mandibular + Maxillary
    4. D
       All of the above
    5. A
       Trigeminal Neuralgia.

Reference:
1. Joshi Murlidhar–Text book of Pain Management 2ndedition Hyderabad India, Joshi Institute of pain 2009.

PREECLAMPSIA & PREGNANCY

Dr. Rajni Kapoor, Professor, Department of Anaesthesiology

A female of age 30 years and 24 wks pregnancy was admitted in Queen Mary Hospital with BP 170/120 mmHg ,persistent headache, epigastric pain, cyanosis,yellow discolouration and her 24 hour urine specimen showed proteins 6 gm % and urine output 400 ml in 24 hours.Platelet count was80,000/cu mm.There was no history of hypertension in past and no air way problem .

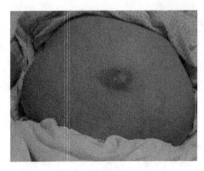

1. What is her probable diagnosis?
    (A) Mild preeclampsia
    (B) Severe preeclampsia
    (C) Gestationalhypertension
    (D) Chronic hypertension
2. What is not associated withits pathogenesis
    (A) Decreased placental perfusion
    (B) Upregulation of cytokines and inflammatory factors
    (C) Excessive activation of coagulation
    (D) Decreased thromboxane and increased prostacyclin
3. Use of MgSO4in control of seizures ineclamptic patient is not associated with
    (A) Vasodilatation and increased cardiac output
    (B) Narrow therapeutic index
    (C) Decreased CNS irritability
    (D) Dcatecholamine release
4. Following antihypertensive not used in pregnancy
    (A) Hydralazine
    (B) Labetalol
    (C) Nitroglycerine
    (D) ACE inhibitor
5. What is untrue about HELLP Syndrome
    (A) Normal blood smear
    (B) Increased liver enzymes
    (C) Low platelet count
    (D) Increased bilirubin

Answers:
1. B
   In mild preeclampsiaBP is <160/110mm of mercury,in gestational hypertension there is no proteinuria and in chronic hypertension there is past history of hypertension
2. D
   There is imbalance of increased thromboxane and decreased prostacyclin in a preeclamptic patient due to high circulating levels of fibronectin and Endothelin because of Endothelin dysfunction
3. D
   Magnesium blunts the response to vasoconstrictors and inhibits catecholamine release after sympathetic stimulation It also increases cardiac output by decreasing systemic vascular resistance.serumlevelbetween 2-3.5mmol/lbeing safe and effective
4. D
   ACE inhibitors can cause congenital malformations
5. A
   Criteria for diagnosing HELLP syndrome is abnormal blood smear,increased level of enzymes and low platelet count.

Reference:
1. Ronald DD. Miller, MD, Complicated Obstetric Conditions Preeclampsia and Eclampsia A Text Book of Anaesthesia by Miller , 7 Edition

PREGNANCY WITH MITRAL STENOSIS

Dr. Rajni Kapoor, Professor, Department of Anaesthesiology

A 25 yrsold unregistered primiwith 36 wks pregnancy was admitted to female hospital with complains of exertionaldyspnoea and decreased foetal movements There is history of rheumatic fever and fleeting type of joint pains in childhood with no subsequent medical follow up. Echo showed mitral valve area > 1 cm2 and Hockey stick appearance of anterior leaflet.There is no past history of heart failure ,sroke and ischemic attack

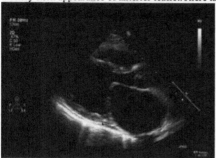

1. What is her probable diagnosis.
   (A) Aortic stenosis
   (B) Severe mitralstenosis
   (C) Mitral regugitation
   (D) Coarctation of aorta
2. The incidence of heart disease in pregnancy in modern era is mostly due to.
   (A) Intrinsic cardiac disease
   (B) Infections
   (C) Congenital heart disease
   (D) Rheumatic heart disease
3. Which cardiovascular change do not occur in normal pregnancy?
   (A) Increased cardiac output
   (B) Increased blood pressure
   (C) Pulmonarycapillarywedge pressure unchanged
   (D) Lt ventricle strokework index unchanged
4. What is untrue about haemodynamic goals of intra operative management of the pregnant patient with mitral stenosis.
   Avoid
   (A) Tachycardia
   (B) Marked increase in SVR
   (C) Marked Increase in Central blood volume
   (D) Increase in pulmonaryvascular resistance
5. What is untrue for giving GA for cesarean section in patient with mitral stenosis?
   Avoid
   (A) Ketamine
   (B) Isoflurane
   (C) Oxytocin
   (D) Phenylephrine

Answers:

1. B
   Hockey stick appearance is characteristic of severe mitral stenosis
2. C
   Decrease in incidence due to intrinsic cardiac disease,infections and rheumaticheart disease is due to their successful treatment
3. B
   Blood pressure is not elevated because peripheral vascular resistance decreases
4. B
   Marked decrease in systemic vascular resistance should be avoided because compensatory increase

in heart rate can result.Elevation of pulmonary vascular resistance is poorly tolerated by these patients.Increased central blood volume can increase load on the heart.

5. D

   If hypotension occurs during GA phenyl ephrine is preferred as it does not cause tachycardia.Ketemine and isoflurane could increase the heart rate.Oxytocin can increase pulmonary vascular resistance

Reference:

1. Robert K. Stoelting M.D Stephen F.Dierdarf,MD Breech Presentation,Fetal Distress and Mitral Stenosis Anaesthesia and coexisting Disease by Yao and Artusio .

COPD

Dr. Zia Arshad, Assistant Professor, Department of Anesthesiology

A 52 year old male was admitted with complain of acute onset breathlessness. His vitals are normal. On auscultation rhonchi were audible Patient is a known case of diabetes and COPD for 20 years. Spirometry reveal FEV_1 is <40%.

1. What will be the next step?
   (A) Short acting B2 Agonist by Metered Dose Inhaler every 20min
   (B) Oral Steroid
   (C) Short acting B2 Agonist + Ipratropium by nebulisation along with IV steroid
   (D) Intubation & Mechanical Ventilation
2. After repeated nebulisation and steroid therapy there was no improvement. (His Blood gases shows PaO_2-55 and $PaCo_2$ 78 mmHg, PH 7.15 and Hco_3-38). The next step would be:-
   (A) Repeat nebulisation
   (B) Reassess the pt after 1 hour
   (C) Admit to ICU
   (D) None of the above
3. Non invasive ventilation is used in the following.
   (A) Unresponsive patient
   (B) Impending cardiac or respiratory failure
   (C) Copious secretion
   (D) Progressive hypercapnia

Answers:

1. C

   Since the patient is having FEV1 less than 40%. So he is having a severe type of severe exacerbation of COPD.
2. C

   Since the patient is having hypoxemia with hypercarbia with respiratory acidosis and it is a life threatening condition, the patient requires admission to ICU.
3. D

   Non invasive ventilation has been most successfully used in acute exacerbation of COPD with progressive hypercapnia.

Reference:

1. Marino P.L. The ICU Book, 4th Edition. Lipincott William and Wilkins, New Delhi, 2014.; 470-479.

HEART FAILURE

Dr. Zia Arshad, Assistant Professor, Department of Anesthesiology

A Patient 60 years old known hypertensive was admitted in ICU as a case of CerebrovascularAccident with right sided hemi paresis 2nd day of admission patient develop dyspnea hypertension, tachycardia. He is suspected to have left sided heart failure.

1. What is the earliest sign of ventricular dysfunction?
   (A) PCWP(Pulmonary Capillary Wedge Pressure)
   (B) HR (Heart Rate)

(C) Stroke Volume

(D) Cardiac index

2. Which one of the following is **CORRECT**?

   (A) Tachycardia offsets the reduction in stroke volume

   (B) Pulonary capillary wedge pressure is not changed in early stages of heart failure

   (C) Earliest sign is the decrease in cardiac output

   (D) None of the above

3. Which among the following is **NOT** correct?

   (A) Diastolic dysfunction is responsible for up to 60% of cases of Heart Failure

   (B) Common case of diastolic Heart Failure is ventilator hypertrophy.

   (C) Heart failure due to diastolic dysfunction is called as heart failure with reduce ejection fraction

   (D) End diastolic volume is the distinguishing feature between systolic & diastolic heart failure

Answers:

   1. A

      Earliest sign of ventricular dysfunction is an increase in cardiac filling pressure that is pulmonary artery wedge pressure.

   2. A

      The filling pressure (PCWP) is the earliest pressure to be raised in heart failure.

   3. C

      The heart failure that is predominantly the result of diastolic dysfunction is called heart failure with normal ejection fraction.

Reference:

1. Marino P.L. The ICU Book, 4th Edition. Lipincott William and Wilkins, New Delhi, 2014.; 240-245.

HYDROCEPHALOUS

Dr. V.K. Bhatia, Professor, Department of Anaesthesiology

A one month old male child was admitted in the hospital with complaints of large head, poor feeding and recurrent vomiting. His examination confirmed the diagnosis of hydrocephalous. CT scan head showed aqueductal stenosis. He was planned for ventriculoperitoneal shunt placement under general anesthesia.

1. Maneuvers leading to increase in intracranial pressure are all except:

   (A) Coughing

   (B) Neck flexion

   (C) Head elevation

   (D) Valsalva maneuver

2. Drugs used to decrease ICP are all except

   (A) Mannitol

   (B) Furosemide

   (C) Acetazolamide

   (D) Phenytoin

3. Clinical features of hydrocephalous in a child does not include:

   (A) Delayed milestone

   (B) Macewen's sign

   (C) Hypoactive reflexes

   (D) 6th nerve palsy

4. Latex allergy is more frequently seen in patient having hydrocephalous associated with:

   (A) Aqueduct stenosis

   (B) Myelomeningocele

   (C) Dandy Walker syndrome

   (D) Arachnoid cyst

5. The following statement regarding intraoperative management of hydrocephalous is correct:

   (A) Use of nitrous oxide is encouraged

   (B) Intraoperative spontaneous ventilation is recommended

   (C) Mild hypocapnia should be maintained

   (D) Volatile anesthetics does not increases ICP

Answers:

   1. C

      Head elevation increases venous return and decreases intracranial pressure.

2. D

   Phenytoin is an antiepileptic.

3. C

   The reflexes are hyperactive in hydrocephalous

4 B

   Latex allergy has been seen associated with meningomyelocoele

5 C

   hypocapnia decreases intracranial pressure

References:

1. Drummond JC, Patel PM. Neurosurgical Anesthesia. In: Miller RD (Eds) Miller's Anesthesia, 7th edition. Elsevier, Philadelhia 2010, pp 2045-2081.
2. Mytra S, Bakshi S, Bhosle S. Hydrocephalous. In Kulkarni AP Objective Anaesthesia Review, 3rd edition. Jaypee, New Delhi 2013, pp 132-140.

POSTERIOR FOSSA SURGERY

Dr. V.K. Bhatia, Professor, Department of Anaesthesiology

A 26 years old female presented with complaints of headache, progressive loss of vision and hearing, weakness in lower limbs and recurrent vomiting. She was examined and investigated and diagnosed to have acoustic neuroma. She was planned for craniotomy and excision of poaterior fossa tumour under general anaesthesia.

1. Irritation of following brainstem areas can result in cardiovascular response except:
   (A) Lower pons
   (B) Cereballarvermis
   (C) Upper medulla
   (D) Extra axial portion of 5th nerve
2. The following cranial nerve is not involved in posterior fossa tumours:
   (A) 1st
   (B) 9th
   (C) 10th
   (D) 12th
3. Following complications can occur in posterior fossa surgery except:
   (A) Bradycardia
   (B) Venous air embolism
   (C) Pneumothorax
   (D) Respiratory failure
4. Airway complication seen in posterios fossa tumours and surgery are due to all except:
   (A) Macroglossia
   (B) Cranial nerve dysfunction
   (C) Depressed sensorium
   (D) Choanal atresia
5. Dysrhythmias seen during posterior fossa surgery is commonly due to:
   (A) Associated cardiac disease
   (B) Brainstem stimulation
   (C) Electrolyte imbalance
   (D) Anesthetic drugs

Answers:

1. B

   Cerebellar vermis is not associated with cardiovascular response

2. A

   1st cranial nerve is not a part of posterior fossa

3. C

   Pneumothorax is not a complication of posterior fossa surgery

4. D

   Choanal atresia is not a cause of airway complication.

5. B

   Brainstem stimulation leads to arrhythmias.

Reference:

1. Drummond JC, Patel PM. Neurosurgical Anesthesia. In: Miller RD (Eds) Miller's Anesthesia, 7th edition. Elsevier, Philadelhia 2010, pp 2045-2081.

SQUINT SURGERY

Dr. Jyotsna Agrawal, Professor, Department of Anaesthesiology

A child, 10 years of age, presented with right sided squint for squint correction surgery under GA. On examination, her cardio-respiratory system was within normal limits.There were no associated congenital anomalies present.There was no family history suggestive of hyperpyrexia present in this child. The child was investigated and all routine investigations were within normal limits. The child was taken up for surgery under GA.

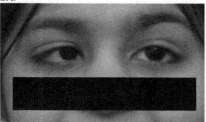

1. Occulocardiac reflex is mediated by:
    (A) Mediated by Optic Nerve and Third Nerve
    (B) Mediated by Oculomotor and Trigeminal Nerve
    (C) Mediated by Optic Nerve and Vagus Nerve
    (D) Mediated by Opthalmic division of Fifth Nerve and Vagus Nerve
2. Occulocardiac reflex is mostly affected by all except:
    (A) Pull on rectus muscle
    (B) Hypercarbia
    (C) Hypoxia
    (D) Hypocapnia
3. Malignant hyperpyrexia is triggered in patients with pre-existing:
    (A) Squint/Ptosis
    (B) Congenital Cataract
    (C) Visual defects
    (D) Retinoblastoma
4. Malignant hyperpyrexia is precipitated under general anaesthesia by using all drugs except:
    (A) Ether
    (B) Halothane
    (C) Vecuronium
    (D) Suxamethonium
5. Signs and symptoms of malignant hyperthermia include all except:
    (A) Elevated Etco2
    (B) Normal pH
    (C) Raised CK and potassium levels
    (D) Muscle rigidity

Answers:

1. D

    Occulocardiacreflex–Reflex was described by Aschner and Dagini so also called Aschner-Dagini reflex. Afferent is mediated by orbital contents to ciliary ganglion viaopthalmic division of Fifth Nerve to sensory nucleus of trigeminal nerve at fourth ventricle. Efferent is via Vagus nerve to heart causing bradycardia, arrhythmia andcardiac arrest. Mostly it is triggered by pull on extraocular muscles –more so bymedial rectus pull than lateral rectus pull.Relieved when surgery is stopped, sometimes it can be caused by local anesthetic infiltrations for Cataract surgery, Strabismus surgery [squint], Enucleation, Blepharoplasty,Enucleation, Periorbital tumor excision.

2. D

    All these causes exaggerated occulocardiac response and can be prevented by atropine or lycopyrrolate premedication.

3. A

    All congenital musculo-skeletal disorders predispose patient to malignant hyperpyrexia. Detailedpatient history and family history should be taken to prevent malignant hyperpyrexia.

4. C

Malignant hyperthermia can be precipitated by Halothane, Isoflurane, Enflurane, Sevoflurane, Desflurane, Suxamethonium, Decamethonium.

5. B

Malignant hyperthermia is a hypercatabolic state causing muscle breakdown, increased temperature, heart rate and increased CO2 production, and acidosis.

Malignant hyperpyrexia is an autosomal dominant genetic character. It is characterized by rigidity after using Suxamethonium and/or Halothane causing:

- Unexplained tachycardia/arrhythmia.
- Tachypnoea.
- Unexplained fall in Po2 and rise in Etco2.
- Metabolic and respiratory acidosis.
- Increase in body temperature above 38.8°C.
- Unexplained serum potassium rise.
- Increased CK levels.
- Rhabdomyolysis causing acute renal failure.
- Myoglobinuria.

Malignant hyperpyrexia should be suspected in patients having:

- Muscle disorder.
- Raised muscle enzyme- CPK levels.
- Electrolyte changes especially potassium and calcium levels.
- History of heat stroke or hyperthermia after exercise.

Treatment:

- Supportive and symptomatic.
- Dantroline – 10mg/kg IV every 5-10 minutes till symptoms are relieved . Continue till three days orally.

Investigation:

- ABG
    o   For acidosis
    o   Serum potassium , calcium
    o   Po2,Pco2
- Coagulation studies PT,PTT

Reference:
1. Miller RD. Miller's Anesthesia. 8th ed. Philadelphia: PA Elsevier Saunders; 2015. p. 1296-1302.

OPEN EYE INJURY

Dr. Jyotsna Agrawal, Professor, Department of Anaesthesiology

An adult male of 45 years of age, presented in emergency. He had a fall and some sharp object hit his eye, one day prior to admission. He was admitted for surgery under GA for repair of perforation. On examination, he is a non-diabetic, non hypertensive and not on any medication. He had no other injury. He is posted for emergency surgery for repair of perforation. He was nil orally for six hours.His routine investigations were within normal range.

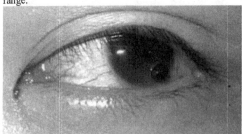

1. Intra-ocular pressure is increased by all except:
   (A) Coughing/straining
   (B) Suxamethonium
   (C) Ketamine
   (D) Hypocapnia

2. Open eye trauma patients may present with:
   (A) Acute changes in IOP
   (B) Vitreous loss
   (C) Retinal detachment
   (D) Glaucoma
3. Anaesthetic problem in open eye injury include all except:
   (A) Full stomach
   (B) Patient with decreased FRC may become hypoxic rapidly
   (C) IOP may be raised
   (D) Increased Etco2 levels
4. Acute ophthalmic emergency include:
   (A) Retinal artery thrombosis
   (B) Chemical burn
   (C) Both (a) and (b)
   (D) Neither (a) nor (b)
5. Sub-acute ophthalmic emergencies include all except:
   (A) Open globe injury
   (B) Lid laceration
   (C) Chronic retinal detachment
   (D) Narrow angle glaucoma

Answers:

1. D
   All the drugs or physiological processes which cause extra-ocular muscle contraction raise intra-ocular pressure.
2. D
   Open eye injury, if small, can lead to rise in IOP, but if large, can lead to vitreous loss and even retinal detachment.
3. D
4. C
   These two conditions can cause blindness within a very short time (minutes-1 hour). Retinal artery thrombosis can also be precipitated by pressure on eyeball by facemask, positioning of patient causing pressure on eyeball or accidental.
5. C
   Chronic retinal detachment is usually present for days to months.

Reference:

1. Miller RD. Miller's Anesthesia. 8th ed. Philadelphia: PA Elsevier Saunders; 2015. p. 2512-2520.

ACUTE RESPIRATORY DISTRESS SYNDROME
Dr. Monica Kohli, Professor, Department of Anaesthesiology

A 56 year old man is admitted to the ICU with ARDS and sepsis following emergency colectomy for mesenteric ischemia. His height is 65 inches; his weight is 285 pounds. On lung protective ventilator settings, his settings are –

Peak inspiratory pressure (PIP) is 35 cm H2O
Plateau pressure (Pplat) is 30 cm H2O
Mean airway pressure (Paw) is 20 cm H2O
Esophageal balloon pressure (Pes) is 17 cm H2O.

1. Transpulmonary pressure (Ptp) is estimated by the formula:
   (A) Paw-Pplat
   (B) PEEP-Pes
   (C) Pplat-Paw
   (D) Paw-Pes
2. The early use of cis-atracurium in severe ARDS is
   (A) Contraindicated in patients with diabetes
   (B) Associated with lower mortality in severe ARDS
   (C) May be facilitated by discontinuation of sedation
   (D) Required with rescue treatment (HFOV, prone positioning, ECMO)

3. Prone Positioning in adult patients with ARDS is associated with:
   (A) Increased radiographic edema
   (B) Reduced pressure ulcer rates
   (C) Increased ventilator associated pneumonia rates
   (D) Reduced mortality in patients with severe hypoxemia
4. Which of the following is not true regarding High Frequency Oscillatory Ventilation (HFOV)?
   (A) Early initiation of HFOV in ARDS is associated with increased survival.
   (B) Decreasing Hertz (decreasing frequency) will increase minute ventilation.
   (C) Improvements in oxygenation may be seen within six hours of therapy.
   (D) Sedation and neuromuscular blockade use are increased with HFOV.
5. The Berlin definition of Severe ARDS includes assessment of which of the following?
   (A) Oxygenation: PaO2/FiO2 < 100 mmHg
   (B) Minute Ventilation: VECORR > 10L/min
   (C) Radiographs: CXR with all 4 quadrants showing pulmonary edema
   (D) Ventilator pressures: Pplat>25 cm H2O

Answers:
1. D
   (Transpulmonary pressure reflects the pressure gradient across the lung opposing alveolar collapse is measured as the difference between alveolar pressure and intrapleural pressure)
2. B
   (The ACURASYS study reported 90-day mortality advantages (30/8% vs. 44.6%) and increased ventilator-free days following 48 hours of neuromuscular blockade versus placebo in early severe ARDS.)
3. D
   (Prone positioning for ARDS attempts to improve shunt by redistributing blood flow away from areas of dependent atelectasis).
4. A
   (Two recent prospective, randomized multicenter trials of HFOV in ARDS revealed no survival benefit and one demonstrated increased mortality.)
5. A
   (The current "Berlin Definition"2 discards the use of the term acute lung injury (ALI) and instead divides ARDS into Mild, Moderate, and Severe categories based on degree of hypoxemia (PaO2/FIO2 ratio 300 mm Hg, 200 mm Hg, and 100 mm Hg,)

References:
1. Talmor D, Sarge T, Malhotra A, O'Donnell CR, Ritz R, Lisbon A, Novack V, Loring SH. "Mechanical Ventilation Guided by Esophageal Pressure in Acute Lung Injury", NEJM 2008; 359:2095-2104
2. Papazian L, Forel J-M, Gacouin A, ET. al., for the ACURASYS Study Investigators. NEJM 2010; 363:1107-16
3. Gattinoni L, Carlesso E, Taccone P, Polli F, Guerin C, Mancebo J. Prone positioning improves survival in severe ARDS: a pathophysiologic review and individual patient meta-analysis. Minerva anestesiologica 2010; 76:448-54
4. Ferguson ND, Cook DJ, Guyatt GH, et. al. for the OSCILLATE Trial investigators and the Canadian Critical Care Trials Group. High-Frequency Oscillation in Early Acute Respiratory Distress Syndrome. NEJM 2013 Feb 28; 368 (9): 795-805
5. Bernard GR, Artigas A, Brigham KL, et al. The American-European Consensus Conference on ARDS.Definitions, mechanisms, relevant outcomes, and clinical trial coordination. American journal of respiratory and critical care medicine 1994; 149:818-24

URETERIC STONE
Dr. Vinita Singh, Professor, Department of Anaesthesiology

A 65 year old male, a known hypertensive for the past 15 years had posterior wall MI for which a bare metal stent was placed in LAD three months back. Since then patient is on low dose aspirin and clopidogrel therapy. Now he has presented with excruciating pain in the right flank radiating to the right groin.
1. What is the most likely diagnosis:
   (A) Right Kidney Stone
   (B) Acute Appendicitis

(C) Right Ureteric Stone

(D) Gastroenteritis

2. What investigation would you perform to confirm the diagnosis:

(A) Plain X Ray Abdomen

(B) Ultrasound Abdomen

(C) Barium Meal

(D) Intravenous pyelography

3. What is the recommendation of ACCP (American College of Chest Physicians) regarding the discontinuation of aspirin and clopidogrel prior to the elective surgery in this patient:

(A) Continue Aspirin and Stop Clopidogrel 7-10 Days Before Surgery

(B) Stop Both Drugs 48 Hours Before Surgery

(C) Stop Aspirin 48 Hours Before and Continue Clopidogrel

(D) Continue both drugs.

4. Patient has to undergo URS and relatively safe anesthetic plan would be:

(A) Epidural Anesthesia

(B) General Anesthesia

(C) Spinal + Epidural Anesthesia

(D) Spinal Anesthesia

5. Bleeding is a major complication of anticoagulant and thrombolytic therapy and typically classified as major and endangering in all except:

(A) Intracranial

(B) Intraoral

(C) Intaocular

(D) Ntraspinal

Answers:

1. C

   Excruciating pain in flank radiating to the groin is suggestive of ureteric stone.

2. D

   Intravenous pyelography is the most sensitive test for the detection of ureteric stone.

3. A

   According to the recommendation of ACCP clopidogrel should be stopped 7-10days before elective surgery and aspirin should be continued because patient is a high risk case of thromboembolic episode and even for perioperative cardiac event.

4. D

   There are least chances of anesthetic complication with spinal (atraumatic) anesthesia alone in this patient.

5. B

References:

1. Douketis JD, Berger PB, Dunn AS, et al. The perioperative management of antithrombotic therapy: American College of Chest Physicians Evidence-Based Clinical Practice Guidelines (8th Edition). Chest 2008; 133: 299S - 339S.

2. Horlocker TT, Wedel DJ, Rowlingson JC, Enneking FK, Kopp SL, Benzon HT, Brown DL, Heit JA, Mulroy MF, Rosenquist RW, Tryba LM, Yuan C. Regional Anesthesia in the Patient Receiving Antithrombotic or Thrombolytic Therapy: American Society of Regional Anesthesia and Pain Medicine Evidence-Based Guidelines (Third Edition). Regional Anesthesia and Pain Medicine 2010; 35(1): 64 – 101.

TURP SYNDROME

Dr. Vinita Singh, Professor, Department of Anaesthesiology

A 72-year-old man, without any coexisting disease, body weight 62 Kg, underwent transurethral resection of prostate under spinal anesthesia, with 2.5 ml of hyperbaric bupivacaine (0.5%). The level extended to the T10, as tested by pin prick. The heart rate at the start of the operation was 80 bpm, blood pressure 140/80 mmHg, normal ECG and spo2 was 98%. The patient was placed in lithotomy position and the TURP surgery was started. The preoperative values for serum sodium was 145 mmol/L, potassium 4.1 mmol/L, creatinine 1.1 mg% and urea 40mg%. The irrigation fluid used by urologist was glycine 1.5%. TURP was performed by monopolar instrument. The total intraoperative bleeding was estimated at 500 ml. The average peroperative blood pressure was 145/85 mmHg and heart rate 85 bpm. During surgery, which lasted for 100 min, the patient had been given

1500 ml normal saline solution by intravenous infusion. Postopertively, after 30 min, patient suddenly developed nausea, vomiting, agitation then rapidly coma, hypoxemia (SpO2 72%), hypotension (60/38 mmHg) and bradycardia (45 bpm). The abdomen and lung auscultation were normal.

1. What is the most likely diagnosis:
    (A) Intracranial Hemorrhage
    (B) Myocardial Ischemia
    (C) Turp Syndrome
    (D) Endotoxemia
2. What investigation would you perform to confirm the diagnosis:
    (A) Serum sodium
    (B) Serum potassium
    (C) Serum urea and creatinine
    (D) Serum Troponin
3. Which irrigating solution can produce electrocardiograhic changes with raised troponin in TURP patients:
    (A) Sorbitol
    (B) Normal saline
    (C) Glycine
    (D) Mannitol
4. All of the following would be included in the treatment regimen of this patient except:
    (A) Diuretic therapy
    (B) Hemodynamic support with vasopressors
    (C) Endotracheal intubation and ventilation
    (D)Hypertonic saline 3%.
5. To prevent this complication all of the following measures can be taken except:
    (A) Laser nucleation or abalation
    (B) Monopolar resection in saline
    (C) Photoselective vaporization
    (D) Reducing the surgical time

Answers:
1. C
   The s/s are suggestive of TURP syndrome.
2. A
   Severe hyponatremia is diagnostic of TURP syndrome.
3. C
4. A
   In a hemodynamically unstable patient, diuretics are not reccommmended.
5. B
   Not monopolar, bipolar resection will reduce the opened venous sinuses so the absorption of the irrigating fluid will reduce.

References:
1. Boukatta B, Sbai H, Messaoudi F, Lafrayiji Z, El Bouazzaoui A, Kanjaa N. Transurethral resection of prostate syndrome: report of a case. Pan African Medical Journal.2013; 14:14.
2. Collins JW, Macdermott S, Brad RA, Keely FX, Timoney AG. The effects of the choice of irrigating fluid on cardiac stress during Transurethral resection of the prostate: A comparison between 1.5% Glycine and 5% glucose. J Urol. 2007;177:1369-73.

Chapter-3

Cardiothoracic and Vascular Surgery

LUNG CANCER

Dr. Shailendra Kumar, Professor, Dr. Archana Mishra, Department of Cardiothoracic
and Vascular Surgery

A 66 year old man came to the hospital with history of chronic cough and haemoptysis. He was a chronic smoker for the last 20 years. There was loss of weight and appetite. Chest X ray was suggestive of right upper lobar mass. CT Scan of the thorax at 2nd rib level is depicted below:

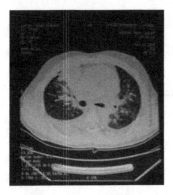

1. What is the most common probable diagnosis
   - (A) Neoplastive pathology
   - (B) Pulmonary tuberculosis
   - (C) Benign lung pathology
   - (D) Bronchietatic lesion
2. What is the most commonly used tool in screening of lung cancer
   - (A) Sputum Evaluation
   - (B) Low dose Helical CT Scan
   - (C) Chest X ray
   - (D) Fluorescence Bronchoscopy
3. Determinants of primary lung neoplastic pathology in screen detected nodule are all except
   - (A) Nodule size
   - (B) Change in size
   - (C) Multiplicity of lesion
   - (D) consistency of the nodule
4. What is the most common histopathological type of Non small cell lung cancer
   - (A) Adenocarcinoma
   - (B) Squamous cell cancer
   - (C) Adenosquamous type
   - (D) Undifferentiated
5. Which is not the common cause of secondary lung metastasis
   - (A) Osteogenic sarcoma
   - (B) Melanoma
   - (C) Breast
   - (D) Oesophagus

Answers:

1. A

   Elderly male with chronic smoking with typical symptoms of loss of weight, chronic cough, and haemoptysis with parenchymal mass lesion is suggestive of neoplastic pathology

2. B

   An ideal screening tool for detecting a disease possesses adequate sensitivity and specificity. Low dose CT Scan has been evaluated by many study groups to be the best way as the screening tool for lung cancer.

3. C

   Multiplicity of the lesions (>6) are generally thought to be low risk for malignancy and more lightly to have inflammatory lung disease

4. A

Historically , histologies associated with heavy smoking use was squamous and small cell carcinomas , squamous cell carcinoma was most commonly diagnosed NSCLC ,but with steady decline in cigarette consumption over the past decades adenocarcinoma has replaced squamous cell carcinoma as the most frequent histologic type in North America,

5. D

Epithelial cancers especially GI cancers are uncommon causes of lung metastasis

References:

1. Goldberg KB NCI Lung Cancer Screening Trial. Cancer Letter. Washington .DC: National Cancer Institute; 2002
2. Bailey & love's 26th edition Malignant Lung Tumours pages 859 to 867
3. Sabiston and Spencer, Surgery of the Chest edition 8, pages 275 to 321
4. Harrison's Principles of Internal Medicine 18th Edition Volume1, page 378

POSTERIOR MEDIASTINAL TUMOUR

Dr. Shailendra Kumar, Professor, Dr. Archana Mishra, Department of Cardiothoracic and Vascular Surgery

A 60 year old lady came to the hospital for gall stone surgery. She was investigated routinely and on chest radiograph, an intra-thoracic right sided opacity was found. Lateral view chest X ray and CT Scan of thorax is shown below:

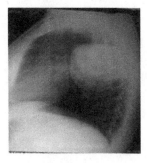 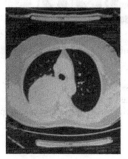

1. What is the probable diagnosis
   (A)Posterior mediastinal mass
   (B)Chest wall mass
   (C)Lung parenchymal mass
   (D)Anterior mediastinal mass
2. What is the most common lesion in posterior mediastinum
   (A)Neurogenic tumour
   (B)Germ Cell tumour
   (C)Brochogenic cyst
   (D)Teratomus
3. Which of the following approach is not used in resection of posterior mediastinal mass
   (A)Cervical
   (B)Paravertebral
   (C)Thoracotomy
   (D)Sternotomy

Answers:

1. A

Chest X ray and CT Scan is suggestive of paraspinal mass which are considered to be posterior mediastinal

2. A

Neurogenic tumours are the most common pathology in the posterior mediastinum

3. D

Sternotomy is used for anterior and middle mediastinal and sometimes for chest wall deformity surgeries

References:
1. Sabiston and Spencer, Surgery of the Chest, edition 8, pages 649 to 660

ANTERIOR MEDIASTINAL TUMOUR

Dr. Shailendra Kumar, Professor, Dr. Archana Mishra, Department of Cardiothoracic
and Vascular Surgery

A 17 year old boy came to the hospital with the symptoms of recurrent cough and difficulty in respiration. On clinical examination there was laboured respiration and hoarseness of voice. There was no peripheral lymphadenopathy and no hepatosplenomagaly on abdominal examination. CT Scan thorax is depicted below:

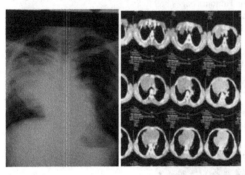

1. What is the most probable diagnosis
   (A) Tracheal mass
   (B) Chest wall mass
   (C) Anterior mediastinal mass
   (D) Rt. Upper lobar apical mass
2. What is the most common anterior mediastinal mass in adult population
   (A) Lymphoma
   (B) Thymus tumour
   (C) Germ Cell tumour
   (D) Fibrous tumour
3. What is the most common thymic lesion in adult
   (A) Thymic hyperplasia
   (B) Thymoma
   (C) Thymic carcinoma
   (D) Thymic carcinoid
4. The most common systemic disease associated with thymoma is
   (A) Cytopanias
   (B) Non thymic malignancies
   (C) Myesthenia gravis
   (D) Pneumatoid arthritis
5. What is the most common site of extra gonadal germ cell tumour
   (A) Anterior mediastinum
   (B) Posterior mediastinum
   (C) Retroperitoneum
   (D) Neck

Answers:
1. C
   CT Scan of the above case is showing anteriorly situated mass in the midline in upper thorax
2. B
   Lesions of the thymus account for approximately 50% of anterior mediastinal masses in adults.
3. B
   Thymomas are the most common thymic tumour and 95% of them are located in anterior medistinum
4. C

Accumulated experience suggests 30% to 50% of thymomas are associated with clinical MG
5.   A
     Anterior mediastinum is the most common location for extra gonadal germ cell tumours which
     account for 15 to 20% of all anterior medistinal masses

References:
1. Sabiston and Spencer, Surgery of the Chest, edition 8, pages 633 to 643

TRACHEO-OESOPHAGEAL FISTULA

Dr. Shailendra Kumar, Professor, Dr. Archana Mishra, Department of Cardiothoracic
and Vascular Surgery

A 23 year old boy came to the hospital with symptom of cough and respiratory distress after taking liquids. His father gave history of engulfing of 50 paisa coin five year back for which he was admitted to a hospital and relieved after assurance that he was all right. He was taking liquid and solid foods normally after that episode. But recently for the last 3 months he developed above mentioned symptoms. The chest radiograph with water soluble contrast oesophagogram was advised which is shown below:

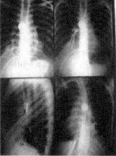

1.   What is the probable diagnosis
     (A) Tracheo- oesophageal fistula secondary to coin impacted in oesophagus
     (B) Coin impacted in trachea leads to trachea oesophageal fistula
     (C) Coin impacted in oesophagus without any fistula
     (D) Coin impacted in trachea without any fistula
2.   Which is the most common type of congenital trachea- oesophageal fistula
     (A) Upper end blind, lower end communicating with trachea
     (B) Upper end communicating , lower end blind
     (C) Communicating both ends
     (D) No communication at all
3.   Most common anomaly associated with congenital TOF is
     (A) Cardiac
     (B) Vertebral
     (C) Renal
     (D) Limb
4.   The treatment goal in congenital repair is division of fistula with end to end esophageal anastomosis . The
     most commonly thoracotomy approach is
     (A) Rt. Posterolateral
     (B) Left Posterolateral
     (C) Rt. Anterolateral
     (D) Left Anterolateral
5.The most common long term complication of repair ofTOF IS
     (A) Tracheomalacia
     (B) Gastro-oesophageal reflux
     (C) Recurrent fistula
     (D) Foreign body impaction

Answers:
1.   A

There is history of coin engulfing and cough on ingestion of fluid. On contrast oesophagogram spillage of contrast is in the bronchus suggestive of fistula formation

2. A
   Oesophageal atrasia with distal TEF constitutes 87.1% of all congenital trachea oesophageal fistulae
3. A
   The most common associated anomaly is congenital heart disease in about a fifth of the patient
4. A
   The standard approach is right posterolateral thoracotomy except in cases of right aortic arch in which approach is through the left thorax
5. B
   Gastro oesophageal reflux is a major concern in patients with EA occurring in as many as 54% of the patients

References:

1. Sabiston and Spencer, Surgery of the Chest edition 8, pages 535 to 545

ATROPHY OF LUNG

Dr. Shailendra Kumar, Professor, Dr. Archana Mishra, Department of Cardiothoracic and Vascular Surgery

A 15 year old girl presented in the department of CTVS with symptom of cough and malaise. Her parents gave history of some foreign body engulfing 10 years back leading to respiratory distress for which she was admitted to a hospital. She was discharged from the hospital after subsidence of symptoms. The girl had recurrent episodes of cough thereafter for 2-3 years. Presently she had symptom of cough and vague pain over the left lower chest wall. CT Thorax been depicted below:

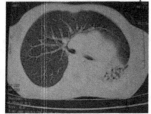

1. What is the most probable diagnosis
   (A) Bronchial atresia of left lower lobe
   (B) Pneumothorax on left side
   (C) Atrophy of left lung with hypertrophy of right lung secondary to forein body impaction in left main bronchus
   (D) Congenital absence of left lung
2. Which of the following is most common congenital abnormality of airway
   (A) Trachea-oesophageal fistula
   (B) Bronchial atresia
   (C) Tracheomalacia
   (D) Tracheal stenosis
3. Horseshoe lung is
   (A) Right and left lung bases are communicating through posterior mediastinum
   (B) Right and left lung bases are communicating through anterior mediastinum
   (C) Right and left upper lobe are communicating through anterior mediastinum
   (D) Right and left upper lobe are communicating through posterior mediastinum

Answers:

1. C
   Obstructed left main bronchus led to atrophy of whole of the left lung. The compensatory hypertrophy of the right lung crossed the midline through anterior mediastinum and occupied most of the left thoracic cavity.
2. A
   TEF is most common abnormality of the trachea occurring in 2.4 per 10,000 births

3. A

    Horse shoe lung is a rare anomaly where right and left lung bases are fused by common tissue extending through the posterior mediastinum anterior to aorta but posterior to heart and oesophagus

References:
1. Sabiston and Spencer, Surgery of the Chest, edition 8, pages 129 to 149

HAMARTOMA LUNG

Dr. Shailendra Kumar, Professor, Dr. Archana Mishra, Department of Cardiothoracic and Vascular Surgery

A 21 year old boy presented in the department of CTVS with cough and recurrent pulmonary infections. The chest radiograph was suggestive of a solitary pulmonary nodular opacity in the right lower lobar area. CECT Scan was advised which suggested solitary 3.8 cm diameter size lesion with calcification in right lower lobe epical segment. CT picture are depicted below:

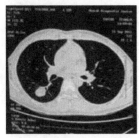

1. What is the most common probable diagnosis
    (A) Hamartoma
    (B) Mucinous gland adenoma
    (C) Infective glanuloma
    (D) Squamus pappiloma
2. Most common benign lung lesion
    (A) Chondroma
    (B) Fibroma
    (C) Hamartoma
    (D) Mucous cystadenoma
3. Which of the following is not a radiologiical feature of hamartoma
    (A) They are peripheral lesions
    (B) They are located mostly in lower lung fields
    (C) They are located in upper lung fields
    (D) The usual size is 1-3
4. Resection of the lesion hamartoma usually needed because of
    (A) Malignant transformations
    (B) recurrent pneumonia
    (C) Haemoptysis
    (D) Cough
5. Which of the following is diagnosis of hamatoma on histological examinations
    (A) Calcifications
    (B) Fibrosis
    (C) Cartilage
    (D) Haematoma

Answers:
1. A

    Solitary peripheral nodule with smooth well circumscribed lesion less than 4cm is suggestive of Hamartoma
2. C

    Hamartoma are the most common benign lung lesions and accout for more than 70% of all non malignant tumours of the lung

3. C
   Hamartomas are peripheral l;esions most often located in lower lung fields
4. A
   Resection is required even after the diagnosis of non malignant disease because of local problems of airway obstruction
5. C
   Cartilage is present in most lesions and is diagnostic of hamartoma

References:
1. Sabiston and Spencer, Surgery of the Chest, edition 8, pages 151 to 155

NHL CHEST WALL

Dr. Shailendra Kumar, Professor, Dr. Archana Mishra, Department of Cardiothoracic and Vascular Surgery

A 75 year old man came to us with slowly growing painless swelling over anterior 3rd and 4th costochondral junction. CECT scan of the chest was suggestive of osteolytic lesion with involvement of adjoining soft tissue. There was associated loss of appetite and weakness without any fever and malaise. The CT Scan picture of the chest are shown below:

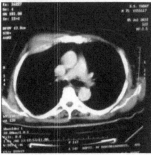

1. Which will be the least probable diagnosis
   (A) Lymphoma
   (B) Osteochondroma
   (C) Chondrosarcoma
   (D) Metastatic sarcoma
2. What will be the first line diagnostic tool in the above case
   (A) Fire needle aspiration cytology
   (B) Incisional biopsy
   (C) Excisional biopsy
   (D) Wait & watch
3. If the needle cytology is non yeilding, then what will be the next appropriate step in this case
   (A) Wide excision of that lesion with reconstruction
   (B) Taking tissue biopsy for institution of appropriate treatment
   (C) Enucleation
   (D) Radiation therapy
4. If tissue diagnosis is NHL, the next step will be
   (A) Staging of the disease
   (B) Chemotherapy
   (C) Radiotherapy
   (D) Surgery
5. The appropriate treatment of chest wall NHL is
   (A) Wide excision
   (B) Chemotherapy
   (C) Radiotherapy
   (D) Surgery and chemotherapy

References:

1. Sabiston and Spencer, Surgery of the Chest, edition 8, pages 379 to 387

CAROTID BODY TUMOUR

Dr. Shailendra Kumar, Professor, Dr. Archana Mishra, Department of Cardiothoracic and Vascular Surgery

A 16 year old girl presented in our OPD with symptoms of slowly growing painless swelling in Rt. Upper neck. On examination a pulsatile 6 cm size mass was felt without any other abnormality including cervical lymphadenopathy. The high resolution ultrasonography was suggestive of a pulsatile mass situated in relation to the divisions of common carotid artery. CT angiogram was advised which is depicted below:

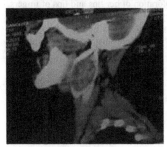

1. What is the most common probable diagnosis
   (A) Lymph node mass
   (B) Carotid aneurism
   (C) Parotid tail lesion
   (D) Carotid body tumour
2. Splaying sign in CECT angiogram suggestive of
   (A) Carotid body tumour
   (B) Carotid aneurism
   (C) High division of common carotid artery
   (D) Carotid body tumour originates from of common carotid
3. Carotid body tumour originates from
   (A) Mesenchymal cell
   (B) Endothelium
   (C) Medial smooth muscle cell
   (D) Neural crest ectoderm
4. The role of carotid body at bifurcation of common carotid artery is
   (A) Monitor blood gases and PH
   (B) Monitor blood pressure
   (C) Secrete vasoactive amines
   (D) Monitor temperature

5. The carotid body tumour is located in
   (A) Medical layer
   (B) Adventitial layer
   (C) Muscular propria layer
   (D) Outside the vessel layer

Answers:
1. D
    The lesion located at bifurcation of common carotid artery and displaying both the branches is suggestive of carotid body tumour
2. A
    Splaying sign is displacing internal and external carotid arteries with lesion in between is suggestive of carotid body tumour
3. D
    Neural ectodermal tissue from the neural crest is the tissue of origin for carotid body tumour
4. A
    Carotid body is sensitive to blood gases and pH in the blood and thus involved in blood gases auto-regulation
5. B
    The carotid body tumour is located in adventitial layer of the common carotid artery

References:
1. Comprehensive vascular and endovascular surgery, 2nd edition ,John W. Hallet, pages 606 to 629

TETRALOGY OF FALLOT
Dr. Vaibhav Jain, SR III, Prof. S. K. Singh, Professor, Department of Cardiothoracic and Vascular Surgery

A 10 year old girl comes to your OPD with the complaints of bluish discoloration of her lips and tips of fingers. Her body weight is less for her age. She also has clubbing of finger and cyanotic spells which are relieved with squatting. She has a ejection systolic murmur in the left third intercostal space. ECG has features of right ventricular hypertrophy. Her chest x-ray shows a small cardiac shadow and diminished pulmonary vascular markings.

1. What is the provisional diagnosis?
   (A) Mitral stenosis
   (B) Ventricular septal defect
   (C) Tetralogy of Fallot
   (D) Tricuspid atresia
2. What is commonly seen in such patients?
   (A) Polycythemia
   (B) Neutropenia
   (C) Anaemia
   (D) Hypokalemia
3. What is the preferred diagnostic test?
   (A) CECT thorax
   (B) Echocardiogram
   (C) ECG
   (D) Chest X-ray
4. What is the definitive management?
   (A) Total Surgical correction
   (B) Only VSD closure
   (C) Watchful observation
   (D) Calcium channel blockers
5. The classical appearance of the cardiomediastinal silhouette on a Chest X-ray is known as
   (A) Boot-shaped heart (coeur en sabot)
   (B) Water bottle appearance
   (C) Box shaped Heart
   (D) Snowman sign
6. A "tet spell" or "blue" spell of tetralogy of Fallot is treated with all of the following except:
   (A) Oxygen
   (B) Knee chest position

(C) Diuretics

(D) Beta blockers

Answers:

1. C

The majority of children with TOF present with some degree of cyanosis. Squatting is a classic behavioral adaptation of older children with TOF, whereby systemic vascular resistance is increased, producing more pulmonary blood flow. The physical examination typically reveals a moderate-intensity midsystolic ejection murmur, heard loudest in the second and third left intercostal space, which may radiate into the axilla. The lung fields usually appear to be oligemic in proportion to the degree of cyanosis.

2. A

Polycythemia is seen in most children with chronic cyanosis.

3. B

Echocardiography has become the most common and usually definitive diagnostic modality for TOF with pulmonic stenosis. Detailed elucidation of the important anatomic features, including the number and location of VSDs, the nature of the RVOT obstruction, the anatomy of the proximal branch pulmonary arteries, and the coronary artery pattern, can be accomplished with a high degree of accuracy.

4. A

TOF is a disease remediable only by surgical intervention, with medical management designed to optimize a patient's surgical candidacy. The goals of surgical therapy are to (1) close intracardiac shunts, (2) provide relatively unobstructed pulmonary blood flow. (3) maintain normal function of the right ventricle

5. A

The classic appearance of the cardiomediastinal silhouette is that of a boot-shaped heart (coeur en sabot). This typical, but not universal, radiographic appearance is caused by right ventricular hypertrophy and tends to become more exaggerated with time as hypertrophy progresses.

6. C

A "tet spell" or "blue" spell is managed by administration of intravenous fluids, sedatives, and oxygen. Placing the infant in a knee-to-chest position can elevate systemic vascular resistance with a resultant increase in pulmonary blood flow. Intravenous beta-blockers such as esmolol and α agonists such as phenylephrine may also be used.

References :

1. Brian W. Duncan. Tetralogy of Fallot with Pulmonary Stenosis. In: Frank W. Sellke, Pedro J. del Nido, Scott J. Swanson (eds.). Sabiston & Spencer surgery of the chest. 8th ed. Philadelphia, PA : Saunders Elsevier;2010. p1881-2.

2. Brian W. Duncan. Tetralogy of Fallot with Pulmonary Stenosis. In: Frank W. Sellke, Pedro J. del Nido, Scott J. Swanson (eds.). Sabiston & Spencer surgery of the chest. 8th ed. Philadelphia, PA : Saunders Elsevier;2010. p1882.

3. Brian W. Duncan. Tetralogy of Fallot with Pulmonary Stenosis. In: Frank W. Sellke, Pedro J. del Nido, Scott J. Swanson (eds.). Sabiston & Spencer surgery of the chest. 8th ed. Philadelphia, PA : Saunders Elsevier;2010. p1882.

4. Brian W. Duncan. Tetralogy of Fallot with Pulmonary Stenosis. In: Frank W. Sellke, Pedro J. del Nido, Scott J. Swanson (eds.). Sabiston & Spencer surgery of the chest. 8th ed. Philadelphia, PA : Saunders Elsevier;2010. p1883-4.

5. Brian W. Duncan. Tetralogy of Fallot with Pulmonary Stenosis. In: Frank W. Sellke, Pedro J. del Nido, Scott J. Swanson (eds.). Sabiston & Spencer surgery of the chest. 8th ed. Philadelphia, PA : Saunders Elsevier;2010. p1882.

6. Brian W. Duncan. Tetralogy of Fallot with Pulmonary Stenosis. In: Frank W. Sellke, Pedro J. del Nido, Scott J. Swanson (eds.). Sabiston & Spencer surgery of the chest. 8th ed. Philadelphia, PA : Saunders Elsevier;2010. p1883.

AORTIC REGURGITATION

Dr. Vaibhav Jain, SR III, Prof. S. K. Singh, Professor, Department of Cardiothoracic and Vascular Surgery

A forty five year old man presented with the complaints of progressive breathlessness since last 3 years. Examination revealed a large volume collapsing pulse; his blood pressure was 160/42 mm of Hg and a early diastolic decrescendo murmur was auscultated on clinical examination. His echocardiogram showed evidence of left ventricular dilatation.

1. What is the provisional diagnosis?
   (A) Mitral stenosis
   (B) Aortic regurgitation
   (C) Tricuspid regurgitation
   (D) Mitral regurgitation
2. What is the preferred diagnostic investigation?
   (A) Chest X-ray
   (B) Echocardiogram
   (C) ECG
   (D) CT-scan
3. Austin flint murmur is produced by aortic regurgitation jet causing fluttering of
   (A) Posterior mitral valve leaflet
   (B) Inter ventricular septum
   (C) Inter atrial septum
   (D) Anterior mitral valve leaflet
4. Ross Procedure entails replacement of patient's Aortic valve with
   (A) Autograft Pulmonary valve
   (B) Allograft Pulmonary valve
   (C) Mechanical Valve
   (D) Bioprosthetic graft
5. What is Quincke's sign ?
   (A) Visible pulsations of the uvula
   (B) Visible pulsation of the retinal arterioles
   (C) Capillary pulsations seen on light compression of the nail bed
   (D) Bobbing of the head with each heartbeat

Answers :

1. B

   Patients with Aortic Regurgitation present with dyspnea on exertion and an early diastolic decrescendo murmur radiating to the ventricular apex. Pulse pressure is widened, with very low diastolic pressure in severe aortic insufficiency.

2. B

   Two-dimensional echocardiography is used to identify underlying aortic valve disease and to measure aortic anular dimension. Valve morphology (cusp number) and apposition of leaflets may be assessed directly as well as by the direction of the regurgitant jet. In addition, echocardiography provides the ability to assess left ventricular function, degree of dilation, and associated hypertrophy. Doppler echocardiography aids in the diagnosis and grading of aortic insufficiency.

3. D

   An Austin Flint murmur is thought to arise from fluttering of the anterior mitral valve leaflet from the aortic insufficiency jet.

4. A

   In Ross procedure the diseased aortic valve is replaced with the patient's own normal pulmonary valve, and a biological valve, usually a pulmonary homograft, is used to replace the pulmonary valve.

5. C

   Quincke's pulse are capillary pulsations observed by lightly compressing the nail beds due to increased pulse pressure in Aortic Regurgitation.

References :

1. Douglas R. Johnston and Joseph F. Sabik III. Acquired Aortic Valve Disease. In: Frank W. Sellke, Pedro J. del Nido, Scott J. Swanson (eds.). Sabiston & Spencer surgery of the chest. 8th ed. Philadelphia, PA : Saunders Elsevier;2010. p1200.
2. Douglas R. Johnston and Joseph F. Sabik III. Acquired Aortic Valve Disease. In: Frank W. Sellke, Pedro J. del Nido, Scott J. Swanson (eds.). Sabiston & Spencer surgery of the chest. 8th ed. Philadelphia, PA : Saunders Elsevier;2010. p1200.
3. Douglas R. Johnston and Joseph F. Sabik III. Acquired Aortic Valve Disease. In: Frank W. Sellke, Pedro J. del Nido, Scott J. Swanson (eds.). Sabiston & Spencer surgery of the chest. 8th ed. Philadelphia, PA : Saunders Elsevier;2010. p1200.

4. Tirone E. David. Surgery of the Aortic Root and Ascending Aorta. In: Frank W. Sellke, Pedro J. del Nido, Scott J. Swanson (eds.). Sabiston & Spencer surgery of the chest. 8th ed. Philadelphia, PA : Saunders Elsevier;2010. p1034.
5. Douglas R. Johnston and Joseph F. Sabik III. Acquired Aortic Valve Disease. In: Frank W. Sellke, Pedro J. del Nido, Scott J. Swanson (eds.). Sabiston & Spencer surgery of the chest. 8th ed. Philadelphia, PA : Saunders Elsevier;2010. p1200.

RHEUMATIC MITRAL STENOSIS

Dr. Vaibhav Jain, SR III, Prof. S. K. Singh, Professor, Department of Cardiothoracic and Vascular Surgery

A thirty year old female patient from a low socioeconomic class came to the hospital with a six year history of breathlessness on exertion, paroxysmal nocturnal dyspnoea, orthopnea, cough and on and off haemoptysis. These symptoms have been gradually progressing. She appears thin built. Examination shows that she has atrial fibrillation and a low-pitched, rumbling diastolic apical heart murmur. She gives a history suggestive of rheumatic fever in her childhood.

1. What is the diagnosis?
   (A) Tricuspid atresia
   (B) Rheumatic Mitral stenosis
   (C) Mitral regurgitation
   (D) Constrictive pericarditis
2. What is the preferred diagnostic investigation?
   (A) Echocardiogram
   (B) Cardiac CTAngiogram
   (C) Cardiac catheterisation
   (D) Chest X- ray
3. Which of the following findings is not usually seen in a case of Rheumatic Mitral Valve stenosis?
   (A) Leaflet thickening
   (B) Commissural fusion
   (C) Leaflet prolapse
   (D) Chordal thickening
4. Papillary muscles attached to Mitral valve are :
   (A) Anterior and Posterior
   (B) Anterior, posterior, and septal
   (C) Anterolateral and Posteromedial
   (D) Anteromedial and Posterolateral
5. Which of the following is not a component of Wilkins score used for Echocardiographic assessment of Mitral valve?
   (A) Leaflet rigidity
   (B) Leaflet prolapse
   (C) Leaflet thickening
   (D) Subvalvular thickening andcalcification

Answers:

1. B

   In developing world chronic rheumatic disease is endemic and remains the most common cause of both mitral regurgitation and stenosis. Symptoms may include fatigue, dyspnea or hemoptysis, new onset of atrial fibrillation, or an embolic event. Auscultatory findings include a loud first heart sound, a diastolic murmur, and an opening snap in some patients. The diastolic murmur is a low-pitched rumble that is heard at the apex of the heart.

2. A

   The diagnostic tool of choice in the evaluation of patients with mitral stenosis is two-dimensional Doppler echocardiography.Echocardiography is used to evaluate the morphology and mobility of the mitral valve leaflets, commissures, and subvalvular apparatus, identifying calcification as well as determining the severity of mitral stenosis by measuring the mitral valve area, the transmitral gradient, and the pulmonary artery pressures.

3. C

   Rheumatic Mitral Valve stenosis is characterised by leaflet thickening, chordal thickening, fusion and shortening, and commissural fusion. Progressive leaflet thickening and commissural fusion eventually producea characteristic "fish mouth" single central opening, with restricted leaflet motion during systole and diastole (Carpentier type IIIa leaflet dysfunction).

4. C

Two papillary muscles arise from the area between the apical and middle thirds of the left ventricular wall. The anterolateral papillary muscle is usually composed of one muscle body and the posteromedial of two muscle bodies. Each papillary muscle provides chordae to both leaflets of Mitral valve.

5. B

Wilkins score, which scores from 0 to 4 for each of four factors: (1) the degree of leaflet rigidity, (2) the severity of leaflet thickening, (3) the amount of leaflet calcification, and (4) the extent of subvalvular thickening and calcification. The maximum score is 16; higher scores indicate more severe anatomic disease.

References:

1. Farzan Filsoufi, Joanna Chikwe, and David H. Adams. Acquired Disease of the Mitral Valve. In: Frank W. Sellke, Pedro J. del Nido, Scott J. Swanson (eds.). Sabiston & Spencer surgery of the chest. 8th ed. Philadelphia, PA : Saunders Elsevier;2010. p1211.

2. Farzan Filsoufi, Joanna Chikwe, and David H. Adams. Acquired Disease of the Mitral Valve. In: Frank W. Sellke, Pedro J. del Nido, Scott J. Swanson (eds.). Sabiston & Spencer surgery of the chest. 8th ed. Philadelphia, PA : Saunders Elsevier;2010. p1211.

3. Farzan Filsoufi, Joanna Chikwe, and David H. Adams. Acquired Disease of the Mitral Valve. In: Frank W. Sellke, Pedro J. del Nido, Scott J. Swanson (eds.). Sabiston & Spencer surgery of the chest. 8th ed. Philadelphia, PA : Saunders Elsevier;2010. p1210.

4. Farzan Filsoufi, Joanna Chikwe, and David H. Adams. Acquired Disease of the Mitral Valve. In: Frank W. Sellke, Pedro J. del Nido, Scott J. Swanson (eds.). Sabiston & Spencer surgery of the chest. 8th ed. Philadelphia, PA : Saunders Elsevier;2010. p1210.

5. Riya S. Chacko, Joseph P. Carrozza Jr., Duane S. Pinto. Interventional Cardiology. In: Frank W. Sellke, Pedro J. del Nido, Scott J. Swanson (eds.). Sabiston & Spencer surgery of the chest. 8th ed. Philadelphia, PA : Saunders Elsevier;2010. p858.

CORONARY ARTERY DISEASE

Dr. Vaibhav Jain, SR III, Prof S. K. Singh, Professor, Department of Cardiothoracic and Vascular Surgery

A fifty year old gentleman has been admitted to the cardiology department with a history of progressive, stable angina not responding to medical management. The patient was ex-smoker. He leads a sedentary type of life, is overweight, has diabetes mellitus -II and also has high cholesterol. He has strong family history heart attacks. A coronary angiogram shows 70 – 80 % occlusion of all three coronary arteries, with good distal vessels with mild LV dysfunction.

1. Which conduit is preferred for bypass of left anterior descending artery?
   (A) Left internal mammary artery
   (B) Right internal mammary
   (C) Reverse saphenous vein graft
   (D) Radial artery
2. Which of the following conduits has the highest long term patency rate?
   (A) Radial artery
   (B) Left internal mammary artery
   (C) Reverse saphenous vein graft
   (D) Gastro Epiploic artery
3. Bilateral Internal Thoracic Artery harvesting should be avoided in all of the following patients EXCEPT
   (A) Diabetes Mellitus
   (B) Obesity
   (C) Severe chronic obstructive pulmonary disease
   (D) Young patients
4. Which of the following clinical test is performed before harvesting Radial artery as a conduit for CABG :
   (A) Hawkins - Kennedy test
   (B) Finkelstein's test
   (C) Watson's test

(D) Allen's test

Answers :

1. A

Nearly all patients should have the left ITA grafted to the left anterior descending artery. In terms of patency, a graft from the left ITA to the left anterior descending artery is the gold standard for all conduits and target vessels.

2. B

The ITA is unique among the arterial conduits in that its muscular media has 6 to 12 elastic lamellae. The subintima lies on the prominent internal elastic lamina, which has few and small fenestrations in contrast to other small arteries, where more and larger fenestrations may allow entry of smooth muscle cells to the subintima and initiate plaque formation. Patency rate for Left ITA is more than 95% at 1 year, 85% to 95% at 10 years, and 88% at 15 years.

3. D

Bilateral ITAs should be considered in young patients, as this procedure is associated with lower reoperation rates, lower late PCI rates, and possible long-term survival benefits.Possible contraindications to bilateral ITAs include emergency operation, diabetes mellitus, obesity, and severe chronic obstructive pulmonary disease for which the patient requires oral or intravenous glucocorticoid therapy.

4. D

Radial artery harvest is avoided in patients with Raynaud's syndrome or on the same side in patients who have had recent radial arterial puncture at the time of preoperative coronary catheterization. It is important both to feel for an ulnar pulse and to perform the Allen test, using a cutoff of 3 seconds, which has a 100% sensitivity for inadequate collateral handcirculation.

References:

1. Hendrick B. Barner. Bypass Conduit Options. In: Frank W. Sellke, Pedro J. del Nido, Scott J. Swanson (eds.). Sabiston & Spencer surgery of the chest. 8th ed. Philadelphia, PA : Saunders Elsevier;2010. p1414.

2. Hendrick B. Barner. Bypass Conduit Options. In: Frank W. Sellke, Pedro J. del Nido, Scott J. Swanson (eds.). Sabiston & Spencer surgery of the chest. 8th ed. Philadelphia, PA : Saunders Elsevier;2010. p1413.

3. Vincent Chan, Frank W. Sellke, and Marc Ruel. Coronary Artery Bypass Grafting. In: Frank W. Sellke, Pedro J. del Nido, Scott J. Swanson (eds.). Sabiston & Spencer surgery of the chest. 8th ed. Philadelphia, PA : Saunders Elsevier;2010. p1375.

4. Vincent Chan, Frank W. Sellke, and Marc Ruel. Coronary Artery Bypass Grafting. In: Frank W. Sellke, Pedro J. del Nido, Scott J. Swanson (eds.). Sabiston & Spencer surgery of the chest. 8th ed. Philadelphia, PA : Saunders Elsevier;2010. p1372.

AORTIC VALVE REPLACEMENT

Dr. Vaibhav Jain, SR III, Prof. S.K. Singh, Professor, Department of Cardiothoracic and Vascular Surgery

A sixty eight year old male farmer gives a history of breathlessness since one year. He also had history of episodes of syncope on exertion and also complains of angina. Examination reveals a crescendo-decrescendo murmur (ejection systolic murmur) that is heard best at the second right intercostal space and radiates to the carotid arteries. Echocardiography showed Severe Aortic stenosis. He underwent Aortic valve replacement with implantation of a Bioprosthetic Aortic prosthesis.

1. Aortic valve area (AVA) may be calculated according to :
   (A) Gorlin's formula.
   (B) Nakata's index
   (C) Z value
   (D) McGoons Index

2. The major advantage of Bioprosthetic valve over Mechanical valve is :
   (A) Long term Durability
   (B) Avoidance of anti coagulation
   (C) More suitable in Younger age groups
   (D) Less incidence of Structural deterioration

3. Tissue fixation in most of the Bioprosthetic valve currently used is achieved with :
   (A) High pressure Glutaraldehyde fixation
   (B) Low pressure Glutaraldehyde fixation
   (C) Pressure fixation
   (D) Amino oleic acid treatment

4. Bundle of His is present below the commissure between :
   (A) Left and Right cusp
   (B) Left and Non coronary cusp
   (C) Right and Non coronary cusp
   (D) Below Non coronary cusp
5. Aortic valve area in severe Aortic stenosis is:
   (A) Less than 2 cm^2
   (B) Less than 1.5 cm^2
   (C) Less than 1 cm^2
   (D) Less than 2.5 cm^2

Answers :

1. A
   Aortic valve area (AVA) may be calculated on Echocardiography according to the Gorlin formula.
   AVA= AVF/ 44.5 √AVG
   where AVF is mean systolic aortic valve flow and AVG is mean systolic aortic valve gradient.
2. B
   Durability remains the Achilles' heel of bioprosthetic valves. A pericardial bioprosthesis is attractive for a middle aged patient who does not want to sacrifice lifestyle for anticoagulation.
3. B
   Low-pressure (<2 mm Hg) and zero pressure glutaraldehyde fixations have been shown tomaintain a more natural collagen alignment and are currently the strategies used in the latest generation of stented bioprostheses.

4. C
   After arising from the atrioventricular node, the bundle of His penetrates the membranous septum, emerging on the surface of the left ventricular septum immediately below the aortic annulus. From a view through the aortic valve, the bundle lies beneath the anulus, just below the commissure between the noncoronary and right coronary leaflet.
5. C
   Noninvasive measurement of aortic valve gradient extrapolated from aortic jet velocity on two-dimensional echocardiography has been shown to be the most reproducible and accurate method of grading aortic stenosis. Aortic stenosis is graded as Severe when valve area is less than 1 cm^2.

References:

1. Douglas R. Johnston and Joseph F. Sabik III. Acquired Aortic Valve Disease. In: Frank W. Sellke, Pedro J. del Nido, Scott J. Swanson (eds.). Sabiston & Spencer surgery of the chest. 8th ed. Philadelphia, PA : Saunders Elsevier;2010. p1196.

2. Edwin C. McGee, Jr., and Gus J. Vlahakes. Valve Replacement Therapy: History, Options, and Valve Types. In: Frank W. Sellke, Pedro J. del Nido, Scott J. Swanson (eds.). Sabiston & Spencer surgery of the chest. 8th ed. Philadelphia, PA : Saunders Elsevier;2010. p1189 & 1192.

3. Edwin C. McGee, Jr., and Gus J. Vlahakes. Valve Replacement Therapy: History, Options, and Valve Types. In: Frank W. Sellke, Pedro J. del Nido, Scott J. Swanson (eds.). Sabiston & Spencer surgery of the chest. 8th ed. Philadelphia, PA : Saunders Elsevier;2010. p1189.

4. Frank A. Pigula. Surgery for Congenital Anomalies of the Aortic Valve and Root. In: Frank W. Sellke, Pedro J. del Nido, Scott J. Swanson (eds.). Sabiston & Spencer surgery of the chest. 8th ed. Philadelphia, PA : Saunders Elsevier;2010. p1943.

5. Douglas R. Johnston and Joseph F. Sabik III. Acquired Aortic Valve Disease. In: Frank W. Sellke, Pedro J. del Nido, Scott J. Swanson (eds.). Sabiston & Spencer surgery of the chest. 8th ed. Philadelphia, PA : Saunders Elsevier;2010. p1197.

VENTRICULAR SEPTAL DEFECT (VSD)

Dr. Vaibhav Jain, SR III, Prof. S. K. Singh, Professor, Department of Cardiothoracic and Vascular Surgery

A five year old boy presented to our OPD with a history of breathlessness while playing and running with his friends. Physical examination revealed a loud, pansystolic murmur best heard at the left sternal border. Chest X-Ray shows increased pulmonary vascular markings. His echocardiography showed a Ventricular Septal Defect of 1.5 cm. size with a Left to Right shunt.

1. Which is the most common type?
   (A) Muscular VSD
   (B) Inlet VSD
   (C) Peri membranous VSD
   (D) Outlet VSD
2. Which is true regarding Eisenmengers syndrome ?
   (A) Results from long standing atrial fibrillation
   (B) Occurs due to Pulmonary hypertension leading to a reversal of shunt
   (C) It is presence of Mitral stenosis with ASD
   (D) It is an indication for urgent VSD closure
3. On a Echocardiography study VSD was found to have a diameter which was 40% of the diameter of Aortic annulus and flow velocity across the defect of 2 m/sec. It can be categorised as :
   (A) Small VSD
   (B) Moderate VSD
   (C) Large VSD
   (D) Very large VSD
4. Papillary muscles arise from :
   (A) Left ventricular side of Interventricular septum only
   (B) Right ventricular side of Interventricular septum only
   (C) From both Left and Right ventricular side of Interventricular septum
   (D) Does not arise from Left or Right ventricular side of Interventricular septum

Answers:

1. C

   Conoventricular defects are located between the conal septum and the ventricular septum. They are centered around the membranous septum and comprise 80% of all VSDs.

2. B

   When pulmonary resistance rises as a result of the development of pulmonary vascular disease, pulmonary blood flow is reduced and the patient appears to improve. However as further increases in PVR occur the classic Eisenmenger complex results. These patients are characterized by fixed pulmonary hypertension, bidirectional shunting, right ventricular hypertrophy, and a normal-sized left ventricle.

3. B

   A moderate defect has a diameter of 33% to 75% of the aortic annulus and flow velocity of 1 to 4 m/s, indicating moderate flow restriction.

4. B

   The left ventricular septum is free of any papillary muscle attachment Two papillary muscles supporting Mitral valve (anterolateral and posteromedial) arise from the area between the apical and middle thirds of the left ventricular wall.

References :

1. Emile A. Bacha. Ventricular Septal Defect and Double-Outlet Right Ventricle. In: Frank W. Sellke, Pedro J. del Nido, Scott J. Swanson (eds.). Sabiston & Spencer surgery of the chest. 8th ed. Philadelphia, PA : Saunders Elsevier;2010. p1850-1.
2. Emile A. Bacha. Ventricular Septal Defect and Double-Outlet Right Ventricle. In: Frank W. Sellke, Pedro J. del Nido, Scott J. Swanson (eds.). Sabiston & Spencer surgery of the chest. 8th ed. Philadelphia, PA : Saunders Elsevier;2010. p1852.
3. Nicholas T. Kouchoukos, Eugene H. Blackstone, Frank L. Hanley, James K. Kirklin. Ventricular Septal Defect. In: Nicholas T. Kouchoukos, Eugene H. Blackstone, Frank L. Hanley, James K. Kirklin (eds.). Kirklin/Barratt-Boyes cardiac surgery: morphology, diagnostic criteria, natural history, techniques, results, and indications.4th ed. Philadelphia, PA : Elsevier Saunders;2013. p1287.
4. Emile A. Bacha. Ventricular Septal Defect and Double-Outlet Right Ventricle. In: Frank W. Sellke, Pedro J. del Nido, Scott J. Swanson (eds.). Sabiston & Spencer surgery of the chest. 8th ed. Philadelphia, PA : Saunders Elsevier;2010. p1849.

POST MYOCARDIAL INFARCTION VSDS

Dr. Vaibhav Jain, SR III, Prof. S. K. Singh, Professor, Department of Cardiothoracic and Vascular Surgery

A seventy year old male businessman complained of severe chest pain for which he was admitted in our institution's cardiology department four days ago. He was diagnosed to have Acute MI and was managed conservatively. His response to conservative management was good and he was being planned for discharge. However during this time he developed severe breathlessness and hypotension and auscultation revealed a pansystolic murmur at the LV apex. Echocardiography showed a Ventricular Septal Rupture.

1. What is the most common location of VSR?
   (A) Anterior
   (B) Posterior
   (C) Basal
   (D) None of the above
2. It is most commonly caused due to occlusion of
   (A) Left circumflex artery
   (B) Left Anterior descending artery
   (C) Right Coronary artery
   (D) Obtuse marginal
3. In VSR situated anteriorly Heart failure commonly seen is :
   (A) Left sided heart failure
   (B) Right sided heart failure
   (C) Both Left and Right sided heart failure occur
   (D) Either Left or Right side heart failure may occur with equal frequency
4. During right heart catheterisation in above mentioned patient which of the following findings is indicative of VSR?
   (A) Step up of oxygen>5% between Right atrium and Pulmonary artery
   (B) Step up of oxygen>9% between Right atrium and Pulmonary artery
   (C) Step down of oxygen>5% between Right atrium and Pulmonary artery
   (D) Step down of oxygen>9% between Right atrium and Pulmonary artery

Answers :

1. A
   Postinfarction VSDs are located most commonly (i.e., in about 60% of cases) in the anteroapical septum as a result of full-thickness anterior infarction.
2. B
   Postinfarction VSDs are located most commonly (i.e., in about 60% of cases) in the anteroapical septum as a result of full-thickness anterior infarction secondary to occlusion of the left anterior descending artery.
3. A
   Left-sided heart failure tends to predominate in anterior VSDs, and right-sided failure predominates in posterior VSDs.
4. B
   The classic technique for distinguishing between acute papillary muscle rupture and postinfarction VSD has been right heart catheterization, during which a greater than 9% stepup in the oxygen saturation between the right atrium and the pulmonary artery is diagnostic of VSD in the appropriate clinical setting.

References :

1. Abeel A. Mangi and Arvind K. Agnihotri. Postinfarction Ventricular Septal Defect. In: Frank W. Sellke, Pedro J. del Nido, Scott J. Swanson (eds.). Sabiston & Spencer surgery of the chest. 8th ed. Philadelphia, PA : Saunders Elsevier;2010. p1449.
2. Abeel A. Mangi and Arvind K. Agnihotri. Postinfarction Ventricular Septal Defect. In: Frank W. Sellke, Pedro J. del Nido, Scott J. Swanson (eds.). Sabiston & Spencer surgery of the chest. 8th ed. Philadelphia, PA : Saunders Elsevier;2010. p1449.
3. Abeel A. Mangi and Arvind K. Agnihotri. Postinfarction Ventricular Septal Defect. In: Frank W. Sellke, Pedro J. del Nido, Scott J. Swanson (eds.). Sabiston & Spencer surgery of the chest. 8th ed. Philadelphia, PA : Saunders Elsevier;2010. p1450.
4. Abeel A. Mangi and Arvind K. Agnihotri. Postinfarction Ventricular Septal Defect. In: Frank W. Sellke, Pedro J. del Nido, Scott J. Swanson (eds.). Sabiston & Spencer surgery of the chest. 8th ed. Philadelphia, PA : Saunders Elsevier;2010. p1450.

ATRIAL SEPTAL DEFECT (ASD)

Dr. Vaibhav Jain, SR III, Prof S. K. Singh, Professor, Department of Cardiothoracic and Vascular Surgery

A local doctor in a village examines an eleven year old schoolgirl for recurrent cold and cough and finds that she has a heart murmur. He then refers her to our cardiology department where examination reveals a systolic murmur at the pulmonary area and a fixed splitting of the second heart sound. Echocardiography was done and revealed an ostium secundum type of large (about 25 mm) atrial septal defect with a left to right shunt.

1. Presence of ASD alongwith Mitral stenosis is known as
   (A) Taussig Bing syndrome
   (B) Brugada syndrome
   (C) Lutembacher syndrome
   (D) Eisenmenger syndrome
2. Which type of Atrial Septal Defect is most commonly seen?
   (A) Ostium Primum
   (B) Ostium Secundum
   (C) Sinus Venosus
   (D) Coronary sinus type
3. Qp : Qs ratio was mentioned in Echocardiogrphy report. It means:
   (A) It is the ratio of Pulmonary blood flow to Systemic flow
   (B) It is the ratio of Pulmonary artery diameter to Diameter of Aorta
   (C) It is the ratio of the orifice area of Pulmonary artery and Aorta
   (D) It is the ratio of pressure in Pulmonary artery to Systemic pressure.
4. Boundaries of Triangle of Koch are formed by all of the following EXCEPT:
   (A) Coronary sinus ostia
   (B) AV node
   (C) Septal leaflet of Tricuspid valve
   (D) Tendon of Todaro
5. Closure of the foramen primum results from the fusion of the
   (A) septum primum and the septum secundum
   (B) septum primum and the endocardial cushions
   (C) septum secundum and the septum spurium
   (D) septum secundum and the endocardial cushions

Answers :

1. C
   Mitral stenosis in association with ASD is known as Lutembacher's syndrome.
2. B
   Secundum ASD occurs in 1 in 1500 live births, accounting for 10% to 15% of congenital heart defects in children and 20% to 40% of defects discovered in adults.
3. A
   Qp : Qs is the ratio of pulmonary-to-systemic flow measured in Echocardiography.
4. B
   Triangle of Koch is demarcated by the tendon of Todaro, the attachment of the septal leaflet of the tricuspid valve, and the orifice of the coronary sinus. The entire atrial component of the axis of atrioventricular conduction tissues is contained within the confines of the triangle of Koch.
5. B
   As the septum primum grows toward the endocardial cushion, the ostium primum is defined. As the ostium primum closes, the ostium secundum forms by the resorption of the cephalad portions of the septum primum.

References:

1. David P. Bichell and Karla G. Christian. Atrial Septal Defect and Cor Triatriatum. In: Frank W. Sellke, Pedro J. del Nido, Scott J. Swanson (eds.). Sabiston & Spencer surgery of the chest. 8th ed. Philadelphia, PA : Saunders Elsevier;2010. p1801.
2. David P. Bichell and Karla G. Christian. Atrial Septal Defect and Cor Triatriatum. In: Frank W. Sellke, Pedro J. del Nido, Scott J. Swanson (eds.). Sabiston & Spencer surgery of the chest. 8th ed. Philadelphia, PA : Saunders Elsevier;2010. p1800.
3. Abeel A. Mangi and Arvind K. Agnihotri. Postinfarction Ventricular Septal Defect. In: Frank W. Sellke, Pedro J. del Nido, Scott J. Swanson (eds.). Sabiston & Spencer surgery of the chest. 8th ed. Philadelphia, PA : Saunders Elsevier;2010. p1450.
4. Andrew C. Cook, Benson R. Wilcox, and Robert H. Anderson. Surgical Anatomy of the Heart. In: Frank W. Sellke, Pedro J. del Nido, Scott J. Swanson (eds.). Sabiston & Spencer surgery of the chest. 8th ed. Philadelphia, PA : Saunders Elsevier;2010. p701.
5. David P. Bichell and Karla G. Christian. Atrial Septal Defect and Cor Triatriatum. In: Frank W. Sellke, Pedro J. del Nido, Scott J. Swanson (eds.). Sabiston & Spencer surgery of the chest. 8th ed. Philadelphia, PA : Saunders Elsevier;2010. p1799.

PATENT DUCTUS ARTERIOSUS

Dr. Vaibhav Jain, SR III, Prof S. K. Singh, Professor, Department of Cardiothoracic and Vascular Surgery

A six and half year old schoolgirl is brought by her parents to our OPD having been referred from a local paediatrician who had noticed a continuous murmur on auscultation. Her mother tells that her child has had a history of recurrent respiratory tract infections since childhood. We advised a 2-D Echo and it was found that the girl was having a Patent Ductus Arteriosus of 8 mm size with L-->R Shunt.

1. In Patent Ductus Arteriosus the ductus connects :
    (A) Left Pulmonary artery with Aorta just proximal to the origin of the left Subclavian artery
    (B) Left Pulmonary artery with Aorta just distal to the origin of the left Subclavian artery
    (C) Right Pulmonary artery with Aorta just distal to the origin of the left Subclavian artery
    (D) Right Pulmonary artery with Aorta just proximal to the origin of the left Subclavian artery
2. Which of the following congenital malformation is commonly associated with the congenital rubella syndrome :
    (A) Coarctation of the aorta
    (B) Tetralogy of fallot
    (C) Patent ductus arteriosus
    (D) Atrial septal defect
3. The ductus arteriosus seals off to produce remnant known as the
    (A) Ligamentum teres
    (B) Ligamentum venosus
    (C) Ligamentum arteriosum
    (D) Falciform ligament
4. First surgical closure of patent ductus arteriosus was performed by :
    (A) Rashkind and Cuaso
    (B) G A Gibson
    (C) Robert E. Gross
    (D) John Gibbon

Answers :

1. B
    The usual isolated PDA connects to the upper descending thoracic aorta 2 to 10 mm beyond the aortic origin of the left subclavian artery. From the aorta, it passes centrally toward the origin of the LPA from the pulmonary trunk, either directly or angling superiorly and hugging the undersurface of the distal aortic arch.
2. C
    Patent Ductus Arteriosus is particularly common when the mother contracts rubella during the first trimester of pregnancy and may then be associated with multiple peripheral pulmonary artery stenoses and renal artery stenosis.
3. C
    Postnatal closure occurs in two stages. The first stage is complete within 10 to 15 hours after birth in full-term infants; smooth muscle in the media of the ductal wall contracts, producing shortening and an increase in wall thickness. The second stage of closure is usually completed by 2 to 3 weeks. It is the result of diffuse fibrous proliferation of the intima, sometimes associated with necrosis of the inner layer of the media, and hemorrhage into the wall. These changes result in permanent sealing of the lumen and produce the fibrous ligamentum arteriosum.
4. C
    The first surgical closure of a PDA was performed by Dr. Robert Gross in 1938 at Boston Children's Hospital.

References :

1. Nicholas T. Kouchoukos, Eugene H. Blackstone, Frank L. Hanley, James K. Kirklin. Patent Ductus Arteriosus. In: Nicholas T. Kouchoukos, Eugene H. Blackstone, Frank L. Hanley, James K. Kirklin (eds.). Kirklin/Barratt-Boyes cardiac surgery: morphology, diagnostic criteria, natural history, techniques, results, and indications.4th ed. Philadelphia, PA : Elsevier Saunders;2013. p1343.
2. Nicholas T. Kouchoukos, Eugene H. Blackstone, Frank L. Hanley, James K. Kirklin. Patent Ductus Arteriosus. In: Nicholas T. Kouchoukos, Eugene H. Blackstone, Frank L. Hanley, James K. Kirklin (eds.). Kirklin/Barratt-Boyes cardiac surgery: morphology, diagnostic criteria, natural history, techniques, results, and indications.4th ed. Philadelphia, PA : Elsevier Saunders;2013. p1346.

3. Nicholas T. Kouchoukos, Eugene H. Blackstone, Frank L. Hanley, James K. Kirklin. Patent Ductus Arteriosus. In: Nicholas T. Kouchoukos, Eugene H. Blackstone, Frank L. Hanley, James K. Kirklin (eds.). Kirklin/Barratt-Boyes cardiac surgery: morphology, diagnostic criteria, natural history, techniques, results, and indications.4th ed. Philadelphia, PA : Elsevier Saunders;2013. p1343.

4. Sitaram M. Emani. Patent Ductus Arteriosus, Coarctation of the Aorta, and Vascular Rings. In: Frank W. Sellke, Pedro J. del Nido, Scott J. Swanson (eds.). Sabiston & Spencer surgery of the chest. 8th ed. Philadelphia, PA : Saunders Elsevier;2010. p1781.

CORONARY ARTERY BYPASS GRAFTING (CABG)

Dr. Vaibhav Jain, SR III, Prof. S. K. Singh, Professor, Department of Cardiothoracic and Vascular Surgery

A sixty seven year old university professor has been referred to us for coronary artery bypass grafting. He gives a history of chest pain on exertion since nearly two years. He is a diabetic (Type-II), has high cholesterol and is an ex-smoker since 2 years. His coronary angiogram was done which Triple Vessel Disease. Echocardiography revealed an ejection fraction of 50%.

1. Commonly used technique for Intraoperative objective Graft Assessment after CABG is:
   (A) intraoperative coronary and graft angiography
   (B) Thermal imaging
   (C) transit-time flow measurement
   (D) MR Angiogram

2. First LITA to LAD bypass operation for Coronary Artery Disease was done by
   (A) Sabiston
   (B) DeBakey
   (C) Kolessov
   (D) Favaloro

3. Stunned myocardium is :
   (A) Hypocontractile segment, with normal perfusion and glucose utilization at rest.
   (B) Decreased perfusion but preserved glucose utilization.
   (C) Reduced perfusion and glucose utilization
   (D) Normally contracting segment with reduced perfusion and glucose utilization

4. Use of which conduit should be avoided in patients with Leriche syndrome :
   (A) Radial artery
   (B) Great saphenous vein
   (C) Lesser saphenous vein
   (D) Left Internal Mammary artery

5. A patient with chronic stable angina complains of chest pain when climbing one flight of stairs. According to Canadian class system he can be categorised under which class?
   (A) Class I
   (B) Class II
   (C) Class III
   (D) Class IV

Answers :

1. C
   The most widely used modality of objective graft assessment is transit-time flow measurement. With this tool, a diastolic- to-systolic perfusion pattern of at least 2:1 for grafts constructed to vessels overlying the left ventricle (such as the LAD and circumflex branches) is a good predictor of patency, and low absolute flow values can be the result of arterial spasm without anastomotic error.

2. C
   In 1964, Kolessov grafted the LITA to the left anterior descending (LAD) artery.

3. A
   Stunned myocardium appears as a hypocontractile segment, with normal perfusion and glucose utilization at rest on Positron Emission Tomography study.

4. D
   Absolute contraindications to the use of an internal thoracic artery include previous damage from penetrating trauma or surgery and documentation of the artery as a major source of collateral perfusion to a lower extremity in patients with Leriche syndrome.

5. C

Severity of angina is typically categorized by the Canadian class system, which differs from the New York Heart Association (NYHA) classification for heart failure.Class IV comprises of patients who complain ofangina occurring with even mild activity. It may occur at rest but must be brief (<15 minutes) in duration. (If the angina is of longer duration, it is called unstable angina.) This implies inability to carry out even mild physical activity.

References :

1. Vincent Chan, Frank W. Sellke, and Marc Ruel. Coronary Artery Bypass Grafting. In: Frank W. Sellke, Pedro J. del Nido, Scott J. Swanson (eds.). Sabiston & Spencer surgery of the chest. 8th ed. Philadelphia, PA : Saunders Elsevier;2010. p1381.

2. Vincent Chan, Frank W. Sellke, and Marc Ruel. Coronary Artery Bypass Grafting. In: Frank W. Sellke, Pedro J. del Nido, Scott J. Swanson (eds.). Sabiston & Spencer surgery of the chest. 8th ed. Philadelphia, PA : Saunders Elsevier;2010. p1368.

3. Vincent Chan, Frank W. Sellke, and Marc Ruel. Coronary Artery Bypass Grafting. In: Frank W. Sellke, Pedro J. del Nido, Scott J. Swanson (eds.). Sabiston & Spencer surgery of the chest. 8th ed. Philadelphia, PA : Saunders Elsevier;2010. p1368-9.

4. Vincent Chan, Frank W. Sellke, and Marc Ruel. Coronary Artery Bypass Grafting. In: Frank W. Sellke, Pedro J. del Nido, Scott J. Swanson (eds.). Sabiston & Spencer surgery of the chest. 8th ed. Philadelphia, PA : Saunders Elsevier;2010. p1372.

5. Nicholas T. Kouchoukos, Eugene H. Blackstone, Frank L. Hanley, James K. Kirklin. Stenotic Arteriosclerotic Coronary Artery Disease. In: Nicholas T. Kouchoukos, Eugene H. Blackstone, Frank L. Hanley, James K. Kirklin (eds.). Kirklin/Barratt-Boyes cardiac surgery: morphology, diagnostic criteria, natural history, techniques, results, and indications.4th ed. Philadelphia, PA : Elsevier Saunders;2013. p361.

Chapter-4

Clinical Haematology

NORMAL HEMATOPOIESIS

Dr. A.K Tripathi, Professor, Department of Clinical Hematology

An 18 year old girl moves from sea level to the height of 2400m by train. The increased requirement for oxygen delivery to tissues stimulates synthesis of renal hormone erythropoietin.

1. Erythropoeitin promotes the survival of early erythroid precursors by which of the following mechanism?
   (A) Altered cell matrix
   (B) Inhibition of apoptosis
   (C) stimulation of globin synthesis
   (D) Enhanced glucose uptake
2. What will be the finding in bone marrow?
   (A) Erythoid hyperplasia
   (B) Myeloid hyperplasia
   (C) Megakaryocytic hyperplasia
   (D) All of the above
3. Exogenous erythropoietin can be used in all of the following except?
   (A) HIV induced anemia
   (B) Iron deficiency anemia
   (C) Anemia of chronic disease
   (D) Myelodysplastic syndrome
4. Least likely Side effect of exogenous erythropoietin is ?
   (A) Hypertension
   (B) Thrombosis
   (C) Progression of cancer
   (D) Seizures

Answers:
1. B
   Erythropoietin promotes survival of early erythroid precursors
2. A
   In response to increased release of erythropoietin bone marrow responds with erythroid hyperplasia
3. B
   All are indications of treatment with erythropoietin except iron deficiency anemia which needs treatment with iron supplements.
4. D
   Progression of hypertension, thrombosis and progression of cancer has been reported with use of erythropoietin.

Reference:
1. Kasper DL, Fauci AS, Houser SL. Anemia and polycythemia .Harrison's Principles of Internal Medicine. 19th Ed. Mc Graw-Hill Education;2015:392-393

HYPOCHROMIC ANEMIAS

Dr. A.K. Tripathi, Professor, Department of Clinical Hematology

A 20 year old male was found to have a Hb -7.8g/dL with reticulocyte count of 0.7%.Peripheral blood film showed microcytic hypochromic picture. Hb A2 and Hb F were 2.4 and 1.2 % respectively. Spleen was palpable. Serum iron and total iron binding capacity were 15mcg/dl and 420 mcg/dl respectively.

1. What is the diagnosis?
   (A) Iron deficiency anemia
   (B) Sideroblastic anemia
   (C) Anemia of chronic disease
   (D) Beta thalassemia
2. What is the treatment of above disease?
   (A) Erythropoeitin
   (B) Oral iron
   (C) pyridoxine
   (D) splenectomy

3. What other peripheral blood findings will be seen in the smear?
   (A) Spherocytes
   (B) leptocytes
   (C) tear drop cells
   (D) basophilic stippling
4. Which of the following is not expected in microcytic hypochromic anemia?
   (A) Reduced serum iron
   (B) Increased total RBC distribution width
   (C) Normal ferritin levels
   (D) Increased TIBC

Answers:
1. A
   Clinical picture and lab parameters are suggestive of iron deficiency anemia. Mild splenomegaly may be found in IDA.
2. B
   Iron deficiency anemia responds with oral iron or IV iron supplementation.
3. B
   Thin pencil shaped cells (leptocytes) are found in peripheral smear of severe IDA. Spherocytes are found in cases of hereditary spherocytosis , autoimmune hemolytic anemia and posttransfusion. Tear drop cells are found in marrow fibrosis and basophilic stippling in thalassemia and megaloblastic anemia.
4. C
   Serum ferritin will be reduced in IDA except conditions where underlying infective or inflammatory process is there.

Reference:
1. Kasper DL, Fauci AS, Houser SL. Iron deficiency and other hypoproliferative anemias.Harrison's Principles of Internal Medicine. 19th Ed. Mc Graw-Hill Education;2015:626-627

HYPOCHROMIC ANEMIAS
Dr. A.K Tripathi, Professor, Department of Clinical Hematology

A 11month old boy exclusively milk fed, born to Sindhi parents presented with complaints of progressive lethargy, irritability and pallor since six months of age. Investigation showed Hb 3.8g/dL, MCV 58fl, MCH 19.4pg. Osmotic fragility test, and HPLC for variant hemoglobin is normal.

1. What is the diagnosis?
   (A) IDA
   (B) Sideroblastic anemia
   (C) Hemoglobin D disease
   (D) Hereditary spherocytosis
2. Which is the next best investigation to confirm the diagnosis?
   (A) Iron studie(B) Bone marrow
   (C) USG abdomen
   (D) Coomb's test
3. What is the treatment of the above disease?
   (A) Iron therapy
   (B) Folic acid
   (C) Pyridoxine
   (D) Phlebotomy
4. Osmotic fragility is normal or decrseased in all of the following except?
   (A) Anemia of chronic disease
   (B) IDA
   (C) Hereditary spherocytosis
   (D) Sideroblastic anemia

Answers:
1. A
   As the child is exclusively milk fed and HPLC for variant hemoglobin is normal, most likely diagnosis is IDA with the above lab values

2. A

Iron studies including serum ferritin will be the best investigations to confirm the diagnosis

3. A

This child will need treatment with iron supplementation till stores are adequate

4. C

In Hereditary spherocytosis osmotic fragility is increased which is useful in diagnosis

Reference:

1. Kasper DL, Fauci AS, Houser SL. Iron deficiency and other hypoproliferative anemias.Harrison's Principles of Internal Medicine. 19th Ed. Mc Graw-Hill Education;2015:626-627

MEGALOBLASTIC ANEMIAS AND OTHER MACROCYTIC ANAEMIAS
Dr. A.K. Tripathi, Professor, Department of Clinical Hematology

A 40 year old female presented with parasthesia in hands and feet and easy fatiguability since two months. Examination showed a smooth tongue with loss of position and vibration sense. General blood picture showed macrocytic picture with hypersegmented neutrohils and Hb-6.0g/dL, TLC-3000/cmm and platelet count-60,000/cmm.

1. What is the probable diagnosis?
   (A) Megaloblastic anemia
   (B) Aplastic anemia
   (C) Acute leukemia
   (D) Hypothyroidism
2. What should be the next investigation?
   (A) Bone marrow examination
   (B) Serum vitamin B12
   (C) Thyroid profile
   (D) Serum iron profile
3. All of the following are associated with decreased serum cobalamine levels except?
   (A) Pregnancy
   (B) Transcobalamin deficiency type 2
   (C) Severe folic acid deficiency
   (D) Large doses of vit c intake

Answers:
1. A

Clinical features and lab findings are suggestive of megaloblastic anemia due to B12 deficiency.

2. B

Estimation of serum B12 levels is confirmatory for B12 deficiency anemia. Marrow will show megaloblastic changes with erythoid hyperplasia.

3. B

Cobalamine levels will be normal in transcobalamin deficiency type-II

Reference:

1. Kasper DL, Fauci AS, Houser SL. Megaloblastic anemias.Harrison's Principles of Internal Medicine. 19th Ed. Mc Graw-Hill Education;2015: 640-644

HAEMOLYTIC ANAEMIAS
Dr. A.K. Tripathi, Professor, Department of Clinical Hematology

A 5 year old child presents with sudden onset bloody diarrhea ,vomiting,hematuria and decrease urine output.BUN level is markedly increased .FDP,D-Dimer and coagulation tests are normal.GBP shows poikilocytes, schistocytes >3/1000rbcs and decrease in number of platelets .Fever and CNS symptoms were not present.

1. What is the most likely diagnosis?
   (A) HUS
   (B) atypical HUS

(C) TTP

(D) DIC

2. Causes of deranged FDP?

    (A) DIC

    (B) TTP

    (C) HUS

    (D) HIT

3. What is the best treatment of above disease?

    (A) steroids

    (B) antibiotics

    (C) plasmapheresis

    (D) Lepirudin

4. Schistocytes are seen in ?

    (A) HUS

    (B)TTP

    (C) DIC

    (D) all of the above

Answers:

1. A

    Microangiopathic anemia (MAHA) in a child with history of diarrhea and renal dysfunction is suggestive of classical HUS. TTP has more of CNS features with fever along with MAHA. DIC will have raised D-Dimers and deranged coagulation profile.

2. A

3. C

    Supportive care and plasmapheresis are the cornerstone of management of TTP-HUS

4. D

    All are well mentioned causes of MAHA.

Reference:

1. Kasper DL, Fauci AS, Houser SL. Hemolytic anemias and anemia due to acute blood loss.Harrison's Principles of Internal Medicine. 19th Ed. Mc Graw-Hill Education;2015:657-658

HEMOLYTIC ANAEMIAS

Dr. A.K. Tripathi, Professor, Department of Clinical Hematology

A 25 year old woman developed severe intermittent pain in her fingers which gets aggravated when exposed to cold. Her fingers turn white and then numb. She had a previous history of mycoplasma pneumonia. She has mild pallor. Direct coombs test was positive. Clinical diagnosis of Reynaud phenomenon was made.

1. What is the clinical diagnosis in above case?

    (A) Cold autoimmune hemolytic anemia

    (B) Warm immune hemolytic anemia

    (C) Paroxysmal cold hemoglobinuria

    (D) Paroxysmal nocturnal hemoglobinuria

2. Causes of Reynaud phenomenon are all except?

    (A) Cold agglutinin disease

    (B) PNH

    (C) Scleroderma

    (D) CREST syndrome

3. In cold agglutinin disease antibody is formed against which antigen on RBCs?

    (A) I antigen

    (B) P antigen

    (C) CD55and CD59

    (D) Rh antigen

4. What is the treatment of choice for above disease?

    (A) Steroids

    (B) Rituximab

    (C) Eculizimab

    (D) Splenectomy

5. Which of the following disease may not be a causative factor?
    (A) Mycoplasma pneumonia
    (B) Waldenstrom macroglobinemia
    (C) CLL
    (D) HCL

Answers:
1. A
    The clinical picture is suggestive of cold autoimmune hemolytic anemia which is further confirmed by positive coombs test. PCH occurs in children and usually following some respiratory infection.PNH is an acquired stem cell disorder characterized by hemolysis, thrombosis and bone marrow failure.
2. B
    Reynaud's phenomenon has been described in all other conditions except PNH
3. A
    In cold agglutinin disease antibodies are formed against carbohydrate I antigen. Antibodies against P antigens are formed in PCH while in Warm antibody type AIHA antibodies are formed against Rh antigen.
4. B
    Rituximab is treatment of choice in cold agglutinin disease. This entity does not respond as well to steroids as Warm antibody type AIHA.
5. D
    All are well mentioned causes of Cold agglutinin disease except Hairy cell leukemia.

Reference:
1. Kasper DL, Fauci AS, Houser SL. Hemolytic anemias and anemia due to acute blood loss.Harrison's Principles of Internal Medicine. 19th Ed. Mc Graw-Hill Education;2015:658-660.

HEMOLYTIC ANEMIAS
Dr A.K. Tripathi, Professor, Department of Clinical Hematology

A 25 year old pregnant lady presents with fever, altered sensorium, echymotic patches all over body, with platelet count <20,000/cmm and fragmented RBCs in peripheral smear. Blood urea-98mg/dl, serum creatinine-2.2mg/dl. S bilirubin-0.8mg/dl, ALT-22U/L, AST-25U/L. PT, APTT and D-dimer levels were normal.

1. What is the most likely diagnosis in the above case?
    (A) TTP
    (B) DIC
    (C) HELLP
    (D) Evans
2. Microangiopathic hemolytic anemia is seen in all except?
    (A) HUS
    (B) ITP
    (C) Malignant hypertension
    (D) TTP
3. Coomb's test will help to rule out which condition in this patient?
    (A) ITP
    (B) Evans syndrome
    (C) HELLP
    (D) TTP
4. What is the treatment of choice in this patient?
    (A) Platelet transfusion
    (B) Plasma exchange
    (C) Eculizumab
    (D) Fresh frozen plasma infusion

Answers:
1. A
    Clinical features and lab parameters are consistent with TTP. DIC is less likely because all the coagulation parameters are normal. HELLP is less likely because liver enzymes are normal. Evans syndrome is autoimmune hemolytic anemia with ITP.

2. B

All are well mentioned causes of MAHA except ITP
3. B

Autoimmune hemolytic anemia and thrombocytopenia is found in Evans syndrome which leads to positive coombs test.
4. B

Plasma exchange is treatment of choice in MAHA due to TTP. Platelet transfusion is generally contraindicated until there is severe bleeding due to thrombocytopenia. FFP can be used when facility of plasma exchange is not available. Eculizumab is used in cases of atypical HUS.

Reference:

1. Guideline British Journal of Haematology, 2003; 120: 556–57

APLASTIC ANAEMIA ,BONE MARROW FAILURE AND IRON OVERLOAD DISORDERS

Dr. A.K. Tripathi, Professor, Department of Clinical Hematology

A patient aged 63 years is diagnosed to have Hb 4gm/dl, TLC 1000/cmm, DLC-Neutrophil 30%, Lymphocyte 70%, platelet count 12,000/cmm. Bone marrow shows hypocellular marrow. HLA compatible sibling is available.

1. Which is the diagnosis in this patient?
    (A) Severe aplastic anemia
    (B) Very Severe aplastic anemia
    (C) Non Severe aplastic anemia
    (D) None of the above
2. What other tests are not indicated in this patient?
    (A) Chromosomal breakage analysis
    (B) MDS panel
    (C) PNH clones
    (D) Both B and C
3. True about severe Aplastic anemia is all except?
    (A) Splenomegaly
    (B) Reticulocytopenia
    (C) Thrombocytopenia
    (D) Neutropenia

Answers:
1. A

This patient has pancytopenia with hypocellular bone marrow biopsy consistent with Aplastic anemia. As absolute neutrophil count is <500 but >200 this qualifies for severe aplastic anemia.
2. A

Chromosomal breakage study is done primarily in younger patients to rule out fanconi anemia which is the most common inherited bone marrow failure syndrome. It is important to rule out MDS and PNH in all elderly cases of pancytopenia.
3. A

Splenomegaly is not a feature of aplastic anemia. Typically these patients have no organomegaly or lymphadenopathy.

Reference:

1. Kasper DL, Fauci AS, Houser SL. Bone marrow failure syndromes including aplastic anemia and Myelodysplasia.Harrison's Principles of Internal Medicine. 19th Ed. Mc Graw-Hill Education;2015:663-667.

APLASTIC ANAEMIA,BONE MARROW FAILURE AND IRON OVERLOAD DISORDERS

Dr. A.K. Tripathi, Professor, Department of Clinical Hematology

A 10 year old boy presented with pallor and mild icterus. Mild Splenomegaly was present . PBF shows macrocytic picture (MCV-120fl) and bone marrow revealed several dyserythropoetic normoblasts showing multinuclearity in erythoblasts in the marrow. Serum bilirurin is 2.5g/dl (Indirect-1.8g/dl). Serum ferritin is 500.

1. What is the most likely diagnosis?
   (A) Erythroleukemia
   (B) Cong. Dyserythropoietic anemia
   (C) Subleukemic leukemia
   (D) Myelodysplastic syndrome
2. Following conditions cause macrocytic anaemia except
   (A) Pernicious anaemia
   (B) Chronic liver disease
   (C) Post hemorrhagic state
   (D) Congenital dyserythropeitic anemia II
3. What may be the least helpful in above case?
   (A) Folvite
   (B) Interferon alpha
   (C) Inj Vitamin B12
   (D) Splenectomy
4. What other test will support your diagnosis except?
   (A) Vitamin B12 level
   (B) HEMPAS positive
   (C) Coomb's positive
   (D) Haptoglobin

Answers:
1. B
   Clinical scenario and marrow findings are suggestive of congenital dyserythropoietic anemia
2. C
   Post hemorrhagic state usually leads to microcytic hypochromic or Normocytic normochromic anemia. Rest all can lead to macrocytic anemia.
3. C
   All have been mentioned as the treatment modalities in these patients except B12 supplementation.
4. D
   Vitamin B12 deficiency will lead to megaloblastic anemia and erythroid hyperplasia, HEMPAS positivity confirms Type II CDA, and coobms positivity confirms autoimmune hemolytic anemia.

Reference:
1. Wickramasinghe SN, Wood WG. Advances in the understanding of the congenital dyserythropoietic anemias. British Journal of Hematol.2005;131:431-46

GENETIC DISORDERS OF HEMOGLOBIN
Dr. A.K. Tripathi, Professor, Department of Clinical Hematology

A 26 year old female presented with mild pallor and moderate hepatosplenomegaly. Her Hb was 9.2g/dL. Her HPLC for variant hemoglobin shows HbA2 6% and fetal Hb of 6.5%, she has not received any blood transfusion till date.
1. What is the diagnosis?
   (A) Thalassemia major
   (B) Thalassemia intermedia
   (C) Hereditary persistence of fetal Hb homozygous state
   (D) Hemoglobin D homozygous state
2. What is the etiology of above diagnosis?
   (A) Decreased beta globin synthesis
   (B) Decreased delta globin synthesis
   (C) Both of the above
   (D) None of the above
3. What other findings will be present in this patient?
   (A) Increased osmotic fragility
   (B) Decreased retic count
   (C) Decreased Hb A2
   (D) Normal to Increased ferritin
4. Most common mutation in Beta thalassemia involves?
   (A) IVS-I-5(G-C)

(B) IVS-I-1(G-T)
(C) 619bp deletion
(D) 317 bp deletion

Answers:

1. B

   Thailassemia trait patients are usually asymptomatic with hemoglobin in almost normal range and mildly elevated HbA2.Thalassemia major will be transfusion dependent since first year of life with severe anemia. HPHF homozygous will have very high levels of HbF and usually asymptomatic. Homozygous HbD will have D peak in HPLC and it is also asymptomatic found in Punjab.

2. A

   Beta thalassemias result from decreased synthesis of beta globin gene.

3. D

   Usually these patients have increased iron absorption from GI tract in response to ineffective erythropoiesis

4. A

Reference:

1. Kasper DL, Fauci AS, Houser SL. Disorders of Hemoglobin.Harrison's Principles of Internal Medicine. 19th Ed. Mc Graw-Hill Education;2015:631-637.

GENETIC DISORDERS OF HEMOGLOBIN

Dr. A.K. Tripathi, Professor, Department of Clinical Hematology

In a febrile 4 year old child with sickle cell disease and a CBC exhibiting a normocytic anemia, absolute leukocytosis and DLC shows > 10% band neutrophis with toxic granulation.

1. You would strongly suspect:
   (A) A viral infection
   (B) Salmonella osteomyelitis
   (C) Streptococcus pneumoniae sepsis
   (D) Tuberculosis
2. Primary defect which leads to sickle cell anemia.
   (A) Abnormality in porphyrin part of haemoglobin
   (B) Replacement of glutamate by valine
   (C) Nonsense mutation
   (D) Substitution of valine by glutamate
3. Which of the following is not seen in chronic case of sickle cell disease?
   (A) hepatomegaly
   (B) cardiomegaly
   (C) pulmonary hypertension
   (D) splenomegaly
4. All are true for sickle cell anemia except?
   (A) fish vertebra
   (B) cholelithiasis
   (C) renal papillary necrosis
   (D)Hypoplastic thumb

Answers:

1. C

   Streptococcal pneumonia sepsis risk is markedly increased in patients with sickle cell anemia. Initially patients smear will show leucocytosis with left shift and toxic granulations.

2. B

   Sickle cell disease (SCD) occurs due to substitution of valine by Glutamic acid at position 6 of beta globin chain. This is an example of single point mutation.

3. D

   Splenomegaly is not a features of sickle cell disease and gets fibrosed and small over due course of time.

4. D

   Hypoplastic thumb and other morphological defects are not a feature of SCD

Reference:
1. Kasper DL, Fauci AS, Houser SL.Disorders of Hemoglobin.Harrison's Principles of Internal Medicine. 19th Ed. Mc Graw-Hill Education;2015:633-635.

HEMOLYTIC ANEMIA: RBC MEMBRANE DEFECT
Dr. A.K. Tripathi, Professor, Department of Clinical Hematology

A 10 year old boy presents with chronic fatigue . Physical examination reveals slight jaundice and splenomaegaly. Laboratory studies showed Hb 11.7g/dL, hematocrit of 32%, total bilirubin of 2.6 mg% and conjugated bilirubin of 0.8gm%. Periperal blood picture show spherocytes. Osmotic fragility test is increased and coombs test is negative.

1. What is the pathogenesis of above disease?
   (A) Erythrocyte cytoskeleton defect
   (B) Erythrocyte membrane defect
   (C) DNA defect
   (D) Enzyme defect.
2. Triad of anaemia,jaundice and splenomegaly is seen in ?
   (A) Felty syndrome
   (B) Hereditary spherocytosis
   (C) MDS
   (D) Hereditary stomatocytosis
3. Osmotic fragility is decreased in all of the following except?
   (A) Iron deficiency anaemia
   (B) Thalesemia
   (C) Hereditary spherocytosis
   (D) Hereditary stomatocytosis

Answers:
1. A
   Hereditary spherocytosis results from defect in membrane proteins like spectrin, ankyrin, Band-3 and Protein 4.2. These proteins are required for integrity of RBC membrane and its pliability. When such cells reach spleen redundant and defective membrane is removed and cells takes shape of a spherocyte.
2. B
   Classical triad has been described in hereditary spherocytosis.
3. C
   Osmotic fragility is increased in HS

Reference:
1. Kasper DL, Fauci AS, Houser SL.Hemolytic anemias and anemias due to acute blood loss .Harrison's Principles of Internal Medicine. 19th Ed. Mc Graw-Hill Education;2015:649-651.

HEMOLYTIC ANEMIA
Dr. A.K. Tripathi, Professor, Department of Clinical Hematology

A couple with the family history of beta thalassemia major in a distant relative have come for counseling. Husband has Hb A2 of 4.8% & wife has Hb A2 2.3%.
1. The risk of having a child with beta thalessemia major is-
   (A) 50%
   (B) 25%
   (C) 5%
   (D) 0%
2. All are true about beta thalessemia trait except-
   (A) Increasd Hb F
   (B) Increased Hb A2
   (C) Microcytosis
   (D) Severe anemia
3. Hb A2 level increased all except-
   (A) Alpha thalessemia

(B) Beta thalessemia
(C) Sickle cell anemia
(D) Megaloblastic anemia

Answers:
1. D
   If one of the parents are normal and other is thal trait the chances of child being thal major is 0% because it is an autosomal recessive inheritance.
2. D
   Severe anemia is not a features of thalassemia trait, infect in thal trait Hb is almost normal or mildly decreased
3. A
   In alfa thalassemia alfa globin chain is decreased so the production of HbA2 ($\alpha2\delta2$) is decreased.

Reference:
1. Kasper DL, Fauci AS, Houser SL. Disorders of Hemoglobin. Harrison's Principles of Internal Medicine. 19th Ed. Mc Graw-Hill Education;2015:637-639.

ACUTE LEUKEMIAS
Dr. S.P.Verma, Assistant Professor, Department of Clinical Hematology

A 40 year old patient presents with a fever and bone pains since 10 days. On investigation Hb was 6 gm/dl, WBC -2000/cmm, with a differential count having 6% blasts. Platelet are reduced to 80,000/cmm. Bone marrow shows hypercellular marrow with 20% blasts. Moderate splenomegaly is present.

1. What is the diagnosis?
   (A) Acute leukemia
   (B) Hairy cell leukemia
   (C) Aplastic anemia
   (D) Megaloblastic anemia
2. Pancytopenia with hypercellular marrow is seen in all except?
   (A) PNH
   (B) Leukemia
   (C) Aplastic anemia
   (D) Hairy cell leukemia
3. These blasts are Myeloperoxidase positive (MPO+).What is the most effective treatment of above disease?
   (A) 7+3 Induction chemotherapy
   (B) Cladirabine
   (C) ATG
   (D) Decitabine

Answers:
1. A
   More than or equal to 20% blast in bone marrow qualifies for acute leukemia diagnosis.
2. C
   Pancytopenia with hypercellular marrow may be seen in all conditions except aplastic anemia where marrow cellularity in biopsy is <25%
3. A
   For AML fit patients initial choice is induction with 7+3 chemotherapy schedule. Seven days of continuous infusion cytarabine and 3 days of bolus daunorubicin.

References:
1. Kasper DL, Fauci AS, Houser SL.Acute Myeloid Leukemia.Harrison's Principles of Internal Medicine. 19th Ed. Mc Graw-Hill Education;2015:679-685.

ACUTE LEUKEMIAS
Dr. S.P.Verma, Assistant Professor,Department of Clinical Hematology

A 17 year old boy presented with fever, lymphnode enlargement and bone pain since 1 month. On investigation he had a TLC of 1,45,000/cmm, with 70% blast on the peripheral smear. Flow cytometry shows Tdt, CD34 and CD19 and CD10 positivity.

1. What is the most likely diagnosis?
    (A) ALL-B cell
    (B) AMl
    (C) NHL with spillover
    (D) ALL-T cell
2. Which are poor prognostic factors in above disease except?
    (A) Age >10 year
    (B) TLC > 50,000/cmm
    (C) Philadelphia positivity
    (D) TEL-AML1, t(12-21)

Answers:
    1. A
        Peripheral blood findings and flowcytometry is suggestive of B –acute lymphoblastic leukemia.Tdt is a marker of prematurity and CD19 and CD10 are b cell markers.
    2. D
        Age <1 year and >10 year, WBC count at diagnosis >50000 and Ph positivity are poor risk factors. TEL-AML-1 is associated with good prognosis. Other good prognosis is hyperdiploidy.

Reference:
    1. Kasper DL, Fauci AS, Houser SL.Malignancies of Lymphoid cells.Harrison's Principles of Internal Medicine. 19th Ed. Mc Graw-Hill Education;2015:701.

ACUTE LEUKEMIAS
Dr. S.P.Verma, Assistant Professor,Department of Clinical Hematology

A 15 year old boy presented with history of gum bleeding, subconjuctival bleed and purpuric rash. Investigation revealed Hb-6.5g/dl, TLC-6000/cmm, platelet count 10,000/cmm. Prothrombin time 22sec(control 13 sec), APTT is 50 sec(Control 32 sec) .Peripheral smear shows atypical cells with auer rods.

1. What is the most likely diagnosis ?
    (A) APML
    (B) AMl-M7
    (C) AML-M0
    (D) AMl-M5
2. Auer rods are generally seen in the following?
    (A) AMl-M0
    (B) AMl-M2
    (C) AMl-M7
    (D) all of the above
3. Which cytogenetic abnormality is commonly seen in above case?
    (A) Flt3-itd
    (B) PML-RARa
    (C) NPM1
    (D) TEL-AML1
4. Initial treatment of above disease includes.
    (A) BMT
    (B) ATRA
    (C) Induction with cytsosine arabinoside and daunorubicin
    (D) MCP841 protocol

Answers:
    1. A
        The clinical presentation is of a leukemia with coagulopathy and cytopenias which fits mostly into APML.,
    2. B
        Auer rodes are also found in AML-M2.
    3. B
        Cytogenetic abnormality in APML is translocation t(15:17) which leads to PML-RARA fusion gene product detected molecularly.

4. B
    There is primarily a block of differentiation in myeloid series at promyelocyte level leading to accumulation of abnormal promyelocytes. ATRA is a differentiating agent which removes the block and leads to normal maturation.

Reference:
1. Kasper DL, Fauci AS, Houser SL. Acute Myeloid Leukemia. Harrison's Principles of Internal Medicine. 19th Ed. Mc Graw-Hill Education;2015:679-687.

MYELOPROLIFERATIVE NEOPLASMS

Dr. S.P.Verma, Assistant Professor, Department of Clinical Hematology

A 55 year old patient with polycythemia vera presents with fever and generalized bodyaches and intense pruritis. On investigation she has decreased white cell count and decreased platelets. She did not require phelobotomy since 3 months. On examination there is massive splenomegaly.

1. What is the likely diagnosis in this case?
    (A) Cellular phase of polycythemia vera(PV)
    (B) Spent phase of PV
    (C) Prefibrotic phase of PV
    (D) Myelofibrosis
2. What is the treatment of choice in this patient?
    (A) Interferon alpha
    (B) Hydroxyurea
    (C) Ruxolitinib
    (D) All of the above
3. Which one of the following is not included in WHO criteria of PV?
    (A) Jak 2STATV617F positivity
    (B) pan myelosis
    (C) High erythropoietin levels
    (D) Increased endogenous erythroid colonies
4. What are the type of megakaryocytic morphology seen in Bone marrow?
    (A) Dwarf megakaryocyte
    (B) Staghorn megakarocyte
    (C) Micro megakarocyte
    (D) Non functional megakarocyte

Answers:
1. B
    Polycythemia vera is a MPN characterized by panmyelosis very high hemoglobin and tendency to progress to spent phase of PV or evolution to acute leukemia. When need for phlebotomy is reduced or anemia develops with progressive splenomegaly and B-Symptoms possibility of going into spent phase should be considered.
2. C.
    This is a case of spent phase of Polycythemia vera where ruxolitinib (JAK2 inhibitor) has been found to be effective as in primary myelofibrosis usually controls spleen size and constitutional symptoms
3. C
    Polycythemia vera is characterized by low or low normal erythropoietin levels
4. B
    Megakaryocytes in polycythemia vera have staghorn appearance. Dwarf megs are found in CML and micromegs in childhood MDS.

Reference:
1. Kasper DL, Fauci AS, Houser SL.Polycythemia vera and other Myeloproliferative neoplasms.Harrison's Principles of Internal Medicine. 19th Ed. Mc Graw-Hill Education;2015:672-674.

MYELOPROLIFERATIVE NEOPLASMS
Dr. S.P.Verma, Assistant Professor, Department of Clinical Hematology

A 60 year old man presented with fatigue, weight loss and heaviness in left hypochondrium for 6 months. The hemogram showed Hb 10gm/dl, TLC-5 lakh/mm, platelet count 4 lakh/mm3, DLC-neutrophil 55%, lymphocytes 4%, monocytes 2%, basophils6%, metamyelocytes 10%, myelocytes 18%,promyelocytes 2%, blast 3%.

1. The most likely cytogenetic abnormality in this case –
   (A) t(1,21)
   (B) t(9,22)
   (C) t(15,17)
   (D) Trisomy 21
2. Most common transcript mutation seen in this condition?
   (A) P190 BCR-ABL
   (B) P210 BCR-ABL
   (C) FL1P1-PDGFRα
   (D) CALR mutation
3. Which is generally not a side effect of Tyrosine kinase inhibitor?
   (A) Fluid retention
   (B) Cytopenia
   (C) Thrombosis
   (D) Muscle cramps

Answers:
1. B
   The peripheral smear findings are very suggestive of Chronic myeloid leukemia which is most common Myeloproliferative neoplasm.
2. B
   It occurs due to reciprocal translocation of BCR region of chromosome 22 to ABL- region of chromosome 9. Shortened chromosome 22 is known as Philadelphia chromosome. This translocation gives rise to BCR-ABL transcript of P210 type which has tyrosine kinase activity
3. C
   Tyrosine kinase inhibitors (TKI'S) are drugs which have targeted potential to control the disease at molecular level. Imatinib is the most commonly used drug which can cause fluid retention, cytopenias and muscle cramps as major side effects.

Reference:
1. Kasper DL, Fauci AS, Houser SL. Chronic Myeloid Leukemia.Harrison's Principles of Internal Medicine. 19th Ed. Mc Graw-Hill Education;2015:687-694.

LYMPHOPROLIFERATIVE DISORDERS
Dr. Pratibha Dhiman, Assistant Professor, Department of Clinical Hematology

A 20 year old female presents with fever ,weight loss, night sweats and painless enlargement of lymphnodes in cervical, axillary and supraclavicular lymph nodes. Biopsy showed atypical mononuclear cells surrounded by clear spaces and binucleate giant cell with prominent acidophilic nucleoli. On immunostaining, these atypical cells were positive for CD15 and CD30 and negative for EMA and CD45.

1. Which of the following is most likely diagnosis?
   (A) Anaplastic large cell lymphoma
   (B) Non Hodgkin lymphoma –DLBCL
   (C) Lymphocyte predominant hodgkin lymphoma
   (D) Nodular sclerosis Hodgkin lymphoma.
2. Which tumors are CD30 positive?
   (A) ALCL
   (B) Hodgkin lymphoma
   (C) Activated lymphocyte
   (D) All of the above
3. Lacunar cells are seen in?
   (A) Nodular sclerosis Hodgkin lymphoma
   (B) Lymphocytic Predominant Hodgkin lymphoma
   (C) Lymphocyte depleted Hodgkin lymphoma

(D) Mixed cellularity
4. EMA positivity is seen in?
   (A) DLBCL
   (B) HL
   (C) CLL
   (D) ALCL

Answers:
1. D
   Nodular sclerosis Hodgkin lymphoma. Patient has B symptoms in the form of fever and weight loss which leads towards diagnosis of lymphoma. The atypical mononuclear cells described are characteristic of Nodular sclerosis Hodgkin Lymphoma.
2. D
   All of the above. ALCL is a type of T cell lymphoma where the large atypical cells with doughnut nuclei express CD30. In Hodgkin lymphoma, Reed Sternberg cells are CD30 positive. Also activated lymphocytes express CD30.
3. A
   Nodular sclerosis Hodgkin lymphoma. Lacunar cells (morphologically different from classical Reed Sternberg cells) are seen in Nodular sclerosis Hodgkin lymphoma.
4. D
   The atypical cells in ALCL manifests EMA i.e Epithelial membrane antigen which is usually positive in solid malignancies.

References:
1. Kasper DL, Fauci AS, Houser SL.Malignancies of Lymphoid cells.Harrison's Principles of Internal Medicine. 19th Ed. Mc Graw-Hill Education;2015:708-709.

LYMPHOPROLIFERATIVE DISORDERS
Dr. Pratibha Dhiman, Assistant Professor, Department of Clinical Hematology

A patient presents to the hospital with complaints of persistent fever and significant weight loss for the past 2 months. On examination he is observed to have cervical and axillary lymphadenopathy.Other examination and investigations are unremarkable. Biopsy from the cervical nodes is performed and returns positive for hodgkin's lymphoma (nodular sclerosis variant)

1. The patient can be staged as having
   (A) IA
   (B) IIB
   (C) IB
   (D) IIA
2. Which one is associated with best prognosis?
   (A) Nodular sclerosis
   (B) Lymphocyte predominance
   (C) Mixed cellularity
   (D) Lymphocyte depletion
3. What is true in this patient
   (A) EBV-
   (B) CD15-, CD30-
   (C) Reticular variant
   (D) Lacunar cells
4. Paraneoplastic cerebellar degeneration is associated with all except?
   (A) Hodgkin's lymphoma
   (B) Thymoma
   (C) Neuroblastoma
   (D) Small cell lung cancer

Answer:
1. B
   Two groups of lymph nodes are involved along with presence of B symptoms.
2. B
   Lymphocyte depletion has the worst prognosis among the category.

3. D

These neoplastic cells are hallmark of nodular sclerosis type of Hodgkin lymphoma.

4. C

All the others can present with paraneoplastic cerebellar involvement.

Reference:

1. Kasper DL, Fauci AS, Houser SL.Malignancies of Lymphoid cells.Harrison's Principles of Internal Medicine. 19th Ed. Mc Graw-Hill Education;2015:708-709.

LYMPHOPROLIFERATIVE DISORDERS

Dr. Pratibha Dhiman, Assistant Professor, Department of Clinical Hematology

CD19 positive, CD22 positive, CD103 positive monoclonal B cells with bright kappa positivity were found to comprise 60% of the peripheral blood lymphoid cells on flow cytometric analysis in a 60 year old man with massive splenomegaly and a total leucocyte count of 3.0×10^9/L.

1. What is the diagnosis?
   (A) CLL
   (B) Mantle cell lymphoma
   (C) HCL
   (D) HCL-V
2. Which are the cytochemical stain used to diagnose this condition?
   (A) Tryptase
   (B) Tartarate resistant acid phosphatase
   (C) Non specific esterase
   (D) Myeloperoxidase
3. Which other CD marker is positive in above case?
   (A) CD11a
   (B) CD11b
   (C) CD11c
   (D) All of the above
4. What is the treatment of choice in this patient?
   (A) Pentostatin
   (B) Interferon alpha
   (C) Purine analogue
   (D) Splenectomy

Answers:

1. C

   It is a B-cell lymphoproliferative disorder affecting adults.Which is characterized by presence of hairy cells in Bone marrow and peripheral smear, usually pancytopenia with massive splenomegaly.

2. B

   Tartarate resistant acid phosphatase. This is a specific cytochemical stain to highlight hairy cells in blood and marrow

3. C

   Markers of B cells, such as CD19, CD20, CD22, CD 103 are positive.

4. C

   Cladrabine remains first line of therapy. Other drugs which can be used are pentostatine, rituximab, fludarabine

Reference:

1. Kasper DL, Fauci AS, Houser SL.Malignancies of Lymphoid cells.Harrison's Principles of Internal Medicine. 19th Ed. Mc Graw-Hill Education;2015:708-709.

LYMPHOPROLIFERATIVE DISORDERS

Dr. Pratibha Dhiman, Assistant Professor, Department of Clinical Hematology

A 62 year old man presented with massive splenomegaly, lymphadenopathy and a total leucocyte count of 18,000/mm3. The flow cytometry showed CD19 positive, CD5 positive, CD23 negative, monoclonal B cells with bright kappa positively compromising 80% of the peripheral blood lymphoid cells.

1. Which translocation is likely to be present in the above condition.
   - (A) t(11,14)
   - (B) t(4,11)
   - (C) t(8,14)
   - (D) t(2,8)
2. How is this condition best differentiated from CLL?
   - (A) Cyclin D1
   - (B) FMC7
   - (C) CD79b
   - (D) All of the above
3. What are good prognostic factors in CLL?
   - (A) Del 13q
   - (B) IgHV unmutated
   - (C) Deletion 17p
   - (D) None

Answers:

1. A

   This translocation is characteristic of Mantle cell lymphoma. The flow cytometric ,report i.e CD19 positive, CD5 positive, CD23 negative, monoclonal B cells with bright kappa positive leads towards a diagnosis of Mantle cell lymphoma.

2. A

   The translocation t(11,14) is identified as cyclin D1, it's presence makes the diagnosis of mantle cell lymphoma clear.

3. A

   Del 13q. Patient with mutated IgH V have a better prognosis . Patients with deletion 17p fare bad in the case of CLL.

Reference:

1. Kasper DL, Fauci AS, Houser SL.Malignancies of Lymphoid cells.Harrison's Principles of Internal Medicine. 19th Ed. Mc Graw-Hill Education;2015:708-709.

MULTIPLE MYELOMA AND REMATED DISORDERS
Dr. A.K.Tripathi, Professor, Department of Clinical Hematology

A 55 year old male complains pain in his back , fatigue & occasional confusion. He admits to polyuria . X- ray evaluation reveals lytic lesion is lumber vertebra. Laboratory studies shows hypoalbuminemia, anemia & thrombocytopenia . monoclonal Ig kappa peak is demonstrated by serum electrophoresis . urinalysis shows 4+ proteinuria . bone marrow biopsy shows 18% plasma cell.

1. What is appropriate diagnosis.-
   - (A) Extramedullary plasmacytoma
   - (B) Multiple myeloma
   - (C) Waldenstrom macroglobinemia
   - (D) CLL
2. True about this disease is all except. –
   - (A) Plasma cell clonal proliferation
   - (B) Common after 50 years of age
   - (C) Amyloidosis can occur
   - (D) Protein cast in urine are made of complete Ig chain
3. Which of following may seen in this condition –
   - (A) Decreased Calcium levels
   - (B) Sclerotic bone lesion
   - (C) Bone deposition
   - (D) Renal failure
4. The following is the least useful investigation in this condition-
   - (A) ESR
   - (B) X-RAY
   - (C) Bone scan
   - (D) Bone marrow biopsy

1. B

   Plasma cell dyscrasias present in older age usually with back pain and symptomatic anemia. On investigations, bony lytic lesions and monoclonal M band are diagnostic of the disease.

2. D

   Protein cast in urine are made of complete Ig chain. Light chain fractions are excreted usually in the urine.

3. D

   Patients presents with features of hypercalcemia and lytic lesions. Sclerotic lesions are part of POEMS syndrome which is a separate entity. Patients present with renal involvement due to tubular injury.

4. C Bone scan is not recommended in the diagnostic work up of multiple myeloma.

Reference:

1. Kasper DL, Fauci AS, Houser SL.Plasma cell disorders.Harrison's Principles of Internal Medicine. 19th Ed. Mc Graw-Hill Education;2015:710-715.

COAGULATION DISORDERS

Dr A.K.Tripathi, Professor, Department of Clinical Hematology

A 15-year-old girl has menorrhagia and tendency to bleed from minor cuts and wounds. Platelet count is normal. PTT and bleeding times are prolonged. Mixing studies revealed normal factor VIII and IX levels. Platelet aggregation studies revealed no aggregation with ristocetin and normal with ADP, collagen and epinephrine.

1. What is the probable diagnosis?
   (A) Bernard Soulier syndrome
   (B) Glanzmann Thrombasthenia
   (C) Von willebrand disease
   (D) Gray platelet syndrome.
2. All of the following conditions are associated with isolated raised APTT except?
   (A) DIC
   (B) VWD
   (C) APLA
   (D) Hemophilia A
3. What is helpful in the above disease?
   (A) Desmopressin
   (B) Platelet transfusion
   (C) Steroids
   (D) Factor transfusion
4. All of the following are associated with normal platelet count except?
   (A) VWD 2B
   (B) VWD 1
   (C) Glanzmann thrombasthenia
   (D) Patient on aspirin therapy

Answers:

1. C

   Von willebrand disease (vWD) which is caused by deficient or defective plasma vWF, is the most common inherited bleeding disorder, affecting as much as 0.1 to 1% of the population.

2. A

   The low level of coagulation factors is reflected by prolonged coagulation screening tests, such as the PT and the aPTT. Hemophilia A and von Willebrand disease presents with increased APTT only. APLA presents with inhibitor to APTT.

3. A

   Most individuals with type 1 vWD and some with type 2 vWD respond to intranasal, intravenous or subcutaneous treatment with desmopressin, which promotes release of stored vWF and raises levels 3- to 6-fold.

4. A

   In many patients with type 2B vWD, thrombocytopenia can develop or worsen with infection, surgery, pregnancy, or treatment with desmopressin.

Reference:
1. Kasper DL, Fauci AS, Houser SL.Disorders od platelets and vessel wall.Harrison's Principles of Internal Medicine. 19th Ed. Mc Graw-Hill Education;2015:730-731.

HAEMATOLOGICAL CHANGES IN SYSTEMIC DISEASES

Dr. A.K.Tripathi, Professor, Department of Clinical Hematology

A 70 year old man presents with UTI and septic encephalopathy with severe anemia .USG shows a hard nodule in left lobe of prostate .PSA was found to be >100ng/ml.GBP shows a leucoerythroblastic picture .

1. What is the likely diagnosis?
   (A) Microangiopathic anemia
   (B) Myelophthisic anemia
   (C) Anemia of chronic disease
   (D) Chronic myeloid leukemia
2. Which investigation should be done next?
   (A) Bone Marrow aspiration
   (B) Bone Marrow Biopsy
   (C) Iron studies
   (D) Serum B12 levels
3. Tumors metastasizing to bone are?
   (A) Breast
   (B) Prostate
   (C) Thyroid
   (D) All of the above
4. Causes of acute myelofibrosis?
   (A) Prostatic cancer
   (B) Breast cancer
   (C) AML-M7
   (D) All of the above

Answers:
1. B
   Myelophthisic anemia. A variety of infiltrative (myelophthisic) processes may be observed. These include malignancies such as small cell lung, breast, and prostate cancers, which not infrequently can appear in advanced stages with marrow involvement.
2. B
   Bone marrow biopsy is the diagnostic investigation for infiltrative disorders.
3. D
   All the malignancies described can infiltrate the bone marrow.
4. D
   Acute myelofibrosis is the representation of infiltration of bone marrow.

Reference:
1. Kasper DL, Fauci AS, Houser SL.Polycythemia vera and other Myeloproliferative neoplasms.Harrison's Principles of Internal Medicine. 19th Ed. Mc Graw-Hill Education;2015:672-674.

BLOOD TRANSFUSION

Dr. A.K.Tripathi, Professor, Department of Clinical Hematology

18 year old boy is rushed to the emergency room in shock following a motor vehicle accident. He is transfused to 5 unit of blood. Following the transfusion patients complains of nausea ,vomiting & chest pain . Laboratory data show elevated indirect serum bilirubin, decreased serum haptoglobin & a positive coomb's test

1. What is the most likely diagnosis
   (A) Autoimmune hemolytic anemia
   (B) Hemolytic transfusion reaction
   (C) DIC
   (D) Microangiopathic hemolytic anemia

2. Most common blood transfusion reaction is-
   (A) Febrile non hemolytic transfusion reaction
   (B) Hemolysis
   (C) Infections
   (D) Electrolyte imbalance
3. All of the following virus transmitted due to blood transfusion except-
   (A) Parvo virus B19
   (B) Hepatitis G
   (C) EB virus
   (D) CMV
4. Which of the following statement about acute hemolytic blood transfusion reaction is true-
   (A) Complement mediated hemolysis
   (B) Type 3 hypersensitivity
   (C) Renal blood flow is always maintained
   (D) Rarely life threatening
5. Which of following investigation should be done immediately to confirm acute hemolytic transfusion reaction –
   (A) Direct coombs test
   (B) Indirect coombs test
   (C) Both
   (D) PT/aPTT

Answers:
   1. B
      Clinical findings are suggestive of major transfusion hemolytic reaction
   2. A
      Febrile non hemolytic transfusion reactions are otherwise the most common reactions during transfusion.
   3. C
      Except EBV all can be transmitted through transfusion
   4. A
      It is an complement mediated lysis of RBC which occurs due to antigen antibody reaction.
   5. B

Reference:
   1. Kasper DL, Fauci AS, Houser SL.Transfusion biology and therapy.Harrison's Principles of Internal Medicine. 19th Ed. Mc Graw-Hill Education;2015:690-692.

Chapter-5
Community Medicine

LOWBIRTH WEIGHT NEWBORN

Dr. Jamal Masood, Professor, Department of Community Medicine

Munni , 25 years old woman is a resident of a village in Block Shahabad, District Hardoi. She has 3 daughters aged 4 ½ years, 3 years and 1 ½ years. When the Accredited Social Health Activist (ASHA) first visited her house she was 7 months pregnant and has not taken antenatal advice. Munni complained of tiredness, giddiness and breathlessness. ASHA noticed that the woman was pale.

ASHA advised Munni to consult the Doctor at Primary Health Centre(PHC).Mother in law of Munni was not convinced to take her to PHC Doctor for checkup as all her three daughters were delivered at home by local dai. After two weeks Munni delivered a male baby at home. Birth weight of the newborn was 1.9 Kg.

1. What is the most likely diagnosis?
    (A) Small for date baby
    (B) Pre term baby
    (C) Malnourished Newborn
    (D) Sick Newborn
2. Risk factor for Low Birth Weight in developing countries is.
    (A) Malnutrition
    (B) Infection
    (C) Unregulated fertility
    (D) All of the above
3. What action should have been taken by ASHA in order to prevent Low Birth Weight ?
    (A) Motivating the pregnant lady to visit sub centre for early registration of pregnancy.
    (B) Ensuring timely antenatal checkup/care by Auxiliary Nurse Midwife(ANM) and motivating lady to follow Antenatal care (ANC) advice.
    (C) Motivating the pregnant lady to take full course of Iron and Folic Acid tabs for prophylaxis
    (D) All of the above
4. The proportion of new borns with low birth weight (less than 2.5 Kg) in India is.
    (A) 28% of live births.
    (B) 33% of live births.
    (C) 40% of live births
    (D) 20% of live births
5. Which of the following statement is **NOT true** ?
    (A) LBW is the single most important factor determining the survival chances of the child.
    (B) The proportion of infants born with LBW is one of the global indicators to monitor
    (C) progress
    (D) LBW does not reflect nutritional and health status of mother
    (E) Approximately two-thirds of all babies of LBW in developed countries are estimated to be preterm

Answers:

1. B

    Babies born before 37 weeks of gestation are known as preterm babies.

2. D

    In the developing countries, adverse prenatal and postnatal development of the child is associated with 3 interrelated conditions :malnutrition, infection and unregulated fertility.

3. D

    The incidence of LBW can be reduced if pregnant women 'at risk' are identified and steps are taken to reduce the risk.

4. A

    Infants who weigh less than 2.5 Kg at birth represent about 28 percent of all live births in India

5. C

    LBW also reflects inadequate nutrition and ill health of the mother

Reference:

1. Park K. Preventive Medicine in Obstetrics, Paediatrics and Geriatrics. In: Park K(ed) Park's Textbook of Preventive and Social Medicine, 21st Edition.,M/sBanarsidas Bhanot Publishers, Jabalpur,India, 2011. p 494-495

ACUTE RESPIRATORY INFECTION

Dr. Jamal Masood, Professor, Department of Community Medicine

Guddi is six month old girl living with her parents in a village of Primary Health Centre(PHC) Dibiyapur District Etawah. During ANM's routine field visit her mother tells the ANM that Guddi has cough and difficulty in breathing for the past two days. On examination it was found that respiratory rate is 60 per minute and chest indrawing is present. Her body temperature is 39 degree C but she is alert. Guddi is malnourished but she is able to drink.

1. What is the most likely diagnosis ?
    (A) Severe Pneumonia
    (B) Pneumonia
    (C) Cold and cough
    (D) No Pneumonia
2. What should the ANM do in this case?
    (A) Treat the patient as per IMNCI (Integrated Management of Neonatal & Childhood Illness) guidelines
    (B) Refer the patient urgently to PHC
    (C) Give cotrimoxazole for 5 days
    (D) Home remedy
3.If the patient is referred to PHC (Primary Health Centre) What should the Medical Officer do in this case ?
    (A) Give cotrimoxazole for 5 days
    (B) Give first dose of injectable chloramphenicol and refer urgently to District Hospital
    (C) Soothe the throat and relieve the cough with a safe remedy
    (D) All of the above
4. What is the sign of severe pneumonia in a child aged 6 months?
    (A) Chest indrawing
    (B) 50 breaths per minute or more
    (C) Stridor in calm child
    (D) Any of the above
5. What is the incidence of pneumonia in children under 5 years of age in developing countries ?
    (A) 25%
    (B) 15%
    (C) 40%
    (D) 5%

Answers:
    1. A
       Severe Pneumonia
    2. B
       Refer the patient Urgently to PHC
    3. B
       Give first dose of injectable chloramphenicol and refer urgently to District Hospital
    4. D
       Any of the above i.e., Chest indrawing/50 breaths per minute /Stridor in calm child
    5. A
       About 25% that is between 20 to 30 percent

References:
    1. Park K.Epidemiology of Communicable Diseases. In:Park K (ed) Park's Text Book of Preventive and Social Medicine,21st Edition, , M/sBanarsidas Bhanot Publishers , Jabalpur,India, 2011,p 158-161.
    2. Ministry of Health & Family Welfare. Integrated Management of Neonatal and Childhood Illness. In : Govt. of India(ed) PHYSICIAN CHART BOOKLET ; 2005 p 12.

DIARRHOEA
Dr. Jamal Masood, Professor, Department of Community Medicine

Samir is 5 months old male baby who lives in a village of Block Harchandpur, District Raebareli. His mother is breastfeeding him. His diarrhoea started last night and he had 8 stools which were very watery. He also vomitted. His mother took him to the local ANM. She first looked for blood and mucus in the stool but could not see any.

As the ANM examines Samir, she finds that the skin pinch goes back slowly, the fontanelle is a little sunken and the eyes are also sunken. Samir does not have fever and he is not vomiting now. His urine output is normal.

1. What is the most likely diagnosis?
    (A) Severe Dehydration
    (B) Some Dehydration
    (C) Persistant Diarrhoea
    (D) Dysentery
2. What should the ANM do in this case?
    (A) Advise mother to continue breastfeeding
    (B) Advise mother to give frequent sips of ORS
    (C) Refer to PHC
    (D) All of the above
3. If the patient is referred to PHC, what should the Medical Officer do in this case ?
    (A) Give extra fluid for Diarrhoea as per plan A
    (B) Give extra fluid for Diarrhoea as per plan B
    (C) Any of the above
    (D) None of the above
4. When should this child be brought to ANM for follow up care ?
    (A) Next day
    (B) After two days
    (C) After three days
    (D) After five days
5. The proportion of deaths due to diarrhoea in children under 5 years of age in India is
    (A) About 5%
    (B) About 12%
    (C) About 18%
    (D) About 20%

Answers:
    1. B
    Some Dehydration
    As per IMNCI guidelines, a child between 2 months to 5 years of age with diarrhoea & two of the following signs will be classified as some dehydration (i) Restless/irritable (ii) Sunken eyes (iii) Drinks eagerly,thirsty (iv) Skin pinch goes back slowly.
    2. D
    All of the above as per IMNCI guidelines
    3. B
    Give extra fluid for diarrhoea as per plan B of IMNCI guidelines
    4. D
    Advise the mother to come for follow up after five days
    5. B
    About 12% --In India acute diarrhoeal disease account for about 13 percent of deaths in under fives (0-5 years age group).

References:
1. Park K.Epidemiology of Communicable Diseases. In:Park K (ed) Park's Text Book of Preventive and Social Medicine,21st Edition, M/sBanarsidas Bhanot Publishers, Jabalpur,India, 2011,p 199-205.
2. Ministry of Health & Family Welfare. Integrated Management of Neonatal and Childhood Illness. In : Govt. of India(ed) PHYSICIAN CHART BOOKLET ; 2005 p 20,26.

MALNUTRITION

Dr. Jamal Masood, Professor, Department of Community Medicine

Roshni has come to Community Health Centre (CHC) Chinhat of District Lucknow for treatment of her one year old son Guddu. She complains that her son is not gaining weight and he suffers from diarrhoea and cold & cough off and on. He had also suffered from Measles two months ago. Medical Officer examined the child and found that his weight is 5 kgs. The child has not been immunized.

1. What is the average normal weight of an Indian boy at the age of one year ?
    (A) 9.0 kgs
    (B) 9.5 kgs
    (C) 10.0 kgs
    (D) 10.5 kgs
2. What is the grade of malnutrition in this child ?
    (A) Mild
    (B) Moderate
    (C) Severe
    (D) None of the above
3. Which of the following conditions might have contributed for development of malnutrition in this child ?
    (A) Measles
    (B) Diarrhoea
    (C) Acute Respiratory Infections
    (D) All of the above
4. This malnourished child should be managed by giving :
    (A) Modified milk diet containing dried skimmed milk 25g +sugar 100g +vegetable oil 30g
    In 1000 ml of warm boiled water in small frequent meals
    (B) Oral cotrimoxazole for 5 days
    (C) Both A and B
    (D) None of the above
5. The proportion underweight children under 5 years of age in India is
    (A) About 48%
    (B) About 25%
    (C) About 33%
    (D) About 20%

Answers:
    1. B
        9.5 kgs as per Integrated Child Development Services (ICDS) growth chart for boys
    2. C
        Severe Malnutrition
    3. D
        All of the above.
    4. C
        Modified milk diet and antibiotic treatment even if the child has no specific signs of infection
    5. A
        At present in India 48 percent children under 5 years age are underweight. This includes 43 percent moderate to severe cases.

References:
1. Park K. Preventive Medicine in Obstetrics, Paediatrics and Geriatrics .In Park K (ed) Park's Textbook of Preventive and Social Medicine, 21st Edition, M/sBanarsidas Bhanot Publishers Jabalpur,India, 2011, P 504-507,
2. Park K. Nutrition and Health. In Park K (ed) Park's Textbook of Preventive and Social Medicine, 21st Edition, M/s Banarsidas Bhanot Publishers Jabalpur India, 2011,p590-592
3. Ministry of Health & Family Welfare. Integrated Management of Neonatal and Childhood Illness In Govt. of India (ed) PHYSICIAN CHART BOOKLET, 2005 p 20,26.
4. Ministry of Health & Family Welfare. Integrated Management of Neonatal and Childhood Illness In Govt. of India (ed) Treat the Child ,2005 p 39-40.

MATERNAL DEATH REVIEW

Dr. Jamal Masood, Professor, Department of Community Medicine

Munni 17 years old had been married for 10 months. She was living with her in-laws in remote village of Block Dhauladevi of District Almora. She was brought by her mother-in-law to the subcentre during 7th month of pregnancy with complaints of headache, dizziness and slight breathlessness. ANM noticed that Munni was pale. She gave her Tetanus Toxoid injection and Iron Folic Acid (IFA) tablets. She assured Munni and her mother-in-law that everything would be alright if she took the tablets regularly.

A few days later she reported back to the ANM with complaints of blurring of vision, severe headache and swelling of feet. The ANM referred her to the PHC to seek the help of the Medical Officer. Mother-in-law of Munni did not take her to PHC. In the meanwhile Munni began to have fits.The family sent for a faith healer to remove evil spirits but the fits continued. The family at this stage got worried and wanted to take her to the hospital but could not arrange for transport. Munni was then taken to the PHC on a cloth stretcher.On reaching the PHC she was found to be unconscious and her Blood Pressure was 170/110. She had not passed urine for 12 hours. The Medical Officer at the PHC referred her to the District Hospital in the PHC vehicle. On the way to the District Hospital Munni again had fits and died before she could reach the hospital.

1. What was Munni suffering from when she first visited the sub centre ?
    (A) Anxiety Neurosis
    (B) Anaemia
    (C) Hypertension
    (D) Hysteria
2. What should the ANM have done in this case during the first visit ?
    (A) Refer the patient to PHC for checkup and management
    (B) Tell the patient regarding danger signs in pregnancy and advice regarding diet &rest
    (C) Motivate the patient for Institutional delivery
    (D) All of the above
3. What should the PHC Medical Officer have given before referring the patient to District Hospital?
    (A) I.V.Fluid
    (B) Antihypertensive drugs
    (C) Sedatives
    (D) All of the above
4. What was the cause of Munni's death ?
    (A) Anaemia
    (B) Exhaustion during transportation
    (C) Eclampsia
    (D) None of the above
5. What role could the family and the community have played in the prevention of this death?
    (A) Marriage at the age of 18 years and first conception at the age of 20 years.
    (B) Early registration of pregnancy and timely & complete antenatal care
    (C) Availability of transport for early referral in case of emergency
    (D) All of the above

Answers:
    1. B
    Anaemia
    2. D
    All of the above
    3. D
    All of the above.
    4. C
    Eclampsia
    5. D
    All of the above

References:
1. Park K.. Preventive Medicine in Obstetrics, Paediatrics and Geriatrics in Park K(ed) Park's Textbook of Preventive and Social Medicine, 21st Edition, M/sBanarsidas Bhanot Publishers, Jabalpur,India,2011, P 514-518.
2. Ministry of Health & Family Welfare. Maternal Death Review Guide Book-Govt. of India,2011.

ANAEMIA IN ADOLESCENT GIRL

Dr. Jamal Masood, Professor, Department of Community Medicine

Rani is a 14 year old girl. Her family comprises of her parents, two brothers and a younger sister. Rani goes to school and also helps her mother in household work. Her normal diet is made up of rice and watery dal twice a day. Vegetables are cooked once a while. As per the social custom in her family, Rani and her sister eat after her father and brothers have eaten. Two months back, she suffered from Malaria and since then has been feeling very weak and is always exhausted. Menarche has also started few months back.

She was brought to the Urban Health Centre, Alambagh, Lucknow after she fainted on her way to school one day. Blood test was done in the Lab of the Urban Health Centre and Haemoglobin was found to be 4g/dl.

1. What is the degree of Anaemia in the Adolescent girl ?
    (A) Mild
    (B) Moderate
    (C) Severe
    (D) Latent
2. Which factor was responsible for development of anaemia in the Adolescent girl ?
    (A) Inadequate diet
    (B) Infection-Malaria
    (C) Menstruation
    (D) All of the above
3. The long term effects of untreated Anaemia in married Adolescent girl may be
    (A) Low birth weight babies
    (B) Maternal mortality
    (C) Pregnancy wastage-Abortion
    (D) All of the above
4. The anaemia in the adolescent girl is to be managed by
    (A) Giving Iron and Folic Acid Tablets
    (B) Balanced Diet rich in Iron
    (C) Deworming every six month
    (D) All of the above
5. The prevalence of Anaemia in Adolescent girls (12-14 years) in India is about
    (A) 68 %
    (B) 55%
    (C) 40%
    (D) 80%

Answers:
    1. C
        Severe Anaemia-According to National Iron plus Initiative, Anaemia in children aged12-14 years is classified as No anaemia (Hb >12 g), Mild Anaemia (Hb 11.0 -11.9 g), Moderate Anaemia (Hb 8.0 – 10.9 g) and Severe Anaemia (Hb <8.0 g)
    2. D
        All of the above
    3. D
        All of the above
    4. D
        All of the above
    5. A
    According to NHFS-3 Prevalence of Anaemia in adolescent girls in the age group 12-14 years Is 68.6 percent.

Reference:
    1. Rashtriya Bal Swasthya Karyakram-Operational Guidelines-Department of Medical, Health & Family Welfare,Uttar Pradesh and National Health Mission Uttar Pradesh, 2013-14, p 22-23.

SEXUALLY TRANSMITTED INFECTION IN MALE
Dr. Jamal Masood, Professor, Department of Community Medicine

Tillu a 25 years old long distance Truck driver attended Suraksha Clinic of King George's Medical University, Lucknow. He complains of painful sores on the penis. He admits to having had unprotected sexual intercourse with a female sex worker. On examination Inguinal lymph nodes were found to be enlarged.

1. What is the most likely syndromic diagnosis ?
   (A) Genital Ulcer Disease Herpetic
   (B) Genital Ulcer Disease Non-Herpetic
   (C) Inguinal Bubo
   (D) None of the above
2. Role of counsellor of Suraksha Clinic in the management of this case is to
   (A) Refer the patient to Integrated Counselling and Testing Centre(ICTC) for HIV Testing and VDRL /RPR Test
   (B) Condom demonstration & counseling for safe sex
   (C) Counselling for partner management
   (D) All of the above
3. Syndromic case management of this case is to be done with
   (A) Kit 1 containing Tab Cefixime and Tab Azithromycin
   (B) Kit 3 consisting of Inj Benzathine penicillin + Tab Azithromycin.
   (C) Kit 5 containing Tab Acyclovir 400mg TDS for 7 days
   (D) Kit 7 containing Tab Azithromycin(single dose) + Cap Doxycycline 100 mg BD X 21 days
4. Genital Ulcer disease is important because
   (A) It is a major cause of infertility
   (B) It may facilitate spread of HIV
   (C) It often causes impotence in men
   (D) It is usually associated with another Reproductive Tract Infection
5. Which of the following Laboratory test is most useful for Sexually Transmitted Infection/Reproductive Tract Infection control in developing countries?
   (A) Screening tests for Syphilis such as RPR or VDRL test
   (B) Gram Stain for Gonorrhoea
   (C) Urine LED (leukocyte esterase dipstick) for white blood cells
   (D) Gonorrhoea culture

Answers:
1. B
   Genital Ulcer Disease Non-Herpetic
2. D
   All of the above
3. B
   Kit 3 consisting of Inj Benzathine penicillin + Tab Azithromycin.
4. B
   It may facilitate spread of HIV
5. A
   Screening tests for Syphilis such as RPR or VDRL test

References:
1. National AIDS Control Programme.Training of doctors to Deliver Quality STI/RTI Services. Resource Material For Trainers, Govt. of India New Delhi 2010 P 29-49,
2. National AIDS Control Organisation.Training of Medical Officers to deliver STI/RTI Services. Participant's Handout, NRHM and NACO, New Delhi, 2012, P 60-93

SEXUALLY TRANSMITTED INFECTION IN FEMALE
Dr. Jamal Masood, Professor, Department of Community Medicine

Sheela a 30 years old Female Sex Worker attended Suraksha Clinic of King George's Medical University, Lucknow after a gap of more than 6 months for check up. She has no complaints but admits to having had unprotected sexual intercourse with a client one month ago .

1. What should be done ?
   (A) Refer her to ICTC for HIV Testing and VDRL Test

(B) Give her Kit 1 containing Tab Cefixime and Tab Azithromycin

(C) Condom demonstration & counseling for safe sex

(D) All of the above

2. Which of the following contributes to the rapid spread of STIs/RTIs ?

    (A) Lack of sufficient laboratory facilities for diagnosis.

    (B) Poor Hygiene

    (C) Lack of effective drugs.

    (D) High risk sexual behaviour

3. In women, the signs and symptoms of STIs/RTIs are often

    (A) More easily recognized than in men

    (B) Less reliable indicators of disease than in men.

    (C) Less likely to become serious than they are in men.

    (D) More likely to affect older women.

4. A woman has cervical mucopurulent discharge and lower abdominal pain with no rebound tenderness or guarding. Which of the following is true?

    (A) She should be referred immediately to a surgeon.

    (B) She should be treated for Pelvic Inflammatory Disease (PID)

    (C) Trichomonas vaginalis is probably the causative organism.

    (D) She is unlikely to have complications unless she is pregnant.

5. Women are more vulnerable to STIs/RTIs infection than men because

    (A) Semen stays in contact with the vaginal wall for a long time.

    (B) Women have less power to negotiate safe sex

    (C) Larger exposed area

    (D) All of the above

Answers:

    1. D

        All of the above

    2. D

        High risk sexual behaviour

    3. B

        Less reliable indicators of disease than in men.

    4. B

        She should be treated for PID

    5. D

        All of the above

References:

1. National AIDS Control Organisation.Training of doctors to Deliver Quality STI/RTI Services. Resource Material For Trainers, Govt. of India New Delhi, 2010, P 29-49,
2. National AIDS Control Organisation.Training of Medical Officers to deliver STI/RTI Services. Participant's Handout, NRHM and NACO, New Delhi, 2012, p 60-93

MALARIA

Dr. Jamal Masood, Professor, Department of Community Medicine

Mahipal Singh a 30 years old man of village Bhanoli of Block Dhauladevi District Almora attended PHC Panuwanaula. He complained of High fever with chills and rigour for last 3 days. He informed the Medical Officer that 10 persons of his village are also suffering from the same problem. Medical Officer immediately prepared Thick and Thin Blood film and sent it to PHC Lab to test for Malaria. PHC Lab confirmed presence of Plaspodium vivax parasite in the blood film. Medical Officer gave treatment to the patient and then proceeded along with his team to investigate the outbreak in village Bhanoli.

1. What treatment should be given to this patient ?

    (A) Chloroquin for 3 days + Primaquin for 14 days under supervision

    (B) Chloroquin for 3 days + Primaquin for 3 days under supervision

    (C) Chloroquin for 3 days + Artesunate for 3 days under supervision

    (D) Chloroquin for 3 days + Primaquin single dose

2. What measures should be taken for control of Malaria outbreak in the affected village?

    (A) Rapid Fever Survey

    (B) Mass Survey

(C) Indoor Residual Spraying

(D) All of the above

3. The insecticide now commonly used for Indoor Residual Spray during outbreaks of malaria is

    (A) DDT

    (B) Pyrethrum

    (C) Malathion

    (D) None of the above

4. How long should the Indoor Residual Spray be carried out in the affected village ?

    (A) One day only

    (B) Five days

    (C) Depends on the decision of Medical Officer

    (D) 7-10 consecutive days or till the residual insecticidal spray in all houses of the locality is completed.

5. When should the First follow up survey of Malaria outbreak be carried out ?

    (A) After one week of completion of remedial measures

    (B) After two weeks of completion of remedial measures

    (C) After three weeks of completion of remedial measures

    (D) After four weeks of completion of remedial measures

Answers:

    1. A

    Chloroquin for 3 days + Primaquin for 14 days under supervision

    2. D

    All of the above as per guidelines

    3. B

    Pyrethrum

    4. D

    7-10 consecutive days or till the residual insecticidal spray in all houses of the locality is completed

    5. C

    After three weeks of completion of remedial measures

References:

1. Government of India. Guidelines for Diagnosis and Treatment of Malaria in India. National Institute of Malaria Research, New Delhi,2011.

DENGUE OUTBREAK

Dr. Jamal Masood, Professor, Department of Community Medicine

Ten cases of confirmed Dengue Fever have been reported from a Medical College Hostel in Uttar Pradesh in October 2014.

1. What is the criteria for declaring Dengue outbreak ?

    (A) One confirmed case of Dengue Fever

    (B) Two or more epidemiologically linked cases

    (C) Five confirmed cases of Dengue Fever

    (D) Ten confirmed cases of Dengue Fever

2. What vector control measures should be taken for control of Dengue outbreak in the affected hostel?

    (A) Environmental management & elimination of mosquito breeding sites

    (B) Community awareness and personal Protection

    (C) Indoor Residual Spraying and Outdoor Fogging

    (D) All of the above

3. The insecticide now commonly used for Indoor Residual Spray during outbreaks of Dengue is

    (A) DDT

    (B) Pyrethrum

    (C) Malathion

    (D) None of the above

4. What preventive measures to be taken to prevent Dengue outbreak in the hostel next year ?

    (A) Application of Temephos in stagnant water on weekly basis to be started in the month of june

    (B) Indoor Space spraying with Pyrethrum2% indoor residual spray to be started in the month of Ma

    (C) Both A & B

    (D) None of the above

5. Biting time of female Aedes Mosquito is
   - (A) Between 9 AM to 12 Noon
   - (B) Between 1PM to 4PM
   - (C) Between 4PM to 7 PM
   - (D) Both A & C

Answers:
1. A
   One confirmed case of Dengue fever
2. D
   All of the above as per guidelines
3. B
   Pyrethrum
4. C
   Both A &B
5. D
   Both A & C

Reference:
1. Government of India. Guidelines for Integrated Vector Management for Control of Dengue/Dengue Haemorrhagic Fever, National Vector Borne Disease Control Programme, Directorate General of Health Services, Ministry of Health & Family Welfare,2006.

Chapter-6

Dermatology, Venereology & Leprosy

PSORIASIS

Dr Swastika Suvirya, Asst. Professor, Department of Dermatology

A 30 year old male patient presented to the dermatology outdoor with multiple well defined erythematous plaques covered with dense white silvery scales over the extensor aspect of extremities including scalp for the last four years. Disease followed a chronically relapsing course with aggravation in winters. He also gave history of pain in the knee and distal interphalangeal joints of hands. On examination there was swelling and tenderness of bilateral knee joints and distal interphalangeal joints of fingers. Auspitz sign was positive on the lesion over the right elbow. Few of the finger nails showed yellowish discoloration, thickening of the nail plate and distal separation of nail plate from nail bed. Histopathological examination of a skin biopsy from the right shin showed parakeratosis associated with focal orthokeratosis and absence of granular layer, Munro microabcess formation and spongiform pustules in the Malpighian layer. There was elongation of rete ridges associated with suprapapillary epidermal thinning.

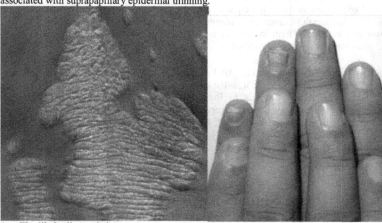

1. The likely diagnosis is:
   (A) Lichen Planus
   (B) Chronic plaque psoriasis
   (C) Pityriasis Rosea
   (D) Pityriasis lichenoides chronic
2. What is the risk of this disease in an offspring if one the parent is affected with the above disease?
   (A) 41%
   (B) 14%
   (C) 6%
   (D) 2%
3. Impetigo herpetiformis is synonym for
   (A) Chronic plaque psoriasis
   (B) Small plaque psoriasis
   (C) Guttate psoriasis
   (D) Pustular psoriasis in pregnancy
4. Following are the nail changes found in patients of above disease except
   (A) Nail pitting
   (B) Oil spots
   (C) Longitudinal striations in the nail
   (D) Onychodystrophy
5. Which of the biological agents used for the treatment of above disease has been withdrawn from market in 2009 due to its side effects of progressive multifocal leukoencephalopathy ?
   (A) Infliximab
   (B) Alefacept
   (C) Efalizumab
   (D) Adalimumab

Answers:
   1. B

Chronic plaque psoriasis is a papulosquamous disorder most likely to appear between the ages of 15-30 years presenting with well defined plaques covered with silvery white scales. Involvement of the DIP joints is characteristic for patients of psoriatic arthritis.

2. B

Risk of psoriasis in an offspring has been estimated to be 41% if both parents are affected, 14% if one parent is affected and 6% if one sibling is affected.

3. D

Impetigo herpetiformis is a variant of pustular psoriasis with onset in the early third trimester of pregnancy. It is often associated with hypocalcemia.

4. C

Nail changes occur in 40% of patients with psoriasis. Nail changes in psoriasis involve nail pitting, oil spots, salmon patches, splinter haemorrhages, subungal hyperkeratosis and onychodystrophy.

5. C

Various biologic agents or biologic response modifiers have been used for the treatment of psoriasis like Infliximab, Etarnecept, Adalimumab, Ustekinumab, Secukinumb,Efalizumab. Efalizumab was withdrawn from the market in 2009 due to reports of progressive multifocal leukoencephalopathy in few treated patients.

References:

1. Sivamani RK, Correa G, Ono Y, Bowen MP, Raychaudhuri SP, Maverakis E. Biological therapy of psoriasis. Indian J Dermatol. 2010; 55(2): 161–70.
2. Griffiths CEM, Barker JNWN. Psoriasis. In: Burns T, Breathnach S, Cox N, Griffiths C, editors. Rook's Textbook of Dermatology. 8th ed. Singapore: Wiley- Blackwell; 2010. p20.1-60.
3. Gudjohnsson JE, Elder JT. Psoriasis. In: Wolff K, Goldsmith LA, Katz SI, Gilchrest BA, Paller AS, Leffell DJ, editors. Fitzpatrick's Dermatology in General Medicine. 7th ed. New Delhi: McGraw Hill Medical; 2008. p169-93.

SEBORRHEIC DERMATITIS

Dr Swastika Suvirya, Asst. Professor, Dr Deepika Aggarwal, Senior Resident,
Department of Dermatology

A 45 year old male presented to the dermatology outdoor with yellowish greasy scales on the medial side of eyebrow, nasolabial fold, retro auricular area and patchy scaling on forehead. Patient gave history of recurrent crusting along the eyelids. Patient also complained of severe itching of the scalp which on examination revealed similar kind of scaling in a diffuse fashion. He complained of his lesions aggravating in winters with partial relief in summers.

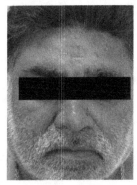

1. Identify the condition
   (A) Seborrheic dermatitis
   (B) Pityriasis rosea
   (C) Lichen nitidus
   (D) Parapsoriasis

2. Sudden confluence of these lesions leading to erythroderma in infants is known as
    (A) DRESS syndrome
    (B) Leiner disease
    (C) Fournier disease
    (D) Netherton's disease
3. Following are the factors involved in the pathogenesis of the disease except
    (A) Increased Seborrhea
    (B) Microbial effects
    (C) Genetic factors
    (D) Autoimmune factors
4. Histological differentiation of classical form of above disease from Aquired Immunodeficiency Syndrome associated disease include all of the following except
    (A) Limited parakeratosis
    (B) Rare necrotic keratinocytes
    (C) Thick walled blood vessels in the dermis
    (D) No interface obliteration
5. All are types of seborrheic dermatitis except:
    (A) Petaloid
    (B) Pityriasiform
    (C) Flexural
    (D) Lichenified

Answers:

1. A
    Seborrheic dermatitis is a papluosquamous disorder presenting with greasy yellowish scales on the scalp, temples, inner part of eyebrows, nasolabial folds, retroauricular areas and V shaped areas of chest and back.

2. B
    Seborrheic dermatitis in infants can lead to erythroderma known as Leiner's disease. It can present in a both familial and non familial form. Familial form is due to deficiency of complement C5 thus leading to defective opsonisation.

3. D
    Pathogenic factors involved in the causation of seborrheic dermatitis include increased sebum production, increased colonisation by *M. furfur*, decreased count of *Propionibacterium acnes*, gene defect in zinc finger protein, neurotransmitter abnormalities, drugs and physical factors.

4. C
    Histological differentiation of classical Seborrheic dermatitis from Aquired Immunodeficiency Syndrome associated seborrheic dermatitis include limited parakeratosis, rare necrotic keratinocytes, no interface obliteration, prominent spongiosis, thin walled vessels in the dermis and rare plasma cells.

5. D
    Pityriasiform, flexural, eczematous, generalised, follicular are all variants of seborrheic dermatitis.

References:

1. Pelvig G, Jansen P. Seborrheic dermatitis. In: Wolff K, Goldsmith LA, Katz SI, Gilchrest BA, Paller AS, Leffell DJ, editors. Fitzpatrick's Dermatology in General Medicine. 7th ed. New Delhi: McGraw Hill Medical; 2008. p219-25.
2. Layton AM. Disorders of Sebaceous Glands. In: Burns T, Breathnach S, Cox N, Griffiths C, editors. Rook's Textbook of Dermatology. 8th ed. Singapore: Wiley- Blackwell; 2010. p42.17-70.

LICHEN PLANUS

Dr Swastika Suvirya, Asst. Professor, Dr Deepika Aggarwal, Senior Resident,
Department of Dermatology

A 20 year old female presents with multiple violaceous flat topped polygonal papules on the limbs and trunk which are intensely itchy. Patient gave history of development of similar lesions at sites of trauma (Koebner's Phenomenon). She also complained of intense burning sensation in the mouth. On closer inspection of the skin lesions, Wickham's Striae were seen. On examination of the oral cavity white reticular lacy pattern was seen on the buccal mucosa. All the twenty nails showed loss of nail plate on examination.

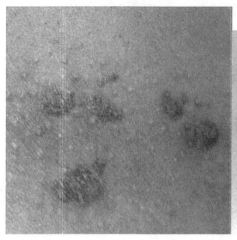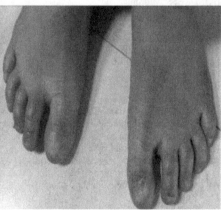

1. Based on the above clinical features which is the characteristic histopathology?
   (A) Band of lymphocyte and histiocyte subepidermally, epidermal thickening with hypergranulosis, saw tooth appearance of rete ridges.
   (B) Hyperplastic epidermis, accentuation of rete ridges with munro micro abscess.
   (C) Spongiosis, parakeratosis, inflammatory cell infiltrate, oedema and vasodilation in the dermis.
   (D) All of the above
2. Graham Little's Feldman syndrome is
   (A) Non scarring alopecia of LP combined with nail thinning in LP
   (B) Hypertrophic Lichen planus in combination with vesiculobullous lichen planus
   (C) Triad of follicular LP of skin, and/or multifocal cicatricial alopecia of scalp and non scarring alopecia of the axilla and pubic area
   (D) None of the above
3. Following are the inducers of photodistributed lichenoid eruptions except
   (A) 5 Fluorouracil
   (B) Tetracycline
   (C) Furosemide
   (D) Penicillamine
4. What are the chances of oral LP transforming into squamous cell carcinoma?
   (A) <1%
   (B) .5-5%
   (C) 0.2-2%
   (D) 1-10%
5. Histopathological features helpful in distinguishing lichenoid drug eruptions from lichen planus include all of the following except
   (A) Presence of abundant plasma cells and eosinophils in the infiltrate
   (B) Focal parakeratoses and hyperkeratosis
   (C) Lymphocytic infiltrate less dense and not band like
   (D) Presence of cytoid bodies in the dermis

Answers:
   1. A
      Lichen planus is a papulosquamous disorder presenting with symmetrical violacoeus flat topped polygonal papules. On histopathological examination epidermal changes include hyperkeratosis, wedge shaped areas of hypergranulosis and elongation of rete ridges resembling saw tooth pattern. Multiple apoptotic cells (Civatte bodies) are seen at dermo epidermal junction. A band like lymphocytic infiltrate is seen in the papillary dermis.
   2. C
      Graham Little Feldman or Graham Little Piccardi Lassueur is a triad of follicular LP of skin, and/or multifocal cicatricial alopecia of scalp and non scarring alopecia of the axilla and pubic area.
   3. D

Photodistributed lichenoid eruptions are caused by 5 FU, Carbamazepine, Tetracycline, Quinidine, Quinine, Thiazide, Furosemide and Ethambutol.
4. B
    It is generally accepted that 0.5-5% of oral LP develop SCC. Risk factors include long standing disease, erosive or atrophic type and tobacco use.
5. D
    Histopathological features helpful in distinguishing lichenoid drug eruptions from lichen planus include presence of abundant plasma cells and eosinophils in the infiltrate, focal parakeratoses and hyperkeratosis , lymphocytic infiltrate less dense and not band like and presence of cytoid bodies high in the stratum corneum.

References:
1. Breathnach SM. Lichen planus and lichenification. In: Burns T, Breathnach S, Cox N, Griffiths C, editors. Rook's Textbook of Dermatology. 8th ed. Singapore: Wiley- Blackwell; 2010. p41.1-17.
2. Pittlekow MR, Doud MS. Lichen planus. In: Wolff K, Goldsmith LA, Katz SI, Gilchrest BA, Paller AS, Leffell DJ, editors. Fitzpatrick's Dermatology in General Medicine. 7th ed. New Delhi: McGraw Hill Medical; 2008. p244-54.

PITYRIASIS RUBRA PILARIS

Dr. Swastika Suvirya, Assistant Professor, & Dr Rohit Kumar Singh, Senior Resident, Department of Dermatology

A 30 year old female patient presented to the outdoor with multiple follicular hyperkeratotic papules all over the body with diffuse yellowish thickening of the palms and soles. On examination nails showed yellowish discoloration and thickening of nail plate. Bi-lateral buccal mucosa appeared white. Hair and nail were normal. Histopathological examination of a skin biopsy taken from the back showed acanthosis, parakeratosis and alternating areas of orthokeratosis and parakeratosis in both horizontal and vertical direction were seen.

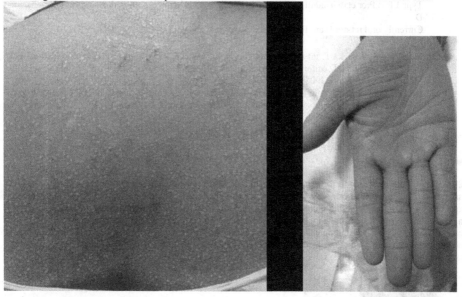

1. The likely diagnosis is:
    (A) Pityriasis Rubra pilaris
    (B) Psoriasis
    (C) Follicular ichthyosis
    (D) Erytrokeratoderma Variabilis
2. The classification scheme used for the above disease is known as
    (A) Pugh Child scheme
    (B) Griffiths and Gonzales-Lopez scheme
    (C) Fischer scheme

(D) None of the above
3. Histopathological criteria used to differentiate P.R.P. from psoriasis are
   (A) Prominent granular layer
   (B) Dilated Capillaries
   (C) Alternate areas of orthokeratosis and parakeratosis
   (D) Prominent granular layer and dilated but not tortuous capillaries
4. Nappes claires or islands of normal skin are seen in which type of P.R.P
   (A) Type I
   (B) TypeII
   (C) TypeIII
   (D) TypeIV
5. The first line therapy in patients with P.R.P. is
   (A) Oral steroids
   (B) Methotrexate
   (C) Biologicals
   (D) Oral retinoids

Answers:
1. A
   Pityriasis rubra pilaris is a papulosquamous disorder presenting in males and females in a equal ratio with a bimodal age distribution in the first and fifth decade of life.
2. B
   P.R.P. is classified according to Griffith and Gonzales-Lopez scheme into six types
3. D
   Prominent granular layer and dilated but not tortuous capillaries help in histopathologically differentiating P.R.P. from psoriasis.
4. A
   Type I P.R.P.or classic adult type is one in which erythroderma is seen with islands of normal skin.
5. D
   Currently oral retinoids are first line therapy for patients with P.R.P.

References:
1. Gerharz DB, Ruzicka T. Pityriasis rubra Pilaris. In: Wolff K, Goldsmith LA, Katz SI, Gilchrest BA, Paller AS, Leffell DJ, editors. Fitzpatrick's Dermatology in General Medicine. 7th ed. New Delhi: McGraw Hill Medical; 2008. p232-6.
2. Disorders of Keratinization. In: Burns T, Breathnach S, Cox N, Griffiths C, editors. Rook's Textbook of Dermatology. 8th ed. Singapore: Wiley- Blackwell; 2010. p19.76-81.

POROKERATOSIS

Dr Swastika Suvirya, Asst. Professor & Dr Deepika Aggarwal, Senior Resident,
Department of Dermatology

A 20 year old male presented to the dermatology outdoor with multiple annular asymptomatic plaques ranging in size from 0.5-2 cm in diameter surrounded by thread like elevated border. On examination multiple annular plaques with hyperkeratotic border were seen on the face and extensor aspect of extremities. There was history of aggravation of these lesions on sun exposure. Mucous membranes, palms soles, hair and nails did not reveal any abnormality. On histopathological examination from a skin biopsy of the face, stratum corneum was hyperkeratotic with a thin column of poorly staining parakeratotic cells- the Cornoid lamella running through the surrounding normal staining cells.

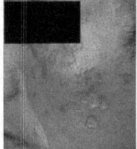

1. Identify the disease
   (A) Psoriasis
   (B) Annular lichen planus
   (C) Porokeratosis
   (D) None of the above
2. Coronoid lamella seen histopathologically in this disease is also seen in other conditions except
   (A) Viral warts
   (B) Nevoid hyperkeratosis
   (C) Actinic Keratosis
   (D) Lichen planus
3. What is first line therapy for the above disease
   (A) Photoprotection and 5-Fu topically
   (B) Topical steroid
   (C) Oral retinoid
   (D) Methotrexate
4. Which of the following types have highest potential for malignant degeneration
   (A) Porokeratosis of Mibelli
   (B) Disseminated superficial actinic porokeratosis
   (C) Punctate porokeratosis
   (D) Linear Porokeratosis
5. Which is the commonest malignancy arising in these lesions
   (A) Basal Cell Carcinoma
   (B) Melanoma
   (C) Squamous Cell Carcinoma
   (D) All of the above

Answers:
1. C

   Porokeratosis is a disorder of keratinisation presenting with hyperkeratotic papules and plaques surrounded by thread like elevated border.
2. D

   Cornoid lamella a column of parakeratotic cells is also seen in viral warts, naevoid hyperkeratosis, actinic keratosis and some forms of ichthyosis.
3. A

   Photoprotection and 5 FU topically remain first line therapy for porokeratosis
4. D

   Linear porokeratosis has highest potential for malignant degerneration
5. C

   Squamous cell carcinoma is commonest malignancy arising in lesions of porokeratosis

References:
1. O'Regan GM, Irwine AD. Porokeratosis. In: Wolff K, Goldsmith LA, Katz SI, Gilchrest BA, Paller AS, Leffell DJ, editors. Fitzpatrick's Dermatology in General Medicine. 7th ed. New Delhi: McGraw Hill Medical; 2008. p442-6.

2. Judge MR, Mclean WHI, Munro CS. Disorders of Keratinization. In: Burns T, Breathnach S, Cox N, Griffiths C, editors. Rook's Textbook of Dermatology. 8th ed. Singapore: Wiley- Blackwell; 2010. p19.90-2.

PEMPHIGUS VULGARIS

Dr Swastika Suvirya, Asst. Professor, Department of Dermatology, Dr Seema Malhotra, Reader, Department of Pedodontics

A 40 year old male presented to outdoor with oral ulceration and multiple bullous lesions all over the body for the last one year. Patient did not give any history of drug intake before the onset of skin lesions. On examination multiple flaccid bullae and erosions were seen all over the body covered with thick crusts at few places. Oral mucosa also showed multiple deep ulcers on tongue and bilateral buccal mucosa. Nikolskys sign was positive and patient had history of being partially relieved on taking oral steroids a few months back. Histopahological examination of a skin biopsy from a fresh bulla showed suprabasal acantholysis in the epidermis. The basal cells showed a "row of Tombstones" appearance. Direct immunoflourescence from the perilesional skin showed staining for IgG autoantibodies throughout the epidermis.

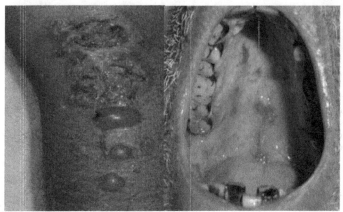

1. Identify the disease
   (A) Pemphigus Vulgaris
   (B) Bullous pemphigoid
   (C) Chronic bullous disease of childhood
   (D) Dermatitis Herpetiformis
2. Senear Usher Syndrome is
   (A) Localised form of pemphigus vulgaris
   (B) Localised form of pemphigus foliaceus
   (C) Drug induced pemphigus
   (D) None of the above
3. The most common cause of death in patients of above disease is
   (A) Cardiac failure
   (B) Respiratory failure
   (C) Renal failure
   (D) Infection
4. Which of the following is an intraepidermal blistering disorder without autoantibodies?
   (A) Linear IgA disease
   (B) Bullous LE
   (C) Familial benign pemphigus
   (D) Cicatricial pemphigoid
5. The most constant clinical feature seen in patients of Paraneoplastic pemphigus is
   (A) Flaccid bullae
   (B) Tense bullae
   (C) Both
   (D) Painful erosive stomatitis resistant to treatment

Answers:

1. A

   Pemphigus vulgaris is an autoimmune blistering disorder of the skin presenting with multiple flaccid blisters and erosions all over the body including buccal mucosa with a mean age of onset of 40-60 years.

2. B

   Senear Usher Syndrome or pemphigus erythematoses is a localised form of pemphigus foliaceus occurring over the malar area of the face.

3. D

   Infection is the commonest cause of death in patients with pemphigus due to the immunosuppressants given for treatment of active disease.

4. C

   Hailey Hailey Disease or Benign Familial Pemphigus is a benign intraepidermal blistering disorder without an autoantibody.

5. D

   Presence of painful extremely refractory stomatitis is the most constant feature of paraneoplastic pemphigus.

References:

1. Stanley JR. Pemphigus. In: Wolff K, Goldsmith LA, Katz SI, Gilchrest BA, Paller AS, Leffell DJ, editors. Fitzpatrick's Dermatology in General Medicine. 7th ed. New Delhi: McGraw Hill Medical; 2008. p459-68.
2. Wojnarowska F, Venning VA. Immunobullous diseases. In: Burns T, Breathnach S, Cox N, Griffiths C, editors. Rook's Textbook of Dermatology. 8th ed. Singapore: Wiley- Blackwell; 2010. p40.1-22.

ALBINISM

Dr Swastika Suvirya, Assistant Professor, Department of Dermatology

A 50 yr old male presented to the outdoor with depigmented skin all over the body and history of blondish hairs since birth. Patient also complained of cutaneous photosensitivity and photophobia. On examination multiple nevi, freckles, lentigenes and actinic keratosis were present all over the body. The colour of his irises was grey.

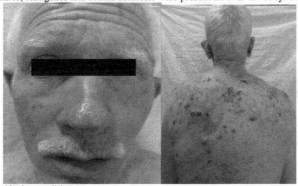

1. Identify the condition
   (A) Vitiligo
   (B) Chemical leucoderma
   (C) Mycosis fungoides
   (D) Albinism
2. Which is the type of albinism in which the patient would develop varying amount of melanin in the hair and skin in the first or second decade of life?
   (A) Oculocutaneous albinism Type 1A (OCA 1A)
   (B) Oculocutaneous albinism Type 1B (OCA 1B)
   (C) OCA 2
   (D) OCA 3
3. Which of the following is the hallmark craniofacial defect found in virtually all patients of Waardenburg Syndrome Type 1?
   (A) Heterochromia iridis
   (B) Premature greying
   (C) Dystopia canthorum
   (D) None of the above
4. Treatment plan for such patients includes all of the following except
   (A) Protection from UV rays
   (B) Ophthalmic consultation
   (C) Use of steroids
   (D) Regular follow up by the dermatologist
5. Complications of albinism include:
   (A) Reduced visual acquity
   (B) Increased risk of cutaneous malignancy
   (C) Both of the above
   (D) Increased risk of pancreatitis.

Answers:

1. D

   Albinism is a congenital disorder of pigmentation in which patient presents with nonpigmented skin and silvery white or yellowish hair colour. Oculocutaneous albinism is subdivided into 4 types.

2. B

   OCA 1B is the type of albinism in which patient would regain some melanin in the hair and skin later in life.

3. C

   Dystopia canthorum or lateral displacement of medial canthi of eye is found in all patients of WS1.

4. C

   All patients of albinism should have ophthalmic consultation, protect themselves from ultraviolet radiation and regular follow up by a dermatologist to look for any malignant condition of the skin.

5. C

   Complications of albinism include reduced visual acuity, early development of cutaneous malignancies like SCC and melanoma.

References:

1. Hornyak TJ. Albinism and other genetic disorders of pigmentation. In: Wolff K, Goldsmith LA, Katz SI, Gilchrest BA, Paller AS, Leffell DJ, editors. Fitzpatrick's Dermatology in General Medicine. 7th ed. New Delhi: McGraw Hill Medical; 2008. p608-16.

2. Anstey AV. Disorders of skin colour. In: Burns T, Breathnach S, Cox N, Griffiths C, editors. Rook's Textbook of Dermatology. 8th ed. Singapore: Wiley- Blackwell; 2010. p58.39-42.

CONGENITAL MELANOCYTIC NEVUS

Dr Parul Verma, Assistant professor, Department of Dermatology

A 22 year old young female had involvement of whole of the right breast in the form of hyper pigmented large plaque with well defined margin. The surface of the lesion was rough and was studded with multiple tiny papules. The lesion was present since birth and was increasing proportionately with the size of the breast. Nipple was retracted and no underlying mass could be felt. On examination there was no axillary lymphadenopathy. Skin biopsy was done to rule out underlying malignancy.

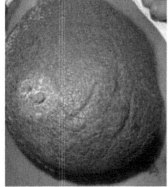

1. What is the most likely diagnosis
   (A) Melanoma
   (B) Melanocytic nevus
   (C) Blue nevus
   (D) Nevus sebaceous
2. When is a melanocytic nevus called giant
   (A) More than 5 cm
   (B) More than 10 cm
   (C) More than 20cm
   (D) More than 30 cm
3. Which malignancy is associated with congenital melanocytic nevus
   (A) Squammous cell carcinoma

(B) Basal cell carcinoma
(C) Melanoma
(D) Rhabdomyosarcoma
4. Best way to manage the above case is
   (A) Excise the lesion
   (B) Ablative laser therapy
   (C) Council the patient and skin biopsy from suspicious area to rule out melanoma
   (D) Topical retinoids

Answers:
1. B
   Deeply pigmented plaque since birth, growing in proportion with age and associated with rugosity is diagnostic of congenital melanocytic nevus.
2. C
   Melanocytic nevus is called giant when it is more than 20 cm in size.
3. C
   Giant congenital melanocytic has increased risk of melanoma specially if associated with satellite lesions.
4. C
   Complete excision is usually not possible in giant lesion. Close follow up such patients should be done to look for any malignant change.

References:
1. Grichnik JM, Rhodes AR, Sober AJ. Benign Neoplasia and Hyperplasia of Melanocytes. In: Wolff K, Goldsmith LA, Katz SI, Gilchrest BA, Paller AS, Leffell DJ, editors. Fitzpatrick's Dermatology in General Medicine. 7th ed. New Delhi: McGraw Hill Medical; 2008. p1099-109.
2. Bishop JAN. Lentigos Melanocytic Naevi and Melanoma. In: Burns T, Breathnach S, Cox N, Griffiths C, editors. Rook's Textbook of Dermatology. 8th ed. Singapore: Wiley- Blackwell; 2010. p54.10-14.

SWEET SYNDROME

Dr Sheena Pandey, Lecturer, Department of Dermatology

A 65 year old female presented with sudden onset of painful red, raised lesions over trunk, upper and lower extremities since last 8 days. Lesions were associated with high grade fever and painful swelling of left ankle and wrist joints. There was no history of loss of sensations, hypopigmented patches, or photosensitivity. There were no accompanying systemic complaints. On examination, brightly erythematous plaques with positive deep dermal tenderness were present all over the body with relative sparing of face. Oral mucosal and genital examination did not reveal any abnormality. On investigations, ESR and C-reactive protein were elevated with no other abnormality in leucocyte counts, liver function and renal function tests. Mantoux reaction was negative. Radiographs of the chest showed fibrocavitary lesion in the upper lobe suggestive of lung malignancy. Histopathology from the lesion showed diffuse neutrophilic infiltration in the dermis with karyorrhexis and papillary dermal edema. Patient was treated with tapering doses of oral corticosteroid with complete resolution of lesions. Patient was referred to oncology for the management of lung malignancy.

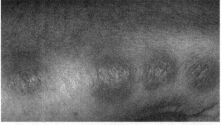

1. What is the most probable diagnosis?
   (A) Erythema nodosum leprosum
   (B) Erythema multiforme
   (C) Acute febrile neutrophilic dermatoses
   (D) Urticarial vasculitis

2. Which of these conditions is not associated with the disease?
   (A) Myeloproliferative diseases
   (B) Pregnancy
   (C) Tuberculosis
   (D) Leprosy
3. Which of these drugs does not have a causative association with this disease?
   (A) Trimethoprim-sulfamethoxazole
   (B) Oral contraceptives
   (C) Erythromycin
   (D) Minocycline
4. Which of these is not the criterion for the diagnosis?
   (A) Elevated ESR
   (B) Excellent response to treatment with systemic steroids
   (C) Joint involvement
   (D) Diffuse dermal neutrophilic infiltratration

Answers:

1. C
   Sweet syndrome (Acute febrile neutrophilic dermatosis) characterizes the abrupt onset of erythematous plaques or nodules, occasionally with vesicles, pustules, or bullae.
2. D
   Acute febrile neutrophilic dermatosis is preceded by a respiratory infection, gastrointestinal infection, or vaccination or associated with inflammatory disease, myeloproliferative disease or malignancy or pregnancy.
3. C
   Oral contraceptives, Trimethoprim-Sulfamethoxazole, Minocycline and All-trans-retinoic acid are responsible for the disease.
4. C
   Sweet syndrome's diagnostic criteria include abrupt onset of erythematous plaques or nodules, diffuse neutrophilic infiltration in the demis with karyorrhexis and papillary dermal edema, preceded by infection, vaccination, or inflammatory disease, myeloproliferative disorder, malignancy or pregnancy, malaise and fever>38 degree Celsius, ESR>20mm, C-reactive protein positive, peripheral leukocytosis, and excellent response to treatment with systemic steroids.

References:

1. Callen JP. Neutophilic dermatoses. Dermatol Clin 2002;20:409.
2. Cohen PR, Kurzrock R. Sweet's syndrome revisited: a review of disease concepts. Int J Dermatol 2003;42:761.

PYOGENIC GRANULOMA
Dr Parul Verma, Assistant professor, Department of Dermatology

A 26 year old male presented with single crusted papule on the cheek. The lesion was present since 6 months, had a narrow base and was covered with haemorrhagic crust. There was history of frequent bleeding on minor trauma. Surrounding skin was normal and rest of the mucocutaneous examination was normal. Radiofrequency ablation with cauterisation of the base was done. On follow up there was mild scarring at the treated site with no reoccurrence.

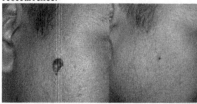

1. What is the most likely diagnosis
   (A) Verruca vulgaris
   (B) Pyogenic granuloma
   (C) Skin tag
   (D) Melanocytic nevus

2. On histopathology pyogenic granuloma shows
   (A) Interface dermatitis
   (B) Suprabasal cleft
   (C) Panniculitis
   (D) Lobular capillary proliferation in dermis
3. Pyogenic granuloma is also known as
   (A) Tufted angioma
   (B) Lobular capillary hemangioma
   (C) cavernous hemangioma
   (D) congenital hemangioma
4. Pyogenic granuloma can be treated with
   (A) Radiofrequency ablation
   (B) Co2 laser ablation
   (C) Surgical excision
   (D) All of the above

Answers:
   1. B
   Solitary red papule, covered with haemorraghic crust with history of requent bleed is characteristic of pyogenic granuloma.
   2. D
   On histopathology there is thinned out epidermis with underlying dermis showing lobulated proliferation of capillary sized vessels in a loose stroma.
   3. B
   The pathological changes shows lobulated capillary proliferation in the dermis.
   4. D
   Co2 laser, Radiofrequency ablation, cryotherapy, surgical excision all can be used as treatment modality.

Reference:
   1 Tara Miller, Ilona J. Frieden. Vascular Tumours. In: Wolff K, Goldsmith LA, Katz SI, Gilchrest BA, Paller AS, Leffell DJ, editors. Fitzpatrick's Dermatology in General Medicine. 7th ed. New Delhi: McGraw Hill Medical; 2008. p 1171-72
   2 E. Calonje. Soft – Tissue Tumours and Tumour – like Conditions. In: Burns T, Breathnach S, Cox N, Griffiths C, editors. Rook's Textbook of Dermatology. 8th ed. Singapore: Wiley- Blackwell; 2010. p56.25-26.

ACNE VULGARIS
Dr Swastika Suvirya, Asst. Professor & Dr Alpna Thakur, Senior Resident,
Department of Dermatology

A 20 year old male patient presented to the outdoor with gradual onset of multiple papules and pustules all over the face, upper chest and back for the last 5 years .On examination multiple open and closed comedones were seen along with papules, pustules and scars.

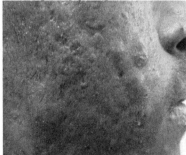

1. Identify the condition
   (A) Milia
   (B) Sebaceous hyperplasia

(C) Staphylococcal folliculitis

(D) Acne vulgaris

2. Which is the only drug available for the above disease supposed to act on all the four pathogenic factors in causation for acne?

(A) Oral antibiotics

(B) Topical clindamycin

(C) Topical benzoyl peroxide

(D) Oral retinoids

3. Which is the only form of acne associated with systemic symptoms of arthralgia?

(A) Acne conglobata

(B) Acne fulminans

(C) Acne excoriee

(D) Acne mechanica

4. A patient with above disease being treated on long term tetracycline comes to us with history of initial relief with the above drugs followed by worsening. On examination multiple pustular lesions were seen on the face. What is the likely diagnosis?

(A) Tropical acne

(B) Acne Aestivialis

(C) Chloracne

(D) Gram negative folliculitis

5. All of the following are involved in the pathogenesis of acne except

(A) Follicular epidermal proliferation

(B) Activity of Propiniobacter acnes

(C) Vasodilation

(D) Inflammation

Answers:

1. D

Acne vulgaris is a common disorder of the pilosebaceous unit seen primarily in adolescents. Presents with lesions like comedones, papules, pustules and nodules.

2. D

Oral retinoids is the group of drug known to act on all the pathogenic factors of acne.

3. B

Acne fulminans is the most severe form of acne accompanied by systemic symptoms.

4. D

Patients being treated with long term antibiotics like tetracycline complain of initial relief followed by worsening of lesions due to colonisation of the lesions with Enterobacter, Klebsiella and Proteus. This phenomena is known as Gram negative folliculitis.

5. C

The following factors are involved in the pathogenesis of acne- Follicular epidermal proliferation, activity of Propiniobacter acnes, inflammation and excess sebum production.

References:

1. Zaenglein AL, Graber EM, Thiboutot DM, Strauss JS. Acne Vulgaris and Acneiform Eruptions. In: Wolff K, Goldsmith LA, Katz SI, Gilchrest BA, Paller AS, Leffell DJ, editors. Fitzpatrick's Dermatology in General Medicine. 7th ed. New Delhi: McGraw Hill Medical; 2008. p690-703.

2. Layton AM. Disorders of Sebaceous Glands. In: Burns T, Breathnach S, Cox N, Griffiths C, editors. Rook's Textbook of Dermatology. 8th ed. Singapore: Wiley- Blackwell; 2010. p42.17-70.

ROSACEA

Dr Swastika Suvirya, Asst. Professor, & Dr Alpna Thakur, Senior Resident,
Department of Dermatology

A 40 year old female presented to the outdoor with multiple papules and pustules on bilateral cheeks for last 5 yrs. She also complained of facial flushing and burning sensation on exposure to sunlight and heat. Patient gave history of aggravation of lesions after intake of spicy foods and hot beverages. On examination multiple papules and pustules were seen on the bilateral malar areas and telengiectasia were visible along the nasolabial folds.

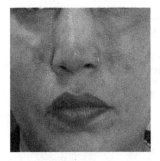

1. Identify the condition
   (A) Papulopustular rosacea (PPR)
   (B) Erythematotelangiectatic rosacea(ETR)
   (C) Phymatous rosacea
   (D) None of the above
2. Following are the triggers for flushing in the disease except
   (A) Hot or cold temperature
   (B) Wind
   (C) Medications
   (D) Pets
3. The treatment plan for patients with above disease include all of the following except
   (A) Topical metronidazole
   (B) Barrier emollients
   (C) Oral cephalosporin
   (D) Pulse dye laser(585 nm)
4. Oral isotretinoin is the first line of treatment for which type of rosacea patients ?
   (A) PPR
   (B) Phymatous rosacea
   (C) ETR
   (D) All of the above
5. Which are the factors involved in the pathogenesis of rosacea?
   (A) Dermal matrix degeneration
   (B) Sun damage
   (C) Colonization by *Demodex folliculorum*
   (D) All of the above

Answers:

1. A
   Papulopustular rosacea presents with papules, pustules, persistent erythema and telangiectasia in males and females after the age of 30 yrs.
2. D
   Triggers for flushing in rosacea include hot or cold temperature, wind, sunlight and alcohol.
3. C
   Treatment for patients with rosacea includes oral therapy like isotretinoin, doxycycline and topical treatments like metronidazole gel and use of vascular lasers.
4. B
   First line treatment for phymatous rosacea is low dose oral retinoids like isotretinoin.
5. D
   Factors involved in pathogenesis of rosacea are dermal matrix degeneration, colonisation by *Demodex folliculorum* and sun damage.

References:

1. Pelle MT. Rosacea. In: Wolff K, Goldsmith LA, Katz SI, Gilchrest BA, Paller AS, Leffell DJ, editors. Fitzpatrick's Dermatology in General Medicine. 7th ed. New Delhi: McGraw Hill Medical; 2008. p703-9
2. Berth-Jones J. Rosacea, Perioral Dermatitis and Similar Dermatoses, Flushing and Flushing Syndromes. In: Burns T, Breathnach S, Cox N, Griffiths C, editors. Rook's Textbook of Dermatology. 8th ed. Singapore: Wiley- Blackwell; 2010. p43.1-9

ALOPECIA AREATA

Dr Swastika Suvirya, Asst. Professor & Dr Alpna Thakur, Senior Resident,
Department of Dermatology

A 10 year old male patient presented to the OPD with multiple round patches of hair loss on the scalp. Patient gave history of similar disease about a year back with spontaneous resolution. On examination there were multiple patches of non scarring alopecia on scalp. All the twenty nails also showed fine pitting. On examination, the skin, teeth and oral mucosa did not reveal any abnormality.

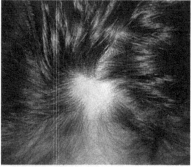

1. The likely diagnosis is:
   (A) Alopecia areata
   (B) Male type baldness
   (C) Tinea Capitis
   (D) Alpoecia Areolaris
2. The following factors are associated with poor prognosis in above disease except
   (A) Ophiasis pattern of hair loss
   (B) Nail involvement
   (C) Loss of body hair
   (D) More than one patch on scalp
3. Trichotillomania can be differentiated from alopecia areata by
   (A) Age of onset
   (B) Sex of patient
   (C) Patches of incomplete hair loss and broken hairs
   (D) Scaling and inflammation of patch
4. The most effective way to treat patchy alopecia areata is
   (A) Oral steroid
   (B) Intralesional steroid injections
   (C) Topical Minoxidil
   (D) Topical anthralin
5. Following are the causes of Anagen effluvium except
   (A) Systemic chemotherapy
   (B) Radiation therapy for head and neck
   (C) Pyrexia
   (D) Mercury intoxiation

Answers:
   1. A
      Alopecia areata presents with multiple patches of non scarring alopecia on scalp and other hair bearing areas. It is associated with nail findings like fine pitting, trachyonychia and onychomadesis.
   2. D
      Factors associated with poor prognosis in alopecia areata include ophiasis pattern, nail pitting, loss of body hair, atopy and onset in early childhood.
   3. C
      Trichotillomania is an O.C.D in which patient pulls his own hair. Can be differentiated from alopecia areata by patches of incomplete hair loss and broken stumps of hair.
   4. B

The most effective way to treat patchy alopecia areata is intralesional steroid injections either with Hydrocortisone Acetate (25mg/ml) or Triamcinolone acetonide (5 or 10 mg /ml).

5. C

Causes of Anagen effluvium are systemic chemotherapy (alkylating agents like cyclophophamide), Radiation therapy for head and neck and mercury intoxication.

References:

1. Messenger AD, Berker DAR, Sinclair RD. Disorders of hair. In: Burns T, Breathnach S, Cox N, Griffiths C, editors. Rook's Textbook of Dermatology. 8th ed. Singapore: Wiley- Blackwell; 2010. p66.1-59
2. Paus R, Olsen EA, Messenger AG. Hair Growth disorders. In: Wolff K, Goldsmith LA, Katz SI, Gilchrest BA, Paller AS, Leffell DJ, editors. Fitzpatrick's Dermatology in General Medicine. 7th ed. New Delhi: McGraw Hill Medical; 2008. p753-78.

PHOTODERMATOLOGY

Dr Swastika Suvirya, Asst. Professor, Department of Dermatology, Dr Alpna Thakur, Senior Resident, Department of Dermatology

A 50 year old female presents with sudden development of burning sensation and redness over sun exposed areas after outdoor activity in the sun for few hours. On physical examination there is diffuse erythema and edema over face, V area of chest and extensors of forearms. There is no history of application of any topical irritants or drug intake in the recent past. Skin biopsy showed epidermal spongiosis with perivascular dermal mononuclear cell infiltrates and edema.

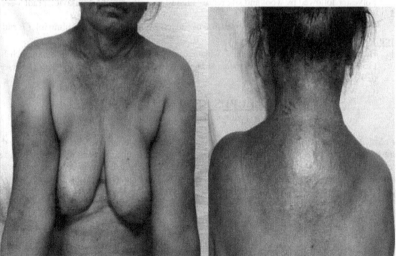

1. What is the likely diagnosis?
   (A) Chronic actinic dermatitis
   (B) Polymorphic light eruption
   (C) Allergic contact dermatitis
   (D) Hydroa Vacciniforme
2. In patients of solar urticaria patients are sensitive to which part of solar spectrum most commonly?
   (A) UV- A rays and Visible light
   (B) UV-B rays
   (C) UV-A and UV-B rays
   (D) Visible light only
3. Following drugs in class of antidepressants are phototoxic agents except
   (A) Amitriptyline
   (B) Imipramine
   (C) Desipramine
   (D) Doxepin

4. Which of the following fibres renders highest protection against sun rays?
   (A) Wool
   (B) Silk
   (C) Rayon
   (D) Polyester
5. Protective effect of a sunscreen against ultraviolet B radiation is measured by
   (A) Sun Protection Factor
   (B) Persistent pigment darkening method
   (C) Sun permeation factor
   (D) Sun promotion factor

Answers:
1. B

   Polymorphic light eruption affects females three times more commonly than males with onset in the first three decades. It presents with polymorphic morphology like papules, papulovesicular, plaque and erythema multiforme kind of lesions. Lesions appear in hours to days after sun exposure.
2. A

   Solar urticaria is a type 1 hypersensitivity reaction in which there is sunlight induced whealing.It is seen most commonly due to UV-A and visible light although can be seen with any combination.
3. D

   Drugs responsible for phototoxicity in antidepressants are Amitriptyline, Imipramine and Desipramine.
4. D

   Polyester followed by wool and silk render highest protection against ultraviolet radiation.
5. A

   Sun protection factor or SPF is a measure of sunscreen protection against ultraviolet B radiation.

Reference:
1. Hawk JLM, Young AR, Ferguson J. Cutaneous Photobiology. In: Burns T, Breathnach S, Cox N, Griffiths C, editors. Rook's Textbook of Dermatology. 8th ed. Singapore: Wiley- Blackwell; 2010. p29.1-24

ACUTE LUPUS ERYTHEMATOSUS
Dr Parul Verma, Assistant professor, Department of Dermatology

A 24 year old female presented with a one month history of multiple erythematous crusted papules and plaques. These were distributed predominantly over photoexposed sites such as face, V area of chest and back. On the face there was sparing of nasolabial fold. History of photosentivity, fever, joint pain was present. On investigation Haemoglobin was 8mg/dl and ANA was positive. Total leucocyte count, platelet count, Chest X-ray and urine routine microscopy was normal. Skin biopsy showed interface changes in the form of vacuolar degeneration and superficial dermal lymphohistiocytic infiltrate.

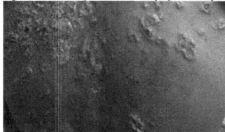

1. What is the most likely diagnosis
   (A) Psoriasis
   (B) Acute lupus erythematosus
   (C) Lichen planus
   (D) Atopic dermatitis
2. Which form of cutaneous lupus erythematosus (LE) is most commonly associated with systemic involvement
   (A) Acute cutaneous LE
   (B) Subacute cutaneous LE

(C) Chronic cutaneous LE
(D) Bullous LE
3. Following are the muco-cutaneous manifestations of lupus erythematosus
   (A) Butterfly rash
   (B) Oral ulcers
   (C) Bullous erruptions
   (D) All of the above
4. Which of the following drugs are associated with drug induced LE
   (A) Procainamide
   (B) Hydralazine
   (C) Isoniazid
   (D) All of the above

Answers:
1. B
   Acute onset maculo-papular rash predominantly in a photodistributed area, sparing of nasolabial fold, associated systemic feature (fever, joint pain) and lab investigations (anemia, positive ANA) supports the diagnosis of lupus erythematosus.
2. A
   Acute cutaneous lupus erythematosus is more commonly associated with life- threatening systemic disease.
3. D
   Cutaneous manifestation of lupus erythematosus can be in the form of malar rash, facial edema, generalised maculo-papular rash (especially in photodistributd area), oral ulcers, scarring alopecia, discoid lupus lesion, bullous lesions, scarring alopecia etc
4. D
   Other drugs which can cause lupus erythematosus include hydrochlorothiazide, calcium channel blockers, phenytoin, minocyclin etc

References:
1   Costner MI, Sontheimer RD. Lupus Erythematosus. In: Wolff K, Goldsmith LA, Katz SI, Gilchrest BA, Paller AS, Leffell DJ, editors. Fitzpatrick's Dermatology in General Medicine. 7th ed. New Delhi: McGraw Hill Medical; 2008. p 1515-35.
2   Goodfield MJD, Jones SK, Veale DJ. The Connective Tissue Diseases. In: Burns T, Breathnach S, Cox N, Griffiths C, editors. Rook's Textbook of Dermatology. 8th ed. Singapore: Wiley-Blackwell; 2010. p51.2-63.

FABRY'S DISEASE

Dr Parul Verma, Assistant professor, Department of Dermatology

A young male presented with multiple erythematous papules distributed predominantly over the trunk. These papules were 1-4mm in size, discrete and some had verrucous surface.Oral mucosa also showed tiny erythematous papules. History of hypohydrosis was present and he had burning-tingling sensations on lower limbs. Other systemic examination was normal. Skin biopsy from the papules showed dilated blood vessels in the dermis. Patient was counselled regarding nature of disease and adviced regular follow up.

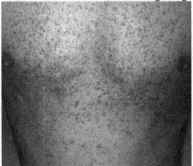

1. What is the most likely diagnosis

(A) Lipoid proteinosis
(B) Fabry's disease
(C) Haemangiomas
(D) Xanthomas
2. Skin lesions present in the given case are known as
(A) Angiokeratoma corporis diffusum
(B) Angiokeratoma of Mibelli
(C) Angiokeratoma circumscriptum
(D) Angiokeratoma of Fordyce
3. Fabry's disease is inherited as
(A) Autosomal dominant
(B) X-linked
(C) Autosomal recessive
(D) None of the above
4. Following enzyme deficiency is found in Fabry's disease
(A) α-galactosidase A
(B) β-glucosidase
(C) α-fucosidase
(D) β-manosidase

Answers:
1. B
   Young male presenting with multiple angiokeratomas especially on trunk, hypohydrosis, paresthesia of limbs, most likely diagnosis is Fabry's disease. Detail examination is important to look for systemic involvement. Typical variants affect skin, eyes, heart, kidney and brain.
2. A
   Multiple punctate, nonblanching, dark red clusters of ectatic blood vessels commonly found in a bathing-trunk distribution are known as angiokeratoma corporis diffusum.
3. B
   Fabry disease is an X-linked lysosomal disorder that leads to excessive deposition of neutral glycosphingolipids in several tissues.
4. A
   Deficiency of alpha-galactosidase A activity leads to lysosomal accumulation of glycosphingolipids.

References:
1. Larralde MM, Luna PC. Fabry Disease. In: Wolff K, Goldsmith LA, Katz SI, Gilchrest BA, Paller AS, Leffell DJ, editors. Fitzpatrick's Dermatology in General Medicine. 7th ed. New Delhi: McGraw Hill Medical; 2008. p 1281-87.
2. Sarkany RPE, Breathnach SM, Morris AAM, Weismann K, Flynn PD. Metabolic and Nutritional Disorders. In: Burns T, Breathnach S, Cox N, Griffiths C, editors. Rook's Textbook of Dermatology. 8th ed. Singapore: Wiley- Blackwell; 2010. p59.36-39.

SCROFULODERMA
Dr. Swastika Suvirya, Asst. Professor, Department of Dermatology

A 25 year old male patient presented to the OPD with plaque on lower part of face studded with ulcers and multiple discharging sinuses for last 8 months. On examination a firm subcutaneous nodule was also present on anterior chest wall .There was history of treatment with several antibiotics for the last six months with no relief. His Mantoux test revealed an induration of 20mm. Haemogram revealed an elevated ESR of 50 mm in the first hour. Histopathology from lesion on face showed multiple caseating granuloma on margins of the sinus with few epitheloid cells and langhans giant cells.

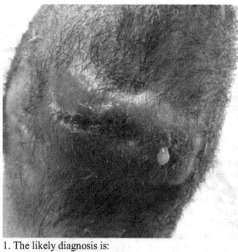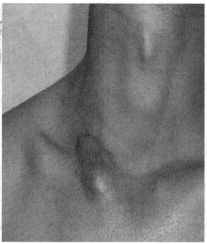

1. The likely diagnosis is:
    (A) Lupus vulgaris
    (B) Acute miliary tuberculosis
    (C) Metastatic tubercular abscess
    (D) Scrofuloderma
2. In developing countries like India Lupus Vulgaris most commonly occurs on which part of the body
    (A) Face and neck
    (B) Acral areas
    (C) Buttocks and trunk
    (D) All of the above
3. Granuloma around the hair follicle is a specific feature of which form of cutaneous tuberculosis
    (A) Papulonecrotic tuberculids
    (B) Lichen scrofulosorum
    (C) Primary inoculation tuberculosis
    (D) Tuberculosis verrucosa cutis
4. Which form of malignancy is most commonly reported in lesions of lupus vulgaris?
    (A) Squamous cell carcinoma
    (B) Basal cell carcinoma
    (C) Melanoma
    (D) Syringocystadenoma papilliferum
5. Which of the following mycobacteria falls under the category of photochromogens?
    (A) *M.marinum*
    (B) *M.kansasii*
    (C) Both
    (D) *M.ulcerans*

Answers:

1. D
    Scrofuloderma is a form of cutaneous tuberculosis which most often presents in parotid, submandibular and supraclavicular areas with multiple ulcers and discharging sinuses.
2. C
    In developing country like India lupus Vulgaris most commonly occurs on buttocks and trunk.In Europeans head and neck are common sites of involvement.
3. B
    Lichen scrofulosorum a lichenoid eruption due to haematogenous spread of mycobacteria is associated with tuberculoid granuloma around hair follicle.
4. A
    Squamous cell carcinoma is the most commonly reported malignancy in lesions of lupus vulgaris.
5. C
    Both M. Marinum and M. Kansasii fall under the category of photocromogens.

References:

1. Tappeiner G. tuberculosis and infections with atypical mycobacteria. In: Wolff K, Goldsmith LA, Katz SI, Gilchrest BA, Paller AS, Leffell DJ, editors. Fitzpatrick's Dermatology in General Medicine. 7th ed. New Delhi: McGraw Hill Medical; 2008. p1768-78.
2. V.M. Yates. Mycobacterial Infections. In: Burns T, Breathnach S, Cox N, Griffiths C, editors. Rook's Textbook of Dermatology. 8th ed. Singapore: Wiley- Blackwell; 2010. p31.1-28.

LEPROMATOUS LEPROSY

Dr Sheena Pandey, Lecturer, Department of Dermatology

A 20 year old male presented with red, raised lesions all over the body since 1 year. There was history of loss of sensations over bilateral upper and lower extremities. He had scar of unnoticed burn injury over right hand. There was no history of light colored skin patches, shooting nerve pains, or ulceration of feet. There was no history suggestive of painful episodes in the existing lesions. On examination, lesions were generalized, ill-defined, erythematous to skin colored, shiny, smooth surfaced plaques involving the face, ear lobes and eyebrows. Superciliary madarosis was present. Bilaterally symmetrical anesthesia to fine touch, hot and cold temperature was present extending from tip of the fingers to the wrist and from tip of the toes to tibial prominence. Bilateral greater auricular, ulnar, median, radial cutaneous, common peroneal and sural nerves were thickened symmetrically, with no evidence of neuritis. There was difficulty in adduction and abduction of fingers, on motor examination. No fixed motor deformity was present in hands and feet. Slit skin smear from the nodules over the eyebrow and the ear lobe showed a bacteriological index of +2. Histopathology showed a diffuse macrophage granuloma involving the entire thickness of the dermis with a clear subepidermal zone. Patient was treated with Multidrug therapy blister pack for multibacillary disease for 1 year.

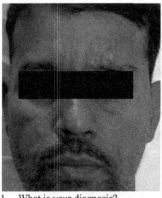 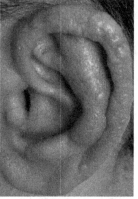

1. What is your diagnosis?
   (A) Borderline lepromatous leprosy
   (B) Lepromatous leprosy
   (C) Tuberculoid leprosy
   (D) Indeterminate leprosy
2. Which of the following is not correct?
   (A) Bacteriological index measures the density of bacilli present in skin smears
   (B) Morphological index measures the solid staining live and dead bacilli
   (C) WHO defines paucibacillary leprosy as 5 or less than 5 lesions
   (D) Multibacillary leprosy is defined as more than 5 lesions by WHO
3. Which of the following treatment will not be given to this patient, as per WHO guidelines?
   (A) Clofazimine 300mg once a month supervised
   (B) Rifampicin 600mg once a month supervised
   (C) Clofazimine 150mg once daily, self-administered
   (D) Dapsone 100mg once daily, self-administered
4. Which of these is not correct for Reversal reaction in leprosy?
   (A) Sudden onset, within 6-24 months of termination of treatment
   (B) Swelling, erythema, and scaling of inactive lesions
   (C) Previously involved nerves become exquisitely tender
   (D) Skin smears are usually positive

Answers:
1. B

    Lepromatous leprosy presents as bilaterally symmetrical, ill defined erythematous, shiny, smooth surfaced, papules and plaques with bilaterally symmetrical peripheral neuropathy.
2. B

    Morphological index measures solid staining live bacilli
3. C

    Clofazimine 50mg is given once daily in MDT-MB
4. D

    Slit skin smears are usually negative in Type 1 Reversal Reaction

References:
1. Sharma VK, Malhotra AK. Leprosy: Classification and clinical aspects. In: Valia RG, Valia AR. IADVL Texbook of Dermatology. 3rd ed. India: Bhalani Publishing House; 2008. p. 2032-69.
2. Girdhar BK. Leprosy: Drug treatment and management of reactions. In: Valia RG, Valia AR. IADVL Texbook of Dermatology. 3rd ed. India: Bhalani Publishing House; 2008. p. 2079-97.

PITYRIASIS VERSICOLOR
Dr Swastika Suvirya, Asst. Professor & Dr Alpna Thakur, Senior Resident,
Department of Dermatology

A 35 yr old male presents with multiple asymptomatic hypo and hyperpigmented macules on the upper chest and back. The lesions showed very fine brawny scales.

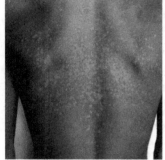

1. Identify the infection and characteristic appearance in KOH
    (A) Tinea corporis. Fragmented hyphae with arthroconidia
    (B) Pityriasis versicolor. Spaghetti and meatball appearance
    (C) Erythrasma with round macroconidia
    (D) Candidiasis. Mass of large arthroconidia
2. Which is the Malassezia species most commonly associated with this infection?
    (A) M. Globosa
    (B) M. Sympodialis
    (C) M. Furfur
    (D) M. Globosa and M. Sympodialis both
3. Woods lamp examination of the above lesion would reveal
    (A) Yellow green fluorescence
    (B) Coral red fluorescence
    (C) Blue fluorescence
    (D) Non fluorescent
4. Following drugs are used for the treatment of this disease except
    (A) Topical selenium sulphide
    (B) Topical ketoconazole
    (C) Oral fluconazole
    (D) Topical steroid
5. Other names for the above disease are:
    (A) Dermatomycosis furfuracea
    (B) Liver spots
    (C) Chromophytosis

(D) All of the above

Answers:
1. B
   Pityriasis versicolor affects young adults usually with lesions on the upper chest, back, trunk and shoulders. It presents as slightly scaly macules that can be hypopigmented, pink or hyperpigmented. Direct examination of the scales using a KOH solution demonstrates a typical hyphae and blastospores in spaghetti and meatball pattern or banana and grapes pattern.
2. A
   M. Globosa is the most commonly isolated Malassezia species in lesions of Pityriasis versicolor
3. A
   One out of three patients of pityriasis versicolor reveal a yellowish fluorescence on woods light examination.
4. D
   P.V. being a superficial mycoses is treated with all local and systemic anti fungal preparations.
5. D
   P.V. is also known as dermatomycosis furfuracea, tinea flavia, tinea versicolor, chromomycosis and liver spots.

References:
1. Hay RJ, Ashbee HR. Mycology. In: Burns T, Breathnach S, Cox N, Griffiths C, editors. Rook's Textbook of Dermatology. 8th ed. Singapore: Wiley- Blackwell; 2010. p36.10-2.
2. Janik MP, Heffernan MP. Yeast infections: Candidiasis and Tinea Versicolor. In: Wolff K, Goldsmith LA, Katz SI, Gilchrest BA, Paller AS, Leffell DJ, editors. Fitzpatrick's Dermatology in General Medicine. 7th ed. New Delhi: McGraw Hill Medical; 2008. p1822-31.

HERPES ZOSTER

Dr Swastika Suvirya, Asst. Professor & Dr Alpna Thakur, Senior Resident,
Department of Dermatology

A 55 year old male presented to the outdoor with sudden onset of vesicular lesions over the face for the last 2 days. On examination, unilateral, grouped vesicles about 2-5mm in diameter, filled with clear fluid were seen involving the side of the forehead, upper eyelid and tip of the nose. The lesions were associated with edema of the upper eyelid, purulent eye discharge, severe pain and burning. On doing a Tzanck test from one of the vesicles, multinucleated giant cells were seen.

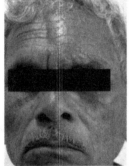

1. What is the likely diagnosis?
   (A) Insect bite
   (B) Pemphigus vulgaris
   (C) Herpes Zoster
   (D) Contact dermatitis
2. Ramsay hunt syndrome is because of involvement of which of the following nerves?
   (A) Facial
   (B) Trigeminal
   (C) Facial and trigeminal both
   (D) Facial and auditory nerves
3. Hutchisons sign in the above disease is indicative of higher chances of
   (A) Neurological manifestations

(B) Auditory involvement

(C) Ocular involvement

(D) None of the above

4. In patients of AIDS with acyclovir resistance in this case following is the drug of choice?

(A) Foscarnet

(B) Valacylovir

(C) Gancyclovir

(D) All of the above

5. Patient of varicella are infectious for what duration?

(A) Till vesicles are erupting

(B) 2 days before disease onset

(C) Febrile period

(D) 2 days before and 5 days after disease onset.

Answers:

1. C

Herpes Zoster presents as unilateral vesicular rash in a dermatomal pattern. It is because of reactivation of varicella zoster virus from sensory ganglion after an initial attack from varicella.

2. D

Ramsay hunt syndrome is one in which there is facial palsy, rash of herpes zoster in the external auditory canal and tinnitus or vertigo. It is because of combined involvement of facial and auditory nerves.

3. C

Hutchisons sign where vesicles involve tip of nose indicate higher chances of ocular involvement.

4. A

Foscarnet is the drug of choice in patients with acyclovir resistance in case of AIDS.

5. D

Patient of varicella is infectious for 2 days before and 5 days after disease onset.

References:

1   Strauss SE, Oxman MN, Schmader KE. Varicella and Herpes Zoster. In: Wolff K, Goldsmith LA, Katz SI, Gilchrest BA, Paller AS, Leffell DJ, editors. Fitzpatrick's Dermatology in General Medicine. 7th ed. New Delhi: McGraw Hill Medical; 2008. p1885-98.

2   Sterling JC. Virus Infections. In: Burns T, Breathnach S, Cox N, Griffiths C, editors. Rook's Textbook of Dermatology. 8th ed. Singapore: Wiley- Blackwell; 2010. p33.22-8.

SCABIES

Dr Swastika Suvirya, Assistant. Professor, Dr Rohit Kumar Singh, Senior Resident, Department of Dermatology

A 20 year old male presents to the dermatology outdoor with 2 week history of itching all over the body. He complains of his itching being aggravated during night. There is history of similar disease in other members of the family. On examination there are multiple excoriated papules seen in the finger webs, axillae, lower abdomen, inner thigh and buttocks. On the genitals, multiple erythematous nodules are seen.

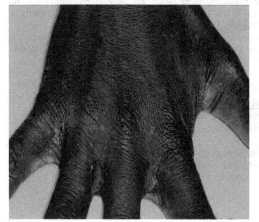 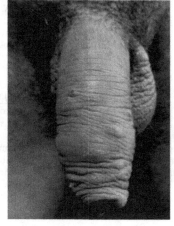

1. Identify the condition
   - (A) Scabies
   - (B) Pediculosis capitis
   - (C) Pityriasis versicolor
   - (D) None of the above
2. Based on the above features which is the treatement of choice for such patients?
   - (A) Oral ivermectin
   - (B) Permethrin 5% topical
   - (C) Combination of oral ivermectin and 5% permethrin topically
   - (D) Malathion .5% topically
3. Oral ivermectin is used in what dose in patients with above disease?
   - (A) 200mcg/kg
   - (B) 100 mcg/kg
   - (C) 50mcg/kg
   - (D) 20mcg/kg
4. What is the number of mites infesting an individual with Norwegian scabies
   - (A) 10-20
   - (B) <25
   - (C) 100-200
   - (D) 1million
5. The treatement of choice in patients with Norwegian scabies is
   - (A) 5% permethrin topically
   - (B) Oral ivermectin
   - (C) Combination of the above
   - (D) Sulphur 6% topically

Answers:

1. A

   Scabies is a disease caused by infestation by a mite known as sarcoptes scabiei var hominis. It presents with characteristic lesions like excoriated papules,nodules in finger webs,lower abdomen,inner thigh and genitalia.

2. B

   Permethrin 5% topically is the treatement of choice for patients with scabies.

3. A

   The only oral drug effective in scabies is ivermectin used in a dose of 200mcg/kg. It is used in a single oral dose which can be repeated in a span of 10-14 days.

4. D

   In Norwegian scabies the no of mites infesting an individual would be a million mites. In normal scabies the number of mites would be less than 10.

5. C

   In Norwegian scabies treatment of choice is a combination of oral ivermectin and permethrin 5% topically both.

References:

1 Stone SP, Goldfarb JN, Baceleiri RE. Scabies, other mites and pediculosis.. In: Wolff K, Goldsmith LA, Katz SI, Gilchrest BA, Paller AS, Leffell DJ, editors. Fitzpatrick's Dermatology in General Medicine. 7th ed. New Delhi: McGraw Hill Medical; 2008. p2029-31.

2 Burns DA. Diseases Caused by Arthropods and Other Noxious Animals. In: Burns T, Breathnach S, Cox N, Griffiths C, editors. Rook's Textbook of Dermatology. 8th ed. Singapore: Wiley-Blackwell; 2010. p38.36-46.

MOLLUSCUM CONTAGIOSUM

Dr Swastika Suvirya, Assistant. Professor & Dr Alpna Thakur, Senior Resident,
Department of Dermatology

A 25 year old female presented to the OPD with multiple asymptomatic papular lesions on the face for last six months. On closer inspection the papules were smooth, shiny with umblication in the centre. Patient had taken treatment from multiple places with no relief and the lesions kept on increasing in size despite therapy.

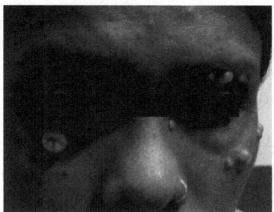

1. What is your diagnosis?
   (A) Herpes labialis
   (B) Warts
   (C) Scabies
   (D) Molluscum contagiosum
2. Giant form of this disease upto 3 cm and multiple facial lesions in adults as in this case is an indicator for?
   (A) Hepatitis B screening
   (B) Hepatitis C screening
   (C) Both of the above
   (D) Human immunodeficiency virus screening
3. Following are the treatment options available for the above disease in this location except?
   (A) Topical cantharidin
   (B) Topical imiquimod
   (C) Topical retinoids
   (D) Podophyllin cream
4. Diagnostic finding histopathologically for the above disease is:
   (A) Copper penny bodies
   (B) Henderson- Patterson bodies
   (C) Negri bodies
   (D) Cowdry bodies
5. A phenomenon associated with the disease is:
   (A) Pseudo Koebner's phenomenon
   (B) Koebner's phenomenon
   (C) Prozone phenomenon
   (D) Raynaud's phenomenon

Answers:

1. D

   Genital molluscum contagiosum is a sexually transmitted infection presenting as multiple smooth shiny papules with central umbilication.

2. D

   Multiple giant facial M.C. lesions in adults is an indicator for H.I.V. testing.

3. A

   Topical cantharidin an extact of blister beetle is not used on face and genital areas because of thinner skin here and chances of severe blistering.

4. B

   Microscopically intracytoplasmic inclusion bodies called Handerson-Paterson body are diagnostic for molluscum contagiosum.

5. A

   Pseudo Koebner's phenomenon is appearance of similar morphological skin lesions along the lines of trauma in infective conditions like verrucae and molluscum contagiosum. It is due to direct transmission of the virus following trauma.

References:
1. Tom W, Friedlander SF. Poxvirus Infections. In: Wolff K, Goldsmith LA, Katz SI, Gilchrest BA, Paller AS, Leffell DJ, editors. Fitzpatrick's Dermatology in General Medicine. 7th ed. New Delhi: McGraw Hill Medical; 2008. p1899-1913.
2. Sterling JC. Virus Infection. In: Burns T, Breathnach S, Cox N, Griffiths C, editors. Rook's Textbook of Dermatology. 8th ed. Singapore: Wiley- Blackwell; 2010. p33.11-14.
3. Kudur MH, Hulmani M. "Pseudo" conditions in in dermatology: Need to know both real and unreal. Indian J Dermatol Venereol Leprol 2012;78:763-73.

LUPUS VULGARIS

Dr Parul Verma, Assistant professor, Department of Dermatology

A young male presented with 15 years history of erythematous plaques on neck and thigh. These plaques were slowly progressive, scaly, firm, infiltrated and left behind scarring at the regresssing edge. There was no significant lymphadenopathy. On diascopy, apple jelly nodules were seen. Family history of tuberculosis was present. Skin biopsy taken from the advancing edge showed epithiloid cell granuloma with giant cells in the dermis.There were no systemic complaints. BCG scar was present and chest X-ray was normal.

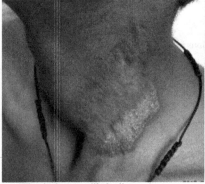 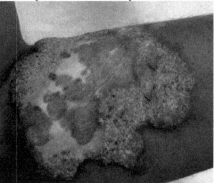

1. What is the most likely diagnosis
   - (A) Scrofuloderma
   - (B) Lupus vulgarism
   - (C) Chromoblastomycosis
   - (D) Mycetoma
2. Following are a type of cutaneous tuberculosis except
   - (A) Tuberculosis verrucosa cutis
   - (B) Scrofuloderma
   - (C) Orificial tuberculosis
   - (D) Lupus profundus
3. Characteristic finding in skin biopsy is
   - (A) Mucinosis
   - (B) Epitheloid cell granulomas
   - (C) Basal cell degeneration
   - (D) Panniculitis
4. Which of the following is a tuberculid
   - (A) Scrofuloderma
   - (B) Tuberculous gumma
   - (C) Lichen scrofulosorum
   - (D) Primary complex like reaction
5. Lupus vulgaris can present as
   - (A) Ulcerative form
   - (B) Vegetating form
   - (C) Tumour like
   - (D) Papular form
   - (E) All of the above

Answers:

1. B

Chronic, progressive infiltrated plaque with areas of scarring is characteristic of lupus vulgaris. Usually it is a solitary lesion but more than one lesion can be present.

2. D

Classification of cutaneous tuberculosis

Host immunity	Method of inoculation	Disease
Naive host	Direct inoculation	Tuberculosis chancre
Multibacillary forms	Contiguous spread	Scrofuloderma
Low host immunity	Autoinoculation	Orificial tuberculosis
	Haematogenous spread	Acute miliary tuberculosis
		Tuberculous gumma(abscess)
Paucibacillary forms	Direct inoculation	Warty tuberculosis
		Lupus vulgaris (some)
	Haematogenous spread	Lupus vulgaris
Tuberculids		Lichen scrofulosorum
		Papulonecrotic tuberculid
		Erythema induratum
		Nodular tuberculid

3. B

The most prominent histopathological feature is formation of tubercles with scanty or absent central caseation, surrounded by epitheloid histiocytes and multinucleate giant cells.

4. C

Refer to table given above.

5. E

Depending on the local tissue response lupus vulgaris can present as Plaque form, Ulcerative and mutilating forms, Vegetating forms, tumour like, Papular and nodular forms.

References:

1 Tappeiner G. Tuberculosis and Infections with Atypical Mycobacteria. In: Wolff K, Goldsmith LA, Katz SI, Gilchrest BA, Paller AS, Leffell DJ, editors. Fitzpatrick's Dermatology in General Medicine. 7th ed. New Delhi: McGraw Hill Medical; 2008. p 1768-75.

2 Yates VM. Mycobacterial Infections. In: Burns T, Breathnach S, Cox N, Griffiths C, editors. Rook's Textbook of Dermatology. 8th ed. Singapore: Wiley- Blackwell; 2010. p31.10-25.

VERRUCA VULGARIS

Dr Parul Verma, Assistant professor, Department of Dermatology

A 25 year old male presented with hyperpigmented papule on the right side of neck. The lesion was present since 6 months, 1.5 cm in size, well defined firm with verrucous surface. It was asymptomatic and gradually increasing in size. Radiofrequency ablation under local anaesthesia was done and there was no reoccurrence on 1 month follow up.

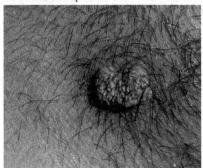

1. What is the most likely diagnosis
   (A) Molluscum contagiosum
   (B) Verruca vulgaris
   (C) Melanocytic nevus
   (D) Seborrheic keratosis
2. Common wart is usually caused by
   (A) HPV 1
   (B) HPV 16,18
   (C) HPV 2,4
   (D) HPV 6,8
3. Following are the high risk type of HPV (associated with cervical dysplasia etc)
   (A) HPV 6
   (B) HPV 11
   (C) HPV 16,18
   (D) HPV 1
4. HPV infection is implicated in following diseases except
   (A) Squammous cell carcinoma
   (B) Epidermodysplasia verruciformis (EDV)
   (C) Basal cell carcinoma (BCC)
   (D) Lupus vulgaris

Answers:
1. B
   A papule with rough, filliform surface is diagnostic of verruca vulgaris or common wart
2. C
   Verruca vulgaris is commonly associated with HPV type 2,4 and less frequently with type 1.
3. C
   HPV 16, 18 classified as high risk type are associated with genital warts & cervical dysplasia.
4. D
   HPV 16, 18 classified as high risk type are associated with genital warts and cervical dysplasia and rarely in cutaneous squammous cell carcinoma. HPV 5 and 8 are associated with EDV. There have been many studies that report detection of low level of HPV DNA in BCC, actinic keratosis, psoriasis and other skin lesions.

References:
1. Androphy EJ, Lowy DR. Warts. In: Wolff K, Goldsmith LA, Katz SI, Gilchrest BA, Paller AS, Leffell DJ, editors. Fitzpatrick's Dermatology in General Medicine. 7th ed. New Delhi: McGraw Hill Medical; 2008. p 1914-18.
2. Sterling JC. Virus Infections. In: Burns T, Breathnach S, Cox N, Griffiths C, editors. Rook's Textbook of Dermatology. 8th ed. Singapore: Wiley- Blackwell; 2010. p33.39-57.

HERPES SIMPLEX

Dr Parul Verma, Assistant professor, Department of Dermatology

A young female presented in our OPD with 1 day history of grouped vesicles with erythematous base present on the leg. Localised mild pain was present but there were no systemic complaints. There was no past history of similar lesion. Examination of oral and genital mucosa was normal. Tzanck smear from the base of the vesicle showed multinucleated giant cells. Patient was started on acyclovir and lesions healed in 7 days.

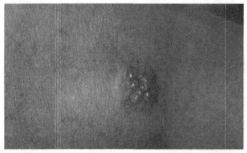

1. What is the most likely diagnosis
   (A) Herpes simplex
   (B) Insect bite
   (C) Herpes zoster
   (D) Contact dermatitis
2. Which side lab procedure is used to diagnose herpes simplex infection
   (A) KOH mount
   (B) WET mount
   (C) Tzanck smear
   (D) Gram stain
3. Wide spread herpes infection can be seen in
   (A) HIV patients
   (B) Patients on chemotherapy
   (C) Patients on steroids
   (D) All of the above
4. Which of the following is true for herpes labialis infection
   (A) Mild infections should be treated with antiviral drugs
   (B) In mild infections no treatment is required
   (C) Is caused only by HSV 1
   (D) Is caused only by HSV 2

Answers:
1. A
   Acute onset grouped vesicles with polycyclic margins are diagnostic of herpes simplex infection.
2. C
   Tzanck smear includes scraping from base of fresh vesicles and staining with giemsa stain to look for multinucleate giant cell which are multinucleated giant keratinocytes.
3. D
   Immunocompromised state can lead to atypical or widespread involvement of herpes simplex infection.
4. B
   Mild herpes labialis heals spontaneously in 5-7 days and usually needs no treatment. It can be caused by HSV1 or HSV 2.

References:
1. Marques AR, Straus SE. Herpes Simplex. In: Wolff K, Goldsmith LA, Katz SI, Gilchrest BA, Paller AS, Leffell DJ, editors. Fitzpatrick's Dermatology in General Medicine. 7th ed. New Delhi: McGraw Hill Medical; 2008. p1873-84.
2. Sterling JC. Virus Infections. In: Burns T, Breathnach S, Cox N, Griffiths C, editors. Rook's Textbook of Dermatology. 8th ed. Singapore: Wiley- Blackwell; 2010. p33.14-22.

HERPES GENITALIS
Dr Sheena Pandey, Lecturer, Department of Dermatology

A 25 year old married, heterosexual male presented with sudden onset of painful fluid filled lesions over external genitalia since 4 days. There was no history of any lesions in oral mucosa or rest of the skin. His wife had similar eruptions consisting of fluid filled lesions and erosions on the vulva, a month ago. He had last sexual exposure with his wife 6 days before the eruption. On examination, coalescing vesicles on a non-erythematous base were present on the shaft of the penis. Rest of the muco-cutaneous examination was normal. No regional lymph nodes were palpable. Tzanck smear from the fluid after rupturing the vesicle showed multinucleate giant cells. Patient was treated with Tablet Acyclovir for 7 days.

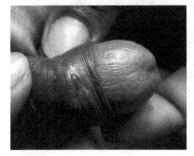

1. What is your most probable diagnosis?
   (A) Chancroid
   (B) Herpes genitalis
   (C) Chancre
   (D) Donovanosis
2. The incubation period for the organism is-
   (A) 3 weeks to 2 months
   (B) 1-2 days
   (C) 5-14 days
   (D) 2-6 months
3. Which of the following is not a sexually transmitted disease?
   (A) Donovanosis
   (B) Bacillary angiomatosis
   (C) Lymphogranuloma venereum
   (D) Molluscum contagiosum
4. Which of these is not a recommended regimen for treatment of this disease?
   (A) Acyclovir 400 mg orally tid for 7-10 days
   (B) Acyclovir 200 mg orally five times daily for 7-10 days
   (C) Famciclovir 500 mg orally tid for 7-10 days
   (D) Valacyclovir 1 g orally bid for 7-10 days

Answers:
   1. B
      Herpes genitalis is characterized by sudden onset of painful vesicles which readily form pustules which rupture and coalesce to form superficial painful ulcers.
   2. C
      The incubation period for herpes simplex virus is 5-14 days.
   3. B
      Bacillary angiomatosis caused by Bartonella hensalae is not a sexually transmitted infection.
   4. C
      Famciclovir 250 mg orally tid is the recommended regimen for treatment of primary episode of Herpes genitalis.

Reference:
   1. Corey L, Wald A. Genital Herpes. In: Homes KK, Mardh PA, Sparling PF. Textbook of sexually transmitted disease. 3rd ed. New York: McGraw Hill; 1999. p. 285-312.

EPIDERMODYSPLASIA VERRUCIFORMIS
Dr. Parul Verma, Assistant professor, Department of Dermatology

A 22 year old male presented with 12 year history of multiple hyperpigmented 2-4mm, flat topped papules, distributed over acral areas and hypopigmented 3-5mm macules distributed over trunk and limbs. The lesions were asymptomatic and gradually increasing in number. There was no family history of similar lesions. Skin biopsy taken from hyperpigmented papule showed epidermal changes in the form of mild acanthosis, keratinocytes containing perinuclear halos with abundant blue-gray cytoplasm. Patient was counselled regarding regarding regular dermatological examination and follow up.

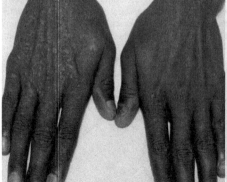

1. What is the most likely diagnosis
    (A) Plane warts
    (B) Epidermodysplasia verruciformis (EDV)
    (C) Pityriasis versicolor
    (D) Dyschromatosis universalis heriditaria
2. Most common HPV types implicated in epidermodysplasia verruciformis are
    (A) Type 1
    (B) Type 5,8
    (C) Type 6,11
    (D) Type 18
3. Patients of epidermodysplasia verruciformis require regular follow up because?
    (A) Risk of internal organ involvement
    (B) Risk of sqammous cell carcinoma
    (C) Risk of eye involvement
    (D) Risk of haematological malignancies
4. Which of the following drugs can be used in epidermodysplasia verruciformis
    (A) Oral retinoids
    (B) Interferon α
    (C) Topical vitamin D analogue
    (D) All of the above

Answers:

1. B
    Combination of plane warts like papules, pityriasis versicolor like lesions in young male strongly supports the diagnosis of Epidermodysplasia verruciformis (EDV). Diagnosis can be confirmed by skin biopsy.
2. B
    More than 20 HPV types have been found in EDV of which type 5 and 8 is commonly found.
3. B
    Dysplastic or malignant change can occur in the lesions, especially on exposed sites commonly as Bowen's disease, Squamous cell carcinoma.
4. D
    Oral retinoids, INF α, topical immunotherapy, topical vitamin D analogue, oral cimitidine has been used in EDV to reduce the number of benign lesions and to prevent malignant change.

Reference:

1. Androphy EJ, Lowy DR. Warts. In: Wolff K, Goldsmith LA, Katz SI, Gilchrest BA, Paller AS, Leffell DJ, editors. Fitzpatrick's Dermatology in General Medicine. 7th ed. New Delhi: McGraw Hill Medical; 2008. p 1918-22.
2. Sterling JC. Virus Infections. In: Burns T, Breathnach S, Cox N, Griffiths C, editors. Rook's Textbook of Dermatology. 8th ed. Singapore: Wiley- Blackwell; 2010. p33.57-60.

CHROMOBLASTOMYCOSIS

Dr Sheena Pandey, Lecturer, Department of Dermatology

A 20 year old farmer presented with itchy dark raised lesions with history of occasional discharge of pus and blood, on right leg since 4 years. Lesions appeared after a thorn injury. On examination, linearly arranged hyperpigmented, hyperkeratotic nodules and plaques with central erosions and crusting were seen on posterior aspect of right leg. Right inguinal lymph nodes were palpable. Potassium hydroxide mount from the scrapings showed thick-walled, dark brown "sclerotic bodies". Skin biopsy on H&E showed pseudoepitheliomatous hyperplasia with intraepidermal abscesses, a dermal granulomatous reaction, and presence of pigmented fungal sclerotic bodies. Radiographs of the chest and the underlying bone did not show any abnormality.

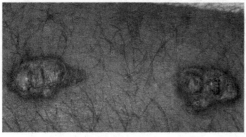

1. What is your diagnosis?
   (A) Sporotrichosis
   (B) Mycetoma
   (C) Tuberculosis verrucosa cutis
   (D) Chromoblastomycosis
2. Which of these is not an organism associated with the infection?
   (A) *Trichophyton mentagrophytes*
   (B) *Fonsacaea pedrosi*
   (C) *Cladosporium carrionii*
   (D) *Phialophora verrucosa*
3. How does the disease spread to the skin?
   (A) Contact of intact skin with the infected skin lesions
   (B) Contact of non-intact skin with infected skin lesions
   (C) Direct inoculation of the organism into the skin
   (D) Spread via lymphatics from systemic infection
4. Sclerotic bodies are commonly known as-
   (A) Asteroid bodies
   (B) Copper pennies
   (C) Cigar bodies
   (D) Gumma
5. Drug of choice in this case is-
   (A) Itraconazole
   (B) Rifampicin
   (C) Amikacin
   (D) Cotrimoxazole

Answers:
1. D
   Chromoblastomycosis is a chronic granulomatous infection, usually of exposed areas, characterized by warty plaques, nodules or cauliflower- like lesions, which may ulcerate.
2. A
   Chromoblastomycosis is caused by brown pigmented fungi such as Fonsacea pedrosoi, Cladosporim carrionii, Phialophora verrucosa. Trichophyton mentagrophytes is a dermatophyte responsible for superficial fungal infection.
3. C
   Infection occurs as a result of introduction of the organisms into the tissues by a thorn, or wooden splinter injury, or abrasion of the skin
4. B
   On histopathology, inflammatory infiltrate is seen with variable pigmented fungal structures called as sclerotic bodies, copper pennies, medlar bodies, muriform cells or fumagoid bodies.
5. A
   The mainstay of treatment is systemic antifungal therapy; itraconazole or terbinafine for 6-12 months. Surgical excision or cryosurgery can be done for isolated or drug resistant lesions.

References:
1. Vijaya D, Kumar BH. Chromoblastomycosis. Mycoses. 2005; 48:82-4.
2. Bonifaz A, Carrasco-Gerard E, Saúl A. Chromoblastomycosis: clinical and mycologic experience of 51 cases. Mycoses 2001; 44:1.

CUTANEOUS LARVA MIGRANS

Dr Sheena Pandey, Lecturer, Department of Dermatology

A 15 year old boy presented with rapidly increasing, slightly itchy linear, red eruptions on dorsum of right foot since a week. It started as tiny, red raised lesions which rapidly increased to form thin, red, tortuous lines with intermittent stinging and pain. History of visit to a public beach before the appearance of the lesions was elicited from the parents. On examination, single, brightly erythematous, non-tender, linear eruption with grouped vesicles was seen on the dorsum of the right foot. Axillary lymph nodes were not palpable. Total leucocyte count was normal with eosinophilia. X ray chest did not reveal any abnormality. Patient was treated with single dose of Ivermectin 12mg with complete resolution of the lesions in few days.

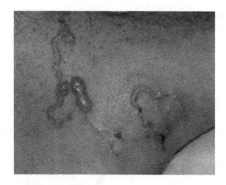

1. What is the diagnosis?
   (A) Scabies
   (B) Tinea manum
   (C) Larva migrans
   (D) Jelly fish dermatitis
2. Which of these organism is responsible for the disease?
   (A) *Trichophyton rubrum*
   (B) *Ancylostoma braziliense*
   (C) *Chironex fleckeri*
   (D) *Dracunculus medinensis*
3. Which of these is not found in Loeffler syndrome?
   (A) Patchy infiltrate of the lungs
   (B) Thrombophlebitis
   (C) Creeping eruption
   (D) Eosinophilia
4. Which of these is not the treatment for the above disease?
   (A) Oral Albendazole
   (B) Oral Ivermectin
   (C) Topical Metronidazole
   (D) Topical Permethrin

Answers:

1. C
   Creeping eruption or larva migrans is a term applied to twisting, windling, linear skin lesions produced by burrowing of larvae.
2. B
   Majority of the cases are caused by penetration by the larvae of a cat and dog hookworm, *Ancylostoma braziliense*. It is acquired from body contact with damp sand or earth that has been contaminated by the excreta of dogs and cats.
3. B
   Loeffler syndrome, consisting of a patchy infiltrate of lungs and eosinophilia as high as 50% in the blood and 90% in the sputum, may complicate creeping eruption.
4. D
   Ivermectin 200ug /kg, given as single 12mg dose and repeated the next day, or Albendazole 400mg/ day for 3 days, are most effective. Topical metronidazole and topical thiobendazole can also be used. If no treatment is given, the larva usually die in 2-8 weeks, with resolution of the eruption.

References:
1. Davies HD, Sakuls P, Keystone JS. Creeping eruption. Arch Dermatol 1993; 129:588.
2. Elgart ML. Creeping eruption. Arch Dermatol 1998; 134:619.

PRIMARY SYPHILIS
Dr Parul Verma, Assistant professor, Department of Dermatology

A 26 year male presented with 7 days history of ulcer on penile shaft. The ulcer was painless, single, well defined and with indurated base. Inguinal lymph nodes were enlarged, 1.5-2 cm in size, firm and shotty. There was history of unprotected premarietal sexual contact 25 days back. There was no history of urethral discharge and perianal examination was normal. Rest of the muco-cutaneous examination was normal. On investigation VDRL was positive (1:16 dilution).

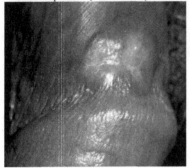

1. What is the most likely diagnosis
   (A) Chancroid
   (B) Herpes genitalis
   (C) Primary chancre
   (D) Donovanosis
2. Which bed side investigation is used to diagnose syphilis
   (A) Gram stain
   (B) Dark field microscopy
   (C) Tzanck smear
   (D) Wet mount
3. Incubation period of syphilis varies from
   (A) 10-14days
   (B) 9-90 days
   (C) 2-5 days
   (D) 5-6 months
4. Primary syphilis is treated with
   (A) Azithromycin 1gm stat
   (B) Inj benzathine penicilline 2.4 million I U stat
   (C) Inj benzathine penicilline 2.4 million I U weekly for 3 weeks
   (D) Cap doxycyclin 100mg twice daily for 14 days.

Answers:
1. C
   Primary syphilis chancre starts as dusky red, painless, non-itchy macule which soon become elevated to form a papule that finally ulcerates. Chancre is round, with well defined regular edges and indurated base.
2. B
   The most specific and easiest means of diagnosing syphilis is dark field microscopy. A positive result on microscopy is definitive evidence of syphilis
3. B
   Incubation period of syphilis is 9 -90 days.
4. B
   Primary, Secondary and Early latent Syphilis is treated with Inj benzathine penicillin 2.4 million units stat.

Reference:
1. Misra RS, Kumar J. Syphilis: Clinical Features and Natural Course. In: Sharma VK, editor .Sexually Transmitted Diseases and HIV/ AIDS. 2nd ed. New Delhi: Viva Books p262-326.

HAEMANGIOMA
Dr Parul Verma, Assistant professor, Department of Dermatology

A 2 month old male infant presented with multiple erythematous, well defined and partially blanchable plaques since birth. These plaques were distributed over trunk and limbs, 2-8 cm in size, increasing in size and were 6 in number. There was no bruit, thrill and no underlying soft tissue swelling. There was no systemic complaints and no limb girth discrepancy. Ultrasound abdomen to look for visceral involvement was normal. Parents were councelled regarding spontaneous resolution of lesions and no specific treatment was given.

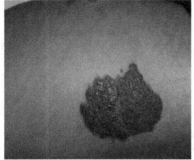

1. What is the most likely diagnosis
   (A) Haemangioma
   (B) Vascular malformation
   (C) Psoriasis
   (D) Lymphangioma
2. Following syndrome is associated with haemangiomas
   (A) PHACE syndrome
   (B) Proteus syndrome
   (C) Sturge Weber syndrome
   (D) K-T syndrome
3. Best way to manage haemangioms in above case
   (A) Treat with oral steroids
   (B) Treat with oral propanolol
   (C) Surgical intervention
   (D) Reassurance and clinical observation
4. Following are the treatment modalities for haemangioms except
   (A) Oral prednisolone
   (B) Oral propranolol
   (C) Topical timolol
   (D) Doxycycline

Answers:

   1. A
      Haemangiomas usually appear within first month of life and its natural progression shows a proliferation phase followed by involution.
   2. A
      PHACE (posterior fossa defects, haemangiomas, arterial anomalies, cardiac defects and eye abnormalities) syndrome is associated with haemangiomas, rest of the 3 syndromes mentioned above are associated with vascular malformations.
   3. D
      Spontaneous resolution is completed in 50% by 5 year, 90% by 9 year.
   4. D
      Oral steroid, prednisolone, topical timolol are known modalities to treat haemangioma whenever indicated.

References:

   1   Boon LM, Vikkula M. Vascular Malformations.In: Wolff K, Goldsmith LA, Katz SI, Gilchrest BA, Paller AS, Leffell DJ, editors. Fitzpatrick's Dermatology in General Medicine. 7th ed. New Delhi: McGraw Hill Medical; 2008. p 1651-60.
   2   Moss C, Shahidullah H. Naevi and other Developmental Defects. In: Burns T, Breathnach S, Cox N, Griffiths C, editors. Rook's Textbook of Dermatology. 8th ed. Singapore: Wiley- Blackwell; 2010. p18.40-52.

Chapter-7

Forensic Medicine & Toxicology

PRECIPITATE LABOUR

Dr. Raja Rupani, Assistant Professor, Department of Forensic Medicine & Toxicology

Dead body of a full term male baby was brought to morgue for PM examination. Mother was alleged to kill the baby. On examination the umbilical cord and placenta were present intact. On examination cyanosis was present on nails & lips, and a contusion of about 2X3 cm was present on scalp. Traces of faecal matter were seen in the trachea. There was no caput succedaneum.

1. What could be the most probable cause of death of baby?
   (A) Head injury
   (B) Choking
   (C) Haemorrhage
   (D) Drowning
2. Medico legally this death is –
   (A) Suicide
   (B) Homicide
   (C) Accidental
   (D) Natural
3. Which of the following term is best suited for this scenario –
   (A) Precipitate labour
   (B) Crib death
   (C) Infanticide
   (D) Caul birth
4. All of the following can be present in this type of birth, except:
   (A) Caput succedaneum
   (B) Tear of umbilical cord
   (C) Staining with faecal matter
   (D) Head injury
5. Which of the following is **not a favourable** condition in this type of birth?
   (A) Roomy pelvis
   (B) Small baby
   (C) Multipara
   (D) Obstructed

Answers:
1. B
    Although any one of the given options may be the cause of death in the present case but present case faecal matter in trachea and presence of cyanosis are suggestive of choking.
2. C
    As the death occurred due to fall in lavatory pan and aspiration of faecal matter, the case is accidental.
3. A
    In precipitate labour all the stages of labour merge and delivery occurs with in short time & baby falls on ground or in lavatory pan.
4. A
    Because caput succedaneum and cephalhematoma are features of obstructed labour, which does not occur in such cases.
5. D
    Because a, b & c facilitate precipitate labour but not obstructed labour.

Reference:
1. Mukherjee J B . Medicolegal aspects of sex and sex related offence. In Karmakar R N (Ed's) *Forensic medicine & Toxicology 4th edition*, Academic Publishers Kolkata 2011, pp.567-695

EXTRADURAL HAEMORRHAGE (EDH)

Dr. Raja Rupani, Assistant Professor, Department of Forensic Medicine & Toxicology

A young male going on bicycle was struck by a car from behind, fell down and lost consciousness. He was taken to the hospital where he regained consciousness. On examination he presented with hemiparesis & dilation of pupil on the opposite side, which was nonreactive to light.

1. Clinically this case appears to be the case of:
    (A) Extradural Haemorrhage
    (B) Subdural Haemorrhage
    (C) Subarachnoid Haemorrhage
    (D) Intracerebral Haemorrhage
2. Extra dural hemorrhage (EDH) is often associated with -
    (A) Concussion
    (B) Lucid interval
    (C) A + B
    (D) None
3. Most common artery involved in EDH due to lateral blow is:-
    (A) Anterior meningeal artery
    (B) Middle meningeal artery
    (C) Posterior meningeal artery
    (D) Meningeal vein
4. Following is true about EDH -
    (A) Seen in children, with pond fracture
    (B) Seen in young adults, with fissured fracture
    (C) Seen in elderly persons, with comminuted fracture
    (D) In all age groups, with any fracture
5. EDH has commonly the following features –
    (A) Venous blood, liquid or semi liquid, in temporo-parietal area
    (B) Arterial blood, oval or circular, in parieto-occipital area
    (C) Arterial & venous, oval or circular, within temporo-parietal area
    (D) Arterial, liquid or semiliquid in frontal area

Answers:

1. A

    As Extra dural hemorrhage (EDH) often follows unconsciousness due to concussion which recovers spontaneously and later cerebral compression, due to EDH presents with these features.

2. C

    Unconsciousness d/t cerebral concussion is followed by spontaneous recovery (Lucid Interval) and is again followed by unconsciousness, is a feature of EDH.

3. B

    Any blow over lateral convexity of head may most commonly injure posterior branch of middle meningeal artery in its posterior coarse across temporo-parietal region.

4. B

    EDH is rare in first 2 years of life d/t greater adherence of dura to skull & is common between 20-40 yrs and in 90% of cases the associated fracture is of fissured type, while SDH is common in children and elderly.

5. C

    EDH is arterial or venous or both and the clot is oval or circular in shape, rubbery in consistency, along the convexity of external surface of brain and usually occurs in temporo- parietal area.

Reference:

1. Mukherjee J B. Injury and its medicolegal aspects. In: Karmakar R N (Ed's)*Forensic medicine & Toxicology , 4th edition*: Academic Publishers, Kolkata,2011, pp 282-498

SUB ARACHNOID HAEMORRHAGE (SAH)

Dr. Raja Rupani, Assistant Professor, Department of Forensic Medicine & Toxicology

A young adult male was brought to the emergency. On examination, the patient was unconscious. Attendants gave the history of sudden onset of intense headache and photophobia. Further examination revealed presence of neck stiffness. On Lumbar puncture, blood tinged CSF mixed with blood was seen coming under pressure.

1. Diagnosis of this case is:
    (A) Extra Dural Hemorrhage
    (B) Sub Dural Hemorrhage
    (C) Sub Arachnoid Hemorrhage
    (D) Intra Cranial Hemorrhage

2. Non traumatic cause of Sub Arachnoid Hemorrhage include all except -
   (A) Rupture of Berry aneurism
   (B) Hypertension / degenerative arterial changes
   (C) Softening of brain due to anoxia
   (D) Severe atheroma/angioma
3. Traumatic causes of Sub Arachnoid Hemorrhage are all, except:
   (A) Rupture of basilar artery due to injury over base of skull.
   (B) Rupture of vertebral artery due to blow over upper side of neck
   (C) Traumatic asphyxia
   (D) Tear in dural venous sinus
4. Whether the bleeding was old or occurred after head injury can be confirmed by the presence of
   ....in the vessel wall and tissues :
   (A) Hemosiderin
   (B) Hemotoidin
   (C) Bilirubin
   (D) Biliverdin
5. Most common site of berry aneurysm is:
   (A) Anterior cerebral artery
   (B) Posterior communicating artery
   (C) Bifurcation of middle cerebral artery
   (D) Vertebral artery

Answers:
1. C
   Blood mixed CSF is suggestive of Subarachnoid haemorrhage which is also suggested by the history
2. C
   It is the cause of intra cerebral haemorrhage while others are causes of SAH
3. D
   Except d, which is a cause of SDH, all others cause SAH
4. C
   As it takes 4 days for hemosiderin to appear, so its presence in the vessel wall and tissues will establish previous leakage as a natural cause and not head injury
5. C
   In 90% of cases Berry aneurysm is found at this site, then followed by a, b and d.

Reference:
1. Mukherjee J B. Injury and its medicolegal aspects. In: Karmakar R N (Ed's)*Forensic medicine & Toxicology , 4th edition* ,Academic Publishers, Kolkata,2011, PP 282-498

DEFENCE WOUNDS
Dr. Raja Rupani, Assistant Professor, Department of Forensic Medicine & Toxicology

Ayoungmale was brought to the mortruary for autopsy. On external examination an elliptical stab wound was seen in the epigastric region. An incised wound (3.5 cm) was seen on right palm, about 4cm above the wrist and all the fingers were incised about 1cm above the base, except thumb. Another incised wound, about 4 cm, bone deep was present on the back of left hand.

1. The above case of stab injury is suggestive of to be:
   (A) Suicide
   (B) Homicide
   (C) Accidental
   (D) None
2. The injuries on palm are indicating of:-
   (A) Accidental incised wounds
   (B) Defence wounds
   (C) Suicidal wounds
   (D) Fabricated wounds
3. Defence wounds are usually present on following areas of body except:-
   (A) Palms and soles

(B) Extensor aspect of forearm
(C) Inner aspect of fore arm, arm and hand
(D) Flexor aspect of arms and legs
4. Defence wounds will be absent in all except –
    (A) If the person is asleep
    (B) If the person is concussed
    (C) Attack from front
    (D) Attack from behind
5. Nature of defence injuries depends on all except –
    (A) Nature of weapon
    (B) Degree of thrust
    (C) Type of attack
    (D) Built of victim

Answers:
1. B
    As stab wound in epigastrium is suggestive of homicide while incised wounds on palms and fingers suggest holding of blade of weapon as a defence phenomenon
2. B
    Injuries on palm occur due to holding of attacking weapon's blade in defence of the victim himself
3. D
    As a, b & c are areas used to stop the attacking weapon in standing or supine position
4. C
    As it is not possible in conditions like a, b & d to hold the weapon during attack
5. D
    Nature of defence injuries depend upon- the nature of weapon, whether sharp cutting or hard blunt, the degree of thurst, and the type of attack, whether stabbing or slashing.

References:
1. Mukherjee J B. Injury and its medicolegal aspects. In Karmakar R N (Ed's)*Forensic medicine & Toxicology, 4th edition*, Academic Publishers, Kolkata, 2011, pp 320-321

PUTREFACTION
Dr. Raja Rupani, Assistant Professor, Department of Forensic Medicine & Toxicology

A dead body was found in a locked room after the complain of foul smell being coming out by nearby residents. On examination face was swollen and distorted with blood stained discharge being coming out from mouth and nostrils. Blisters were present over different parts of the body with patchy dark greenish discolouration present all over the body.

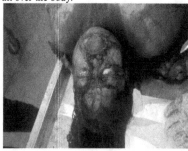

1. Above given features are suggestive of:
    (A) Burn
    (B) Asphyxia
    (C) Putrefaction
    (D) Poisoning
2. Most probable cause of blood stained discharge from mouth and nostrils in this case is
    (A) Poisoning
    (B) PM purge

(C) Strangulation

(D) Pulmonary edema

3. Features of antemortem blisters are:

(A) Presence of inflammatory fluid in side

(B) Base is white

(C) Red ring around the margin absent

(D) Presence of gas in the blister

4. Estimated time since death in the above case is :

(A) About one day

(B) 2-3 days

(C) 5-7 days

(D) >7 days

5. Which of the following is true regarding the order of the putrefaction in organs from earliest to last?

(A) Larynx and trachea> stomach and intestine > heart > prostate and uterus

(B) Larynx and trachea > prostate and uterus > heart > stomach and intestine

(C) Stomach and intestine >Larynx and trachea > prostate and uterus > heart

(D) Prostate and uterus > stomach and intestine > heart > larynx & trachea

Answers:

1. C

In dead bodies, putrefactive gases produced by bacteria, have foul smell and they also produce features of bloating , blisters & purging (d/t pressure effects). Colour changes are also due to sulphmethaemoglobin, formed by these bacteria.

2. B

Pressure effects of putrefactive gases in abdomen cause pressure over diaphragm, compressing lungs and heart & rupture of pulmonary vasculature, causing haemorrhage and blood stained discharge or P. M. Purging.

3. A

Antemortem blister contains inflammatory fluid rich in albumen, base of blister is congested and red ring is present around the margin; while b, c & d are features of P.M. blisters.

4. B

Colour changes d/t sulphmethaemoglobin starts in 1-2 days (earlier in summers) and spreads all over body & effects of putrefactive gases are noticed in 2-3 days (earlier in summers).

5. C

The first putrefactive change occurs in larynx and trachea, heart putrefies later than stomach and intestine, while prostrate and uterus being the fibromuscular organs putrefy last.

References:

1. Mukherjee J B. Death and its medicolegal aspects. In Karmakar R N (Ed's)*Forensic medicine & Toxicology* , 4th edition ,Academic Publishers, Kolkata,2011, pp 219-281

STARVATION

Dr. Raja Rupani, Assistant Professor, Department of Forensic Medicine & Toxicology

A beggar was found dead along road side and the body was brought by the police for autopsy examination. On examination the body showed general emaciation. Eye and cheek were shrunken. Abdomen was scaphoid with prominent ribs. Muscles atrophied and all organs reduced in size and all organs reduced in size and weight, except GB which was distended.

1. These findings are suggestive are suggestive of:

(A) Hypothermia

(B) Hyperthermia

(C) Starvation

(D) Septicaemic shock

2. Death in case of starvation may occur due to any of the following except:

(A) Exhaustion

(B) Circulatory failure

(C) Liver failure

(D) Infection

3. Pathological findings in case of starvation can be all except:
   (A) Brown atrophy of heart
   (B) Atrophy of brain
   (C) Centrilobular necrosis of liver
   (D) Granular degeneration of muscle fibres
4. Symptoms of starvation in a patient include all, except
   (A) Cardiovascular insufficiency
   (B) Diarrhoea and dysentery followed by constipation
   (C) Offensive odour before death
   (D) Occasionally delusions and hallucinations
5. Blood examination in case of starvation will reveal all, except:
   (A) ↓ protein
   (B) ↓ chloride
   (C) ↓ non protein nitrogen
   (D) ↑ urea

Answers:
   1. C
       Chronic starvation results in loss of weight, cachexia, absence of fat & atrophy of muscles and organs.
   2. C
       Death in starvation occurs d/t exhaustion, circulatory failure (d/t brown atrophy of heart) or intercurrent infection. Liver is atrophied and may show necrosis d/t protein deficiency.
   3. B
       In starvation there is reduction in size and weight of all organs except brain which is pale & soft, while a, c and d are features of starvation
   4. B
       In starvation constipation is usual, but towards death, diarrhoea and dysentery are common
   5. C
       Non – protein nitrogen is raised in starvation.

References:
   1. Mukherjee J B. Injury and its medicolegal aspects. In Karmakar R N (Ed's) *Forensic medicine & Toxicology* , 4th edition ,Academic Publishers, Kolkata,2011, pp 484-487

ALCOHOL
Dr. Shiuli, Lecturer, Department of Forensic Medicine & Toxicology

An episode of mass causality was reported from a village after drinking adulterated liquor. Those who survived had severe abdominal pain, cardiac depression, muscular weakness and visual disturbance.
1. What could be the possible adulterant?
   (A) Chloroform
   (B) Methanol
   (C) Diethyl ether
   (D) Methyl barbitone
2. Which is true regarding the absorption of ethyl alcohol?
   (A) 20% absorbed from stomach, 80% absorbed from small intestine
   (B) 80% absorbed from stomach, 20% from small intestine
   (C) Habituation increases the rate of absorption
   (D) Drinks mixed with carbonated soda decrease absorption
3. Toxicity of methyl alcohol is due to:
   (A) Acetaldehyde
   (B) Glycoaldehyde
   (C) Acetophenone
   (D) Formaldehyde
4. All of the following clinical syndromes can be seen in a chronic alcoholic except:
   (A) Confusional insanity
   (B) Korsakoff psychosis
   (C) Churg strauss syndrome
   (D) Delirium tremens

5. Principle of breath alcohol testing devices:
   (A) Chemical reaction involving alcohol that produces colour change.
   (B) Detects alcohol by infra red spectroscopy.
   (C) Detects chemical reaction involving alcohol by fuel cell.
   (D) All of the above

Answers:

1. B
   Methanol is used as adulterant in denatured alcohol
2. A
   20% of ethyl alcohol is absorbed from stomach and rest 80% from small intestine.
3. D
   Toxicity of methyl alcohol is due to its metabolite formaldehyde
4. C
   Churg strauss syndrome is an auto immune condition that causes vasculitis in persons 5.with history of allergy. Rest all are seen in persons with chronic alcohol abuse.
5. D
   All the given options are principle in various types of breath alcohol testing devices.

References:

1. Sage W. Wiener (2006). Toxic alcohols. In Lewis S. Nelson, Neal A. Lewin, Mary Ann Howland, Robert S. Hoffman, Lewis R. Goldfrank, Neal E. Flomenbaum (Eds.).:Goldfrank's*Toxicologic Emergencies* New York, NY: 9th edition , Tata Mc Graw Hill, pp1400 – 1410.

ALUMINIUM PHOSPHIDE

Dr. Shiuli, Lecturer, Department of Forensic Medicine & Toxicology

A young, 18 years male presented to emergency department with history of "rice tablet" ingestion. He was complaining of vomiting, diarrhea, ataxia, paresthesia, tremors and diplopia. There was hypotension which was refractory to dopamine therapy.

1. What could be the rice tablet?
   (A) Organophosphorus insecticide
   (B) Aluminium phosphide
   (C) Sodium chlorate
   (D) Zinc phosphide
2. What is the mechanism of action of aluminium phosphide as poison?
   (A) GABA antagonism
   (B) Liberation of phosphine gas
   (C) Sodium channel blocking
   (D) Inhibition of acetyl choline esterase
3. Mechanism of toxicity at cellular level are all except:
   (A) Reaction with cytochrome C, inhibiting mitochondrial O2 uptake
   (B) Blockage of oxidative phosphorylation
   (C) Lipid peroxidation
   (D) Generation of reactive oxygen species
4. Aluminium phosphide poisoning causes all, except:
   (A) Cardiogenic shock
   (B) Hypovolemic shock
   (C) Peripheral circulatory failure
   (D)Neurogenic shock
5. All are true regarding the PM findings in case of Aluminium phosphide poisoning, except:
   (A) Garlic odour
   (B) Blood stained froth
   (C) PM Caloricity
   (D) Congested organs

Answers:

1. B
   Aluminium phosphide is available in market as dark brown or grayish green tablets popularly known as rice tablets.
2. B

Liberation of phosphine gas
3. D
   No reactive oxygen species are generated, instead reactive hydroxyl radicals are generated
4. D
   Neurogenic shock is not seen in case of aluminium phosphide poisoning
5. C
   Postmortem caloricity i.e. rise of body temperature after death is not a feature of aluminium phosphide poisoning.

Reference:

1. Aggarwal A. In:Agricultural Poisons. Text book of Forensic Medicine & Toxicology, Avichal Publishing Company New Delhi 2014, 1ˢᵗ edition: pp598 – 612.

BURN

Dr. Shiuli, Lecturer, Department of Forensic Medicine & Toxicology

A charred body was recovered from a burn accident site with injuries over the head as shown in the picture.

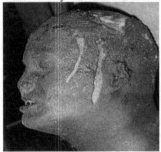

(photo Courtesy :Forensic Pathology Bernard Knight)

1. What is the most probable cause of the injury?
   (A) Post mortem injury caused by heat
   (B) Ante mortem assault
   (C) Putrefactive changes
   (D) Postmortem artifact
2. Regarding a burn which is true?
   (A) The adult formulae using rule of nine cannot be used in children
   (B) Scalds cause charring of skin
   (C) Trickle pattern is seen in dry burns
   (D) The rule of nine can be used in every adult irrespective of body wt.
3. All are true regarding ante mortem burn, except:
   (A) Line of redness present around the burn
   (B) Blisters contain air and clear fluid
   (C) Soot particles present in trachea
   (D) Carboxyhemoglobin present in blood
4. All of the following can be the cause of death in case of burn, except:
   (A) Neurogenic shock
   (B) Cardiogenic shock
   (C) Hypovolemic shock
   (D) Septicaemic shock
5. A patient has sustained burns to anterior chest and anterior abdomen. Using rule of nine, how much body surface area is affected?
   (A) 9%
   (B) 18%
   (C) 27%
   (D) 36%

Answers:
   1. A

Heated skin contracts markedly and splits often appear. This may lead inexperienced observers to suspect ante mortem wounds

2. A

The adult formula using "rule of nine" for calculating the burned area does not apply to infants whose body proportions are different from adults

3. B

Blisters of ante mortem burn contain serous fluid. Air filled blisters are characteristic of post mortem burn

4. B

Death can be caused in a burn victim by neurogenic shock due to pain, hypovolemic shock due to loss of fluid and later due to septicaemic shock as a result of spreading infection from the wounds

5. B

As per rule of nine, anterior chest + anterior abdomen is equal to 9% + 9% = 18%

Reference:

1. Knight B, Saukko P . Burns & scalds. In: *knight's Forensic Pathology*, Edward Arnold Ltd, London2004,3rd edition pp281- 295.

CANNABIS

Dr. Shiuli, Lecturer, Department of Forensic Medicine & Toxicology

A 35 years old male was arrested by the police while he was trying to commit suicide after killing his neighbour over some petty issue and stabbing two more. The subject was very lean and thin looked anaemic. His family members gave the history of some kind of drug abuse.

1. Which of the following term best describes the above condition?
   (A) Run amok
   (B) Risus sardonicus
   (C) Cocaine bugs
   (D) Cock walk

2. What is the most probable substance of abuse leading to above condition?
   (A) Alcohol
   (B) Cocaine
   (C) Cannabis
   (D) LSD

3. Which of the following is not a form of cannabis?
   (A) Ganza
   (B) Charas
   (C) Smack
   (D) Hashish

4. What is the specific antidote for cannabis?
   (A) Methylene blue
   (B) Dimercaprol
   (C) Sodium thiosulphate
   (D) No specific antidote

5. The principal constituents of cannabis responsible for its poisonous effects are:
   (A) THC
   (B) Tyramine
   (C) Canthradine
   (D) Aflatoxin

Answers:

1. A

Running amok is the homicidal mania developed under the influence of long continued use of cannabis

2. C

Cannabis is usually used in India as Ganja, Bhang, Charas (Hashish). Also known as Marijuana in America. Smack is another name for Heroine, a form of Morphine

3. C

As already explained in answer 1, long continued use of cannabis induces running amok

4. D

No specific antidote exists for cannabis. Treatment in case of cannabis poisoning is mainly symptomatic

5. A

The principal constituents responsible for its poisonous effects are – Cannabinol, Cannabidiol and THC (tetra hydro cannabinol)

Reference:

1. Michael A. McGuigan (2006).Cannabinoids. In Lewis S. Nelson, Neal A. Lewin, Mary Ann Howland, Robert S. Hoffman, Lewis R. Goldfrank, Neal E. Flomenbaum (Eds.), *Toxicologic Emergencies* New York, NY: Tata Mc Graw Hill.9th edition pp.1177 – 1184

CYANIDE POISONING

Dr. Shiuli, Lecturer, Department of Forensic Medicine & Toxicology

A male, 46 years old, overweight unexpectedly died during night. There was no history of any disease. He just emitted a loud scream, staggered into chair and died. Bloody froth was found dribbling out of his mouth. The standard toxicology screen, for common exposures such as narcotics and carbon monoxide, was clear. On autopsy, all viscera was congested, trachea contained blood stained froth, lungs edematous and post mortem staining of cherry red colour

1. What could be the possible cause of death
   (A) Heart failure
   (B) Cyanide poisoning
   (C) Organ phosphorus poisoning
   (D) Carbon monoxide poisoning
2. Which of the following can cause cyanide poisoning
   (A) Almonds
   (B) Cherry
   (C) Processed cassava
   (D) Apricot
3. Chronic exposure to cyanide is not associated with
   (A) Uterine carcinoma
   (B) Thyroid disorders
   (C) Tropical ataxic neuropathy
   (D) Tobacco amblyopia
4. At autopsy, the cyanide poisoning case will show the following features, except:
   (A) Characteristic bitter lemon smell
   (B) Congested organs
   (C) The skin may be pinkish or cherry red in colour
   (D) Erosion and haemorrhages in oesophagus and stomach
5. Which of the following antidotes is NOT used in cyanide poisoning:
   (A) Dicobalt EDTA
   (B) Hydroxycobalamine
   (C) Sodium nitrite
   (D) Dimercaprol

Answers:

1. B

Cyanide poisoning deaths are characterized by being abrupt & sudden, bloody froth from mouth, edematous lungs and cherry red PM staining.

2. C

Linamarin is the major cyanogenic glycoside in cassava roots. If processing is inefficient, linamarin and cynohydrin, the immediate product of hydrolysis of linamarin, remain in the food.

3. A

Chronic exposure to cyanide may result in insidious syndromes including tobacco amblyopia, tropical ataxic neuropathy, and Leber hereditary optic neuropathy.

4. A

Bitter almond smell is seen in cyanide poisoning cases not bitter lemon.

5. D

Dimercaprol is not used to treat cyanide poisoning.

Reference:
1. Christopher P. Holstege, Gary E. Isom, Mark A. Kirk (2006). Cyanide and Hydrogen Sulphide. In Lewis S. Nelson, Neal A. Lewin, Mary Ann Howland, Robert S. Hoffman, Lewis R. Goldfrank, Neal E. Flomenbaum (Eds.), *Toxicologic Emergencies* New York, NY: Tata Mc Graw Hill.9th edition pp 1678 – 1694.

DNA FINGER PRINTING
Dr. Shiuli, Lecture, Department of Forensic Medicine & Toxicology

Results from a single locus probe DNA fingerprint analysis for a man and woman and their four children are shown in the autoradiograph

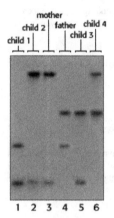

1. Which child is **least likely** to be the biological offspring of this couple?
   (A) Child 1
   (B) Child 2
   (C) Child 3
   (D) Child 4
2. Which of the following can be isolated from naturally shed hair?
   (A) Nuclear DNA
   (B) Mitochondrial DNA
   (C) Both of the above
   (D) None of the above
3. Each individual has a unique DNA fingerprint as individuals differ in
   (A) Number of minisatellites
   (B) Location of minisatellites
   (C) Size of minisatellites
   (D) All of these
4. DNA fingerprint pattern of a child is
   (A) Exactly similar to both the parents
   (B) Similar to father's DNA
   (C) Similar to mother's DNA
   (D) 50% similar to father & rest similar to mother
5. DNA fingerprinting relies on identifying minisatellites which are
   (A) Repetitive coding short DNA sequences
   (B) Repetitive non-coding short DNA sequences
   (C) Repetitive coding and non coding short DNA sequences
   (D) Non repetitive non coding short DNA sequences

Answers:
1. B

   If we match the locus in the given figure, child 2 has matching locus with the mother only, while all other have matching locus with both the parents. Thus child 2 seems to be related to mother but not to father (least likely the biological offspring of the couple)
2. B

   In a naturally shed hair, it is very unlikely to get nuclear DNA, but mitochondrial DNA which is present in abundance in a cell can be isolated. Nuclear DNA can be isolated from a plucked hair
3. D
4. D

   DNA fingerprint pattern of a child is 50% similar to mother and rest to father as half of the chromosomes (read DNA) comes from mother and rest from father
5. B

   More than 60% of the human genome sequence consists of intergenic non coding sequence located between genes. These contain large quantities of various types of repetitive DNA. One type is called minisatellite DNA.

Reference:
1. Li Richard(2008), Introduction to human genome.In: Forensic Biology Taylor & Francis group, 1st edition,Abingdon, pp 185 – 196.

LEAD

Dr. Shiuli, Lecturer, Department of Forensic Medicine & Toxicology

A man, 40 yrs was brought to the physician with complaints of abdominal colic, constipation, joint pain and decline in mental functioning and memory loss. There was no history of any chronic illness or occupational exposure. But the wife told that he has been using an ancient pewter mug which he bought from a local antique shop, for his drink

1. What could be the possible cause of the symptoms?
   - (A) Diabetic neuropathy
   - (B) Gout
   - (C) Lead poisoning
   - (D) Mercury poisoning
2. True about Lead colic is:
   - (A) Aggravated by pressure
   - (B) Relieved by pressure
   - (C) Not related to pressure
   - (D) More common in males
3. Blue lines on gum can be seen in all, except:
   - (A) Copper poisoning
   - (B) Lead poisoning
   - (C) Arsenic poisoning
   - (D) Bismuth poisoning
4. Which of the following is the lab finding in a case of lead toxicity:
   - (A) Pus cells in urine
   - (B) Basophilic stippling of RBC's
   - (C) Thrombocytopenia
   - (D) Sickle cell RBC's
5. Treatment of lead poisoning includes all except:
   - (A) Penicillamine
   - (B) Ca EDTA
   - (C) Desferoxamine
   - (D) BAL

Answers:
1. C

   Pewter is an alloy of tin (85 – 90%) as the main component and other metals like copper, antimony and bismuth and less commonly lead especially in lower grades of pewter. Pewter was used in

ancient times and used to be the chief tableware. Thus using pewter for drinking purpose for long can cause chronic lead poisoning.
2. B
Lead colic is characteristically relieved by pressure.
3. C
Blue line on gums is seen in: lead, copper sulphate, bismuth, silver, mercury.
4. B
Basophilic stippling
5. C
Desferroxamine

Reference:
1. Fred M. Henretig (2006). Lead. In :Lewis S. Nelson, Neal A. Lewin, Mary Ann Howland, Robert S. Hoffman, Lewis R. Goldfrank, Neal E. Flomenbaum (Eds.), *Toxicologic Emergencies* New York, NY: Tata Mc Graw Hill. 9th edition , pp1266 – 1283.

OPP

Dr. Shiuli, Lecturer, Department of Forensic Medicine & Toxicology

A 16 year old boy was brought to casualty with the history of some poison ingestion. The boy was restless & anxious. There was excessive salivation, lacrymation (red colored tears), profuse sweating, abdominal pain & diarrhea. Pupils were constricted and non reactive. Bradycardia and hypotension were also noted.

1. What is the most probable poisonous substance taken
   (A) Aluminium phosphide
   (B) Zinc phosphide
   (C) Organo phosphorus compound
   (D) Naphthalene
2. What could be the possible cause of red tears?
   (A) Blood in tears
   (B) Porphyrin
   (C) Dyes
   (D) Artefact
3. What is the pharmacological action of the poison in question?
   (A) Depression of cerebellum and motor cortex
   (B) Inhibition of acetyl choline esterase
   (C) Myocardial damage
   (D) Depression of bone marrow
4. All of the following can be used in the management of the above patient **except**
   (A) Atropine
   (B) Neostigmine
   (C) Pralidoxime
   (D) Artificial respiration
5. Most poisonous organophosphorus compound is:
   (A) Tetraethyl pyrophosphate
   (B) Hexaethyl pyrophosphate
   (C) Parathion
   (D) Malathion

Answers:
1. C
   Organophosphorus compound
2. B
   Presence of Porphyrin is the cause of red tears
3. B
   Inhibition of acetylcholine esterase resulting in rise of acetylcholine concentration is the mechanism of action
4. B
   OPP compounds act by increasing acetylcholine, so neostigmine is not to be given in the treatment.
5. A

Tetraethyl pyrophosphate is the most toxic while hexaethyl pyrophosphate is the least toxic organophosphorus compound.

Reference:

1. Michael Eddleston, Richard Franklin Clark (2006). Insecticides: Organic Phosphorus Compounds And Carbamates . In: Lewis S. Nelson, Neal A. Lewin, Mary Ann Howland, Robert S. Hoffman, Lewis R. Goldfrank, Neal E. Flomenbaum (Eds.), *Toxicologic Emergencies* New York, NY: Tata Mc Graw Hill,9th edition ,pp.1450 – 1466

SNAKE BITE

Dr. Shiuli, Lecturer, Department of Forensic Medicine & Toxicology

A man was working in the fields when he felt like he was bitten by some insect, though could not find or see anything. After few hours, he noticed his eyelids drooping and there was abdominal pain and blurring of vision.

1. What could be possible cause of his symptoms?
   (A) Scorpion bite
   (B) Anaphylactic reaction
   (C) Krait bite
   (D) Centipede bite
2. First aid after snake bite should include:
   (A) Immobilization of affected limb
   (B) Incision and washing of the bite
   (C) Suction of the bite area
   (D) Bandaging proximal to the bite area to prevent spread of toxin
3. Which of the following snakes is **not** included in the big four snakes of India?
   (A) King Cobra
   (B) Common Cobra
   (C) Common Krait
   (D) Russel's viper
4. Krait venom is:
   (A) Neurotoxic
   (B) Vasculotoxic
   (C) Myotoxic
   (D) All of the above
5. Viper bite is characterized by all except:
   (A) Bleeding from the bite site
   (B) Progressive paralysis
   (C) Coagulopathy
   (D) DIC

Answers:

1. A
   Krait bite often presents with minimal or no local signs and there is usually little or no pain
2. A
   Immobilization of the affected limb with the help of splint
3. A
   King cobra. The big four are – common cobra, common krait, saw scaled viper and russel's viper
4. A
   Krait and cobra belong to family elapidae and have neurotoxic venom
5. B
   Viper venom is vasculotoxic, characterized by features of incoagulable blood.

Reference:

1. Michael Eddleston, Richard Franklin Clark (2006), Neal A. Lewin, Mary Ann Howland, Robert S. Hoffman, Lewis R. Goldfrank, Neal E. Flomenbaum (Eds.). In: Snakes and other reptiles .Goldfrank's *Toxicologic Emergencies* New York, NY: Tata Mc Graw Hill,9th edition pp.1601-1611

STRYCHNINE

Dr. Shiuli, Lecturer, Department of Forensic Medicine & Toxicology

A child was brought to ED with markedly rigid and stiff muscles and arched body. Child was conscious with orientation to time, place & person. Parents gave the history of convulsion and also told that the child was seen chewing some disc like seeds while playing.

1. What could be the possible cause of child's condition?
    (A) Epileptic fits
    (B) Tetanus
    (C) Hysterical state
    (D) Nux vomica
2. What is the mechanism leading to this condition?
    (A) Inhibitory action on glycine
    (B) Inhibitory action on GABA
    (C) Excitatory action on glycine
    (D) Excitatory action on GABA
3. Feature of strychnine poisoning include all the following, **except:**
    (A) Convulsions
    (B) Cyanosis
    (C) Opisthotonus posture
    (D) Loss of consciousness
4. All is true regarding the management in the above case, **except:**
    (A) Induce emesis
    (B) Give activated charcoal
    (C) Barbiturates
    (D) Cooling with ice water
5. All is true in case of autopsy in the above case, **except:**
    (A) PM Caloricity
    (B) Cyanosis
    (C) Congested organs
    (D) Cherry coloured PM staining

Answers:
1. D
    Nux vomica is a tree native to tropical asia with characteristic disc like, grayish brown seeds.
2. A
    Glycine is one of the major inhibitory neurotransmitter in the spinal cord. Strychnine affects the binding glycine to a chloride channel thus having an inhibitory action on glycine.
3. D
    Strychnine poisoning is differentiated from generalized seizures by the presence of a normal sensorium
4. A
    Inducing emesis is absolutely contraindicated because of the risk of aspiration and loss of airway control following rapid onset of muscle contractions.
5. D
    Cherry coloured PM staining is seen in case of CO poisoning.

Reference:
1. Yiu-cheung Chan (2006). Strychnine. In: Lewis S. Nelson, Neal A. Lewin, Mary Ann Howland, Robert S. Hoffman, Lewis R. Goldfrank, Neal E. Flomenbaum (Eds.), *Toxicologic Emergencies*) New York, NY: Tata Mc Graw Hill, pp 1445 – 1447

VASO VAGAL SYNCOPE

Dr. Shiuli, Lecturer, Department of Forensic Medicine & Toxicology

A 14-year-old boy got into a fight with his elder brother and received blows against the chest and abdomen. The young boy fell down senseless on the floor and had a spasm. An ambulance was called, but he was declared dead on arrival to the hospital. An autopsy revealed no external injuries on the chest and abdomen. There was no evidence of preexisting disease.

The internal examination was completely unremarkable .No cerebral lesion no pericardial lesion. The heart was intact without any petechiae or anatomical alteration. No fat emboli. Microscopic examination of representative sections of all vital organs disclosed no abnormality.

1. What could be the possible cause of death?
    (A) Physiological changes associated with fight (↑ cardiac rate, ↑ BP, ↑ Catecholamines)
    (B) Cerebral concussion
    (C) Vasovagal syncope
    (D) Hypovolemic shock
2. What is the manner of death?
    (A) Homicide
    (B) Suicide
    (C) Accidental
    (D) None of the above
3. Vasovagal syncope is an example of
    (A) Neurogenic shock
    (B) Hypovolemic shock
    (C) Septicemic shock
    (D) Cardiogenic shock
4. What is the mechanism in vasovagal syncope?
    (A) Vagal inhibition
    (B) Vagal stimulation
    (C) Parasympathetic stimulation
    (D) Both b & c
5. What are the specific autopsy findings in vasovagal syncope?
    (A) Congestion
    (B) Petechiae
    (C) Goose Bumps
    (D) No Specific Findings

Answers:
    1. C
       Vasovagal syncopecan be triggered by sudden blows on the abdomen
    2. C
       Accidental– as the blows were unintentional
    3. A
       Neurogenic shock results from decreased vasomotor activity or increased parasympathetic discharge. Vasovagal syncope results when there is strong emotional reaction. This results in stimulation of parasympathetic nervous system thus decreasing the activity of heart and peripheral resistance.
    4. D
       Vagal stimulation and parasympathetic stimulation
    5. D
       There is no specific postmortem finding. Negative findings and history helps in making the diagnosis

Reference:
    1. Knight B, Saukko P (2004).Fatal Pressure on Neck,In: knight's Forensic Pathology,3rd edition Edward Arnold Ltd, London, pp 336-340

CRIMINAL ABORTION
Dr. Sangeeta Kumari, Lecturer, Department of Forensic Medicine & Toxicology

A young 25 years unmarried female was brought to the mortuary for autopsy. On detailed external and internal examination she was pale and findings suggestive of recent pregnancy like breast changes were present, vulva was bruised & blood clot was present in vagina. On internal examination there was excoriation & bruising of upper part of vagina. A punctured wound was present on fundus of uterus.

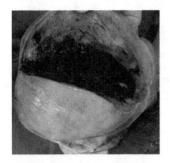

1. What is the most probable diagnosis-
    (A) Septicemia
    (B) Pelvic inflammatory disease
    (C) Criminal abortion
    (D) Air embolism
2. **True** about "Abortion sticks"
    (A) 12-18 cm long
    (B) Twig of calatropis , nerium odorum, cerebra thevatia or plumbago rosea used.
    (C) Induces uterine contractions
    (D) All of above
3. Ground for MTP in case of Pregnancy due to Rape :
    (A) Humanitarian
    (B) Social
    (C) Therapeutic
    (D) Health
4. True about MTP Act, 1971:
    (A) Consent of husband compulsory
    (B) Women needs proof of her age
    (C) Professional secrecy not to be maintained
    (D) MTP act is extremely liberal but it does not state that it is 'abortion on demand'
5. Emmenagogues:
    (A) Increases uterine contractions
    (B) Produce or increase menstrual flow
    (C) Acts indirectly on uterus producing congestion of pelvic organs.
    (D) Causes partial separation of placenta.

Answers:
    1. C
        Criminal abortion is the illegal act of expulsion of the products of conception when unskilled abortionist can cause local injury, uterine rupture and even death of the patient
    2. D
        Abortion sticks are 10 to 15 cm long thin pieces of wood or irritant plants which induces uterine contraction
    3. A
        When pregnancy is caused by rape
    4. D
        The medical termination of pregnancy act is said to be a permissive law but not a law of abortion on demand
    5. B
        Produce or increase menstrual flow

References:
    1. Mukherjee J B, Medicolegal aspects of sex and related offences. In: Karmakar R N (Ed's) *Forensic medicine & Toxicology*, 4th edition: Academic Publishers, Kolkata 2011: pp 567- 695.

DROWNING

Dr. Sangeeta Kumari, Lecturer, Department of Forensic Medicine & Toxicology

A 14 years female was missing from her house since morning. Her body recovered from Gomti River at mid night. The following day postmortem examination was done and following findings were observed –whole body swollen, face bloated & white froth coming from mouth & nostrils. On opening the chest cavity lungs appeared voluminous, bulky and on section trachea was filled with continuous column of froth. All the organs were found congested.

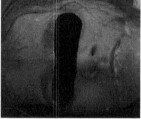

1. Most probable diagnosis:
    (A) Drowning
    (B) Putrefaction
    (C) Hanging
    (D) Hydrocution
2. Surest sign of **'Antemortem drowning'**
    (A) Washerwomen's hands & feet
    (B) Petechial haemorrhages in eyes
    (C) Gettler's Test
    (D) Oedema aquosum
3. Histological findings in cases of drowning:
    (A) Acute dilatation of alveoli.
    (B) Extension, elongation & thinning of septas
    (C) Compression of alveolar capillaries
    (D) All of above.
4. True about **'Hydrocution'**
    (A) Sudden blow of water upon the abdomen .
    (B) Sudden rise in arterial pressure & vagal output
    (C) Mild alcoholic intoxication
    (D) All of above.
5. True about "Cutis anserine " seen in drowning:
    (A) Antemortem phenomena
    (B) Commonly seen in India
    (C) Produced by rigor mortis
    (D) It is a "reaction phenomena"

Answers:
1. A
    Trachea filled with continuous column of froth and bulky lungs along with congested organs point towards drowning as the most probable diagnosis
2. C
    Gettler's test i.e. difference in chloride content between the right and left side of heart of more than 5% indicates antemortem drowning
3. D
4. D
5. D
    Cutis anserine is the puckered appearance of skin immersed in cold water, due to contraction of erector pilorum muscles

Reference:
1. Mukherjee J B, Violent Asphyxial Deaths. In: Karmakar R N (Ed) *Forensic medicine & Toxicology*,4th edition: Academic Publishers, Kolkata 2011: pp 499-566

CHOKING

Dr. Sangeeta Kumari, Lecturer, Department of Forensic Medicine & Toxicology

An unconscious person was brought to the emergency. Attendants gave the history that while having dinner the person grabbed his neck and suddenly collapsed. On examination he was found dead. On autopsy, alcoholic smell was coming from mouth. On internal examination, food bolus was seen in trachea. No other significant findings were seen:

1. What is the most probable diagnosis
   (A) Myocardial infarction
   (B) Café-coronary
   (C) Gagging
   (D) Mugging
2. The term **'Café coronary'** coined by:
   (A) Swann & spafford
   (B) Dr. Roger Haugen
   (C) Prinsloo & Gordon
   (D) R.V Verrier.
3. Cause of death in Choking:
   (A) Asphyxia
   (B) Vagal inhibition
   (C) Laryngeal spasm
   (D) All of above.
4. What is true about management of choking:
   (A) Heimlich maneuver
   (B) Tracheostomy
   (C) Blow on the back of sternum
   (D) All of above.
5. Choking is usually indicated by :
   (A) Universal distress signal
   (B) Coughing
   (C) Cyanosis
   (D) Sudden collapse

Answers:
1. B
   Café coronary is a condition met with, when a fatty intoxicated alcoholic, while taking his meal suddenly coughs and collapses and dies suddenly
2. B
3. D
   Death can occur in choking due to asphyxia or vagal inhibition or laryngeal spasm.
4. A
   Heimlich maneuver is an emergency technique for dislodging an obstruction from a person's windpipe by applying pressure over the epigastrium.
5. A
   A person with airway obstruction will probably clutch his throat. This clutching action is natural, but it has been adopted as the universal distress signal for choking. This sign alerts other people that the problem is an airway obstruction

Reference:
1. Mukherjee J B, Violent Asphyxial Deaths. In: Karmakar R N (Ed) *Forensic medicine & Toxicology*, 4th edition: Academic Publishers, Kolkata 2011: pp 499-566

HANGING

Dr. Sangeeta Kumari, Lecturer, Department of Forensic Medicine & Toxicology

A male prisoner, 35 years old died in the police custody. He was brought for postmortem examination. On external examination no signs of injuries or struggle were seen. Dried saliva dribbling marks were seen from angle of mouth. A ligature mark was seen on neck which was oblique, non-continuous, grooved, parchmentised and knot present on occipital region. Glove & stocking pattern of lividity was seen over extremities.

On internal examination, below the ligature mark subcutaneous tissue was dry, white, hard & glistening and all internal organs were found congested.

1. This case would be best categorized as:
   (A) Typical hanging
   (B) Atypical hanging
   (C) Judicial hanging
   (D) Incomplete hanging
2. All are findings suggestive of **"Antemortem Hanging "**, except:
   (A) Glove & Stocking lividity
   (B) Dribbling of saliva from angle of mouth
   (C) Discharge of fecal matter & urine.
   (D) Cyanosis over finger tips, nailbeds & lips.
3. True about **"Judicial Hanging"**
   (A) Unlawful homicide
   (B) Fracture vertebrae of C2- C3
   (C) Type of incomplete hanging
   (D) Not a form of judicial execution in India
4. True about "Custodial Death"
   (A) Reporting of custodial death within 24 hours.
   (B) Postmortem to be conducted by board of doctors
   (C) Elongated X shaped incision on back for subcutaneous tissue dissection for blunt injuries.
   (D)All of above.
5. Lynching is:
   (A) Practiced in North America
   (B) Homicidal hanging
   (C) Practiced by white people on Negroes
   (D) All of above.

Answers:

1. A
   Typical hanging is a form of hanging where the point of suspension is over the centre of occiput
2. A
   Glove and stocking lividity can be seen even in post mortem hanging
3. B
   Judicial hanging comes under lawful homicide where a long drop causes fracture dislocation of cervical vertebrae usually 3/4 or 2/3
4. D
   All the options are true for custodial death.
5. D
   Lynching was a method of homicidal hanging practiced in South America by white coloured people on Negroes charged of committing rape on a white girl

Reference:

1. Mukherjee J B, Violent Asphyxial Deaths. In: Karmakar R N (Ed) *Forensic medicine & Toxicology*, 4th edition: Academic Publishers, Kolkata 2011: pp 499-566

SEXUAL ASSAULT

Dr. Sangeeta Kumari, Lecturer, Department of Forensic Medicine & Toxicology

Naked body of a 35 years female was recovered from a sugarcane field and was brought to the mortuary for autopsy. On external examination finger nail marks were present over face & neck, a bruise 7cm x 6cm present over the right thigh. On genital examination labia majora & minora were bruised and blood clot was present in the vaginal. On internal examination a subdural haematoma present below the left temple.

1. From the above finding it appears to be a case of
   (A) Smothering
   (B) Strangulation
   (C) Sexual assault
   (D) Head injury

2. **"Unlawful sexual contact"** which lead to death or resulting in persistent vegetative state of victim is punished under section-
   (A) 376 A
   (B) 376 B
   (C) 376 C
   (D) 376 D
3. Age of female for giving consent for sexual intercourse as per Indian law is:
   (A) 16 years
   (B) 18 years
   (C) 21 years
   (D) 14 years
4. Which of the following shall not constitute Rape, as per Indian law:
   (A) Touching of Penis with labia majora without consent
   (B) Medical procedure or intervention without consent in emergency situation
   (C) Sexual intercourse by a man with his own wife, if she is less than 15 yrs
   (D) Sexual intercourse when wife is living separately from husband under a decree of judicial separation
5. Which of the following is a test done to detect vaginal cells during investigation for rape
   (A) Lugol's iodine test
   (B) Acro reaction test
   (C) Precipitin test
   (D) Barberio's test

Answers:
   1. C
       A naked body along with genital injury indicates this most probably to be a case of sexual assault
   2. A
       376 A
   3. B
       Age for giving consent for intercourse has recently been increased to 18 years which was 16 years previously
   4. B
   5. A
       Lugol's iodine test is done to detect the squamous epithelial cells from the vaginal epithelium which might be present on glans. These cells turn brown when exposed to the vapours of lugol's iodine .

Reference:
   1. Mukherjee J B, Medicolegal aspects of sex and sex related offence . In: Karmakar R N (Ed) *Forensic medicine & Toxicology*, 4th edition: Academic Publishers, Kolkata 2011: pp 567-695

SMOTHERING
Dr. Sangeeta Kumari, Lecturer, Department of Forensic Medicine & Toxicology

A 37 years old female was brought in the casualty with history of snake bite. After examination she was declared dead and sent to mortuary. On external examination 3 pin-point marks found on the left foot which were alleged to be fang marks but no swelling or erythema was seen around the marks. Bruises were present on nose & both cheeks and laceration was seen on the inner side of lower lip. Also bruises were present on both the wrists and right ankle. On opening, no swelling or tissue reaction was seen below the alleged fang marks. All the organs were found congested.

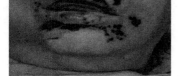

1. What is the most probable cause of death-
    (A) Blunt force injury
    (B) Respiratory arrest due to snake bite
    (C) Manual strangulation
    (D) Smothering
2. Bruise can be differentiated from postmortem lividity by-
    (A) On incision blood oozes out & can be easily washed off
    (B) On incision clotted blood & cannot be washed off
    (C) Blanches on application of pressure
    (D) Overlying tissue not damaged.
3. Hyoid fracture is most commonly seen in
    (A) Hanging
    (B) Ligature strangulation
    (C)Throttling
    (D) Mugging
4. "Spanish Windlass Technique"is used as a method of legal execution in
    (A) India
    (B) USA
    (C) Turkey
    (D) Ukraine
5. "Pseudo strangulation" is seen in
    (A) Obese
    (B) Infant
    (C) Person wearing tight collar.
    (D) All of above.

Answers:

1. D
    Smothering is a form of suffocation, where death is caused by closure of mouth and nostrils either by hand or any clothing, mud, sand or paper
2. C
    Colour of lividity blanches on application of pressure and reappears on release while pressure has no appreciable change on bruise
3. C
    Fracture of hyoid is the most diagnostic finding of throttling
4. C
    Spanish windlass is a device for tightening a rope, cable or other constricting device by twisting it using a stick as a lever. It was a form of judicial executing once practiced in Spain and Turkey
5. D
    Bands of contact flattening in the skin of the neck may simulate strangulation mark. These can be seen in an obese subject or a plump well nourished infant or if a dead body lies with a tight fitting collar band.

Reference:

1. Mukherjee J B, Violent Asphyxial Deaths. In: Karmakar R N (Ed) *Forensic medicine & Toxicology*, 4th edition: Academic Publishers, Kolkata 2011: pp 499-566

FOOD POISONING

Dr. Sangeeta Kumari, Lecturer, Department of Forensic Medicine & Toxicology

A 45 year old man working as a clerk in an office presents to the emergency department at 6pm with history of nausea, vomiting, diarrhea and abdominal colicky pain. On examination, there was no fever or any other finding. He told that he has taken fried rice in morning.

1. What is the likely etiology of above case?
    (A) Clostridium perfringens
    (B) Salmonella species
    (C) Shigella species
    (D) B.Cereus
2. Food borne illnesses are most commonly caused by
    (A) Bacterial contamination
    (B) Viral contamination

(C) Fungal contamination

(D) All of the above

3. Which of the followings may cause abdominal cramp,fever and bloody diarrhea?

    (A) Salmonella species

    (B) B.Cereus

    (C) Clostridium perfringens

    (D) S.aureus

4. All cause intoxication except?

    (A) S.aureus

    (B) B.Cereus

    (C) Clostridium botulinum

    (D) Salmonella species

5. Which of the following cause neurological symptoms?

    (A) Salmonella species

    (B) E.Coli

    (C) B.Cereus

    (D) Clostridium botulinum

Answers:

1. D

    B.Cereus produce exo-toxin

2. A

    Bacterial Contamination lead to 75 to 80% illnesses

3. A

    Salmonella species cause abdominal cramp,fever and bloody diarrhea

4. D

    Option a,b,c, causes intoxication while Salmonella species causes infection

5. D

    Clostridium botulinum

Reference:

1. Michael G. Tunik .Food Poisoning. In : Goldfrank's Toxicologic Emergencies,9th Edition. Mc Graw Hill, pp 668-675.

AGE ESTIMATION

Dr. Mousami Singh, Assistant Professor, Department of Forensic Medicine & Toxicology

A young female was brought by police for medico legal age estimation after an FIR was lodged by girl's father that his 16 year old daughter was abducted. On examination, 32 teeth were present in oral cavity and secondary sexual characteristics were well developed. On radiological examination, medial end of clavicle, lower end of radius and 3rd & 4th segment of body of sternum were fused; while 1st & 2nd segment were not fused.

1. What will be the approximate age in this case?

    (A) 12 – 14 yrs

    (B) 14 -16 yrs

    (C) 16 – 18 yrs

    (D) 20 – 25 yrs

2. At what age skull vault suture start fusing?

    (A)14 – 15 yrs

    (B) 24 – 25 yrs

    (C) 34 – 35 yrs

    (D) 44 – 45 yrs

3. Germination of teeth occurs during intra-uterine life for:

    (A) Temporary teeth

    (B) Permanent teeth

    (C) Germination occur after birth

    (D) A & B both

4. Most reliable method of age estimation is :

    (A) Stature

    (B) Weight

(C) Radiology of bones

(D) Secondary sexual characters

5. Calcification of roots of 3rd molars is absent in X ray. The presumed age is:

    (A) 12 to 14 year

    (B) 20 to 25 year

    (C) 25 to 30 year

    (D) 30 to 35 year

Answers:

    1. D

    2. C

    3. D

    4. C

    5. B

    Eruption of third molar is very irregular. They usually erupt by 17 to 25 years. Hence presences of all the third molars indicate that the subject is over 18 years of age, but their absence gives no certain idea about age. If the X-Ray shows no calcification of the roots of third molar, it is presumed that the age is below 25 years. If calcification is found to be complete, then the age can be presumed to be atleast 25 years. In general, complete calcification of the roots of teeth takes place within 3 to 4 years of their eruption.

Reference:

    1. Mukherjee JB, Personal identification, In: KarmarKar RN (Ed) forensic Medicine & Toxicology, 4th edition: Academic publishers, Kolkata 2011;pp 122-127

EMBOLISM

Dr. Mousami Singh, Assistant Professor, Department of Forensic Medicine & Toxicology

A 25 years female was brought for autopsy. On history she had 3 month pregnancy and has undergone recent D & C. On external examination no significant findings were found. And on internal examination lungs were congested and on sectioning of lung were showing multiple, minute fat globules. On dissection of heart a large 2cm x 2cm fat globule was seen in right ventricle, uterus was enlarged. Blood clots were present inside the uterus.

1. Most probable cause of death.

    (A) Septicaemia

    (B) Haemorrhagic shock

    (C) fat embolism

    (D)Vagal inhibition

2. Pulmonary embolus differentiated from postmortem clot by-

    (A) Are found often branched & frequently curled

    (B) Moist,smooth & rubbery in feel

    (C) Loosely or not at all attached to vessel wall

    (D) No line of Zahn

3. All are Causes of Fat embolism except-

    (A) Bone & fatty tissue injury

    (B) Osteomyelitis

    (C) Barotraumas

    (D) Faulty technique of giving intravenous injection

4. Amount of air sufficient to cause fatal air embolism

    (A)100-120 cc

    (B) 200-220cc

    (C) 300-320cc

    (D) 400-420 cc

5. Diagnosis of Fat embolism confirmed by microscopic examination of frozen sections stained by -

    (A) Haemalum and Sudan III

    (B) Scharlach R

    (C) Osmic acid

    (D) All of the above

Answers:

    1. C

Crushing or blunt force injuries and fracture of long bones destroys fat cells producing liquid fat which get forced into the torn vessels specially into veins in the vicinity of injury.The force of impact, muscular spasm and raised local pressure at the site of injury being greater than the venous pressure, will force the released fat into the injured veins and thus fat embolism will occur.

2.   A
3.   D
4.   A
5.   D

References:
1.   Mukherjee J B,Injury and its Medicolegal Aspects. In: Karmakar R N (Ed) *Forensic medicine & Toxicology*, 4th edition: Academic Publishers, Kolkata 2011: pp 442-445
2.   Sydney Smith SIR ,Injury. In:Taylor'principles and practice of medical jurisprudence :J.&A. Churchill 1956.P.241

FABRICATED WOUND

Dr. Mousami Singh, Assistant Professor, Department of Forensic Medicine & Toxicology

A 27 year old married female lodged FIR against her in laws, husband & sister in law that they injured her by giving electric current on different parts of body. She was brought for medicolegal examination after 15 days of incident. On examination we found (1) Three healed scar marks of superficial injury on left thigh 6.5 cm above left knee joint (2) Three healed scar marks of superficial injury on right thigh 9cm above right knee joint (3) Three linear healed scar marks of superficial injury irregularly present on left arm 19cm.below left acromian process.(4) Three linear healed marks of superficial injury were present over front of right arm 14cm below right acromian process. (5) A linear abrasion on medial side of right leg was present 9cm below right knee joint .Scab was present over the wound.(6) Three linear healed marks of superficial injury were present on left leg; all 19cm below left knee joint. History did not correlate with the age and feature of injuries. The characteristic features of electrical injuries were absent.

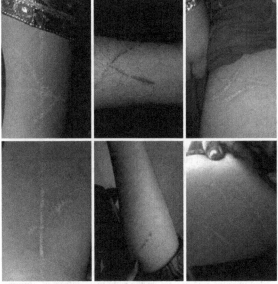

1. Electrical injury are characterized by-
    (A) Crater with pale floor
    (B) Metallization
    (C) Charring
    (D) All of the above
2. Characterstics feature of fabricated wound is/are-
    (A) Multiple & superficial
    (B) Parallel & mirror image pattern
    (C) On accessible areas

(D) All of the above

3. Most common type of fabricated wound is-
    (A) Incised
    (B) Burn
    (C) Contusion
    (D) Firearm
4. Which of the following fact is true about homicide wound
    (A) Multiple in number
    (B) Incised wound
    (C) Over Vital parts
    (D) Presence of tentative cuts
5. All are true about acroreaction test except-
    (A) It demonstrate metallization
    (B) Applicable for exit marks
    (C) Definite evidence of electrical burn
    (D) In this test skin is treated with acid
6. Histological examination of skin of entry wound reveals all except-
    (A) No effect on epidermal cells
    (B) Presence of microblisters
    (C) Presence of vacuolation
    (D) Collagen stains blue in ordinary H & E stains

Answers:
    1. D
        Electrical entry wound is characterized by crater,produced due to melting of keratin.keratin melts due to endogenous heat generated while paleness of floor is caused by ischaemia and coagulation of blood.
    2. D
    3. A
    4. C
    5. B
        Acroreaction test is a microchemical test for metals.it is applicable for entry marks.
    6. A
        The epidermis is elevated with microblisters developing with in the squamous epithelium as well as in the external horny layer.These blisters result from the cooking effect on the tissues.cells are separated in the form of sharp splits.this pattern is known as vacuolation.

References:
1. Reddy N, Murty OP, Thermal Deaths .In: The essentials of forensic medicine and toxicology 32nd edition: K.Suguna Devi 2013:pp 314-318
2. Aggarawal A ,Electrical injuries,Atomspheric Lightening,Radiaion Injuries. In:Textbook of forensic medicine and toxicology,1st edition:Avichal publishing company2014: pp 316-323
3. Mukherjee J B, Violent Asphyxial Deaths. In: Karmakar R N (Ed) *Forensic medicine & Toxicology*, 4th edition: Academic Publishers, Kolkata 2011: pp 401-405
4. Sydney Smith SIR ,Injury. In:Taylor'principles and practice of medical jurisprudence :J.&A. Churchill 1956 ,pp 407-419

FIRE ARM INJURIES
Dr. Mousami Singh, Assistant Prof, Department of Forensic Medicine & Toxicology

A 38 year old male was found dead in his bedroom with gun tightly clutched in his right hand. On examination, a large irregular stellate shaped wound with everted margins was present on the right mastoid region. Burning and blackening were present around the wound while track was cherry red in color.

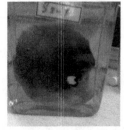

1. At what distance the firearm was discharged-
    (A) Contact shot
    (B) Close shot
    (C) Near shot
    (D) Distant shot
2. Primary and secondary markings on a metal bullet can be used for-
    (A) Identification of weapon
    (B) To know the range of firing
    (C) Severity of tissue damage
    (D) To know the time of crime
3. The most sophisticated and qualitative tool for detecting minute traces of gun shot residues on body of suspect-
    (A) SEM-EDXA
    (B) FAAS
    (C) Harrison and Gilroys test
    (D) Dermal nitrate test
4. Which of the following fact suggest, that the death was suicidal in nature-
    (A) Gun tightly clutched in right hand
    (B) Stellate shaped
    (C) Everted margin
    (D) Cherry red color
5.Which of thefollowing feature is suggestive of contact wound-
    (A) Inverted edge
    (B) Everted edge caused by gases
    (C) Burning and singeing of hair
    (D) Tattooing

Answers:
    1. A
        Appearance of entry wound is influenced by range of firing.
    2. A
    3. A
        As a gun is fired, the GSR comprising chemical substances that burn and produce gases providing the velocity for the bullet, and metals such as antimony, barium, copper etc.are also sprayed out and get deposited on the hands, clothes and even on the face of the person.In this gunshot residues are removed from the body using adhesive lifts.The material removed is scanned with SEM for the gunshot residues particles.The X-ray analysis capability is used to identify the chemical elements in each of the particles.the test is positive up to 12 hours after firing.
    4. A
    5. B

References:
    1. Reddy N, Murty OP, Mechanical Injuries .In: The essentials of forensic medicine and toxicology 32nd edition: K.Suguna Devi 2013:pp 198-228
    2. Mukherjee J B, Mechanical Asphyxial. In: Karmakar R N (Ed) *Forensic medicine & Toxicology*, 4th edition: Academic Publishers, Kolkata 2011: pp 338-373

INFANTICIDE

Dr. Mousami Singh, Assistant Professor, Department of Forensic Medicine & Toxicology

A dead body of a 16 day old male infant was brought to the mortuary for autopsy.It was claimed that death occurred after giving oral polio vaccine. Autopsy surgeon enquired the parents about the incidence and it was revealed that the father was out for work and the mother was alone so she gave the child to his aunt to take care. The aunt came after 20 min. with a dead child and said that the child suddenly stopped responding. The mother rushed to the hospital where the child was declared dead. On examination, no significant external finding was present. On internal examination hematoma was found in between duramater and arachnoid.

1. What will be the most probable cause of death-
    (A) Subdural hemorrhage
    (B) Subarachnoid hemorrhage
    (C) Extradural hemorrhage
    (D) Intracerebral hemorrhage

2. Most common artery involved in extradural hemorrhage caused due to blow over forehead-
    (A) Middle meningeal artery
    (B) Anterior ethmoidal artery
    (C) Sagittal sinus
    (D) Transverse sagittal sinus
3. A women delivered child when she was standing. The child fell down due to tear of umbilical cord. The most
    common site of tearing of umbilical cord is at the-
    (A) Fetal end
    (B) Maternal end
    (C) Middle
    (D) Not specifc
4. A minimum fall of _____ cm. can cause fracture of skull-
    (A) 25
    (B) 45
    (C) 35
    (D) 55
5. Head moulding during labour in newborn may cause subdural hemorrhage due to rupture of-
    (A) Middle meningeal artery
    (B) Circle of willis
    (C) Vein of galen
    (D) Superior saggital sinus

Answers:
    1. A
        As oral polio vaccine is a safe remedy. No cases of mortality has been reported yet.In internal
        examination hematoma found in subdural space so most probable cause of death is subdural
        hemorrhage due to some blunt trauma or fall.
    2. B
        The vessel injured in extradural hemorrhage depends upon the site of trauma.A blow over forehead
        involves the anterior ethmoidal artery.
    3. A
        Tearing of cord commonly occurs at the foetal end than at the maternal end and rarely at middle.
    4. B
        A minimum fall of 45 cm.can cause of fracture of skull. The average distance of the female
        genitals from the ground in erect position is 75 cm.The average length of the umbilical cord is 50
        cm.
    5. C
        Subdural hematoma may occur in newborn due to head moulding during labour due to rupture of
        vein of galen or tentorial tear usually in posterior fossa and massive in amount.

References:
    1. Reddy N, Murty OP,Regional Injuries.In: The essentials of forensic medicine and toxicology 32nd
        edition: K.Suguna Devi 2013:pp 245-249
    2. Mukherjee J B,Injuries and its Medicolegal Aspects. In: Karmakar R N (Ed) *Forensic medicine &
        Toxicology*, 4th edition: Academic Publishers, Kolkata 2011: pp 401-405

SULPHURIC ACID
Dr. Mousami Singh, Assistant Professor, Department of Forensic Medicine & Toxicology

A young male was brought to emergency with complaints of severe pain in mouth, throat, and stomach. Mucosa
of mouth and lips were swollen and covered with brownish black necrotic membrane. The saliva dribbling from
mouth was causing brownish discolouration of the skin. Patient gave history of drinking something from a glass
bottle which he thought of as soft drink.

1. What could be the possible liquid in the bottle?
    (A) Ammonia solution
    (B) Sulphuric acid
    (C) Caustic soda
    (D) Carbolic acid
2. Which of the following is not true regarding management in the above case:
    (A) Use of strong alkalies should not be done

(B) Stomach wash with stomach tube should be done

(C) Emetics should not be given

(D) Morphine can be given to relieve the pain

3. All of the following can cause death in the above case, except:

(A) Shock

(B) Perforation

(C) Spasm or edema of glottis

(D) Hepatic failure

4. If immediate death occurs in this case, all the following can be seen during autopsy, except:

(A) Stomach looks like soft, spongy mass.

(B) Perforation of stomach

(C) Stricture oesophagus

(D) Upper GI is inflamed and swollen.

5. Throwing of acid over the face or body of someone with the intention of disfiguration comes under which IPC:

(A) Sec 335

(B) Sec 375

(C) Sec 326

(D) Sec 354

Answers:

1. B

Sulphuric acid causes necrosis and brownish black discoloration of mucosa

2. B

Stomach tube should not be used in case of any caustic poisoning as it can cause perforation of an already softened git

3. D

Hepatic failure is not a cause of death in case of sulphuric acid poisoning

4. C

Stricture oesophagus is a long term sequel of sulphuric acid poisoning, not seen in immediate death.

5. C

Acid throwing or vitriolage comes under sec 326 IPC.

Reference:

1. Jessica A. Fulton . Caustics. In: Goldfrank's *Toxicologic Emergencies* , 9th edition: Tata Mc Graw Hill, pp 1364 – 137155

Chapter-8

Geriatric Mental Health

ALZHEIMER'S DISEASE

Dr. Shailendra M. Tripathi, Assistant Professor, Department of Geriatric Mental Health

A 72 year old gentleman, retired science teacher in a higher secondary school was brought in the OPD with history of progressive loss of memory over the last two years. Specifically he would read the newspaper or magazine and forget what he had read. For last eight months he would immediately forget what was said. His son noticed his financial records to be in mess. Most recently he was lost his way while coming from his relative's house hardly one mile away from his house. There is no history of previous stroke, depression, diabetes mellitus or hypertension. His physical examination is normal. Mental status testing reveals normal affect. Mini Mental State Examination was 19/30. The detailed higher mental function assessment revealed abnormality in memory and new learning ability followed by calculation and constructional ability. His MRI brain reveals diffuse cerebral atrophy. His complete blood count, electrolyte, glucose, thyroid function test were within normal limits.

1. What is the most likely diagnosis?
   (A) Dementia due to Frontotemporal degeneration
   (B) Dementia due to Alzheimer's disease
   (C) Dementia due to Lewy body disease
   (D) Dementia due to Vascular disease
2. The most important risk factor for dementia due to Alzheimer's disease is
   (A) Obesity
   (B) Smoking
   (C) Age
   (D) Hypertension
3. The most frequent first symptom in Alzheimer's disease is:
   (A) Memory impairment
   (B) Naming difficulties
   (C) Visuospatial abilities
   (D) Executive dysfunction
4. The mutations in genes on chromosomes **NOT** associated with risk of Alzheimer's disease is:
   (A) 1
   (B) 7
   (C) 14
   (D) 21
5. The most common gene associated with the risk of Alzheimer's disease is:
   (A) Sortilin-1
   (B) APOE-4
   (C) presenilin-1
   (D) presenilin-2

Answers :

1. B
   This case shows the typical features seen in Dementia due to Alzheimer's disease
2. C
   Age is the single most important risk factor in Alzheimer's dementia with rates doubling every decade after age of 60 and almost 50% of over 80 year olds suffer from AD
3. A
   Memory impairment is seen first in patients with Alzheimer's disease
4. B
   Mutations on chromosome 7 are associated with Fronto temporal dementia
5. B
   APO E-4 is the most common gene associated with the risk of Alzheimer's disease

References:

1. Blazer DG, Steffens DC. Textbook of Geriatric Psychiatry, 4th Edition, American Psychiatric Publishing, Inc, Washington, DC 2009. Pp247-249.
2. Tripathi M. Dementia Decoded. Kontentworx, New Delhi, 2014. Pp137-144.

FRONTO-TEMPORAL DEMENTIA

Dr. Priti Singh, Assistant Professor, Department of Geriatric Mental Health

A 60 year old shop assistant attended the Memory clinic with family members concerned regarding change in his behavior with increased aggressiveness and severe change in his social manner over the last 2 years. He was initially treated for agitated depression but gradually his condition continued to worsen. He was also sacked from his job after series of unacceptable behavior including making lewd remarks at customers and staff. He was also noted to be hoarding items for no reason and engaging in purposeless activities. His wife described a significant change in his eating habits and increased preference for sweets with inappropriate lack of social inhibition in public. On examination the patient denied any problems and his MMSE was 27/30. CT Scan Head showed significant atrophy of frontal lobes.

1. What is the most likely diagnosis?
   (A) Dementia due to Frontotemporal degeneration
   (B) Dementia due to Alzheimer's disease
   (C) Dementia due to Lewy body disease
   (D) Dementia due to Vascular disease
2. Incidence of Fronto-Temporal Dementia is:
   (A) equal to that of Alzhiemer's disease in elderly
   (B) equal to that of Alzhiemer's disease in the young onset dementia
   (C) higher than Alzhiemer's Dementia in the Young onset dementia
   (D) Lower than Alzhiemer's Dementia in the Young onset dementia
3. Which of the following in NOT a type of Frontotemporal dementia:
   (A) Behavioural variant
   (B) Logopenic variant
   (C) Semantic variant
   (D) Progressive non fluent aphaisa
4. Which statement of the following regarding Fronto temporal dementia is TRUE:
   (A) It is more common in females
   (B) It is more common above the age of 60 yrs
   (C) with the onset of Semantic Dementia, speech becomes more effortful and agrammatic
   (D) with the frontal variant, day to day memory is relatively unaffected
5. Which neurological condition is associated with Fronto temporal dementia:
   (A) Multiple Sclerosis
   (B) Parkinson's disease
   (C) Guillian Barre
   (D) Motor neuron disease

Answers :

1. A
   Fronto-temporal dementia of the behavioural variant presents with early onset behavioural changes commonly mistaken for a functional mental illness.
2. D
   Fronto-Temporal dementia is more common in the younger age group but the incidence is still only 13% compared to that of 31% in Alzheimer's Dementia in the Young.
3. B
   Logopenic Dementia is a variant of Alzhiemer's disease which presents primarily with Language impairment
4. D
   In behavioural variant of Fronto temporal dementia, memory is usually well preserved in the early stages of illness.
5. D
   The rate of dementia in MND is much higher than expected, with up to 10% of patients with MND show features of dementia. These patients typically have an aggressive course of illness.

References:

1. Vincent Deramecourt, Florence Lebert and Florence Pasquier. Fronto Temporal Dementia. In: Tom Denning, Alan Thomson. Oxford Textbook of Old age Psychiatry. 2nd ed. Oxford: Oxford University Press; 2013. p 480- 490
2. Jefferies K, Agrawal N. Early-onset dementia. Adv Psychiatr Treat. 2009 Sep 1;15(5):380–8.

NEUROPSYCHIATRIC ASPECTS OF PARKINSON'S DISEASE
Dr. Priti Singh, Assistant Professor, Department of Geriatric Mental Health

A 76 year old retired railway officer presented with a gradual deterioration of his memory with recent onset of sleep disturbance with periods of lashing out his arms and screaming in his sleep. His wife was also concerned about periods where she described him seeing imaginary children and animals and would insist that his wife bring them into the house. The patient had a known history of Parkinson's disease(PD) for 5 years and was on regular treatment. On examination, his MMSE was 20/30 loosing significantly in the memory and visuo-spatial scores. MRI brain showed age related atrophy with some ischemic demyelination in sub-cortical areas.

1. Which of the following is the most common neuropsychiatric disorder in Parkinson's disease:
   (A) Depression
   (B) Psychosis
   (C) Impulse control disorders
   (D) Dementia
2. Which one of the following statements is FALSE about Psychosis in PD:
   (A) The most frequent psychotic phenomenon in PD is visual hallucinations
   (B) Visual hallucinations are generally associated with treatment with dopaminergic drugs
   (C) The most common delusions in PD are grandiose in nature
   (D) The prevalence of psychotic phenomenon in PD is 30-40%
3. Which of the following is TRUE regarding treatment of psychosis in PD?
   (A) The first step in treatment of psychosis in PD is to increase dose of dopaminergic drugs
   (B) The antipsychotic drug with the highest evidence in treatment of psychosis in PD is clozapine
   (C) Atypical antipsychotics are not associated with worsening of motor symptoms of PD
   (D) There is no evidence that cholinesterase inhibitors have any role in treatment of psychosis in PD
4. Which one of the following statements is FALSE about Cognitive impairment in PD:
   (A) 20-30% patients with PD will eventually also be diagnosed with Dementia
   (B) In patients with PD a reduced speed of information processing is usually seen
   (C) Both limbic/ paralimbic and pre-frontal areas are involved in dementia of PD
   (D) Cholinesterase inhibitors are not useful in improving cognition in PD
5. There is an evidence base for which one of the following drug groups being effective in the symptomatic treatment of dementia in Parkinson's disease?
   (A) Nootropics
   (B) Cholinesterase inhibitors
   (C) Cholinergic drugs
   (D) Dopamine agonists

Answers:
1. A
   Depression is the commonest neuropsychiatric condition in Parkinson's disease with up to 50% of patients of PD suffering from this condition
2. C
   Delusions of Paranoia are the most common delusions seen in PD
3. C
   Most Anti-psychotic medication have anti dopaminergic properties and tend to worsen the motor symptoms of PD
4. D
   There is some evidence that Cholinesterase inhibitors may improve psychotic symptoms presenting in PD although no large studies exist in this area

5. B
   There is good evidence that cholinesterase inhibitors are useful in improving cognitive deficits in Dementia with PD

References:

1. Ehrt U, Aarsland D. Psychiatric aspects of Parkinson's disease. Curr Opin Psychiatry. 2005 May;18(3):335–41.
2. Aarsland D, Ballard C, Rongve A, Broadstock M, Svenningsson P. Clinical trials of dementia with Lewy bodies and Parkinson's disease dementia. Curr Neurol Neurosci Rep. 2012 Oct;12(5):492–501.
3. Ravina B, Putt M, Siderowf A, Farrar JT, Gillespie M, Crawley A, et al. Donepezil for dementia in Parkinson's disease: a randomised, double blind, placebo controlled, crossover study. J Neurol Neurosurg Psychiatry. 2005 Jul;76(7):934–9.

ELECTROCONVULSIVE THERAPY

Dr. Priti Singh, Assistant Professor, Department of Geriatric Mental Health

An 80 year old widower was admitted to hospital with severe reduction in interaction with others, minimal food and water intake and persistent low mood with several nihilistic ideations. He had received treatment with various antidepressants in the last 6 months but did not show much improvement. It was decided to commence him on Electroconvulsive therapy and within 4 sessions of this treatment the patient made significant recovery.

1. ECT would not usually be the first line treatment in the following conditions:
   (A) Paranoid Schizophrenia
   (B) Bipolar affective disorder with depression
   (C) Mania
   (D) Major depressive disorder
2. The highest rates of remissions are seen in which one of the following conditions:
   (A) Mania
   (B) Major depression, psychotic subtype
   (C) Unipolar depression without psychosis
   (D) Treatment resistant depression
3. The rates of remission after ECT treatment is
   (A) 30%
   (B) 40%
   (C) 50%
   (D) 75%
4. Which of the following statements is FALSE regarding Cognitive adverse effects of ECT treatment
   (A) Electrode placement is the single most important factor in cognitive adverse effects
   (B) Anterograde amnesia is a natural consequence of the post-ictal phase of ECT
   (C) ECT can cause permanent brain damage
   (D) Retrograde amnesia can occur in some cases but most patients recover these memories within six months
5. Which of the following is a contraindication for ECT treatment
   (A) Age
   (B) Cognitive impairment
   (C) Lack of Consent
   (D) Comorbid diagnosis of epilepsy

Answers:

1. A
   ECT is not routinely used as first line in treatment of Paranoid Schizophrenia
2. B
   The highest rates of remission with ECT are seen with Major depression with psychosis
3. D
   The overall remission rate for ECT treatment is around 75%

4. C
   ECT may cause retrograde amnesia in a few minority patients but does not cause any brain damage.
5. C
   There are no absolute contraindications for ECT but a valid consent is necessary for treatment

References:

1. Heijnen WT, Birkenhäger TK, Wierdsma AI, van den Broek WW. Antidepressant pharmacotherapy failure and response to subsequent electroconvulsive therapy: a meta-analysis. J Clin Psychopharmacol. 2010 Oct;30(5):616–9.
2. Ottosson J-O, Odeberg H. Evidence-based electroconvulsive therapy. Acta Psychiatr Scand. 2012 Mar;125(3):177–84.

MARCHIAFAVA- BIGNAMI DISEASE

Dr. Shailendra M. Tripathi, Assistant Professor, Department of Geriatric Mental Health

A 61 year old chronic alcoholic, presented with 7 days history of speech disturbances and gait abnormality. 3 days prior to the admission he had seizures and altered sensorium. He had been consuming average 300 ml of alcohol for last 30 years. There was no history of vaccination or prior fever. Examination revealed signs of malnutrition but no signs of liver failure. Signs of meningeal involvement were absent. Motor examination revealed normal power in all limbs with increased tone and brisk reflexes with extensor planter bilaterally. Gait was wide based and spastic. MRI brain shows hyperintense lesion in central portion of corpus callosum. EEG suggested diffuse slowing. All other blood and CSF parameters were normal.

1. What is most likely diagnosis?
   (A) Delirium tremens
   (B) Alcoholic dementia
   (C) Marchiafava bignami disease
   (D) Wernicke- korsakoff syndrome
2. Hallmark of the Marchiafava Bignami Disease is:
   (A) Acute demyelination of corpus callosum
   (B) Atrophy of the mid brain
   (C) Atrophy of mammillary bodies
   (D) Enlargement of the third ventricles
3. Following can be manifestation of Marchiafava Bignami disease EXCEPT:
   (A) Left hand anomia
   (B) Apraxia
   (C) Agraphia
   (D) Hemineglect
4. Following is NOT TRUE regarding Marchiafava Bignami disease?
   (A) Moderate atrophy of posterior callosal region
   (B) Severe atrophy of anterior callosal region
   (C) Diminished signal intensity with gadolinium involvement in corpus callosum on T1W images
   (D) Increased brain metabolism in frontal and parietal region
5. What is the treatment of Marchiafava Bignami disease?
   (A) 500 mg/day of Thiamine daily IM for 14 days then once weekly for 1 month
   (B) 1000 mcg of methylcobalamine once daily for 5 days.
   (C) 5 mg of folic acid once daily
   (D) 6.67 mg of pyridoxine thrice daily

Answers:

1. C
   The case summary highlights important clinical features of Marchiafava bignami disease
2. A
   Acute demyelination of corpus callosum is hallmark of this disease
3. D
   Hemi neglect is not usually seen in Marchiafava bignami disease

4. D

Brain metabolism in frontal and parietal region is not increased

5. A

Intensive replacement of Thiamine is the main stay treatment of this condition

References:

1. Tripathi M. Dementia Decoded. Kontentworx, New Delhi, 2014. pp89-92.

LATE ONSET MANIA

Dr. Shailendra M. Tripathi, Assistant Professor, Department of Geriatric Mental Health

A 72-year-old married Muslim male, farmer by occupation, presented with history of five days duration with complaints of unduly cheerful mood, over-talkativeness, aggressive behavior and decreased sleep. There was no past or family history of any medical or psychiatric illness. There was no history of any substance abuse/dependence or any history of drug use. There was no associated history of any loss of consciousness, forgetfulness, head injury, or urinary / fecal incontinence. He was well adjusted premorbidly. Mental status examination at the time of presentation revealed an authoritative elderly male with adequate grooming and hygiene, increased psychomotor activity, elated affect, ideas of grandiosity and insight Grade I/V. His mini mental status examination revealed a score of 26/30.

1. What is the most likely diagnosis?
   - (A) Very Late onset schizophrenia like psychosis
   - (B) Late onset Depression
   - (C) Late onset Mania
   - (D) Late onset schizophrenia

2. Compared to onset in Younger age group late onset mania in elderly people is characterize by:
   - (A) Stronger genetic loading
   - (B) Lesser frequency of cerebral pathology
   - (C) More mixed picture than classic manic presentation
   - (D) Higher rates in women

3. Which of the following is **NOT** true regarding late life bipolar disorder?
   - (A) Mortality rate is higher than expected to the population norms
   - (B) Substance abuse is less common than the younger patients with bipolar disorder
   - (C) Quality of life score higher than the normal controls
   - (D) Existence with neurological disorders is more consistent finding

4. Following is **NOT** true regarding late life bipolar disorder in comparison to normal controls :
   - (A) Larger hippocampal volume
   - (B) Smaller caudate nucleus
   - (C) Decreased total brain volume
   - (D) Right hemisphere lesion

5. Side effects of Valproate imperative to Geriatric patients are following **except:**
   - (A) Cardiotoxicity
   - (B) Hepatotoxicity
   - (C) Pancreatitis
   - (D) Thrombocytopenia

Answers:

1. C

   The case describes classical features of Late Life Mania

2. C

   Late Life Mania tends to present with atypical symptoms and a more mixed picture than classic manic presentation

3. B

Substance abuse is as common in Late Life Mania as in than of younger patients with bipolar disorder
4. C
There are no significant changes in the brain volumes in Late life mania patients as compared to controls
5. A
Cardiotoxicity is not commonly reported with valproate treatment

Reference:

1. Blazer DG, Steffens DC. Textbook of Geriatric Psychiatry, 4th Edition, American Psychiatric Publishing, Inc, Washington, DC 2009. Pp301-309.

VERY LATE-ONSET SCHIZOPHRENIA LIKE PSYCHOSIS

Dr. Shailendra M. Tripathi, Assistant Professor, Department of Geriatric Mental Health

A 72-year-old Hindu widow was brought by her son in a rather distraught state. Since the last 8 weeks, she repeatedly complained to her son that her daughter-in-law was "out to get her." She was certain that her daughter-in-law was poisoning her food. Frequent quarrels ensued at home. She further added that there were "voices" of unfamiliar men, who commented on all her daily activities. Two weeks ago, she was seen trying to strangulate herself in order to make the voices stop. Sleep eluded her. No significant past history. She was premorbidly described as suspicious and introvert. She was physically well, at ease, oriented and expressive. Persecutory, along with partition delusions were present in which she believed that daughter-in-law, would transgress the walls of her room and kill her at night. Third person auditory hallucinations with sinister content were present continuously. Her mini-mental status examination (MMSE) score was 28/30. Magnetic resonance imaging (MRI) brain showed age related cortical atrophy.

1. What is the most likely diagnosis?
   (A) Very Late onset schizophrenia Like psychosis
   (B) Late onset Depression
   (C) Late onset Mania
   (D) Late onset schizophrenia
2. Which of the following is NOT true regarding Very late onset schizophrenia like psychosis in comparison to Early onset Schizophrenia
   (A) Female Preponderance
   (B) More negative symptoms
   (C) Progressive cognitive Deterioration
   (D) Lower genetic loading
3. Which of the following is **true** regarding Very late onset schizophrenia like psychosis in comparison to Early onset Schizophrenia
   (A) Relative lack of thought disorder
   (B) Lower risk of Tardive dyskinesia
   (C) Early childhood maladjustment
   (D) Neurodevelopmental process
4. Which of the following is Not true regarding Very late onset schizophrenia like psychosis in comparison to late onset Schizophrenia
   (A) More brain structural abnormalities
   (B) Evidence of neurodegenerative process
   (C) Family history of schizophrenia
   (D) Both genders equally affected
5. Which of the following class of drugs are used in treatment of Very late onset schizophrenia?
   (A) Tricyclic Antidepressants
   (B) First Generation Antipsychotics
   (C) Second Generation Antipsychotics

(D) Acetyl Cholinesterase inhibitors

Answers:

1. A
   The case highlights the common presentation of Very Late onset schizophrenia Like psychosis
2. B
   Negative symptoms are less common in Very Late onset schizophrenia Like psychosis
3. A
   Thought disorder is less common in Very Late onset schizophrenia Like psychosis
4. C
   There is no evidence of genetic loading in Very Late onset schizophrenia Like psychosis
5. C
   Second Generation Antipsychotics are most commonly used in treatment

Reference:

1. Blazer DG, Steffens DC. Textbook of Geriatric Psychiatry, 4th Edition, American Psychiatric Publishing, Inc, Washington, DC 2009. 319-320.

CREUTZFELDT- JACOB DISEASE

Dr. Shailendra M. Tripathi, Assistant Professor, Department of Geriatric Mental Health

A 60 year old male vegetarian presented with three months history dizziness without fever or headache. Three weeks prior to hospital admission, he had behavioural disturbances in the form of irritability, agitation, confusion and irrelevant speech. He complained of blurred vision and needed assistance in activities of daily living. He was disoriented with loss of memory for recent events. He had rigidity in all four limbs with normal deep tendon reflexes and flexor planter response. Over the next four weeks of hospitalization the cognitive function worsened gradually with no fluctuation in between. Terminally he had myoclonic jerks. Routine hematological and biochemical profile including thyroid functions and Vitamin B-12 levels were normal. CSF analysis was normal. He was sero-negative for HIV and VDRL. FLAIR sequences of MRI show hyper-intense signals in caudate nucleus and focal areas of cortical ribbon in insular and occipital region. EEG revealed periodic sharp wave discharges over a low background activity.

1. What is the most likely diagnosis?
   (A) Progressive multifocal leukoencephalopathy
   (B) Hashimoto's encephalopathy
   (C) Dementia due to Lewy body disease
   (D) Creutzfeldt- Jacob disease
2. Which of the following is NOT a human prion disease?
   (A) Creutzfeldt - Jacob disease
   (B) Familial fatal insomnia
   (C) Bovine spongiform encephalopathy
   (D) Gerstmann-Straussler-Sheinker syndrome
3. Which of the following is NOT a characteristic of Creutzfeldt- Jacob disease?
   (A) Periodic sharp wave discharges over slow background
   (B) "Hot cross bun" sign
   (C) Pulvinar sign
   (D) Cortical ribbon sign
4. Following are considered pathognomic of the Creutzfeldt- Jacob disease EXCEPT:
   (A) Frontal intermittent rhythmic delta activity on EEG
   (B) Elevated 14-3-3 protein in CSF
   (C) Bilaterally symmetrical hyperintensities in basal ganglia and thalamus
   (D) Spongiform changes in brain biopsy
5. Typical time from onset to death in Creutzfeldt- Jacob disease is:
   (A) 1-3 months
   (B) 6-9 months

(C) 12-15 months

(D) 18-21 months

Answers:

1. D

   The described clinical presentation is classical for Creutzfeldt- Jacob disease
2. C

   Bovine spongiform encephalopathy also known as mad cow disease is a neurodegenerative disease seen in cattle
3. B

   "Hot cross bun" sign is seen in Multiple system atrophy
4. A

   Periodic sharp wave complexes are typical in EEG of patients suffering from Creutzfeldt- Jacob disease
5. B

   General typical survival rate is about 6-9 months

References:

1. Blazer DG, Steffens DC. Textbook of Geriatric Psychiatry, 4th Edition, American Psychiatric Publishing, Inc, Washington, DC 2009. Pp252-253.
2. Tripathi M. Dementia Decoded. Kontentworx, New Delhi, 2014. Pp235-254.

END OF LIFE CARE IN GERIATRIC MENTAL HEALTH

Dr. Priti Singh, Assistant Professor, Department of Geriatric Mental Health

A 85 year old lady with severe dementia, osteoarthritis, hypertension and diabetes mellitus is admitted to the hospital for the fourth time in two months with fever, diminished oral intake and acute confusion. She was diagnosed with delirium and treated successfully. Despite this the patient continues to present with several chronic difficulties including severe pain in bilateral knee joints, reduced mobility, swallowing difficulties and double incontinence. The treating medical team considered the aspects of effective end of life palliative care for the patient and a care plan was prepared for management in the community.

1. Which one of the following is <u>NOT TRUE</u> regarding anxiety and depressive symptoms in the terminally ill?
   (A) Anxiety and depressive symptoms in terminally ill are more prominent than in those with chronic illnesses
   (B) Delirium may mimic depression or anxiety disorders
   (C) Hospital Anxiety and Depression scale may assist in diagnosis
   (D) Organic causes for clinical presentations need not always be ruled out
2. Which of the following is not a stage of the process for the personal journey towards death, as described by Elisabeth Kübler-Ross
   (A) Anger
   (B) Bargaining
   (C) Denial and shock
   (D) Emptiness
3. Which of the following is NOT TRUE regarding care of the terminally ill patient
   (A) Religious issues are irrelevant in the acute management of patients
   (B) Decision making must be a multi-disciplinary approach involving patients and their care givers
   (C) It is inappropriate to over investigate and aggressively treat every symptom
   (D) Physical and mental comfort along with overview on quality of life must always be a priority
4. In the psychological management of patients with terminal illness:
   (A) Only current issues of management must be discussed
   (B) Overall care issues including need for palliative care should not be routinely discussed
   (C) Full prognosis and management plan should be discussed with patients and their care givers
   (D) Denial of diagnosis by patient or care givers should be confronted
5. As per the Endicott criteria, which one of the following is NOT a symptom of depression in terminally ill
   (A) Feelings of worthlessness or excessive or inappropriate guilt

(B) Social withdrawal or decreased talkativeness
(C) Reactive mood to environmental events
(D) Recurrent thoughts of death or suicide

Answers:

1. A
   Anxiety and depressive symptoms in terminally ill are just as prominent than in those with chronic illnesses
2. D
   Emptiness is not a stage of the process for the personal journey towards death, as described by Elisabeth Kübler-Ross
3. A
   Religious sentiments of patients and care givers must always be considered and in cooperated in the care plan
4. C
   Full diagnosis and prognosis with available care options must be discussed with patients/care givers and the decision-making must be a multi disciplinary process
5. C
   Mood is usually unreactive to the environment

References:

1. Breitbart W, Jacobsen PB. Psychiatric symptom management in terminal care. Clin Geriatr Med. 1996 May;12(2):329–47.
2. Jaiswal R, Alici Y, Breitbart W. A comprehensive review of palliative care in patients with cancer. Int Rev Psychiatry Abingdon Engl. 2014 Feb;26(1):87–101.
3. Asghar-Ali AA, Wagle KC, Braun UK. Depression in terminally ill patients: dilemmas in diagnosis and treatment. J Pain Symptom Manage. 2013 May;45(5):926–33.

HUNGTINTON'S DISEASE

Dr. Priti Singh, Assistant Professor, Department of Geriatric Mental Health

A 59 year old lawyer was brought by his son to the hospital due to his growing concerns regarding his father's behavior. Over the last 2 years he had lost his job, become reckless with his finances and severed relationship with most of his friends. He had previously been a meticulous and hard working professional and socially very polite. Along with this drastic change in his behavior the son was concerned that his father had been gradually deteriorating in his abilities to plan and manage even daily activities of living. On examination he was shabbily dressed and had a prominent unsteady gait with choreo-athetoid movements and scored 15/30 on MMSE with significant frontal dysexecutive functioning.

1. Huntington's disease (HD) is a rare genetic disorder that is
   (A) Autosomal recessive
   (B) Autosomal dominant
   (C) X linked recessive
   (D) X linked dominant
2. In HD, the genetic abnormality is with the Trinucleotide CAG repeat expansion with ____number of repeat size:
   (A) 10 or less
   (B) 25 or more
   (C) 36 or more
   (D) 50 or more
3. The following statement is FALSE regarding Mood symptoms associated with HD:
   (A) The incidence of depression is likely to be as high as 50% in HD
   (B) Mania is very commonly seen in HD
   (C) Irritability and anxiety symptoms are very common in HD
   (D) Around 5% of patients of HD have psychotic symptoms

4. The Following statement is FALSE with regards to treatment of Huntington's disease:
   (A) SSRI's are first line in treatment of Depression associated with HD
   (B) Tetrabenazine is indicated in treatment of motor symptoms like chorea
   (C) Dopamine agonists may be tried to treat dystonia and parkinsonism like features of HD
   (D) Irritability and impulse control issues respond well to pharmacological interventions
5. The following statement is TRUE regarding the Cognitive impairment in HD:
   (A) Cognitive impairment is identical to that seen in Alzheimer's disease
   (B) Aphasia is common
   (C) Semantic memory impairment is common
   (D) Organic denial is common

Answers:

1. B
   HD is an Autosomal dominant disorder with defect on the HD gene on the (P) arm of chromosome 4
2. C
   36 or more CAG repeats are indicative of HD and more than 40 repeats indicate that the person will definitely develop HD if they live long enough
3. B
   Mania is usually not associated with HD
4. D
   Irritability and Impulse disorders may respond minimally to SSRI's but there is no significant evidence for pharmacological treatment with may class
5. D
   Organic denial refers to the lack of insight into the level of disability in patents with HD due to cognitive impairment

References:

1. Senile Dementias, Pre-Senile Dementias and Pseudo-dementia. Organic psychiatry: the Psychological Consequences of Cerebral Disorder [3rd edition] (1998) W A Lishman, Blackwell Science, Oxford.
2. El-Nimr G, Barrett K. Huntington's disease: GP guide to clinical management. *The Prescriber 2006;* 17(10): 23–31.

TREATMENT OF LATE LIFE DEPRESSION

Dr. Priti Singh, Assistant Professor, Department of Geriatric Mental Health

A 62 year old man was brought to the casualty after being discovered by his wife in an unconscious state. He had slashed his wrists and requested the medical emergency team to not treat him. His wife gave a history of low mood, reduced pleasure in any activity and sleep disturbances. There was no other past psychiatric history. He also suffered from a stroke about 1 year ago and was receiving treatment for hypertension. The gentleman was admitted for further evaluation and a diagnosis of Late Life Depression was made.

1. Which of the following classes of drugs are most associated with electrolyte imbalance
   (A) SSRI's
   (B) Tricyclic antidepressants
   (C) SNRI's
   (D) Agomelatine
2. Which one of the following statements is TRUE regarding treatment of late life depression:
   (A) SSRI's are better options for patients at risk of falls
   (B) CBT is not as effective as antidepressant treatment in moderately severe cases.
   (C) Venlafaxine is effective in treating severe depression
   (D) ECT is a good option for patients presenting with severe depression with psychosis
3. Vascular depression is often associated with:
   (A) Psychotic symptoms
   (B) Suicidal symptoms
   (C) Apathy like symptoms

(D) Somatic symptoms

4. One of the following statements is FALSE regarding ECT treatment for late life depression
    (A) ECT is often better tolerated than multiple courses of antidepressants.
    (B) Bifrontal ECT offers the best chance of reducing cognitive disturbance with ECT without compromising efficacy.
    (C) Lithium has the best evidence base for the prevention of relapse after ECT.
    (D) Headache and memory loss are the most commonly reported side effects

5. The approach of 'start slow go slow' does not apply when treating with the following antidepressant
    (A) Escitalopram
    (B) Mirtazepine
    (C) Venlafaxine
    (D) Agomelatine

Answers:

1. A
   SSRI's are associated with a significantly high risk of hyponatremia
2. C
   Venlafaxine is indicated for moderate to severe depression especially if there is a poor response to first line antidepressants
3. C
   Vascular depression is associated with apathy like symptoms
4. B
   Bifrontal ECT does not reduce the chances of cognitive disturbance
5. D
   Agomelatine may be started and increased to full dose by day two of treatment

References:

1. Alan Thomson.Depression in older people.Tom Denning, Alan Thomson. Oxford Textbook of Old age Psychiatry. 2nd ed. Oxford: Oxford University Press; 2013. p 545-570
2. Alexopoulos GS. Depression in the elderly. Lancet Lond Engl. 2005 Jun 4;365(9475):1961–70.
3. Heijnen WT, Birkenhäger TK, Wierdsma AI, van den Broek WW. Antidepressant pharmacotherapy failure and response to subsequent electroconvulsive therapy: a meta-analysis. J Clin Psychopharmacol. 2010 Oct;30(5):616–9.

DELIRIUM

Dr. Anil Kumar, SR-I, Prof. S.C Tiwari, HOD, Department of Geriatric Mental Health

A 70 years old man was brought to the out-patient department of Geriatric Mental health. Family members complained of forgetfulness in the patient for 2 years which was gradually progressive. For the past 1 week the patient started to complain of burning micturation, increased frequency of micturation and for the past 5 days he was unable to identify family members and his house. He wouldn't sleep at night and appeared to play with the bed sheet and talked irrelevantly. He was unable to follow the commands and was constantly uttering same answers for different questions. After admission he was diagnosed with dementia with delirium with U.T.I and low serum sodium (125 meq/L).

1. Which of the following is not an alternative name for delirium?
    A) Acute Confusional State
    B) I.C.U Psychosis
    C) Acute and Transient Psychotic Disorder
    D) Sundowning
2. Which of the following is not a risk factor for the development of delirium?
    A) Elderly population
    B) Dementia
    C) Hospitalization in I.C.U
    D) Good Mobility
3. Most Common EEG finding in delirium is:
    A) Diffuse fast activity in the background
    B) Diffuse slow activity in the background

C) Focal fast activity in left Cerebral hemisphere
D) Focal Slow activity in the left cerebral hemisphere
4. Most common neurochemical change in delirium is?
   A) Decrease in Acetylcholine
   B) Decrease in Dopamine
   C) Decrease in Glutamate
   D) Increase in GABA
5. Which tool is not used to assess delirium?
   A) Mini- Mental Status examination
   B) Confusion Assessment method
   C) Memorial delirium Rating scale
   D) Hamilton depression rating scale

Answers:

1. C
   Acute and transient psychotic disorder is not a type of delirium
2. D
   Good mobility is not a risk factor for Delirium
3. B
   Diffuse slow activity in the background
4. A
   Decrease in Acetylcholine is reported to be the commonest neurochemical change
5. D
   Hamilton depression rating scale is used to assess depression

References:

1. Kumar L, Solai K. Delirium. In: Kaplan & Sadock's Comprehensive Textbook of Psychiatry. 9th ed. Sadock BJ & Sadock VA (eds) Philadelphia: Lippincott Williams & Wilkins.2009

BEREAVEMENT

Dr. Shailendra M. Tripathi, Assistant Professor, Department of Geriatric Mental Health

A 70 year old female was brought by her son to the Out patients clinic with concerns regarding her mental health. The patient's husband had suddenly expired 15 days ago. Her son, who lived abroad was concerned that she had been behaving abnormally and did not show much emotional reactivity to his death. She had recently started saying that her husband was alive and that she could see him at times. Her sleep was very erratic and she had been sleeping only 2-3 hours at night.

1. The following symptom or reaction, still present a year after bereavement, is a likely feature of normal, uncomplicated grief:
   (A) Trouble accepting the loss as real
   (B) Extreme bitterness or anger related to the loss
   (C) Hypnagogic hallucinations of the lost person
   (D) Feeling stunned/shocked by the loss.
2. Which one of the following is FALSE regarding the neurobiology of grief:
   (A) The 'loss process' in the dual process model involves periods of relative calm when the bereaved person can pay attention to immediate responsibilities.
   (B) Separation distress can vary from individual to individual depending on known factors such as gender and culture.
   (C) Hypnagogic hallucinations disappear on arousal.
   (D) Acute grief can impair functioning of beta lymphocytes.
3. The following still present a year after bereavement, is a likely identification reaction:
   (A) Hypnopompic/hypnogogic hallucinations
   (B) Trouble accepting the real loss
   (C) Feeling stunned and shocked
   (D) Hypochondriacal conditions in which the bereaved person develops symptoms. resembling the illness of the person who has died.

4. Which of the following is NOT associated with increased risk of psychological problems after bereavement?
    (A) Anxious/ambivalent attachment to mother in childhood.
    (B) Family perceived as unhelpful
    (C) Timely but unexpected death.
    (D) Sudden unexpected death
5. Shear's complicated grief treatment <u>DOESNOT</u> include the following:
    (A) use of the dual process model to focus attention on the loss and restoration components of grieving
    (B) 'Memory questionnaire' used to identify positive and negative memories
    (C) 'Motivational enhancement therapy' to identify goals and monitor progress.
    (D) Causing a Cathartic response to release hidden emotions

Answers:
    1. C
        Hypnagogic hallucinations of the lost person even after one year of event may be normal
    2. A
        This describes the 'restoration process'. The loss process involves episodic 'pangs of grief' in which the bereaved person is preoccupied with memories of the loss event and of the lost person, experiencing intense separation distress.
    3. D
        Identification reaction can be normal in bereavement
    4. C
        Timely but unexpected death is associated with the least abnormal grief reaction
    5. D
        Causing a cathartic response is not a part of Shear's complicated grief treatment

Reference:
    1. ZISOOK S, SHEAR K. Grief and bereavement: what psychiatrists need to know. *World Psychiatry 2009;* 8:p67–74.

DEMENTIA WITH LEWY BODIES (DLB)
Dr. Shailendra M. Tripathi, Assistant Professor, Department of Geriatric Mental Health

A 60 year old hindu male from Unnao, Uttar Pradesh presented with 7 year history of REM Sleep Behaviour Disorder(RBD) and two years history of cognitive dysfunction in the form of visuospatial disturbances, apathy, difficulty in execution, planning and calculation. He developed visual hallucinations like seeing cattle for last three years. One year later he gradually developed slowness, took longer time for activities of daily living and gait became slow. The parkinsonism was mild and symmetric. There were no tremors. MMSE was 16/30. Detailed cognitive assessment revealed frontal and parietal lobe dysfunction. On examination he had mild distal cogwheel rigidity and bradykinesia. Biochemical and hematological parameters were within normal limits. MRI brain showed diffuse cerebral atrophy.

1. What is most likely diagnosis?
    (A) Dementia due to Frontotemporal degeneration
    (B) Dementia due to Alzheimer's disease
    (C) Dementia due to Lewy body disease
    (D) Dementia due to Vascular disease
2. All the following are core features of dementia with Lewy bodies **EXCEPT:**
    (A) Fluctuating cognition
    (B) Visual hallucination
    (C) REM sleep behavior disorder
    (D) Spontaneous Parkinsonism
3. Which of the following is **NOT TRUE** regarding differentiating Dementia with Lewy bodies (DLB) to Alzheimer's disease (AD)?
    (A) Presence of psychiatric symptoms at onset is good discriminator of DLB from AD

(B) Visual hallucinations are more specific (99%) parameter for differentiating DLB from AD in early stages

(C) Presence of cognitive dysfunction in beginning is good discriminator of DLB from AD

(D) Visuo-spatial dysfunction is most sensitive (74%) parameter for differentiating DLB from AD in early stages

4. All are the following are suggestive feature of Dementia with Lewy bodies **EXCEPT:**
   (A) REM sleep behavior disorder
   (B) Severe neuroleptic sensitivity
   (C) Low dopamine transporter uptake in basal ganglia
   (D) Presence of systematized delusions

5. The classification difference between Dementia with Lewy bodies and Parkinson's Disease Dementia (PDD) is:
   (A) In DLB, motor symptoms are first to appear
   (B) In PDD, memory symptoms are first to appear
   (C) To diagnose DLB, parkinsonian motor features must appear after atleast 1 year of diagnosis
   (D) To diagnose DLB, parkinsonian motor features must appear after at least 1 year before the diagnosis

Answers:

1. C
   The case study highlights important clinical aspects of Lewy body dementia
2. C
   REM sleep behaviour disorder may be seen in DLB but is not a corefeature
3. C
   Cognitive dysfunction is seen early in both Alzheimer's dementia and Lewy body dementia
4. D
   Low dopamine transporter uptake in basal ganglia is not suggestive of Lewy body dementia
5. C
   Symptomatology of DLB and PDD may clinically overlap but for diagnosis of DLB, parkinsonian motor features must appear at least 1 year of diagnosis

References:

1. Blazer DG, Steffens DC. Textbook of Geriatric Psychiatry, 4th Edition, American Psychiatric Publishing, Inc, Washington, DC 2009. pp250-251.
2. Tripathi M. Dementia Decoded. Kontentworx, New Delhi, 2014. pp164-181.

RECURRENT DEPRESSION

Dr.Nisha Mani Pandey, Assistant Professor, Department of Geriatric Mental Health

A 65 years old female known case of repeated depressive episodes referred for psychological assessment and therapeutic interventions. She was feeling low energy, unable to engage herself in pleasurable activities. On detailed assessment it was found that she started believing that people don't like her, they are gradually fade up with her illness and she also feels that life is not worth. Her self-defeating thoughts were weakened and self-affirming thoughts and beliefs were strengthened.

2. Patients with repeated depressive episodes characterized as-
   (A) Depressive episode
   (B) Recurrent depressive disorder
   (C) Bipolar affective disorder, current episode mild or moderate depression
   (D) Dysthymia

2. Which kind of assessment tools is appropriate for evaluating severity of depression-
   (A) Neuro-psychological battery
   (B) Geriatric depression scale (GDS)
   (C) The Hamilton rating scale for depression (HAM-D)
   (D) Beck depression inventory

3. Which of the following therapies is the best option in such patients
   (A) Validation therapy

(B) Cognitive behavior therapy (CBT)

(C) Reminiscence therapy

(D) Supportive therapy

4. Before imparting CBT the process of gathering information in relation to subjects current problem done through-

(A) Case conceptualization

(B) Situation analysis

(C) Belief system

(D) Activating event

5. CBT in elderly most often needs:

(A) Competency

(B) Ability

(C) Activeness

(D) Collaborative approach

Answers:

1. B

Recurrent depressive disorder is characterized by repeated episodes of depression as specified in depressive episodes without any history of mood elevation and over activity.

2. C

The Hamilton Depression Rating Scale (HAM-D) is a useful tool to assess the level of severity in patients of depression, it is widely used for assessing the severity of depression before, during, and after treatment by a clinician.

3. B

Benefits from CBT to older adults reported approximately similar as in younger adults. It needs specific adaptations to the therapy strategies and process to maximize treatment gains with older clients, although the core ingredients of CBT remain the same when working with older adults.

4. A

Before starting CBT the therapist need to recognize the constellation of (interacting) components that contribute to the individual's current problems, which is done through case conceptualization process.

5. D

Collaborative strategies/ approach (more than one therapist and involvement of care givers) help in identifying and changing of maladaptive cognitions and thinking pattern.

References:

1. WHO. The ICD-10 Classification of Mental and Behavioural Disorders-clinical descriptions and diagnostic guidelines. World Health Organization, Geneva, Indian Edition 2004. P124

2. Hamilton M. A rating scale for depression, Journal of Neurology, Neurosurgery, and Psychiatry 1960.23:p56-62.

3. Karlin BE. Cognitive Behavioral Therapy With Older Adults In: Sorocco KH, Lauderdale S (eds.). Cognitive Behavior Therapy with Older Adults- Innovations Across Care Settings. 2011 by Springer Publishing Company, LLC; 2011. p1.

4. Persons JB. Case formulation-driven psychotherapy. Clinical Psychology:Science and Practice, 2006. 13;167–170.

COGNITIVE IMPAIRMENT

Dr. Nisha Mani Pandey, Assistant Professor, Department of Geriatric Mental Health

A 69-years-old, widowed, graduate female referred to the department with complaints of forgetfulness, irritability and suspiciousness. Gradually her ability to perform daily task worsen. On Mini Mental State Examination (MMSE) she obtained a score of 22; she failed to perform on items of recall and serial subtraction. Despite medication training was provided to her care for giving her verbal commands and modeling with admiration to perform her day to day tasks.

1. The lady is suffering from which of the following condition:
   (A) Alzheimer's Dementia
   (B) Fronto- temporal Dementia
   (C) Levy body dementia
   (D) Mild cognitive impairment
2. MMSE is a 30 point scale and less than ….. score refer to significant decline
   (A) 25
   (B) 24
   (C) 23
   (D) 26
3. The inability to plan and perform consequential tasks like dressing, cooking etc. is :
   (A) Impairment of daily living
   (B) Impairment in intelligence
   (C) Impairment in executive functions
   (D) Impairment in memory
4. Executive dysfunction is associated with which of the following area of brain.
   (A) The neocortex
   (B) The pre frontal cortex
   (C) The Corpus collasum
   (D) The cerebellum
5. Providing verbal commands and reward to facilitate a positive desired behaviour is an example of :
   (A) Classical conditioning
   (B) Operant conditioning
   (C) Validation therapy
   (D) Modelling

Answers:

1. A

   Evidence of memory impairment specially registration, storage and retrieval of information is the commonest presentation in Alzheimer's dementia

2. C

   As per Folstein's MMSE norms, a score of 23 or less is indicative of Dementia

3. C

   Executive functioning involves the ability to show initiative, planning, organization, monitoring and problem solving skills

4. B

   The anterior part of frontal lobe of brain including the pre frontal cortex is involved in executive functioning

5. A

   Classical conditioning involves providing a regular stimulus to facilitate or inhibit a particular behaviour

References:

1. WHO. The ICD-10 Classification of Mental and Behavioural Disorders-clinical descriptions and diagnostic guidelines. World Health Organization, Geneva, Indian Edition 2004. p47.
2. Folstein MF, Folstein SE, McHugh PR. Mini-mental state. A practical method for grading the cognitive state of patients for the clinician". *Journal of Psychiatric Research* 1975. 12 (3): 189–98.

Chapter-9

Medicine

OSTEOPOROSIS
Dr. Madhukar Mittal, Associate Professor, Medicine

A 68 year female presents with low back pain. There is no radiation of pain to the lower limbs. There is no history of trauma. Her son feels that she has lost height. There is past history of left hip fracture due to fall in bathroom 4 years back. There is no history of smoking or alcohol intake. Menopause was attained at the age of 45 years. On physical examination, her weight is 74 kg and height 150 cm. Her blood pressure is 160/80 mm of Hg with respiratory rate of 18 per min. Cardiac, respiratory examination is normal. X-ray spine shows wedge compression fracture of L1 vertebra.

1. What is the probable cause for her vertebral fracture?
   (A) Osteogenesis imperfecta
   (B) Osteomalacia
   (C) Osteoporosis
   (D) Osteopetrosis
2. What would be next line of investigation to confirm her cause for fracture?
   (A) QCT
   (B) DXA
   (C) Heel Ultrasound
   (D) 25(OH)D
3. Which is NOT a common site for fracture in a postmenopausal female?
   (A) Colles'
   (B) Hip
   (C) Vertebrae
   (D) Tibia
4. Which one of the following statements is correct?
   (A) Glucocorticoid use can lead to the above clinical condition
   (B) Severe Vitamin D deficiency causes rickets in adults
   (C) Estrogen deficiency leads to increased bone formation
   (D) Low BMD is reported as A, B and C scores

Answers:
   1. C
   Osteomalacia occurs due to vitamin D deficiency and presents with bony pains, proximal muscle weakness and psuedofractures. Osteogenesis imperfecta is a genetic disorder occurring usually in childhood, with bluish sclera and recurrent fractures. Osteopetrosis is again a genetic disorder. Vertebral fracture in a postmenopausal female is most commonly due to Osteoporosis.
   2. B
   Gold standard test for assessing Bone Mineral Density (BMD) is a DXA scan. Three machines in common use are Hologic, Lunar and Norland. Heel USG may be used for screening in peripheral centers and is not specific. QCT is used in research settings. 25(OH)D levels would be useful to detect Osteomalacia.
   3. D
   The common sites for low-trauma fractures in Osteoporotic patients are Hip, vertebra and wrist (Colles').
   4. A
   Secondary causes for Osteoporosis include hypogonadism (estrogen and testosterone deficiency in females and males respectively) and drugs like glucocorticoids. Rickets is a disease of children. BMD is reported as T and Z scores.

Reference:
   1. Lindsay R, Cosman F.Osteoporosis. In: Longo DL, Fauci AS, Kasper DL, Hauser SL, Jameson JL, Loscalzo J (Eds)Harrison's Principles of Internal Medicine,18th edition. McGraw Hill, New Delhi 2012, pp3120

ACROMEGALY
Dr Madhukar Mittal, Associate Professor, Medicine

A 39 year female presents with recurrent headaches. For the past 4 years her menses have stopped. Physical examination shows coarse facial features, frontal bossing and large hands and feet. Her blood pressure is 130/80 mm of Hg with respiratory rate of 16 per min. Cardiac, respiratory examination is normal. MRI brain shows:

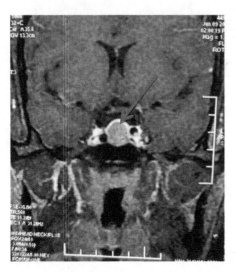

1. In order to diagnose her condition, what would be the appropriate screening test?
   (A) Random growth hormone
   (B) Serum IGF-1
   (C) 24-hour urinary free cortisol
   (D) Serum prolactin
2. What is her most likely diagnosis?
   (A) Acromegaly
   (B) Cushing's disease
   (C) Prolactinoma
   (D) Primary Ovarian failure
3. Which is NOT a pituitary hormone?
   (A) Prolactin
   (B) Cortisol
   (C) Growth hormone
   (D) TSH
4. Which one of the following statements about pituitary adenomas is NOT correct?
   (A) Pituitary adenomas frequently have distant metastasis
   (B) They are the most common cause of pituitary hormone hypersecretion and
       hyposecretion syndromes in adults
   (C) Pituitary adenomas are benign neoplasms
   (D) Plurihormonal tumors can occur

Answers:
   1. B
      IGF-1 is used as a screening test for GH hypersecretion syndromes. Random GH is not useful for diagnosing GH hypersecretion due to variability in secretory rates over 24 hours. 24 hr urinary cortisol would be used for Cushings disease and prolactin levels would be useful in a case of proalctinoma.
   2. A
      With the presenting clinical features, the diagnosis is Acromegaly.
   3. B
      Cortisol is secreted from the adrenal cortex (predominantly from zona fasciculata). Rest are all anterior pituitary hormones.
   4. A
      Pituitary adenomas are commonly benign neoplasms with local invasion. Multiple hormones can be secreted from these tumors although nonfunctional tumors are the most common subtype.

Reference:
   1. Melmed S, Jameson JL.Disorders of the Anterior Pituitary and Hypothalamus.In: Longo DL, Fauci AS, Kasper DL, Hauser SL, Jameson JL, Loscalzo J (Eds) Harrison's Principles of Internal Medicine, 18th edition.McGraw Hill,New Delhi 2012,pp2893

HYPOGLYCEMIA
Dr Madhukar Mittal, Associate Professor, Medicine

A 35 year nurse presents with complaints of recurrent episodes of weakness and feeling faint during work hours but never have these episodes occurred at home. Blood sugars tested several times during those episodes were detected to be low (45-55mg/dl). Her symptoms improved on taking sugar or juice. She is not a known diabetic and is otherwise healthy. Family history is contributory for diabetes mellitus in father who is on Insulin. Physical examination shows that her blood pressure is 120/80 mm of Hg with respiratory rate of 18 per min. Cardiac, respiratory and other systemic examination is normal.

1. What is the first hormone to change as a defense against hypoglycemia?
    (A) Glucagon
    (B) Insulin
    (C) Cortisol
    (D) Adrenaline
2. In order to diagnose her condition, what would be the appropriate test?
    (A) Serum cortisol
    (B) Fasting insulin and glucose
    (C) Fasting insulin, glucose and C-peptide
    (D) Insulin, glucose and C-peptide when she has symptoms
3. What is her most likely diagnosis?
    (A) Insulinoma
    (B) Exogenous insulin intake
    (C) Pancreatic malignancy
    (D) Hirata syndrome
4. Which one of the following statements about hypoglycemia in diabetes mellitus is NOT correct?
    (A) Metformin and DPP-4 inhibitors cause more frequent hypoglycemia than sulfonylureas
    (B) Hypoglycemic unawareness can occur with recurrent episodes of hypoglycemia
    (C) Mild hypoglycemia should be treated with 25% dextrose
    (D) Chronic renal failure and chronic liver disease predispose to hypoglycemia

Answers:
1. B
    Hypoglycemia induces a counter-regulatory rise in hormones in the body to maintain blood sugar levels (Glucagon, Adrenaline, Cortisol and Growth Hormone). However even before that, the initial reaction is for insulin secretion to be decreased.
2. D
    Blood sample taken for Insulin glucose and C-peptide during the episode of symptoms would be most appropriate to confirm the diagnosis.
3. B
    Factitious hypoglycemia is common in medical and health personnel. The person is a young female with father being on insulin. All the episodes of fainting occurring during work hours only, is another key pointer.
4. C
    In the management of diabetes mellitus, commonly implicated oral drugs for hypoglycemia include sulfonylureas. Taken alone, metformin and DPP-4 inhibitors do not cause hypoglycemia. Chronic renal failure and chronic liver disease leads to reduction in dose requirement of antihyperglycemic agents and patients may have more frequent hypoglycemic episodes. In mild hypoglycemia, patients are conscious and able to treat themselves for hypoglycemia; usually oral glucose, sugar, toffee intake followed by a meal is sufficient.

Reference:
1. Cryer PE, Davis SN. Hypoglycemia. In: Longo DL, Fauci AS, Kasper DL, Hauser SL, Jameson JL, Loscalzo J (Eds) Harrison's Principles of Internal Medicine, 18th edition. McGraw Hill, New Delhi 2012,pp3003

HYPOGONADISM: KLINFELTER SYNDROME
Dr Madhukar Mittal, Associate Professor, Medicine

A 28 year male presents for infertility. He has been married for the past 7 years. He and his wife have been trying to conceive a child for the past 4 years but with no success. He was referred to Endocrinology after semen analysis showed no sperms. Physical examination shows that he is tall with a sparse beard. His blood pressure is 130/80 mm of Hg with respiratory rate of 16 per min. Cardiac, respiratory examination is normal. Bilateral gynecomastia is present and he has bilateral small testes.

1. What is the next line of tests to be ordered in this patient?
   (A) Serum TSH, T4, T3
   (B) Serum Urea, Creatinine
   (C) Serum Prolactin, Testosterone, FSH/LH
   (D) Serum Androstenedione, 17-OH progesterone
2. In order to diagnose his condition, what would be the appropriate test?
   (A) Karyotype
   (B) MRI brain for pituitary
   (C) Mammogram
   (D) USG of scrotum
3. What is his most likely diagnosis?
   (A) Turner syndrome
   (B) Noonan syndrome
   (C) Kallman syndrome
   (D) Klinefelter syndrome
4. Which one of the following statements about infertility is NOT correct?
   (A) Infertility is defined as the inability to conceive after 12 months of unprotected sexual intercourse.
   (B) Both male and female factors contribute to infertility
   (C) For infertility treatment, option includes adoption.
   (D) Etiology can be ascertained in more than 90% of men with suspected male factor infertility

Answers:

1. C
   Initial hormonal evaluation in an azoospermic male who has eunnuchoid habitus and poor secondary sexual characteristics would include serum testosterone, prolactin, LH and FSH.
2. A
   Azoospermic male who has eunnuchoid habitus and poor secondary sexual characteristics with gynecomastia suggests a diagnosis of Klinefelter syndrome. 47 XXY is the karyotype. MRI brain would be required if we are dealing with a case of hypogonadotropic hypogonadism. USG scrotum helps to rule out local pathology and may be indicated in obstructive azoospermia. Hypogonadism is not a presentation of obstructive azoospermia.
3. D
   Discussion as above in point 2. Klinefelter's syndrome is the most common chromosomal disorder associated with testicular dysfunction and male infertility.
4. D
   40-50% of male infertility is due to idiopathic causes. Factors for infertility are 58% female, 25% male and 17% unexplained.

References:

1. Hall JE. The Female Reproductive system, Infertility, and Contraception. In: Longo DL, Fauci AS, Kasper DL, Hauser SL, Jameson JL, Loscalzo J (Eds) Harrison's Principles of Internal Medicine, 18th edition. McGraw Hill, New Delhi 2012,pp3028
2. Bhasin S, Jameson JL. Disorders of the Testes and Male reproductive System. In: Longo DL, Fauci AS, Kasper DL, Hauser SL, Jameson JL, Loscalzo J (Eds) Harrison's Principles of Internal Medicine, 18th edition. McGraw Hill, New Delhi 2012,pp3010

AN ALCOHOLIC PATIENT PRESENTING WITH FATIGUE AND EXERTIONAL BREATHLESSNESS

Dr. S P Verma, Assistant Professor, Department of Medicine

A 24 year old male presented with history of fatigue and exertional breathlessness for 1 month and altered behavior for 2 days. He is a chronic alcoholic and vegetarian. His hemogram shows Hb-6 gm%, TLC-2500 and differentials N70L25M3E1 with platelet count 70,000/cmm. His RBC parameters show MCV-125 fl, MCH-33 and MCHC – 36.

1. All investigations are helpful in diagnosis of B12 deficiency
   (A) Serum B12 levels

(B) Serum Homocystein
(C) Serum Methylmalonic acid levels
(D) Serum lactate dehydrogenase

2. The above mentioned patient peripheral smear shows Macroovalocytes, hypersegmented neutrophils and Howell Jolly bodies. Hypersegmented neutrophils are found in all of these conditions except-
   (A) Vitamin B12 deficiency
   (B) Treatment with hydroxyurea
   (C) Iron deficiency anemia
   (D) Aplastic anemia

3. You have diagnosed the patient as Anemia due to B12 deficiency and started Intramuscular vitamin B12 injections. All are the complications patient can develop after initiation of treatment **Except-**
   (A) Hypokalemia
   (B) Hypocalcemia
   (C) Allergic reactions
   (D) Local pain and irritation

4. This patient stopped treatment after 6 months and was asymptomatic for 1 year. Recently he has developed similar symptoms for last 2 months. All are probable causes of recurrent B12 deficiency except-
   (A) Pernicious anemia
   (B) Malabsorption syndrome
   (C) Ileal resection
   (D) Nutritional deficiency

Answers:

1. D
   Serum LDH levels are done to see ineffective erythropoiesis. LDH levels may be elevated in various conditions of hemolysis, ineffective erythropoiesis and Lymphomas/leukemias. Rest all options have diagnostic significance in B12 deficiency.

2. D
   Megaloblastic anemia, Iron deficiency anemia and treatment with hydroxyurea and antifolates are known to cause neutrophil hypersegmentation.

3. B
   With start of B12 supplementation there is rapid proliferation of cells in bone marrow and potassium in redistributed inside the cell causing serum potassium levels to fall. Allergic and anaphylactic reactions are known to occur with inj Vitamin B12.

4. D
   Nutritional deficiency develops after 2-3 years of complete absence of B12 in diet. Rest all are well known factors for recurrent B12 deficiency

References:

1. Longo D, Fauci A, Kasper DL, Hauser SL, Jameson JL, Loscalzo J, editors. Harrison's principles of internal medicine. 18th ed. New York: McGraw Hill: 2012. P. 646. Hematopoietic disorders. vol 1.
2. S M Lewis, B J Bain,I bates editors. Dacie and Lewis Practical Haematology.10th ed. Churchill Livingstone: 2010. P105.Red cell morphology in health and disease.

A PATIENT PRESENTING WITH PALLOR, JAUNDICE WITH HEPATOSPLENOMEGALY

Dr. S P Verma, Assistant Professor, Department of Medicine

Eight year old Mr. A was referred to hematologist for investigating the cause of recurrent episodes of severe pain, pallor, jaundice and hepatosplenomegaly. His hemogram showed Hb-8 gm/dl, TLC 24000 DLC=N78L20M2E0, and platelets-1.5 lakh. Peripheral smear showed Normocytic normochromic RBC, anisopoikilocytosis and few sickle cells and target cells

1. All of these are methods to diagnose sickle cell disease **Except**?
   (A) Sickling test
   (B) Hb electrophoresis
   (C) High performance liquid chromatography
   (D) Betke test

2. All of the following complications can be seen in Sickle cell disease **Except**?
   (A) Stroke
   (B) Acute Chest syndrome

(C) Painful crises

(D) Pancreatitis

3. All are modalities of treatment in sickle cell anemia **Except**?

    (A) Packed red cell transfusion

    (B) Prophylactic antibiotics

    (C) Hydroxyurea

    (D) Stem cell transplantation

4. Mechanism of action of Hydroxyurea in management of sickle cell disease is?

    (A) Elevates HbA2

    (B) Elevates HbF

    (C) Elevates HbA

    (D) Decreases HbA2

Answers:

  1. D

    Betke test is done to detect fetal hemoglobin (HbF). Sickling test is done to demonstrate increased sickling in hypoxemic condition. Hb electophoresis and HPLC are the initial standard methods to diagnose hemoglobinopathies.

  2. D

    Acute chest syndrome, painful crises and strokes are well known complications in Sickle cell disease. Other manifestations are priapism, ocular and renal complications. Pancreatitis is not a known complication in sickle cell disease.

  3. B

    Bone marrow transplantation is the only cure available for sickle cell disease. Hydroxyurea is used to raise fetal Hemoglobin levels as it is protective against sickling. Blood transfusion is needed for anemia as well as prevention of stroke in children and adolescents. No role of regular prophylactic antibiotics.

  4. B

    Hydroxyurea elevates fetal hemoglobin.

Reference:

  1. Longo D, Fauci A, Kasper DL, Hauser SL, Jameson JL, Loscalzo J, editors. Harrison's principles of internal medicine. 18th ed. New York: McGraw Hill: 2012. P. 638. Hematopoietic disorders. Vol 1.

DEEP VEIN THROMBOSIS DURING PREGNANCY

Dr. S P Verma, Assistant Professor, Department of Medicine

A 34 year old woman presents to hematology OPD with history of recurrent 3rd trimester abortions. She developed left lower limb deep vein thrombosis during last pregnancy. Her hemogram shows Hb 9 gm/dl, TLC - 4500/cmm and platelet count of 60000/cmm.

1. What is the most probable diagnosis?

    (A) Chromosomal abnormalities

    (B) Syphilis

    (C) Antiphospholipid antibody syndrome

    (D) Takayasu arteritis

2. All are included in Diagnostic criterias of APLA **except?**

    (A) Lupus anticoagulant

    (B) Anti beta2 glycoprotein antibody

    (C) Anticardiolipin antibody

    (D) Antinuclear antibody

3. What should be the treatment strategy in this patient ?

    (A) Indefinite anticoagulation to target INR-2.0-3.0

    (B) Low dose aspirin or no therapy

    (C) Strict control of vascular risk factors

    (D) Hydroxychloroquine

4. APLA syndrome **Except**?

    (A) CNS thrombosis

    (B) DVT

(C) Mesentric artery thrombosis

(D) Deep hematoma

Answers:

1. C

This patient has classical manifestations of APLA syndrome. In congenital anomalies abortions are usually in the first trimester. Syphilis is rare nowadays and abortions have progressive duration and DVT is not a usual feature.

2. D

ANA is not primary investigation in diagnosis of APLA syndrome

3. A

In a patient of APLA syndrome who developed thrombotic event lifelong anticoagulation with INR range of 2-3 is indicated

4. D

Bleeding manifestations are not common in APLA. Rarely it happens when antibodies against coagulation factors are formed or severe thrombocytopenia develops.

Reference:

1. David Keeling, Ian Mackie, Garry W. Moore et al.Guidelines on the investigation and management of antiphospholipid syndrome. British Journal of Haematology 2012. 157, 47-58

A CASE PRESENTING WITH GUM BLEEDING

Dr. S P Verma, Assistant Professor, Department of Medicine

A 70 year old patient presents to Hematology OPD with history of fever and bleeding (gum bleeding and purpura) for last 1 month. His hemogram shows Hb-7.8, TLC-2400 with differential count N70L25M4E1 and Platelet count of 30000/cmm. MCV-86 fl, MCH, MCHC and RDW are within normal limits. Examination does not show any lymphadenopathy and organomegaly.

1. All of the following are the possibilities in this patient **Except**?
   (A) Aplastic anemia
   (B) Myelodysplastic syndrome
   (C) Aleukemic leukemia
   (D) Megaloblastic anemia
2. Aleukemic leukemia is defined as?
   (A) Absence of blast in bone marrow
   (B) Absence of blast in peripheral smear
   (C) Absence of blast in peripheral smear with presence of >20% blast in bone marrow
   (D) Presence of>20% blast in peripheral smear with absence of blast in bone marrow
3. All of the following statements are true about Acute Myeloid Leukemia Except?
   (A) Myeloperoxidase (MPO) is the lineage marker of Myeloid blasts
   (B) CD13,CD33,CD117 are myeloid markers used in flowcytometry to detect myeloid linease
   (C) Granulocytic sarcomas are most commonly found in AML-M6 subtype
   (D) AML-M2 has better prognosis
4. All are true about cytogenetics in AML **Except**?
   (A) t(8:21) has bad prognosis
   (B) inv-16 has good prognosis
   (C) Complex karyotype has poor prognosis
   (D) Normal karyotype is considered as intermediate risk

Answers:

1. D

Pancytopenia with history of significant bleeding and fever for 1 month duration and normal MCV is very less likely to be megaloblastic anemia. All other conditions can present with these findings

2. C

Aleukemic leukemia means absence of blast in peripheral blood but in bone marrow >20% blast will be there to qualify for WHO criteria for diagnosis of acute leukemia

3. D

Granulocytic sarcoma is found most commonly in M4,M5 type of acute myeloid leukemia.MPO is a lineage determining marker and CD13,CD33 ,CD117 are other myeloid markers. Sometimes CD13 and CD33 can be aberrantly expressed on lymphoid blasts and they are not lineage specific.
4. A

t(8:21) is associated with good prognosis. Other good prognostic AML are inv16, t(16:16) and t(15:17)

Reference:

1. Longo D, Fauci A, Kasper DL, Hauser SL, Jameson JL, Loscalzo J, editors. Harrison's principles of internal medicine. 18th ed. New York: McGraw Hill: 2012.P.905. Hematopoietic disorders. Vol 1.

BRONCHIECTSIS
Dr. Shyam Chand Chaudhary, Associate Professor, Department of Medicine

A 48 year old male presented with the chief complaints of fever since past 6 months, cough with purulent expectoration for 3 months and breathlessness for 15 days. He is a chronic smoker (smoking index-300). He had past history of hospitalization due to pneumonia 5 years back which required mechanical ventilation. For last 5 years he had several episodes of cough with expectoration and fever requiring frequent consultations.

1. All of the following could be the possible causes of cough with purulent expectoration **except**.
    (A) Chronic bronchitis
    (B) Bronchiectasis
    (C) Lung abscess
    (D) Idiopathic Pulmonary Fibrosis

On examination his vitals are stable. He has clubbing but no cyanosis or peripheral edema. Chest examination reveals bilateral rhonchi and coarse leathery crepitations in right lung fields. His chest radiograph reveals tram track appearance in right lung fields.

2. What would be the next investigation in this patient?
    (A) Contrast enhanced CT scan of the chest
    (B) High resolution CT scan of the Chest
    (C) Bronchoscopy with bronchoalveolar lavage
    (D) Pulmonary function test

3. All of these are the expected CT scan findings in this case **except**
    (A) Signet ring sign
    (B) Tree in bud appearance
    (C) Bronchial wall thickening
    (D) Ground glass opacification

4. What would be the most appropriate empirical treatment to start in this patient besides chest physiotherapy:
    (A) Antifungal
    (B) Steroids
    (C) Antibiotics
    (D) Diethyl carbamazepine

5. All of the following can be the possible complications of this disease **except**
    (A) Hemoptysis
    (B) Empyema
    (C) Secondary amyloidosis
    (D) Left ventricular failure

Answers:

1. D

    A persistent cough that is productive of purulent sputum occurs in chronic bronchitis, bronchiectasis, and a variety of other suppurative disorders including lung abscess.[1]Idiopathic Pulmonary Fibrosis may present as an incidental finding in an otherwise asymptomatic individual but more typically presents with progressive breathlessness and a non-productive cough.[2]

2. B

    In view of the previous history of pneumonia and the symptoms of chronic cough with purulent expectoration, digital clubbing, coarse leathery crepitations on auscultation and tram track appearance on chest radiograph the diagnosis of bronchiectasis should be considered. High resolution CT (HRCT) Chest is more specific for bronchiectasis and is the imaging modality of choice for confirming the diagnosis.[3]

3. D
HRCT chest findings of bronchiectasis include airway dilation (detected as parallel "tram tracks"or as the"signet-ring sign"-a cross-sectional area of the airway with a diameter at least 1.5 times that of the adjacent vessel), lack of bronchial tapering (including the presence of tubular structures within 1 cm from the pleural surface), bronchial wall thickening in dilated airways, inspissated secretions (e.g., the"tree-in-bud"pattern), or cysts emanating from the bronchial wall.[3]

4. C
The treatment of bronchiectasis includes control of active infection and improvements in secretion clearance and bronchial hygiene so as to decrease the microbial load within the airways and minimize the risk of repeated infections.[3]

5. D
Recurrent infections can result in injury to superficial mucosal vessels, with bleeding and, in severe cases, life-threatening hemoptysis.[3] Other complications include empyema, lung abscess, pneumothorax, cor pulmonale, respiratory failure, secondary amyloidosis and metastatic brain abscesses.[4]

References:

1. Taichman DB, Fishman AP. Apporach to the patient with respiratory symptoms. In: Fishman AP, Elias JA, Fishman JA, Grippi MA, Senior RM, Pack AI, editors. Fisman's pulmonary diseases and disorders, 4th ed. New York: Mc Graw-Hill Medical Publishing Division; 2008. p. 387-426.
2. Reid PT, Innes JA. Respiratory disease. In: Walker BR, Colledge NR, Ralston SH, Penman ID, editors. Davidson's principles and practice of medicine, 22nd ed. London: Churchill Livingstone Elsevier; 2014. p. 644-731.
3. Baron RM, Barshak MB. Bronchiectasis. In: Kasper DL, Fauci AS, Hauser SL, Longo DL, Jameson L, Loscalzo J, editors. Harrison principles of internal medicine, 19th ed. New York: Mc Graw-Hill Medical Publishing Division; 2015. p. 1694-1696.
4. Gupta D. Suppurative Pleuro-Pulmonary Diseases: Bronchiectasis, Lung Abscess and Empyema. In: Shah SN, Anand MP, Billimoria AR, Kamath SA, Karnad DR, Munjal YP. et al., editors. API Textbook of Medicine 8th ed. Mumbai: Urvi computographics;2008. p. 373-375.

BRONCHIAL ASTHMA

Dr. Shyam Chand Chaudhary, Associate Professor, Department of Medicine

A 22 year young woman presents to the emergency room with chief complaints of acute onset of breathlessness for the past 2 hours. She also gives a history of wheeze. She had past history of repeated similar episodes of breathlessness from last 6 years with exacerbations in winter. She also had history of eczema since childhood. Her family history is significant for allergies in her mother. Her vitals are stable except for a respiratory rate of 28/min. Bilateral polyphonic rhonchi are auscultated diffusely over the chest.

1. What would be the investigation of choice to diagnose the ailment she is suffering from?
   (A) Chest X-ray
   (B) HRCT Thorax
   (C) Pulmonary function tests
   (D) Sputum examination

This patient has an unremarkable Chest X ray. On pulmonary function test her FEV_1 is 35% and the FEV_1/FVC ratio is 45% of the predicted values.

2. This set of spirometric values can be encountered in all of the following settings except
   (A) Chronic Bronchitis
   (B) Bronchiectasis
   (C) Bronchial asthma
   (D) Interstitial lung disease

3. The reversibility of bronchoconstriction can be demonstrated by all of the following except
   (A) $\geq12\%$ increase in FEV_1 following administration of a trial of corticosteroids
   (B) $> 20\%$ diurnal variation on ≥3 days in a week for2 weeks on PEF diary
   (C) $\geq15\%$ decrease in FEV_1 after 6 mins of exercise
   (D) ≥100 mL increase in FEV_1 following administration of a bronchodilator

4. The acute management of this patient includes all except
   (A) Inhaled corticosteroids
   (B) Inhaled short acting bronchodilators
   (C) Omalizumab

(D) Infusion of aminophylline

5. All of the following statements regarding asthma are correct **except**
   (A) Refractory asthma patients are resistant to inhalation therapy
   (B) Corticosteroid resistant asthma is defined by a failure to respond to a high dose of oral prednisolone
   (C) Brittle asthma is characterized by chaotic variations in lung function despite taking appropriate therapy
   (D) Aspirin sensitive asthma is seen in atopic individuals with a early onset of the disease

Answers:

1. C

   Asthma is a syndrome characterized by airflow obstruction that varies markedly, both spontaneously and with treatment. Patients with asthma commonly suffer from other atopic diseases, particularly allergic rhinitis (in 80%) and atopic dermatitis (eczema). The characteristic symptoms of asthma are wheezing, dyspnoea, and coughing. Typical physical signs are inspiratory, and to a greater extent expiratory, rhonchi throughout the chest, and there may be hyperinflation. The diagnosis of asthma is usually apparent from the symptoms of variable and intermittent airways obstruction, but is usually confirmed by objective measurements of lung function. Simple spirometry confirms airflow limitation with a reduced FEV_1 and FEV_1 /FVC ratio and PEF.[1]

2. D

   The initial pulmonary function test obtained is spirometry. A diminished forced expiratory volume in 1 second (FEV_1)/forced vital capacity (FVC) (often defined as less than 70% of predicted value) is diagnostic of obstruction. The obstructive pathophysiology is seen in asthma, COPD, and bronchiectasis.[2]

3. D

   Reversibility of bronchoconstriction in asthma is demonstrated by a >12% and 200-mL increase in FEV_1 15 minutes after an inhaled short-acting β 2 -agonist or in some patients by a 2 to 4 week trial of oral corticosteroids (OCS) (prednisone or prednisolone 30–40 mg daily), > 20% diurnal variation on ≥ 3 days in a week for 2 week s on PEF diary and ≥ 1 5 %d ecrease in FEV_1 after 6 mins of exercise.[2&3]

4. C

   The acute treatment of Asthma consists of bronchodilators, inhaled corticosteroids, inhaled short acting beta agonists, inhaled anticholinergics, and systemic corticosteroids. Omalizumab is an antibody to IgE which improves asthma control over a period of 3 to 4 months. This treatment has been shown to reduce the number of exacerbations in patients with severe asthma and may improve asthma control. Omalizumab is usually given as a subcutaneous injection every 2–4 weeks.[1]

5. D

   Aapproximately 5% of asthmatics are difficult to control despite maximal inhaled therapy defined as refractory asthma. Some of these patients will require maintenance treatment with oral corticosteroids. Complete resistance to corticosteroids is extremely uncommon and is defined by a failure to respond to a high dose of oral prednisone/prednisolone (40 mg once daily over 2 weeks).

   Brittle asthma patients show chaotic variations in lung function despite taking appropriate therapy. Some patients (type 1) may require oral corticosteroids or, at times, continuous infusion of β 2 - agonists, whereas others (type 2) are difficult to manage as they do not respond well to corticosteroids and with inhaled bronchodilators. The most effective therapy is subcutaneous epinephrine.

   A small proportion (1–5%) of asthmatics becomes worse with aspirin and other COX inhibitors. Aspirin-sensitive asthma is usually preceded by perennial rhinitis and nasal polyps in non atopic patients with a late onset of the disease. Aspirin, even in small doses, characteristically provokes rhinorrhea, conjunctival irritation, facial flushing, and wheezing. All nonselective COX inhibitors should be avoided, but selective COX2 inhibitors are safe to use when an anti-inflammatory analgesic is needed. Aspirin-sensitive asthma responds to usual therapy with ICS.[1]

References:

1. Peter J. Barnes. Asthma. In: Kasper DL, Fauci AS, Hauser SL, Longo DL, Jameson L, Loscalzo J, editors. Harrison principles of internal medicine, 19th ed. New York: Mc Graw-Hill Medical Publishing Division; 2015. p. 1669-1681.
2. Kritek P, Choi AMK. Approach to the Patient with disease of the respiratory system. In: Longo DL, Kasper DL, Jameson L, Fauci AS, Hauser SL, Loscalzo J, editors. Harrison principles of internal medicine, 18th ed. New York: Mc Graw-Hill Medical Publishing Division; 2012. p. 1661-1663.
3. Reid PT, Innes JA. Respiratory disease. In: Walker BR, Colledge NR, Ralston SH, Penman ID, eds. Davidson's principles and practice of medicine, 22nd ed. London: Churchill Livingstone Elsevier; 2014. p. 644-731.

CHRONIC OBSTRUCTIVE PULMONARY DISEASE
Dr. Shyam Chand Chaudhary, Associate Professor, Department of Medicine

A 55 year old male presented to the Medical Outpatient Department with the chief complaints of progressively increasing dyspnoea on exertion for the past 2 years. There is no history of rhinorrhoea, sneezing or any allergic disorders. He is a chronic smoker with 40 pack years of smoking and he quit 3 years back. On general examination vitals are stable with respiratory rate of 28/min. Accessory muscles of respiration are prominent and pursed lip breathing is present. Chest reveals bilaterally decreased intensity of breath sounds and polyphonic rhonchi all over the chest. Upper border of Liver dullness is present in 7th intercostal space.

1. All of the following are the components of Chronic Obstructive Pulmonary Disease **except**
   (A) Chronic Bronchitis
   (B) Emphysema
   (C) Bronchial Asthma
   (D) Small Airway Disease
2. This patient undergoes a pulmonary function test analysis and his results are as follows:FEV_1=40% of predicted, FEV_1/FVC=60% of predicted with absence of reversibility. According to GOLD classification this patient can be classified as
   (A) Stage I COPD
   (B) Stage II COPD
   (C) Stage III COPD
   (D) Stage IV COPD
3. All of the following are the components of BODE Index, used in prognostication of Chronic Obstructive Pulmonary Disease **except**
   (A) FEV1/FVC ratio
   (B) Distance walked in 6 min
   (C) MRC dyspnoea Scale
   (D) Body mass index
4. Regardinglong-term domiciliary oxygen therapy (LTOT) in COPD all are true **except**
   (A) The aim of the therapy is to increase the PaO2 to at least 60 mmHg or SaO2 to at least 90%.
   (B) It improves survival in patients with COPD complicated by severe hypoxaemia (PaO2 < 55 mmHg).
   (C) It should be used in patients with PaO2 of 55–60 mmHg plus pulmonary hypertension, peripheral oedema or nocturnal hypoxaemia.
   (D) It should be used at least 15 hours/day at 2–4 L/min to achieve a PaO2 > 60 mmHg with unacceptable rise in PaCO2.
5. Lung Volume Reduction Surgery (LVRS) in COPD is contraindicated in all of the following conditions **except**
   (A) Patients with an FEV_1<20% of predicted and diffusely distributed emphysema on CT scan
   (B) Significant pleural disease
   (C) Pulmonary artery systolic pressure <45 mmHg
   (D) Congestive heart failure

Answers:
1. C
   Chronic obstructive pulmonary disease (COPD) is defined as a disease state characterized by airflow limitation that is not fully reversible. COPD includes *emphysema,* an anatomically defined condition characterized by destruction and enlargement of the lung alveoli; *chronic bronchitis,* a clinically defined condition with chronic cough and phlegm; and *small airways disease,* a condition in which small bronchioles are narrowed.[1]
2. C
   The HallImark of COPD is airflow obstruction and pulmonary function testing shows reduction in FEV 1 and FEV 1 /FVC ratio. With worsening disease severity, lung volumes may increase, resulting in an increase in total lung capacity, functional residual capacity, and residual volume. The degree of airflow obstruction is an important prognostic factor in COPD and is the basis for the Global Initiative for Lung Disease (GOLD) redundant classification. Patients are graded as per GOLD criteria (table).[1]

GOLD Stage	Severity	Spirometry
I	Mild	FEV_1/FVC <0.7 and $FEV_1 \geq$ 80% predicted
II	Moderate	FEV_1/FVC <0.7 and $FEV_1 \geq$ 50% but <80% predicted
III	Severe	FEV_1/FVC <0.7 and $FEV_1 \geq$ 30% but <50% predicted
IV	Very Severe	FEV_1/FVC <0.7 and FEV_1<30% predicted

3. A

    COPD has a variable natural history but is usually progressive. The prognosis is inversely related to age and directly related to the post-bronchodilator FEV_1. Additional poor prognostic indicators include weight loss and pulmonary hypertension. Recent study has suggested that a composite score (BODE index) comprising the body mass index (B), the degree of airflow obstruction (O) in the form of FEV_1, a measurement of dyspnoea (D) in the form of MRC dyspnoea scale and exercise capacity (E) in the form of distance walked in 6 min, may assist in predicting death from respiratory and other causes.[2]

4. D

    Long-term home oxygen therapy (LTOT) improves survival in selected patients with COPD complicated by severe hypoxaemia (arterial PaO_2 less than 55 mmHg). Arterial blood gases measured in clinically stable patients on optimal medical therapy on at least two occasions 3 weeks apart and LTOT should be initiated if:

    a. PaO_2< 55 mmHg irrespective of $PaCO_2$ and FEV1 < 1.5 L

    b. PaO_2 55–60 mmHg plus pulmonary hypertension, peripheral oedema or nocturnal hypoxaemia

    Use at least 15 hrs/day at 2–4 L/min to achieve a PaO_2 60 mmHg or SaO_2 to at least 90% without unacceptable rise in $PaCO_2$.[2]

5. C

    Lung volume reduction surgery (LVRS) should not be done if patients have significant pleural disease, a pulmonary artery systolic pressure >45 mmHg, extreme deconditioning, congestive heart failure, or other severe comorbid conditions. Patients with an FEV_1<20% of predicted and either diffusely distributed emphysema on CT scan or diffusing capacity of lung for carbon monoxide (DL_{CO}) <20% of predicted have an increased mortality rate after the procedure and thus are not candidates for LVRS. The anatomic distribution of emphysema and post-rehabilitation exercise capacity are important prognostic characteristics. Patients with upper lobe–predominant emphysema and a low post-rehabilitation exercise capacity are most likely to benefit from LVRS.[1]

References:

1. Reilly JJ, Silverman EK, Shapiro SD. Chronic Obstructive Pulmonary Disease. In: Kasper DL, Fauci AS, Hauser SL, Longo DL, Jameson L, Loscalzo J, editors. Harrison principles of internal medicine, 19th ed. New York: Mc Graw-Hill Medical Publishing Division; 2015. p. 1700-1707.
2. Reid PT, Innes JA. Respiratory disease. In: Walker BR, Colledge NR, Ralston SH, Penman ID, editors. Davidson's principles and practice of medicine, 22nd ed. London: Churchill Livingstone Elsevier; 2014. p. 644-731.

PNEUMONIA

Dr. Shyam Chand Chaudhary, Associate Professor, Department of Medicine

A 43 year old man presented with the chief complaints of pyrexia and breathlessness from the past 3 days. The pyrexia is high grade associated with chills and rigors relieved only on taking medications. He also reports cough with expectoration from the past 2 days. The expectoration is purulent and approximately a cupful in a day, not associated with blood. He is a nonsmoker and without any comorbidities. On general examination he is tachypnoeic having RR=36/min, PR= 120/min and BP=114/70 mmHg. He is febrile (101.4⁰F) and chest examination reveals dull note on percussion in right sided infraaxillary, Infrascapular and mammary areas. On auscultation bronchial breath sound, coarse crepitations and increased vocal resonance are found in the corresponding areas.

1. What would be the provisional diagnosis in this patient?
    (A) Lung abscess
    (B) Bronchiectasis

    (C) Pneumonia

    (D) Empyema

2. What is the next investigation you would like to proceed with in this patient?

    (A) Chest X ray

    (B) Blood culture

    (C) Pulmonary function tests

    (D) Sputum examination

Investigations reveal: Hb-11.0 gm%, TLC-18000/mm^3 with polymorph of 95%, Platelet count-1.5 lakh/mm^3. His random blood sugar-116 mg/dl, blood urea-5 mmol/L, serum creatinine-0.7 mg/dl and a normal urine examination. Chest X ray reveals homogenous opacity in right lower lung field.

3. All of the following are included in the CURB-65 criteria for determining the site of patient care **except:**

    (A) Confusion

    (B) Serum uric acid

    (C) Age ≥65 years

    (D) Respiratory rate ≥30/min

4. The empirical outpatient therapy for this patient includes all of the following **except:**

    (A) Oral Azithromycin

    (B) Oral Levofloxacin

    (C) Oral Clarithromycin

    (D) Oral Doxycycline

5. The following are known complications of this condition **except:**

    (A) Pleural effusion

    (B) Lung abscess

    (C) Multiple organ dysfunction syndrome

    (D) Lung carcinoma

Answers:

1. C

    Pneumonia is an infection of the pulmonary parenchyma. Patient is frequently febrile with tachycardia or may have a history of chills and/or sweats. Cough may be either nonproductive or productive of mucoid, purulent, or blood-tinged sputum. Gross hemoptysis is suggestive of community acquired MRSA pneumonia. Depending on severity the patient may be able to speak in full sentences or may be very short of breath. If the pleura is involved the patients may experience pleuritic chest pain. Up to 20% of patients may have gastrointestinal symptoms such as nausea, vomiting, and/or diarrhea. Other symptoms may include fatigue, headache, myalgias, and arthralgias. Findings on physical examination vary with the degree of pulmonary consolidation and the presence or absence of a significant pleural effusion. An increased respiratory rate and use of accessory muscles of respiration are common. Palpation may reveal increased or decreased tactile fremitus, and the percussion note can vary from dull to flat, reflecting underlying consolidated lung and pleural fluid, respectively. Crackles, bronchial breath sounds, and possibly a pleural friction rub may be heard on auscultation.[1]

2. A

    Sensitivity and specificity of the findings on physical examination are less, averaging 58% and 67%, respectively. Therefore, chest radiography is often necessary to differentiate CAP from other conditions. Gram's Stain and Culture of Sputum: Even in cases of proven bacteremic pneumococcal pneumonia, the yield of positive cultures from sputum samples is 50%. Blood Cultures: Only ~5–14% of cultures of blood from patients hospitalized with CAP are positive.[1]

3. B

    CURB-65 criteria, is used to decide the site of care in pneumonia patients. The CURB-65 criteria include five variables: confusion (C); urea >7 mmol/L (U); respiratory ≥30/min (R); blood pressure, systolic ≤90 mmHg or diastolic ≤60 mmHg (B); and age ≥ 65 years (65). Patients with a score of 0, among whom the 30-day mortality rate is 1.5%, can be treated outside the hospital. With a score of 2, the 30-day mortality rate is 9.2%, and patients should be admitted to the hospital. Among patients with scores of ≥3, mortality rates are 22% overall; these patients may require admission to an ICU.[1]

4. B

    The empiric antibiotic regimen recommended by the Infectious Disease Society of America and the American Thoracic Society for individuals who are previously healthy and have not received antibiotics in the prior 3 months is either doxycycline or a macrolide such as azithromycin or clarithromycin. In outpatients with significant medical comorbidities or antibiotics within the previous 3 months, the suggested antibiotic therapy is either a respiratory fluoroquinolone or a beta lactam plus a macrolide.[1]

5. D

Common complications of severe CAP include respiratory failure, shock and multiorgan failure, coagulopathy, and exacerbation of comorbid illnesses. Three particularly noteworthy conditions are metastatic infection, lung abscess, and complicated pleural effusion. Metastatic infection (e.g., brain abscess or endocarditis), although unusual, deserves immediate attention by the physician, with a detailed workup and proper treatment. Lung abscess may occur in association with aspiration or with infection caused by a single CAP pathogen such as CA-MRSA, P. aeruginosa, or (rarely) S. pneumoniae.[1]

Reference:

1. Mandell LA, Wunderink RG. Pneumonia. In: Kasper DL, Fauci AS, Hauser SL, Longo DL, Jameson L, Loscalzo J, editors. Harrison principles of internal medicine, 19th ed. New York: Mc Graw-Hill Medical Publishing Division; 2015. p. 803-13.

COR PULMONALE

Dr. Shyam Chand Chaudhary, Associate Professor, Department of Medicine

A 55 year old man who is a chronic smoker for the past 30 years presents to the emergency room with complaints of increased breathlessness and generalized body swelling. On examination: Blood Pressure -146/90 mmHg, PR-110/min, bilateral pitting type pedal oedema is present up to knees and neck veins are engorged. Chest reveals-bilateral rhonchi, tender hepatomegaly on abdominal examination. On CVS examination a holosystolic murmur is auscultated at the left parasternal border which increases in intensity with inspiration. ECG finding reveals p-pulmonale.

1. What is the most probable diagnosis in this case
    (A) Hypertensive heart failure
    (B) Cor pulmonale
    (C) Acute exacerbation of chronic obstructive pulmonary disease
    (D) Chronic renal failure
2. Following are the manifestations of cor pulmonale **except**
    (A) Prominent V waves in JVP
    (B) Cyanosis
    (C) Holosystolic murmur at apex of the heart
    (D) Tender hepatomegaly
3. All the following are causes of chronic cor pulmonale **except**
    (A) Chronic obstructive pulmonary disease
    (B) Chronic pulmonary thromboembolic disease
    (C) Cystic fibrosis
    (D) Hypertensive heart failure
4. What is the most common cause of right sided heart failure?
    (A) Secondary to left sided heart failure
    (B) Chronic bronchitis
    (C) Bronchiectasis
    (D) Emphysema
5. What is the emergency treatment you would like to institute in this patient
    (A) Emergent hemodialysis
    (B) IV diuretics, IV bronchodilators and nebulization
    (C) Rapid lowering of blood pressure using IV nitroglycerine
    (D) Anticoagulants, antiplatelet drugs, long acting vasodilators

Answers:

1. B

Cor pulmonale (pulmonary heart disease), is defined as dilation and hypertrophy of the right ventricle in response to diseases of the pulmonary vasculature and/or lung parenchyma. Historically, this definition has excluded congenital heart disease and those diseases in which the right heart fails secondary to dysfunction of the left side of the heart. Once patients with chronic pulmonary or pulmonary vascular disease develop cor pulmonale, the prognosis worsens.

The symptoms of chronic cor pulmonale generally are related to the underlying pulmonary disorder. Dyspnea, the most common symptom, is usually the result of the increased work of breathing

212

secondary to changes in elastic recoil of the lung (fibrosing lung diseases), altered respiratory mechanics (e.g., overinflation with COPD), or inefficient ventilation (e.g., primary pulmonary vascular disease). Orthopnea and paroxysmal nocturnal dyspnea are rarely symptoms of isolated right HF and usually point toward concurrent left heart dysfunction. Rarely, these symptoms reflect increased work of breathing in the supine position resulting from compromised diaphragmatic excursion. Abdominal pain and ascites that occur with cor pulmonale are similar to the right-heart failure that ensues in chronic HF. Lower-extremity edema may occur secondary to neurohormonal activation, elevated RV filling pressures, or increased levels of carbon dioxide and hypoxemia, which can lead to peripheral vasodilation and edema formation.

Signs of cor pulmonale include, tachypnea, elevated jugular venous pressures with prominenet$v$ as a result of tricuspid regurgitation, hepatomegaly, and lower-extremity edema. Other cardiovascular signs include an RV heave palpable along the left sternal border or in the epigastrium. The increase in intensity of the holosystolic murmur of tricuspid regurgitation with inspiration ("Carvallo's sign") may be lost eventually as RV failure worsens. Cyanosis is a late finding in cor pulmonale.[1]

2. C

Kindly refer to explanation of question number 1.

3. D

Although chronic obstructive pulmonary disease (COPD) is the most important cause, any disease that affects the pulmonary vasculature or parenchyma can lead to cor pulmonale.[1]

4. A

The most common cause of right-heart failure is not pulmonary parenchymal or vascular diseases but left heart failure.[1]

5. B

The primary treatment goal of cor pulmonale is to target the underlying pulmonary disease, since this will decrease pulmonary vascular resistance and lessen RV afterload. Most pulmonary diseases that lead to chronic cor pulmonale are advanced and therefore are less amenable to treatment. General principles of treatment include decreasing work of breathing by using noninvasive mechanical ventilation and bronchodilation, as well as treating any underlying infection. Adequate oxygenation (oxygen saturation 90–92%) and correcting respiratory acidosis are vital for decreasing pulmonary vascular resistance and reducing demand on the RV.

Diuretics are effective in RV failure, and indications are similar to those for chronic HF. One caveat of chronic diuretic use is to avoid inducing contraction alkalosis and worsening hypercapnia. Pulmonary vasodilators can effectively improve symptoms through modest reduction of pulmonary pressures and RV afterload when isolated pulmonary arterial hypertension is present.[1]

Reference:

1. Douglas LM, Chakinala M. Heart Failure and Cor pulmonale. In: Longo DL, Kasper DL, Jameson L, Fauci AS, Hauser SL, Loscalzo J, editors. Harrison principles of internal medicine, 18th ed. New York: Mc Graw-Hill Medical Publishing Division; 2012. p. 1901-1915.

PANCYTOPENIA

Dr K K Sawlani, Associate Professor, Department of Medicine

A 32 year old male presented with history of malaise, weakness and breathlessness on exertion for 20 days. There was no history of diabetes or hypertension. On examination there was pallor, mild icterus, no Lymphadenopathy, pulse 96/ min and regular, BP 138/66 mm Hg. Examination of chest and Cardiovascular System was normal. Abdominal examination revealed mild splenomegaly.

Investigations revealed

Hb-	8.5 g/dL
TLC	3600/cumm (P62 L38 M0 BO)
Platlet count	72000/cumm
MCV	116 fL
MCH	34 pg
Urea	24 mg%
Creatinine	0.8 mg%
Serum bilirubin	2.8 mg/dL (Indirect 1.9mg/dl)
SGPT	32 U/L
SGOT	26 U/L
ALP	116 U/L

1. All of the following are causes of pancytopenia with cellular marrow except
   (A) Systemic lupus erythematosus
   (B) Vitamin B12 deiciency
   (C) Mylelopthhthisis
   (D) Fanconi's anemia
2. Causes of aplastic anemia include all except
   (A) HIV infection
   (B) Paroxysmal nocturnal hemoglobinuria
   (C) Pregnancy
   (D) Brucellosis
   Peripheral blood smear examination of this patient is given below

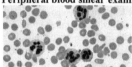

3. What is the probable cause of pancytopenia in this patient
   (A) Leukemic leukemia
   (B) Myelofibrosis
   (C) Aplastisc anemia
   (D) Vitamin B12 deficency
4. All of the following findings can be present due to ineffective erythropoiesis (hemolysis within the marrow) except
   (A) Increased serum lactate dehydrogenase
   (B) Raised urinary urobilinogen
   (C) Reticulocytosis
   (D) Decreased haptoglobins
5. All of the following are causes of megaloblastic anemia except
   (A) Hydroxyurea
   (B) Cyclosporine
   (C) Cytosine arabinoside
   (D) 6-mercaptopurine
6. Which of the following finding can differentiate between folate deficiency or cobalamin deficiency when facilities for blood levels of these two is not available
   (A) Megaloblastic bone marrow
   (B) Increased homocysteine
   (C) Increased methyl malonic acid(MMA)
   (D) Increased indirect bilirubin

Answers:
1. D
   Causes of pancytopenia with hypocellular bone marrow include aplastic anemia, Constitutional aplastic anemia (Fanconi anemia, dyskeratosis congenita), and some myelodysplasia and rera aleukemic leukemia. SLE, Vitamin B12 deficiency and myeopthisis are causes of pancytopenia with cellular bone marrow.[1]
2. D
   Acquired causes of aplastic anemia are secondary to radiation and drugs, Viruses (EBV, non A non B non C hepatitis, parvovirus B19 virus, HIV -1), Immune diseases, Paroxusmal nocturnal hemoglobinuria, pregnancy and idiopathic. Inherited causes of aplastic anemia include Fanconi's anemia, dyskeratosis congenital, Shwachman-Diamond syndrome, reticular dysgenesis.[1]
3. D
   PBS shows hypersegmented neutrophils. Probable cause in this case is Vitamin B12 dficiency. Pancytopenia, raised MCV and MCH, indirect hyperbilirubinemia and hypersegmented neutrophils in peripheral smear examination are present in Vitamin B12 deficiency.[2]
4. C
   Ineffective erythropoiesis (hemolysis within the marrow) can cause increase in serum LDH, increased indirect bilirubin, raised urinary urobilinogen, decreased haptoglobins and positive urinary hemosiderin. Reticulocytosis present in other haemolytic conditions is not seen in vitamin B12 deficiency.[2,3]
5. B

Causes of megaloblastic anemia are cobalamin and folate deficiency, antifolate drugs (methotrexate), independent of cobalamin and folate deficiency (some cases of acute myeloid leukemia, myelodysplasia, orotic aciduria, therapy with drugs interfering with synthesis of DNA eg. cytosine arabinoside, hydroxyurea, 6-mercaptopurine, azidothymidine(AZT). Later will not respond to cobalamin and folate therapy.[2]

6. C

Megaloblastic bone marrow and indirect bilirubin are present in both folate and cobalmin deficiency. Serum homocysteine deficiency is raised in both early cobalamin and folate deficiency but methylmalonate is raised only in cobalamin deficiency.[2,3]

References:

1. Young SN. Bone Marrow Failure Syndromes Including Aplastic Anemia and Myelodysplasia. In: Kasper DL, Fauci AS, Hauser SL, Longo DL, Jameson JL, Loscalzo J. editors. Harrison's Principles of Internal Medicine. 19th edition. New Delhi: McGraw Hill; 2015. p. 662-672.
2. Hoffbrand AV. Megaloblastic Anemias. In: Kasper DL, Fauci AS, Hauser SL, Longo DL, Jameson JL, Loscalzo J. editors. Harrison's Principles of Internal Medicine. 19th edition. New Delhi: McGraw Hill; 2015. p. 640-649.
3. Watson HG, Craig JLO, Manson LM. Blood Disease. In: Walker BR, Colledge NR, Ralston SH, Penman ID, editors. Davidson's Principles and Practice of Medicine .22nd edition. London: Churchill Livingstone Elsevier; 2014. p. 1024.

MASSIVE LEFT-SIDED PLEURAL EFFUSION

Dr K K Sawlani, Associate Professor, Department of Medicine

A 56 year old male, non smoker was admitted to the hospital with a chief complaint of shortness of breath for 3 weeks. He had history of low grade fever for 15 days.

General examination revealed polar, mild tachycardia, BP- 126/84 mm Hg. There was no icterus and lymphadenopathy. Chest examination revealed decreased movements on left side, stony dullness and absent breath sounds on left side.

The CXR showed a large left-side pleural effusion.

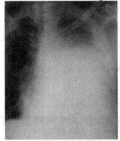

1. All of the following possibilities can be considered in this case except
   (A) Para pneumonic effusion
   (B) Hepatic hydrothorax
   (C) Tuberculous pleuritis
   (D) Effusion secondary to malignancy
2. All of the following criteria are met if effusion is exudative except
   (A) Pleural fluid protein/ Serum fluid protein > 0.5
   (B) Pleural fluid LDH/ Serum fluid LDH > 0.6
   (C) Pleural fluid LDH more than two thirds normal lower limit for serum LDH
   (D) Difference between the protein levels in pleural fluid and serum < 3.1 g/dL

   The patient denied any history of cough, he had decreased appetite for 15 days and was not sure about loss of weight.

   His pleural fluid examination report revealed

   Colour   Pale yellow
   Protien   5.6 g/dL (serum protein 7.2 g/dL)
   LDH   256 U/L (serum LDH 210 u/L)
   Pleural fluid ADA 16 U/L

   The cytology of pleural fluid was positive for malignant cells.

3. All of the following findings can be present in malignant pleural effusion except
   (A) Hemorrhagic pleural effusion
   (B) Raised pleural fluid amylase
   (C) Low pleural fluid glucose < 60 mg/dL
   (D) Raised interferon γ > 320 pg/ml
4. Which of the following findings favours diagnosis of tuberculous pleural effusion?
   (A) Positive Skin test (Mantaux test)
   (B) Pleural fluid ADA > 10 U/L
   (C) Raised interferon γ >140 pg/ml
   (D) Low pleural fluid glucose < 40 mg/dL
5. All of the following cause > 75% of all malignant pleural effusions except
   (A) Lung carcinoma
   (B) Breast carcinoma
   (C) Mesothelioma
   (D) Lymphoma

Answers:

   1. B
      Parapneumonic effusion, malignant effusion and tuberculous peritonitis are causes of exudative effusion. Hepatic hydrothorax occurs in about 5% of patients with cirrhosis and ascites and fluid is transudative. The fluid passes through pore in the diaphragm into pleural cavity. It is usually right sided and large effusion enough to produce dyspnea.

   2. C
      Exudative pleural effusions meet at least one of the following criteria, whereas transudative pleural effusions meet none:
      a. Pleural fluid protein/serum protein >0.5
      b. Pleural fluid LDH/serum LDH >0.6
      c. Pleural fluid LDH more than two-thirds normal **upper limit** for serum
      25% of transudates can be classified as exudates by these criteria. If the patient is clinically thought to have a condition producing a transudative effusion, the difference between the protein levels in the serum and the pleural fluid should be measured. If this gradient is >31 g/L (3.1 g/dL), the exudative categorization by these criteria can be ignored because almost all such patients have a transudative pleural effusion.

   3. D
      In malignant effusion the pleural fluid is an exudate, and its glucose level may be reduced if the tumor burden in the pleural space is high. Some malignant effusions have high amylase levels and may be hemorrhagic, high interferon gamma is helpful in diagnosis of tuberculous effusions(> 140 pg/mL).

   4. C
      Patients with tuberculous pleuritis present with fever, weight loss, dyspnea, and/or pleuritic chest pain. The pleural fluid is an exudate with predominantly small lymphocytes. The diagnosis is established by adenosine deaminase >40 IU/L or interferon gamma > 140 pg/mL. Diagnosis can also be established by culture/ PCR of the fluid, biopsy of pleura or thoracoscopy. Low pleural fluid glucose may be present in empyema and malignant effusions.

   5. C
      Lung carcinoma, breast carcinoma, and lymphoma are the three tumors that cause >75% of all malignant pleural effusions. Most patients present with dyspnea, out of proportion to the size of the effusion. In mesothelioma the chest radiograph reveals a pleural effusion, generalized pleural thickening, and a shrunken hemithorax

Reference:

   1. Light RW. Disorders of the Pleura and Mediastinum. In: Kasper DL, Fauci AS, Hauser SL, Longo DL, Jameson JL, Loscalzo J. editors. Harrison's Principles of Internal Medicine. 19th edition. New Delhi: McGraw Hill; 2015. p. 1716-1719.

A CASE OF EPISODIC WEAKNESS

Dr K K Sawlani, Associate Professor, Department of Medicine

A 22 year old male presented to emergency department with complaints of weakness of all four limbs for 1 day. He had similar episode about 6 months back and weakness recovered within 48 hrs after treatment. On examination patient was conscious, oriented, cranial nerve examination was normal, motor power was diminished in all four limbs (proximal> distal), sensory examination was normal. He had tachycardia and blood pressure was 142/74 mm Hg.

He had also giving history of excessive sweating.

1. All of the following can cause episodic generalized weakness except
   - (A) Hyperkalemia
   - (B) Myasthenia gravis
   - (C) Transient ischemic attacks of brainstem
   - (D) Gullain Barre syndrome

   Investigations revealed

Hb	13g/dL,
TLC	8600/cumm(P62 L38 M0 BO),
Platlet count	3.5 lacs /cumm,
MCV	84fL,
MCH	34 pg,
Urea	24 mg%,
Creatinine	0.8 mg%,
Serum bilirubin	1.9mg/dL (Indirect0.9mg/dL),
SGPT	34 U/L,
SGOT	28 U/L,
ALP	119 U/L
TSH	0.01 µIU/ml
Serum sodium	138 meq/L
Serum potassium	2.2 m meq/L

2. All of the following are causes of hypokalemia except
   - (A) Vitamin B 12 therapy
   - (B) Hypomagnesemia
   - (C) Mineralocrticoid excess
   - (D) Trimethoprim ingestion
3. In hypokalemic periodic paralysis mutations can occur in all of the following except
   - (A) Potassium channel gene
   - (B) Calcium channel gene
   - (C) Sodium channel gene
   - (D) Magnesium channel gene
4. All of the following statements are true regarding hypokalemic periodic paralysis (hypoKPP)except
   - (A) Episodic weakness with onset after age 25 years
   - (B) In type 1 HypoKPP mutations are present in calcium channel gene
   - (C) In type 2 HypoKPP mutations are present in sodium channel gene
   - (D) HypoKPP type 1 is the most common form
5. All of the following are true regarding thyrotoxic periodic paralysis except
   - (A) Onset below 25 years of age
   - (B) It occurs more in men
   - (C) Attacks abate with treatment of underlying thyroid condition
   - (D) Attacks are provoked by meals high in carbohydrate and sodium

Answers:

1. D

   Hyperkalemia, myasthenia gravis and transient ischemic attacks of the brainstem can cause episodic weekness besides Electrolyte disturbances (e.g., hypokalemia, hyperkalemia, hypercalcemia, hypernatremia, hyponatremia, hypophosphatemia, hypermagnesemia), Channelopathies (periodic paralyses), Transient global cerebral ischemia, Multiple sclerosis and Lambert-Eaton myasthenic syndrome. Generalized episodic weakness is not a feature of G B Syndrome.[1]

2. D

   Trimethoprim, amiloride, triamterene and pentamidine cause hyperkalemia due to inadequate excretion of potassium. ACE inhibitors ARBs, spironolactone, eplerenone also cause hyperkalemia.[2]

3. D

   HypoKPP type 1 patients have mutations in the voltage-sensitive, skeletal muscle calcium channel gene, *CALCL1A3*). HypoKPP type 2 arises from mutations in the voltage-sensitive sodium channel gene (*SCN4A*). In either instance, the mutations lead to an abnormal gating pore current that predisposes the muscle cell to depolarize when potassium levels are low. Some cases of thyrotoxic HypoKPP are caused by genetic variants in a potassium channel (Kir 2.6).[3]

4. A

Episodic weakness with onset after age 25 is almost never due to periodic paralyses, with the exception of thyrotoxic periodic paralysis. Type 1 hypoKPP is the most common form, is inherited as an autosomal dominant disorder with incomplete penetrance. Approximately 10 % of patients have type 2 hypoKPP.[3]

5. A

Episodic weakness with onset after age 25 is almost never due to periodic paralyses, with the exception of thyrotoxic periodic paralysis. Clincal presentation of thyrotoxic periodic paralysis resemble those of primary HypoKPP. Attacks are provoked by high carbohydrate and sodium consumption and may occur with rest after frolonged exercise. Attacks of thyrotoxic periodic paralysis resemble those of primary HypoKPP.

References:

1. Aminoff MJ. Neurologic Causes of Weakness and Paralysis. In: Kasper DL, Fauci AS, Hauser SL, Longo DL, Jameson JL, Loscalzo J. editors. Harrison's Principles of Internal Medicine. 19th edition. New Delhi: McGraw Hill; 2015. p. 154-157.
2. Mount DB. Fluid and Electrolytes Disturbances. In: Kasper DL, Fauci AS, Hauser SL, Longo DL, Jameson JL, Loscalzo J. editors. Harrison's Principles of Internal Medicine. 19th edition. New Delhi: McGraw Hill; 2015. p. 295-312.
3. Amato AA, Brown RH. Muscular Dystrophies and Other Muscle Diseases. In: Longo DL, Fauci AS, Kasper DL, Hauser SL, Jameson JL, Loscalzo J. editors. Harrison's Principles of Internal Medicine. 18th edition. New Delhi: McGraw Hill; 2012. p. 3487-3509.

ACUTE PANCREATITIS

Dr Vivek Kumar, Associate Professor, Department of Medicine

A 40 yr old female seeked evaluation for complaint of severe epigastric abdominal pain radiating to back more intense on lying supine and is relieved to an extent on sitting and bending forward. Pain was associated with nausea and vomiting and a feeling of abdominal distension.On examination, pulse rate was 106/min and Blood pressure was 80/60mmHg and epigastric tenderness was present along with localized guarding and rest of the examination was normal .Investigations revealed, Hb-11 g/dl, total leukocyte count-17,600/mm3, Platelet count-70,000/mm3, random blood sugar - 86mg/dl.The kidney function test and liver function test were normal.

1. What is the possible diagnosis?
   (A) Acid peptic disease
   (B) Acute pancreatitis
   (C) Cholecystitis
   (D) Intestinal obstruction
2. Which laboratory test would you order to confirm diagnosis?
   (A) Serum amylase and lipase
   (B) Serum procalcitonin
   (C) Liver function tests
   (D) D-dimer
3. Imaging modality of choice in this case?
   (A) CECT abdomen
   (B) MRI abdomen
   (C) Colonoscopy
   (D) Endoscopy
4. What is the possible etiology in this case?
   (A) Idiopathic
   (B) Gall stone
   (C) Alcohol
   (D) Sphincter of oddi dysfunction

Answers:

1. B

   Patient presents with the classical pattern of epigastric pain which is radiating to back and gets relieved on sitting up, these points favours the diagnosis of acute pancreatitis.
2. A

Serum amylase and lipase are the biochemical tests used for the diagnosis of acute pancreatitis. Values greater than three times the upper limit of normal virtually clinch diagnosis.

3. A

Imaging modality of choice is contrast enhanced CT of abdomen. It is best done three to five days into hospitalization as it might not possible to distinguish interstitial and necrotizing pancreatitis on day of admission. Pancreas is not well visualizwd by ultrasound of abdomen by virtue of it being a retroperitoneal structure.

4. B

Worldwide the most common cause of pancreatitis is gallstone disease followed by alcohol.

Reference:

1. Greenberg NJ, Conwell DL, Wu BU, Banks PA. Acute and Chronic Pancreatitis, in Harrison's principles of internal medicine, 18th ed, Longo et al (eds). New York, Mc Graw-Hill, 2012, pp 2631-39.

WHIPPLE'S DISEASE

Dr Vivek Kumar, Associate Professor, Department of Medicine

A 40 years old male seeked evaluation for chronic diarrhea and weight loss for the past 5 yrs. Stool were reported to be foul smelling greasy and bulky. Patient has developed migratory large joint pain over the last 3 months. Patient's brother also complains that the patient is having difficulty in remembering things. On examination right knee joint is swollen and tender and bilateral pedal edema was present. Rest of the examination was normal.On investigation, the hemoglobin was 10.1 g/dl and kidney function test were normal .Liver function test revealed a serum total protein of 5.1 mg/dl albumin of 3.1 mg/dl.

1. What is the possible diagnosis in this case?
    (A) Celiac disease
    (B) Whipple's disease
    (C) Tropical sprue
    (D) IBS
2. How would you confirm the daignosis?
    (A) Intestinal biopsy
    (B) Stool for microscopic examination
    (C) Anti-ttg antibody
    (D) D-xylose test
3. What would you find on biopsy?
    (A) PAS positive macrophages
    (B) Mycobacterium avium
    (C) Mastocytes
    (D) Amyloid deposit
4. What is the treatment?
    (A) Trimethoprim-sulphamethoxazole
    (B) Anti-tuberculous therapy
    (C) Sulphasalazine
    (D) Steroids

Answers :

1. - B

The diagnosis of whipple's disease is suggested by multisystem disease in presence of diarrhea and steatorrhea. Patient presents with migratory polyarthritis and memory deficits which are known extraintestinal complications of whipple's disease.

2. A

Diagnosis of whipple's disease is confirmed by tissue biopsy. Anti-TTG is used for diagnosis of celiac disease and d-xylose test is used for diagnosis of proximal small intestine as a cause of malabsorption.

3. A

The presence of PAS positive macrophages containing the characteristic small bacilli point towards diagnosis. The presence of *Tropheryma whipplei* outside them acrophages is a more important indicator of active disease than its presence inside the macrophage.

4. A

The treatment is prolonged course of antibiotic. The current drug of choice is double strength trimethoprim/sulfamethoxazole for approximately 1 year.

Reference:

1. Binder HJ: Disorders of absorption, in Harrison's principles of internal medicine, 18th ed, Longo et al (eds). New York, Mc Graw-Hill, 2012, pp 2474.

WILSONS DISEASE

Dr Vivek Kumar, Associate Professor, Department of Medicine

A 16 years old boy was brought to the out patient department with chief complaints of abnormal movements of hand with unusual posturing of body since last 2 yrs. He had a history of 2 episodes of jaundice 4 years back. On examination, patient was conscious and oriented, icterus was present and dystonic posture of right upper limb and trunk was noted. The cranial nerves, motor,sensory and other system examination was normal. The hemogram and kidney function test were normal and serum Bilirubin was 4.2mg/dl with a predominance of indirect fraction, the SGPT was 64 IU/dl and SGOT was 42 IU/dl.

1. What is your possible diagnosis?
   (A) Wilson's disease
   (B) Hemochromatosis
   (C) Hepatic encephalopathy
   (D) Alpha 1 anti trypsin deficiency
2. How you will confirm diagnosis?
   (A) 24 hour urinary copper
   (B) Serum ceruloplasmin
   (C) Ferritin levels
   (D) Transferring saturation
3. What is the treatment of choice?
   (A) Zinc
   (B) Phlebotomy
   (C) Zinc + Tetrathiomolybdate
   (D) Penicillamine
4. What would you not find in this case?
   (A) Kayser-fleischer ring
   (B) Sunflower cataract
   (C) Seizure
   (D) Motor weakness

Answers:

1. A
   Icterus and neurological involvement in the form of dystonia in a adolescent male, point towards the diagnosis of Wilsons disease.
2. A
   24 hour urinary copper is the non-invasive test employed in the diagnosis of Wilson's disease. Values >100mcg in symptomatic patient are diagnostic. .
3. C
   Treatment of choice in this case would be zinc and tetrathiomolybdate.
4. D
   Kayser-fliescher ring (copper deposits in the descement membrane of cornea), Sunflower catart and seizures are known complications of Wilson's disease. Motor wekness and sensory abnormalities do not occur in Wilson's disease .

Reference:

1. Brewer GJ: Wilson's disease, in Harrison's principles of internal medicine, 18th ed, Longo et al (eds). New York, Mc Graw-Hill ,2012, pp 3188-90.

MASSIVE PROTEINURIA

Dr. Satyendra Kr. Sonkar, Associate Professor, Department of Medicine

A 42 year male, type 2 diabetic mellitus, detected 2 years ago, presented with chief complaints of generalized body swelling and frothy urine for the past 3 months. On examination, vital was normal and bilateral pedal edema was present. In the urine examination, protein was 4+ with no active sediment. Biochemistry investigations showed, fasting lipid profile- triglycerides-325 mg/dl , total cholesterol- 240 mg/dl, LDL- 180 mg/dl,fasting blood sugar- 120mg/dl, PP-180 mg/dl, S. prot-4.5 gm/dl, s.alb- 2.0 gm/dl, s urea- 40 mg/dl and s.creatinine-1.0 mg/dl.

1. What is most likely diagnosis?
   (A) Nephritic syndrome
   (B) Nephrotic syndrome
   (C) Acute kidney injury
   (D) Chronic kidney disease
2. Nephrotic range of proteinuria in adult is-
   (A) < 500 mg/day
   (B) 500 mg-2g/day
   (C) >2 g/day
   (D) >3 g/day
3. What is the least likely cause of nephrotic syndrome in adults?
   (A) Minimal change disease(MCD)
   (B) FSGS
   (C) MPGN
   (D) Membranous nephropathy
4. What is the most likely secondary cause of nephrotic syndrome in above patient?
   (A) Lymphoma
   (B) Diabetic nephropathy
   (C) Amyloidosis
   (D) Lupus nephritis
5. On fundus examination there was no evidence of retinopathy, on further investigations HbA1c was 7%. What would be the next step for diagnosis and further management of the above patient?
   (A) USG for renal size
   (B) Renal biopsy
   (C) Anti- Nuclear antibody
   (D) HIV, HCV, HbsAg

Answers:
1. B
   Nephrotic syndrome classicaly presents with heavy proteinuria, minimal hematuria, hypoalbuminemia, hypercholesterolemia, edema and hypertension.
2. D
   Nephrotic range of proteinuria is greater than 3gm/d which may be whithout clinical manifestation.
3. A
   Minimal change disease (MCD) sometimes known as nil lesion, causes 70-90% of nephrotic syndrome in childhood but only 10-15% of nephrotic syndrome in adults.
4. B
   Proteinuria in frank diabetic nephropathy can be variable ranging from 500mg-25gm/d and is often associated with nephrotic syndrome.
5. B
   In patients with diabetes, albuminuria occurs after 5-10 years of the onset of diabetes. In the presence of other clinical or serological data in diabetic patient and here duration of diabetes is short, renal biopsy is indicated for further management.

Reference:
1. Julia B.Lewis, Eric G Neilson: Glomerular disease, in Harrison's Principles Of Internal Medicine, 18th ed, Longo et al (eds). New York, McgrawHill, 2012,pp 2337-2348.

CHRONIC KIDNEY DISEASE PRESENTING WITH ALTERED SENSORIUM

Dr. Satyendra Kr. Sonkar, Associate Professor, Department of Medicine

A 50 yr male of chronic kidney disease, for the past 5 yrs presented with episode of GTCS in Emergency Department. Patient was uncoscious and there was no neurogical deficit. Patient's pulse was 100/min, respiratory rate 28/min and blood pressure 190/100 mm Hg. Patient's investigation showed: Hemoglobin 7.0gm/dl, S. Urea -196mg/dl, creatinine 9.2mg/dl, blood sugar-110mg/dl , pH-7.2, HCO_3-16 mEq/l, S. Na- 139 mEq/l, S. K-6.5 mEq/l, S. ca-7.0mg/dl, phoshorus-6 mg/dl and urine showed 2+ proteinuria.

1. What could be the likely cause of GTCS and coma in above patient?
   (A) Uremic encephalopathy
   (B) Hypocalcemia
   (C) Hypoglycemia
   (D) Hyponatremia
2. All of the followings are the complications of chronic kidney disease in above patient except
   (A) Anemia
   (B) Metabolic acidosis
   (C) Coma
   (D) Proteinuria
3. Medical management of hyperkalemia are all except
   (A) I.V. calcium gluconate
   (B) Glucose insulin infusion drip
   (C) I. V. mannitol
   (D) Intravenous Sodium bicarbonate
4. All the clinical abnormalities can be corrected by patient undergoing dialysis and related therapy except
   (A) Coma
   (B) Hyperkalemia
   (C) Dialysis disequilibrium syndrome
   (D) Metabolic acidosis
5. What is the leading cause of death in patients with chronic kidney disease?
   (A) Mineral bone disease
   (B) Cardiovascular disease
   (C) Abnormal homeostasis
   (D) Infection

Answers:
1. A
   Patient's GTCS and Coma is due to uremia as there is no hypoglycemia or hyponatremia in this patient.[1]
2. D
   Proteinuria is not the complication but a disease manifestation of CKD whereas all other given above are hematological, acid base disorder and neurological complication due to uremia in CKD patients. [1]
3. C
   Except mannitol all the above are given for medical management of hyperkalemia.[2]
4. C
   Dialysis disequilibrium syndrome is itself a complication of hemodialysis. [1]
5 B
   Cardiovascular disease is the leading cause of mortality and morbidity in CKD patients.[1] .

References:
1. Joanne M Bargmann, Karl Skorecki: Chronic Kidney Disease, in Harrison's Principles Of Internal Medicine, 18th ed, Longo et al (eds). New York, McgrawHill, 2012, pp 2311-14
2. David B Mount: Fluid and electrolyte disorders, in Harrison's Principles Of Internal Medicine, 18th ed, Longo et al (eds). New York, McgrawHill, 2012, pp358

DECREASED URINE OUTPUT FOLLOWING CAESARIAN SECTION
Dr. Satyendra Kr. Sonkar, Associate Professor, Department of Medicine

A 24 year female developed high grade fever with chills on second day of caesarian section. Patient was started on IV Ceftriaxone & Gentamycin. After 1 day patient developed breathlessnes and decrease in urine output and then transferred to medicine ward. On examination patient was drowsy and pulse was 110/min , B.P. 90/60mm Hg, pedal edema was present with B/L crepts in chest. Investigations revealed– Hb-10.1gm/dl, Total Leukocyte Count-35000/mm³(N-90%,L-10%), platelet- 46000/mm³, S. urea-100mg/dl , creatinine -5.1mg/dl, urine protein-absent , no pus cells/no RBC. Arterial blood gas analysis- pH 7.1 & HCO3- 16mEq/l, S. Na- 130 mEq/l. S. K-5.9 mEq/l.
1. What is the most likely pathology?
   (A) Chronic kidney disease
   (B) Acute kidney injury

(C) Nephritic syndrome

(D) Ecclampsia

2. All of the following may be contributing factors for above pathology except

    (A) Sepsis

    (B) Drug

    (C) Hypotension

    (D) Bladder outlet obstruction

3. Indications of dialysis in this patient are all of the following except

    (A) Hyperkalemia

    (B) Neutrophilia

    (C) Oliguria

    (D) Acidosis

4. Which would be the best modality of renal replacement therapy in above patient ?

    (A) Hemodialysis

    (B) Peritoneal dialysis

    (C) CRRT/ SLED

    (D) CAPD

5. All are true about outcome and prognosis for above patient except

    (A) Low risk for progressive chronic kidney disease if patients recovers and discharged

    (B) Upto 10% may develop ESRD end stage renal disease

    (C) Above patient has bad prognosis

    (D) Post discharge patient requires supervision for aggressive prevention of secondary kidney disease.

Answers:

    1. B

    Acute kidney injury is due to sudden impairment of kidney function resulting in retention of nitrogenous and other waste products.

    2. D

    The above patient has sepsis as evidenced by leukocytosis and there is hypotension also. Patient received gentamycin which is nephrotoxic. Hence all the above are contributing factors of acute kidney injury in the above patient.

    3. B

    Except neutrophilia all others are indications for dialysis in above patient.

    4. C

    To treat hemodynamically unstable patients without inducing the rapid shifts of volume, osmolarity and electrolytes Continuous Renal Replacement Therapy (CRRT)/Slow Low Effective Dialysis (SLED) is the best modality of treatment.

    5. A

    Survivors of an episode of AKI requiring temporary hemodialysis,however, are at extremely high risk for progressive chronic kidney

Reference:

1. Sushrut S. Waiker, Joseph Bonventre: Acute Kidney Injury, in Harrison's Principles Of Internal Medicine, 18th ed, Longo et al (eds). New York, McgrawHill, 2012, pp 2293-3308

CUSHING'S SYNDROME

Dr Arvind Mishra, Professor, Department of Medicine

A 38 year old female came w,ith complaints of with gain, fatigue, amenorrhoea and acne over face for past 3 months. On examination BP- 160/90 mmHg, weight- 92 kg, hairs on face, purple stretch marks over abdomen and weakness of proximal muscles were present.

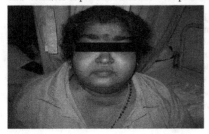

1. What is the diagnosis of this patient .
   (A) Cushing syndrome
   (B) Hypothyroidism
   (C) Addison's disease
   (D) Hypercalcemia
2. Which is not the test for confirmation of diagnosis in this patient
   (A) 24 hr urinary cortisol
   (B) Dexamethasone overnight test
   (C) 8:00 am plasma cortisol level
   (D) Low dose dexamethasone test
3. In case this patient would be ACTH- Dependent cushing syndrome, which of the following could not be a cause
   (A) Pituitary adenoma
   (B) Ectopic ACTH production by carcinoid tumor
   (C) Hypothalamic adenoma
   (D) Adrenocortical carcinoma
4. Drug not used preoperatively to control cortisol excess in very severe overt cushing syndrome is
   (A) Metyrapone
   (B) Ketoconazole
   (C) Mitotane
   (D) Mitomycin

Answers:
1. A
2. C
3. D
4. D

   Cushing's syndrome reflects a constellation of clinical features that result from chronic exposure to excess glucocorticoids of any etiology. The disorder can be ACTH-dependent or ACTH-independent as well as iatrogenic. The term *Cushing's disease* refers specifically to Cushing's syndrome caused by a pituitary corticotrope adenoma. Cushing's syndrome.

Table 342-1 Causes of Cushing's Syndrome		
Causes of Cushing's Syndrome	**Female:Male Ratio**	**%**
ACTH-Dependent Cushing's		**90**
Cushing's disease (= ACTH-producing pituitary adenoma)	4:1	75
Ectopic ACTH syndrome (due to ACTH secretion by bronchial or pancreatic carcinoid tumors, small cell lung cancer, medullary thyroid carcinoma, pheochromocytoma and others)	1:1	15
ACTH-Independent Cushing's	4:1	**10**
Adrenocortical adenoma		5-10
Adrenocortical carcinoma		1%
Rare causes: PPNAD, primary pigmented nodular adrenal disease; AIMAH, ACTH-independent massive adrenal hyperplasia; McCune-Albright syndrome		

Signs and symptoms of cushing's disease includes weight gain, fatigue, amenorrhoea, acne, hirsutism, purple stretch marks, proximal muscle weakness. Screening of cushings syndrome is done by overnight dexamethasone test.Confirmation is done by low dose dxamethasone test and differentiation between pituitary secreteted ACTH and ACTH producing tumors is done by high dose dexamethasone test. Medical treatment of cushings disease consists of metyrapone, ketoconazole,etomidate and mitotane.

Reference:
1. Arlt W. Disorders of the Adrenal Cortex, In : Longo DL, Fauci AS, Kasper DL, Hauser SL, Jameson JL et. Al (eds) .*Harrison's principles of internal medicine* ; 18(2)New York, MacGraw Hill Medical Publishing division;2012 .p 2945-2949.

THYROTOXICOSIS

Dr Arvind Mishra, Professor, Department of Medicine

A 40 year old female patient came to medicine OPD with complaint of palpitation, weakness, weight loss, sweating and oligomenorrhoea for past 3 months. On examination PR-140/min, regular, Respiratory rate-28/min, moist skin, fine tremors in hands were present. Cardiovascular examination revealed normal heart sounds and absence of any murmur.

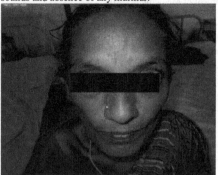

1. What could be the most probable diagnosis?
   (A) Pheochromocytoma
   (B) Thyrotoxicosis
   (C) Anxiety neurosis
   (D) Dilated cardiomyopathy
2. What will be the expected thyroid profile in this patient?
   (A) ↓FT3,↓FT4,↑TSH
   (B) ↓FT3,↓FT4,normal TSH
   (C) ↑ FT3,↑ FT4, normal TSH
   (D) ↑ FT3,↑ FT4, ↓TSH
3. Which of the following drug could not be of any help in the medical management of this patient
   (A) Propylthiouracil
   (B) methimazole
   (C) Carbimazole
   (D) Metyrapone
4. Inadequately treated severe thyrotoxicosis can sometimes presents as
   (A) Myxoedema coma
   (B) Addisonian crisis
   (C) Thyroid storm
   (D) Acute respiratory failure

Answers:
1. B
2. D
3. B
4. C

Thyrotoxicosis is defined as the state of thyroid hormone excess and is not synonymous with *hyperthyroidism*, which is the result of excessive thyroid function. However, the major etiologies of thyrotoxicosis are hyperthyroidism caused by Graves' disease, toxic MNG, and toxic adenomas.

Signs and signs of thyrotoxicosis includes tachycardia, diarrhea, palpitations, weight loss,gynaecomastia, oligomenorrhea, warm moist skin, proximal myopathy

In Graves' disease, the TSH level is suppressed and total and unbound thyroid hormone levels are increased.T*hyroid storm*, is rare and presents as a life-threatening exacerbation of hyperthyroidism, accompanied by fever, delirium, seizures, coma, vomiting,. Thyrotoxic crisis is usually precipitated by acute illness (e.g., stroke, infection, trauma, diabetic ketoacidosis), surgery (especially on the thyroid), or radioiodine treatment of a patient with partially treated or untreated hyperthyroidism.

The main *antithyroid drugs* are the thionamides, such as propylthiouracil, carbimazole, and the active metabolite of the latter, methimazole. All inhibit the function of TPO, reducing oxidation and organification of iodide. These drugs also reduce thyroid antibody levels by mechanisms that remain unclear.

Reference:
1. Jameson JL, Weetman AP, Disorders of the thyroid gland.In : Longo DL, Fauci AS, Kasper DL, Hauser SL, Jameson JL et. Al (eds) *Harrison's principles of internal medicine*. 18(2) .Newyork, Mac Graw Hill Medical Publishing division;2012,p.2922-2927.

HYPOTHYROIDISM
Dr Arvind Mishra, Professor, Department of Medicine, KGMU

A 28 year old female came with history of swelling over entire body, dry skin, alopecia, cold intolerance and menorrhagia for past 5 months. On examination BP-140/90, PR-64/min, pallor, puffiness of face, non-pitting pedal edema with delayed relaxation of ankle jerks were present.

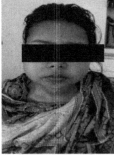

1. What could be the diagnosis of this patient
    (A) Nephrotic syndrome
    (B) Hypothyroidism
    (C) Angioneurotic edema
    (D) Constrictive pericarditis
2. Thyroid profile of this patient will be
    (A) ↓FT3,↓FT4,↑TSH
    (B) ↓FT3,↓FT4,normal TSH
    (C) ↑ FT3,↑ FT4, ↓TSH
    (D) ↑ FT3,↑ FT4, normal TSH
3. Anemia in this patient will be predominantly
    (A) Normocytic normochromic
    (B) Microcytic hypochromic
    (C) Macrocytic
    (D) Dimorphic
4. Best single investigation to assess efficacy of thyroid replacement therapy in this patient
    (A) FT3,FT4
    (B) FT4
    (C) Total T4
    (D) TSH

Answers:
> 1. B
> 2. A
> 3. C
> 4. D
>   A normal TSH level excludes primary (but not secondary) hypothyroidism. If the TSH is elevated, an unbound T4 level is needed to confirm the presence of clinical hypothyroidism, but T_4 is inferior to TSH when used as a screening test, because it will not detect subclinical hypothyroidism.anemia is usually normocytic normochromic type.

Reference:
1. Jameson JL, Weetman AP, Disorders of the thyroid gland.In : Longo DL, Fauci AS, Kasper DL, Hauser SL, Jameson JL et. Al(eds) *Harrison's principles of internal medicine*.18(2) .New York, Mac Graw Hill Medical Publishing division; 2012, p. 2918-2922.

ACUTE MYOCARDIAL INFARCTION

Dr Jitendra Singh, Senior Resident, Department of Medicine, KGMU, Lucknow &
Dr Anju Dinkar, Senior Resident, Department of Microbiology, SGPGIMS

A 50 years old male presented to emergency department with complaints of vomiting and diaphoresis. He was known case of type 2 diabetes mellitus and taking oral hypoglycemic agents regularly. He had no history of hypertension. On examination there was no pallor or icterus and Blood Pressure was 84/60mmHg. His urine input was adequate. His investigations revealed–Hb 13.2gm/dl, TLC 11, 800/mm3, PC 3.8 Lac/mm^3, Random Blood Sugar 98mg/dl. His Serum electrolytes, Liver function test, renal function test and Coagulation profile were within normal range. Serum Troponin T was 0.18ng/ml (elevated). ECG was like this-

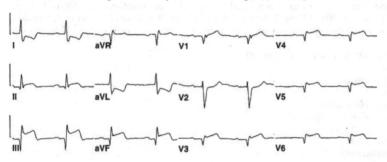

1. What is your probable diagnosis?
   (A) Septic Shock
   (B) Acute Myocardial Infarction
   (C) Anxiety Disorder
   (D) Hypoglycemia
2. Which are most appropriate investigations to establish diagnosis?
   (A) ECG and Troponin T
   (B) CT Scan Head and RBS
   (C) ECG and CBC
   (D) RBS and Pro BNP
3. In this case scenario which is most important step of management?
   (A) Give a broad spectrum antibiotic and iv fluid.
   (B) Loading with Aspirin and Clopidrogrel 300mg each then 75/75 mg HS daily and IV fluids.
   (C) 25%D 100ml solution and Dopamine infusion.
   (D) DNS fluid and Anxiolytics.

Answers:
1. B
   On the basis of complaints, differential diagnosis of above case may be myocardial infarction and hypoglycemia. RBS is normal which rules out hypoglycemia.
2. A
   Increased troponin level confirms acute myocardial infarction. ECG shows ST segment elevation in lead II, III and aVF which suggests acute inferior wall MI. Aspirin is essential in the management of patients with suspected STEMI and is effective across the entire spectrum of acute coronary syndromes.
3. B
   Rapid inhibition of cyclooxygenase-1 in platelets followed by a reduction of thromboxane A2 levels is achieved by buccal absorption of a chewed 160–325-mg tablet in the Emergency Department. This measure should be followed by daily oral administration of aspirin in a dose of 75–162 mg. It is clearly mention that up to one-half patient with acute inferior wall MI shows evidence of parasympathetic hyperactivity (bradycardia/and or hypotension). When these patients are treated with IV fluid, hypotension is readily reversed in majority of patients.

Reference:
1. Antman EM, Loscalzo J. ST Segment Elevation Myocardial Infarction. In: Longo DL, Fauci AS, Kasper DL, Hauser SL, Jameson JL, Loscalzo J et al., editors. Harrison's Principles of Internal Medicine. 18th Ed. New York: McGraw Hill; 2012:2021-35.

HYPONATREMIA

Dr Jitendra Singh, Senior Resident, Department of Medicine, KGMU, Lucknow
Dr Anju Dinkar, Senior Resident, Department of Microbiology, SGPGIMS, Lucknow

A 49-year old female with history of hypertension visits a General Practitioner with complaint of nausea vomiting and lethargy for few days. She was taking antihypertensive medicines (telmisartan 40mg with hydrochlorthiazide 12.5mg OD) regularly. Her general examination was unremarkable and BP was 124/80 mmHg. So General Practitioner prescribed her pentaprazole with domperidone and advised her some investigations. In the same evening she was presented to emergency department with complaint of altered behavior. There was no history of fever. On examination there was neither icterus or pallor nor any focal deficit. Dehydration was present. There was no sign of meningeal irritation. Her investigations were–Hb 14.1 gm/dl, TLC 8000/mm^3, PC 4.2 Lac/mm^3, RBS 102mg/dl, Serum sodium 115mmol/L and Serum potassium 4.1mmol/L. Her Liver function test, renal function test and coagulation profile were normal. ECG and CT head were unremarkable.

1. What is most appropriate cause of altered behavior?
    (A) Cerebral stroke
    (B) Myocardial infraction
    (C) Hyponatremia
    (D) Hypertensive encephalopathy.
2. What are risk factors of above diagnosis?
    (A) Hydrochlorthiazide and vomiting.
    (B) Telmisartan and vomiting
    (C) Telmisartan and headache
    (D) Hydrochlorthiazide and headache
3. What is suitable management in this case?
    (A) IV Normal saline is treatment of choice.
    (B) IV 3% NaCl is treatment of choice.
    (C) Oral fluid and antibiotics are better.
    (D) IV 3% NaCl and oral antibiotics.

Answers:
1. C
    It is a case of hyponatremia. Normal BP and CT Head rules out cerebral stroke and hypertensive encephalopathy.
2. A
    She is taking diuretic (hydrochlorthiazide) for hypertension. Thiazides and vomiting both are common causes of hyponatremia.
3. A
    Once diagnosis is established, next step is to classify patient as hypovolemia, euvolemia or hypervolemia because management varies with hydration status of body. This is case of hypovolemic hyponatremia which will better respond to intravenous hydration with normal saline. Patient has complaint of nausea and vomiting and is not fully conscious so intravenous fluid is indicated not oral.

Reference:
1. Parikh C, Berl T. Disorders of Water Metabolism. In: Floege J, Johnson RJ, Feehally J, Editors. Comprehensive Clinical Nephrology. 4th ed. Saunders, Elsevier Inc; 2010:100-17.

NEPHROTIC SYNDROME

Dr Jitendra Singh, Senior Resident, Department of Medicine, KGMU, Lucknow
Dr Anju Dinkar, Senior Resident, Department of Microbiology, SGPGIMS, Lucknow

A 34 years old male presented with complaints of generalized body swelling for three months. Swelling started from face and progressed gradually to all over body. His past medical history was not significant. He had no history of diabetes, hypothyroidism and malabsorption. There was no history of paroxysmal nocturnal dyspnoea. General examination was normal except bilateral pedal oedema. BP was 118/80 mmHg. His investigations showed Hb 13.2 gm/dl, TLC 8400 m^3, PC 3.1 Lac/mm^3 and RBS 94mg/dl. Serum electrolytes, liver function test, thyroid function test and coagulation profile were within normal limits. Serum Urea and S. Creatinine were 22 mg/dl and 0.7mg/dl respectively. X-ray chest revealed right sided minimal pleural effusion and USG abdomen detected no abnormality. ECG was normal.

1. Which is most probable diagnosis of this case?
   (A) Membranous nephropathy
   (B) Pericardial effusion
   (C) Hypertensive heart failure
   (D) Chronic kidney disease.
2. Which are most appropriate investigations to establish diagnosis in this case?
   (A) 24 hours urinary protein and Renal Biopsy
   (B) S. Urea, S. Creatinine and Renal Biopsy
   (C) 2D Echocardiography and Renal Biopsy
   (D) S. Urea, S. Creatinine and 2D Echo
3. Which of following is most common cause of death in these patients?
   (A) Hypertension.
   (B) Deep Venous Thrombosis
   (C) Myocardial infarction
   (D) Sepsis

Answers:
   1. A
   There is loss of urinary protein more than 3.5 gm per day which defines nephrotic syndrome. The common cause of nephrotic syndrome at this age is Membranous Nephropathy.
   2. A
   Sonography of abdomen shows normal study. Kidney Biopsy is mainstay to confirm diagnosis.
   3. D
   Nephrotic patients are more prone to bacterial infection and sepsis is most common cause of death.

Reference:
   1. Floege J, Feehally J. Introduction of Global Disease: Clinical Presentations. In: Floege J, Johnson RJ, Feehally J, Editors. Comprehensive Clinical Nephrology. 4th ed. Saunders, Elsevier Inc; 2010:193-207.

CHRONIC KIDNEY DISEASE
Dr Jitendra Singh, Senior Resident, Department of Medicine
Dr Anju Dinkar, Senior Resident, Department of Microbiology, SGPGIMS

A 40 years old and 64 kg weight male patient present to emergence department with breathlessness, generalized body swelling and decrease urine output for four month. Pallor is present. Auscultatory findings are bilateral chest crepitations and pericardial rub. He has past history of multiple blood transfusions. His USG revealed bilateral contracted kidney. Arterial blood gas analysis (ABG) reveals– pH 7.12, Na+ 138 mmol/L, K+ 7.6 mmol/L, Glucose 100mg/dl, pCO_2 28 mmHg, pO_2 84 mmHg, HCO_3^- 12.0 mmol/L. He has investigations showing hyperphosphatemia and hyperuricemia. His Serum Urea and S. Creatinine were 112 mg/dl and 8.0 mg/dl respectively.

1. What is most probable diagnosis of this case?
   (A) Hypothyroidism
   (B) Chronic Kidney Disease
   (C) Hemolytic Anemia
   (D) Dilated cardiomyopathy
2. What is ABG interpretation?
   (A) Metabolic Acidosis
   (B) Metabolic Alkalosis
   (C) Respiratory Acidosis
   (D) Respiratory Alkalosis
3. Which of the following are indications for early start on hemodialysis?
   (A) Uremic Pericarditis and hyperkalemia
   (B) Decrease Urine Output and hyperkalemia
   (C) Metabolic Acidosis and hyperuricemia
   (D) Uremic Pericarditis and decrease urine output
4. What is the stage of Chronic Kidney Disease on the basis of GFR?
   (A) Stage 2
   (B) Stage 3
   (C) Stage 4
   (D) Stage 5

5. What is most common cause of End Stage Renal Disease (ESRD)?
   (A) Hypertension
   (B) Diabetes Mellitus
   (C) Sepsis
   (D) Glomerulonephritis
6. Which of following is not a manifestation of CKD?
   (A) Hyperkalemia
   (B) Anemia
   (C) Hypouricemia
   (D) Hypocalcemia
7. Which of the following is most common cause of mortality in Dialysis dependent patients?
   (A) Ventricular Fibrillation
   (B) Pulseless Electrical Activity
   (C) Asystole
   (D) Valvular Disease
8. Which diet is not recommended for this patient?
   (A) Fruit juice and Soup
   (B) Milk Products and Ice cream
   (C) Pulses
   (D) Sweets
9. Who is the near relative for renal transplantation?
   (A) Father and Daughter
   (B) Spouse and Aunty
   (C) Father and Uncle
   (D) Uncle and Aunty

Answers:

1. B

   Chronic kidney disease (CKD) encompasses a spectrum of different pathophysiologic processes associated with abnormal kidney function and a progressive decline in glomerular filtration rate. Clinical feature of above case are suggestive of Chronic Kidney Disease. It is defined as kidney damage or glomerular filteration rate (GFR) below 60ml/1.73m2 for 3 months or more irrespective of the cause.[1]

2. A

   ABG interpretation shows low pH, low HCO_3^- (primary change) and decreased $PaCO_2$ (secondary change). It is Metabolic Acidosis.[2]

3. A

   Indications for early start on hemodialysis are intractable fluid overload, intractable hyperkalemia, malnutrition due to uremia, uremic neurological dysfunction, uremic serositis and functional deterioration otherwise unexplained.[3]

4. D

   GFR is calculated by using Cockroft-Gault formula which is as- Ccr = (140-Age) × Weight / 72 × Scr. After calculation GFR comes 11.11. it fits in stage 5. A widely accepted classification, based on guidelines of the National Kidney Foundation [Kidney Dialysis Outcomes Quality Initiative (KDOQI)], CKD is classified into 5 stages on the basis of GFR.

GFR (mL/min per 1.73 m^2)	>90^a	90^b	60–89	30–59	15–29	<15
Stage	0	1	2	3	4	5

^{a}With risk factors for CKD (see text). ^{b}With demonstrated kidney damage (e.g., persistent proteinuria, abnormal urine sediment, abnormal blood and urine chemistry, abnormal imaging studies.[4]

5. B

   Diabetes accounted for 44% of incident US ESRD patients.

6. C

   Hyperkalemia, Anemia, Hypocalcemia, Hyperphosphatemia, Hyperurecemia etc are manifestations of CKD.

7. A

   Cardiac arrest occurring in hemodialysis centres found predominant rhythm was Ventricular Fibrillation (66%), followed by Pulseless Electrical Activity (23%) and Asystole (10%).[5]

8. A

Fruit juice and soup are potassium rich diet so avoid because patient already has developed hyperkalemia which may be dangerous to life.

9. A

The Act currently in Section 2 sub section (i) defines the term "near relative" to mean spouse, son, daughter, father, mother, brother or sister. As the law stands today, any individual who wishes to donate his or her organs for a recipient, who comes in the category of "near relatives" of the donor, can do so without the case being routed through the Authorization Committee. A suggestion has been made that the definition of the term 'near relative' should be expanded to include grandparents, grand children, uncles and aunts all of whom are related by blood to the recipient. After view of the experts, it is proposed to modify the definition of 'near relative' in Section 2, only to the extent of including grandparents and grand children.[6]

References:

1. Bello A et al. Epidemiology and Pathophysiology of Chronic Kidney Disease. In: Floege J, Johnson RJ, Feehally J, Editors. Comprehensive Clinical Nephrology. 4th ed. Saunders, Elsevier Inc; 2010:907-18.
2. Biff F et al. Metabolic Acidosis. In: Floege J, Johnson RJ, Feehally J, Editors. Comprehensive Clinical Nephrology. 4th ed. Saunders, Elsevier Inc; 2010:155-67.
3. Rayner HC, Imai E. Approach to Renal Replacement Therapy. In: Floege J, Johnson RJ, Feehally J, Editors. Comprehensive Clinical Nephrology. 4th ed. Saunders, Elsevier Inc; 2010:1019-30.
4. Bargman JM, Skorecki K. Chronic Kidney Disease. In: Longo DL, Fauci AS, Kasper DL, Hauser SL, Jameson JL, Loscalzo J et al., editors. Harrison's principles of internal medicine. 18th ed. New York:McGraw Hill; 2012, p2308-22
5. Stenvinkel P et al. Cardiovascular Disease in Chronic Kinney Disease. In: Floege J, Johnson RJ, Feehally J, Editors. Comprehensive Clinical Nephrology. 4th ed. Saunders, Elsevier Inc; 2010:935-50.
6. Government of India. Transplantation of Human Organs Act, 1994. 1994. Central Act 42 of [cited 2015 April 18] Available from: http://wwwmedindianet/tho/thobill1asp.

PULMONARY THROMBOEMBOLISM

Dr. K.K. Gupta , Associate Professor, Department of Medicine

A 50 year old women presents to the emergency room with acute onset shortness of breath, light headedness and chest pain. She recently had visited her parents out of country by flight for about 12 hours each way. Two days ago, she developed mild calf pain and swelling, but she thought that this was not unusual after having been sitting with her legs dependent for the recent trip. On arrival to the emergency room, she is noted to be tachypneic and diaphoretic. Her vital signs are as follows: blood pressure 86/58 mm Hg, heart rate 114 beats /min, respiratory rate 28 breaths /min, oxygen saturation of 92% on room air, weight 84 kg. The lungs are clear bilaterally. Cardiovascular examination shows a regular tachycardia without murmurs, rub or gallop. There is pain in the right calf with the dorsiflexion of the foot and the right leg is more swollen when compared to the left. An arterial blood gas measurement shows a pH of 7.52, PCO_2 25 mmHg and PO_2 68 mmHg. Kidney and liver function test are normal.

1. What is the most likely cause in this patient?
   (A) Acute Respiratory Distress Syndrome
   (B) Myocardial Infarction
   (C) Pulmonary Thromboembolism
   (D) Pleuritis
2. Which is the most frequent symptom of this disease?
   (A) Syncope
   (B) Pleuritic pain
   (C) Dyspnea
   (D) Haemoptysis
3. What is the most frequent ECG finding in this diease?
   (A) S1Q3T3 pattern
   (B) P pulmonale
   (C) Sinus tachycardia
   (D) Right axis deviation
4. What is best investigation to be done in this patient for diagnosis?
   (A) D- Dimer Assay
   (B) Multidetector CT angiography

(C) Doppler Ultrasound

(D) ECG

5. False positive D-dimer assay is seen in all except?

   (A) Pneumonia

   (B) Myocardial Infarction

   (C) Pregnancy

   (D) DVT

6. What is the treatment of choice in case of Massive Pulmonary Embolism in shock?

   (A) Low molecular weight heparin

   (B) Thrombolytic therapy

   (C) Aggressive fluid resuscitation

   (D) Anticoagulation and Thrombolytic therapy

Answers:

1. C

   Venous thromboembolism (VTE) includes deep venous thrombosis and pulmonary embolism. DVT patients usually presents with history of cramps in the lower calf that persists for several days and becomes more uncomfortable as the time progress.

   ### Clinical decision rule for pulmonary embolism

Clinical variable	Score
1. Sign and symptoms of DVT	3.0
2. Alternative diagnosis less likely than PE	3.0
3. Heart rate >100	1.5
4. Immobilization >3 days; surgery within 4 wks	1.5
5. Prior PE/DVT	1.5
6. Hemoptysis	1.0
7. Cancer	1.0

   ### High clinical likelyhood of PE if point score exceeds 4.

   This patient is having total score of 7.5 (3.0+3.0+1.5), that suggest Pulmonary Thromboembolismis the most likely diagnosis.

2. C

   Dyspnoea is the most common symptom of PE, and tachypnea is the most common sign. Dyspnoea, syncope, hypotension, or cyanosis indicates a massive PE, whereas pleuritic pain, cough, or hemoptysis often suggests a small embolism situated distally near the pleura.

3. C

   The most frequently cited abnormality, in addition to sinus tachycardia, is the S1Q3T3 sign: an S wave in lead I, a Q wave in lead III, and an inverted T wave in lead III .S1Q3T3 sign is relatively specific sign to PE but not sensitive.

4. B

   Chest CTwith intravenous contrast is the principal imaging test for the diagnosis of PE. Multidetector-row spiral CT acquires all chest images with≤1 mm of resolution during a short breath hold. This generation of CT scanners can image small peripheral emboli. Sixth-order branches can be visualized.

   A normal or nearly normal chest x-ray often occurs in PE. Abnormalities on x-ray include focal oligemia (**Westermark's sign),** a peripheral wedged-shaped density above the diaphragm (**Hampton's hump),** and an enlarged right descending pulmonary artery (**Palla's sign).**

5. D

   The D-dimer assay is a useful 'rule out' test. More than 95% patient having normal D-dimer (< 500ng/ml) do not have pulmonary embolism. The D-dimer assay is non specific test. False positive D-dimer assay can be seen in myocardial infarction, pneumonia, sepsis, cancer, post operative state and those in second and third trimester of pregnancy.

6. D

   Primary therapy consists of clot dissolution with thrombolysis or removalof PE by embolectomy. Anticoagulation with heparin and warfarin or placement of an inferior vena caval filter constitutes secondary prevention of recurrent PE rather than primary therapy.

Reference:

1. Goldhaber SZ. Deep Venous Thrombosis and Pulmonary Thromboembolism. In: Longo DL, Fauci AS, Kasper DL, Hauser SL, Jameson JL, Loscalzo J. editors. Harrison's Principles of Internal Medicine. 18th edition. New Delhi: McGraw Hill; 2012. p. 2170-2177.

WHEEZE
Dr. Kauser Usman, Associate Professor, Department of Medicine

A 55 year old man presents with episodic wheezing and breathlessness. His wheezing is often accompanied by dry cough which worsens at night, as well as with exertion. There is no history of chest pain, orthopnea, sneezing, rhinorrhea or hemoptysis. He is smoker for last 25 years but has reduced in frequency for last 2 years. On physical examination, his blood pressure is 140/70 mm of Hg and dyspneic with respiratory rate of 22 per min. He is awake and neck examination shows no engorged veins or neck mass. Cardiac examination was normal. Chest examination revealed polyphonic rhonchi with prolonged expiratory phase. His chest x ray showed normal sized heart and the lung fields are clear but hyperinflated.

1. What is the most probable diagnosis in the above patient?
   (A) Left ventricular failure
   (B) Emphysema
   (C) Chronic bronchitis
   (D) Bronchial asthma
2. Which of the following is **not** a common cause of polyphonic wheezing?
   (A) Left ventricular failure
   (B) Chronic obstructive pulmonary disease
   (C) Bronchial asthma
   (D) Endobronchial lesions
3. What would be the next line of investigation for confirmation of the diagnosis?
   (A) CT thorax
   (B) Pulmonary function tests
   (C) 2D echocardiography
   (D) Arterial blood gas analysis
4. Which one of the following statement is **not** correct?
   (A) Rhonchi with prolonged expiratory phase are present in mild bronchial asthma
   (B) Rhonchi may be both expiratory and inspiratory in bronchial asthma
   (C) Rhonchi may be absent in severe bronchial asthma
   (D) Rhonchi are not heard in left ventricular failure

Answers:
1. B
   The most important clue is hyper inflated lung fields on chest X-ray.(1)
2. D
   Tumors or any obstruction in the passage of bronchus presents as monophonic wheeze.
3. B
   The hallmark of emphysema (COPD) is airflow obstruction which can be demonstrated by Pulmonary function tests , reduction in FEV_1 and FEV_1/FVC.(3)
4. D
   Rhonchi are heard in left ventricular failure due to interstitial edema often referred to as cardiac asthma[1]

References:
1. Schwartzstein RM. Dyspnea. In: Longo DL, Kasper DL, Jameson L, Fauci AS, Hauser SL, Loscalzo J, eds. Harrison Principles of Internal Medicine, 18th ed. New York: Mc Graw-Hill Medical Publishing Division; 2012:279.
2. Simon. C, Everitt H., Dorp.F.V, Burkes M. Respiratory medicine, Chapter 11, Oxford Handbook of General Practice, Oxford University Press, p298.
3. Reilly j. ,Silverman E.K., Shapiro S.D , Chronic Obstructive Pulmonary Disease In: Longo DL, Kasper DL, Jameson L, Fauci AS, Hauser SL, Loscalzo J, eds. Harrison Principles of Internal Medicine, 18th ed. New York: Mc Graw-Hill Medical ublishing Division;2156.

CHRONIC COUGH
Dr. Kauser Usman, Associate Professor, Department of Medicine

A 52 year old man presents with a 5 month history of daily nonproductive cough which worsens at night. He often has to clear his throat frequently. There is no history of fever, breathlessness or wheezing, hemoptysis, heartburn, water brash. Patient is nonsmoker but a known hypertensive for 5 years and being treated with metoprolol and amlodipine. On examination his blood pressure is 156/90 mm of Hg in right arm sitting position.

His chest is clear on auscultation and cardiac examination is unremarkable. There is some clear nasal discharge on posterior pharyngeal wall.

1. What is the most probable diagnosis in the above patient?
   (A) Gastro esophageal reflux disease
   (B) Post nasal drip
   (C) Left ventricular failure
   (D) Bronchial asthma
2. What would be the next step for confirmation of diagnosis in this patient?
   (A) Chest X ray
   (B) Per speculum nasal examination
   (C) Esophageal manometry
   (D) 2D echocardiography
3. Which of the following cause of chronic cough is **not** common?
   (A) Asthma
   (B) Bronchitis
   (C) Endobronchial lesions
   (D) Gastro esophageal reflux disease
4. What one of the pharmacological agent would be useful in the above patient?
   (A) Antibiotics
   (B) Diuretics
   (C) Bronchodilators
   (D) Nasal decongestants

Answers:

1. B
   Post-nasal drainage of any etiology can cause cough as a response to stimulation of sensory receptors of the cough-reflex pathway in the hypopharynx or aspiration of draining secretions into the trachea. Clues to this etiology include symptoms of post-nasal drip, frequent throat clearing, and sneezing and rhinorrhea

2. B
   On speculum examination of the nose, one may see excess mucoid or purulent secretions, inflamed and edematous nasal mucosa, and or nasal polyps; in addition, one might visualize secretions or a cobblestoned appearance of the mucosa along the posterior pharyngeal wall.

3. C
4. D
   Therapy for post-nasal drainage depends on the presumed etiology (infection, allergy, or vasomotor rhinitis) and may include systemic antihistamines; antibiotics; nasal saline irrigation; and nasal pump sprays with corticosteroids, antihistamines, or anticholinergics.

Reference:

1. Kritek P. and Fanta C. Cough and Hemoptysis. In: Longo DL, Kasper DL, Jameson L, Fauci AS, Hauser SL, Loscalzo J, eds. Harrison Principles of Internal Medicine, 18th ed. New York: Mc Graw-Hill Medical Publishing Division; 2012: p283-284.

SEPTICEMIC SHOCK
Dr. D. Himanshu, Assistant Professor, Department of Medicine

A 14 year old male presented to the emergency department with complaints of fever (high grade) and sore throat for four days. Three days later he developed rash predominantly involving lower limbs and trunk and developed alteration of consciousness since one day. On examination patient was febrile, temperature, 103.8F, pulse rate was 130/min and blood pressure was 60/40. His extremities were cold and cyanosed. The rash was involving the trunk and lower limbs, confluent and necrotic in appearance. His blood pressure did not improved despite adequate fluid resuscitation and inotropic support but improved after a dose of 1mg/kg of Hydrocortisone. He was started on gram-negative antibiotic coverage along with steroids and improved significantly over a period of next seven days.

1. Which of the following is **least** common cause of fever with rash in this patient?
   (A) Viral exanthems
   (B) Enteric fever
   (C) Fungal infection
   (D) Drug reactions
2. What is the most probable diagnosis of the patient?

234

(A) Gram negative septicemic shock

(B) Waterhouse friedrichson syndrome by meningococcal infection

(C) Fitz hugh Curtis syndrome by gonococcal infection

(D) Hypovolemic shock by upper gastrointestinal bleeding

3. Which of the following statement best describes the cause of shock in the above patient?

(A) Disseminated intravascular coagulation

(B) Bilateral adrenal gland hemorrhage

(C) Gram negative septicemia

(D) Dysfunction of vasomotor centre due to raised Intra-cerebral tension

4. What is the investigation of choice for diagnosis in the above patient?

(A) Blood culture for infective organism

(B) 2D ECHO for infective endocarditis

(C) USG abdomen for intra-abdominal fluid collection

(D) Upper GI endoscopy for gastric hemorrhage

5. Which of the following is not included in the definition of Systemic Inflammatory Response syndrome?

(A) fever (oral temperature >38°C) or hypothermia (<36°C)

(B) tachypnea (>24 breaths/min)

(C) tachycardia (heart rate >90 beats/min) or bradycardia (<50 beats/min)

(D) leukocytosis (>12,000/L), leucopenia (<4,000/L)

Answers:

1. C

   Fungal infections donot commonly present as fever with rash.(1)

2. B

   Along the spectrum of presentations of meningococcal disease, the most common clinical syndromes are meningitis and meningococcal septicemia.In fulminant cases, death may occur within hours of the first symptoms. Occult bacteremia is also recognized and, if untreated, progresses in two-thirds of cases to focal infection including meningitis or septicemia, thus patient may land into hypotension, shock and coma like stage reffered to as Waterhouse friedrichson syndrome. (2)

3. B

   Bilateral adrenal gland hemorrhage lead to insufficiency of minerelo and glucocorticosteroids causing shock like state. (2)

4. A

   Although meningococcal disease is often diagnosed on clinical grounds, in suspected meningococcal meningitis or meningococcemia, blood should routinely be sent for culture to confirm the diagnosis and to facilitate public health investigations; blood cultures are positive in up to 75% of cases. (2)

5. C

   Bradycardia is not mentioned in diagnostic guidelines of SIRS.(3)

References:

1. Kaye E.T , Kaye K.M. Fever and rash. In: Longo DL, Kasper DL, Jameson L, Fauci AS, Hauser SL, Loscalzo J, eds. Harrison Principles of Internal Medicine, 18th ed. New York: Mc Graw-Hill Medical Publishing Division; 2012: p149-156.

2. Anderw J. Pollard. Meningococcal infection. In: Longo DL, Kasper DL, Jameson L, Fauci AS, Hauser SL, Loscalzo J, eds. Harrison Principles of Internal Medicine, 18th ed. New York: Mc Graw-Hill Medical Publishing Division; 2012: p1214-1217.

3. Robert S. Munford. Severe sepsis and septic shock. In: Longo DL, Kasper DL, Jameson L, Fauci AS, Hauser SL, Loscalzo J, eds. Harrison Principles of Internal Medicine, 18th ed. New York: Mc Graw-Hill Medical Publishing Division; 2012:p2223.

COMPLICATED MALARIA

Dr. D. Himanshu, Assistant Professor, Department of Medicine

A 36 year old female presented in the emergency room in a delirious state with history of high grade fever for five days. On examination she was pale and icteric. Her husband also informed that she had missed her last two periods. A pregnancy test was performed and it came positive.

Her laboratory examination showed the following:

- TLC: 12000 cells/ cmm
- DLC: N 90 L8 M2

- S. bil – Total 6.8 mg/dl, SGPT- 240 IU/L, SGOT 200IU/L
- Blood Urea 121mg/dL   S. Creatinine- 3.2mg/dl
- Electrolytes- normal

A provisional diagnosis of Malaria was kept.

1. Which of the following investigations would have the highest sensitivity among the following for diagnosing Malaria?
   (A) Blood smear thin film
   (B) Blood smear thick film
   (C) Rapid Diagnostic test (RDT) antibody based
   (D) Rapid Diagnostic test (RDT) antigen based

A peripheral capillary blood smear was taken and the slide showed the following picture Courtesy: CDC, Atlanta. USA

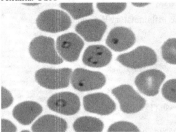

2. What is your diagnosis?
   (A) Plasmodium vivax gametocyte phase
   (B) Plasmodium falciparum gametocyte phase
   (C) Plasmodium falciparum asexual phase
   (D) Plasmodium vivax asexual phase

3. What is the drug of choice for treating this patient as per 2014 guidelines by National Vector Borne Disease Control Programm?
   (A) Artemether
   (B) Artesunate
   (C) Chloroquine
   (D) Quinine

Answers:

1. B

   Malaria diagnosis can be made by blood films, Rapid Diagnostic Tests (RDT) and PCR. Blood smears and RDTs are easily available. The blood smears are in turn of two types, thick smears and thin smears. Thin smears are useful in identifying the species of malaria whereas the thick smear has higher sensitivity in diagnosing malaria. The thick film can detect even if the parasitemia is as less as 20 parasites/microLwhere as RDTs cannot detect if parasitemia is less than 100 parasites/microL. (1)

2. C

   This is a thin blood smear showing multiply-infected rbcs, some appliqué forms and some classic "head phone" form of several of the infected red blood cells. Plasmodium falciparum rings have delicate cytoplasm and one or two small chromatin dots. Rbcs that are infected are not enlarged; multiple infection of RBCs is more common in P. falciparum than in other species. Occasional appliqué forms (rings appearing on the periphery of the rbc) can be present. (2)

3. D

   As per the current 2014 guidelines by National Vector Borne Disease Control Programme for complicated malaria, the treatment is divided into two parts the Initial 48 hours and the follow up phase. In the initial 48 hours there are four regimens which have been described based on the usage of Quinine, Artesunate, Artemether and Arteether. Apart from quinine all others are not recommended for usage in first trimester for pregnancy. Our patient has presented with complicated malaria and is in first trimester of pregnancy. Therefore the drug of choice here as per as current Indian guidelines is quinine.(3)

References:

1. Hopkins H. Diagnosis of malaria. Oct. 2014 Available from URL:http://www.uptodate.com

2. DPDx - Laboratory Identification of Parasitic Diseases of Public Health Concern. Laboratory diagnosis of Malraia. Atlanta (GA) USA. Center for Disease Control. Available from URL:http://www.cdc.gov/dpdx/
3. National Institute of Malaria Research. Guidelines for Diagnosis and Treatment of Malaria in India 2014. National Vector Borne Disease Control Programme.New Delhi. India.Available from URL:http://www.mrcindia.org/Diagnosis of Malaria pdf/Guidelines 2014.pdf

ACUTE HEPATITIS

Dr, Ajay Kumar, Assistant Professor, Department of Medical Gastroenterology

A 66 year old man with a history of jaundice for 15 days and past history of alcohol intake and ischemic heart disease undergoes liver function tests and results show: total bilirubin 3.6 mg/dl, direct 2.2 mg/dl, SGOT 116 IU/ml, SGPT 156 IU/ml, SALP 136 IU/ml.

1. What is the next line of investigation?
   (A) Review drug list
   (B) Upper G.I. Endoscopy
   (C) Liver Biopsy
   (D) USG Abdomen
2. What is the condition best known as
   (A) Chronic hepatitis
   (B) Obstructive jaundice
   (C) Acute hepatitis
   (D) Cirrhosis
3. Which of the following not included in differential diagnosis
   (A) Viral hepatitis
   (B) Drug induced hepatitis
   (C) Periampullary carcinoma
   (D) Choledocholelithiasis
4. Which of the following drug may be the most probably caused the condition
   (A) Amiodarone
   (B) Methotruxate
   (C) Metformin
   (D) Pioglitazone

Answers:

1. A
   Before any investigation, review of drug list is the most important step in this case as a cause of abnormal LFT.
2. C
   In this case, both transaminases are elevated and alkaline phosphatase is normal which represent hepatocellular injury(hepatitis) lasting 15 days. So best nomenclature for this condition will be acute hepatitis.
3. C
   In this case serum ALP levels are not raised, which is not in favour of obstructive jaundice caused by periampullary carcinoma. Acute CBD obstruction by stone may cause picture like acute hepatitis.
4. A
   Amiodarone use is accompanied in 15 to 50 % patients by modest elevations in serum aminotransferase levels that may remain stable or diminish despite continuation of the drug.

References:

1. Daniel et al. Evaluation of liver function, Harrison's Principles of Internal Medicine, volume 2, 18th edition, New York, McGraw Hill Medical, 2012, Page 2528-29
2. Jules LD et al. Acute viral hepatitis, Harrison's Principles of Internal Medicine, volume 2, 18th edition, New York, McGraw Hill Medical, 2012, Page 2562-64
3. Norton J. G. et. al. Diseases of gall bladder and bile ducts, Harrison's principles of internal medicine, volume 2, 18th edition, New York , Mac Graw Hill Medical, 2012, page 2624-2625
4. Jules et al. Toxic and drug induced hepatitis, Harrison's Principles of Internal Medicine, volume 2, 18th edition, New York, McGraw Hill Medical, 2012, Page 2564

ACUTE INFECTIVE DIARRHEA

Dr. Ajay Kumar, Assistant Professor, Department of Medical Gastroenterology

An eight year old previously healthy girl is brought to the emergency department with 1 week of diarrhoea and running nose. The patient had two episodes of bloody diarrhoea on the day of presentation. Examination showed temperature 99°F, PR 110/ min, BP 86/ 50 mmHg, left hypochondriac and epigastric tenderness with voluntary guarding. Few bowl sounds are heard. A rectal examination reveals bright red blood on finger. Laboratory tests result show haemoglobin 10.2 g/dl, platelets count 60,000/ml, serum creatinine 3.2 mg/dl, amylase 840 IU/L, lipase 1200IU/L, total and direct bilirubin 3.9 & 2.5 mg/dl, peripheral smears shows schistocytes.

1. Which is not present in this case
   (A) Acute gastroenteritis
   (B) Acute kidney injury
   (C) Shock
   (D) Pneumonia
2. Most probable etiologic agent of the condition is
   (A) Shigella
   (B) E. coli
   (C) Rotavirus
   (D) Clostridium difficile colitis
3. Most common cause of travellers' diarrhea
   (A) Shigella
   (B) E. coli
   (C) Rotavirus
   (D) Clostridium difficile colitis
4. Which of the following is not a complication of acute infectious diarrheal illness.
   (A) Irritable bowel syndrome
   (B) Reactive arthritis
   (C) Dubin Johnson Syndrome
   (D) Hemolytic-uremic syndrome

Answers:

1. D
   The details given in case summary have all the possible diagnosis except pneumonia.
2. A
   Although rotavirus infection is common in children but shigella is major cause of dysentery present in this case.
3. A
   Enterotoxigenic E. coli is the most common cause of travellers' diarrhea.
4. C
   All are the complications of acute diarrheal illness except Dubin Johnson Syndrome which is a syndrome of hereditary hyperbilirubinemia.

References:

1. Regina CL et al, Acute infectious diarrheal diseases and bacterial food poisoning, Harrison's principles of internal medicine, volume 1, 18th edition, New York, McGraw Hill Medical, 2012, Page 1084-1086
2. Philippe S et al, Shigellosis, Harrison's principles of internal medicine, volume 1, 18th edition, New York, McGraw Hill Medical, 2012, Page 1281-1285.
3. Regina CL et al, Acute infectious diarrheal diseases and bacterial food poisoning, Harrison's principles of internal medicine, volume 1, 18th edition, New York, McGraw Hill Medical, 2012, Page 1087 (table 128-3)
4. Regina CL et al, Acute infectious diarrheal diseases and bacterial food poisoning, Harrison's principles of internal medicine, volume 1, 18th edition, New York, McGraw Hill Medical, 2012, Page 1087 (table 128-2)

ISCHEMIC HEPATITIS

Dr. Ajay Kumar, Assistant Professor, Department of Medical Gastroenterology

A 65 year old man present to the emergency department in unconscious state. His pulse was 72/min, irregularly irregular, BP 172/100 mmHg. His left sided limbs were not moving even on painful stimuli. His stat test were normal except AST/ALT 1570 & 128 IU/L.

1. Which is not present in this case
   (A) Stroke
   (B) HTN
   (C) Hepatitis
   (D) Gastroenteritis
2. Which is the most likely cause of hepatitis in this case:
   (A) Acetamenophen overdose
   (B) Acute alcoholic hepatitis
   (C) Ischemic hepatitis
   (D) Viral hepatitis
3. Which test is not indicated in this case:
   (A) ECG
   (B) CT head
   (C) HBsAg
   (D) Amylase
4. All may cause acute hepatitis except:
   (A) Isoniazid
   (B) Halothane
   (C) Levetiraceton
   (D) Zidovudine

Answers:

1. D
   Gastroenteritis has not been described in symptoms.
2. C
   Striking elevations- i.e. aminotransferases> 1000 U/L occur almost exclusively in disorders associated with extensive hepatocellular injury such as 1. Viral hepatitis, 2. Ischeamic liver injury, 3. Toxin and drug induced liver injury.
3. D
   The case summary mentioned above has features suggestive of stroke, arrhythmia and acute hepatitis but not acute pancreatitis. So all except amylase is indicated in this case.
4. C
   All other drugs except levetiracetam are known to cause acute hepatitis, which one of most liver safe antiepileptic.

References:

1. Daniel S. P. et al. Evaluation of liver function, Harrison's principles of internal medicine, volume 2,18th edition, New York, McGraw Hill Medical, 2012, pp 2526- 2529, ii) Daniel HL et al, Approach to a patient with neurologic disease, Harrison's principles of internal medicine, 18th edition, New York, McGraw Hill Medical, 2012, Page 3233-3239
2. Table 369-9, Harrison's principles of internal medicine, 18th edition, New York, McGraw Hill Medical, 2012, Page 3265.
3. Daniel HL et al, Approach to a patient with neurologic disease, Harrison's principles of internal medicine, 18th edition, New York, McGraw Hill Medical, 2012, Page 3233-3239
4. Jules L. D., Toxic and drug induced hepatitis, Harrison's principles of internal medicine, volume 2, 18th edition, New York, McGraw Hill Medical, 2012. Page 2558.

WERNIKE'S ENCEPHALOPATHY

Dr. Shobhit Shakya, Senior resident, Department of medicine

A 60 year old man, chronic alcoholic for last 20 years brought to medical emergency trauma centre after he was found wandering road side in undergarments and shoes. When asked about the circumstances that led him to this state in hospital, he initially said that some men had thrashed him and robbed. When enquired again after 25 minutes, he does not recall attending doctor and states that he was thrown out of house by his wife without clothing. His son reports that he frequently seems confused and makes up stories all the time regarding his behavior. Patient also complaints of burning pain and tingling sensations in his legs that is present all the time. He has no history of psychiatric illness. He is clerk and employed. However, he lost his job due to his alcoholism 3 years back. He usually drinks 1.5 liters of country made alcohol daily but denies recent alcohol intake. On physical examination, he is confused and oriented to name only. Vital signs are except sinus tachycardia. He has bilateral symmetric sensory neuropathy with stocking-glove distribution. Deep tendon reflexes are depressed. His gait is broad based and ataxic. He also had fine resting tremors.

1. What is the most likely cause of patient's current condition?
   (A) delirium tremens
   (B) acute alcohol intoxication
   (C) thiamine deficiency
   (D) Alzheimer's disease with Parkinsonism.

2. Which of the following is not true about actions of alcohol?
   (A) alcohol inhibits NMDA receptors
   (B) alcohol inhibits GABAa receptors
   (C) increased serotonin actions and upregulation of receptors
   (D) Inhibition of uptake of adenosine.

3. Chronic alcohol intake can lead to deficiency of all vitamins except:
   (A) vitamin A
   (B) vitamin B1 (thiamine)
   (C) vitamin E
   (D) Folate

4. Korsakoff's syndrome in alcoholics is predisposed by the deficiency of:
   (A) acetylketolase deficiency
   (B) transketolase deficiency
   (C) aldolase deficiecncy
   (D) galactokinase deficiency

5. Which of the following are the features of Wernike's syndrome?
   (A) Ataxia
   (B) Ophthalmoperesis
   (C) Encephalopathy
   (D) all of the above

Answers:

1. C:
   Alcohol interferes with the absorption of thiamine and with synthesis of thiamine pyrophosphate. When thiamine deficiency is suspected , it must be replenished whenever carbohydrate is administered., as failure to do so can precipitate lactic acidosis. thiamine deficiency in its earliest stages produces anoxia and nonspecific symptoms. Prolonged deficiency results in beriberi, which is often characterised as wet or dry. In patients with wet beriberi, cardiovascular symptoms predominate while in dry beriberi symptoms are primarily neurologic with symmetric peripheral sensory and motor neuropathy, and diminished reflexes. Alcoholics have CNS findings that are frequently missed and are attributable to alcoholism.[1]

2. B
   Alcohol acutely enhances actions ɣ -aminobutyric acid(GABA$_A$) receptors and inhibits N-methyl –D- aspartate(NMDA) receptors.[2]

3. C
   Alcohol in general is associated with decreased intake of nutrients and may be asociated with malabsorption or impaired storage, common vitamin deficiency includes thiamine, folate, niacin, vit B6, vit. C, vit. A, rarely vit. B12(abundant in food). Dietary Defeciency of vit. E does not occur (only in prolonged malabsorption and genetic abnormalities in vit. E metabolism or transport)[2]

4. B
   Because transketolase enzyme requires thiamine for action.[1,2]

5. D
   Wernicke encephalopathy manifests as horizontal nystagmus, ophthalmoplegia, cerebellar ataxia and mental impairement. When memory loss with confabulation presesnt its called Wernicke-Korsakoff syndrome.[2]

References:

1. Russell MR, Suter PM. Nutrion: Vitamin and Trace Mineral Deficiency and Excess: Vitamins. In: Fauci AS, Braunwald E, Kasper DL, Hauser SL, Longo DL, Jameson JL, et al., editors. Harrison's principles of internal medicine. 18th ed. New York: McGraw Hill; 2012:594-7.
2. Schuckit MA. Alcohol and Drug Dependency: Alcohol and Alcoholism. In: Fauci AS, Braunwald E, Kasper DL, Hauser SL, Longo DL, Jameson JL, et al., editors. Harrison's principles of internal medicine. 18th ed. New York: McGraw Hill; 2012:3546-7.

BRONCHIAL ASTHMA

Dr. Shobhit Shakya, Senior resident, Department of Medicine

A 35 year old woman with moderate persistent asthma, with no other comorbities.

1. What is the first line of therapy?
   (A) beta2- adrenergic agonists
   (B) inhaled corticisteroids
   (C) anticholinergics
   (D) theophyllins

   Above patient now has been under good control for 5 months salbutamol inhaler for symptomatic control once a week. She awakens at night thrice monthly with asthma symptoms, but has no difficulty in exercise. She also takes LABA (salmeterol)(50 mcg/puff) with fluticasone (100 mcg/puff)inhaler twice daily.Her FEV1 is 84% of her personal best.

2. What is the best next step in management?
   (A) As the salbutamol usage suggests poor control, add montelukast.
   (B) Discontinue salmeterol
   (C) Discontinue fluticasone
   (D) Decrease fluticasone to 50mcg/puff twice a day.

   20 Years later patient progressed to severe persistent asthma requiring oral prednisone at 7.5mg daily with high dose inhaled corticosteriodes, long acting bronchodilators and montelukast to control her symptoms. Now she is planned for omalizumab therapy.

3. Which of the following is best necessary step prior to initiating omalizumab.?
   (A) discontinuation of oral prednisolone
   (B) Present level of immunoglobin E >200 IU/L (IgE).
   (C) Presence of sensitivity to a perennial aeroallergen
   (D) Switching oral to parenteral prednisolone.

4. Omalizumab is given in bronchial asthma by which route?
   (A) Intravenous
   (B) Intramuscular
   (C) Subcutaneous
   (D) Aerosol

5. All are used in treatment of refractory asthma, except:
   (A) theophylline
   (B) oral corticosteroids
   (C) omalizumab
   (D) anti-TNF(Tumor necrosis factor) therapy.

Answers:

1. B

   Inhaled corticosteriods are the first-line therapy for persistent asthma.

2. B

   A step down in asthma therapy can be considered when an individual has been clinically stable for 3-6 months.factors pointing towards appropriate asthma control are day time symptoms≤2 per week, nighttime symptoms≤2 per months, use of resque inhaler ≤2 per week, FEV $_1$ and PEFR≥80%. When stepping down its important to consider dosing.as dose of fluticasone is already low, it would not be recommended to reduce its dose. At this point, best course of therapy would be to stop LABA.

3. C

   Omalizumab is a blocking antibody that binds to and neutrilizes circulating immunoglobin E (IgE) to inhibit IgE – mediated reactions.it has been shown that treatment with omalizumab decreases the number of exacerbations and decrease the dose of oral/ inhaled corticosteriods.elevations in serum IgE are frequently seen in asthmatics. Omalizumab can be considered in individuals whose IgE ranges from 30 to 700 IU/L.

4. C

   Omalizumab given as subcutaneus injections every 2-4 week in hospital setting because minor risk of anaphylactic reactions.

5. D

   Anti- TNF therapy is ineffective in severe asthma and should not be used.

Reference:

1. Barnes PJ. Diseases of the Respiratory System: Asthma. In: Fauci AS, Braunwald E, Kasper DL, Hauser SL, Longo DL, Jameson JL, et al., editors. Harrison's principles of internal medicine. 18th ed. New York: McGraw Hill; 2012:2109-14.

MALNURTITION

Dr. Shobhit Shakya, Senior resident, Department of medicine

A 20 year old woman with anorexia nervosa undergoes surgery for cholangitis wth cholelithiasis. After surgery patient developed acute respiratory distress syndrome and put on ventilator. Her lab investigations are: TLC= 4100/mcL, Hb=10 gm/dl, albumin= 2.0 g/dl, total protein= 5.0 g/dl.

1. Which of the following is true regarding the etiology and treatment of malnutrition in this patient?
    (A) patient has marasmus and nutritional support should be started slowly
    (B) Patient has kwashiorkor and nutritional support should be aggressive
    (C) Patient has marasmic kwashiorkor, kwashiorkor predominant and nutritional support should be aggressive.
    (D) Patient has marasmic kwashiorkor, marasmus predominant and nutritional support should be started slowly.
2. All of the following factors are used to determine the patient's caloric needs except:
    (A) Age
    (B) Weight
    (C) Gender
    (D) Albumin
3. What body mass index individual is considered underweight?
    (A) 19.5 kg/m2
    (B) 20 kg/m2
    (C) 16 kg/m2
    (D) 18.5 kg/m2
4. All of the following statements regarding enteral feeding in critically ill patients are true Except:
    (A) Enteral feeding increases splanchnic blood flow
    (B) Enteral feeding stimulates secretion f gastrointestinal hormones and neuronal activity to promote trophic gut activity.
    (C) Enteral feeding decreases IgA antibody release.
    (D) In enteral feeding the risk of aspiration pneumonia can be reduced by feeding directly into the jejunum beyond the ligament of treitz.
5. Which of the following statements regarding skinfold thickness measurement is not true?
    (A) Measurement of skinfold thickness is useful for estimating body fat stores.
    (B) Skinfold thickness measurements not helpful in discrimination of fat mass from muscle mass.
    (C) Most convenient site is triceps skinfold and it is generally representative of body's overall fat level.
    (D) Thickness of<3mm is suggestive of complete fat stores' exhaustion.

Answers:
1. C
    Protien energy malnutrition includes two major types: marasmus and kwashiorkor. The prompt differentiation is important as it directly affects treatment. The patient in question belongs to marasmic kwashiorkor because of anorexia nervosa, stress in form of surgery and starvation.[1] The patient had prolonged starvation with kwashiorkor(as shown by reduced level of proteins). Hence, kwashiorkor is predominant in this case and aggressive nutritional therapy is indicated.[1,2]

2. D
    Patients basal energy expenditure (BEE) is calculated by the Harris-Benedict equation. The factors that are used for determining BEE are age, gender weight and height.[1]

3. A
    Normal BMI ranges between 18.5 to 24.9 kg/m^2 .BMIs $\leq$18.5 kg/m^2 considered underweight.Severe malnutrition is expected when BMI reaches below 16kg/m^2 .[1]

4. C
    It is always important to give a portion of the nutritional support in the form of enteral nutrition. It's particularly important in maintaining the overall health of GIT. Enteral feedings improve splanchnic blood flow and stimulate neuronal activity to prevent ischemia and ileus. Also, it maintains the

immunologic function of the gut as they stimulate the secretion of IgA and hormones to promote trophic activity of the gut.[3]

5. B

Skinfold thickness is helpful in discrimination of fat mass from muscle mass. It is san useful tool in estimation of body fat stores as nearly half of body fat is in subcutaneous plane. midarm muscle circumference (MAMC) is also an important tool , especially to estimate skeletal muscle mass.[1]

References:

1. Heimburger DC. Nutrition: Malnutrition and Nutritional Assessment. In: Fauci AS, Braunwald E, Kasper DL, Hauser SL, Longo DL, Jameson JL, et al., editors. Harrison's principles of internal medicine. 18th ed. New York: McGraw Hill; 2012:605-11

2. Walsh BT, Attia E. Nutrition: Eating Disorders. In: Fauci AS, Braunwald E, Kasper DL, Hauser SL, Longo DL, Jameson JL, et al., editors. Harrison's principles of internal medicine. 18th ed. New York: McGraw Hill; 2012:636-639.

3. Bistrian BR, Driscoll DF. Nutrition: Enteral and Parenteral Nutrition Therapy. In: Fauci AS, Braunwald E, Kasper DL, Hauser SL, Longo DL, Jameson JL, et al., editors. Harrison's principles of internal medicine. 18th ed. New York: McGraw Hill; 2012:614.

METHANOL POISONING

Dr. Shobhit Shakya, Senior resident, Department of medicine

45 years male was brought to us in emergency department with complains of epigastric pain, myalgia blurring of vision and worsening consciousness, all starting within 8 hours of drinking country liquor from a nearby shop. On examination patient was drowsy and was hyperventilating.ABG of this patient was as follows: PH-7.1, PCO_2-14, PO2-93, GLU-119, Na^+-134, K^+-6.1, HCO3$^-$-5.3, Lac-2.3 with Osm.Gap-22.One family member and a few other villagers were having similar complaint and they also gave history of taking alcohol from same shop. A provisional diagnosis of acute methanol toxicity was made.Patient was intubated and was kept on mechanical ventilator and other supportive medications.

1. Which of the following are the causes of high anion gap metabolic acidosis?
    (A) Diarrhea
    (B) Ureterosigmoidoscopy
    (C) Renal tubular acidosis type 2
    (D) Methanol poisoning
2. Which of the following is the cause of normal anion gap metabolic acidosis?
    (A) Salicylate poisoning
    (B) Starvation
    (C) Renal tubular acidosis
    (D) Alcohol
3. All of the following can be used in management of acute methanol poisoning except?
    (A) Ethanol
    (B) Fomepizole
    (C) Sodium bicarbonate
    (D) Activated Charcoal
4. Which of the following is not a feature of methanol poisoning?
    (A) Anion gap metabolic acidosis
    (B) Snow field vision with central scotoma on fundoscopy
    (C) Oxalate crystals in urine
    (D) Basal ganglia hemorrhage
5. Blindness in methanol poisoning is due to?
    (A) Direct damage due to Methanol
    (B) Formaldehyde
    (C) Formic acid.
    (D) Fomepizole therapy.

Answers:

1. D

Few importantcauses of High anion gap metabolic acidosis are as follows:
*   Lactic acidosis
*   Ketoacidosis
    - Diabetic
    - Alcoholic

- Starvation

Toxins such as ethylene glycol, methanol, salicylates, propylene glycol, pyroglutamic acid etc.

2. C

Few important causes of Non-Anion-Gap metabolic acidosis are as follows:

Gastrointestinal bicarbonate losses. Diarrhea, External pancreatic or small-bowel drainage, Ureterosigmoidostomy, jejunal loop, ileal loop etc.

Renal acidosis eg. Distal (classic) RTA (type 1) Proximal RTA (type 2)Generalized distal nephron dysfunction (type 4 RTA) etc.

Drugs -Potassium-sparing diuretics (amiloride, triamterene, spironolactone) ACE-Is and ARBs, Nonsteroidal anti-inflammatory drugs, Cyclosporine and tacrolimus etc.

3. D

Charcoal does not absorb significant amounts of MeOH and should not be used as it has a high risk of aspiration in acutely intoxicated patients.4-Methylpyrazole , Fomepizole; an alcohol dehydrogenase

antagonist is FDA approved for the treatment of MeOH toxicity. Folinic acid to increase the metabolism of formate can also be given. Ethyle Alcohol delyas metabolism of MeOH to its toxic metabolites by competing for alcohol dehydrogenase and can be used in situations in which fomepizole is unavailable. Hemodialysis is indicated for anMeOH level that exceeds 50 mg/dL, severe and resistant acidosis, renal failure, or visual symptoms.

4. C

Clinical Presentation:

Early stage: Early after ingestion mild CNS depression or headache evolve, but profound obtundation or inebriation can occur as well. Early symptoms are directly cause by methanol prior to metabolism.

Late stage: After a latent period of about 14-18 hours,severe anion gap metabolic acidosis without significant lactate or ketone concentration develops.Formate accumulation within the retina and optic nerve fiber causes snow field vision ,blurred vision,visual field defects or blindness .Visual field testing may reveal central scotoma and other visual field defects.Other CNS symptoms during the late phase are lethargy,convulsion,delirium and coma.Basal ganglia hemorrhage with dyskinesia and hypokinesia has been observed.Abdominal complains include nausea ,vomiting,pain and acute pancreatitis.Oxalate crystels in urine is a feature of ethylene glycol poisoning.

5. C

The toxicity of MeOH is due to its conversion by alcohol dehydrogenase to formaldehyde and then by acetaldehyde dehydrogenase to formic acid.Formate accumulation within the retina and optic nerve fiber causes snow field vision, blurred vision,visual field defects or blindness.

References:

1. Eliza S, Schwarz E, Mullins ME. Toxicology, Methanol. In Godara H, editor. The Washington manual of medical therapeutics.34th ed.Lippincott Wiliamsand Wilkins; 2013. P.1060-4
2. Thomas D, DuBoseJr, Acidosis and alkalosis. In: Fauci AS, Braunwald E, Kasper DL, Hauser SL, Longo DL, Jameson JL, et al., editors. Harrison's principles of internal medicine. 18th ed. New York: McGraw Hill; 2012:363-70.

A CASE OF DIABETES WITH HYPERTENSION

Dr. Munna Lal Patel, Assistant Professor, Department of Medicine

A 74-year-old man with T2DM for 7 years was referred with gradually worsening renal impairment (eGFR 21 mL/min). His HbA1C was 6.3% on oral hypoglycemic agents with no vascular complications. Other medical history included hypertension and obstructive sleep apnoea. Urine examination did not show any proteinuria; kidneys were small-sized on ultrasonography.

1. Which of the following is not a risk factor for of end stage renal disease
   (A) Smoking
   (B) Atherosclerosis
   (C) Normal birth weight
   (D) Older age
2. Which of the following is preferred method for diagnosis of disease progression.
   (A) USG abdomen
   (B) Urine examination
   (C) Kidney biopsy
   (D) Blood investigation

3. To prevent disease progression in this case optimal blood pressure should be.
    (A) ≤ 130/80 mmHg
    (B) ≤ 110/70 mmHg
    (C) ≤ 120/76 mmHg
    (D) ≤ 140/80 mmHg
4. Nephritic syndrome consist of all of the following except
    (A) Hematurea
    (B) Hypertension
    (C) Proteinuria
    (D) small-sized kidneys
5. Malignant hypertension leads to all of the following except
    (A) Fibrinoid necrosis
    (B) Thrombotic microangiopathy
    (C) Normal urinary protein
    (D) Acute renal failure

Answers:

1. C

    Risk factors for end stage kidney disease include smoking, hypercholesterolemia, duration of hypertension, low birth weight and preceding renal injury.

2. C

    In absence of proteinuria preferred method to diagnose disease progression is kidney biopsy to see the early changes within glomerulus.

3. A

    Treating hypertension is the best way to avoid progressive renal failure; most guideline recommended lowering blood pressure to 130/80 mmHg if there is preexisting diabetes or kidney disease.

4. D

    Nephritic syndrome is a triad of hematurea, hypertension and proteinuria with normal sized kidneys.

5. C

    Malignant hypertension leads to fibrinoid necrosis of small blood vessel, thrombotic microangiopathy, a nephritic urinalysis and acute renal failure.

Reference:

1. Julia B.Levis, Eric G. Neilson, Glomerular diseases: In: Longo DL, Fauci AS, Kasper DL, Hauser SL, Jameson JL, Loscalzo J. editors. Harrison's Principles of Internal Medicine. 18th edition pp no. 2352

A CASE OF NEPHROTIC SYNDROME

Dr. Munna Lal Patel, Assistant Professor, Department of Medicine

A 18 years boy admitted in medical emergency with gradual onset generalized swelling all over the body with breathlessness. There was no history of decreased urine output. On examination normal blood pressure, no pallor/ hypertension was present. There was no history of jaundice, hematemesis or maelena. On systemic examination B/L decreased breath sound was present and cardiovascular examination was within normal limit.

1. Which of the following investigation should be done on priority.
    (A) Urine examination
    (B) X- Ray chest PA view
    (C) Automated count
    (D) All of the above
2. Which of the following is most appropriate clinical diagnosis
    (A) Nephritic syndrome
    (B) Nephrotic syndrome
    (C) Chronic liver disease
    (D) All of the above
3. Nephrotic syndrome classically present with all of the following except
    (A) Heavy proteinuria
    (B) Minimal hematurea
    (C) Hypertension
    (D) Hypotension

4. Complication of nephrotic syndrome are all of the following except
   - (A) Cardiovascular disease
   - (B) Venous thrombosis
   - (C) Thyroid dysfunction
   - (D) Mood alteration
5. First line of immunosuppressive therapy in idiopathic nephrotic syndrome is
   - (A) Azathioprime
   - (B) Cyclophosphamide
   - (C) Serolimus
   - (D) Prednisolone

Answers:
1. A

   In young boy with gradual onset generalized swelling all over the body with breathlessness without history of decreased urine output with normal blood pressure and no pallor/ hypertension was present with normal cardiovascular system examination priority investigation is urine examination.

2. B

   Nephrotic syndrome classically present with gradual onset generalized swelling all over the body with breathlessness without any history of decreased urine output in young age.

3. D

   Nephrotic syndrome classically present with heavy proteinuria, minimal hematuria, hypoalbuminemia, hypercholesterolemia, edema and hypertension.

4. D

   Complication of nephrotic syndrome include cardiovascular disease, Venous thrombosis, thyroid dysfunction and end stage renal disease.

5. D

   First line of immunosuppressive therapy in idiopathic nephrotic syndrome is prednisolone at 1.2mg/kg body weight with dietary protein restriction.

Reference:
1. Julia B.Levis, Eric G. Neilson, Glomerular diseases: In: Longo DL, Fauci AS, Kasper DL, Hauser SL, Jameson JL, Loscalzo J. editors. Harrison's Principles of Internal Medicine. 18th edition pp no. 2345

A CASE OF DIABETIC PATIENT WITH SEIZURE
Dr. Munna Lal Patel, Assistant Professor, Department of Medicine

A 40 year old male diabetic patient with renal dysfunction presented with shock in medicine emergency department, having recurrent seizures, decreased urine output, with altered behaviour. He was on metformin therapy for diabetes.

1. Most common cause of shock in this patient.
   - (A) Arrhythmia
   - (B) Gastritis
   - (C) Neurogenic
   - (D) Septicemia
2. What is target blood pressure in this patient
   - (A) 120-139/<90 mmHg
   - (B) 130-149/<90 mmHg
   - (C) 120-129/<90 mmHg
   - (D) 130-139/<90 mmHg
3. Can Metformin be used in this patient.
   - (A) Nephrotoxic
   - (B) Causes hypoglycemia
   - (C) Renal safe
   - (D) Used with insulin
4. How is CKD classified
   - (A) Based on eGFR
   - (B) Based on serum creatinine
   - (C) Based on ultrasonography
   - (D) Based on blood urea

5. Seizures in CKD patients is explained by
   (A) Hypoglycemia
   (B) Hypocalcemia
   (C) Hypomagnesimia
   (D) All of the above

Answers :
   1. A
       Hyperkalemia in chronic kidney disease patients causes arrhythmia and hence shock.
   2. A
       Target blood pressure in CKD is 120-139/<90 mmHg
   3. A
       Metformin is renal safe can be given.
   4. A
       According to KDIGO guidelines 2012 CKD classified by eGfr.
   5. D
       Causes of seizure in CKD is hypoglycemia , hypocalcemia, hypomagnesemia, uremia.

Reference:

   1. Julia B.Levis, Eric G. Neilson, Glomerular diseases: In: Longo DL, Fauci AS, Kasper DL, Hauser SL, Jameson JL, Loscalzo J. editors. Harrison's Principles of Internal Medicine. 18th edition,vol. 2, pp no. 2308, 2295,2317.

MULTIPLE SCLEROSIS
Prof V Atam, Department of Medicine

A 37-year-old woman with progressive multiple scleroses is being admitted for intravenous glucocorticoid therapy. She was diagnosed with multiple sclerosis 10 years ago after presenting with bilateral decreasedvisual acuity. She had an abnormal MRI at that time. She has been hospitalized approximately seven times since presentation, each time because of increasing bilateral lower extremity weakness and decreased sensation manifested as a heavy feeling, waxing and waning generalized fatigue, bilateral hand tingling and speech changes. She has also had bilateral optic neuritis and one transient episode of aphasia in the past. For the past 2 years she has been on cyclophosphamide and methylprednisolone, initially every 4 weeks, and now every 6 weeks, with the last treatment 1 month ago. Interferon therapy was tried but failed. For one weekprior to admission, the patient has had worsening bilateral lower extremity weakness/heaviness, increased fatigue.She also complaint of high grade fever with rigors, abdominal pain dysuria and urinary incontinence. Physical examination of this patient was as follows:
PR: 102/min,BP 158/94mmHg,Chest: NAD,CVS: S_1S_2 normal, no added sounds, Abdomen: Soft, +BS, wears a diaper,CNS: Fully conscious, no neck rigidity, unable to stand and walk, Motor: Upper Limbs: NAD,Lower Limbs-Spastic, Right; power 3/5,Left;Power2/5,DTR +++,Planter: Extensor, Sensory: Normal.

1. Which of the following is not a feature of multiple sclerosis?
   (A) Onset between ages 15 and 50.
   (B) Internuclearophthalmoplegia
   (C) Worsening with elevated body temperature
   (D) Deficit developing within minutes
2. Which of the following is a poor prognostic factor in multiple sclerosis?
   (A) Female sex
   (B) Early age of onset
   (C) Early impairment of sensory pathways
   (D) Secondary progressive form of disease.
3. All of the following are true regarding bladder dysfunction in MS except?
   (A) Symptomatic bladder dysfunction occurs in about 5-6% of the patients.
   (B) Severity of bladder dysfunctions is unrelated to the disease.
   (C) Anticholinergic medications are better used in patients with hyperreflxic bladder without outlet obstruction.
   (D) Anticholinergic medications are used in combination with α sympathetic blocking agent in patientswithhyperreflxic bladder with outlet obstruction.
4. Which of the following is not a paraclinical evidence in multiple sclerosis diagnosis?
   (A) OligoclonalIgG bands in CSFor elevated IgG index.
   (B) Delayed and well preserved waveform in VEP.
   (C) Single gadolinium enhancing brain or cord lesion is considered as positive MRI.

(D) OligoclonalIgM bands in CSFor elevated IgM index.
5. Which drug has following mechanism of action: Stimulation of anti-inflammatory cytokines production and inhibition of synthesis and transport of matrix metaloproteinnases.
  (A) Fingolimod
  (B) Intravenous immunoglobulin
  (C) Glatiramer
  (D) IFN-β
  (E) Natalizumab

Answers:

1. D

Explanation: The clinical features of MS reflect the multifocal areas of CNS injury. The high degree of variability and the difficulty in predicting the course and severity make MS one of the most puzzling CNS diseases. Following is a table summarizing clinical features typical of MS. Table also summarizes clinical features not suggestive of MS.

Clinical Features Suggestive of Multiple Sclerosis	Clinical Features Not Suggestive of Multiple Sclerosis
Onset between ages 15 and 50	Onset before age 10 or after age 60
Involvement of multiple areas of the CNS	Involvement of the PNS
Optic neuritis	Hemianopsias
Lhermitte sign	Rigidity, sustained dystonia
Internuclear ophthalmoplegia	Cortical deficits such as aphasia, apraxia, alexia, neglect
Fatigue	Deficit developing within minutes
Worsening with elevated body temperature	Early dementia

CNS, Central nervous system. PNS, peripheral nervous system.

2. D

Explanation: MS appears to follow a more benign course in women than in men. Onset at an earlyage is a favorable factor. Relapsingform of the disease is associatedwith a better prognosis than progressive disease. Among initial symptoms, impairmentof sensory pathways has been found in several studies to be a favorable prognostic feature, whereas pyramidaland particularly brainstem and cerebellar symptomscarry a poor prognosis.

3. A

Explanation: Symptomatic bladder dysfunction occurs at some time during the course of MS in 50% to 80% of patients. The severity of bladder symptoms is unrelated to the duration of the disease but often parallels the severity of other myelopathic symptoms. Differentiating between bladder spasticity and hypotonia is important before initiating therapy, because different therapies are employed for each condition. Initial steps in managing bladder dysfunction include fluid management, timed voiding, and the use of a bedside commode. Anticholinergic medications are often used for patients with a hyperreflexic bladder without outlet obstruction. Detrusor hyperreflexia with outlet obstruction may respond to antispasticity medications, or anticholinergics in combination with α-sympathetic blocking agents

4. D

Explanation: OligoclonalIgG bands in CSFor elevated IgG index and not theelevatedIgM index is a paraclinical evidence for diagnosing MS

5. D

Explanation:

IFN-β is a class I interferon whoseefficacy in MS probably results from its immunomodulatory properties, including (1) downregulating expression of MHC molecules on antigen-presenting cells, (2) inhibiting proinflammatory and increasing regulatory cytokine levels, (3) inhibition of T cell proliferation, and (4) limiting the trafficking of inflammatory cells in the CNS.

Glatiramer acetate is a synthetic, random polypeptide composed of four amino acids (l-glutamic acid, l-lysine, l-alanine, and l-tyrosine). Its mechanism of action may include (1) induction of antigen-specific suppressor T cells; (2) binding to MHC molecules, thereby displacing bound MBP; or (3) altering the balance between proinflammatory and regulatory cytokines.

Natalizumabis a humanized monoclonal antibody directed against the α₄ subunit of $\alpha_{4\beta1}$ integrin, a cellular adhesion molecule expressed on the surface of lymphocytes. It prevents lymphocytes from binding to endothelial cells, thereby preventing lymphocytes from penetrating the BBB and entering the CNS.

Fingolimod is a sphingosine-1-phosphate (S1P) inhibitor and it prevents the egress of lymphocytes from the secondary lymphoid organs such as the lymph nodes and spleen. Its mechanism of action is probably due, in part, to the trapping of lymphocytes in the periphery and the prevention, thereby, of lymphocytes reaching the brain. However, because S1P receptors are widely expressed in the CNS tissue and because fingolimod is able to cross the BBB, it may also have central effect.

References:

1. Maria KH, Fred DL, Aaron EM, Samia JK. Multiple Sclerosis and Other Inflammatory Demyelinating Diseases of the Central Nervous System, In:Daroff RB editior. Bradley's Neurology in Clinical Practice. 6th ed. Elsevier Saunders ;2012 . p.1284-1308.
2. Stephen L. Houser Douglas S. et al, Multiple Sclerosis and Other Demyelinating Diseases, In, Longo, editor. Harrison's principles of internal medicine. 18th ed. McGraw Hill ; 2012.p.3395-3407

Chapter-10

Microbiology

STREPTOCOCCUS B SEPSIS IN A NEONATE

Dr. Mastan Singh, Professor & Head, Microbiology

A two days old baby born at home was admitted in the neonatal intensive care unit with the complaints of fever, difficulty feeding and lethargy (limpness and hard to wake up the baby). Pediatrician suspected sepsis and advised blood culture.

1. What may be the causative organism of early onset septicemia?
   - (A) Group B Streptococcus
   - (B) Escherichia coli
   - (C) Listeria monocytogenes
   - (D) Any of the above
2. Which of the following is not a risk factor to get infection with vaginal Group B Streptococcus
   - (A) Prematurity < 37 weeks
   - (B) Premature rupture of Membrane >18 hours
   - (C) Positivity for group B Streptococcus in previous pregnancy
   - (D) Primipara
3. Which of the following is a Group B Streptococcus
   - (A) Streptococcus mitis
   - (B) Streptococcus agalactiae
   - (C) Streptococcus pneumonia
   - (D) Streptococcus zooepidemicus
4. Antimicrobial of choice to treat group B Septicemia is:
   - (A) Vancomycin
   - (B) Ampicillin + aminoglycoside
   - (C) Metronidazole + aminoglycoside
   - (D) Ceftriaxone
5. Prevention of early onset group B Streptococcus infection includes:
   - (A) Antiseptic wipe of vagina at delivery
   - (B) Intrapartam antibiotic
   - (C) Isolation of baby from mother
   - (D) Avoid breast feeding

Answers:

1. D

   Septicemia in the first 7 days of life is predominantly caused by Group B Streptococcus, *Escherichia coli, Listeria monocytogenes*. Other enterobacteriaceae and hospital associated organisms are occasionally implicated.

2. C

   Risk factors associated with GBS neonatal infection include delivery at less than 37 weeks of gestation, GBS bacteruria, intrapartum fever or intra-amniotic infection, rupture of membranes for 18 hours or longer before delivery, maternal age younger than 20 years and a history of previous miscarriage.

3. B

   Group A Streptococcus is *S. pyogenes*.
   Group B Streptococcus is *S. agalactiae*.

4. B

   Empirical treatment is ampicillin (150mg/kg/day) + an aminoglycoside as *Listeria monocytogenes* is resistant to most cephalosporins. Once infection with GBS is confirmed then penicillin G (200,000 U/kg/day) is given for a total duration of 10 days.

5. B

   Intrapartum prophylaxis with penicillin G (5million units stat; then 2.5 million units 4hourly till delivery) is recommended for prevention of early onset GBS disease.

Reference:

1. Edwards MS, Baker CJ. *Streptococcus agalactiae*. In: Mandell GL, Bennett JE, Dolin R, eds. Mandell, Douglas, and Bennett's Principles and Practice of Infectious Diseases. 7th ed. Philadelphia, Pennsylvania: Churchill Livingstone Elsevier; 2010:2655-2666.

DIPHTHERIA
Dr. Mastan Singh, Professor & Head, Microbiology

An 8 years male child came with low grade fever and difficulty in breathing. He appears toxic. On examination a thick, dirty gray membranous covering is present over the tonsils. It is firmly adherent and bleeds on removal. Tonsils are not much enlarged.

1. The most likely diagnosis is
   (A) Membranous tonsillitis
   (B) Diphtheria
   (C) Candidiasis of tonsil
   (D) Agranulocytosis
2. Grayish covering :
   (A) Is made of intact squamous epithelium
   (B) Usually does not extend beyond tonsil
   (C) Causative agent is present in the membranous covering
   (D) Grey shade of covering is due to pigment
3. All are true for *Corynebacterium diphtheriae* EXCEPT
   (A) Highly invasive
   (B) Toxinogenic
   (C) Only lysogenic strains can cause diphtheria
   (D) Non-spore forming
4. Following test helps best in diagnosis of diphtheria
   (A) Demonstration of bacteria in the lesion.
   (B) IgM in serum
   (C) Antigen detection in serum
   (D) Shick intra-dermal test
5. All are true for Diphtheria toxin EXCEPT
   (A) Polypeptide
   (B) Interferes with Protein Synthesis
   (C) Reach the target organ through circulation
   (D) Non-antigenic

Answers:
1. B
   The classical diphtheritic pseudomembrane presents as a dirty grey, adherent membrane which bleeds on removal with little or no local discomfort. In the other conditions pus points and membrane consisting of inflammatory cells and necrotic debris may be seen, and is painful on removal.
2. C
   The grey pseudomembrane composed of fibrin, leukocytes, erythrocytes, dead respiratory epithelial cells, and organisms. The membrane can extend widely up to the tracheobronchial tree. *Corynebacterium diphtheriae* does not produce any pigment.
3. A
   Diphtheriae is a non-sporing, non motile, Gram positive bacilli and is essentially a non invasive bacteria. Lysogeny with a toxin gene carrying β-phage is necessary for toxin production and virulence.
4. A
   Diagnosis of diphtheria is confirmed by isolation on culture of a toxigenic strain of *C. diphtheriae* from the local lesion. Serological testing for antigen and antibody is not useful for diagnosis of acute cases. Shick's intradermal test is used to determine susceptibility to diphtheria.
5. D
   Diphtheria toxin is locally produced, circulates throughout the body and acts on a wide variety of tissues (heart muscles, nerves and kidneys). It is a polypeptide composed of two segments: B (binds to specific receptors) and A (active segment). Segment A causes inactivation ofEF2 present in eukaryotic cells but not in bacteria. This inhibits protein synthesis and results in cell death. Diphtheria toxin and toxoid are both highly antigenic stimulating production of protective antibodies.

Reference:
1. Macgregor RR. *Corynebacterium diphtheriae*. In: Mandell GL, Bennett JE, Dolin R, eds. Mandell, Douglas, and Bennett's Principles and Practice of Infectious Diseases. 7th ed. Philadelphia, Pennsylvania: Churchill Livingstone Elsevier; 2010:2687-2693.

SPOTTED FEVER RICKETTSIOSIS

Dr. Mastan Singh, Professor & Head, Microbiology

A 12 years male was admitted in the pediatric ward with a history of 10 days fever, rash, persistent headache, myalgia and occasional vomiting. The rash appeared on day 3 of the illness and spread from the trunk to the extremities. The lesions progressed from macules to maculopapules to petechiae. Subsequently the child developed delirium.

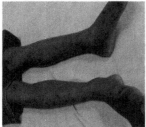

1. What is the most likely diagnosis?
   (A) Enteric Fever
   (B) Chicken Pox
   (C) Spotted fever Rickettsiosis
   (D) Scarlet Fever
2. The Commonest vector for Spotted fever Rickettsiosis is
   (A) Tick
   (B) Anopheles
   (C) Body louse
   (D) Aedes
3. Causative agent of Spotted fever is
   (A) *Rickettsia mooseri*
   (B) *Rickettsia rickettsii*
   (C) *Rickettsia akari*
   (D) *Rickettsia prowazekii*
4. Following tests are helpful in diagnosis EXCEPT:
   (A) IgM capture ELISA
   (B) Haemagglutination inhibition
   (C) Weil Felix Test
   (D) Complement Fixation test
5. Treatment of choice is:
   (A) Metronidazole
   (B) Doxycycline
   (C) Acyclovir
   (D) Interferon

Answers:
1. C
   Spotted fever rickettsiosis presents with fever and rash (after 3-5days of fever).
2. A
   Ticks are the vector for Rocky Mountain Spotted Fever (RMSF), Indian Tick Typhus and Boutonneuse fever.
3. B
   Causative agent is *R. rickettsii*.
4. B
   Weil-felix test is traditional heterophile antibody test with varying specificity and sensitivity. CFT and ELISA are useful in diagnosing specific rickettsial diseases especially RMSF. Haemagglutination Inhibition is not used as Rickettsia is not a haemagglutinating organism.
5. B
   Treatment of choice is Doxycycline 100mg every 12 hourly for 7 days

Reference:

1. Walker DH. *Rickettsia rickettsii*. In: Mandell GL, Bennett JE, Dolin R, eds. Mandell, Douglas, and Bennett's Principles and Practice of Infectious Diseases. 7th ed. Philadelphia, Pennsylvania: Churchill Livingstone Elsevier; 2010:2499-2507.

MDR TUBERCULOSIS

Dr. Amita Jain, Professor, Department of Microbiology

A 45 year old man presenting with fever, weight loss, cough and hemoptysis for more than 4 weeks presented in outpatient clinics. He gave history of taking antitubercular treatment two years ago for a period of three months, for similar kind of complaints. On examination of available prescription it was noted that he was treated with first line antitubercular drugs. He had stopped the treatment once his symptoms were relieved. Sputum tested positivefor acid fast bacilli.

1. What is your most probable provisional diagnosis in this case, based on available history?
    (A) Drug sensitive Tuberculosis
    (B) MDR Tuberculosis suspect
    (C) Miliary tuberculosis
    (D) XDR tuberculosis
2. What should be the next step for management of the present case as per Revised National Tuberculosis Control Program (RNTCP) guidelines 2014?
    (A) Manage as MDR TB, without further laboratory investigation
    (B) Test for Rifampicin resistance, if positive manage as MDR TB
    (C) First manage as Drug sensitive TB and subsequently as MDR TB, if there is no response
    (D) MDR TB is not curable.
3. MDR TB is defined as resistance to
    (A) More than three antitubercular drugs
    (B) All first line antitubercular drugs
    (C) INH and Rifampicin, irrespective of resistance to any other antitubercular drug
    (D) INH, Rifampicin, quinolones and injectable antitubercular drugs.
4. What is the most common risk factor in development of MDR TB?
    (A) Mismanagement of drug sensitive tuberculosis
    (B) Natural prevalence of MDR strains
    (C) A new mycobacterial strain
    (D) None of the above

Answers:

1. B
    MDR TB is a man made problem; inadequate treatment is one of the most important risk factor for emergence of MDR strains. Approximately 15% (range 11-19%) of patients with history of treatment in past, have MDR TB. (Ref 1 page 7)
2. B
    MDR TB is a laboratory based diagnosis. Rifampicin resistance is taken as a laboratory marker of MDR TB. Laboratory confirmation of rifampicin resistance in *Mycobacterium tuberculosis* isolate from a suspect of MDR TB is mandatory for establishing the diagnosis. Radiology has no role in diagnosing MDR TB. RNTCP has implemented DOTS PLUS program for management of MDR TB cases all over the country using second line drugs.(Ref 1 page 18)
3. C
    MDR tuberculosis is defined as resistance to both INH and Rifampicin, irrespective of resistance to any other anti-tubercular drug. (Ref 2)
4. A
    Drug resistance in *Mycobacterium tuberculosis* occurs due to chromosomal mutations. Development of multi drug resistance in occurs by selection of resistant strains due to antibiotic pressure created by inappropriate use of antitubercular drugs as seen in this patient (untimely termination of therapy). (Ref 3 page 43)

References:

1. TB INDIA 2014 Revised National TB Control Programme ANNUAL STATUS REPORT (pg 29)
2. www.tbcindia.nic.in
3. Guidelines for PMDT in India - May 2012

INFLUENZA A/PANDEMIC H1N1

Dr. Amita Jain, Professor and Dr. Bhawna Jain, Department of Microbiology

A 24 years old female presented with chief complaints of acute onset high grade fever for the last 2 days, along with dry cough, rhinorrhea, headache and body ache, during an Influenza outbreak time. There was no past history suggestive of any chronic illness. There was no history of travel outside the country and of direct contact with patients having similar complaints. On auscultation, chest was bilaterally clear with vesicular breath sounds. No crepts or rhonchi were audible.

1. What can be the most probable provisional diagnosis?
   (A) Asthma
   (B) Lobar pneumonia
   (C) Pulmonary tuberculosis
   (D) Influenza
2. Which is the most appropriate sample to be collected for laboratory confirmation of Influenza?
   (A) Bronchoalveolar lavage (BAL)
   (B) Throat swab/ Nasal swab
   (C) Blood
   (D) Lung biopsy tissue
3. Which is the common route of transmission of Influenza virus?
   (A) By sexual route
   (B) Parenteral
   (C) By droplets
   (D) Oral
4. Influenza A/pandemic H1N1 virus is a novel virus which was
   (A) result of gradual accumulation of mutations
   (B) a reassortment of swine human and avian influenza viruses
   (C) a reassortment of swine and avian influenza viruses
   (D) a reassortment of swine and human influenza viruses

Answers:

1. D

    Since there was already an epidemic of Influenza in the locality, Influenza becomes an obvious diagnosis. Diseases like pneumonia and asthma usually presents with crepitations/ wheeze/ rhonchi. URTIs present with sudden onset of fever, cold and cough and can have several causes including influenza.

2. B

    Since in this situation cause of epidemic is already established, it may not be necessary to establish diagnosis in each case. However, for URTI the ideal sample is throat swab or nasal swab. BAL and lung biopsy tissue are taken in case of lower respiratory tract involvement. Viremia is transient so blood is usually not a good sample for virus detection. Antibodies determination is also not recommended.

3. C

    All respiratory viruses spread via respiratory route. Hence to protect an individual, social distancing, hand hygiene, cough etiquettes, chemoprophylaxis (if advised) and vaccination can be helpful.

4. B

    2009 flu pandemic was a global outbreak of a new strain of a influenza A virus subtype H1N1 officially named the "novel H1N1" / pdm H1N1 first identified in April 2009 commonly called "Swine flu" combining components of swine, avian and human influenza viruses.

References:

1. Influenza virus: A brief overview. Tanushree Dangi, Amita Jain 2012. Proceedings of Indian Nation Academy of Science 82(1):111-121
2. http://www.cdc.gov/flu/professionals/antivirals/summary-clinicians.htm
3. World Health Organization 2002. Manual on animal influenza diagnosis and surveillance, WHO/CDS/CSR/ NCS2002.2.
4. World Health Organization. Acute respiratory infections: Influenza. 2007 http://www.who.int/vaccine_research/diseases/ari/en/index.html. Accessed 15 March 2011.

ENCEPHALITIS SYNDROME

Dr. Amita Jain, Professor and Dr. Parul Jain, Department of Microbiology

A 13 year old male, resident of district Sultanpur, presented on 10th of illness day with complaints of moderate to high grade fever and severe headache, without chills, rigor, rash, photophobia, vomiting or diarrhea. Four days ago patient had an episode of generalized tonic clonic seizures. Since then he has altered sensorium. The patient has no previous history of seizures. On examination the patient has no signs of meningeal irritation and a Glasgow coma scale E3V2M5. His peripheral blood examination revealed hemoglobin of 6.2 g/dl, total leucocyte count 18,370/mm^3 (Neutrophils 44%, Lymphocyte 46% and Monocytes 7%), platelet count 55,000/mm^3, serum sodium levels 135.8 mmol/L and serum potassium levels 4.79 mmol/L. Examination of the cerebrospinal fluid showed leucocyte count 40cells/μl, predominantly lymphocytes, proteins 56 mg/dl and glucose 35mg/dl.

1. What is the syndromic diagnosis of the patient?
   (A) Acute encephalitis syndrome
   (B) Acute Meningitis
   (C) Septicaemia
   (D) Acute Sepsis
2. What is the most common causative agent of AES in Uttar Pradesh?
   (A) Japanese Encephalitis virus
   (B) Herpes Simplex Virus
   (C) Hemophilus influenzae
   (D) Enteroviruses
3. What is the sample of choice for establishing the etiological diagnosis of AES?
   (A) Serum
   (B) Cerebrospinal fluid
   (C) Nasal/ Throat swab
   (D) Stool
4. Which of the following describes the JEV vaccination campaign in India?
   (A) SA 14-14-2 strain to children between 1 to 15 years of age
   (B) SA 14-14-2 strain to adults >15 years of age
   (C) Beijing 1 strain to children between 1 to 15 years of age
   (D) Beijing 1 strain to adults >15 years of age
5. Which of the following are not a WHO-recommended compound/ formulation for control of mosquito larvae in container habitats for Vector Borne Disease control?
   (A) Temephos
   (B) Novaluron
   (C) Bacillus thuringiensis israelensis
   (D) Oil of lemon eucalyptus

Answers:

1. A
   According to World Health Organization (WHO) the definition of Acute encephalitis syndrome is: "a person of any age, at any time of year with the acute onset of fever and a change in mental status (including symptoms such as confusion, disorientation, comatose, or inability to talk) and/or new onset of seizures (excluding simple febrile seizures)".

2. A
   Japanese encephalitis (JE) is a mosquito-borne viral infection and remains the most common cause of viral encephalitis in Uttar Pradesh (UP). From 2003 to 2009, a total of 19,644 cases and 4331 deaths were reported due to JEV in UP.

3. B
   The standard for establishing the etiology of AES is to detect pathogen specific IgM or nucleic acid in CSF.

4. A
   Following the massive outbreak of JE in 2005 in the districts of Eastern Uttar Pradesh and the adjoining districts of Bihar, vaccination campaigns were carried out in 11 of the highest risk districts of the country in 2006, 27 districts in 2007, 22 districts in 2008 and 30 districts in 2009. A single dose of SA14-14-2 vaccine was given to children between the age group of 1 to 15 years.

5. D
   WHO recommends use of Organophosphates eg. Pirimiphos-methyl and Temephos; Insect growth regulators eg. Diflubenzuron, rs-methoprenee, Novaluron and Pyriproxyfen; and Biopesticides eg. *Bacillus thuringiensis israelensise* and Spinosad for Dengue vector control.

References:

1. CNS Infections.Edited by Garcia-Monco JC. Published by Springer.
2. Japanese encephalitis surveillance standards. From WHO-recommended standards for surveillance of selected vaccine-preventable diseases [updated January 2006] Available from:http://www.path.org/files/WHO_surveillance_standards_JE.pdf
3. WHO Regional Office for Southeast Asia. Comprehensive guidelines for prevention and control of dengue and dengue haemorrhagic fever. Revised and expanded version. SEARO Technical Publication Series, New Delhi, India 2011.

RSV INFECTION IN SMALL CHILD

Dr. Amita Jain, Professor and Dr. Bhawana Jain, Department of Microbiology

A previously healthy, 4-month-old boy presented to the emergency department with rhinorrhea and tachypnea for the past 4 days. Fever developed during the night. He had no vomiting or diarrhoea. He had no cough, but his mother reported that when he breathes, his chest sounds. He has been recently exposed to other sick children at his daycare center. He was born at 34 weeks and 5 days prematurely. His birth weight was 2.3kg. His height, weight, and head circumference are all at the 50th percentile. His immunizations are up to date to 4 months. There are no smokers at home. Mother is a known asthmatic. Clinical and radiological examination suggests bronchiolitis and the child is admitted for management.

1. Which is the most suggestive etiological virus?
    (A) Rhinovirus
    (B) Parainfluenza virus
    (C) Influenza virus
    (D) Respiratory syncytial virus
2. Which one of the following is a risk factor for acquiring this infection?
    (A) Prematurity at the time of birth
    (B) Attending day care center
    (C) Low birth weight
    (D) All of the above
3. Which one of the following is the correct sequence of laboratory tests in order of their sensitivity that may be used to detect this virus?
    (A) IFA > serology > nucleic acid detection > culture
    (B) Serology > nucleic acid detection > culture > IFA
    (C) Nucleic acid detection > IFA > culture > serology
    (D) IFA > culture > nucleic acid detection > serology
4. Which of the following statements is not true in reference to human Respiratory Syncytial Virus (HRSV)?
    (A) In infants, 25–40% of HRSV infection results in lower respiratory tract involvement, including pneumonia, bronchiolitis, and tracheobronchitis
    (B) HRSV is member of family Paramyxoviridae of order Mononegavirales and is the nonsegmented negative-strand RNA virus
    (C) HRSV is so named because its replication in vitro leads to the fusion of neighboring cells into large multinucleated syncytia
    (D) HRSV is transmitted primarily by contaminated food or water
5. Which of the following is not used for HRSV treatment?
    (A) Ribavirin
    (B) Oseltamivir
    (C) Palivizumab
    (D) Bronchodilators

Answers:

1. D
    Rhinovirus and Parainfluenza viruses commonly cause symptoms of common cold. Influenza virus usually causes mild influenza like illness, while RSV is mainly responsible for lower respiratory tract illness like pneumonia and bronchiolitis.(ref1)
2. D
    HRSV is a major respiratory pathogen of young children, prematurity and low birth weight is predisposing factors. The attack rates approach 100% in settings such as day-care center.(ref2)
3. C
    Rapid antigen tests, especially IFA, are more sensitive than culture. Nucleic acid detection is most sensitive. Serology is useful only for epidemiologic studies. (ref 3)

4. D

HRSV is transmitted primarily by close contact with contaminated fingers or fomites and by self-inoculation of the conjunctiva or anterior nares. (ref2)

5. B

Ribavirin is an antiviral drug that is licensed for use by inhalation for severe RSV bronchiolitis. The anti-RSV antibody palivizumab, reduces the number of RSV cases requiring hospitalization for at-risk infants by 55% if given prophylactically. Bronchodilators have been used widely, including β2 agonists, nebulized epinephrine, and antimuscarinics such as ipatropium bromide (ref 4)

References:

1. Knipe, David M.; Howley, Peter M. Fields Virology, 5th Edition, Copyright Â©2007 Lippincott Williams & Wilkins, p. 1619-1620.
2. Harrison's Principles of Internal Medicine, 18 edition (e book), Copyright © The McGraw-Hill Companies. Chapter 186. Common Viral Respiratory Infections
3. Mandell, Douglas, and Bennett's principles and practice of infectious diseases / [edited by] Gerald L. Mandell, John E. Bennett, Raphael Dolin.—7th ed., p. 260
4. Tregoning JS, Schwarze J. Respiratory Viral Infections in Infants: Causes, Clinical Symptoms, Virology, and Immunology. Clinical Microbiology Reviews, Jan. 2010, p. 74–98

PARVOVIRUS INFECTION

Dr. Amita Jain, Professor and Dr. Parul Jain, Department of Microbiology

A 12 year old male presented with mild to moderate, off and on fever and easy fatigability for the past one month and some bleeding from the mouth for the past two days. On examination there was severe pallor. There was no rash, organomegaly or lymphadenopathy. His blood picture showed a haemoglobin of 4.9 gm/dl, total leucocyte count of 3950/mm³ (Neutrophils 5%, Lymphocytes 93%, Monocytes 1%) and platelet count of 56000/mm³. His liver and kidney function tests were normal. In view of the pancytopenia with normal biochemical parameters, he underwent a bone marrow study. The marrow aspirate smears were particulate with increased cellularity. There was myeloid prominence (M: E= 8:1) with normal and orderly maturation. Severe erythroid hypoplasia was noticed with giant proerythroblasts being the only recognizable erythroid cells. Intranuclear viral inclusions and "dog ear" like outpouchings were observed in the giant proerythroblasts.

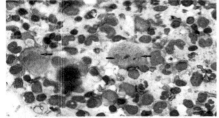

1. What is the most probable diagnosis?
   (A) Human Parvovirus B19 infection
   (B) Epstein Barr virus infection
   (C) Guillain Barre Syndrome
   (D) Measles virus infection
2. What other laboratory tests are done for diagnosing Human parvovirus B19 infection?
   (A) Anti-B19V IgM antibodies
   (B) Anti-B19V IgG antibodies
   (C) B19V-DNA detection
   (D) All of the above
3. Human parvovirus B19 is:
   (A) Enveloped, single stranded DNA virus
   (B) Enveloped, double stranded DNA virus
   (C) Non Enveloped, single stranded DNA virus
   (D) Non Enveloped, double stranded DNA virus
4. The mode of transmission of B19V is:
   (A) Respiratory route

(B) Parenteral, through blood transfusion

(C) Transplacental

(D) All of the above

5. Which of the following is an indication for starting specific intravenous immunoglobulin (IVIG) therapy for B19V infection?

(A) Mild febrile illness

(B) Transient aplastic crisis

(C) Persistent anemia in immuno-compromised children

(D) Reticular rash

Answers:

1. A

Most patients infected with B19V are asymptomatic or develop mild, non specific flu-like symptoms following which children may develop the classic "slapped cheek" rash or erythema infectiosum. Patients with underlying hemoglobinopathies may experience transient aplastic crisis. In immunocompromised hosts persistent infection may manifest as pure red cell aplasia or chronic anemia. B19V can have significant marrow aplastic effects even in immunocompetent individuals. The typical bone marrow aspirate findings are marked myeloid prominence, abnormally large proerythroblasts with classic intranuclear viral inclusions, cytoplasmic vacuolation and fuzzy "dog ear" like out pouching.

2. D

Anti-B19V IgM and IgG antibodies can be determined by ELISA, radioimmunoassay or immunofluorescence. IgM and IgG antibodies can be detected about 10-12 days and 2 weeks respectively after initial infection. PCR for detection of B19V- DNA from serum is available.

3. C

B19V is a small non-enveloped virus of family Parvoviridae, with a genome consisting of linear single-stranded DNA of approximately 5.6 kb.

4. D

The B19V can be transmitted through exposure to infected respiratory droplets, through blood transfusion and vertically from mother to fetus, though respiratory route is the most common mode of transmission.

5. C

Treatment of B19V infection is usually supportive and does not require treatment with specific immunoglobulins (IVIG). However, its use may be considered in immunocompromised patients presenting with pure red cell aplasia/ chronic anemia.

References:

1. Berns K, Parrish CR. 2007. Parvoviridae. In: Knipe DM, Howley PM, editors Fields Virology. Lippincott William & Wilkins. P 2438–2477.

2. Cennimo DJ. Parvovirus B19 infection. Edited by Steele RW. URL: emedicine.medscape.com/article/961063-clinical

LEPROSY

Dr Amita Jain, Professor Department of Microbiology

Fifty years old male, attended the skin (Dermatology) OPD with complaints of Hypo-pigmented patches and loss of cutaneous sensations in affected areas in both the arms. On examination total number of lesions was three, and there was presence of thickened ulnar nerve. No other finding was present. No one else in his family had similar complaints. Patient was referred for slit skin smear examination which showed presence of occasional AFB in skin and nasal smears (as shown in picture).

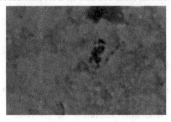

1. Most probable diagnosis is:
   (A) Cutaneous Tuberculosis
   (B) Leprosy
   (C) Atypical mycobacteriosis
   (D) Actinomycosis
2. A case of leprosy with good cell mediated immunity usually presents as following form of disease:
   (A) Lepromatous
   (B) Tuberculoid
   (C) Indeterminate
   (D) Borderline
3. Based on clinical examination this case will be classified as:
   (A) Multibacillary Leprosy
   (B) Paucibacillary Leprosy
   (C) Indeterminate Leprosy
   (D) Borderline Leprosy
4. Which of the following description suits lepra bacilli best?
   (A) Acid-fast rod-shaped organism, extracellular, often grouped together like bundles of cigars
   (B) Acid-fast rod-shaped organism, chiefly in masses within the lepra cells (globi), often grouped together like bundles of cigars or arranged in a palisade
   (C) Acid-fast rod-shaped organism, chiefly intracellular in Chinese letter form
   (D) Acid-fast rod-shaped organism, extracellular, Chinese letter form
5. Gerhard Henrik Armauer Hansen's contribution to Microbiology was;
   (A) First identified *M. leprae* as the cause of leprosy in 1873
   (B) First identified *M. tuberculosis* as a cause of TB in 1895
   (C) First identified *B. anthracis* as a cause of Anthrax in 1872
   (D) First identified that small pox is a contagious disease

Answers:

   1. B
   2. B
       Patients of Leprosy with good CMI usually presents as pausibacillary form, have very few or no Bacilli in lesions and show presence of well formed granuloma in skin biopsy (tuberculoid form). Patients with poor CMI presents as multibacillary form, have very several Bacilli/ globi in lesions without well formed granuloma in skin biopsy (Lepromatous form)
   3. B
       Clinically Paucibacillary Leprosy is 1-5 skin patches with definite sensory loss or any one nerve trunk affected by leprosy. Multibacillary leprosy is 6 or more skin patches with definite sensory loss or 2 or more nerve trunks affected by leprosy or 5 skin patches and 1 nerve trunk which mean 6 lesions. Classification is important to decide the course and number of medicines to be prescribed.
   4. B
       Lepra bacilli are acid-fast rod-shaped organism with parallel sides and rounded ends closely resembles the tubercle bacillus, occurs in large numbers in the lesions of lepromatous leprosy, chiefly in masses within the lepra cells, often grouped together like bundles of cigars or arranged in a palisade. Chains are never seen. Most striking are the intracellular and extra-cellular masses, known as globi, which consist of clumps of bacilli in capsular material.
   5. A
       Gerhard Henrik Armauer Hansen was a German physician who first identified M*ycobacterium leprae* as the cause of leprosy in 1873.

Reference:

   1. http://nlep.nic.in/index.html

KALA AZAR
Dr. Vimla Venkatesh, Professor, Department of Microbiology

Ramprasad, a 22 year old, from Sirohi village, Varanasi district, is brought to the OPD with a history of fever with chills, loss of weight and fatigue over the last few weeks. He was treated with traditional medicines and a course of antibiotics in his village, but continued to deteriorate. On examination important clinical findings included a grossly enlarged spleen and hepatomegaly. Preliminary laboratory investigations revealed anaemia with a hemoglobin of 5.5 gm/dl, a lowered total leucocyte count of 3000 cell/cumm and the differential count showed a lymphocytic predominance. The clinician strongly suspects Kala Azar.

1. The likely causative agent of Kala Azar in India is
   (A) *Leishmania infantum*
   (B) *Leishmania tropica*
   (C) *Leishmania donovani*
   (D) *Leishmania chagasi*

2. The investigation most likely to yield a positive result is a
   (A) Blood smear examination
   (B) Splenic aspirate examination
   (C) Bone marrow examination
   (D) Lymph node aspirate examination

3. If you wish to advise that other cases of fever in the region be screened with a suitable field test for Kala Azar, you would recommend a
   (A) rk39 based RDT
   (B) HRP2 based RDT
   (C) IFAT(Indirect immunofluorescent antibody test)
   (D) DAT (Direct agglutination test)

4. The recommended culture media for isolating the parasite is
   (A) Diamond's medium
   (B) NNN medium
   (C) Fletcher's medium
   (D) BHI medium

5. The parasite form obtained on culture in biphasic media would be:
   (A) Amastigotes
   (B) Promastigotes
   (C) Amastigotes and Promastigotes
   (D) Amoeboid forms

Answers:

1. C
   Leishmania donovani. In India *L. donovani* is the prevalent species and transmission is from man to man (anthroponotic), through the sandfly vector *Phlebotomus argentipes*. In other countries the disease may be anthroponotic or zoonotic and the subspecies involved may be *L. infantum* or *L. donovani*.

2. B
   Splenic aspirates, though requiring a higher degree of expertise (to avoid bleeding complications) gives the highest yield of parasites on examination of Giemsa stained smears and on culture. Amastigocytes are typically found within macrophages (and most easily identified in large numbers within cells rather than when lying singly extracellularly.

3. A
   The rk39 antigen test (based on a 39 amino acid conserved fragment of the kinesin protein of *L. Infantum*) is a newly recommended test for screening for antibodies in visceral leishmaniasis and is recommended as a field screening test under the national programme. HRP2 is an antigen detection test for falciparum malaria. IFAT and DAT are antibody detection tests for kala azar but can only be performed in well equipped laboratories.

4. B
   The NNN medium and its modifications are used to cultivate the Kinetoplastida including *Leishmania* species. Diamond's medium and it's modification are used for cultivating another human flagellate *T. vaginalis*, Fletcher's medium contains rabbit serum and used to cultivate leptospires, Leishmania do not grow in routine bacterial blood culture media like BHI.

5. B
   Promastigotes. In the body, the demonstrable form of the parasite is the amastigote form, while on culture in biphasic media like NNN we obtain the promastigote form of *L. Donovani*.

References:

1. http://nvbdcp.gov.in/Doc/Guidelines%20on%20use%20of%20rK39_rapid%20diagnostic%20kit.pdf accessed 28/01/2015
2. Lumsden WHR, Burns S, McMillan A. Protozoa. In: Collee JG, Fraser AG, Marmion BP, Simmons A, eds. Mackie &Mac Cartney practical medical microbiology. 14th ed. New York: Churchill Livingstone, 1996: 721-754 (725, 739).

3. Longo DL ,Fauci AS, Kasper DL, Hauser SL, , Jameson JL, Loscalzo J et al., editors. Harrison's principles of internal medicine. 18th ed. New York: McGraw Hill; 2012 (chapter 212 online ed)

HIV SCREENING EARLY DIAGNOSIS

Dr. Vimla Venkatesh, Professor, Department of Microbiology

Rakesh, a 28 year long haul truck driver, attends the integrated counseling and testing centre (ICTC) in his home district, requesting that he be tested for HIV, a disease he has recently read about in hoardings at his truck stops. He tells the counselor that he has been feeling feverish for the last 1-2 months.On being assessed for risk behavior, he says he practices safe sex, but has doubts about the quality of the condoms he uses.

1. What type of HIV screening test will be performed in the ICTC as per the national AIDS control programme.
   (A) HIV Rapid test
   (B) HIV Western blot
   (C) HIV p24 assay
   (D) HIV cDNA PCR

2. If a screening test for HIV is positive, the sample is tested further to confirm the diagnosis. The strategy adopted as per the national AIDS control programme in India, is to test samples further by:
   (A) HIV cDNA PCR
   (B) HIV Western blood
   (C) Two more rapid tests
   (D) Three more rapid tests

3. The antigen used in many HIV rapid tests and ELISA's is
   (A) gp160/gp36
   (B) p10
   (C) p17
   (D) gp105/gp36

4. The HIV virus is a
   (A) DNA virus
   (B) Segmented RNA virus
   (C) Double stranded RNA virus
   (D) Retrovirus

5. The subtype of the HIV virus prevalent in India is
   (A) A
   (B) B
   (C) C
   (D) D

6. The window period for most HIV antibody tests is generally
   (A) 2 days
   (B) 7 days
   (C) 12 weeks
   (D) 24 weeks

7. The test of choice to detect HIV positivity in a 3 month old infant is
   (A) HIV ELISA
   (B) HIV Western blot
   (C) HIV p24 assay
   (D) HIV cDNA PCR

Answers:

1. A

   As per current guidelines, screening for HIV at all ICTC's in India is by Rapid HIV tests. High quality rapid tests for HIV have been show to have performance characteristics equivalent to ELISA and have the additional advantages including quick turnaround times. This ensures same day reporting for clients; hence rapid tests have been recommended by the WHO in resource constrained settings.

2. C

   This is called strategy III, where a first positive HIV antibody test is confirmed by two additional rapid antibody tests on the same sample. All three tests should use either different antigens or must be based on a different test principle. This is a strategy devised by WHO-NACO to ensure a high

positive predictive value of a positive test result, in populations with relatively low prevalence of HIV(<10%).
3. A
By including gp36, the test kit is able to detect antibodies to HIV-2 in addition to HIV-1. As infection with HIV-2 is prevalent in India(the quantum of such infection is unclear, but it is likely to be <3% from reported figures) and also leads to the AIDS, testing for HIV in India needs to include HIV-2.
4. D
Both HIV 1&2 belong to the Retroviridae family, subfamily Orthoretrovirinae, genus Retrovirus.
5. C
6. C
7. D

References:
1. http://naco.gov.in/upload/Policies%20&%20Guidelines/5GUIDELINES%20FOR%20HIV%20TE STING.pdf accessed
2. WHO recommendations on the diagnosis of hiv infection in infants andchildrenhttp://whqlibdoc.who.int/publications/2010/9789241599085_eng.pdf?Ua=1
3. Thushan de Silva& Robin A. Weiss. HIV-2 goes global: an unaddressed issue in Indian anti-retroviral programmes. Indian J Med Res 132;2010: 660-662

HPV AND PREVENTION OF CERVICAL CANCER
Dr. Vimla Venkatesh, Professor, Department of Microbiology

Fifteen year old Shruthi is brought by her mother, Meena to the gynecology OPD. Shruthi's grandmother had been detected with a carcinoma about ten years back, when she presented with spotting between periods and lower abdominal pain. Meena has recently heard about a new vaccine which may protect her daughter from this type of cancer and has come for advice. The doctor takes Shruthi's history and finds that she attained menarche three years ago and is not sexually active. She also notes that Shruthi has two female siblings, 13 and 11 years old. The doctor advises a course of vaccination for all three girls.

1. What is the likely carcinoma that Shruthi's grandmother had been diagnosed with
    (A) Cervical cancer
    (B) Hepatic carcinoma
    (C) Ovarian cancer
    (D) Bladder cancer
2. Which virus has been strongly associated with this cancer
    (A) Human Herpes Virus 8
    (B) Human Papilloma Virus
    (C) Hepatitis C virus
    (D) Epstein Barr Virus
3. The vaccine is recommended to be given in
    (A) Sexually active women over 21 years of age only
    (B) Sexually active women after menopause
    (C) Girls before the onset of sexual activity
    (D) Girls less than 2 years of age
4. The recommended vaccination dose is
    (A) One dose
    (B) Two doses
    (C) Three doses
    (D) One dose and booster every 5 years
5. The current vaccines contains two or more of the virus subtypes
    (A) 6,11,16,18
    (B) 1,2,4,7
    (C) 5,8,9,12
    (D) 11,16, 88,92

Answers:
1. A

Cervical cancer. This cancer has been the most common cancer in Indian women, accounting for 16% of all cancers in urban cancer registries in 2005

2. B

Several serotypes of HPV, especially type 16 and 18 are strongly associated with cervical cancer. All the other viruses noted are also oncogenic viruses. While most HPV infections are self-limited, persistent infections are implicated in onccogenesis, causing cervical cancer in women as well as other anogenital and oropharyngeal cancers in women and men.

3. C

The HPV vaccine appears to have the greatest protective effect if given before the onset of sexual activity and acquisition of sexually transmitted HPV infections. The recommended age for vaccination is 11-12 years. Older persons between 13-26 years may also be vaccinated

4. C

3 doses- 0, 1-2 and 6 months, 0.5 ml i.m. per dose.

5. A

Two noninfectious HPV vaccines based on recombinant L1 protein are licensed for use in the United States. Quadrivalent HPV vaccine (types 6,11,16,18) (Gardasil, Merck and Co, USA) is licensed for use in females and males aged 9 through 26 years. Bivalent HPV vaccine (Types 16,18) (Cervarix, GlaxoSmithKline, Rixensart, Belgium) is licensed for use in females aged 9 through 25 years.. Both bi- and quadrivalent vaccines are marketed in India, and are recommended by the Indian Academy of Pediatrics but not included in the Universal Immunization programme.

Reference:

1. Nandakumar A, Ramnath T, Chaturvedi M. The magnitude of cancer cervix in India. Indian J Med Res 130: 2009: 219-221.
2. Bonnez W, Reichman RC. Papillomaviruses. In: Mandell GL, Bennett JE, Dolin R, eds. Mandell, Douglas, and Bennett's Principles and Practice of Infectious Diseases. 7th ed. Philadelphia, Pennsylvania: Churchill Livingstone Elsevier; 2010:2035-2049.
3. Human Papillomavirus Vaccination Recommendations of the Advisory Committee on Immunization Practices (ACIP) accessed at www.cdcgov / mmwr / preview / mmwrhtml / rr6305a1.html.

SEVERE MALARIA PRESENTING AS CEREBRAL MALARIA

Dr. Vimla Venkatesh, Professor, Department of Microbiology

Varsha, a 8 year old child is referred from the primary health centre near her village in Lakhimpur district, to the emergency unit of a tertiary care centre, with a history of high grade fever since the last 2 days and convulsions and unresponsiveness since morning. On examination she has a temperature of 104 degree Celsius, a GCS of 8 and a palpable spleen. The clinician suspects a parasitic infection and orders a rapid test. The blood smear examination stained by leishman stain is shown:

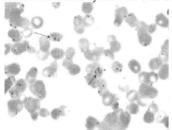

1. The rapid test ordered by the clinician is most likely:
   (A) HRP-2 antigen test
   (B) Aldehyde test
   (C) Rk39 antibody test
   (D) RPR test
2. The parasite detected by this test and seen on the blood smear is:
   (A) *Plasmodium falciparum*
   (B) *Wuchereria bancrofti*
   (C) *Babesia microti*

(D) *Trypanosoma brucei*
3. The parasite form that helps to confirm the species includes
    (A) Accole forms
    (B) Schuffner's dots
    (C) Maltese cross appearance
    (D) Microfilariae
4. The vector which is commonly responsible for transmission of this parasite is
    (A) *Phlebotomus argentipes*
    (B) *Anopheles culicifacies*
    (C) *Culex tritaeniorhynchus*
    (D) *Aedesaegypti*
5. The empirical treatment likely to be started is
    (A) Artesunate
    (B) Miltefosine
    (C) Amphotericin
    (D) Chloroquine

Answers:

1. A
    The clinical features suggest severe malaria caused by *P. falciparum* and the HRP-2 antigen is specific to P*lasmodium falciparum*. The HRP-2 rapid test is sensitive in quickly screening for *P. falciparum* malaria infection in finger prick or EDTA anticoagulated blood specimens, with results available in a few minutes. The aldehyde and Rk39 tests screen for antibodies in kala azar and VDRL is a non specific test used to screen for syphilis.
2. A
    P. falciparum ring forms within RBC's.
3. A
    Accole forms are trophozoites of *P. falciparum* found on the edge of the red blood cells. Accole forms are of three types-common, rim and displaced. Schuffner's dots are seen in RBC's parasitized by *P. vivax*. The maltese cross appearance is typically seen in RBC's when parasitized by *Babesia* spp. Microfilaria are seen in *W. bancrofti* infections.
4. B
    In India *Anopheles culicifacies* is the predominant species among the 6 anophiline species implicated in transmitting malaria. *A. culicifacies* is responsible for the transmission of 60-70% and *A. fluviatilis*, 15-20% new cases of malaria.
5. A
    Injectable artemisinin derivatives like artesunate/artemether is recommended for initiating therapy(including empirical) for severe malaria in India. However therapy must be continued as artemisinin combination therapy (ACT)with artemisinin plus long acting antimalarials like sulfadoxine-pyrimethamine or amodiaquine, lumefantrine, mefloquineetc as artemisinin monotherapy is NOT recommended due to the high possibility of emergence of resistant strains. Miltefosine and Amphotericin are used in treatment of kala azar. Chloroquine is used for treatment of P vivax malaria in areas where resistance has not been demonstrated.

References:

1. http://nvbdcp.gov.in/Doc/Guidelines%20for%20Diagnosis2011.pdf accessed 30/01/2015
2. http://nvbdcp.gov.in/Doc/Guidelines%20on%20use%20of%20rK39_rapid%20dia20kit.pdfaccessed 28/01/2015
3. http://ukneqasmicro.org.uk/parasitology/images/pdf/BloodParasitology/MalariaSpecies/Plasmodium Falciparum.pdf (ans 3)
4. Guidelines for Indoor Residual Spray (IRS) : http://nvbdcp.gov.in/iec.html : accessed on 15 April 2015
5. Longo DL ,Fauci AS, Kasper DL, Hauser SL, , Jameson JL, Loscalzo J et al., editors. Harrison's principles of internal medicine. 18 th ed. New York: McGraw Hill; 2012 (chapter 210, 212 online ed)

NEUROLOGICAL DEFICIT IN JAPANESE ENCEPHALITIS

Dr. Vimla Venkatesh, Professor, Department of Microbiology

5 year old Shyam a resident of district Maharajganj, Uttar Pradesh is brought to the neurology department with persistent apathy, dullness and loss of power in his left lower limb. He had been recently admitted for a week for a febrile illness with convulsions and loss of consciousness and had received ventilator support. The parents have misplaced his discharge and investigative reports. The neurologist wants to rule out Japanese Encephalitis infection as a cause of the neurological sequel.

1. The laboratory test which could be ordered by the clinician are
    (A) Anti-JE IgM antibodies in CSF
    (B) Anti-JE IgM antibodies in serum
    (C) Both the above
    (D) Neither
2. The JE virus is a:
    (A) Flavivirus
    (B) Bunyavirus
    (C) Herpesvirus
    (D) Orthmyxovirus
3. The recently launched indigenous Indian JE vaccine is a
    (A) Live attenuated vaccine
    (B) Inactivated Vero-celled derived vaccine
    (C) Killed vaccine
    (D) Oral inactivated vaccine
4. The vector which is commonly responsible for transmission of this virus is
    (A) *Phlebotomus argentipes*
    (B) *Anopheles culicifacies*
    (C) *Culex tritaeniorhynchus*
    (D) *Aedes aegypti*
5. Antiviral medication has proven efficacy in improving prognosis in one of the following viral encephalitis:
    (A) Herpes Simplex encephalitis
    (B) Japanese Encephalitis
    (C) West Nile encephalitis
    (D) Enterovirus encephalitis

Answers:

1. C
    IgM antibodies are found in CSF and serum. Presence in CSF is considered a more definitive sign of CNS infection; the antibodies are present from a few days post infection and may be detected for 3 months or longer.
2. A
3. B
    The Jenvac is a newly marketed indigenous JE vaccine prepared using a JE virus isolated in Kolar by the National Institute of Virology. It is administered in two i.m. doses given 28 days apart and has shown high long lasting protection.
4. C
5. A
    Intravenous acyclovir (10 mg/kg q8h; 30 mg/kg per day) is given for 10 days or until HSV DNA is no longer detected in CSF for the treatment of HSV encephalitis. No specific antiviral therapy is recommended for the other encephalitis.

References:

1. http://www.wpro.who.int/immunization/documents/Manual_lab_diagnosis_JE.pdf
2. http://nicd.nic.in/writereaddata/linkimages/je3038660088.pdf
3. http://www.bharatbiotech.com//pdf/Jenvac%20Pack%20Insert.pdf
4. http://www.cdsco.nic.in/SMPC/Bharat%20Biotech%20_%20JE.pdf
5. http://jid.oxfordjournals.org/content/early/2015/01/18/infdis.jiv023.long
6. Longo DL ,Fauci AS, Kasper DL, Hauser SL, , Jameson JL, Loscalzo J et al., editors. Harrison's principles of internal medicine. 18 th ed. New York: McGraw Hill; 2012 Online chapter 179

PERTUSSIS
Dr. Vimala Venkatesh, Professor, Department of Microbiology

An 18 month old child is brought to the O.P.D. by his mother, with a history of uncontrolled coughing fits for the last few days. The child is waking up several times a night with episodes of violent cough. The child's face turns red during the coughing fit and each episode is followed by a peculiar breathing sound and vomiting. The illness started with a running nose, cough and mild fever about two weeks back. The mother says this is her second child, the older child is of school going age and had a similar episode of cold and cough, but is now improving. Both children were home births and neither has received any vaccination. A blood examination in the child reveals a total leucocyte count of 18,600 cells per mm, with 72 per cent lymphocytes.

1. The likely diagnosis in this child is an infection with which of the following organisms:
    (A) *Corynebacterium diphtheriae*
    (B) *Bordetella pertussis*
    (C) *Legionella pneumophilia*
    (D) Influenza virus
2. The set of investigations that can be ordered in the child to make a definitive diagnosis is a
    (A) Blood culture and PCR on a blood sample
    (B) Nasopharyngeal swab culture and PCR on a nasopharyngeal swab
    (C) Blood culture and urine culture
    (D) Nasopharyngeal swab culture and PCR on a blood sample
3. All the following statements regarding prevention of this infection are true **EXCEPT**:
    (A) Whole cell killed vaccine given 3 times 4-6 weeks apart, followed by booster doses is protective
    (B) Acellular vaccine given 3 times 4-6 weeks apart, followed by booster doses is protective
    (C) Live vaccine given before one year of age followed by five yearly boosters
    (D) Vaccination of health care workers with an acellular vaccine is recommended
4. The following statements are true for the aetiological agent
    (A) Gram positive, motile, strict aerobe
    (B) Greyish white, bisected pearl or mercury drop colony appearance
    (C) It grows best on charcoal containing media
    (D) The toxin produced has an important role in pathogenesis
5. The disease pertussis is characterized by: all EXCEPT
    (A) An incubation period of 5-21 days
    (B) Reservoir of infection is dogs
    (C) Catarrhal, paroxysmal and convalescent stages
    (D) Prolonged duration of illness, 6-10 weeks in children

Answers:
1. B
    Prolonged cough, an inspiratory whoop, post-tussive vomiting, leucocytosis with lymphocytosis clinically suggest pertussis caused by *Bordetella pertussis*. Lack of vaccination and history of contact with a possible case are other pointers.
2. B
    The organism does not enter the circulation, blood and urine cultures are unlikely to yield the organism. Culture, especially in the early phase and PCR are sensitive and specific for the detection of *B. pertussis* infections.
3. C
    Both whole cell and acellular vaccines provide good protection. Whole cell may be marginally more effective but also has more side effects. No live vaccines are available for immunization against *B. pertussis*. Infected adults transmit the infection and post vaccination immunity wanes over several years, hence it is advocated that health care workers in hospitals and ambulatory care settings be vaccinated.
4. A
    B. pertussis is a gram negative bacilli, non motile, strict aerobe
5. B
    B. pertussis is human pathogen with no animal reservoirs. *B. bronchiseptica*, which causes kennel cough in dogs may occasionally transmit to humans and cause respiratory and systemic disease in the immunocompromised (HIV, cystic fibrosis patients).

Reference:
1. Pertussis: Epidemiology and Prevention of Vaccine-Preventable Diseases: The Pink Book: Course Textbook - 13th Edition (2015): Accessed at http://www.cdc.gov/vaccines/pubs/pinkbook/pert.html

CRYPTOCOCCAL MENINGITIS

Dr. Gopa Banerjee, Professor and Dr. Prashant Gupta, Department of Microbiology

A 48-year-old male previously diagnosed with AIDS was admitted to the medicine department with chief complaints of high-grade fever and moderate to severe headache since last15 days associated with multiple episodes of vomiting, and altered sensorium for four days. Neck rigidity and Kernig's sign were positive. CT scan of the brain with contrast showed mild hydrocephalus without any mass lesions and inflammation of basal meninges. Lumbar puncture was remarkable for an opening pressure of 460mm H2O. Cerebrospinal fluid (CSF) examination revealed 80 cells, predominantly lymphocytes; with protein of 54.7 mg/dl and glucose of 28 mg/dl (corresponding blood glucose was 136 mg/dl). India ink preparation of the CSF showed characteristic predominant round budding yeast cells ranging from 5-20µm in size with distinct halos.

1. Suggest the clinical diagnosis of condition
   (A) Cryptococcal meningitis
   (B) Pyogenic meningitis
   (C) Tubercular meningitis
   (D) Japanese Encephalitis
2. Most common cryptococcal species causing meningitis in AIDS patient is
   (A) *Cryptococcus neoformans*
   (B) *Cryptococcus albidus*
   (C) *Cryptococcus laurentii*
   (D) *Cryptococcus gatii*
3. In the clinical laboratory, *C. neoformans* can be readily differentiated from other yeasts on the basis of following tests
   (A) India ink preparation
   (B) Rapid urease test
   (C) Detecting laccase activity
   (D) All of the above
4. Following is true about *C. gatii*
   (A) Most commonly isolated from pigeon droppings
   (B) Associated with the river red gum trees (*Eucalyptus camaldulensis*)
   (C) Most commonly associated with AIDS patients
   (D) Contains strains with serotype A & D
5. All of the following factors are related to poor prognosis of cryptococcal meningitis in AIDS **EXCEPT**
   (A) High burden of yeast in India ink
   (B) High polysaccharide antigen titre
   (C) Raised intracranial pressure
   (D) Strong inflammatory response in the CSF

Answers:
1. A
   Diagnosis of Cryptococcal meningitis is based on the clinical features of meningitis and capsulated yeast present in India ink preparation of the CSF.
2. A
   Most common Cryptococcal species causing meningitis in AIDS patients is *C. neoformans*. Only a small measurable portion of cases with AIDS have been reported to be caused *by C. gattii*.
3. D
   There are three direct tests that predict that a yeast may be C. neoformans. First, placing the yeast into an India ink preparation may reveal encapsulation of the yeast. The capsule is generally better seen in direct clinical specimens from the host and may not be as apparent in wet mounts made from in vitro cultures. Second, a rapid urease test is positive in most *Cryptococcus* species. *Cryptococcus* spp., unlike *Candida* spp., possess urease, an enzyme that hydrolyzes urea to ammonia and increases the ambient pH. A positive urease test can be detected within minutes. Third, *C. neoformans* possess prominent laccase enzyme. This enzyme allows the conversion of diphenolic compounds into melanin.This is detected by inoculating the specimen in the media containing nigerseed (birdseed), caffeic acid, or dopamine. Yeast colonies that turn brown to black on these special agars are identified as melanin-positive.
4. B
   C. neoformans has frequently been isolated from soil contaminated by guano from birds (esp. pigeon). Unlike C. neoformans, C. gattii has never been cultured from bird guano. C. gattii has frequently been isolated from river red gum trees (Eucalyptus camaldulensis) and forest red gum trees (*Eucalyptus tereticornis*). Most common Cryptococcal species causing meningitis in AIDS

patients is C. neoformans. Only a small measurable portion of cases with AIDS have been reported to be caused by *C. gattii*. *C. neoformans* strains had been grouped into two varieties that included five serotypes based on capsule structure. C. neoformans var. neoformans and *C. neoformans var. grubii* included strains with serotypes D, A, and AD, and *C. gattii* contained strains with serotypes B and C.

5. D

A poor prognosis in cryptococcal meningitis is indicated by a strongly positive India ink examination, a high polysaccharide antigen titer and a poor inflammatory response in the CSF (e.g. less than 20 cells/μL). It is clear from natural history studies in patients with AIDS that the risk of infection dramatically increases as total CD4 lymphocyte counts drop below 50 to 100 cells/μL of blood. In these patients, the paucity of inflammatory cells at the site of infection, such as the subarachnoid space, is impressive.

References:

1. Perfect RJ. *Cryptococcus neoformans*. In: Mandell GL, Bennett JE, Dolin R, eds. Mandell, Douglas, and Bennett's Principles and Practice of Infectious Diseases. 7th ed. Philadelphia, Pennsylvania: Churchill Livingstone Elsevier; 2010:3287-3303.

TINEA PEDIS

Dr. Gopa Banerjee, Professor, Dr. Prashant Gupta, Department of Microbiology

A 48 year old male farmer presented with pruritic, scaly soles and painful fissures between the toes. Both the feet were affected. Scrapping of the scaly lesions was done using No. 15 blade and was examined in direct 10% KOH mount. On microscopy numerous irregular, branched andseptate fungal hyphae were found.

1. The clinical condition is called
   (A) Tinea nigra
   (B) Tinea corporis
   (C) Tinea pedis
   (D) Tinea capitis
2. Tinea pedis is most commonly caused by
   (A) *Trichophyton rubrum*
   (B) *Trichophyton mentagrophyte*
   (C) *Microsporum gypseum*
   (D) *Epidermophyton flocossum*
3. Following is an anthropophilicdermatophyte
   (A) *Trichophyton mentagrophyte varmentagrophyte*
   (B) *Trichophyton rubrum*
   (C) *Microsporum canis*
   (D) *Microsporum gypseum*
4. Which of the following usually infects skin and hair and not the nails
   (A) *Trichophyton rubrum*
   (B) *Microsporum audounii*
   (C) *Epidermophyton flocossum*
   (D) *Trichophyton mentagrophyte*
5. Hair perforation test is used to differentiate between
   (A) *Trichophyton mentagrophyte and Trichophyton rubrum*
   (B) *Microsporum canis and Microsporum equinum*
   (C) *Epidermophyton flocossum and Epidermophyton stockdaleae*
   (D) *Both A & B*

Answers:

1. C

Tinea pedis is the term used for a dermatophyte infection of the soles of the feet and the interdigital spaces. Tinea corporis is disease of glaborous (non-hairy) skin of the body. Tinea capitis is the infection of shaft of scalp hairs. Tinea nigra is infection of horny layer of epidermis characterized by painless brown to black, pigmented non-scaly, macular patches usually affecting palms and rarely soles. It is caused by pigmented (dematiaceous or phaeoid) fungi i.e *Hortae werneckii* and *Stenella araguata*.

2. A

Tinea pedis is most commonly caused by *Trichophyton rubrum*.

3. B

The fungal species exclusively affecting humans are known as anthropophilic while those inhabiting domestic and wild animals as well birds are called zoophilic. A third group, frequently isolated from soil is known as geophilic. *T. mentagrophyte* is an anthropophilic dematophyte but one of its variety *T. mentagrophyte var mentagrophyte* is a zoophilic fungi. *M. canis* generally affects canines (cats and dogs), human beings gets accidently infected. *M. gypseum* is a geophilic fungi.

4. B

The *Trichophyton* species usually infect skin, hair and nails. *Microsporum* species infect skin and hair and not nails. *Epidermophyton* species infect skin as well as nails but not hair.

5. D

Hair perforation test is done to differentiate the growth of some dermatophytes growing in culture media. The test is positive when dermatophyte species show wedge shaped perforation in sterilized prepubertal or infant hair. This test is positive in *T. mentagrophyte* and *M. canis* and negative in *T.rubrum* and *M. equinum.*

References:

1. Chander J. Dermatophytoses In: Text book of Medical Mycology. 3rd ed. New Delhi: India.Mehta Publishers; 2009:122-246.
2. Chander J. Tinea nigra In: Text book of Medical Mycology. 3rded. New Delhi: India.Mehta Publishers; 2009:106.
3. Chander J. Conventional Mycological Techniques In: Text book of Medical Mycology. 3rded. New Delhi: India. Mehta Publishers; 2009:522.

CANDIDIASIS

Dr. Gopa Banerjee, Professor, Department of Microbiology

A 61 year old male on treatment for acute myeloid leukemia was admitted to the hospital with fever, cervical lymphadenopathy and other nonspecific symptoms. Examination of his tongue revealed a white thick patch. Microscopy of a swab collected from the patch showed gram positive yeast like cells, presumptively identified as *Candida* species. His blood culture was also positive for *Candida* spp.

1. How will you confirm the species identification of Candida.
   (A) Germ tube test
   (B) Urease test
   (C) Melanin production
   (D) All of the above
2. What are the non cultural detection methods for Candida.
   (A) Candida manan assay
   (B) Candida heat labile antigen assay
   (C) D-inositol assay
   (D) 1.3 beta-D glucan assay
   (E) All of the above
3. Describe treatment of the infection caused by *Candida* spp
   (A) Azoles
   (B) Nystatin
   (C) Amphotericin B
   (D) All of the above

Answers:

1. A
2. E
3. D

Reference:

1. Pfaller MA, Pappas PC, Wingard JR. Invasive fungal pathogen. Current epidemiological trends clinical infectious Disease 2006; 43:53-14.

STREPTOCOCCUS PYOGENES SORE THROAT AND SEQUEL

Dr Jyotsna Agarwal, Professor, Department of Microbiology

A 7 year old girl presented with throat pain, difficulty in swallowing & fever for 2 days. On examination she was afebrile, submandibular nodes were tender & enlarged. Oral cavity showed enlarged tonsils with exudates.

Throat swab was collected for culture and she was advised warm saline gargles and a course of antibiotics and was asked to come after3 days for re-evaluation. She presents again after a month with slowly progressing painful swelling of both knee & ankle joints for 5 days and breathlessness& palpitations since yesterday. Parents admitted to not having given the antibiotic as was advised. Upon examination there was bilateral swelling of large joints. Doctors are thinking of acute rheumatic fever.

1. Which of the following is most commonly associated with a sore throat
   (A) *Staphylococcus aureus*
   (B) *Haemophilus* spp.
   (C) *Streptococcus pyogenes*
   (D) *Streptococcus pneumoniae*
2. How are beta hemolytic streptococci classified?
   (A) Runyon classification
   (B) Lancefield classification
   (C) Kauffman white scheme
   (D) None of the above
3. How does a group A streptococcus lead to Rheumatic heart disease
   (A) Molecular mimicry
   (B) Bacteria infects the heart valve
   (C) Bacterial toxin damage heart
   (D) Any of the above mechanism
4. *Streptococcus pyogenes* can be differentiated from other beta haemolytic Streptococci on the basis of
   (A) Bacitracin sensitivity
   (B) Erythromycin sensitivity
   (C) Novobiocin sensitivity
   (D) Penicillin sensitivity
5. Which of the following test(s) may be helpful in diagnosis of Acute Rheumatic fever
   (A) Anti-DNAse B test
   (B) Rapid streptococcal antigen test
   (C) Throat culture
   (D) All of the above

Answers:
1. C
   Although, respiratory viruses are the most common cause of acute pharyngitis (namely rhinoviruses and coronaviruses). Acute bacterial pharyngitis is typically caused by S. pyogenes.
2. B
   Lancefield classification for beta hemolytic streptococci is based on C carbohydrate antigen on the bacterial cell wall
3. A
   Apart from factors related to organism (certain M serotypes of *S. pyogenes*) and host factors; currently it is believed that the initial damage to the heart valve is due to cross-reactive antibodies attaching at valve endothelium, leading to subsequent inflammation and tissue damage.
4. A
   S. pyogenes is Group A beta hemolytic streptococci and it is sensitive to bacitracin unlike other beta hemolytic streptococci in groups B, C D etc.
5. D
   Dr. T. Duckett Jones in 1944 developed a set of criteria to help in diagnosis of ARF. It was revised in 1992, based on which WHO has laid down guidelines for diagnosis of ARF. Apart from major and minor manifestations, it includes supporting evidence of an antecedent group A streptococcal infection.

References:
1. Mandell, Douglas, and Bennett's Principles and Practice of Infectious Diseases, 7th Edition. Volume 2, part III, section F, chapter 199. Publisher: Churchill Livingstone.
2. Harrison's Principles of Internal Medicine (Harrison online), 18th Edition, Part 8, Section5, Chapter 136& chapter 322Publisher McGraw-Hill.

STREPTOCOCCUS PYOGENES AND ACUTE GLOMERULONEPHRITIS AS SEQUELA

Dr. Jyotsna Agarwal, Professor, Department of Microbiology

5 year old boy has a skin infection which the local doctor diagnosed as pyoderma. Parents did not seek any treatment for the skin condition. A month later, the boy starts passing dark colored urine &becomes lethargic and anorexic. On examination he is afebrile, has bilateral pitting pedal edema, high blood pressure. Urine examination reveals: proteinuria ++, Hematuria++ with red cell casts. Doctor is suspecting Post Streptococcal Acute Glomerulonephritis

1. Post streptococcal acute glomerulonephritis is associated with
   (A) Group A streptococci
   (B) Group B streptococci
   (C) Group C streptococci
   (D) Non beta hemolytic streptococci
2. What is the attack rate of AGN following throat or skin infection with Nephritogenic   streptococci
   (A) 1%
   (B) 15%
   (C) 50%
   (D) All of them develop AGN
3. Which of the following help (s) in confirming diagnosis of Post Streptococcal Acute   Glomerulonephritis
   (A) ASO titers
   (B) Impetigo
   (C) Renal biopsy
   (D) All of the above
4. What is the Prognosis of PSGN in children?
   (A) >90% recover completely
   (B) >90% develop renal failure
   (C) Majority end up with chronic glomerulonephritis
   (D) Rapidly fatal

Answers:
   2. A
       Skin and throat infections with certain beta hemolytic group A streptococci (nephritogenic strains) precedes glomerular disease
   2. A
   3. D
       The diagnosis of PSAGN is based on history, clinical findings and evidence of antecedent streptococcal infection demonstrated by serology. Also if renal biopsy is performed, demonstration of diffuse proliferative glomerulonephritis with subepithelial deposits helps in confirming the diagnosis.
   4. A
       Long-term prognosis in children is excellent and more than 90% of children with PSAGN make uneventful recovery

References:
   1. Mandell, Douglas, and Bennett's Principles and Practice of Infectious Diseases, 7th Edition. Volume 2, part III, section F, chapter 199. Publisher: Churchill Livingstone.
   2. Harrison's Principles of Internal Medicine (Harrison online), 18th Edition, Part 8, Section5, Chapter 136. Publisher McGraw-Hill.

INFECTIVE ENDOCARDITIS

Dr. Jyotsna Agarwal, Professor, Department of Microbiology

A 29-years-wo man reported to the hospital with low grade fever, myalgia & fatigue of 3 weeks duration. Upon examination: her temperature was 100.2oF, spleen was palpable &a systolic cardiac murmur was heard. Echo cardiogram confirmed atrial septal defect. She gave history of dental treatment at a clinic 1 week prior to have taken ill. Suspecting infective endocarditis, two sets of blood cultures were taken.

1. Which organism is most likely to be isolated from blood culture specimen?
   (A) *Salmonella typhi*
   (B) *Shigella dysentriae*

(C) Viridans Streptococcus
(D) *Vibrio cholera*
2. All are true for viridans streptococci EXCEPT
    (A) Organism of low virulence
    (B) Part of normal flora of mouth
    (C) Most are beta hemolytic
    (D) Some species may be associated with dental caries
3. How is Viridans streptococci differentiated from *Pneumococcus*, another alpha hemolytic streptococci?
    (A) Sensitivity to optochin
    (B) Bile solubility
    (C) Quellung reaction
    (D) All of the above
4. Which of the following may help in diagnosis of infective endocarditis
    (A) Jones criteria
    (B) Dukes criteria
    (C) Dukes classification
    (D) None of the above

Answers:

1. C
   Viridans streptococci are part of the normal microbial flora of our oral cavity. Viridans streptococci have been more frequently associated with endocarditis in patients with preexisting heart conditions.
2. C
   They are considered as bacteria of low virulence. Most are either alpha hemolytic or non-hemolytic. Certain species of viridans streptococci, eg. *S. mutans*, are strongly associated with development of dental caries
3. D
   Streptococcus pneumoniae (Pneumococcus) is optochin sensitive, soluble in bile and gives Quellung reaction
4. B
   Dukes Criteria are a highly sensitive and specific diagnostic criteria, developed on the basis of clinical, laboratory, and ECG findings.

References:

1. Mandell, Douglas, and Bennett's Principles and Practice of Infectious Diseases, 7th Edition. Volume 2, part III, section F, chapter 203. Publisher: Churchill Livingstone
2. Harrison's Principles of Internal Medicine, 18th Edition, Part 8, Section5, Chapter136. Publisher McGraw-Hill.

STREPTOCOCCAL MENINGITIS IN A NEONATE

Dr Jyotsna Agarwal, Professor, Department of Microbiology

4 day old baby was brought to the emergency by the parents. Baby was born through normal vaginal delivery, at 36 weeks gestation and birth weight was 2.1kg. She developed listlessness & focal seizures since morning. On examination he has bulging fontanels. Lumbar puncture was performed which revealed elevated cell count. Diagnosis of neonatal meningitis is made

1. Endogenous infections are those infections which are caused by
    (A) One's own normal flora
    (B) Microbes from hospital environment
    (C) Bacteria that have been ingested into the gut
    (D) Endotoxin producing bacteria
2. Identify sterile (microbe-free) anatomical site from list
    (A) Vagina
    (B) Urethra
    (C) Rectum
    (D) Bladder
3. Which of the following is most likely associated with neonatal meningitis
    (A) Enterococcus

(B) Group B Streptococcus

(C) Staphylococcus aureus

(D) Meningococcus

4. Group B streptococci can be differentiated from other beta hemolytic streptococci by

    (A) Inability to Hydrolyse hippurate

    (B) Sensitivity to bacitracin

    (C) Production of CAMP factor

    (D) PYR positivity

Answers:

    1.   A

        Endogenous infections are due to one's own body flora

    2.   D

        In Urinary tract, only the distal part of urethra is colonized by normal flora, rest is microbe free

    3.   B

        Neonatal meningitis is commonly caused by bacteria found in mother's vagina. Group B streptococci frequently colonize genital tract in women. Others are being E. coli and *Listeria monocytogens*.

    4.   C

        Group B streptococci are beta hemolytic and can be differentiated from other beta hemolytic streptococci by their ability to hydrolyze hippurates, resistance to bacitracin, and a positive CAMP test. Pyrrolidonyl Arylamidase (PYR) test is used for presumptive identification of group A beta-hemolytic Streptococci and Enterococci. It is negative for group B streptococci

References:

    1.   Mandell, Douglas, and Bennett's Principles and Practice of Infectious Diseases, 7th Edition. Volume 2, part III, section F, chapter 202. Publisher: Churchill Livingstone

    2.   Harrison's Principles of Internal Medicine, 18th Edition, Part 8, Section5, Chapter 136. Publisher McGraw-Hill

STAPHYLOCOCCAL FOOD POISONING

Dr. Jyotsna Agarwal, Professor, Department of Microbiology

24 year old man presents in emergency with 3 episodes of vomiting, associated retching and abdominal pain for last 2 hours. He gives a history of having eaten a cream bun at a local bakery in the morning. On examination he is afebrile. He does not appear dehydrated. Vitals are stable. He is admitted with a presumptive diagnosis of Staphylococcal food poisoning. Patient is admitted for observation

1. All but one are toxins liberated by *Staphylococcus aureus*

    (A) Toxic shock syndrome toxin

    (B) Exfoliative toxin

    (C) Enterotoxin

    (D) Pyrogenic toxin

2. All are likely associated with Staphylococcal food poisoning, EXCEPT

    (A) Improper handling& storage of cooked food

    (B) Milk & dairy products

    (C) Extensive diarrhea

    (D) Generally good prognosis

3. All is true for enterotoxin released by *S. aureus* EXCEPT

    (A) It is easily destroyed by acidic pH in stomach

    (B) It is heat stable

    (C) It can act as super antigen

    (D) It is preformed in the contaminated food

4. All but one is true for Staphylococcal food poisoning

    (A) Epidemic in nature

    (B) Absence of fever

    (C) Rapid onset

    (D) Feco-oral transmission

Answers:

    1.   D

Toxic shock syndrome toxin, Exfoliative toxin and Enterotoxins are produced by *S. aureus*. Pyrogenic toxin is produced by *Streptococcus pyogenes*.

2. C

Staphylococcal food poisoning is caused by food handlers colonized with in enterotoxin producing *S. aureus* stains. Commonly associated with food preparations involving lot of handling and food rich in protein and generally has good prognosis

3. A

Enterotoxin released by *S. aureus* is pre formed in the contaminated food, is resistant to both the heat and the acidic pH in stomach. By heating the contaminated food, bacteria will be destroyed but toxin already formed will remain unaffected. Enterotoxin can act as super antigen

4. D

Staphylococcal food poisoning have short incubation period and are epidemic in nature. Fever is not a prominent symptom.

References:

1. Mandell, Douglas, and Bennett's Principles and Practice of Infectious Diseases, 7th Edition. Publisher: Churchill Livingstone Volume 1, part II, section J; and Volume 2, part III, section F, chapter 195.
2. Harrison's Principles of Internal Medicine, 18th Edition, Part 8, Section5, Chapter 135. Publisher McGraw-Hill

ANTIBIOTIC ASSOCIATED DIARRHEA

Dr. Jyotsna Agarwal, Professor, Department of Microbiology

A 53 year old man was admitted to the hospital with fever and cellulitis of right leg following an injury about a week ago. He is a known diabetic. Upon investigations his TLC was 12600/cmm and random blood glucose was 356 mg/dL with predominant increase in polymorphonuclear leucocytes. Patient was started on clindamycin and admitted for blood sugar management. Patient's condition improved and he was discharged on day 3 and was asked to return for a follow up after 3 days. Patient came back after 10 days and this time he was admitted with profuse diarrhea and abdominal cramps for last 2 days. Patient admitted to still taking clindamycin he was prescribed for leg wound.

1. What is the likely diagnosis in this patient?
   (A) Food Poisoning
   (B) Enteric fever
   (C) Antibiotic associated diarrhea
   (D) Cholera
2. What is the most likely etiology?
   (A) *Clostridium botulinum*
   (B) *Clostridium difficile*
   (C) *Campylobacter jejuni*
   (D) *Campylobacter coli*
3. Which of the following investigations may help in confirming the diagnosis?
   (A) Stool culture for *C. difficile*
   (B) Assay for *C. difficile* toxin in stool
   (C) Lower GI endoscopy
   (D) All of the above
4. Which of the following describes the pathogenesis of this infection
   (A) Disruption of normal colonic flora by antibiotic
   (B) Colonization by toxigenic *C. difficile*
   (C) Toxin causing mucosal injury and inflammation
   (D) All of the above
5. Which would be the most effective practice in prevention of spread of this infection in hospital
   (A) Hand wash with soap and water
   (B) Alcohol based hand rub
   (C) Prophylactic therapy with metronidazole
   (D) Prophylactic therapy with Vancomycin

Answers:

1. C

   Although almost all antibiotic classes have been associated with antibiotics associated diarrhea (AAD), those most commonly implicated are clindamycin, penicillins, cephalosporins, and fluoroquinolones. Additional factors are advanced age and severity of underlying illness.

2. B

   Other pathogens with possible association with AAD are *Clostridium perfringens*, *Staphylococcus aureus* and *Candida*.

3. D

   Anaerobic culture for *C. difficile* can be done on selective media (Cycloserine, cefoxitin, and fructose agar). However, ELISA for toxin detection in stool, being more rapid is used more often. Endoscopy as a diagnostic test is usually reserved for special situations. *C. difficile* most often causes a nonspecific colitis in severe cases however, distinct pseudomembranous plaques can be seen at lower GI endoscopy.

4. D

   In animal studies, it has been demonstrated that normal flora *en masse* confers resistance to *C. difficile* colonization. Disruption in this microbial ecosystem with antibiotics is a prerequisite to establish *C. difficile* disease. Bacteria produce two very potent exotoxins: A and B which damage the colonic mucosa.

5. B

   Intestinal carriage rates of toxigenic *C. difficile* in healthy adults are reported to be < 10%. It may increase up to 20% among hospitalized adults. Majority of disease causing organisms is acquired from exogenous sources. Bacterial spores are responsible for transmission of infection. Alcohol is not effective in killing spores. For treatment of mild to moderate cases metronidazole is recommended and oral vancomycin is used for severe cases of AAD.

Reference:

1. Mandell, Douglas and Bennett's Priciples and Practice of Infectious Diseases, 7th Edition, Volume 1, Part II, Section J, Chapter 96: Antibiotic associated colitis. Churchill Livingstone, PA. pages 1375-1387

BRUCELLOSIS

Dr. Rajkumar Kalyan, Department of Microbiology

A 55 year old slaughter house worker, presented with a history of fever, headache, myalgia, chills, drenching night sweats and swelling in his neck and groin over the last few weeks. The fever was low to moderate grade with an evening spike. The onset of symptoms was gradual. On physical examination he had enlarged cervical and inguinal lymph nodes and mild hepatosplenomegaly. A peripheral blood count shows leucopoenia with relative lymphocytosis. Blood cultures on prolonged incubation in a biphasic medium yielded a gram negative cocco-bacillus without bipolar staining. The isolate was oxidase and urease positive.

1. Which of the following microorganisms is the most likely etiological agent?
   (A) *Francisella tularensis*
   (B) *Salmonella typhi*
   (C) *Brucella mellitensis*
   (D) *Mycobacterium bovis*

2. Milk ring test is used to identify which of the following infections?
   (A) Bubonic plague
   (B) Bovine tuberculosis
   (C) Salmonellosis
   (D) Brucellosis

3. What is the cardinal manifestation of human brucellosis ?
   (A) Vomiting and diarrhoea
   (B) Lymphadenopathy
   (C) A fluctuating pattern of fever
   (D) Myalgia

4 Which of the following species of *Brucella* requires 5-10% CO2 for their growth in laboratory?
   (A) *Brucella suis*
   (B) *Br. melitesis*
   (C) *Br. canis*
   (D) *Br. abortus*

5. Vaccination for human against brucellosis is done with following species:
   (A) *Br. suis*
   (B) *Br. canis*
   (C) *Br. melitensis*
   (D) *Br. abortus*

Answers:

1. C

   Myalgia and drenching night sweats point towards the diagnosis of brucellosis. Abattoir workers are at risk. Mycobacterium bovis is not isolated in usual bacterial culture media. *Salmonella typhi* is oxidase and urease negative. *Fransicella tularensis* shows bipolar staining.

2. D

   The test is performed by adding 30 μl of antigen to a 1 ml volume of whole milk that has been stored for at least 24 hours at 4°C. The milk/antigen mixtures are incubated at 37°C for 1 hour. A strongly positive reaction is indicated by formation of a dark blue ring above a white milk column.

3. C

   Human brucellosis is known for presenting with protean manifestations. However, irregular fever is almost always present

4. D

   CO_2 required for the growth of *B. abortus*.

5. D

   B. abortus strain 19BA was used in the former USSR and China.

References:

1. Buchanan TM, Faber LC, Feldman RA. Brucellosis in the United States, 1960-1972. An abattoir-associated disease. Part I. Clinical features and therapy. Medicine (Baltimore) 1974; 53 :403-13.
2. Gotuzzo E. Brucellosis. In: Tropical Infectious Diseases. Principles, Pathogens & Practice, Guerrant RL, Walker DH, Weller PF (Eds), Churchill Livingstone, Philadelphia 1999.P.498.
3. World Health Organization 1997 The Development of New/Improved Brucellosis Vaccines: Report number: WHO/EMC/ZDI/98.14, p.10.

ADULT GONOCOCCAL OPTHALMITIS

Dr. Rajkumar Kalyan, Department of Microbiology

A 21 year old boy attended the ophthalmic department at a tertiary care centre complaining of pain and redness of his right eye, accompanied by a thick yellow discharge, for the last three days. He had consulted a private ophthalmologist who prescribed tobramycin eye drops. There was no improvement with regular use of the local antibiotic. On questioning the patient admitted to having some purulent urethral discharge a few days, for which he took some medicines from a local practitioner.

Two conjunctival swabs were collected, one for gram staining and one for culture. A microphotograph of the Gram stained direct smear is shown below. The patient was admitted and treated with injectable ceftriaxone, and his eye cleared dramatically. The culture on chocolate blood agar grew fastidious gram-negative diplococci that fermented glucose but not maltose. On questioning the patient admitted to having some purulent urethral discharge a few days, for which he took some medicines from a local practitioner.

Fig1. Gram staining of eye discharge

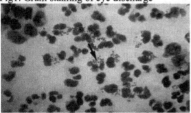

1. Based on the above history the most likely organism is:
   (A) *Streptococcus pneumonia*
   (B) *Neisseria meningitides*
   (C) *Chlamydia trachomatis*
   (D) *Neisseria gonorrhoeae*
2. The most likely source from which this organism entered the patient's eye is :
   (A) His unwashed hands after touching a toilet seat
   (B) A public swimming pool

(C) His unwashed hands after touching his genitalia.

(D) Kissing his girl friend

3. Which one of the following is characteristic of *N. meningitidis* but not *N. gonorrhoeae* ?

(A) Ferment glucose but not maltose

(B) Oxidase-positive

(C) Contains a polysaccharide capsule

(D) Most isolates show resistance to penicillin

4. Ocular prophylaxis with 1% silver nitrate is given to neonates against which of the following organism?

(A) *N. meningitidis*

(B) *N. gonorrhoeae*

(C) *N. subflava*

(D) *N. sicca*

5. Virulence of *Neisseria gonorrhoeae* is due to

(A) Cell wall

(B) Cell membrane

(C) Pili

(D) Protein I

Answers:

1. D

This patient had adult gonococcal conjunctivitis. Topical therapy with antibiotic drops is inadequate to treat gonococcal conjunctivitis. *Streptococcus pneumoniae* is a gram positive diplococci. *N.meningitidis* ferments maltose also. Chlamydial conjunctivitis not fit in gram staining findings..

2. C

It is most probable that this patient transferred the N gonorrhoeae to his eye after contaminating them with urethral discharge. Gonococci do not survive very well on inanimate objects or in the environment. Facial skin is seldom involved with gonorrhoea.

3. C

N.meningitidis contains a polysaccharide capsule,

4. B

Ocular prophylaxis with 1% silver nitrate in the first hour after birth has generally been recommended to prevent opthalmia neonatorum.[1]

5. C

Pili are nonflagellar surface appendages and mediate highly specific initial attachment of gonococci to genital epithelial cells.

References:

1. Sanjay Ram, Peter A. Rice. Gonococcal infections. In: Dan L. Longo, et al (ed).Harrison's Principles of Internal Medicine 18th edition New York McGraw-Hill Professional Publishing 2011, p.1223.

WEIL'S DISEASE

Dr. Rajkumar Kalyan, Department of Microbiology

A 25- year old male, municipality worker by occupation, presented with high grade fever, oliguria, darkening of urine, malaise, myalgia and mild headache, progressing over the last 10 days. He says he felt better 3-4 days back but his condition then worsened and he has been coughing blood over the last two days On physical examination he had conjunctival suffusion, pallor, jaundice and painful mild hepatomegaly. Laboratory results showed a raised level of C-reactive protein , relative neutrophilia, a marked increase in the level of liver transaminases and increased levels of serum urea and creatinine. Chest radiograph is suggestive of pulmonary haemorrhage. He is admitted to the hospital and started on IV penicillin. Culture and serology reports are pending.

1. The most probable diagnosis in this case is?

(A) Malaria

(B) Typhoid fever

(C) Leptospirosis

(D) Dengue fever.

2. Which of the following organism is transmitted to the human primarily by contact with urine and is a zoonotic?

(A) Treponema

(B) Leptospira

(C) Borrelia

(D) Bacillus

3 Which serogroup of Leptospirainterrogans is responsible for Weil's disease ?
   (A) Australis
   (B) Canicola
   (C) Hebdomadis
   (D) Icterohaemorrhagiae

4. All of the following statements about leptospirosis are true, except :
   (A) Infection acquired by direct contact with infected urine
   (B) Mortality is 5 - 15% in severe cases.
   (C) Antibodies are detectable within three days of infection.
   (D) IV penicillin is recommended for treatment of severe cases

5. Leptospira are easily cultured from :
   (A) Bood
   (B) CSF
   (C) Urine
   (D) None of the above

Answers:
1. C
   The most characteristics findings in leptospirosis includes conjunctival suffusion, renal failure, tender liver and marked increase in the levels of liver transaminases, serum urea and creatinine.
2. B
   Leptospira transmitted to human by direct or indirect contact with water contaminated by urine of carrier animals.
3. D
   Weil's disease is caused by *Leptospira interrogans*, serovar *icterohaemorrhagiae* or *Copenhageni*.
4. C
   Antibodies are usually detectable in the serum towards the end of first weak after onset but this may be delayed until the second week.
5. D
   Leptospira are difficult to culture. Diagnosis is usually confirmed by serology.

References:
1. JosephM.Vinetz .Leptospirosis In: Dan L. Longo, (ed) et al.Harrison's Principles of Internal Medicine 18th edition New York McGraw-Hill Professional Publishing 2011, p.1394-95.
2. Edward A., Hodder, Staughton. Leptospirosis. Topley and Wilson's Principles of Bacteriology, Virology and Immunity. 8th edn. Vol. 3, 619, 1990.
3. JoyceD.Coghlan; Leptospira, Borrelia, Spirillum In; J. Geraldcollee et al.(ed), Mackie and McCartney Practical medical microbiology 14th edition, Churchill Livingstone 1996, p 562.
4. Shieh WJ, et al. Chapter 49- Leptospirosis. In: Guerrant RL et al (ed). Tropical Infectious Diseases: Principles, Pathogens, and Practice. 2001, Charlottesville: Churchill Livingstone, pp. 547-555.

ACANTHAMOEBA KERATITIS IN CONTACT LENS USER
Dr. Prashant Gupta, Department of Microbiology

A 24 years old female patient presented with complaints of pain, redness and watering in right eye since five days. The patient is a contact lens wearer who has been using disposable soft contact lenses for the past 3 months. Three weeks prior to presentation, the patient began to develop cloudy vision, photophobia and pain in the right eye. On examination the vision in right eye was 6/36 and in the left eye was 6/12. The right eye showed a large epithelial defect with ring infiltrates in the center of cornea measuring 3mm vertically. The cornea was scrapped with surgical blade and a wet mount was prepared. On microscopy 10-25 μm round cyst like structures were seen. Outer wall of these appeared to be wrinkled and fibrous and inner wall was polygonal. The cysts contained a single nucleus.

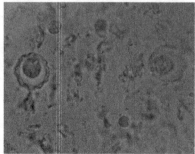

1. The most likely diagnosis is
   (A) Acanthamoeba keratitis
   (B) Staphylococcal keratitis
   (C) Fungal keratitis
   (D) Herpes simplex keratitis
2. All are free living amoeba EXCEPT
   (A) *Acanthamoeba* spp.
   (B) *Nagleria fowleri*
   (C) *Balamuthia mandrallis*
   (D) *Entamoeba histolytica*
3. Clinical syndromes caused by free living amoebas are
   (A) Primary amoebic meningoencephalitis (PAM)
   (B) Granulomatous amebic encephalitis (GAE)
   (C) Amoebic keratitis
   (D) All of the above
4. Following is true regarding route of entry of Acanthamoeba
   (A) Enters through the lower respiratory tract or through ulcerated or broken skin
   (B) Enter through the olfactory neuroepithelium
   (C) Enters through blood stream
   (D) All of the above
5. Mainstay of therapy for Acanthamoeba keratitis (AK) is
   (A) Corticosteroids
   (B) Topical chlorhexidine (0.02%) and polyhexamethylenebiguanide (PHMB, 0.02%)
   (C) Miltefosine
   (D) Intravenous pentamidine and oral itraconazole

Answers:

1. A

   Keratitis, uveitis and corneal ulceration have been associated with *Acanthamoeba* spp. Infections have been seen in both hard and soft contact lens wearers. Particular attention has been paid to soft lens disinfection systems, including homemade saline solutions. *Acanthamoeba* cysts are usually round (10-25 μm), double walled with single nucleus. Corneal ring infiltrates are most consistently associated with Acanthamoeba keratitis. Though they can be also be found in *Pseudomonas aeruginosa* or *Moraxella*, herpes simplex virus, fungi, and varicella-zoster virus infections, as well as immunity-related conditions like rheumatoid arthritis.

2. D

   Distinct from other pathogenic protozoa such as *Entamoeba histolytica*, these free living organisms have no known insect vectors, no human carrier states of epidemiologic importance, and little relationship between poor sanitation and transmission.

3. D

   Four distinct clinical syndromes are caused by the free-living amoebas that infect humans: (1) primary amoebic meningoencephalitis (PAM); (2) granulomatous amoebic encephalitis (GAE); (3) disseminated granulomatous amoebic disease (e.g., skin, pulmonary, and sinus infection); and (4) amoebic keratitis (AK). PAM is caused by *Naegleria fowleri*.GAE is caused by *Acanthamoeba* spp., *B. mandrillaris*, and *Sappinia* spp. Disseminated granulomatous amoebic disease involving the skin, lungs, or sinuses but without CNS infection with *Acanthamoeba* and *Balamuthia* have also been reported. *Acanthamoeba* spp. also cause a subacute to chronic keratitis that is most often associated with contact lens use or corneal trauma, with rare reports of cases occurring after radial keratotomy.

4. A

   Acanthamoeba spp. and *Balamuthia mandrillaris* enter through the lower respiratory tract or through ulcerated or broken skin causing granulomatous amebic encephalitis (GAE) in individuals with compromised immune system. *Naegleria fowleri* enters through the olfactory neuroepithelium causing primary amebic meningoencephalitis (PAM) in healthy individuals.

5. B

   Topical chlorhexidine or PHMB with or without adjuvant pentamidine or other agent should be applied every hour for the first several days. Treatment is then tapered based on the clinical response. Medical therapy may fail or require adjunctive surgical therapy. The use of corticosteroids in AK is controversial.

References:

1. Protozoa. Amoeba (Other body fluids) *Acanthamoeba* spp. *Balamuthia mandrillaris*, Sappiniadiploidea. In: Garcia LS. Practical guide to diagnostic parasitology. 2nd ed. Washington DC: ASM Press 2009; 326-327.
2. Wallang BS, Das S, SharmaS, Sahu SK, Mittal R. Ring Infiltrate in Staphylococcal Keratitis. J Clin Microbiol. 2013; 51: 354–355.
3. Koshy AA, Blackburn BG, Singh U. Free living amoebas. In: Mandell GL, Bennett JE, Dolin R, eds. Mandell, Douglas, and Bennett's Principles and Practice of Infectious Diseases. 7th ed. Philadelphia, Pennsylvania: Churchill Livingstone Elsevier; 2010:3427-3436.

NOCARDIA SPP. IN CHRONIC OBSTRUCTIVE PULMONARY DISEASE

Dr. Prashant Gupta, Department of Microbiology

An 85-year-old man was admitted to the medical intensive care unit with a 10-day history of severe breathlessness, fever and cough. The patient was known to have chronic obstructive pulmonary disease and had been receiving corticosteroids in the preceding 18 months. He had been treated for tuberculosis 2.5 years previously. On examination he was febrile, tachycardicand had tachypnea with a respiratory rate of 46/min. Auscultation revealed bilateral crepitation's and wheeze. Chest radiograph revealed patchy infiltrates on rightlung. The patient developed respiratory depression andwas mechanically ventilated. The sputum and endotracheal aspirate (ET) showed predominant branching, beaded, weakly acid fast filamentous bacilli.

Figure: Photomicrograph of endotracheal aspirate showing acid fast, filamentous, branching bacteria (×1000).

1. Based on the patients clinical presentation and findings in sputum and ET aspirate samples which of the following statement is true?
   (A) Patient is suffering from pulmonary tuberculosis
   (B) Patient is suffering from pulmonary nocardiosis; Nocardia is mostly weakly acid fast
   (C) Pulmonary actinomycosis is a common infection and they are mostly weakly acid fast.
   (D) Clinical manifestations and sputum examination is consistent with anaerobic infection
2. Aerobic nocardiform actinomycetes include all EXCEPT
   (A) Mycobacteria
   (B) Corynebacteria
   (C) Nocardia
   (D) Actinomyces
3. Main stay of therapy for the treatment of Nocardia infection is
   (A) Sulphonamides
   (B) Penicillins

(C) Aminoglycosides

(D) Floroquinolones

4. Mycolic acid of *Nocardia* contains

    (A) 60-80 carbon atoms

    (B) 22-36 carbon atoms

    (C) 40-60carbon atoms

    (D) 5-10carbon atoms

5. Most common mode of entry of Nocardia is

    (A) Inhalation

    (B) Contaminated food

    (C) Direct inoculation by trauma

    (D) Feco-oral

Answers:

1. B

Nocardia spp. is weakly acid-fast, filamentous branching aerobic actinomycetes causing superficial and deep-seated infections, usually in the immunocompromised host. COPD, especially when associated with steroid therapy, is significantly associated with pulmonary nocardiosis. Actinomyces are non-acid fast anaerobic and microaerophilic organisms.

2. D

Aerobic nocardiform actinomycete includes the genera *Mycobacteria, Corynebacteria, Nocardia, Rhodococcus, Gordona* and *Tsukamurella*. Actinomyces are anaerobic or microaerophilic bacteria.

3. A

Sulphonamides have been the main stay of therapy since their introduction in the 1940s, have substantially improved the outcomes. Trimethoprim-sulfamethoxazole is currently the preferred drug among sulphonamides for the treatment of Nocardia infections.

4. C

Mycolic acids are most characteristic cell wall components in bacteria belonging to the order Actinomycetales and contribute to the physiological properties of cell walls such as acid fastness and hydrophobicity. Mycobacteria generally possess C60 to C80 acids, whereas Nocardia and Rhodococci possess shorter chain homolog's such as C40 to C60.

5. A

Inhalation of the bacteria is considered to be the most common mode of entry, which is supported by the observation that majority of infections caused by Nocardia involve the lung.

References:

1. Sorrell TC, Mitchell DH, Iredell JR et al., Nocardia species. In: Mandell GL, Bennett JE, Dolin R, eds. Mandell, Douglas, and Bennett's Principles and Practice of Infectious Diseases. 7th ed. Philadelphia, Pennsylvania: Churchill Livingstone Elsevier; 2010:3199-3207.

2. Russo TA. Agents of Actinomycosis. In: Mandell GL, Bennett JE, Dolin R, eds. Mandell, Douglas, and Bennett's Principles and Practice of Infectious Diseases. 7th ed. Philadelphia, Pennsylvania: Churchill Livingstone Elsevier; 2010:3209-3219.

3. Tomiyasu I. Mycolic acid composition and thermally adaptive changes in Nocardiaasteroids. Journal of bacteriology1982: 828-837.

4. Spelman D. Microbiology, epidemiology, and pathogenesis of nocardiosis. In: UpToDate, Post TW (Ed), UpToDate, Waltham, MA. (Accessed on May 28, 2015.)

CRYPTOSPORIDIAL DIARRHEA

Dr. Prashant Gupta, Department of Microbiology

A 58 year female presents with severe diarrhea since last 1 week. She is a known case of renal failure who underwent cadaveric renal transplant 1 month before. Patient was on Tacrolimus 3 mg/day, Mycophenolatemofetil 2 g/day and Prednisolone 10mg/day as maintenance therapy since transplant. She does not have fever, chills, gastrointestinal bleeding, or vomiting. The physical examination shows diffuse abdominal tenderness (without signs of peritoneal irritation). The examination of a stool sample using a modified acid-fast smear revealed several pink to red round structures of 4 to 6 µm size.

Figure: Modified acid fast smear of stool sample showing 4-6 µm size round red structures

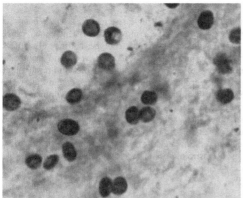

1. Based on the patients clinical presentation and findings in stool samples which of the following statement is true?
   (A) Patient is most likely suffering from cryptosporidiosis
   (B) Clinical manifestations and stool examination is consistent with cryptococcal infection.
   (C) Patient is most likely suffering from isosporiasis
   (D) Patient is most likely suffering from intestinal tuberculosis; an intestinal biopsy must be performed to confirm the diagnosis
2. Following statement is true regarding pathogenesis of Cryptosporidium species EXCEPT
   (A) Organisms are primarily localized in large intestine
   (B) Organisms are found within parasitophorous vacuoles in the microvillus layer of epithelial cells
   (C) Heavier infection may be associated with extraintestinal manifestation.
   (D) CD4+ T cells play a key role in the control of human cryptosporidiosis.
3. Following is true about the genus Cryptosporidium
   (A) Most human isolates belong to a single species, *C. parvum*
   (B) Belongs to subphylum Apicomplexa
   (C) Human infections are caused by sporozoites
   (D) To complete its life cycle Cryptosporidium requires two or more hosts
4. Most important way to prevent cryptosporidiosis in immunocompromised patients
   (A) Prophylaxis with azithromycin
   (B) Good hygiene, such as handwashing and proper disposal of contaminated material
   (C) Chlorination of water
   (D) Filtration of water
5. Most appropriate treatment for cryptosporidiosis is
   (A) Trimethoprim-sulphamethoxazole
   (B) Nitazoxanide
   (C) Metronidazole
   (D) Albendazole

Answers:

1. A

   Modified acid fast stained stool sample showing 4 to 6 μm size oocysts is caused by cryptosporidium spp. These oocysts contain four sporozoites. *Isospora belli* oocyst is up to 35 μm in size and is also acid fast; it is best identified in wet mount preparations. The infective oocyst of *Isospora* contains two sporocysts, each with four sporozoites.

2. A

   Cryptosporidium spp. is primarily localized in distal part of small intestine (e.g., terminal ileum, proximal colon) and is found within parasitophorous vacuoles in the microvillus layer of epithelial cells. However, in immunodeficient hosts, the parasites have been identified throughout the gut, in the biliary tract, and even in the respiratory tract. Respiratory tract involvement is often asymptomatic, but may also manifest as bilateral pulmonary infiltrates with dyspnea. Patients with low CD4 counts may also present with acalculous cholecystitis, sclerosing cholangitis, or pancreatitis. CD4+ T cells play a key role in the control of human cryptosporidiosis. In patients with HIV infection, cryptosporidiosis is self-limited in individuals with CD4 cell counts higher than 180/μL, chronic in patients with CD4 cell depletion to less than 100/μL, and fulminant in some of those with counts less than 50/μL.

3. B

Initially most human isolates were thought to belong to a single species, *C. parvum* but now molecular studies have identified various other species of Cryptosporidium which may cause infection in human beings. *C. parvum* is now designated as bovine genotype, but may also infect human beings. By contrast, the human genotype, now termed *C. hominis,* is found mainly in humans and is rarely infectious for cattle or mice, but can infect gnotobiotic pigs and rarely other species. The genus Cryptosporidium consists of a group of protozoan parasites within the protist subphylum Apicomplexa. The life cycle of Cryptosporidium can be completed within a single host. Infection is caused by ingestion of oocysts, they undergo excystation in the small bowel, and release four banana-shaped motile sporozoites that attach to the epithelial cell wall. The sporozoites mature asexually into meronts, which release merozoites intraluminally. These can reinvade host cells, resulting in autoinfection, or can undergo sexual maturation to form new oocytes which can excyst within the host gastrointestinal tract or can pass out into the environment. Oocysts are infectious and can remain viable for many months at a wide range of temperatures.

4. B

Good hygiene, such as hand washing and proper disposal of contaminated material, are the most important ways to prevent infection. Oocysts are resistant to most standard purification techniques, including filtration and chlorination. Prophylaxis for Cryptosporidium is not routinely recommended.

5. B

Most appropriate treatment for the cryptosporidial diarrhea is nitazoxanide. Nitazoxanide is a synthetic nitrothiazolyl salicylamide derivative and an antiprotozoal agent. Drug of choice for the diarrhea associated with *Isospora belli* is trimethoprim-sulfamethoxazole.

References:

1. White AC. Cryptosporidium. In: Mandell GL, Bennett JE, Dolin R, eds. Mandell, Douglas, and Bennett's Principles and Practice of Infectious Diseases. 7th ed. Philadelphia, Pennsylvania: Churchill Livingstone Elsevier; 2010:3547-3560.
2. Davies AP, Chalmers RM. Cryptosporidiosis. BMJ 2009; 339:b4168.
3. Leder K, Weller PF. Treatment and prevention of cryptosporidiosis. In: UpToDate, Post TW (Ed), UpToDate, Waltham, MA. (Accessed on May 28, 2015.)
4. White AC. Nitazoxanide: An important advance in antiparasitic therapy. Am. J. Trop. Med. Hyg 2003; 68; 382-383.

Chapter-11

Neurology

JAPANESE ENCEPHALITIS

Dr. Rakesh Shukla, Professor, Department of Neurology

A 20 years old man, resident of Gorakhpur presented in the post-monsoon period with a 4-5 days history of headache, fever with chills, anorexia and nausea without vomiting. A day prior to admission he had recurrent seizures followed by altered sensorium. The patient responded to simple verbal commands, and was moving all the 4 limbs in response to a painful stimulus. Neck rigidity was present. There was no papilloedema. CSF examination revealed a pressure of >250 mm of water, cells were 10/mm³, predominantly lymphocytes, proteins 100 mg/dL and glucose 60 mg/dL with a corresponding serum glucose of 100 mg/dL. CSF smear examination was negative for Gram's stain, Zeihl Nelson stain and India ink preparation. The MRI brain shows :

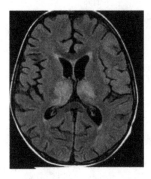

1. What is the most likely diagnosis:
   (A) Tuberculous meningitis
   (B) Japanese encephalitis
   (C) Herpes simplex encephalitis
   (D) Dengue encephalitis
2. The most important vector for JE virus is transmission of the
   (A) Culex tritaeniorrhynchus
   (B) Culex bitaeniorrhynchus
   (C) Aedes japonicus
   (D) Mansonia uniformis
3. The virulence of the JE virus is determined by
   (A) Capsid protein
   (B) Membrane protein
   (C) Envelope protein
   (D) Non-structural proteins
4. The most reliable technique for laboratory diagnosis of JE is
   (A) IgM capture ELISA
   (B) Haemagglutination inhibition
   (C) Complement fixation
   (D) Indirect immunofluoroscence
5. JE vaccination in endemic areas is indicated in all of the following, EXCEPT:
   (A) Children of 1-2 years of age
   (B) Elderly above 65-70 years age
   (C) Travellers visiting rural areas
   (D) Laboratory workers potentially exposed to viruses

Answers:

1. B
   Bilateral thalamic involvement in a patient with encephalitis in an endemic area is suggestive of JE.
2. A
   Culex tritaeniorrhynchus is the most important vector for JE virus transmission.
3. C

The envelope protein has a major role in determining the virulence of JE virus and a single amino acid substitution may result in loss of virulence or neuroinvasion.

4. A

    IgM capture enzyme-linked immunosorbent assay (ELISA) is the most reliable method for laboratory diagnosis of JE and has a sensitivity and specificity of 90%.

5. B

    Immunisation is the only effective measure for long-term prevention against JE.

Reference:

1. Misra UK, Kalita J (Eds). Japanese encephalitis. In: Diagnosis and Management of Neurological Disorders. Wolters Kluwer Health, Lippincott Williams & Wilkins, New Delhi 2011, pp 1-20.

CARPAL TUNNEL SYNDROME

Dr. Rakesh Shukla, Professor, Department of Neurology

A 45 years old right handed woman presented with a 2 years history of tingling and numbness in both upper limbs, worse on the right side. The pain was triggered by doing household chores like kneading the floor, washing clothes, holding a book and driving a two-wheeler. She would often wake up in the night from sleep because of numbness in the hands which was relieved by vigorously rubbing or shaking her hands. There was no weakness in the hands. There is a past history of fracture right humerus 5 years back. Tapping over the palmar aspect of the wrist produced a tingling sensation in both the hands.

1. What is the most likely diagnosis:
    (A) Carpal tunnel syndrome
    (B) Cervical spondylosis
    (C) Thoracic outlet syndrome
    (D) Tardy ulnar nerve palsy
2. What investigation would you perform to confirm the diagnosis
    (A) MRI cervical spine
    (B) X Ray of both hands
    (C) Nerve conduction studies
    (D) Ultrasonography
3. Median motor nerve conduction studies will show
    (A) Prolonged distal latency
    (B) Reduced conduction velocity
    (C) Decreased CMAP amplitude
    (D) All of the above
4. The most common and specific sign of carpal tunnel syndrome is
    (A) Positive Tinel's sign
    (B) Positive Phalen's sign
    (C) Atrophy of thenar eminence
    (D) Weakness of thumb abduction
5. All of the following are true with respect to splinting of the wrist in the treatment of carpal tunnel syndrome, EXCEPT
    (A) They are effective in 60% of patients
    (B) It does not involve any risk
    (C) Custom designed splints are better
    (D)They are designed to maintain neutral wrist position

Answers:

1. A

    Episodic numbness and pain in the affected hand mostly at night, relieved by shaking the affected hand is suggestive of CTS.

2. C

    Nerve conduction studies have a sensitivity of 85% and specificity of 95% in detecting median neuropathy at the wrist.

3. A

    The electrophysiological hallmark of CTS is focal slowing of conduction at the wrist, resulting in prolongation of the latencies of both motor and sensory fibres.

4. B

Phalen's sign is present in 80-90% of patients with CTS with rare false positives.
5. C
There is no additional benefit derived from custom-designed splints or from daytime wear.

References:

1. Arnold WD, Elsheikh BH. Entrapment neuropathies. In: Barohn RJ, Dimachkie MM, Evans RW (Eds) Peripheral Neuropathies. Neurol Clin 2013; 31: 405-24.
2. Preston DC, Shapiro BE (Eds). Median neuropathy at wrist. In: Electromyography and Neuromuscular Disorders: Clinical-Electrophysiological correlations, 2nd edition Elsevier: Butterworth-Heinemann, Philadelphia 2005, pp. 255-79.

GUILLAIN BARRE SYNDROME

Dr. Rakesh Shukla, Professor, Department of Neurology

A 20 years old man presented with a history of backache by pain in both calves. Over the next 2 weeks he developed progressive difficulty in getting up from the squatting position, combing his hair and feeding himself. The patient was afebrile, vital signs including pulse, respiration and blood pressure were normal. Neurological examination revealed normal mental status and cranial nerves. Power was grade 4- to 4+ (MRC grading) in all four limbs, proximal weakness was more than distal. Deep tendon reflexes were not elicitable. Sensory examination was normal.

1. The most likely diagnosis is
   (A) Guillain Barre syndrome
   (B) Polymyositis
   (C) Cord compression
   (D) Periodic paralysis
2. The following features make the diagnosis of Guillain Barre syndrome doubtful EXCEPT:
   (A) Asymmetrical weakness
   (B) Well demarcated sensory level
   (C) Persistent bladder-bowel dysfunction
   (D) Less than 10 mononuclear cells/mm^3 in CSF
3. Which infective agent is most commonly associated with Guillian Barre syndrome
   (A) Epstein Barr virus
   (B) Mycoplasma pneumonia
   (C) Cytomegalo virus
   (D) Campylobacter jejuni
4. The best electrodiagnostic predictor of a poor outcome in Guillain Barre syndrome is
   (A) Low mean CMAP amplitude
   (B) Presence of fibrillation potential
   (C) Profound slowing of conduction velocities
   (D) Absent F waves and H reflex
5. The preferred immunotherapeutic modality for treatment is
   (A) Intravenous immunoglobulin
   (B) Intravenous methylprednisolone
   (C) Oral corticosteroids
   (D) Mycofenolate

Answers:

1. A
   Symmetrical weakness in two or more limbs with areflexia is suggestive of GB syndrome.
2. D
   The presence of CSF pleocytosis (less than 50 cells/mm^3) is not incompatible with the diagnosis of GBS.
3. D
   Campylobacter jejuni enteritis is the most common identifiable antecedent infection and precedes axonal GBS in up to 33% of patients.
4. A
   Low distal CMAP amplitude (<20% of the lower limit of normal at 3 to 5 weeks) is the best single predictor of a poor outcome or prolonged course.
5. A

Intravenous immunoglobulin (IVIg) hastens recovery from GBS and is equivalent to plasma exchange. Oral corticosteroids and intravenous methylprednisolone are not recommended.

References:
1. Dimachkie MM, Barohn RJ. Guillain Barre syndrome and variants. In: Barohn RJ, Dimachkie MM, Evans RJ (Eds) Peripheral Neuropathies. Neurol Clin 2013; 13: 491-510.
2. Preston DC, Shapiro BE (Eds). Polyneuropathy. In: Electromyography and Neuromuscular Disorders: Clinical-Electrophysiological Correlations, 2nd edition. Elsevier: Butterworth-Heinemann, Philadelphia 2005, pp 389-420.

TRIGEMINAL NEURALGIA
Dr. Ajay Pawar, Senior Resident, Department of Neurology

A 45 years old male presented with complaints of episodes of severe lancinating pain on left side of the face for past 2 years. Pain was restricted to left side of face, including lips, gums and cheeks. Though the duration of pain in each episode was very short, lasting for few seconds only, however pain was of intense severity and patient described it as 'paroxysmal and excruciating'. Pain episodes used to occur during the day as well as night and was characteristically triggered by movement of the affected area while speaking, chewing or smiling. Patient reported to have some trigger zones on face and teeth, which when touched, used to stimulate the pain episode. Common activities of daily routine which used to stimulate the trigger zones were washing the face and brushing the teeth. General physical as well as neurological examination did not reveal any abnormality.

1. What is the most likely diagnosis?
    (A) Trigeminal neuralgia
    (B) Trigeminal neuropathy
    (C) Hemifacial spasm
    (D) Complex tics
2. Which investigation is a must in the diagnostic approach to the patient?
    (A) MRI Brain
    (B) NCCT Head
    (C) Facial nerve conduction studies with blink reflex
    (D) Trigeminal nerve conduction studies
3. Tic Douloureux is –
    (A) Trigeminal neuralgia
    (B) Cluster headache
    (C) Paroxysmal hemicrania
    (D) SUNCT
4. What is correct in relevance to trigeminal neuralgia-
    (A) Sometimes, objective sensory loss may be demonstrated.
    (B) Pain is least common in ophthalmic division of Trigeminal nerve
    (C) children are affected primarily
    (D) Presence of trigger zones is atypical for trigeminal neuralgia.
5. Cluster-tic is an other name for
    (A) Migraine
    (B) Cluster headache
    (C) SUNCT
    (D) Cluster headache with trigeminal neuralgia

Answers:
1. A
    Trigeminal neuralgia has episodic symptoms while trigeminal neuropathy has persistent symptoms.
2. A
    MRI Brain is a must be done in a case of trigeminal neuralgia to rule out the secondary causes of trigeminal neuralgia such as an aberrant vessel at the Trigeminal root entry zone.
3. A
    Tic Douloureux is another name for trigeminal neuralgia.
4. B
    Ophthalmic division of trigeminal nerve is least involved in trigeminal neuralgia. An essential feature of Trigeminal neuralgia is that objective signs of sensory loss cannot be demonstrated on examination.
5. D

Cluster-tic is another name for cluster headache with trigeminal neuralgia.

References:
1. Longo F, Kasper,Hauser. Harrison's principles of internal medicine. volume 2.chapter 376. 18th ed: McGraw Hill Education; 2011.

LENNOX-GASTAUT SYNDROME (LGS)

Dr. Anand Kumar Verma, Senior Resident, Department of Neurology

An 8 years old boy presented in Neurology clinic with history of episodes of stiffening of arms, legs and trunk, upward turning of eyeballs which occurs for few seconds on several times during sleep from last 18 months. Pt.'s father told that he had recurrent falls on ground from last 12 months. Patient used to fall suddenly on ground due to loss of body tone and immediately stand up again. These falls occur many times a day and he was injured many times. He had also intermittent episodes of tonic clonic movements of both upper limbs and lower limbs from last 6 months. His father added that despite taking many drugs these abnormal movements were not well controlled. Patient had also history of decrease school performance and he did not prefer to play games with his friends. There was perinatal history of birth asphyxia and delayed cry. Mile stones were also delayed. There was no past history of any CNS infection or head injury. Family history was also not significant. Physical examination was normal except several injury scar marks on body. On neurological examination there was abnormalities in mental status function. Other neurological examination was within normal limits. On investigation, MRI brain showed diffuse atrophy and gliosis. On electroencephalography (EEG) there was generalized slow spike and wave discharges(<2.5 Hz).

1. What is the diagnosis–
    (A) Juvenile myoclonic epilepsy (JME)
    (B) Lennox-Gastaut syndrome (LGS)
    (C) Landau Kleffner syndrome (LKS)
    (D) Autsomal dominant nocturnal frontal lobe epilepsy(ADNFLE)
2. Many children with Lennox-Gastaut syndrome may have past history of
    (A) Infantile spasm
    (B) Febrile seizure
    (C) Myoclonus
    (D) Epilepsia partialis continua
3. Seizures in LGS
    (A) Very good response to drugs
    (B) Complete remission occurs with time
    (C) Tend to be drug resistant
    (D) Do not require treatment
4. Most common seizure type in LGS
    (A) Atonic
    (B) Atypical absence
    (C) Generalized tonic-clonic
    (D) Tonic

Answers:
1. B
    Multiple seizure types, mental regression and generalized slow spike-and-wave discharges (<2.5 Hz) on electroencephalography (EEG) is triad of Lennox-Gastaut syndrome (LGS).
2. A
    18-50% of patients having infantile spasm (salaam attacks) will develop Lennox-Gastaut syndrome or some other form of symptomatic generalized epilepsy in later part of life.
3. C
    A variety of therapeutic approaches are used in LGS, ranging from antiepileptic drugs to diet and surgery. Unfortunately, much of the evidence supporting these approaches is not robust, and treatment is often ineffective.
4. D
    Over three-fourths of LGS patients monitored with prolonged sleep or video EEG recordings have been reported to have tonic seizures.

References:
1. Commission on Classification and Terminology of the International League Against Epilepsy. Proposal for revised classification of epilepsies and epileptic syndromes. Epilepsia. 1989 Jul. Aug;30(4):389-99.
2. Ohtsuka Y, Amano R, Mizukawa M, Ohtahara S. Long-term prognosis of the Lennox-Gastaut syndrome. Jpn J Psychiatry Neurol. Jun 1990;44(2):257-64.
3. Zupanc ML.Infantile spasms.Expert Opin Pharmacother. Nov 2003;4(11):2039-48.
4. Van Rijckevorsel K. Treatment of Lennox-Gastaut syndrome: overview and recent findings. Neuropsychiatr Dis Treat. Dec 2008;4(6):1001-19.
5. Markand ON. Lennox-Gastaut syndrome (childhood epileptic encephalopathy). J Clin Neurophysiol. 2003;20:426-441.

STROKE AND THROMBOLYSIS

Dr. Anand Kumar Verma, Senior Resident, Department of Neurology

A 60 years old man presented to Emergency Department with weakness in right upper limb and right lower limb from last one hour . Onset of weakness was sudden while coming from his field in morning time. He was also not able to speak but able to understand what was told to him. There was no history of trauma ,fever, headache, nausea, vomiting, seizure, altered consciousness, bladder bowel involvement. He had history of facial asymmetry but no history of features suggestive of any other cranial nerve involvement. There was past history of diabetes mellitus and hypertension from last 5 years and he was taking amlodipine 5 mg and metformin 500 mg daily but from last 2 month he was on irregular treatment. Patient was also chronic bidi smoker. There was no past history of prior stroke ,head injury, any major surgery in preceding 14 days, any GI bleeding in preceding 21 days or recent myocardial infarction. On examination BP-170/90 mm Hg and PR-86/min regular. Patient was conscious and GCS was E4VaM6.He had Broca's aphasia. There was UMN right sided facial palsy. Power in left side was normal and in both right UL and right LL power was 2/5.Plantar in right side was extensor and in left side it was flexor .Sensory examination was normal. On cardiovascular examination S1 and S2 were normal and there was no murmur. CT scan was done immediately and it was found to be normal. Random blood sugar was 350 mg%. platelets-1.75 lakh/mm^3·, hematocrit-30% , PT(INR) and aPTT were normal. Patient had acute ischemic stroke and was treated with IV recombinant tissue plasminogen activator(rtPA) and there was rapid recovery of patient. Diabetes and hypertension were controlled by insulin and appropriate antihypertensive .

1. Which of the following is NINDS IV r-tPA inclusion criteria for thrombolysis
    (A) Onset of symptoms to drug administration is <3 hours
    (B) Onset of symptoms to drug administration is < 4.5 hours
    (B) Onset of symptoms to drug administration is < 6 hours
    (D) Onset of symptoms to drug administration is < 8 hours
2. Which of the following is NINDS IV r-tPA exclusion criteria for thrombolysis
    (A) CT scan showing no hemorrhage or edema of >1/3 of the MCA territory
    (B) Age >18 years
    (C) Glucose 450mg/dl
    (D) A deficit measurable on the NIHSS(National Institutes of Heart Stroke Scale)
3. Which of the following is not a recombinant tissue plasminogen activator(rtPA)
    (A) Alteplase
    (B) R
    (C) T
    (D) Streptokinase
4. Not a risk factor for stroke
    (A) Hypertension
    (B) Young age
    (C) Diabetes
    (D) Smoking

Answers:
1. A

The National Institute of Neurological Disorders and Stroke rt-PA Stroke Study Group(NINDS 1 and 2 trial) showed that treatment with intravenous t-PA within three hours of the onset of ischemic stroke improved clinical outcome at three months.

2. C

Glucose <50 or >400 mg/dl is contraindication for thrombolysis.

3. D

rtPA is manufactured using recombinant biotechnology techniques. Streptokinase is an enzyme produced by several species of streptococci. Clinical trials of streptokinase were halted prematurely because of unacceptably high rates of hemorrhage, and this agent should not be used.

4. B

Advancing age is risk factor for stroke not young age.

References:

1. Adams HP Jr t al.Guidelines for the early management of adults with ischemic stroke.Stroke38;1655,2007.
2. The National Institute of Neurological Disorders and Stroke rt-PA Stroke Study Group. Tissue plasminogen activator for acute ischemic stroke. N Engl J Med.. 1995;333:1581-1587.

DUCHENNEMUSCULAR DYSTROPHY (DMD)

Dr. Gaurav BL Lachuriya, Senior Resident, Department of Neurology

A, nine years male right handed resident of Unnao district studying in 4th standard, presented with chief complaints of difficulty in running and walking since last 5 years, not able to make up with children of same age while playing and also had frequent episodes of falls while playing. Parents also noticed that patient had difficulty in standing from floor and uses support of both upper limb while standing. Patient also had difficulty in climbing upstairs initially, uses support of both upper limb and side wall initially but not able to do the same currently. On enquiry parents also told that patient started walking late without support at 18 months of his age. On examination, blood pressure was 100/70 mm Hg, pulse rate 72/min regular. Higher mental function was normal. Cranial nerve examination was normal. In motor examination, tone was normal, muscle power was decreased in all 4 limbs, proximal > distal. Gower's sign was positive. Sensory examination was normal. Reflexes were normal. Routine blood investigations like complete blood count, serum electrolytes, renal function test and liver function test were normal. Creatine phosphokinase was 8100 IU/L. ECG and 2D Echo were showing a feature of cardiomyopathy. Patient was treated with oral prednisone 0.75 mg/kg body weight. No significant improvement was seen after 2 months of treatment.

1. What is the most likely diagnosis
   (A) Duchenne muscular dystrophy
   (B) Sarcoglycanopathy (LGMD2C)
   (C) Calpainopathy (LGMD2A)
   (D) Oculopharyngeal dystrophy
2. Duchenne muscular dystrophy is
   (A) Autosomal dominant
   (B) Autosomal recessive
   (C) X linked dominant
   (D) X linked recessive
3. Valley sign is seen in
   (A) Duchenne muscular dystrophy
   (B) Sarcoglycanopathy (LGMD2C)
   (C) Calpainopathy (LGMD2A)
   (D) Oculopharyngeal dystrophy
4. The most frequent cause of death in DMD
   (A) Heart failure
   (B) Respiratory insufficiency and chest infection
   (C) Intracranial pathology
   (D) Ventricular fibrillation
5. Dose of oral prednisone in DMD treatment is
   (A) 0.3 mg/kg
   (B) 0.75 mg/kg
   (C) 1.0 mg/kg

(D) 1.5 mg/kg

Answers:
1. A
   Duchenne muscular dystrophy
2. D
   X linked recessive
3. A
   Duchenne muscular dystrophy
4. B
   Respiratory insufficiency and chest infection
5. B
   0.75 mg/kg

References:
1. Moxley RT 3rd, Pandya S, Ciafaloni E, Fox DJ, Campbell K Change in natural history of Duchenne muscular dystrophy with long-term corticosteroid treatment: implications for management.J Child Neurol. 2010 Sep;25(9):1116-29. doi: 10.1177/0883073810371004. Epub 2010 Jun 25.
2. Patterson V, Morrison O, Hicks E. Mode of death in Duchenne muscular dystrophy. Lancet 1991;337:801-802.

MULTIPLE MONONEUROPATHY (HANSEN'S DISEASE)
Dr. Gaurav BL Lachuriya, Senior Resident, Department of Neurology

A, 32 year old male is right handed, studied till 8th standard, farmer by occupation resident of Sitapur district presented with complaints of numbness and weakness of right upper limb below elbow since 1 year and numbness in upper aspect of left foot since last 6 months with intermittent slippage of slipper from left foot since 6 months. On examination, blood pressure was 110/70 mm Hg, pulse rate 78/min regular. Two hypaesthestic hypopigmented patches were present on chest. Right ulnar nerve and left common peroneal nerve were thickened. Higher mental function was normal. Cranial nerve examination was normal. In motor examination, tone was normal. There was weakness in right hand fingers adduction, abduction and finger flexion of 4th and 5th fingers with clawing of right hand and weakness of dorsiflexion and inversion of left foot. Power was normal in all other joints in all range of motion. Pinprick, temperature and touch sensation were lost in right hand in medial two fingers and dorsum of left foot. Remaining sensory examination was normal. Reflexes were normal. Cerebellar examination was normal. Routine blood investigations like complete blood count, serum electrolytes, renal function test and liver function test were normal. Slit smear examination shows lepra bacilli. Nerve conduction study showed right ulnar and left common peroneal sensorimotor axonal neuropathy.

1. What is the most likely diagnosis
   (A) Leprosy
   (B) Tuberculosis
   (C) Vasculitis
   (D) HIV
2. Hansen's disease is caused by:
   (A) Mycobacterium tuberculosis
   (B) Mycobacterium leprae
   (C) Mycobacterium kansasi
   (D) Mycobacterium cheloni
3. Paucibacillary leprosy is characterized by:
   (A) 5 or fewer lesions
   (B) 4 or fewer lesions
   (C) 3 or fewer lesions
   (D) 2 or fewer lesions
4. Erythema nodosum leprosum is same as:
   (A) Type 1 reaction
   (B) Type 2 reaction
   (C) Lucios phenomenon
   (D) None of the above

5. Type 2 reaction occurs in:
   (A) Borderline tuberculoid leprosy
   (B) Borderline leprosy
   (C) Lepromatous leprosy
   (D) All of the above
6. Most common cranial nerve involved in leprosy:
   (A) Fifth cranial nerve
   (B) Sixth cranial nerve
   (C) Seventh cranial nerve
   (D) Eight cranial nerve

Answers:
   1. A
      Leprosy
   2. B
      Mycobacterium leprae
   3. A
      5 or fewer lesions
   4. B
      Type 2 reaction
   5. C
      Lepromatous leprosy
   6. C
      Seventh cranial nerve

References:
   1. D. M. Scollard,* L. B. Adams, T. P. Gillis, J. L. Krahenbul, R. W. Truman, and D. L. Williams. ClinMicrobiol Rev. Apr 2006; 19(2): 338–381.
   2. Gopinath D, Thapa DM, Jaishankar TJ. A clinical study of the involvement of cranial nerves in leprosy. Indian J Lepr 2004; 76:1-9.

TUBEROUS SCLEROSIS
Dr. Imran Rizvi, Senior Resident, Department of Neurology

A 15 year old female was brought to Neurology outpatient department with the complaints of abnormal jerky movements of the body since the age of 5 years and poor scholastic performance. On detailed enquiry the parents described these abnormal movements as tonic spasm of all four limbs and neck along with uprolling of eyeballs for a few seconds; these tonic spasms were followed by jerky movements of all four limbs which continued for about 2 minutes. Patient often developed urinary incontinence and tongue bite during these episodes. She remained drowsy and confused for about ten minutes following such episodes. These episodes occur at a frequency of 1-2 episodes every 6 months. Regarding poor scholastic performance her mother told that she was not doing well at school and was not able to pass in fifth grade since last 3 years. She was very shy and did not mix and play with girls of her age and even needed assistance for dressing. She was the only child of non-consanguineous marriage; she was born at full term through normal vaginal delivery. There was no significant past medical history and the parents denied any delay in developmental milestones. Neither of the parents or any blood relatives had any history of intellectual disability or seizures. On general examination we noted discrete, papular lesions over cheeks, nose and chin in a symmetrical fashion suggesting adenoma sebaceum (Figure 1A). Irregular, elevated areas with an orange peel texture and rubbery consistency were observed over the lower back suggestive of Shagreen patches (Figure 1B). Hypopigmented oval or leaf shaped spots were present on left forearm suggesting ash leaf macules. She was conscious, cooperative and well oriented. Her speech was normal. Her intelligence quotient (IQ) as determined by formal testing was 58. All her cranial nerves, motor and sensory system were normal, there were no signs of meningeal irritation. Routine investigations were with in normal limits, contrast enhanced CT scan showed a heterogeneous lesion at foramen of Monro with significant contrast enhancement and dilatation of bilateral lateral ventricles suggestive of subependymal giant cell astrocytoma.

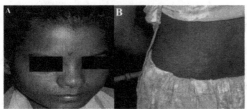

Figure 1 A: Siscrete, papular lesions over cheeks, nose and chin in a symmetrical fashion suggesting adenoma sebaceum or facial angiofibroma. 1 B: Irregular, elevated areas with an orange peel texture and rubbery consistency over lower back suggesting Shagreen patch.

1. What is the most likely diagnosis?
   (A) Tuberous sclerosis
   (B) Neurofibromatosis
   (C) Struge Weber syndrome
   (D) None of the above

2. Tuberous sclerosis is a multisystem disorder which is inherited as?
   (A) Autosomal dominant
   (B) Autosomal recessive
   (C) X linked dominant
   (D) X linked recessive.

3. Shagreen patches are typically seen over which part of body?
   (A) Face
   (B) Forearms.
   (C) Lumbosacral area.
   (D) Chest.

4. Which type of seizures occur in tuberous sclerosis?
   (A) Infantile spasm
   (B) Generalized
   (C) Myoclonic
   (D) All of the above.

5. Vogt's triad in tuberous sclerosis consists of all of the following except.
   (A) Seizures.
   (B) Mental retardation.
   (C) Shagreen patch.
   (D) Adenoma sebaceum.

Answers:

1. A
2. A

   autosomal dominant. Tuberous sclerosis complex (TSC) is a multisystem, autosomal dominant disorder affecting children and adults. It is caused due to mutation of any of two genes TSC1 or TSC2. TS1 gene is located on 9q34 and encodes hamartin, TSC2 is located on 16p13 and encodes for tuberin. [1]

3. C

   Lumbosacral area. Shagreen patches are irregular, elevated areas of varying size with an orange peel texture and rubbery consistency, they are typically found on lumbosacral area and other dorsal surfaces. [2]

4. D

   All of the above. Any type of seizure from infantile spasm, myoclonic seizures, simple/complex partial seizures to generalized tonic clonic seizure can occur in patients with TSC. Seizures are difficult to control even with polytherapy with antiepileptic drugs. [3]

5. C

References:

1. Crino PB, Nathanson KL, Henske EP. Medical progress, the Tuberous Sclerosis Complex. N Engl J Med 2006;355:1345-56.
2. Rosser T, Panigrahy A, McClintock W. The Diverse Clinical Manifestations of Tuberous Sclerosis Complex: A Review. Semin Pediatr Neurol. 2006;13:27-36.
3. Thiele EA. Managing epilepsy in tuberous sclerosis complex. J Child Neurol 2004;19:680-6.

LATERAL MEDULLARY SYNDROME

Dr. Neeraj Kumar, Assistant Professor, Department of Neurology

A 65 year male presented with sudden onset hoarseness of voice, dysphagia and nasal regurgitation. Patient also has swaying to left side on walking and facial deviation to right. Patient was known case of hypertension for 9 years and smoker for 25 years. There was no history of headache, vomiting, fever, diplopia, visual loss, palpitation, chest pain and previous such episodes. No significant family history. On general examination, blood pressure is 170/110 mmHg, pulse rate 78/min regular. Higher mental function was normal with dysarthric speech. Cranial nerve examination revealed normal vision and ocular movements. Mild left eyelid ptosis, miosis and nystagmus were present. Decreased sensations over left side of face and LMN type facial palsy was present. Uvula was deviated to right with decreased palatal movement on left side and absent ipsilateral gag reflex. Motor examination showed normal power and intact deep tendon reflexes. Sensory examination showed decreased touch, vibration and position sense on left side and decreased pain on right half of body. Impaired left sided cerebellar signs and swaying to same side. Other system examinations were normal. Blood investigations revealed impaired lipid profile with normal blood sugar, electrolytes and counts. Brain MRI showed T2 and T2 flair hyper intense lesion on left lateral medulla with restriction in DWI image also suggestive of ischemic stroke(Figure). Cardiac evaluation of ECG and 2D-Echo were normal. Carotid Doppler study showed bilateral 30% luminal narrowing with unruptured plaque on left side. Four- vessel angiography was not performed.

Patient was put on Ryle's tube feeding and prescribed antiplatelet agent with atorvastatin. Blood pressure was controlled on ACE inhibitors with diuretic. Patient gradually improved and became independent after 2 months.

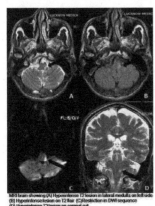

MRI brain showing (A) Hyperintense T2 lesion in lateral medulla on left side (B) Hyperintense lesion on T2 flair (C)Restriction in DWI sequence (D) Hyperintense T2lesion on coronal cut

1. Lateral medullary syndrome can occur with occlusion of
   (A) Vertebral artery
   (B) Posterior inferior cerebellar artery
   (C) Both (a) & (b)
   (D) None
2. Lateral medullary syndrome, features are all except
   (A) Ipsilateral numbness of face
   (B) Ipsilateral Horners syndrome
   (C) Contralateral decreased pain sensation over half body
   (D) Contralateral paralysis
3. Medullary syndromes are all except
   (A) Wallenberg's syndrome
   (B) Dejerine syndrome
   (C) Opalski syndrome
   (D) Weber syndrome

Answers:

1. C
   Occlusion of any of five vessels may be responsible for Lateral medullary syndrome: (1)vertebral (2) posterior inferior cerebellar (3),(4),(5)superior, middle, or inferior lateral medullary artery.[1,2]
2. D
   Lateral medullary syndrome spares pyramidal tracts and thus there is no weakness. Rest of the features are due to involvement of descending tract and nucleus of trigeminal nerve, descending sympathetic tract and spinothalamic tract.[1,2]

3. D

    Weber syndrome is a midbrain syndrome featuring oculomotor nerve palsy with contralateral hemiparesis. Opalski syndrome is a rare variant of lateral medullary syndrome involving pyramidal tract and causing ipsilateral weakness[2,3].

References:

1. Balami JS, Chen RL, Buchan AM. Stroke syndromes and clinical management. QJM : monthly journal of the Association of Physicians. 2013;106(7):607-15.
2. Fauci AS, Longo DL, Jameson JL, Hauser SL, Loscalzo J, Kasper DL. Harrison's principles of internal medicine. 18th ed. New York: McGraw Hill, Health Professions Division; 2012.p.220-223.
3. Parathan KK, Kannan R, Chitrambalam P, Aiyappan SK, Deepthi N. A Rare Variant of Wallenberg's Syndrome: Opalski syndrome. Journal of clinical and diagnostic research. 2014; 8(7): MD05–MD06.

NEUROCYSTICERCOSIS WITH SEIZURE

Dr. Neeraj Kumar, Assistant Professor, Departmentof Neurology

A 15 years boy presented with 3 episodes of right sided tonic clonic movements with secondary generalisation lasting for 3-4 minutes. The patient notices twitching movement starting from right foot and then involving whole of the right side with neck turning, generalisation, frothing, uprolling of eyes and loss of consciousness. There is also history of Todd's palsy once on right side lasting less than 24 hours. There is no history of headache, vomiting, fever, diplopia, visual loss, dysphagia, hearing abnormality, head injury. There is no other type of seizure and no family history. General examination was normal without any neurocutaneous markers. Nervous system examination was normal without any cranial nerve or sensorimotor deficit. Other system examination was also normal. Routine blood investigations were normal. Serum Elisa for neurocysticercosis was positive. MRI brain showed single hyperintense cyst with hypointense eccentric dot in left frontal region on T2 sequence. SPGR contrast showed ring enhancing lesion. EEG of the patient showed localized spike and sharp discharges over left fronto-parietal region.

Patient was given steroid for short duration and oxcarbazepine. No albendazole was given. Patient is asymptomatic on follow up after 6 months with proper drug compliance.

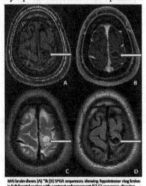

MRI brain shows (A) & (B) SPGR sequences showing hypointense ring lesion in left frontal region with contrast enhancement (C) T2 sequence showing hyperintense cyst with hypointense dot like scolex (D) T2 flair also shown scolex.

1. Maximum edema is present in which stage of neurocysticercosis
    (A) Vesicular
    (B) Colloidal
    (C) Granular Nodular
    (D) Calcified

2. Most common presentation of neurocysticercosis is
    (A) Headache
    (B) Seizure
    (C) Vision loss
    (D) Limb weakness

3. Which statement is false regarding neurocysticercosis
    (A) T. solium cysticerci causes neurocysticercosis
    (B) Definite diagnosis can be made by MRI showing scolex

(C) Intraventricular lesions are usually larger than parenchymal lesions

(D) Albendazole has to be given in all cases

Answers:

1. B

   Vesicular cysticerci elicit little inflammatory reaction. In contrast, colloidal cysticerci show more inflammatory reaction and edema. Later granular nodular lesion has decreased edema.[1]

2. B

   More than three-quarters of symptomatic NCC patients present with seizure or epilepsy. Headache is present in approximately one-third of NCC patients.[1,2]

3. D

   Albendazole is relatively contraindicated in calcified lesion, multiple   lesions, brainstem lesion and ocular lesion.[3,4]

References:

1. Del Brutto OH. Neurocysticercosis: A review. Scientific World Journal 2012. 2012:159821.
2. Carabin H, Ndimubanzi PC, Budke CM, et al. . Clinical manifestations associated with neurocysticercosis: a systematic review. PLoS Negl Trop Dis. 2011;5(5):e1152
3. Prasad KN, Prasad A, Verma A, Singh AK. Human cysticercosis and Indian scenario: a review. Journal of biosciences. 2008;33(4):571-82.
4. Nash TE, Garcia HH. Diagnosis and treatment of neurocysticercosis. Nat Rev Neurol. 2011;7: 584–94.

SECONDARY HYPOKALEMIC PARALYSIS

Dr. Rajan N. Ingole, Senior Resident, Department of Neurology

A 48 year old female patient was admitted with complaint of acute epigastric pain, diarrhea and vomiting (3-4 episodes per day), her serum lipase was 358 u/l, serum amylase was 513 u/l and serum potassium was 3.6 mmol/l. CT abdomen was suggestive of acute pancreatitis and she was managed conservatively. Two days later she started complaining of weakness in both lower limbs which progressed to involve her both upper limbs, neck muscle and trunk muscle over next 12 hours. She had hyporeflexia in all four limbs, plantars were flexor and sensory examination was normal. Her repeat serum potassium was 2.6 mmol/l and NCV was normal.

1. All of the following are true regarding hypokalemic periodic paralysis except:
   (A) Attacks are often provoked by meals high in carbohydrates
   (B) Usually affects proximal limb muscles more than distal.
   (C) Weakness may take as long as 24 hours to resolve
   (D) Ocular and bulbar muscles are most likely to get affected

2. Hypokalemia periodic paralysis is a:
   (A) Potassium channel disorder
   (B) Sodium channel disorder
   (C) Calcium channel disorder
   (D) Mitochondrial myopathy

3. Preferred vehicle for IV potassium administration is
   (A) 5% Dextrose
   (B) 0.9% Normal saline
   (C) Mannitol
   (D) Ringer lactate

Answers:

1. D

   Weakness usually affects proximal limb muscles more than distal. Ocular and bulbar muscles are less likely to be affected. Respiratory muscles are usually spared but when they are involved, the condition may prove fatal.

2. C

   Sodium channel disorders are hyperkalemic periodic paralysis and paramyotonia congenita. Potassium channel disorder is Andersen-Tawil syndrome, where as hypokalemic periodic paralysis is a calcium channel disorder.

3. C

   Administration of potassium in a glucose solution should be avoided because it may further reduce serum potassium levels. Mannitol is the preferred vehicle for administration of IV potassium.

References:
1. Raymond T Chug, Daniel K Podlosky. Muscular dystrophies and Other Muscle Diseases.Chap387 Harrison's Principles of Internal Medicine.Edt Braunwald,Fauci,Kasper McGraw Hill 18Edi Page3504.
2. Raymond T Chug, Daniel K Podlosky. Muscular dystrophies and Other Muscle Diseases.Chap387 Harrison's Principles of Internal Medicine.Edt Braunwald,Fauci,Kasper McGraw Hill 18Edi Page3504.
3. Raymond T Chug, Daniel K Podlosky. Muscular dystrophies and Other Muscle Diseases.Chap387 Harrison's Principles of Internal Medicine.Edt Braunwald,Fauci,Kasper McGraw Hill 18Edi Page3505.

LEFT THALAMIC BLEED

Dr. Rajan N. Ingole, Senior Resident, Department of Neurology

A 55 year old female patient, a known case of hypertension and diabetes mellitus was admitted with history of sudden onset weakness in right half of body associated with pain over right half of body without any history suggestive of cranial nerve involvement. There was no history of headache, vomiting, seizure or loss of consousness. Patient was conscious, oriented and her blood pressure was 190/100 mm of Hg. On neurological examination she had sensory-motor right hemiparesis without cranial nerve involvement.

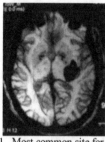 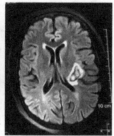

1. Most common site for hypertensive IC bleed is
   (A) Cerebellum
   (B) Pons
   (C) Thalamus
   (D) Putamen
2. Contralateral prominent sensory deficit is a feature of
   (A) Occipital bleed
   (B) Putaminal bleed
   (C) Thalamic bleed
   (D) None of the above
3. All of following are correct in IC bleed except
   (A) Keep cerebral perfusion pressure above 60 mm Hg
   (B) Most cerebellar bleed s > 3 cm diameter require surgical evacuation
   (C) "Dot sign" portends increased mortality
   (D) Glucocorticoids are helpful for reducing edema

Answers:
1. D
   The putamen is the most common site for hypertensive hemorrhage, and the adjacent internal capsule is usually damaged. Other common site for hypertensive intraparenchymal bleed are thalamus, cerebellum, and pons.
2. C
3. D
   If the hematoma causes marked midline shift of structures with consequent obtundation, coma, or hydrocephalus, osmotic agents coupled with induced hyperventilation can be instituted to lower ICP, glucocorticoids are not helpful for the edema from intracerebral hematoma.

References:
1. Raymond T Chug, Daniel K Podlosky. Cerebrovascular Diseases.Chap370 Harrison's Principles of Internal Medicine.Edt Braunwald,Fauci,Kasper McGraw Hill 18Edi Page3294.
2. Raymond T Chug, Daniel K Podlosky. Cerebrovascular Diseases.Chap370 Harrison's Principles of Internal Medicine.Edt Braunwald,Fauci,Kasper McGraw Hill 18Edi Page3295.

3. Raymond T Chug, Daniel K Podlosky. Cerebrovascular Diseases.Chap370 Harrison's Principles of Internal Medicine.Edt Braunwald,Fauci,Kasper McGraw Hill 18Edi Page3298.

Chapter-12

Obstetrics & Gynaecology

PRETERM LABOUR
Dr. Amita Pandey, Professor, Department of Obstetrics & Gynaecology

Mrs AN, 33 year old G4P1A2L0 reported in your OPD at 31 weeks pregnancy with pain in abdomen for 2 days. Pain was intermittent in nature and associated with hardening of uterus. Fetal movements were perceived normally. On P/A examination fundal height was 30 weeks, lie longitudinal, presentation cephalic, FHR 132/min regular, one uterine contraction felt in 10 mins. P/V examination revealed cervical dilatation of 2 cm, effacement of 80% and presenting part was high up.

1. The most common genital tract infection causally related to preterm labor is
    (A) Trichomonas vaginalis
    (B) Group B streptococci
    (C) Bacterial vaginosis
    (D) Chlamydia trachomatis
2. The best way to predict Preterm labor is
    (A) Cervical changes on P/S examination
    (B) Vaginal swab C/S
    (C) Transvaginal evaluation of cervical length
    (D) Abdominal USG for funneling of internal os
3. Which of the following is NOT a risk factor for Preterm labour?
    (A) Poor dental hygiene
    (B) Vaginal infection
    (C) Previous history of Preterm delivery
    (D) Previous surgery for endometriosis
4. Corticosteroids should not be given in this case if there is associated
    (A) Rupture of membranes
    (B) Severe pre-eclampsia
    (C) Intra uterine fetal death
    (D) Abnormal fetal Doppler study
5. Which is the most preferred tocolytic if decision is taken to prolong pregnancy
    (A) Nifedipine
    (B) Ritodrine
    (C) Indomethacin
    (D) Micronized progesterone

Answers:
1. C
    Bacterial vaginosis is the commonest genital infection known to cause preterm labor. Group B Streptococcal infection though associated with preterm labor but a causal link has not been established[1]
2. C
    cervical length evaluation by Transvaginal USG is more accurate in predicting preterm labor[1]
3. D
    Poor dental hygiene, vaginal infection & previous history of Preterm delivery are common risk factors for Preterm labor[1]
4. C
    Corticosteroids are administered for enhancing fetal lung maturity, hence not needed in case of Intra uterine death[1]
5. A
    Nifedipine is the first line of drug recommended for tocolysis[1]

Reference:
1. Cunningham FG, Leveno KJ, Bloom SL, Spong CY, Dashe JS, Hoffman BL et al. Williams Obstetrics 24th edition. USA: Mc Graw Hill Education; 2014.

GESTATIONAL TROPHOBLASTIC DISEASE
Dr Amita Pandey, Professor, Department of Obstetrics & Gynaecology

Mrs LM, 23 year old G2P0+1+0+0 presents in your OPD with history of vaginal bleeding for 2 days following amenorrhea of approximately 3 months. She is not sure of her LMP. On examination her PR is 90/min, BP-150/90 mm Hg, pallor +. Office dipstick test showed 3+ proteinuria. On P/A examination the fundal height was

24 weeks, fetal parts were not palpable and fetal heart sound was not audible on hand held Doppler. P/S revealed 1+ vaginal bleeding with a closed cervical os. USG shows uterine cavity filled with cystic space occupying lesions.

1. What is the most probable diagnosis?
   (A) Gestational hypertension
   (B) Gestational trophoblastic disease
   (C) Spontaneous abortion
   (D) Abruptio placentae
2. Which of the following tests is essential before proceeding to treat this patient?
   (A) Serum TSH
   (B) CT pelvis
   (C) Serum β HCG
   (D) Urine pregnancy test
3. What is the treatment of choice in this patient?
   (A) Dilatation & evacuation
   (B) Hysterotomy
   (C) Hysterectomy
   (D) I/M Methotrexate
4. Follow up advice to this patient on discharge should include :
   (A) Weekly Serum β HCG
   (B) Weekly USG for Ovarian cyst
   (C) Weekly LFT
   (D) Monthly chest Xray
5. Which chromosomal pattern is most common in this case?
   (A) Triploid 69, XXY, extra chromosomes of paternal origin
   (B) Triploid 69, XXY, extra chromosomes of maternal origin
   (C) Diploid 46, XX, all chromosomes of paternal origin
   (D) Diploid 46, XX, all chromosomes of maternal orig
6. Which histopathologic feature is most characteristic of this condition?
   (A) Marked villous scalloping with stromal trophoblastic inclusions
   (B) Generalized swelling of chorionic villi with diffuse trophoblastic hyperplasia with diffuse marked atypia in implantation site tyrophoblast
   (C) Varying sized chorionic villi
   (D) Focal mild atypia of implantation site trophoblast

Answers:

1. B
   Gestational trophoblasic disease (complete hydatidiform mole) as evident by the typical snow storm appearance on USG[1]
2. C
   Serum β HCG is a diagnostic & prognostic marker to confirm diagnosis and to assure remission and facilitate early detection of recurrence[1]
3. A
   Dilatation & evacuation is the preferred procedure to empty the uterus[1]
4. A
   Weekly Serum β HCG is mandatory till 3 normal values are obtained[1]
5. C
   Complete moles usually have a 46,XX karyotype and the molar chromosomes are derived entirely from paternal origin[1]
6. B
   Complete hydatidiform moles have no identifiable embryonic tissue. The chorionic villi have generalized swelling and diffuse trophoblastic hyperplasia. The implantation site trophoblast has diffuse marked atypia. [1]

Reference:

1. Cunningham FG, Leveno KJ, Bloom SL, Spong CY, Dashe JS, Hoffman BL et al. Williams Obstetrics 24th edition. USA: Mc Graw Hill Education; 2014.

POLYCYSTIC OVARIAN SYNDROME

Dr. Amita Pandey, Professor, Department of Obstetrics & Gynaecology

Miss S, an 18 year old unmarried girl has reported in your OPD with history of oligomenorrhoea. She menstruates every 3-4 months but the amount of bleeding is normal. She is obese and is very anxious about increased facial hair.

1. Which of the following is NOT needed to confirm the diagnosis of PCOS?
   (A) Persistent oligomenorrhoea
   (B) Hirsutism
   (C) Acne PCO morphology or USG

2. Which of the following investigation is NOT needed in this patient?
   (A) Serum Prolactin
   (B) Total testosterone
   (C) Fasting Insulin
   (D) 75g GTT

3. Which of the following drugs can be given to her to best manage her condition?
   (A) Estrogen & Progesterone
   (B) Estrogen & Cyproterone acetate
   (C) Medroxy progesterone acetate
   (D) Metformin

4. Miss S got married but has not been able to conceive in 2 years. You have found that anovulation is the factor responsible for her infertility. Which of thefollowing drug would you prescribe her?
   (A) Clomiphene citrate
   (B) Aromatase inhibitor
   (C) Gonadotropins
   (D) GnRH analogues

5. Miss S conceived following infertility treatment. During pregnancy she should be rigorously monitored for
   (A) Raised LH
   (B) Hyperprolactinemia
   (C) Gestational Diabetes
   (D) Hypo thyroidism

6. Mrs S is now 52 year old. She is obese and is taking oral hypoglycemic agents for to monitor diabetes mellitus. Routine evaluation of which of the following is recommended her?
   (A) FSH/LH
   (B) Ovarian size
   (C) Endometrial thickness
   (D) Urinary proteins

Answers:

1. D

   As per the AE-PCOS 2009 criteria, only presence of hyperandrogenism & ovulatory dysfunction is needed for diagnosis of PCOS in adolescent girls.

2. C

   Fasting insulin level is not indicated in women with PCOS.

3. B

   As the patient is having oligomenorrhoea & hirsuitism, estrogen & cyproterone acetate is the treatment of choice

4. A

   Chronic anovulation in PCOS responds will to clomphene citrate

5. C

   Women with PCOS are more prone to develop GDM & hence should be monitored for it by early blood sugar screening

6. C

   PCOS is a hyperestrogenic state & hence carries a risk of endometrial hyperplasia

Reference:

1. Azziz R, Carmina E, Dewailly D, Kandarakis ED, Morreale HFE, Futterweit W et al. The androgen excess and PCOS society criteria for the polycystic ovary syndrome: The complete task force report. Fertility Sterility 2009, Vol 91(2): 456-488.

HYPERTENSIVES DISORDERS IN PREGNANCY
Dr. Anjoo Agarwal, Professor, Department of Obstetrics & Gynaecology

A 30 yrs old lady, P0+0, married for 1 year presented at 28 wks of pregnancy with complaint of headache for 1 day. On examination her BP is 150/90 mmHg, urine albumin is negative, non dependent edema is absent. Investigations revealed a platelet count of 1.5 lac/cu mm, uric acid 4.5 mg%, SGOT – 62 IU/lit, SGPT – 56 IU/lit, S. creat – 0.9mg%

1. What is your provisional diagnosis?
   (A) Pre eclampsia without severe features
   (B) Severe pre eclampsia
   (C) HELLP syndrome
   (D) Gestational Hypertension
2. How will you manage?
   (A) Fortnightly antenatal visits
   (B) Weekly antenatal visits
   (C) Twice weekly antenatal visits
   (D) Hospitalization
3. What other investigation will you do?
   (A) NST and USG and Doppler
   (B) NST and USG
   (C) USG and Doppler
   (D) USG
4. How frequently will you repeat Lab investigation
   (A) Monthly
   (B) Fortnightty
   (C) Weekly
   (D) Daily
5. After 2 wks her BP is 170/100 mmHg and urine albumin is 2++ positive, platelet count is 1.4 lac/cu mm, uric acid 3.6 mg%, SGOT – 65 IU/lit, SGPT – 62 IU/lit, S.creat 0.95 mg%, How will you manage
   (A) Magnesium sulphate + Antihypertensives + Termination of Pregnancy
   (B) Magnesium sulphate + Termination of Pregnancy
   (C) Antihypertensives + Termination of Pregnancy
   (D) Magnesium sulphate + Antihypertensives + Feto Maternal Monitoring

Answers:
1. D
   Diagnosis is gestational hypertension as urine albumin is negative and all biochemical parameters are within normal limits
2. D
   Hospitalization is advisable as she is having associated headache. If headache subsides with rest and analgesics she may be managed on outpatient basis
3. D
   Only ultrasound is required. Doppler is indicated only if there is associated fetal growth restriction. Fetus is too preterm for NST and only half of fetuses before 30 weeks exhibit accelerations in response to fetal movements.
4. C
   Weekly monitoring by urinary protein and serum biochemistry is recommended by ACOG
5. D
   She is now a case of severe preeclampsia and requires Magnesium sulphate for 24 hrs. Antihypertensives must be started as systolic BP is 170 mmHg predisposing to intracerebral haemorrhage. Termination of pregnancy is not indicated as period of gestation is only 30 wks.

References:
1. Cunningham FG, Leveno KJ, Bloom SL, Spong CY, Dashe JS, Hoffman BL et al. Williams Obstetrics. 24th edition. USA: Mc Graw Hill Education; 2014.
2. Gabbe SG, Niebyl JR, Simpson JL, Landon MB, Galan HL, Jauniaux ERM et al. Obstetrics-Normal and Problem Pregnancies. 6th edition. New Delhi: Elsevier; 2013.

BREECH PREGNANCY

Dr. Anjoo Agarwal, Professor, Department of Obstetrics & Gynaecology

A 25 years old G2P1+0, previous term normal delivery, alive and healthy presented with 38 weeks pregnancy and pain in abdomen full. On examination, she is found to have a singleton complete breech pregnancy with an estimated fetal weight of 2.6-2.7 kg. She is in early labour with mild uterine contractions, cervical dilatation of 3-3.5 cm, membranes intact, breech at -2 station, pelvis gynaecoid, adequate

1 . If you are senior gynecologist managing case, how will you manage?
   (A) Emergency Caesarean section
   (B) Augmentation of labour and leave for vaginal delivery
   (C) Spontaneous labour and leave for vaginal delivery
   (D) Attempt External cephalic version
2. What is the Zatuchni Andros score of this patient?
   (A) 3
   (B) 4
   (C) 5
   (D) 6
3 Which of the following is **NOT** a factor in deciding mode of delivery?
   (A) Flexion of fetal head
   (B) Facilities for anesthesia and caesarean section
   (C) Race of mother
   (D) Presence of IUGR
4 . During breech delivery what action will you take once the inferior angle of scapula   is visible?
   (A) Lovset's maneuver
   (B) Bringing down of arms
   (C) Classical maneuver
   (D) Pinard's maneuver
5. When will you make attempts to deliver the fetal head
   (A) Shoulders are delivered
   (B) Arms are delivered
   (C) Hairline of fetus is visible
   (D) Neck of fetus is visible

Answers:

1. D
    As the person managing the case is a senior gynecologist so he/she is expected to be trained in all methods of management. As the perinatal mortality and morbidity is lower for a cephalic presentation so ECV is the preferred option as patient is in early labour. Emergency caesarean section is associated with increased maternal mortality and morbidity

2. D
    Zatuchni Andros score is 6

Zatuchni Andros System			
Factor	0	1	2
Parity	Nullipara	**Multipara**	Multipara
Gestational Age	39	**38**	37
Estimated fetal weight	8lb	7-8lb	**7 lb**
Previous Breech	**No**	One	Two
Dilatation	2	**3**	4 or more
Station	-3 or greater	**-2**	-1 or less

3. C
    Race of mother is not involved

4. B
    Lovset's and Classical maneuver are used for extended arms while Pinard's maneuver is for bringing down the legs in frank breech

5. C
    Attempts to deliver head before hairline is visible are associated with increased risk of spinal cord injury

Reference:

1. Gabbe SG, Niebyl JR, Simpson JL, Landon MB, Galan HL, Jauniaux ERM et al. Obstetrics- Normal and Problem Pregnancies. 6th edition. New Delhi: Elsevier; 2013.

TRANSVERSE LIE

Dr. Anjoo Agarwal, Professor, Department of Obstetrics & Gynaecology

A 28 yr old G4P3+0 presents as a case of 36 wks pregnancy with pain in abdomen. On examination she has a fundal height of 32 wks with transversely ovoid uterine contour. Head is felt in left iliac fossa and pelvic grip is empty. Fetal heart sounds are 140/min regular. No uterine contractions are felt

1. What is your diagnosis regarding the presentation of the fetus?
   (A) Breech presentation
   (B) Cephalic presentation with high floating head
   (C) Brow presentation
   (D) Shoulder presentation
2. Which of the following is **NOT** a common complication of this presentation?
   (A) Cord prolapse
   (B) PPROM
   (C) Abruptio placentae
   (D) Obstructed labour
3. If ECV fails at this stage when would you like to admit the patient?
   (A) Keep her hospitalized
   (B) At 37 wks
   (C) At 38 wks
   (D) At 39 wks
4 . If elective caesarean section is done in this case, what difficulties will you face?
   (A) Lower segment will not be well formed
   (B) Difficulty in delivering placenta
   (C) Difficulty in controlling PPH
   (D) Difficulty in pushing down bladder
5. If the gravid woman comes late in labour with hand lying out of introitus and intrauterine fetal death how will you manage?
   (A) Craniotomy
   (B) Internal podalic version
   (C) External cephalic version
   (D) Evisceration

Answers:

1. D
   The uterus is transversely ovoid and head is in left iliac fossa, pelvic grip is empty so it is a case of transverse lie or shoulder presentation.

2. C
   Cord prolapse along with PPROM is common in transverse lie as presenting part is not well fitting in the pelvic inlet. As there is no mechanism of labour in transverse lie so if patient goes into labour unsupervised than obstructed labour and rupture uterus is common.

3. A
   Due to the high risk of cord prolapsed it is recommended that elective hospitalization permits observation and early recognition and provides proximity to immediate care.

4. A
   In case of transverse lie as the lower pole is empty so lower segment is not well formed

5. D
   Craniotomy is done in cases of cephalic presentation. There is no role of internal podalic version in singleton pregnancy in modern obstetrics. External cephalic version is not possible with hand prolapsed. As fetus is dead so vaginal delivery by evisceration is preferred.

Reference:

1. Gabbe SG, Niebyl JR, Simpson JL, Landon MB, Galan HL, Jauniaux ERM et al. Obstetrics- Normal and Problem Pregnancies. 6th edition. New Delhi: Elsevier; 2013.

ABNORMAL UTERINE BLEEDING

Prof Nisha Singh, Professor, Department of Obstetrics & Gynaecology

A 45 year old P1+0 presents with heavy bleeding at prolonged intervals since 6 months. Prior cycles were regular. On clinical examination, she is pale, vitals are stable, abdomen is soft, cervix healthy, uterus normal size with bilateral fornices free.

1. What is the most probable diagnosis?
   (A) Fibroid uterus
   (B) Anovulatory perimenopausal bleeding
   (C) Cervical carcinoma
   (D) Adenomyosis
2. What investigation is required to find the cause of bleeding?
   (A) Abdominal Ultrasonography
   (B) Hemoglobin
   (C) Cervical biopsy
   (D) Trans vaginal sonography
3. If transvaginal sonography reveals a normal size uterus with normal myometrium & thickened endometrium, what is the next line investigation?
   (A) Endometrial biopsy
   (B) Cervical biopsy
   (C) CT scan abdomen & pelvis
   (D) MRI abdomen & pelvis
4. What is he most common finding on endometrial biopsy in such cases?
   (A) Endometrial carcinoma
   (B) Complex hyperplasia with atypia
   (C) Complex hyperplasia without atypia
   (D) Simple hyperplasia without atypia
5. What is the treatment if histology shows hyperplasia without atypia?
   (A) Hysterectomy
   (B) Combination Pills
   (C) Cyclical Progesterone therapy
   (D) Chemotherapy

Answers:

1. B
   Since the cycles are prolonged, cervix is healthy and uterus is normal in size, anovulatory bleeding is most probable diagnosis. This happens mostly in adolescents (puberty) or perimenopausal women.
2. D
   A transvaginal ultrasonography is the non-invasive test to detect uterine abnormality missed by clinical examination particularly endometrial thickening; commonly seen in anovulatory bleeding.
3. A
   Endometrial biopsy is required to confirm the histological pathology in all women above 40 years because of high risk of carcinoma and hyperplasia.
4. D
   Simple hyperplasia without atypia is most common abnormality in comparison to the other options
5. C
   Since Simple hyperplasia without atypia is caused by unopposed estrogen exposure, it should be treated with cyclical Progesterone therapy. Moreover, the condition has minimal (1%) risk of endometrial cancer.

Reference:

1. Seshadri L. Abnormal uterine bleeding in "Essentials of Gynaecology". India : Wolters Kluwer; 2011

FIBROID UTERUS

Prof Nisha Singh, Professor, Department of Obstetrics & Gynaecology,

A 40 year old P4+0 presents with heavy menstrual bleeding for last 2 years. Clinical examination reveals pallor. Vitals are stable. Abdomen is soft but a supra pubic firm mass is felt in midline equivalent to 14 weeks gravid uterus. Pelvic examination reveals a healthy cervix & vagina with uterus firm nodular irregular & equal to 14 weeks gravid uterus. The specimen obtained is shown below.

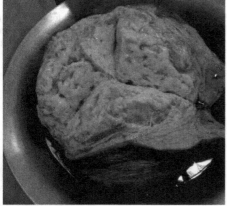

1. What is your clinical diagnosis?
    (A) Fibroid uterus
    (B) Adenomyosis
    (C) Ovarian tumor
    (D) Uterine cancer
2. How will you confirm your diagnosis?
    (A) CT scan
    (B) MRI
    (C) Ultrasonography
    (D) X-ray abdomen
3. What is the treatment of choice for this patient?
    (A) Myomectomy
    (B) Hysterectomy
    (C) Radiotherapy
    (D) Chemotherapy
4 . What type of fibroid is seen in the picture of hysterectomy specimen obtained?
    (A) Subserosal
    (B) Intramural
    (C) Submucus
    (D) All the above
5. What is risk of malignant change in this tumor?
    (A) <1%
    (B) 10%
    (C) 20%
    (D) 30%

Answers:

1. A
    History of menorrhagia with an enlarged nodular uterus is highly suggestive of a fibroid uterus
2. C
    Ultrasound is a costeffective, non invasive, easily available and accurate investigation to confirm the diagnosis of fibroid uterus
3. B
    Since the patient is 40 year old, para 4, symptomatic and has multiple fibroids; hysterectomy is the best option for her.
4. B
    It is a solitary large intramural fibroid.
5. A
    Malignant transformation of fibroids is rare seen in <1% cases.

Reference :

1. Seshadri L. Abnormal uterine bleeding in "Essentials of Gynaecology". India : Wolters Kluwer; 2011

OVARIAN TUMOR

Prof. Nisha Singh, Professor, Department of Obstetrics & Gynaecology

A 55 yrs old postmenopausal woman presented with abdominal distension & loss of appetite for last 2 months. On examination she looked sick but vital were stable. Abdomen was distended fluid thrill present. There was a cystic to firm mass arising from the pelvis measuring 10 X 15 cm with side to side mobility. On PV examination uterus was normal in size & abdominal mass was felt through the right fornix. CA-125 was 500mIU/ml. On laparotomy, there was no ascites or peritoneal deposits and specimen obtained was as shown below.

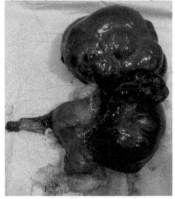

1. What is the clinical diagnosis of the case?
    (A) Fibroid uterus
    (B) Ovarian tumor
    (C) Abdominal tuberculosis
    (D) Portal hypertension
2. What is the primary investigation of choice for diagnosis of this case?
    (A) Ultrasonography
    (B) Doppler study
    (C) X ray abdomen
    (D) CA 125
3. The confirmatory diagnosis of malignant ovarian tumor is obtained by
    (A) Ultrasonography
    (B) CT scan
    (C) MRI
    (D) Histopathology
4. Ovarian tumor is primarily treated by
    (A) Surgery
    (B) Chemotherapy
    (C) Radiotherapy
    (D) Immunotherapy
5. What is the surgical stage of the case based on the specimen obtained on laparotomy?
    (A) I
    (B) II
    (C) III
    (D) IV

Answers:
1. B
   Abdominal ascites with solid/cystic tumor in postmenopausal women is suggestive of an Ovarian tumor
2. A
   Ultrasound of abdomen and and pelvis is the primary investigation to confirm the ovarian tumor and ascites. In addition it gives some information about benign/malignant status of the tumor.
3. D
   Final confirmation of type of tumor is obtained by histopathological examination
4. A

An exploratory laparotomy is primary requirement for surgicopathological staging and treatment of the disease

5. A

It is stage I surgically because only one ovary is involved on gross examination. Final staging will be done after histopathological evaluation of the specimen and cytological evaluation of the ascitic fluid.

Reference:

1. Seshadri L. Abnormal uterine bleeding in "Essentials of Gynaecology". India : Wolters Kluwer; 2011

INCOMPLETE ABORTION

Dr. Pooja Gupta, Assistant Professor, Department of Obstetrics & Gynecology

Mrs. A, is 20 years old P_{1+1} presents with vaginal bleeding following amenorrhea of 3 months. On examination her blood pressure is 110/70 mmHg pulse rate is 100bpm, temperature is 37°C and respiratory rate is 20/minute. Abdominal examination is unremarkable. Vaginal examination shows heavy bleeding with clots. Products of conception are visualized in the cervix, cervical os is open, uterus is 8 weeks size with no adnexal or cervical motion tenderness.

1. What is the most likely diagnosis:
    (A) Threatened abortion
    (B) Inevitable abortion
    (C) Incomplete abortion
    (D) Missed abortion.

2. Based on your diagnosis what is the treatment of choice in your patient
    (A) MVA
    (B) Suction evacuation followed by gentle check curettage
    (C) Dilatation and curettage
    (D) Conservative management

3. Mrs. A has recovered well from procedure and is fit to be discharged. All below mentioned warning signs must be explained to her except,
    (A) Cramping
    (B) Excessive and prolonged bleeding
    (C) Fever with chills or malaise
    (D) Urinary incontinence

4. What is the most common chromosomal anomaly which causes spontaneous Ist trimester abortion.
    (A) Autosomal trisomy
    (B) Triploidy
    (C) Monosomy X
    (D) Tetra ploidy

5. The best known immunologic cause of 2nd trimester abortion is
    (A) Antiphospholipid antibody syndrome
    (B) Maternal thrombophilias
    (C) Autoimmune antibodies
    (D) Alloimmune antibodies

6. How can you confirm your diagnosis
    (A) Pervaginum examination
    (B) Per rectal examination
    (C) USG lower abdomen and pelvis
    (D) CT pelvis

Answers:

1. C

    In incomplete abortion, the abortion has occurred but the process is incomplete. The cervical os is open and products of conception are partly expelled.

2. B

    Suction curettage is performed to evacuate the uterus in cases of incomplete abortion. It is important to use blunt curette to avoid risk of uterine perforation and synaechiae formation.

3. D

Infection and sepsis, uterine perforation, incomplete evacuation and bleeding per vaginum are common complications of the procedure, so the patient is explained about the warming signs on discharge.

4. A

Autosomal trisomy- This non dysfunctional defect is found in approximately 60% of blighted ova with abnormal karyotype. This trisomy predominantly affects chromosomes 16, 21 & 22.

5. A

The best known cause of second trimester losses is antiphospholipid antibody syndrome.

6. C

By pelvic ultrasound any retained products inside uterine cavity can be visualized, simultaneously adenexa can also be assessed if ectopic pregnancy is suspected.

References:

1. Daftary S N. , Chakravarti S. Holland and Brews Manual of obstetrics. 3rd edition. New Delhi: Elsevier; 2013.
2. Arias F, Daftary S N, Bhide A G. Practical guide to high risk pregnancy and delivery. 3rd edition. New Delhi: Elsevier; 2008.

SEPTIC ABORTION

Dr. Pooja Gupta, Assistant Professor, Department of Obstetrics & Gynaecology

Mrs. B, a 20 years old P4+1 presents with vaginal bleeding, fever with chills, vomiting and pain in abdomen for 4 days following amenorrhea of 2 months. There is history of insertion of some abortifacient into vagina by dai 4 days back. She is mildly pale, temperature is 38.5°C, pulse rate is 120 bpm, blood pressure is 100/60 mmHg and respiratory rate is 24/minute. Her lower abdomen is tender. On vaginal examination a foul smelling, blood stained discharge is present. Cervical os is dilated and products of conception felt at the os. The uterus is 8 weeks size tender and fornices are extremely tender

1. What is the most likely diagnosis
   (A) Induced septic abortion
   (B) Missed abortion
   (C) incomplete abortion
   (D) Threatened abortion.
2. The following are the common organisms involved in the infection except.
   (A) E. coli
   (B) Clostridium tetani
   (C) Klebsiella
   (D) N. Gonorrhoea
3. The first line investigations for the above condition is all except.
   (A) Complete blood count and urinalysis
   (B) High vaginal swab culture and sensitivity
   (C) H1N1
   (D) Kidney function test and liver function test
4. The appropriate management of this condition is:
   (A) Resuscitation of patient and broad spectrum IV antibiotics.
   (B) Resuscitation of patient, broad spectrum IV antibiotics and evacuation of products.
   (C) Evacuation of products directly.
   (D) Explorative laparotomy
5. The complications of this condition may be all except
   (A) Generalized septicaemia
   (B) Pelvic abscess
   (C) Bladder and bowel injury
   (D) Gestational trophoblastic disease
6. Grade 3 septic abortion includes
   (A) Involvement of the endometrium and myometrium
   (B) Involvement of adenoma and pelvic structures
   (C) Generalized peritonitis
   (D) Involvement of endometrium only.

Answers:

1. A

Since amenorrhea, vaginal bleeding along with fever and foul smelling discharge are present and there is history of dai-handling it is most likely a case of septic abortion.

2. B
    The common organisms involved in septic abortion are Aerobic- E. Coli, Pseudomonas, β hemoloytic streptococci, E. faecalis, Anaerobic Bacteroids, clostridium, neisseria gonorrhoea, chlamydia trachomatis.
3. C
    The investigations usually done in this condition are CBC and urinalysis, blood urea, s. creatinine, serum electrolyte, high vaginal swab, blood culture, S. fibrin degradation products, pelvic ultrasound, radiograph of abdomen & radiograph of chest.
4. B
    Shock is treated aggressively, urine output is monitored, close monitoring of vitals of patient, simultaneously broad spectrum IV antibiotics are started followed by evacuation of products.
5. D
    Septicaemia, intraabdominal abcess, pelvic abscess and bladder bowel injury can be complication of septic abortion.
6. C
    Grade-I – involves endometrium and myometrium.
    Grade-II- involves the adenexa and pelvic structures.
    Grade-III- Generalized peritonitis

Reference:

1. Daftary S N. , Chakravarti S. Holland and Brews Manual of obstetrics. 3rd edition. New Delhi: Elsevier; 2013.

PROLAPSE OF UTERUS

Dr. Pooja Gupta, Assistant Professor, Department of Obstetrics & Gynaecology

A 35 years old P_{3+0} (2 living) presented to our OPD with chief complaints of something coming out of vagina for the past three months. All her previous deliveries were full term normal deliveries, conducted in squatting position at home by dai. Her last delivery was 3 years back. There is history of resumption of routine physical activity immediately after delivery and inter-delivery interval is 1½-2 years. There is no history of chronic cough, constipation or any urinary complaints. Fig. 1 shows the clinical findings of the lady.

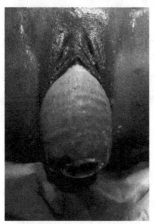

1. What is the most likely clinical diagnosis as shown in Fig. 1.
    (A) III° uterine prolapse with cystocele and rectocele
    (B) Inversion of uterus
    (C) Cervical fibroid polyp
    (D) Vaginal cyst

2. What is the type of ulcer present over the cervix as shown in Fig. 2

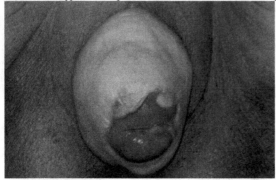

(A) Apthous ulcer
(B) Decubitus ulcer
(C) Carcinomatous ulcer
(D) Circumoral erosion

3. What is the staging of the prolapse according to Baden Walker halfway classification if the above picture has been taken on maximum straining?
(A) 1
(B) 2
(C) 3
(D) 4

4. Expectant management of prolapse includes all except
(A) Pelvic floor exercises
(B) Pessary treatment
(C) Treatment of chronic diseases
(D) Nutritional therapy

5. What is the surgery of choice is this patient
(A) Ward Mayo's hysterectomy
(B) Fother gill repair (Manchester Operation)\
(C) Shirodhkar's operation
(D) Leforts repair

6. Delancy level I support of genital tract include all except
(A) Uterosacral ligament
(B) Cardinal ligament
(C) Pelvic fascias and paracolpos
(D) None of the above

Answers:

1. A
   1° degree – cervix descends into vagina
   2° degree – cervix descends upto vulva
   3° degree – cervix protrudes outside vaginal orifice
   Anterior vaginal wall
   Upper 2/3rd cystocele
   Lower 1/3rd urethrocele
   Post vaginal wall
   Upper 1/3rd enterocoele
   Lower 1/3rd rectocele

2. B
   Ulceration of the prolapsed tissue is caused by friction, congestion and circulatory changes in the dependent portion of the prolapse into the vagina and daily packing heals the ulcer in a week or two.

3. D
   Balden walker halfway classification
   Stage I – Cervix descends halfway upto hymen
   Stage II – Cervix descends upto hymen

Stage III – Cervix descends halfway past hymen

Stage IV – Maximum prolapse

4. D

Pelvic floor exercises, weight loss, treatment of chronic disease, physical therapy cessation of smoking and estrogen therapy are all considerations in the conservative management of pelvic organ prolapse.

5. B

This operation preserves menstrual and child bearing functions. It is suitable for women under 40 years who are desirous of retaining their menstrual and reproductive functions.

6. C

Delancy introduced three level system of support

Level I – Uterosacral and cardinal ligament

Level II – Palvic fascias and paracolpos

Level III – Levator ani muscle

References:

1. Padubidri V G, Dasftary S N. Hawkins & Bourne Shaw's. Text book of Gynaecology. 15th edition. New Delhi: Elsevier; 2011.
2. Rock J A, Jones III H. W. Telinde's operative gynecology. 10th edition. New Delhi: Wolters Kluwer; 2008.

TRAUMATIC PPH

Dr. Pushplata Shankwar, Professor, Department of Obstetrics & Gynaecology

A 24 yrs old G1P0+0 was admitted in the labor room of a district hospital in 1st stage of labor. She had normal progress of labor and delivered a 4 kg healthy female baby & placenta was expelled in toto. After delivery there was continuous fresh bleeding per vaginum. On examination pallor was ++, PR 110/ min, BP 80 systolic. On abdominal examination, uterus was hard & well contracted. On exploration of birth canal, there were multiple lacerations in vagina, & cervix was also torn at 3'o clock position.

1. The most appropriate diagnosis based on given situation is-
   (A) Third stage PPH with anemia in shock
   (B) Traumatic PPH with anemia in shock
   (C) Atonic PPH with anemia in shock
   (D) Mixed PPH in shock
2. The definitive immediate management of the patient will include
   (A) Packing of genital tract
   (B) IV fluids & repair of cervical tear & vaginal lacerations
   (C) Repair of cervical tear & packing of vagina
   (D) Blood transfusion & packing of vagina
3. This is the picture* of above patient with progressive swelling after 4 hours of delivery with rising pulse rate, what is the diagnosis and its management?

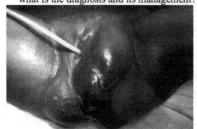

Figure * for question -3
   (A) Vulvo-vaginal hematoma needs drainage
   (B) Vulval hematoma needs ice packing of vulva and blood transfusion.
   (C) Vulvo-vaginal hematoma needs drainage, hemostatic sutures, vaginal packing and blood transfusion.
   (D) Vulval hematoma needs conservative management and blood transfusion.
4. Most probable Cause of traumatic PPH in this patient is-
   (A) Good size baby
   (B) Application of fundal pressure

(C) Episiotomy

(D) Premature bearing down

5. All the following precautions must be taken to avoid traumatic PPH EXCEPT

    (A) Fundal pressure in good sized baby.

    (B) Indicated Episiotomy

    (C) Avoid Premature bearing down

    (D) Rule out cephalo pelvic disproportions

Answers:

1. B

    Patient is having features of shock, anemia and birth canal injuries.

2. B

    Patient needs resuscitation as she is in shock and repair of lacerations to arrest hemorrhage.

3. C

    This is the picture showing huge vulvo-vaginal hematoma with deteriorating pulse, so it should be explored ,drained and hemostatic sutures to be applied along with replacement of blood.

4. A

    Most obvious cause seems to be vaginal delivery of macrosomic baby.

5. A

    No evidence has been found for use of Fundal pressure, so it is not recommended in any vaginal delivery.

Reference:

1. Cunningham FG, Leveno KJ, Bloom SL, Spong CY, Dashe JS, Hoffman BL et al. Williams Obstetrics 24th edition. USA: Mc Graw Hill Education; 2014.

ATONIC PPH

Dr. Pushplata Shankwar, Professor, Department of Obstetrics & Gynaecology

Mrs X, P2+0 referred from PHC was brought in emergency room with complaints of excessive bleeding per vaginum following delivery of a full term 3.5 kg female baby one hour back. On examination, she was severely pale, dyspnoic, PR-120/mt, BP- 70 systolic. On abdominal examination the uterus was flabby, soft, with no other organomegaly. On local examination fresh bleeding was seen coming through os, no tear or laceration was seen in cervix, vagina or perineum.

1. What is your provisional diagnosis?

    (A) Third stage PPH in shock.

    (B) Traumatic PPH with anemia in shock

    (C) Atonic PPH with severe anemia in shock

    (D) Primary PPH with DIC in shock

2. All the following steps should be done to resuscitate the patient EXCEPT

    (A) SHOUT for help

    (B) Establish 2 wide bore IV lines.

    (C) O2 inhalation & Foley's catheterization

    (D) Propped up position

3. What management should not be done as 1st line of management-

    (A) Oxytocics

    (B) β Lynch suturing

    (C) Uterine massage

    (D) Prostaglandins

4. Following are the surgical techniques used to manage atonic PPH EXCEPT

    (A) Aortic compression

    (B) β Lynch suturing

    (C) Cho-Cho stitches

    (D) Uterine artery ligation

5. What suturing technique is depicted in the photograph?

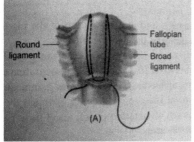

Figure for ques.-5
(A) Choo-Choo stitches
(B) Square sutures
(C) β Lynch suture
(D) Modified β Lynch suture

Answers:
1. C
   Patient is having tachycardia and hypotension and uterus is flabby not contracted, so she is a case of atonic PPH in shock
2. D
   Patient is aldeady in shock, and propped up position will hamper the blood flow to the brain.
3. B
   B Lynch suturing is a surgical procedure which needs opening of abdomen, so it has to be done if medical management fails.
4. A
   Aortic compression is a conservative management of PPH.
5. C
   This picture is showing technique of B-Lynch suturing.

Reference:
1. Cunningham FG, Leveno KJ, Bloom SL, Spong CY, Dashe JS, Hoffman BL et al. Williams Obstetrics 24th edition. USA: Mc Graw Hill Education; 2014.

PREGNANCY WITH ANEMIA
Dr. Pushplata Shankwar, Professor, Department of Obstetrics & Gynaecology

A 26 yrs old G4P3+0 (all home deliveries) came in emergency room with complaints of shortness of breath & generalized weakness for one week following 8 month amenorrhea. On examination she was ill looking, severely pale, dyspnoic with anasarca and raised JVP. Chest examinations showed basal crepts. RR was 32/min. and on room air SPO2 was 90%. PR was 120/min, BP 120/60 mmHg. Per abdominal findings revealed abdominal wall edema & 32 wks pregnancy with cephalic presentation.

1. What is your provisional diagnosis?
   (A) Pregnancy with severe anemia in shock.
   (B) 32 wks pregnancy with ana sarca
   (C) 32 wks pregnancy with congestive heart failure with severe anemia
   (D) 32 wks pregnancy with CHF with preeclampsia in pulmonary edema.
2. In which position would you like to keep the patient when you admit her?
   (A) Trenelenberg position
   (B) Knee chest position
   (C) Dorsal lithotomy position
   (D) Propped up position
3. What is the best time of delivery in such condition?
   (A) At 34 wks after steroids coverage
   (B) Once the patient is out of danger
   (C) After Hb% reaches 11gm%
   (D) Spontaneous delivery at term

4. The most reliable investigation to know the type of anemia is
   (A) General Blood Picture
   (B) Hb electrophoresis
   (C) Total iron binding capacity
   (D) S. Ferritin
5. The peripheral smear shows a microcytic hypochromic picture, what is the diagnosis?
   (A) Iron Deficiency
   (B) B12 Deficiency
   (C) Folic acid Deficiency
   (D) Ascorbic acid Deficiency

Answers:
1. C
   Patient is having raised JVP and basal crepts with severe anemia indicating CHF.
2. D
   Patient is in congestive heart failure so she should be kept in propped up position.
3. D
   If the anemia is corrected optimally and pregnancy is otherwise uncomplicated, then it is recommended that patient should be left for spontaneous delivery at term.
4. A
   GBP is the best investigation to know for type of anemia as it gives information about the morphology and type of cells.
5. A
   A microcytic hypochromic picture on peripheral smear suggest Iron deficiency anemia. It may also be seen in Thalassemia.

Reference:

1. Cunningham FG, Leveno KJ, Bloom SL, Spong CY, Dashe JS, Hoffman BL et al. Williams Obstetrics 24th edition. USA: Mc Graw Hill Education; 2014.

IMPERFORATE HYMEN
Dr. Rekha Sachan, Professor, Department of Obstetrics & Gynaecology

A 18 years old unmarried female presented with chief complaints of not having attained menses with cyclical spasmodic pain in lower abdomen. For last 3 months she also noticed a lump in lower abdomen. On per abdominal examination, there was a suprapubic lump arising from pelvis of 14 weeks of size gravid uterus. On local examination, there was a tense bluish bluging membrane at introitus. On external examination, genitalia were normal and she had well developed secondary sexual characters.

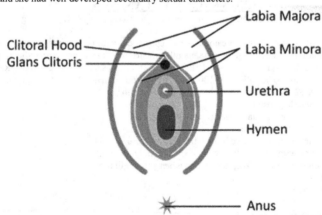

1. What is the most likely diagnosis?
   (A) Secondary amenorrhoea
   (B) Cryptomenorrhoea
   (C) Oligomenorrhoea
   (D) Menouria

2. Which one is the confirmatory test to diagnose this disease?
   (A) Ultrasonography
   (B) Hysteroscopy
   (C) Serum CA-125 level
   (D) Hysterosalpingography
3. What is the probable cause of this problem?
   (A) Absent vagina
   (B) Transverse vaginal septum
   (C) Imperforate hymen
   (D) Absent uterus
4. Which one of the following is the treatment option in the above case.
   (A) Laparotomy
   (B) Hysterectomy
   (C) Cruciate incision and drainage
   (D) Hormonal therapy
5. All are the mullerian anomalies **EXCEPT**:
   (A) Bicornuate uterus
   (B) Uterus didelphys
   (C) Absent uterus
   (D) Non canalization of lower 1/3 of vagina
6. Which one of the following anomalies is commonly associated with mullerian agenesis?
   (A) Wolffian duct anomalies
   (B) Ovarian anomalies
   (C) Hepatobiliary anomalies
   (D) Cardiac anomalies

Answers:

1. B

   Cryptomenorrhoea is the condition in which normal menstruation is present but due to imperforate hymen blood collects inside vaginaand appears as bluish bulging membrane at the level of introitus.

2. A

   Ultrasonography gives accurate idea about the presence of uterus and ovaries and collection of blood within the cervical and vaginal canal.

3. C

   In imperforate hymen, due to collection of blood, hymenal membrane bulges out and bluish appearance is due to collection of old blood.

4. C

   Simple cruciate incision has to be given on most prominent bulging point to facilitatedrainage of old collected blood.

5. D

   All anomalies are due to mullerian fusion defect or absence of development but noncanalisation of lower 1/3 of vagina due to incomplete development of Sinovaginal bulb. Lower1/3 of vagina develops from sinovaginal bulb.

6. A

   Wolffian duct anomalies are most commonly associated with mullerian anomalies because development of both of them takes place simultaneously

Reference:

1. Padubidri V G, Dasftary S N. Hawkins & Bourne Shaw's Text book of Gynaecology. 16th edition. New Delhi: Elsevier; 2011.

ENDOMETRIOSIS

Dr. Rekha Sachan, Professor, Department of Obstetrics & Gynaecology

A 24 years old nulliparous woman, married for more than 5 years presented in Gynae OPD with chief complaints of persistent chronic pain in lower abdomen. She also had pain just before the menses which got relieved with start of menses and was taking treatment for infertility. Her per abdominal examination was insignificant. P/S examination revealed a bluish nodule in posterior fornix. Per vaginal examination showd uterus was of normal size with restricted mobility and a right adenexal mass 5X5cm, firm to cystic in consistency. A nodularity was felt in pouch of doughlas.

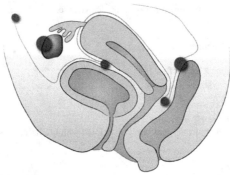

1. What is the most likely diagnosis?
   (A) Tuberculosis
   (B) Endometriosis
   (C) Ovarian malignancy
   (D) Adenomyosis
2. Which type of dysmenorrhoea is present in this case:
   (A) Congestive dysmenorrhoea
   (B) Spasmodic dysmenorrhoea
   (C) Membranous type of dysmenorrhoea
   (D) None of the above
3. Which one of the following is the most reliable confirmatory test for diagnosis of endometriosis:
   (A) Ultrasonography
   (B) Laparoscopy
   (C) Hysteroscopy
   (D) Serum CA-125 levels
4. All are the conservative treatment options of endometriosis **EXCEPT**
   (A) Fulgration
   (B) Drainage of Endometrioma
   (C) Hysterectomy with bilateral Salpingoeopherectomy
   (D) GnRH analogue
5. Following are the probable causes of infertility in this case **EXCEPT**
   (A) Blockage of fallopian tube
   (B) Distortion of anatomy
   (C) Anovulatory cycles
   (D) Defect in ovum

Answers:
   1. B
      Most likely diagnosis is endometriosis because persistant chronic pelvic pain with dysmenorrhoea with adenexal lump and nodule in pouch of douglous usually present in endometriosis.
   2. A
      This is congestive type dysmenorrhoea because in this type of dysmenorrhoea, pain because of congestion and it is relieved after start of menses.
   3. B
      Ultrasonography is the most reliable test by which we can see the collection within the cervix and vagina.
   4. C

Hysterectomy with bilateral Salpingooopherectomy is the definitive treatment option, rest are conservative treatment,

5. D

In endometriosis infertility is because of distortion of anatomy and blockage of tubes but it never causes defect in ovum.

Reference:

1. Padubidri V G, Dasftary S N. Hawkins & Bourne Shaw's Text book of Gynaecology. 16th edition. New Delhi: Elsevier; 2011.

PELVIC INFLAMMATORY DISEASE (PID)
Dr. Rekha Sachan, Professor, Department of Obstetrics & Gynaecology

A 27 year old P2+0, presented to gynae OPD with c/o pain in lower abdomen & foul smelling discharge for 2 months. She also had complain of burning on micturition. She had IUCD insertion 3yr back which was removed 1month back for similar complaint. She has no h/o weight loss, loss of appetite or hypomenorrhoea. Husband has no complaint. On perspeculum examination circumoral cervical erosion with greenish white discharge was present. On pervaginal examination cervix was forward, uterus was retroverted, normal size, tender, bilateral fornices were tender.

1. What is the clinical diagnosis of this case?
   (A) Vaginitis
   (B) Cervicitis
   (C) Tuberculosis
   (D) PID
2. All of the following are causative organisms of PID **EXCEPT**
   (A) Neisserria gonorrhea
   (B) Chlamydia trachomatis.
   (C) Mycobacterium Bovis
   (D) Gardenella vaginalis
3. Clinical feature of PID include all **EXCEPT**
   (A) Severe abdominal pain.
   (B) Vaginal discharge
   (C) Fever
   (D) Gastroenteritis
4. Long term complications of PID include all **EXCEPT**
   (A) Pelvic abscess.
   (B) Ectopic pregnancy
   (C) Infertility
   (D) Urinary retention.
5. First line treatment of chlamydial infection includes
   (A) Doxycycline
   (B) Cefixime
   (C) Levofloxacin
   (D) Cefotaxime

Answers:

1. B

Clinical diagnosis of this case is pelvic inflammatory disease as all other conditions involving only lower genital tract.

2. C

Mycobacterium Bovis is responsible for tuberculosis in cattle.

3. D

Gastroenteritis is not a clinical feature of PID.

4. D

Urinary retention is not a long term complication of PID.

5. A

As per CDC Guideline doxycycline is the first line treatment for PID.

Reference:
1. Padubidri V G, Dasftary S N. Hawkins & Bourne Shaw's Text book of Gynaecology. 16th edition. New Delhi: Elsevier; 2011.

THIRD STAGE OF LABOR

Dr. Renu Singh, Professor, Department of Obstetrics & Gynaecology

A 25 year old primigravida had full term pregnancy. She was complaining of pain lower abdomen with watery discharge per vaginum. On her way to hospital she delivered a female baby. On arrival in the labor room, the newborn is lying with an unseparated placenta and umbilical cord.

1. In which stage of labor the woman was admitted in the labor room?
   (A) First stage
   (B) Second stage
   (C) Third stage
   (D) Fourth stage

2. What is the normal duration (in minutes) of this stage of labor?
   (A) 10
   (B) 15
   (C) 20
   (D) 25

3. The commonest method of placental separation amongst following is
   (A) Central separation
   (B) Marginal separation
   (C) Umbilical separation
   (D) Peripheral separation

4. Which one of the following is not a sign of placental separation?
   (A) Firm and globular uterus
   (B) Gush of blood from vagina
   (C) Apparent shortening of umbilical cord
   (D) Apparent lengthening of umbilical cord

5. The oxytocic of choice in above mentioned case is
   (A) Methyl ergometrine
   (B) Oxytocin
   (C) Syntometrine
   (D) Carboprost

Answers:

1. C
   The third stage begins after the birth of the baby and ends with expulsion of the placenta.

2. B
   The third stage of labor lasts for about 15 minutes.

3. A
   As there is retraction of the uterus after the baby is born; the placental bed is reduced to one third its size. The placenta itself remains unchanged and therefore the shearing effect starts separating the placenta and causes retroplacental bleeding from torn vessels of intervillous space which separate the placenta further.

4. C
   The signs of placental separation are: (1) a gush of blood from vagina; (2) lengthening of the cord outside the vulva; (3) rise in the height of the fundus which occurs as the placenta fills up the collapsed lower segment, the uterus becomes firm and globular

5. B
   Oxytocin is the drug of choice for active management of third stage of labor.

Reference:
1. Daftary S N, Chakravarti S. Holland and Brews Manual of Obstetrics. 3rd edition. New Delhi: Elsevier; 2011..

NEWBORN RESUSCITATION

Dr. Renu Singh, Professor, Department of Obstetrics & Gynaecology

Mrs X, 39 weeks multigravida was admitted in labor room with complaints of pain abdomen & discharge per vaginum. On examination she was full term with good uterine contractions, head 0/5 palpable, and FHR of 90 beats per minute. On per vaginal examination the cervix was fully dilated, effaced with vertex at + 4 station. There was no moulding or caput, but liquor was thick meconium stained. She delivered a non vigorous male baby, meconium stained with heart rate of 60 bpm.

1. One of the following is a primary measure of adequate neonatal ventilation
   (A) Improvement in heart rate
   (B) Pink extremities
   (C) sPo2 of 80%
   (D) chest wall movement
2. Endotracheal intubation may be indicated at several points during neonatal resuscitation except
   (A) If BMV is ineffective
   (B) During chest compressions
   (C) vigorous meconium stained newborn
   (D) Non vigorous meconium stained newborn
3. The recommended compression to ventilation ratio in neonatal resuscitation is
   (A) 2:1
   (B) 3:1
   (C) 4:1
   (D) 5:1
4. The recommended dose(mg/kg per dose) and route of epinephrine in neonatal resuscitation
   (A) 0.01-0.03,IV
   (B) 0.01-0.03,IM
   (C) 0.03-0.05,1V
   (D) 0.05-0.1,IV
5. Recommended method of confirming ET placement is
   (A) Condensation in ET
   (B) Chest movement
   (C) Equal breath sounds on auscultation
   (D) Exhaled CO_2 Detection

Answers:
1. A
   Increase in heart rate is the most sensitive indicator of a successful response to neonatal resuscitation
2. C
   A meconium stained vigorous newborn does not requires endotracheal intubation
3. B
   The recommended compression to ventilation ratio in neonatal resuscitation is 3:1[90 compressions :30 ventilations]
4. A
   The recommended dose & route of epinephrine in neonatal resuscitation is 0.01 -0.03 mg/kg per dose, intravenously
5. D
   Detection of exhaled Co2 confirms endotracheal tube placement

Reference:
1. Daftary S N, Chakravarti S. Holland and Brews Manual of Obstetrics. 3rd edition. New Delhi: Elsevier; 2011.

NEWBORN INJURIES

Dr. Renu Singh, Professor, Department of Obstetrics & Gynaecology

Mrs X, 38weeks multigravida was admitted in labor room with complaints of pain abdomen with discharge per vaginum. On examination she was full term with good uterine contractions, head 0/5 palpable, and FHR of 90 beats per minute, irregular . On per vaginal examination the cervix was fully dilated, effaced with vertex at + 4 station. There was no molding but liquor was thick meconium stained. She delivered a non vigorous male baby, meconium stained with heart rate of 60 bpm following instrumental (forceps) delivery. After few hours of delivery there was a huge swelling on the newborn's head .

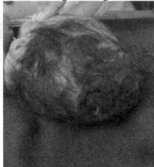

1. Which one of the following is suspected in the above mentioned newborn?
   (A) Cephalhematoma
   (B) Moulding
   (C) Caput succedaneum
   (D) Craniosynostosis
2. All the following are causes of newborn injury except
   (A) Prolonged latent labor
   (B) Instrumental delivery
   (C) Precipitate labor
   (D) Difficult labor
2. Following feature is not associated with caput succedaneum
   (A) Present at birth
   (B)Limited by suture lines
   (C)Resolves spontaneously
   (D) Prolonged labor
4. Following is not a feature of cephalhematoma
   (A) Subperiosteal in location
   (B) Limited by suture lines
   (C) Appears at birth
   (D) Feels soft at centre
5. What is the recommended management in a newborn with cephalhematoma
   (A) Incision and drainage
   (B) Aspiration of blood
   (C) Conservative
   (D) Vigorous massage

Answers:
   1. A
      Cephalhematoma develops because of development of subperiosteal hematoma, here in this case after forceps delivery.
   2. A
      The causes of newborn injury are; prolonged difficult labor; instrumental delivery; precipitate labor; prolonged latent labor is not a cause of newborn injury.
   3. B
      Caput succedaneum is a soft tissue swelling/edema, that is not limited by suture lines,is present at birth and resolves in first few hours of birth.
   4. C
      Cephalhematoma is subperiosteal in location, is limited by suture lines, feels soft at centre,and is never present at birth. It appears few hours after birth.
   5. C
      The cephalhematoma appears within a few hours of birth and get absorbed gradually over 6 to 12 weeks

Reference:
   1. Daftary S N, Chakravarti S. Holland and Brews Manual of Obstetrics. 3rd edition. New Delhi: Elsevier; 2011.

PLACENTA PREVIA

Dr. Sabuhi Qureshi, Professor, Department of Obstetrics & Gynaecology

Mrs X, 26year old woman, G2 P1 L1, unbooked, unsupervised pregnancy, reported to the emergency of a PHC with bleeding per vaginum for 6 hours following amenorrhea of 8 months. On examination, she was conscious, oriented and responding to verbal commands. Skin was cold, pallor +++, pulse rate – 120 per minute, feeble, B.P- 80/60 mm of mercury, respiratory rate – 30/ minute. On per abdominal examination, uterus was 32 weeks (fundal height), longitudinal lie, cephalic presentation, head high floating, fetal heart absent, uterus was relaxed. Local examination of the external genitalia was normal, blood stains were seen on thigh and legs. On per speculum examination, blood clots were seen in vagina, bleeding was coming from os, cervix vagina was healthy.

1. Based on the clinical scenario, what is the provisional diagnosis?
   (A) Abruptio placentae.
   (B) Rupture uterus.
   (C) Labour with heavy show.
   (D) Placenta previa.

3. Following are the prerequisites of Macafee and Johnson regimen (Expectant management) EXCEPT-
   (A) Good general condition of the mother, Hb > 10gm/dl.
   (B) Absence of active vaginal bleeding
   (C) Gestation more than 37 weeks.
   (D) Good fetal condition as assessed by USG and NST.

3. Following are indications of "Double set up examination" in a case of placenta previa EXCEPT-
   (A) USG facility not available
   (B) Inconclusive USG report
   (C) USG reveals type I and II placenta previa
   (D) USG reveals type IV and III placenta previa.

4. Stallworthy's sign is associated with-
   (A) Fetal malpresentation
   (B) Fetal tachycardia
   (C) Fetal bradycardia
   (D) Fetal congenital malformation

5. Which of the following is contraindicated in a patient with placenta previa-
   (A) Abdominal palpation
   (B) Ultrasonography
   (C) Per vaginal examination
   (D) Cardiotocography

Answers:

1. D

   The diagnosis is placenta previa (ante partum haemorrhage) as the patient has bleeding per vaginum which is painless. On examination, relaxed uterus with high floating head and on per speculum examination, blood clots in vagina support the diagnosis of ante partum haemorrhage due to placenta previa.

2. C

   The aim of Macafee and Johnson regimen (Expectant management) is to prolong the pregnancy till the fetus is reasonably mature, if possible till term without compromising maternal condition in a centre with round the clock facility of caeserean section and blood transfusion

3. D

   Per vaginal examination is normally contraindicated in placenta previa. In few conditions double set up examination is done i.e. is performed in operation theatre keeping things ready for caesarean section. Vaginal examination conclusively confirms the clinical diagnosis and degree of placenta previa.

4. C

   Fetal bradycardia occurs on pressing the head down into the pelvis and its prompt recovery on release of pressure is suggestive of low lying placenta specially of posterior type.

5. C

   Per vaginal examination can cause life threatening hemorrhage in placenta previa and is therefore contraindicated.

References:

1. Sharma JB. Text book of obstetrics. Avichal publishing company. Sirmour (HP). 2014.

2. Cunningham FG, Leveno KJ, Bloom SL, Spong CY, Dashe JS, Hoffman BL et al. Williams Obstetrics 24th edition. USA: Mc Graw Hill Education; 2014.

ABRUPTIO PLACENTAE

Dr. Sabuhi Qureshi, Professor, Department of Obstetrics & Gynaecology

Mrs X, 26year old woman, G-2 P1 L1, unbooked, unsupervised pregnancy, reported to the emergency of a PHC with pain in abdomen and bleeding per vaginum for 6 hours following amenorrhea of 7 months. On examination, she was conscious, oriented and responding to verbal commands. Skin was cold, pallor +++, pulse rate – 120 per minute, feeble, B.P- 80/60 mm of mercury, respiratory rate – 30/ minute. On per abdominal examination, uterus was 36 weeks (fundal height), longitudinal lie, cephalic presentation. Uterus was tense and tender. Fetal heart sound was absent. Local examination of the external genitalia was normal, blood stains seen on thigh and legs. On per speculum examination, blood stained liquor was seen coming from os, cervix and vagina were healthy.

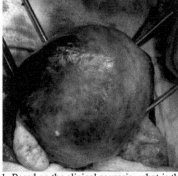

1. Based on the clinical scenario, what is the provisional diagnosis?
   (A) Abruptio placentae.
   (B) Rupture uterus.
   (C) Labour with heavy show.
   (D) Placenta previa.
2. Identify the pathology seen in the photograph.
   (A) Blue uterus
   (B) Unicornuate uterus
   (C) Couvelaire uterus
   (D) Didelphus uterus
3. Which of the following is NOT a risk factor for placental abruption?
   (A) Nulliparity
   (B) Polyhydroamnios
   (C) Preclampsia
   (D) Cocaine abuse
4. The incidence of abruption placentae is-
   (A) 1 in 100 deliveries
   (B) 1 in 200 deliveries
   (C) 1 in 300 deliveries
   (D) 1 in 400 deliveries
5. All of the following are complications of abruption placentae EXCEPT-
   (A) Haemorrhagic Shock
   (B) Coagulopathy
   (C) Renal failure
   (D) Respiratory failure

Answers:
   1. A
       The provisional diagnosis is abruption placentae as there is history of bleeding per vaginum with pain in abdomen. On examination, fundal height is more than period of amenorrhea, uterus being tense and tender support diagnosis of antepartum haemorrhage due to abruption placentae.

2. C

Couvelaire uterus is seen in the photograph.

3. A

Polyhydramnios ,Preeclampsia, Cocaine abuse, Increased parity are risk factors for placental abruption. Ref- Obstetrical haemorrhage chapter of Williams

4. B

Ref- Obstetrical haemorrhage chapter of Williams

5. D

Haemorrhagic Shock, Coagulopathy, Renal failure are all complications of abruption placentae. Respiratory failure is not a complication of same.

References:

1. Sharma JB. Text book of obstetrics. Avichal publishing company. Sirmour (HP). 2014.
2. Cunningham FG, Leveno KJ, Bloom SL, Spong CY, Dashe JS, Hoffman BL et al. Williams Obstetrics 24th edition. USA: Mc Graw Hill Education; 2014.

RUPTURE UTERUS

Dr. Sabuhi Qureshi, Professor, Department of Obstetrics & Gynaecology

Mrs X, 26 year old, G5 P4 L4, unbooked, unsupervised pregnancy, reported to the emergency of a PHC with pain in abdomen for one day with cessation of pain, bleeding per vaginum for 6 hours following amenorrhea of 9 months. On examination, she was conscious, oriented and responding to verbal commands. Skin was cold, pallor +++, pulse rate – 120 per minute, feeble, B.P- 80/60 mm of mercury, respiratory rate – 30/ minute. On per abdominal examination, uterine contour was not felt, fetal parts were felt superficially. Abdomen was tender. Fetal heart sound was absent. Local examination of the external genitalia was normal, blood stains seen on thigh and legs. On per speculum examination, blood clots in vagina, bleeding coming from os, cervix vagina healthy.

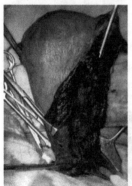

1. What is the provisional diagnosis?
   (A) Abruptio placetae
   (B) Placenta previa
   (C) Rupture uterus
   (D) Vasa previa.

2. Following are causes of rupture uterus EXCEPT
   (A) Obstructed labour
   (B) Difficult instrumental delivery.
   (C) Severe Preclampsia
   (D) External trauma.

3. Following are signs of rupture uterus EXCEPT
   (A) Hypertension
   (B) Non reassuring fetal heart rate.
   (C) Severe pallor
   (D) Abdomen is tender.

4. Incidence of uterine rupture in India is
   (A) <1 per 1000 births
   (B) 2 per 1000 births
   (C) 4 per 1000 births

(D) 7 per 1000 births

5. Following are complications of rupture uterus EXCEPT-
  (A) Maternal mortality
  (B) Couvelaire uterus
  (C) Vesicovaginal fistula
  (D) Perinatal mortality

Answers:
  1. C
      The provisional diagnosis is rupture uterus as patient has bleeding per vaginum with pain in abdomen followed by cessation of pain. On examination, loss of uterine contour with fetal parts being felt superficially and tenderness in abdomen support the diagnosis of rupture uterus.
  2. C
      Obstructed labour,Difficult instrumental delivery, External trauma are causes of rupture uterus. Severe Preclampsia does not lead to rupture uterus.
  3. A
      As a result of rupture uterus, hypotension occurs due to haemorrhage
  4. A
      Antepartum Haemorrhage. Text book of Obstetrics- J B Sharma. Avichal publishing company. First edition 2014.
  5. B
      Couvelaire uterus is seen in abruption placentae. Rest are complications associated with rupture uterus.

References:
  1. Sharma JB. Text book of obstetrics. Avichal publishing company. Sirmour (HP). 2014.
  2. Cunningham FG, Leveno KJ, Bloom SL, Spong CY, Dashe JS, Hoffman BL et al. Williams Obstetrics 24th edition. USA: Mc Graw Hill Education; 2014.

RECURRENT PREGNANCY LOSS
Dr. Seema Mehrotra, Associate Professor, Department of Obstetrics & Gynaecology

A 30 years old female G5P0+4, presented in the antenatal OPD with 16 weeks pregnancy with abdominal discomfort . She gave a past H/o recurrent pregnancy loss between 14 to 18 weeks of gestational age. On examination there was no pallor, PR 88/min, BP 130/80 mm Hg, no pedal edema, her fundal height was 16 wks. Perspeculum examination revealed the following picture-

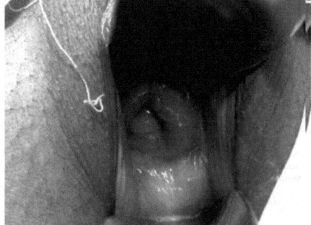

1. What is the most likely diagnosis?
  (A) Vaginal Cyst
  (B) Cervical incompetence
  (C) Cervical fibroid
  (D) Cervical cyst

2. Following are the causes of 2nd trimester pregnancy loss except
   - (A) Parental chromosomal abnormality
   - (B) Septate uterus
   - (C) Fibroid uterus
   - (D) Cervical incompetence
3. The ideal method for diagnosing cervical incompetence condition during pregnancy is
   - (A) Passage of No 8 Hegar cervical dilator
   - (B) Hysterosalpingography
   - (C) Hysteroscopy
   - (D) Trans vaginal sonography
4. Treatment of choice for cervical incompetence is
   - (A) Amputation of cervix
   - (B) Cervical cerclage
   - (C) Cauterization of cervix
   - (D) Conization of cervix
5. The most commonly performed procedure for cervical incompetence in pregnancy is
   - (A) Lash & Lash operation
   - (B) Robinson's operation
   - (C) Forthergill operation
   - (D) Mc Donalds operation

Answers:

1. B

   The pictures shows dilated cervical OS with bulging membranes suggesting of cervical incompetence

2. A

   Parental chromosomal abnormality most common balanced translocation is responsible for first trimester abortion. Risk of miscarriage is > 25%

3. D

   Trans-vaginal sonography is the ideal method to detect early incompetence during pregnancy. A cervical length less than 30 mm & an internal OS diameter more than 20 mm is suggestive of cervical incompetence. Option A&B are used to diagnose cervical incompetence during non pregnant state.

4. B

   Cervical Cerclage is the treatment of choice for cervical incompetence which makes cervix competent by use of a stitch.

5. D

   Mc Donalds operation is the most commonly performed procedure for cervical incompetence during pregnancy Lash & lash operation for cervical incompetence is done in non pregnant state Forthergill repair is the operation for prolapsed uterus Robinson's procedure is the operation for inversion uterus using abdominal approach

References:

1. Sharma JB. Text book of obstetrics. Avichal publishing company. Sirmour (HP); 2012.
2. Cunningham FG, Leveno KJ, Bloom SL, Spong CY, Dashe JS, Hoffman BL et al. Williams Obstetrics 24th edition. USA: Mc Graw Hill Education; 2014.

GESTATIONAL DIABETES MILLITUS

Dr. Seema Mehrotra, Associate Professor, Department of Obstetrics & Gynaecology

A 32 year old G4P1+2 (none alive) presented in the antenatal OPD with 26 wks pregnancy. On examination there was no pallor, PR 88/min, BP-130/86 mmHg. Systemic examination was with in normal limits. Obstetical examination revealed fundal height of 30 wks, abdomen was tense, breech presentation, FHS-136/ min. Investigation – Hb-10 gm/Blood group- A+ve, viral markers were negative, Blood sugar (2hrs after 75 gm of glucose) -198 mg%

1. What is the likely diagnosis?
   - (A) Pre-eclampsia
   - (B) Gestational hypertension
   - (C) Gestational diabetes mellitus
   - (D) Intrauterine growth restriction

2. Gestational diabetes is diagnosed when blood sugar 2 hours after 75 gm of glucose is
   - (A) > 110mg/dl
   - (B) >120mg/dl
   - (C) >130mg/dl
   - (D) >140mg/dl
3. Following are the risk factor for the development of gestational diabetes mellitus except?
   - (A) Age > 30 yrs
   - (B) Family history of diabetes mellitus
   - (C) Previous still birth
   - (D) Previous history of small for date baby
4. Most common maternal complication in pregnancy with diabetes mellitus is
   - (A) Anaemia
   - (B) Polyhydroammios
   - (C) Oligohydroammios
   - (D) Intrauterine growth restriction
5. Most specific fetal congenital malformation seen in diabetes during pregnancy is
   - (A) Gastroschisis
   - (B) Omphalocele
   - (C) Sacral agenesis
   - (D) Cystic hygroma
6. The infant of the diabetic mother is at increased risk of
   - (A) Anaemia
   - (B) Hypoglycemia
   - (C) Hypermagnesemia
   - (D) Hyperglycemia

Answers:

1. C

   According to DIPSI guidelines plasma glucose > 140mg% 2 hr after 75 gm of glucose is diagnostic of gestational diabetes mellitus.

2. D

   Gestational Diabetes Mellitus is diagnosed when blood sugar 2 hrs after 75 gm of glucose is >140mg%

3. Previous history of macrosomic baby is the risk factor rather than small for date baby. Other risk factors in history age over 30 yrs. Past history of GDM, Unexplained perinatal loss Family history of diabetes mellitus, BOH, Prior history of macrosomic baby. Previous still birth. Previous fetal anomalies.

4. B

   Most common maternal complication seen in pregnancy complicated with diabetes mellitus is polyhydramnios seen in 25-50% of the women followed by pre-eclampsia seen in 25% of the woman.

5. C

   Sacral agenesis is the most specific congenital malformation seen in diabetes during pregnancy. Other common congenital malformation seen in pregnancy with diabetes are neural tube defects, cardiovascular defects, renal anomalies, duodenal & anorectal atresia.

6. B

   Hypoglycemia, blood glucose < 45mg/dl occurs due to hyperplasia of fetal β islet cells & related to maternal blood glucose (>145 mg/dl) during labour. Other complication include hypocalcemia, hypomagnesemia, hyperbilirubinemia, RDS & polycythemia.

References:

1. Cunningham FG, Leveno KJ, Bloom SL, Spong CY, Dashe JS, Hoffman BL et al. Williams Obstetrics 24th edition. USA: Mc Graw Hill Education; 2014.
2. Sharma JB. Text book of obstetrics. Avichal publishing company. Sirmour (HP); 2012.

NST

Dr. Seema Mehrotra, Associate Professor, Department of Obstetrics & Gynaecology

A 26 years old woman G1P0+0 was admitted in labour room with diagnosis of 37 weeks pregnancy with labour pains. Her BP was110/70mmHg, PR 88/min. There was no pallor, systemic examination was within normal limits. Obstetrical examination revealed FH- 36 weeks, Cephalic presentation, head 5/5 at brim, uterine contraction present (1-2 in 10 min) FHS 140/min, liquor was adequate & estimated fetal weight was approximately 2. 8 KG .On P/S examination there was no leaking or bleeding. On P/V examination OS -2.5 cm ,Cx- 30-40% effaced, head at - 5 station, membranes present and pelvis was adequate

Cardiotocography (CTG) was done. The image of the trace in given below

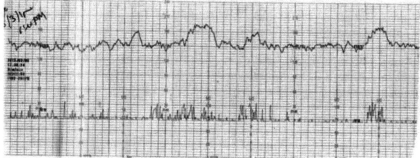

1. Following statement is true regarding cardiotography. It is a
   (A) Graphic recording of fetal heart rate is response to uterine contractions.
   (B) Graphic recording of fetal breathing in response to uterine contractions
   (C) Graphic record of fetal tone in response to uterine contractions
   (D) Graphic record of fetal movement in response to uterine contractions
2. Following are the components of CTG trace except
   (A) Baseline fetal heart rate
   (B) Baseline variability
   (C) Uterine contractions
   (D) Amniotic fluid index
3. In the given trace the baseline fetal heart rate is
   (A) 120 bpm
   (B) 130 bpm
   (C) 140 bpm
   (D) 150 bpm
4. In the given trace beat to beat variability is
   (A) 2-5 bpm
   (B) 5-10 bpm
   (C) 10-20 bpm
   (D) 20-30 bpm
5. Considering the interpretation of normal/ reassuring CTG following statement is false
   (A) Baseline fetal heart rate should be between 120-160 bpm
   (B) Baseline variability should be < 5 beats per min
   (C) There should be no decelerations
   (D) Two or more acceleration of fetal heart rate of > 15 beats/ min lasting for at least 15 sec within a 20 min period
6. Considering all the components of CTG, the given CTG is
   (A) Normal/ Reassuring
   (B) Suspicious
   (C) Pathological/ Non reassuring
   (D) None of the above

Answers:
   1. A
      CTG is based on the response of the fetal heart rate to uterine contraction. It is believed that fetal oxygenation will be transiently worsened by uterine contraction halting uterine blood flow which can be tolerated by a healthy fetus.
   2. D
      Aminotic fluid index is a part of biophysical profile & not CTG
   3. D

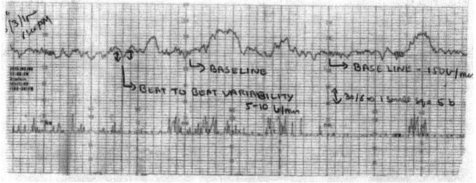

4. B
5. B
   Baseline variability should be > 5 bpm
6. A

References:

1. Cunningham FG, Leveno KJ, Bloom SL, Spong CY, Dashe JS, Hoffman BL et al. Williams Obstetrics 24th edition. USA: Mc Graw Hill Education; 2014.
2. Sharma JB. Text book of obstetrics. Avichal publishing company. Sirmour (HP); 2012.

INFERTILITY

Dr. Smriti Agrawal, Associate Professor, Department of Obstetrics & Gynaecology

A 28 years old woman presented to the OPD with history of inability to conceive for 6 years. She has been cohabiting since then & has regular menstrual cycles with no other concomitant illness. Investigations reveal a normal semen examination of her husband. Her HSG shows the following picture

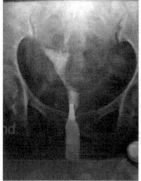

1. HSG Shows
   (A) Uterine cavity is normal with bilateral patent tubes
   (B) Uterine cavity is normal with bilateral fimbrial block
   (C) Uterine cavity is normal with bilateral cornual block
   (D) Uterine cavity small with bilateral blocked tubes
2. What is the confirmatory test for tubal blockade?
   (A) Sonosalpingography
   (B) Diagnostic laproscopy
   (C) Laparoscopic Chromopertubation
   (D) Hysteroscopy
3. The therapeutic option for proximal tubal block include all **EXCEPT**
   (A) Transfallopian tube catheterization
   (B) Bilateral cornual implantation

332

(C) Invitro fertilization
(D) Intrauterine insemination
4. The possible causative organism for this condition are all **EXCEPT**
    (A) Mycobacterium Tuberculosis
    (B) Neisseria gonorrhea
    (C) Chlamydia trachomatis
    (D) Salmonella typhi
5. Which of the most diagnostic test for genital tuberculosis?
    (A) Endometrial aspirate for mycobacterium tuberculosis
    (B) Tuberculin skin testing
    (C) Antibodies against mycobacterium tuberculosis
    (D) Chest X-ray

Answers:

1. C
    The basic investigation that should ideally be performed before starting any infertility treatment are
    Semen analysis, Confirmation of ovulation, Tubal patency
    Tubal factor accounts for 25-35% of cases of infertility. HSG (Hysterosalpnigography) involves instillation of radio opaque dye (urograffin 76%) under fluoroscopy to visualize uterine cavity, fallopian tube architecture, & tubal patency. The sensitivity & specificity of HSG for bilateral tubal patency is 86.5% & 79.8% & for bilateral tubal occlusion is 90% & 97% respectively.
2. C
    Laparoscopic chromopertubation is the gold standard test for tubal patency
3. D
    Proximal tubal blockade can be treated by proximal tubal catheterization bilateral cornual implantation, Invitro fertilization. Intrauterine insemination requires patent tubes.
4. D
    Chlamydia trachomatis & Neisseria gonorrhea are common pathogens associated with PID & in infertility mycobacterium tuberculosis also leads to tubal blockade
5. A
    Genital TB is diagnosed by endometrial aspirate for mycobacterium tuberculosis. Tuberculin skin testing has poor sensitivity (55%) to diagnose genital TB. Antibodies testing is not recommended Chest X ray is used to detect if pulmonary TB is also present along with genital TB.

Reference:

1. Bereck J S. Bereck Novak's Gynaecology. 15th edition. Gurgaon: Wolters Kluwer; 2012.

PARTOGRAM OF NORMAL LABOR
Dr. Smriti Agrawal, Associate Professor, Department of Obstetrics & Gynaecology

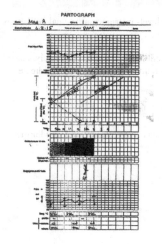

Mrs A 28 yrs old primigravida at 39 wks pregnancy in labour admitted to labor room at 8 am. The partogram is plotted as below

1. What should be the management at admission?
   (A) Reassure the patient with no further monitoring required
   (B) Reassure the patient with regular monitoring & PV examination every 4 hrs
   (C) Reassure the patient with regular monitoring & PV examination every 2 hrs
   (D) Start oxytocin infusion
2. After 4 hours, PV examination shows cervical dilation of 9 cm & head at 0 station Her FHR is 140 beats per minute with clear liquor. What is the next management?
   (A) Increase oxytocin infusion
   (B) Shift for LSCS in view of slow progress of labor
   (C) Shift for instrumental vaginal delivery
   (D) Allow for further progress of labor
3. If FHR after 2 hours decreases to 60 bpm & the station of the head is +3 with thick meconium stained liquor, What should be the next management?
   (A) Stop oxytocin & give uterine relaxant
   (B) Shift for LSCS
   (C) Shift for instrumental vaginal delivery
   (D) Allow for spontaneous vaginal delivery
4. Describe the contractions at 6 cm cervical dilatation
   (A) 3 contraction of <20 s duration
   (B) 3 contraction of 20-40 s duration
   (C) 3 contraction of >40 s duration
   (D) 4 contraction of >40 s duration
5. How is head plotted at partogram
   (A) Perabdominal examination every hour
   (B) Pervaginal examination every hour
   (C) Perabdominal examination every 4 hourly
   (D) Pervaginal examination every 4 hourly

Answers:
1.   B
      Partogram involves graphic representation of the labor events including maternal vitals & cervical assessment, descent of head, uterine contractions their frequency & duration
      It involves maternal pulse rate, uterine contraction, FHR assessment every 30 min. Cervical assessment should be done pervaginally every 4 hrs.
2.   D
      Since the patient has progressed well & her partograph line is to the left of alert line with normal fetal heart rate & good uterine contraction, patient can be left for spontaneous progress of labor.
3.   C
      The dilatation after 2 hours is full & as the station is at +3 level- instrumental vaginal delivery is attempted.
4.   B
      Slanting line in the boxes indicates the duration of contraction 20-40 sec & completely shaded boxes indicates contraction lasting more than 40 sec. The number of boxes shaded indicate the number of contraction in 10 min.
5.   C
      Descent of head is also plotted every 4 hrs per abdominally & not pervaginally.

Reference:
1.   Mathai M, Sanghvi H, Guidotti R J. Managing complications in pregnancy and childbirth : A guide for midwives and doctors. 2nd edition. WHO 2002.

PARTOGRAM OF ABNORMAL LABOR

Dr. Smriti Agrawal, Associate Professor, Department of Obstetrics & Gynaecology

Mrs B 30 yrs old Gravida 3 with previous 2 term vaginal deliveries at 40 wks 2 day pregnancy admitted to labor room at 5 cm cervical dilatation & head 5/5 palpable above brim. The partogram is plotted below. She had leaking per vaginum for last 7 hours.

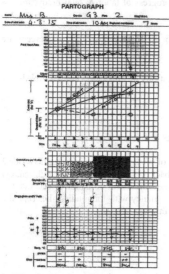

1. What is the plan of management at admission?
   (A) Watch for spontaneous progress of labor
   (B) Start oxytocin infusion
   (C) Do PV examination every 1 hr for progress of labour
   (D) Shift for LSCS as head 5/5 palpable
2. At 2 PM cervix is 7 cm dilated & head 4/5 palpable above brim. Next plan of management is
   (A) Shift for LSCS due to slow progress of labour
   (B) Continue to keep the patient hydrated & continue oxytocin infusion
   (C) Only hydrate the patient
   (D) Increase oxytocin infusion till patient delivery
3. On evaluation at 7 cm cervical dilatation, what factors are not present
   (A) Liquor is meconium stained
   (B) Fetal Heart rate 130-140 bpm
   (C) Absence of moulding of fetal head
   (D) Head 5/5 palpable
4. At 6 PM, cervix is 8 cm dilated with head 4/5 palpable above brim. What should be the next management?
   (A) Continue oxytocin infusion till delivery
   (B) Stop oxytocin infusion till delivery
   (C) Repeat PV after 2 hrs for further management
   (D) Shift for LSCS
5. What is the cause of abnormal labor?
   (A) Slow progress of labor
   (B) Uterine inertia
   (C) Obstructed labor
   (D) Rupture uterus

Answers:
   1. B
      Partogram is plotted only in active labor. If woman admitted to labor room at > 4 cm cervical dilatation, it should be plotted at the corresponding number or alert line. Oxytocin is initiated as the uterine contractions are < 20 sec duration.
   2. B

The patient shows slow progress of labor & with good uterine contraction & normal fetal heart rate. Partograph line is between alert & action line. Patient to be reevaluated to confirm fetal position & rule out cephalopelvic disproportion. If there is no contraindication keep the patient hydrated & continue oxytocin infusion to watch further progress of labor.

3. A
4. D

As the partograph line has crossed action line with poor progress of labor & fetal bradycardia is present, shift for cesarean section.

5. C

Presence of grade 3 moulding with poor progress of labor & no change in cervical descent are features suggestive of obstructed labor.

Reference:

1. Mathai M, Sanghvi H, Guidotti R J. Managing complications in pregnancy and childbirth : A guide for midwives and doctors. 2nd edition. WHO 2002.

PPROM

Dr. SP Jaiswar, Professor, Department of Obstetrics & Gynaecology

25 years G_3P_{2+0} with 32 weeks pregnancy came to hospital with history of watery discharge per vaginum for 2 hrs. She has two full term normal vaginal deliveries 5 years and 3 years back with alive and healthy children. On examination, her general examination was normal, Pulse, temp, BP were normal with no pallor or oedema. On obstetric examination- fundal height was corresponding to 30 weeks pregnancy with longitudinal lie, cephalic presentation and normal fetal heart sound. P/S- Clear fluid seen coming through OS.

1. What is your diagnosis
   (A) Preterm labor
   (B) Pre labor rupture of membrane
   (C) Preterm Prelabor rupture of membrane
   (D) Patient is having urinary incontinence
2. Incidence of PROM is
   (A) 2-8%
   (B) 8-10%
   (C) 10-12%
   (D) 12-15%
3. What is the commonest cause of PROM
   (A) Unstable lie
   (B) Polyhydramnios
   (C) Weakness of chorion and amnion
   (D) Incompetent cervix
4. How will you manage this case
   (A) Expectant management
   (B) Antibiotics
   (C) Antibiotics and cortico steroids then induction of labor
   (D) Induction of labor
5. What complication may occur due to prolonged PPROM
   (A) A Chorio amnionitis
   (B) B IUGR
   (C) C Meconium Aspiration Syndrome
   (D) D Malpresentation

Answers:

1. C
    PPROM
    As her pregnancy is less than 37 weeks and she has come with history of leaking.
2. C
    2-8%
    PPROM is 2-4% while PROM is 8%
3. C
    Weakness of chorion and amnion, it may be due to inflammatory causes or developmental anomalies.

4. C

   Antibiotics and corticosteroids as pregnancy is less than 34 weeks.
5. A

   Chorio amnionitis – due to infection

Reference:

1. Daftary SN, Chakravarti S. Manual of obstetrics Updated edition of the classic Holland & Brews Manual of Obstetrics. 3rd edition. New Delhi:Elsevier;2011.

ECLAMPSIA

Dr. SP Jaiswar, Professor, Department of Obstetrics & Gynaecology

A 26 years primigravida with 34 weeks pregnancy came to hospital from a remote area in altered sensorium with history of recurrent convulsions for last six hours. She was complaining of severe headache, nausea, vomiting, epigastric pain before onset of convulsion. She did not receive any antenatal checkup except two doses of tetanus toxoid. On general examination she was responding to deep stimuli, had frothing from mouth with tongue bite. Blood pressure was 160/110 mm of Hg. On obstetrical examination- fundal height was 34 weeks with cephalic presentation and normal fetal heart rate .She was not in labor. On investigation- her Hb% 10 gm% with thrombocytopenia present in GBP with deranged LFT and KFT and urine albumin +++

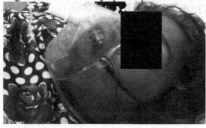

1. What is the most likely diagnosis?
   - (A) Epilepsy
   - (B) Encephalitis
   - (C) Eclampsia
   - (D) Meningitis
2. Which is not a feature of HELLP syndrome?
   - (A) Thrombocytopenia
   - (B) Eosinophillia
   - (C) Raised liver enzyme
   - (D) Haemolytic anaemia
3. Preferred anti- convulsant drugs used in Eclampsia patients is-
   - (A) Phenytoin
   - (B) Magnesium sulphate
   - (C) Diazepam
   - (D) Lytic cocktail
4. Which antihypertensive is the drug of choice in eclampsia-
   - (A) Labetalol
   - (B) Metoprolol
   - (C) Alphamethyl dopa
   - (D) Lisinopril
5. Following should be checked before giving next dose of Magnesium Sulphate EXCEPT-
   - (A) Urinary output
   - (B) Respiratory rate
   - (C) Pulse rate
   - (D) Patellar reflex

Answers:

1. C

   Eclampsia

As the patient is pregnant, has high blood pressure and history of seizures, the most probable diagnosis is eclampsia
2. B
   HELLP syndrome is a variant of severe pre-eclampsia comprising of Hemolysis, Elevated liver enzyme & Low Platelet count
3. B
   Magnesium sulphate is the drug of choice because it does not affect fetus, it is safe for mother and newborn.
4. A
   Labetalol it is more effective & has less side effects and available in both oral & parenteral preparation.
5. C
   Pulse rate is not affected by magnesium level in blood.

Reference:
1. Daftary SN, Chakravarti S. Manual of obstetrics Updated edition of the classic Holland & Brews Manual of Obstetrics. 3rd edition. New Delhi:Elsevier;2011.

ABNORMAL PEURPERIUM
Dr. SP Jaiswar, Professor, Department of Obstetrics & Gynaecology

24 Years Primipara delivered a 3 kg live male baby. The delivery was conducted by dai at home two days back. She came to hospital with history of high grade fever with chills. There is also history of leaking per vaginum for 3 days before delivery she had no antenatal checkup & received only two injections of tetanus toxoid.
On examination- temperature was 104^0 F , pulse rate 120/min, BP 110/80 mm of Hg pallor+, uterus 20 weeks size, tender, lochia foul smelling with vulval and perineal laceration. On investigation Hb% 8 gm, TLC18000 cell/3mm, P_{74}, L_{20}, E_6, M_0, KFT,LFT normal.

1. What is your provisional diagnosis
    (A) Urinary tract infection
    (B) Malaria
    (C) Puerperal sepsis
    (D) Typhoid
2. What is the commonest organism responsible for the puerperal sepsis
    (A) Doderlein bacili
    (B) Escherichia Coli
    (C) Streptococcus group
    (D) Fungi
3. Which important investigation should be sent before starting the antibiotics
    (A) Hb, TLC, DLC
    (B) Urine Culture
    (C) Lochia culture
    (D) Blood culture
4. What antibiotics should be started immediately till report of culture comes
    (A) Ampicilline
    (B) Cefetriaxone
    (C) Gentamycin
    (D) Cefetriaxone, Gentamycin, Metronidazole
5. Antibiotic should be continued till -
    (A) Patient becomes afebrile
    (B) 48 hours after patient becomes afebrile
    (C) 5 days patient becomes afebrile
    (D) 7 days patient becomes afebrile

Answers:
1. C
   Puerperal sepsis
   As she is having history of prolonged leaking, delivery at home by dai and lochia foul smelling with increased TLC
2. C
   Streptococcus group

They are present in vagina and cervix as endogenous infection anaerobic streptococci, streptococcus haemolyticus as directly or hematogenous from throat.

3. C

Lochia culture because Lochia is foul smelling, showing signs of infection.

4. D

Broad spectrum antibiotics should be started to cover Gram positive, Gram negative and anaerobic bacteria.

5. B

Antibiotic should be continued till 48 hrs after patient become afebrile.

Reference:

1. Daftary SN, Chakravarti S. Manual of obstetrics Updated edition of the classic Holland & Brews Manual of Obstetrics. 3rd edition. New Delhi:Elsevier;2011.

CAESAREAN SECTION
Dr. Sujata, Professor, Department of Obstetrics & Gynaecology

Mrs X, 24 yrs old G1P0+0 admitted at 38 weeks pregnancy with C/o pain in abdomen for 2 days. On P/A-Fundal Heightc full term, cephalic presentation, FHS-110/min, irregular. Non stress Test (NST) shows loss of beat to beat variability, no acceleration & no deceleration. On P/V examination Cervix 2 cm dilated 30-40% effaced, membranes were present.

1. What will be the best management option for above patient?
   (A) Expectant management
   (B) Cesarean section
   (C) Augmentation of labour and vaginal delivery
   (D) Augmentation of labour and forcep delivery

2. Absolute indication for cesarean section is
   (A) Dystocia
   (B) Breech presentation
   (C) Fetal distress
   (D) H/o previous rupture of uterus

3. During cesarean section, how will you identify the lower segment of uterus:
   (A) Loose attachment of visceral peritoneum
   (B) Dilated venous sinus
   (C) Thinness of lower segment as compared to the upper segment
   (D) Deflection of uterine artery towards upper segment

4. In which condition 'VBAC' is possible
   (A) Previous classical cesarean section
   (B) H/o vaginal bleeding is present in pregnancy
   (C) Breech presentation in previous pregnancy
   (D) H/o contracted pelvis in previous pregnancy

5. Which is the most common intraoperative complication during LSCS
   (A) Anesthetic complications
   (B) Extention of uterine incision
   (C) Bladder andurethral injuries
   (D) Gastrointestinal injuries

Answers :

1. B

   Caesarean section because irregular fetal heart rate & non reactive NST shows intrauterine fetal jeopardy.

2. D

   H/O previous repair of rupture uterus chances of dehiscence of uterine scar in normal delivery is to high so elective caesarean section is recommended.

3. A

   Identification of loose attachment of visceral peritoneum (uterovesical fold) over lower segment of uterus identifies the lower uterine segment.

4. C

   breech presentation in previous pregnancy is not contraindication to VBAC.

5. B

   Extension of uterine incision in difficult delivery of head is the most common complication

Reference:
1. Cunningham FG, Leveno KJ, Bloom SL, Spong CY, Dashe JS, Hoffman BL et al. Williams Obstetrics 24th edition. USA: Mc Graw Hill Education; 2014.

ECTOPIC PREGNANCY

Dr. Sujata, Professor, Department of Obstetrics & Gynaecology

Mrs X, 28 years old G1P0+0, presented with 8 weeks amenorrhea with pain in lower abdomen and H/o fainting attacks. On examination pallor +++, BP-80/40mnHg, Pulse 110/min. Tenderness +nt in lower abdomen. On P/S examination slight bleeding through os. On P/V examination marked cervical movement tenderness was present, the exact size of uterus could not be assessed. On USG marked fluid was present in pouch of douglas.

1. What is the most probable diagnosis?
   - (A) Ruptured ovarian cyst
   - (B) Ruptured ectopic pregnancy
   - (C) Red degeneration of fibroid
   - (D) Pelvic abscess
2. First diagnostic test in case of ruptured ectopic pregnancy
   - (A) Culdocentesis
   - (B) Serial β-HCG
   - (C) Transvaginal USG
   - (D) Serum Progesterone
3. In which part of fallopian tube is ectopic pregnancy most common?
   - (A) Ampulla
   - (B) Isthmus
   - (C) Infundibulum
   - (D) Interstitial
4. Medical treatment of ectopic pregnancy is contraindicated if
   - (A) h/o previous ectopic pregnancy
   - (B) Sac size is 3 cm
   - (C) Serum β HCG level < 3000IU/L
   - (D) Presence of fetal heart activity
5. In a nulliparous women treatment of choice in ruptured ectopic pregnancy is
   - (A) Salpingo-oophorectomy
   - (B) Linear salpingostomy
   - (C) Partial Salpingectomy and end to end anastomosis
   - (D) Subtotal hysterectomy

Answers:
1. B
   The classical H/Oacute abdominal pain with fainting attackandcollapse associated with feature of intraabdominal hemorrhage in women of child bearing age is ruptured ectopic pregnancy unless proven otherwise
2. C
   The diagnostic feature of transvaginal USG are absence of intrauterine pregnancy, adnexal mass separated from ovary,fluid in pouch of douglus and sometime cardiac activity in unruptured ectopic pregnancy
3. D
   Ampulla is wildest portion (5 cm in length) of fallopian tube, so more chance to occur ectopic pregnancy in this part.
4. D
   Presence of fetal heart activity because there is increased risk of tubal rupture
5. C
   Salpingectomy and end to end anastomosis.

Reference:
1. Cunningham FG, Leveno KJ, Bloom SL, Spong CY, Dashe JS, Hoffman BL et al. Williams Obstetrics 24th edition. USA: Mc Graw Hill Education; 2014.

PUBERTY MENORRHAGIA

Dr. Sujata, Professor, Department of Obstetrics & Gynaecology

A 15 years old unmarried girl is brought to the clinic with c/o bleeding per vaginum for 20 days following 4 months amenorrhea. She attained menarche at 12 years of age. Her prior menstrual cycles were irregular, she menstruated for 10-15 days every 2-3 months. She complains of weakness. On examination pallor ++ and on local examination bleeding P/V present.

1. What is the most likely diagnosis
   - (A) Puberty menorrhagia
   - (B) Endometriosis
   - (C) Normal menstrual cycle
   - (D) Pelvic congestion syndrome
2. All of the following will be first line investigations in this patient EXCEPT:
   - (A) Haemogram
   - (B) Platelet count
   - (C) EUA(examination under anasthesia)
   - (D) USG
3. Most common cause of puberty menorrhagia is
   - (A) Bleeding disorders
   - (B) Anovulation
   - (C) Endometriosis
   - (D) Malignancy
4. All of the following are common treatment options for puberty menorrhagia EXCEPT:
   - (A) Progesterone
   - (B) Estrogen and progesterone
   - (C) Surgery
   - (D) Danazole
5. A patient with amenorrhea had bleeding after giving progesterone. This implies all of the following EXCEPT
   - (A) Sufficient estrogen production
   - (B) Ovulatory cycles
   - (C) Patient outflow tract
   - (D) Intact endometrium

Answers:
1. A
   Puberty menorrhagia in which adolescents have irregular period following menarche due to anovulatory cycles
2. C
   First line investigations are noninvasive to rule out common causes. EUA is done only is bleeding persist & no cause can be found.
3. B
   Anovulation is the commonest cause in earlier age(1-5 yr) of menarche due to dysfunction of H-P-O axis
4. C
   Puberty menorrhagia is mainly due to hormonal imbalance so medical treatment with hormone is more effective unless proven otherwise
5. B
   As it indicate normal H-P-O axis and uterus is sufficiently primed with estrogen.

Reference:
1. Padubidri V G, Dasftary S N. Hawkins & Bourne Shaw's. Text book of Gynaecology. 15th edition. New Delhi:Elsevier; 2011.

HEART DISEASE IN PREGNANCY

Dr. Uma Singh, Professor, Department of Obstetrics & Gynaecology

A 25 year old woman Mrs R, gravida 1 para 0, presented with 32 weeks of pregnancy with breathlessness on her day to day activities for past 15 days. She had history of fever with joint pains in childhood. On examination her pulse rate was 108/ min, BP 120/80, mild pallor, pedal edema and there was mid diastolic murmur at the apex of the heart. The obstetric examination suggested 32weeks size live fetus in longitudinal lie and cephalic presentation.

1. What is the clinical diagnosis?
   - (A) Pregnancy with anaemia
   - (B) Pregnancy with URTI
   - (C) Pregnancy with rheumatic heart disease
   - (D) Pregnancy with preeclampsia
2. All are the critical periods during pregnancy when the patient may go in heart failure EXCEPT
   - (A) 6-8 weeks of pregnancy
   - (B) 20-24 weeks of pregnancy
   - (C) 30-34 weeks of pregnancy
   - (D) Immediately delivery
3. Patient with cardiac disease is comfortable at rest but gets breathless by minimal physical activity. She is in NYHA
   - (A) Class 4
   - (B) Class 3
   - (C) Class 2
   - (D) Class 1
4. Third stage of labour in patients with heart disease has to be actively managed by
   - (A) 10 unit oxytocin IM
   - (B) 10 units of oxytocin IV
   - (C) 0.2 mg of ergometrine IM
   - (D) 0.2 mg of ergometrine IV
5. The method of contraception which is contra indicated in woman with heart disease is
   - (A) Barrier method
   - (B) Ligation by mini laparotomy
   - (C) Depot medroxy progesterone acetate
   - (D) Combined oral pills

Answers:

1. C

   Rheumatic infection in childhood presents as valvular disease in adults which often in women becomes apparent during pregnancy. The commnest is mitral stenosis which is diagnosed by mid diastolic murmur

2. B

   During pregnancy due to hemodynamic and cardiovascular changes which are more at certain periods in pregnancy, there is risk of cardiac failure with heart disease. These critical period are 6-8 weeks and 30-34 weeks of pregnancy, second stage of labour, immediately after delivery and second week of puerperium.

3. B

   NYHA class of patient is according of symptoms, occurring in relation to physical activity.
   Class 1- Uncompromised, no symptom on ordinary activity
   Class 2- Slightly compromised, symptom on ordinary activity
   Class 3- markedly compromised, symptom on less than ordinary activity but not at rest
   Class 4- severely compromised symptom at rest.

4. B

   Ergometrine is contraindicated as it leads to strong uterine contraction and hence sudden overloading of heart resulting in cardiac failure IV bolus of oxytocin is avoided due to the sudden hypotension it may cause.

5. D

   Combined oral pills are contraindicated in women with heart desease as they can precipitate thrombo embolism.

References:

1. Cunningham FG, Leveno KJ, Bloom SL, Spong CY, Dashe JS, Hoffman BL et al. Williams Obstetrics 24th edition. USA: Mc Graw Hill Education; 2014.
2. Sharma JB. Text book of obstetrics. Avichal publishing company. Sirmour (HP). 2012.

CARCINOMA CERVIX

Dr. Uma Singh, Professor, Department of Obstetrics & Gynaecology

Mrs R, a 52 year old, para 4 presents with foul smelling discharge per vaginum for past 4 months. She attained menopause 3 years back and her menstrual history preceding menopause was normal. However on asking she does give history of post coital bleeding for past 6 months. On examination her general condition is fair except for mild pallor and all systems are within normal limits. On per speculum examination there is an irregular, friable growth replacing the cervix, measuring 3X3 cms. The vaginal walls are normal. On pervaginum examination same growth was felt to be soft and irregular, uterus is anteverted normal size and parametrium is free of any involvement. The per rectal examination confirms these findings.

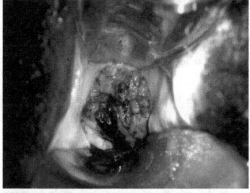

1. What is the probable clinical condition?
   (A) Cervical Polyp
   (B) Uterine fibroid
   (C) Carcinoma Cervix
   (D) Uterine inversion
2. What investigation is required to confirm the diagnosis?
   (A) Cervical biopsy
   (B) Ultra Sonography
   (C) MRI
   (D) Colposcopy
3. What is the stage of the disease?
   (A) Ia_1
   (B) Ia_2
   (C) Ib_1
   (D) Ib_2
4. What is the treatment of choice for this stage of disease
   (A) Radical Hysterectomy
   (B) Radiotherapy
   (C) Chemotherapy
   (D) Chemoradiation
5. Cancer cervix in micro invasive stage, in a young woman who wants to preserve uterus for fertility purpose, can be treated by
   (A) Large loop excision of transformation zone
   (B) Radical trachelectomy
   (C) Extrafascial Hysterectomy
   (D) Radical Hysterectomy

Answers:

1. C

An irregular, friable growth in elderly age group women, associated with foul smelling discharge, most commonly is due to carcinoma cervix. History of postcoital bleeding adds to the probability of its being malignancy.

2. A

Histopathological examination of cervical biopsy specimen will confirm the diagnosis. Colposcopy is not indicated if growth is seen on cervix. Imaging methods like ultrasonography and MRI can suggest extent of disease spread but disease can be confirmed only by HPE.

3. C

According to FIGO staging of cancer cervix, disease strictly confined to cervix, visible to naked eye examination is categorized in stage Ib. Further if the size of the lesion does not exceed 4 cm, it is of stage Ib1 but if it exceeds 4 cm it is of stage Ib2

4. A

Cancer cervix, stage Ib_1 can be optimally treated by radical hysterectomy which includes removal of uterus, tubes and ovaries of both sides, upper one third of vagina, parametrium and pelvic lymphadenectomy. Radiotherapy can be advised if the woman is not fit for surgery or if surgical facility or skill is not available.

5. B

Radical trachelectomy can be done if the disease is in FIGO (stage Ia_2)or stage Ib_1 and fertility has to be preserved. This includes removal of cervix, with vaginal cuff (2cm) along with paracervical tissue. This can be done by laparoscopic, vaginal or open abdominal route. A close follow-up is required.

Reference:

1. Berek J S. Berek & Novak's Gynaecology. 15th edition. New Delhi: Wolter Kluwer; 2012.

PREINVASIVE LESIONS OF CERVIX

Dr. Uma Singh, Professor, Department of Obstetrics & Gynaecology

A 32 year old, nulliparous woman, sex worker by profession is motivated to undergo cytological screening by Pap smear by an NGO. Cytological report according to Bethesda system suggests high grade squamous intraepithelial lesion (HSIL)

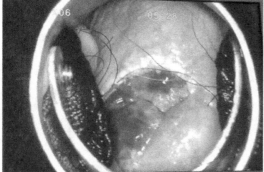

1. HSIL reported in pap smear examination should be followed by
   (A) Repeat cytology
   (B) Colposcopy
   (C) Conization
   (D) Hysterectomy
2. Colposcopic examination findings which suggest high grade lesion are
   (A) Acetowhite area with irregular, blurred margins
   (B) Acetowhite area with fine punctuation
   (C) Acetowhite area with coarse punctuation
   (D) Acetowhite area away from SCZ
3. Which virus has been reported to be associated with causation of cancer cervix?
   (A) HPV

(B) HSV
(C) HCV
(D) CMV

4. Cervical Intraepithelial Neoplasia III should be treated by
   (A) Chemical cautery
   (B) Large loop excision of transformation zone
   (C) Conization
   (D) Hysterectomy

5. Following is true with reference to cervical intraepithelical neoplasia (CIN)
   (A) 50% of CIN 1 progress to CIN II
   (B) 50% of CIN 2 progress to CIN III
   (C) 20% of CIN II progress to invasive cancer
   (D) 20% of CIN III progress to invasive cancer

Answers:

1. B

   HSIL is a cytological report and should always be followed by histological confirmation. Colposcopy helps in visualizing the cervix under illumination and magnification hence biopsy can been taken from appropriate site. This helps in correct management of premalignant lesions of cervix.

2. C

   Colposcopic examination can delineate areas showing metaplastic and dysplastic changes. Dense acetowhite area near SCJ with sharp margins, and or coarse punctuation, coarse mosaic or abnormal blood vessels, suggests high grade lesion.

3. A

   Human Papilloma Virus has been reported to play an important role in development of malignant changes in cervical epithelium and is found to be present in almost 99% cases of CIN and invasive cancers. HPV types with high oncogenic risk are types 16, 18,31, 33, 35, 45, 56. Clinical application of this fact is HPV testing for early detection and HPV vaccine for primary prevention

4. B

   Large Loop Excision of Transformation Zone (LLETZ) can remove cervical tissue up to a depth of 10 mm hence is ideal for treatment CIN III. The tissue received can be subjected to histopathological examination for further confirmation and to rule out focal invasive disease.

5. D

   Natural history of CIN suggests that there is high rate of regression of CIN to normal and this rate of regression is 60% - CIN I, 40% - CIN II, 30% - CIN III –. It is important to note that progression to invasive cancer is only < 1% in CIN 1, 5% in CIN II and 20% in CIN III. This understanding is helpful in appropriate management and in avoiding unnecessary over treatment.

Reference:

1. Berek J S. Berek & Novak's Gynaecology. 15th edition. New Delhi: Wolter Kluwer; 2012.

CONTRACEPTION

Dr. Urmila Singh, Professor, Department of Obstetrics & Gynaecology

Mrs X a 27 year old mother of two children, last delivery 2 year back, visits family planning OPD for contraception. She has history of menorrhagia and dysmenorrhoea. There is no other significant systemic and chronic illness and no history of any medication. Her BP is 120/70 mm Hg, BMI 27 kg/m^2, Hb 10 gm%. On perspeculum and pervaginal examination no abnormality is present.

1. Which of the following contraceptive is contraindicated for Mrs. X?

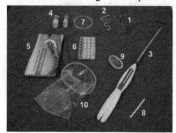

2. Which of the following is non steroidal contraceptive?
   (A) Combined Oral Pills
   (B) Mini Pills
   (C) Centchroman
   (D) Triphasic contraceptive pills
3. One of the following is NOT a barrier method of contraceptive
   (A) Femshield
   (B) Today
   (C) Lactational Amenorrhoea method
   (D) Spermicidal gel
4. Mrs X opts Depot injection what is the dose and route of injection DMPA
   (A) 150 mg intramuscular 2 monthly
   (B) 150 mg subcutaneous 3 monthly
   (C) 200 mg intramuscular3 monthly
   (D) 150 mg intramuscular 3 monthly
5. All of the following are only progestogen contraceptive EXCEPT
   (A) Norplant
   (B) LNG IUS
   (C) Nuva Ring
   (D) Norethisteron Enanthate
6. Which of the following is NOT an acceptable time to insert an IUCD
   (A) 20 min after expulsion of placenta
   (B) 36 hours postpartum
   (C) 2 weeks postpartum
   (D) 6 weeks after delivery

Answers:

1. 1 & 2
   Dysmenorrhoea and menorrhagia are side effects of copper T
   1. Copper T
   2. Lippe's Loop
   3. LNG – IUD
   4. Depot injection
   5. Progestogen only pill
   6. COC's
   7. NUVA Ring
   8. Subdermal Implant
   9. Male Condom
   10. Femshield
2. C
   Centchroman is a synthetic non steroidal contraceptive. It is taken 30 mg on 1st day of menses then taken twice weekly for 12 weeks and weekly thereafter
3. C
   LAM is a natural method of contraception. It is appropriate for 6 months, postpartum women who are fully breastfeeding their infants and are amenorrhoeic
4. D
   DMPA (Depomedroxy Progesteron Acetate) it is given 150 mg deep intramuscular three monthly
5. C
   NUVA Ring, a soft vaginal ring contains both estrogen and progesterone. It releases 15μg of ethinyl estradial and 120 μg of etonogestrel daily over a period of 21 days.
6. C
   Increase risk of uterine perforation after 48 hrs to less than 6 weeks postpartum period.

References:

1. Sharma JB. Text book of obstetrics. Avichal publishing company. Sirmour (HP). 2012.
2. Padubidri V G, Dasftary S N. Hawkins & Bourne Shaw's. Text book of Gynaecology. 15th edition. New Delhi: Elsevier; 2011.

FEMALE STERILIZATION (LIGATION)

Dr. Urmila Singh, Professor, Department of Obstetrics & Gynaecology

A 32 years old mother of 3 children, last delivery 1 year back, has come to family planning OPD for permanent contraception. Her menstrual cycle is normal and last menstrual period was 5 days back. She has no significant medical and surgical history. On examination no pallor pulse 80/min, BP 110/70 mm Hg systemic examination, perspeculum and pervaginal examination are within normal limit, Hb 11 gm%, random blood sugar 110mg/dl.

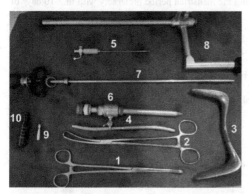

1. The above instruments shown in photograph are used in which technique of female sterilization
   - (A) Minilaparotomy
   - (B) Postpartum ligation
   - (C) Laparoscopic ligation
   - (D) Vaginal ligation
2. Ideal time for tubal ligation operation
   - (A) Follicular phase
   - (B) Luteal phase
   - (C) Premenstrual phase
   - (D) Ovulatory phase
3. Ideal gas for creation of pneumoperitoneum in laparoscopic ligation
   - (A) Carbon dioxide
   - (B) Nitrous oxide
   - (C) Oxygen
   - (D) Air
4. Technique used in Laparoscopic ligation is
   - (A) Pomeroy's
   - (B) Banded by silastic ring
   - (C) Madlender
   - (D) Uchida
5. Following are the methods of tubal occlusion in laparoscopic sterilization EXCEPT
   - (A) Falope ring
   - (B) ESSURE Microinsert
   - (C) Filshie clip
   - (D) Electro coagulation
6. The site of the occlusion of fallopian tube must be
   - (A) 2-3 cm from uterine cornua
   - (B) 2-3 cm from fimbrial end
   - (C) 5-6 cm from uterine cornua
   - (D) 2cm from ampullary end

Answers:
   1. C
      1. Sponge holder
      2. Valsellum
      3. Speculum
      4. Dilater

5. Veres needle
6. Trochar and Cannula
7. Laparocator
8. Laparoscope
9. Falope ring and loader
10. Pusher

2. A

The ideal time for tubal ligation is following the menstrual period preferably with in 7-10 days of period in follicular phase

3. A

CO_2 is safer than air and nitrous oxide and oxygen. Which can cause air embolism and accidental explosion respectively.

4. B

Silastic ring (Falope ring) made of silicon rubber with 5% barium sulphate. It is radio opaque.

5. B

ESSURE Microinsert occluds the cornual end of fallopian tube. It is inserted with the help of hysteroscope.

6. A

It is highly reversible if needed

Reference:
1. Sharma JB. Text book of obstetrics. Avichal publishing company. Sirmour (HP); 2012.

HIV POSITIVE PREGNANCY
Dr. Urmila Singh, Professor, Department of Obstetrics & Gynaecology

Mrs Y 26 years old G1P0+0 with 4 months pregnancy has come to PPTCT centre and diagnosed to be asymptomatic HIV +ve with pregnancy. She has no previous history of infection, chronic illness and medication. On general examination no pallor, pulse 86/min, BP 120/76 mmHg, wt 50 kg, no oedema. Systemic examination is with normal limit. On clinical examination and USG, she has 16 wks pregnancy. Her antenatal investigations revealed Hb 11 gm%, blood group A +ve, VDRL non reactive, complete urine examination – no abnormality detected and CD_4 count is 500 cells/mm^2.

1. Which of the following is the first step in sequence of care in PPTCT program?
    (A) HIV counseling and testing
    (B) CD_4 assessment and baseline lab test
    (C) Care support and treatment
    (D) ART centre linkage
2. Newly initiated ART eligibility criteria for HIV positive pregnant woman
    (A) Life long ART, irrespective of WHO clinical stage and irrespective of CD_4 count
    (B) Irrespective of WHO clinic stage and CD_4 count < 350 cells/ mm^2
    (C) WHO clinical stage 3and 4 irrespective of CD_4 count
    (D) WHO clinical stage 1 and 2 and CD_4 < 500 cells/ mm^2
3. Choice of ART regimen for HIV positive pregnant women who is not on ART
    (A) Zidovudine + Lamivudine + Nevirapine
    (B) Zidovudine + Lamivudine + Efaviranz
    (C) Tenofovir + Lamivudine + Efaviranz
    (D) Tenofovir + Lamivudine + Zidovudine
4. Which of the following obstetrical risk factor influencing PTCT?
    (A) Vaginal cleaning
    (B) Rupture of membrane < 2 hours
    (C) Cesarean section
    (D) Instrumental delivery and episiotomy
5. Mrs Y opts for breastfeeding post delivery. How long the new born should continue on ARV prophylaxis (NVP)
    (A) Till 6 weeks
    (B) Till 9 weeks
    (C) Till 12 weeks
    (D) Till she continue breast feeding

6. Mrs Y baby is weighing 3 kg. What is the dose of syrup Nevirapine in ml/ once a day
   (A) 0.2 ml/kg
   (B) 1 ml
   (C) 1.5 ml
   (D) 2 ml
7. When to start cotrimaxazol prophylactic therapy (CPT) to HIV exposed infant of Mrs. Y
   (A) Immediate after birth
   (B) 4 weeks after birth
   (C) 6 weeks after birth
   (D) 8 weeks after birth

Answers:

1. A
   First step in PPTCT program is pretest counseling, testing and post test counseling
2. A
   If woman has diagnosed HIV positive during pregnancy and want to continue pregnancy. ART should be started irrespective to CD_4 count, WHO clinical stage and gestational age and continue life long
3. C
   Tenofovir + Lamivudine + Efaviranz (TLE)
   Efaviranz is not contraindicated in Ist trimester
4. D
   Instrumental deliveries and episiotomy should be avoided if needed forceps preferred over ventouse
5. A
   If duration between ART initiation and delivery is less than 24 weeks and woman opts for exclusive breast feeding then NVP ARV to baby for 12 weeks
6. C
   Baby weight < 2 kg dose of NVP 0.2 ml/kg once a day
   Baby weight 2-2.5 kg dose is 1 ml/ once a day
   Baby weight > 2.5 dose is 1.5 ml once a day and continue minimum for 6 weeks
7. C
   CPT to exposed infant should be started at 6 weeks of age and continue till 18 months

Reference:

1. Kumari G, Kanchar A, Rao R, Rewari B B, Rani M N, Sivalenka S. Updated guidelines for prevention of parent to child transmission (PPTCT) of HIV using multi drug anti-retrovoiral therapy in India. New Delhi. Dec 2013.

RH INCOMPATIBLE PREGNANCY

Dr Vinita Das, Professor & Head, Department of Obstetrics & Gynaecology

Mrs S.K 25 yr old primigravida comes for consultation in OPD at 5 months gestation. Her Hb is 12gm%, she is O Rh negative, her BP is 120/70 mm of Hg, viral markers are negative and her husband's blood group is Rh positive. She has been advised indirect coomb's test which comes negative.

1. At what gestational age should she be advised administration of Rh IG
   (A) 20 weeks
   (B) 24 weeks
   (C) 28 weeks
   (D) 32 weeks
2. Following are additional indication for the antepartum administration of RhIG **EXCEPT** (Level A scientific evidence by ACOG)
   (A) Spontaneous or elective abortion
   (B) Threatened abortion/ H.mole
   (C) Ectopic pregnancy
   (D) CVS/FBS/ Aminocentesis
3. When Anti D is administered to a antenatal woman at 28 weeks, a repeat dose is unnecessary if delivery occurs less than - weeks (unless a large FMH is detected at the time of delivery)
   (A) 3 weeks
   (B) 6 weeks
   (C) 9 weeks

(D)   12 weeks
4.   After delivery newborn had Rh positive blood group. Some how Rh IG was inadvertently omitted after
     delivery, recommendations have been made to administer it as late as how many days after delivery
     (A)   14 days
     (B)   28 days
     (C)   42 days
     (D)   56 days
5.   Once postpartum administration of Rh IG is undertaken the Anti D antibody screen may remain positive
     upto how much time
     (A)   6 month
     (B)   12 month
     (C)   18 month
     (D)   24 month

Answers:

1.   C
     If there is no evidence of Anti D allo immunization in the Rh negative woman the patient should
     receive 300 μg of Rh IG at 28 wks of gestation. This will help in declining back ground
     incidence of Rh D allo immunization in antenatal period from 2% to 0.1%.
2.   B
     These are level C evidence. Most expert agree that such events also warrant strong
     considerations for use of Rh IG (Rh Anti D)
3.   A
     Half life of Rh IG is approx 23-26 days, 15% to 20% of patients receiving it at 28 weeks have a
     very low anti D titre at term (usually 2 to 4). So to maintain adequate serum level of RhIG, if
     delivery occurs after 3 weeks of RhIG administration a repeat dose post partum is necessary.
     The rule of thumb should be to administer RhIG, when in doubt, rather than to with hold it.
4.   B
     Recommendation have been made to administer as late as 28 days after delivery
5.   A
     Antibody is serum is positive up to 6 months. Anti D persisting after 6 months is likely to be the
     result of sensitization

Reference:

1.   Gabbe SG, Niebyl JR, Simpson JL, Landon MB, Galan HL, Jauniaux ERM et al. Obstetrics-
     Normal and Problem Pregnancies. 6th edition. New Delhi: Elsevier; 2013.

TWIN GESTATION – MONOCHORIONIC TWINNING
Dr Vinita Das, Professor & Head, Department of Obstetrics & Gynaecology

Mrs PK, 25 yrs female presents in obstetric clinic with 2 months amenorhoea. Her obstetric USG shows 9 wks
pregnancy, one gestational sac with a thin dividing membrane & two fetuses.

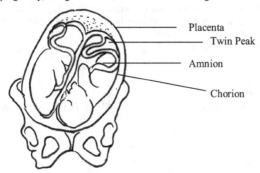

Placenta

Twin Peak

Amnion

Chorion

1.   At 11-14 weeks gestation, repeat USG report comments about the absence of "Twin Peak Sign" What is
     the diagnosis?
     (A)   Monochorionic monoamniotic twin
     (B)   Monochorionic diamniotic twin

(C) Dichorionic diamniotic twins

(D) None of the above

2. The risk of Monozygotic twin pregnancy is dependent & affected by

(A) Maternal age

(B) Family history

(C) Race

(D) None of the above

3. What is the spontaneous rate of MZ twins

(A) 0.4%

(B) 0.8%

(C) 1.2%

(D) 1.6%

4. Which one of the following statement is false in relation to causes of MZ twinning

(A) MZ twinning has been induced by delayed fertilization in rabbits & by iatrogenic hypoxia in mice

(B) MZ twinning may be due to damage to inner cell mass leading to two separate points of regrowth & splitting of the fertilized ovum

(C) MZ twinning in human is a non teratogenic event

(D) MZ twinning in human include fertilization of an "old" ovum with a more fragile zona pellucida or inadequate cytoplasm

5. "Stuck Twin appearance" on USG in late second trimester confirms diagnosis of

(A) Monochorionic diamniotic gestation

(B) Monochorionic monoamniotic gestation

(C) Dichorionic diamniotic gestation

(D) None of the above

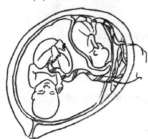

Answers:

A MZ twin pregnancy is created by the fertilization of one egg by one sperm & then subsequent spontaneous cleavage of the fertilized ovum. MZ twin are at higher risk for adverse outcomes than the DZ twins.

1. B

Twin peak sign is a triangular projection of tissue extending beyond the chorionic surface of placenta. This tissue is insinuated between the layers of the inter twin membrane, wider at the chorionic surface & tapering at the point at some distance inward from that surface. This space exists only in dichorionic pregnancies. Twin peak sign cannot occur in monochorionic placentation because the single continuous chorion does not extend into the potential inter amniotic apace of the monochorionic, diamniotic twin membrane.

2. D

MZ twinning rates are constant across all variables, with the exception of assisted reproduction

3. A

Spontaneous rate of MZ twinning in general population is 0.4%, studies have reported that rate may be more than 10 fold higher in pregnancies conceived by ART

4. C

It is proposed that MZ twinning in human is a teratogenic event

5. A

Stuck twin sign is present in monochorionic diamniotic gestation. The dividing membrane may not be seen because severe ologohydramnios causes them to be closely opposed to the fetus in that sac. This results in stucked twin appearance. In this trapped fetus remains firmly held against the uterine wall despite changes in maternal position. In many cases, a small portion of the dividing membrane can be seen extending from a fetal edge to the uterine wall.

Reference:
1. Gabbe SG, Niebyl JR, Simpson JL, Landon MB, Galan HL, Jauniaux ERM et al. Obstetrics-Normal and Problem Pregnancies. 6th edition. New Delhi: Elsevier; 2013.

EARLY PREGNANCY

Dr. Yashodhara Pradeep Prof. Dept of Obstetrics and Gynecology KGMU

Mrs X, 21 year old G0 married 3 months ago complaints of amenorrhea approximately 6 weeks with nausea and occasional vomiting usually in the morning with frequency of micturition, fatigue and breast swelling.

1. Which one of the following is most appropriate test to diagnose pregnancy in this case?
   (A) Serum beta hCG
   (B) Urinary beta hCG
   (C) Ultrasound
   (D) Pelvic examination
2. She revisits after 15 days with complaints of persistent excessive vomiting.
   All of the following are causes of this EXCEPT
   (A) Cholecystitis
   (B) Pyelonephritis
   (C) Reflux oesophagitis
   (D) Thyrotoxicosis
3. The daily supplementation of folic acid in pregnant women.
   (A) 0.4 mg
   (B) 0. 5 mg
   (C) 0.6mg
   (D) 4mg
4. Mrs X is pregnant and develops spotting how will you confirm the viability of pregnancy-
   (A) Serum beta hCG
   (B) Ultrasound
   (C) Hegar Sign
   (D) Presence of nausea
5. On transvaginal ultrasound fetal cardiac activity can be usually detected by gestational age of
   (A) 5 weeks
   (B) 6weeks
   (C) 7 weeks
   (D) 7.5 weeks

Answers:

1. B
   In this case the most appropriate test for detection of pregnancy is urinary beta hCG. It can be detected by 8-9 days after ovulation (hCG 12.5 mIU /mL). Most UPT kits can detect hCG levels of 100 mIU/mL. It is simple cost effective test for the diagnosis of pregnancy[1].

2. C
   Women presenting with persistent excessive vomiting the possibility of underlying disease like cholecystitis, pyelonephritis & thyrotoxicosis should be ruled out. Reflux esophagtiis causes heart burn not the vomitting[1]

3. C
   The DRI for folic acid in pregnant women is 0.6mg. The daily dose of folic acid in women with previously affected child is 4mg /day.   For prevention of NTD folic acid should be started 4 weeks prior to pregnancy and should be continued through first trimester. The requirement of folic acid for all women in child bearing age is 0.4 mg (CDC)[2]

4. B
   In case of spotting / bleeding p/v the viability of fetus in first trimester should be confirmed with Ultrasound, demonstration of cardiac activity. Urinary beta hCG confirms qualitative presence of chorionic activity, Hegar sign is softening of isthmus so body and neck of uterus felt separately. Nausea is a symptom not a sign of viability of fetus

5. B
   On TVS the cardiac activity of embryo is usually detected by 6weeks of GA when embryo measures 5mm, trans abdominal ultrasound can detect it by 7weeks.

References :
1. Cunningham FG, Leveno KJ, Bloom SL, Spong CY, Dashe JS, Hoffman BL et al. Williams Obstetrics. 24th edition. USA: Mc Graw Hill Education; 2014.
2. Gabbe SG, Niebyl JR, Simpson JL, Landon MB, Galan HL, Jauniaux ERM et al. Obstetrics-Normal and Problem Pregnancies. 6th edition. New Delhi: Elsevier; 2013.

MENOPAUSE

Dr. Yashodhara Pradeep Prof. Obstetrics & Gynecology

A 50 year old G4P4 presents with complaints of amenorrhea for 12 months and occasional hot flashes, lethargy & fatigue. She had one cesarean delivery followed by three vaginal deliveries. She has no family history of type two diabetes, hypertension, her recent report of pap smear HPVDNA16, 18 are negative.

1. The years prior to menopause that encompass the change from normal ovulatory cycles to cessation of menses are known as
   (A) Climacteric
   (B) Perimenopause transition
   (C) Menopause
   (D) Premature menopause

2. The protocol for preventive Health screening for healthy menopausal women complete history and physical examination between 40- 55 years should be done at every.
   (A) 5 Years
   (B) 3Y
   (C) 3-5 Y
   (D) 1-2 Y

3. The minimum preventive health screening protocol for healthy postmenopausal women should include Height, Weight, BMI, Blood sugar, TSH, Lipid profile, B.P., Pap smear and Mammography. It should be done.
   (A) Annually
   (B) Biannually
   (C) Every 3years
   (D) Every 5 Years

4. All of the following cancers are common in menopausal age group **Except**
   (A) Breast
   (B) Cervix
   (C) Ovarian
   (D) Lungs

5. Which one of the following is not a risk factor for osteoporosis?
   (A) Obesity
   (B) Hyperthyroid
   (C) Premature menopause
   (D) Prior fracture

Answers:

1. B
   The perimenopausal transitional years is marked by menstrual irregularities. Menopause is characterized by amenorrhea for one year. Climasteric an older more general and less precise term includes perimenopausal transition, menopause to the postmenopausal years. Premature menopause when menopause occurs before 40 years of age.

2. A
   Preventive health screening of healthy menopausal women complete medical history and physical examination should be done every 5 years, at about age 40, 45, 50 and 55

3. A
   Preventive health screening of healthy menopausal women to prevent or early detection of non communicable diseases cervical and breast cancers for compression of morbidities should be done annually[1]

4. D
   The incidence of various cancers in menopausal women in decreasing order is cervical cancer, breast cancer, ovarian cancer & lungs.

5. A

Bone mass is greater in black and obese women and less in white and thin and sedentary women[1]. Premature menopause and Hyperthyroidism is risk factor for osteoporosis[1].

References:

1. Fritz MA, Speroff L. Clincal Gynecologic Endocrinolgy and Infertility.8th edition. Philadelphia PA19103:Wolters Kluwer and Lipincott Williams &Willkins; 2011.
2. Berek SJ. Berek&Novak's Gynecology. 14th Edition. Philadelphia PA19106 : Lippincott Williams&Wilkins; 2007.

PELVIC MASS

Dr. Yashodhara Pradeep , Prof obstetrics & Gynecology

A 21 year old unmarried woman presents with sudden onset of severe pain in lower abdomen associated with vomiting. She looks ill T 99.4°F, pulse 106/min, B.P. 110/70, RR 18/min, On P/A examination an anterior 10 cm firm, tender mass is palpate guarding and rebound tenderness present. P/S, P/V not done, P/R tender swelling on left side of uterus. Pelvic ultrasound shows normal uterus left adnexa with unilocular thick wall cyst highly Echogenic with areas of calcification and acoustic enhancement. Investigations CBC show leucocytosis 11000 rest of biochemistry is with in normal limit.

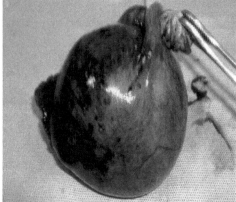

1. What is the Most probable cause of acute abdomen in this patient:
   (A) Acute appendicitis
   (B) Tuboovarian abscess
   (C) Ovarian torsion
   (D) Ruptured cyst
2. This case is managed with laparotomy, What are the structures removed and the surgical procedure is known as.
   (A) Ovarian cystectomy
   (B) Ovariotomy
   (C) Salpingo-oopherectomy
   (D) Cholecystectomy
3. Most common ovarian tumour in young age group is:
   (A) Dysgerminoma
   (B) Dermoid
   (C) Mucinous cystadenoma
   (D) Fibroma
4. All is true about dermoid cyst of ovary EXCEPT:
   (A) It is teratoma
   (B) X- Ray is diagnostic
   (C) Invariably turns to malignancy
   (D) Contains sebaceous material and hair
5. Most common tumour to undergo ovarian torsion is:
   (A) Benign cystic teratoma
   (B) Epithelial cell carcinoma
   (C) Endodermal sinus tumour

(D) Brenner's tumour

6. In this case the primary investigation to confirm the diagnosis
   (A) USG
   (B) USG Colour Doppler
   (C) CTd
   (D) MRI

Answers

1. C

   Young woman presenting with acute onset of symptoms with tender mass lying anterior to uterus, acute appendicites will have Macburney's tenderness, tuboovarian abscess will have and subacute presentation for last few days to few weeks associated with fever and toxic look, ruptured ovarian cyst may present with shock and mass will disappear on USG there will be free fluid in pelvis.

2. C

   The structures removed are ovary and tube surgical procedure known as salpingo-oopherectomy, ovarian cystectomy is removal of only ovarian cyst, ovariotomy is removal of whole diseased ovary, Cholecystectomy is removal of gallbladder

3. B

   The most common ovarian tumor in young reproductive age group is benign mature teratoma (5-10% of all cystic tumors of the ovary), followed by dysgerminoma 3-5%, fibroma 3%, mucinous cyst adenoma is common in age group 30-60 years[1]

4. C

   Dermoid cyst is innocent ovarian tumors in only 1.7% cases may turn malignant eg. epidermoid carcinoma or sarcomatous changes, It is a germ cell mature benign teratoma, The diagnosis can be made on X ray due to presence of teeth and bone.

5. C

   The benign cystic teratoma is most common ovarian tumor to undergo torsion due to high fat content they float in abdominal cavity and prone to twist, other common tumors undergo torsion are pedunculated fibroid paraovarian cyst and broad ligament fibroid.

6. B

   On USG dermoid cyst can be identified by presence of highly Echogenic sebaceous material, calcifications and acoustic shadowing due to presence of teeth and bone. The doppler USG can tell about the blood flow which may be absent in cases of torsion ovary. CT and MRI are high end investigations.

References:

1. Berek SJ. Berek&Novak's Gynecology. 14th Edition.Philadelphia: Lippincott Williams&Wilkins; 2007.
2. Bhatla N. Jeffcoate's Principles of Gynecology, Revised & Updated International from Fifth Edition London:Arnold; 2001.

Chapter-13

Opthalmology

BILATERAL CONGENITAL 6TH NERVE PALSY

Dr Siddharth Agrawal, Assistant Professor, Department of Ophthalmology

A two year old boy was brought to the clinic with in turning of both the eyes since birth. The examination showed eso deviation of 50 PD. There was limitation of abduction in both the eyes. No palbebral aperture changes were noted on attempted abduction.

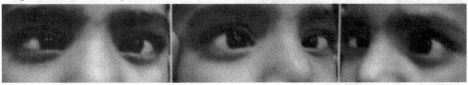

1. What is the most probable diagnosis?
   - (A) Essential infantile esotropia
   - (B) Congenital B/L sixth nerve Palsy
   - (C) Nystagmus blockade syndrome
   - (D) Strabismus fixus
2. Which of the following comes in the differential diagnosis of the above presentation?
   - (A) Essential infantile esotropia
   - (B) Nystagmus blockade syndrome
   - (C) Strabismus fixus
   - (D) All of the above
3. Following are the characterstics of essential infantile esotropia EXCEPT
   - (A) Large angle deviation
   - (B) High Refractive error
   - (C) No limitation of movement
   - (D) Inferior oblique overaction
4. Following are the characterstics of nystagmus blockade syndrome except
   - (A) Begins in early childhood and is associated with esotropia
   - (B) Nystagmus is reduced with fixating eye in adduction
   - (C) Esotropia decreases in abduction
   - (D) Limitation of movement in abduction

Answers:
1. B

   In essential infantile esotropia -no abduction limitation. Nystagmus blockade syndrome -EOM full. Strabismus fixus – globe retraction is seen
2. D

   In all conditions large angle esotropia is seen
3. B

   In essential infantile esotropia one gets large angle esotropia, cross fixation, associated B/L IO overaction (68%) DVD (50%), no limitation of movement
4. D

   Begins in early childhood and is associated with esotropia , Nystagmus is reduced with fixating eye in adduction , Esotropia decreases in abduction , no limitation of movements.

Reference:
1. Sharma P. Strabismus simplified . 2nd edition. New Delhi: CBS Publication; 2013; Chapter 7:p. 90-101.

PARTIAL 3RD CRANIAL NERVE PALSY

Dr Siddharth Agrawal, Assistant Professor, Department of Ophthalmology

This 10 year old boy presented with a chin up posture and marked left hypertropia. He was involved in a road traffic accident a year ago in which he sustained head injury but no fracture of facial bones. He never wore glasses and his vision was fine prior to the accident. Examination showed no gross refractive error. On straightening the head, the left was markedly hypertropic to 35 PD. There was no movement of the eye downwards beyond the primary. Adduction was slightly limited while abduction and intorsion was full. There was no evidence of intraocular trauma. Fundus was normal.

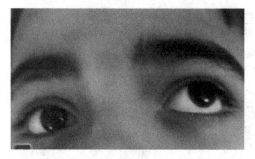

1. What is the most probable diagnosis?
   (A) Inferior division palsy of third nerve
   (B) Superior division palsy of third nerve
   (C) Total third nerve palsy
   (D) Can be any of the above.
2. Levator Palpebrae Superioris muscle is supplied by
   (A) Inferior division of third nerve
   (B) Superior division of third nerve
   (C) Both the divisions
   (D) Third nerve along with sympathetic nerve
3. Pupil sparing 3rd nerve paralysis is seen in
   (A) Aneurysm
   (B) Diabetes
   (C) Uncal herniation
   (D) Basal meningitis
4. Surgical management (if required) for incomitant squint following nerve palsy in planned after
   (A) 2month
   (B) 4 month
   (C) 6 month
   (D) 8 month

Answers:
   1. A
       Inferior division of nerve supplies MR, IR, IO. Thus causing the limitation of movements
   2. B
       Superior division supplies the LPS and SR
   3. B
       Medical lesions like HTN, DM spare pupil
   4. C
       Spontaneous improvement ceases after 6 months

Reference:
   1. Kanski JJ, Bowling B . Clinical ophthalmology - A systemic approach: 7th edition. New York: Elsevier;2011; Chapter 19: 830-3.

ESSENTIAL INFANTILE ESOTROPIA
Dr Siddharth Agrawal, Assistant Professor, Department of Ophthalmology

A 2 year old child presented to us with inward deviation of right eye noticed by parents at 6 months of age. On examination freely alternating large angle esotropia (~60 PD) was observed. No significant refractive error was found. Fundus examination revealed no abnormality.

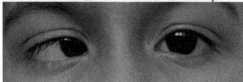

1. What is the most likely diagnosis?
   - (A) Essential infantile esotropia
   - (B) Duane's retraction syndrome
   - (C) Myaesthenia gravis
   - (D) None of the above
2. What is the most likely age group for manifestation of essential infantile esotropia?
   - (A) At birth
   - (B) 4-6 months
   - (C) After 2 years
   - (D) Any of the above
3. Which of these is not a feature of essential infantile esotropia?
   - (A) Large angle esotropia
   - (B) Free alternation
   - (C) High refractive error
   - (D) No neurological defect
4. Medial recti surgery gives more effect than the lateral recti for each mm in the ratio:
   - (A) 1:2
   - (B) 3:2
   - (C) 1:1
   - (D) 2:1
5. Long standing esotropia with limitation of abduction can be differentiated from a 6th nerve palsy with the help of:
   - (A) Doll's eye movements
   - (B) Optokinetic nystagmus
   - (C) Both
   - (D) None

Answers:
1. A

   Essential infantile esotropia is the most common cause of nonaccomodative esodeviation in children.
2. B

   The most likely age group for manifestation of essential infantile esotropia is 4-6 months.
3. C

   Refractive error does not contribute to esodeviation in essential infantile esotropia.
4. B

   Medial recti surgery gives more effect than the lateral recti for each mm in the ratio of 3:2
5. C

   Long standing esotropia with limitation of abduction can be differentiated from a 6th nerve palsy with the help of both doll's eye movements and optokinetic nystagmus.

Reference:
1. Sharma P: Strabismus simplified. 2nd edition. New Delhi: CBS Publishers, 2013, Chapter 7, pp 90-95.

CONGENITAL PTOSIS
Dr Siddharth Agrawal, Assistant Professor, Department of Ophthalmology

A 3 year old boy presented with drooping of right upper lid. His mother stated that it has been present since birth and has remained stationary. No diurnal variation. No other ocular or systemic complaint.

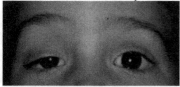

1. What is the most likely diagnosis?
   - (A) Congenital myogenic ptosis
   - (B) Myaesthenia gravis
   - (C) Acquired ptosis
   - (D) None of the above

2. What are the attachments of levator palpebrae superioris muscle?
   (A) Medial and lateral palpebral ligaments
   (B) Skin and tarsal plate
   (C) Fornices
   (D) All of the above
3. Which of these is NOT a component of blepharophimosis syndrome?
   (A) Ptosis
   (B) Epicanthus inversus
   (C) Entropion
   (D) Lateral ectropion
4. Which of these is not a feature of congenital myogenic ptosis?
   (A) Poor levator function
   (B) Increased palpebral aperture on downgaze
   (C) Absence of lid crease
   (D) Increase in drooping by evening
5. Which of these is correctly matched?
   (A) Mild ptosis- Frontalis sling surgery
   (B) Severe ptosis- Fasanella Servat procedure
   (C) Normal margin reflex distance (MRD1)- 4mm
   (D) Good LPS action- 10mm

Answers:

1. A
   Drooping of eyelid since birth is congenital ptosis
2. D
   LPS muscle has five attachments: Medial and lateral palpebral ligaments, upper and lower fornices, tarsal plate and skin
3. C
   Ptosis, epicanthus inversus, lateral ectropion and telecanthus are the main features of blepharophimosis syndrome.
4. D
   Increase in drooping of eyelid by evening is a feature of myasthenia gravis.
5. C
   Mild ptosis- Fasanella Servat procedure
   Severe ptosis- Frontalis sling surgery
   Normal margin reflex distance (MRD1)- 4 mm
   Good LPS action- 16 mm

Reference:

1. Kanski JJ, Bowling B. Clinical Ophthalmology – A systemic approach. 7th edition. New York: Elsevier; 2011, Chapter 1, pp 39-43.

SUB RETINAL GROWTH

Dr Sandeep Saxena, Professor, Department of Ophthalmology

A 27-year old male presented for refraction. Best-corrected visual acuity (BCVA) both eyes were 6/12 OD and 6/9 OS. Slit lamp biomicroscopy of the anterior segment was unremarkable. Fundus examination of the left eye was unremarkable. The right eye examination revealed four juxtapapillary yellow white glistening calcified lesions of various sizes (Figure 1). A+B Scan ultrasonography revealed multiple hyperechogenic lesions on the optic nerve head. Autofluorescence imaging of the right optic nerve head showed increased autofluorescence of the nodular mass.Three-dimensional spectral domain optical coherence tomography (3D SD-OCT) (Carl Zeiss Meditec Inc., CA, U.S.A.), optic disc cube 200x200 advanced visualization was performed. Comprehensive physical and dermatological examination did not reveal features of phacomatoses. Brain magnetic resonance imaging, abdominal ultrasound and audiometry were unremarkable. In the absence of any known treatment,the patient was not subjected to any management.

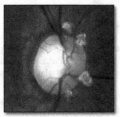 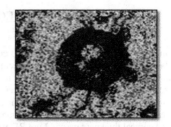

1. Provisional diagnosis of the case is:
   (A) Retinoblastoma
   (B) Toxocara
   (C) amelanotic choroidal melanoma
   (D) retinal astrocytoma
2. True statement among the following :
   (A) Most often located in outer layers of retina
   (B) Associated with phacomatoses
   (C) On fluorescein angiography intrinsic tumour vascularization is highlighted in early phase of angiogram
   (D) Needs urgent treatment.
3. True regarding clinical presentation are all except:
   (A) Tends to arise in early childhood
   (B) Predilection for male sex
   (C) Tuberous sclerosis is principle risk factor
   (D) Can cause non rhegmatogenous retinal detachment.
4. Systemic association to be looked for:
   (A) Tuberous sclerosis
   (B) Pinealoblastoma
   (C) Cavernous haemangioma
   (D) Melanoma
5. Aggressive cases are treated with :
   (A) Photodynamic therapy
   (B) Intravitreal chemotherapy
   (C) Peribulbar steroids
   (D) Laser therapy

Answers:
   1. D
      retinal astrocytoma
   2. C
      On fluorescein angiography intrinsic tumour vascularization is highlighted in early phase of angiogram
   3. B
      Predilection for male sex
   4. A
      Tuberous sclerosis
   5. A
      Photodynamic therapy

References:

1. Williams R, Taylor D. Tuberous sclerosis. *SurvOphthalmol.* 1985; 30:143–54.
2. Ulbright TM, Fulling KH, Helveston EM. Astrocytic tumours of the retina. Differentiation of sporadic tumours from phakomatoses-associated tumours. *Arch Pathol Lab Med.* 1984;108:160–63.
3. Reeser FH, Aaberg TM, Van Horn DL. Astrocytichamartoma of the retina not associated with tuberous sclerosis. *Am J Ophthalmol.* 1978; 86:688–98.
4. Shields C, Benevides R, Materin M et al. Optical coherence tomography of retinal astrocytichamartoma in 15 cases. Ophthalmology. 2006; 113:1553–57.
5. Lessell S, Kuwabara T. Retinal neuroglia. Arch Ophthalmol1963; 70:671-78.
6. Watanabe T, Raff M. Retinal astrocytes are immigrants from the optic nerve. Nature 1988; 332:834-37.

MEGALOCORNEA

Dr. Arun Sharma, Associate Professor, Department of Ophthalmology

A 3 month old patient named Gayatri came to our tertiary care centre with her parents complaining of enlarged eyeballs since birth and searching movements of eyes at 3 months of age. Parents consulted a local ophthalmologist for the above complaints He made a diagnosis of bilateral congenital glaucoma (buphthalmos) and referred her for glaucoma surgery to our centre.

Examination under anaesthesia was done at our centre documented the following findings:

Corneal diameter of both eyes were 12.5 mm vertical; 13 mm horizontal.

Central corneal thickness was 542 μm RE & 566 μm LE.

Intra-ocular pressure was 14 mmhg RE & 16 mm hG LE.

Cornea was clear of both eyes.

Optic nerve head showed no glaucomatous change.

High myopia was present: -6D in RE & -8D LE (causing the searching movements).

Diagnosis of bilateral megalocornea was made. This is a non-progressive sporadic / autosomal condition. Only refractive error needs correction.

She is under follow-up for last 5 years.

All parameters are stationary.

No evidence of glaucoma is present.

No searching movements of eyes.

Glasses are being used constantly.Child was saved from an unnecessary surgical intervention.

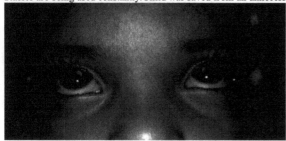

1. What should be the corneal diameter for the diagnosis of megalocornea?
   (A) >15mm
   (B) >10mm
   (C) ≥13mm
   (D) <17mm

2. The most common cause of megalocornea-
   (A) Traumatic
   (B) Developmental
   (C) Inflammatory
   (D) Neoplastic

3. Incidence of megalocornea in male and female-
   (A) male=female
   (B) male<female
   (C) male>female
   (D) None of the above

4. Mutation in which of the following chromosome is found in megalocornea:-
   (A) xp23
   (B) xq23
   (C) xp20
   (D) xq20

5. Most common complication of megalocornea-
   (A) Glaucoma
   (B) Refractive error
   (C) Early cataract
   (D) Lens subluxation

   Megalocornea is a rare congenital disorder characterized by horizontal corneal diameter≥ 13mm in absence of raised intraocular pressure. Most commonly the disease is developmental inherited – predominantly X- linked. (X – Linked recessive)
2. B
   Explanation with answer 1
3. C
   Since the disease has X-linked recessive pattern of inheritance, it is more common among males
4. B
5. B
   Megalocornea occurs alone but may occasionally be associated with dysgenesis of iris, lens or ciliary body and iris megalophthalmos. Commonly the patient with magalocornea presents with refractive error.

References:
1. Sihota R, Tandon R (editors). Parsons' diseases of the eye; Elsevier, New Delhi. 21st edition
2. Kanski JJ, Bowling B. Clinical Ophthalmology – A systemic approach. 7th edition. New York: Elsevier; 2011

SEBACEOUS GLAND CARCINOMA UPPER EYELID

Dr. Apjit Kaur, Professor, Department of Ophthalmology

A 47 year old , non- diabetic female of urban dwelling, presented with a painless, slowly progressive nodule on the right upper eyelid since one year. It was associated with foreign body sensation right eye, of recent onset. No lymphadenopathy was identified.

On examination, a smooth, non-tender, non-mobile nodule, continuous with the tarsal plate but free from overlying skin, was palpable on the right upper eyelid. On eversion the palpebral surface showed a nodular, vascularized, friable growth.

Fine needle aspiration cytology was consistent with sebaceous gland carcinoma.

Total excision of mass with safe margin was performed under local anaesthesia. Eyelid reconstruction was done using Cutler Beard Procedure stage 1 and 2.

Histopathology was consistent with sebaceous gland carcinoma of eyelid.

The patient is asymptomatic till current two year follow up.

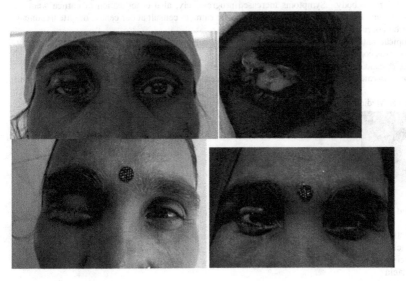

1 Masquerade presentation in eyelid neoplasia is common clinical feature of
  (A) Sebaceous gland carcinoma
  (B) Squamous cell carcinoma
  (C) Basal cell carcinoma
  (D) Malignant melanoma
2 Blepharoconjunctivitis, recurrent chalazion may be misdiagnosis for
  (A) Sebaceous gland carcinoma
  (B) Squamous cell carcinoma
  (C) Basal cell carcinoma
  (D) Malignant melanoma
3 Procedure of choice for eyelid reconstruction is dependent on
  (A) size of defect
  (B) age of the patient
  (C) both A and B
  (D) type of tumor morphology

Answers:
  1 A

    Masquerade presentation is commonest with Sebaceous gland carcinoma

  2 B

    Blepharoconjunctivitis and recurrent chalazion are masquerade presentations of sebaceous gland carcinoma

  3 C

    Increased age is associated with decreased elastic tissue of the skin, thus large defects can be reconstructed with locally available tissue.

Reference:
  1. Albert and Jakobiec, Principles and practice of Ophthalmology, Section X111, second edition, Philadelphia, WB Saunders Company.

CORNEAL ULCER
Dr. Arun Sharma, Associate Professor, Department of Ophthalmology

A 46 years old patient named Kalawati developed pain, redness, watering of RE 1 month back. There was no history of trauma or foreign body. Symptoms increased progressively; also opacification of cornea went on increasing. She was already treated for bacterial ulcer when she came to consult at our centre, despite treatment, perforation of ulcer had occurred. Hypopyon was still present.

Treatment: The topical antibiotics were changed to fortified cefazoline & fortified tobramycin 1 hourly. Supportive treatment was continued.

Cyano-acrylate glue & bandage contact lens application was done.

Blood investigations revealed a Hb% of 7 gm which had been overlooked previously hence the fulminant course.

Patient was referred to Medicine department for management of anaemia.

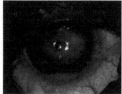

Corneal ulcer healed faster.

1. Which drug instiilation in eye leads to formation of white corneal percipitates?
  (A) Moxifloxacin
  (B) Tobramycin
  (C) Ciprofloxacin
  (D) Gatifloxacin

2. Which bacteria can penetrate intact corneal epithelium?
   (A) Staphylococcus
   (B) H.influenza
   (C) Pseudomonas
   (D) Diptherioid
3. In which type of herpes simplex keratitis topical steroids are given?
   (A) Epithelial keratitis
   (B) Disciform keratitis
   (C) Necrotizing stromal keratitis
4. Ring abscess is seen in which type of keratitis?
   (A) Bacterial
   (B) Viral
   (C) Fungal
   (D) Acanthamoeba
5. At what endothelial cell count corneal edema develops?
   (A) 2600 cells/mm
   (B) 1500 cells/mm
   (C) 1000 cells/mm
   (D) 500 cells/mm

Answers:
1. C
   The difference in tear film pH and metabolism of ciprofloxacin eye drop (~4.5) leads to precipitation of any and formation of white precipitates
2. B
   Increased virulence of H. influenzae is the reason for penetration through intact cornea. Other organisms include N. gonorrhea, and N. meningitides and C. diphtheria.
3. B
   Disciform keratitis is a hypersensitivity reaction to viral protein and is treated with topical antibiotics.
4. D
   Acanthamoeba keratitis is classically results in ring shaped lesions in later stages.
5. D
   With reductions in endothelial cell counts, the activity of Sodium potassium pump is reduced and when this count reduces ≤ 500 cells/ mm, corneal edema occurs.

References:
1. Sihota R, Tandon R (editors). Parsons' diseases of the eye; Elsevier, New Delhi. 21st edition
2. Kanski JJ, Bowling B. Clinical Ophthalmology – A systemic approach. 7th edition. New York: Elsevier; 2011,

INFANTILE CAPILLARY HEMANGIOMA
Dr. Apjit Kaur, Professor, Department of Ophthalmology

Two months old male child, born of a full term normal delivery at hospital, to a primi, was brought with complains of a progressively increasing mass over the right eyelid. The child was unable to open the eye. No abnormality was noticed in other parts of the body.The child had normal milestones and feeding.

On examination a diffuse non-pulsatile, mass with prominent vascular markings was seen involving the left upper eyelid, extending onto the forehead. There was no change in size on crying. Instrument assisted retraction of left upper eyelid normal eyeball.

CT scan revealed an intensely enhancing irregular (vascular) mass in the left eyelid with extension in the extraconal space, mainly superiorly.

Clinico-radiological diagnosis of Congenital Infantile Capillary Hemangioma was made.

The child was put on oral corticosteroid therapy in accordance with weight, along with antacid and calcium supplementation.

The mass regressed over a period of eight weeks. During this period, parents were explained regarding Amblyopia therapy for the left eye.

Follow up visits revealed minimal vascular prominence in the area of the lesion.Palpebral aperture height is adequate.

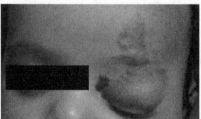

Infantile capillary heamangioma , extending over eyelid , forehead and into the orbit

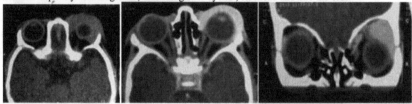

CT scans showing enhancing lesions in the left orbit and eyelid

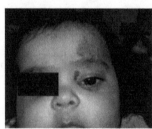

Clinical photograph showing regressed lesion and good palpebral opening

1. In its natural course, untreated Infantile capillary hemangioma of eyelid
   (A) is always progressive
   (B) may undergo spontaneous regression
   (C) always undergoes spontaoneous regression
   (D) Is biphasic , with periods of growth few years apart
 2. Oral corticosteroid therapy is indicated for infantile hemangioma of eyelid when
   (A) associated with orbital extension
   (B) lesion is progressive
   (C) lesion of the eyelid is extensive
   (D) all of the above
3. Indication for early treatment of infantile hemagioma of eyelid is
   (A) Cosmetic
   (B) Prevent amblyopia
   (C) both A and B
   (D) associated conjunctival   extension

Answers:
   1   B
       Infantile capillary hemangioma may undergo spontaneous regression.
   2   D
       Lesions that are large, progressive or have orbital extension, are treated with oral steroids.
   3   B
       Prevention of Amblyopia is the indication for early treatment.

Reference:
   1.   Albert and Jakobiec, Principles and practice of Ophthalmology, Section X111, second edition,
        Philadelphia, WB Saunders Company.

ORBITAL CAVERNOUS HEMANGIOMA

Dr. Apjit Kaur, Profesor, Department of Ophthalmology

A 27 year female presented with history of progressive drooping of left upper eyelid associated with a painless mass she could feel in the upper part of left eyelid since nearly two years. She had no visual symptoms.

On examination, she had mechanical ptosis caused by a palpable soft to firm mass in the left superior. Left eyeball was hypotropic and elevation was restricted. There were no signs of Optic nerve compression.

CT scan revealed a well circumscribed enhancing mass in the left superior orbit causing moulding of the roof of orbit.

FNAC showed blood , and no cytological conclusion was drawn.

The mass was excised in toto under general anaesthesia using the sub-brow approach.

Histopathology was consistent with cavernous hemangioma.

Post-opoeratively the patient developed ptosis LUL that was corrected under local anesthesia using silicon sling. The patient is asymptomatic with good cosmesis till three years of follow-up

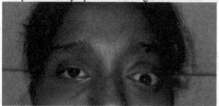

Mechanical ptosis and dystopia of left eyeball

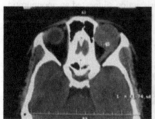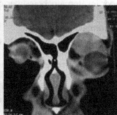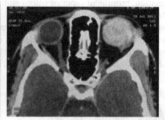

CT Scan showing well circumscribed enhancing mass in the left superior orbit causing moulding of the roof of orbit.

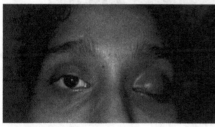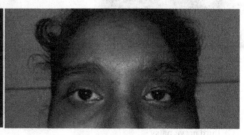

Post operative severe ptosis   Ptosis correction using frontalis sling procedure

1. Moulding of orbital bones is a feature of the following lesion
   (A) benign,Short duration
   (B) benign long duration
   (C) malignant short duration
   (D) all malignant masses
2. Orbital tonometry is used to asses
   (A) consistency of retrobulbar lesion
   (B) intra ocular pressure
   (C) vascularity of tumor
   (D) size of retrobulbar mass

3. Treatment of choice for solitary orbital cavernous hemangioma
    (A) surgical excision
    (B) intralesional sclerosing agent
    (C) External beam radiotherapy
    (D) Any one of the above

Answers:
    1. B
        Because benign lesions cause pressure of long duration
    2. A
        Because backward pressure suggests consistency.
    3. A
        Because well capsulated lesion.

Reference:
    1. Albert and Jakobiec, Principles and practice of Ophthalmology, Section X111,second edition, Philadelphia, WB Saunders Company.

SENILE PTOSIS WITH ECTROPION
Dr. Apjit Kaur, Profesor, Department of Ophthalmology

65 years female, presented with progressive drooping of right upper eyelid since 3months. She associated it with excessive crying due to a tragic event.The was no history of diurnal variation, diplopia or any other systemic disease.

On examination, prominent superior sulcus and poor levatorpalpebraesuperioris action suggested an aponeurotic ptosis. She also had lateral ectropion of the left lower eyelid along with horizontal eyelid laxity. Her bells phenomenon, corneal sensation and tear film were normal.

Ptosis correction was done by re attachment of disinserted aponeurosis and ectropion correction done by lateral tarsal sling procedure in the same sitting under local anesthesia.

Good post op recovery of eyelid movement and ectropion correction were gained.

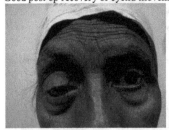
Pre-operative RUL ptosis and RLL ectropion

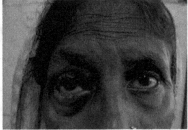
Post operative good RUL elevation and normal RLLposition

1. Pathophysiology of Senile ptosis is
    (A) weakening of muscle fibres of Levator palpebrae superioris(LPS)
    (B) disinsertion of LPS aponeurosis
    (C) third nerve palsy
    (D) weakening of orbital septum
2. Horizontal eyelid laxity of lower eyelid leads to
    (A) Ectropion
    (B) Entropion
    (C) Blepharochalasis
    (D) Dermatochalasis
3. Lateral canthal sling surgery is used to correct
    (A) horizontal lid laxity
    (B) vertical eyelid laxity
    (C) retractor disinsertion
    (D) all of the above

Answers:

1.   B

    Involutional changes affect the levator aponeurosis which becomes weak/ partially or totally disinserted at its attachment. Its reattachment results in correction of ptosis

2.   A

    Horizontal lid laxity leads to lengthening of the horizontal eyelid length, thus causing the lower eyelid to droop away and cause ectropion

3.   A

    Lateral canthal sling procedure results in reattaching the lower eyelid, after shortening to its appropriate length

References:

1.   Albert and Jakobiec, Principles and practice of Ophthalmology, Section X111,second edition, Philadelphia, WB Saunders Company.

PRIMARY NARROW ANGLE GLAUCOMA

Dr. S K Bhasker, Professor, Department of Ophthalmology

A 38 year old male presented with diminution of vision for 4 years. The diminution of vision was gradual in onset and was progressive in nature. This was associated with occasional headache, heaviness in head and colored haloes around a bright light (more in the evening). After sleep or on taking rest the patient was relieved of symptoms. History of frequent change of glasses was also present.

On examination the visual acuity was 6/24 in both eyes. The disc size was small with the cup to disc ratio being 0.5 (OD) and 0.7 (OS). On pachymetry central corneal thickness was 530☐ in both eyes. Intra ocular pressure at time of examination was 16 and 18 mm of Hg in right and left eyes respectively. Goniscopy showed occludable angles. Medications were prescribed but patient was not compliant. Finally trabeculectomy was performed in both eyes with interval of 2 months.

Postoperative photographs are shown below.

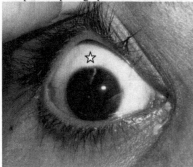 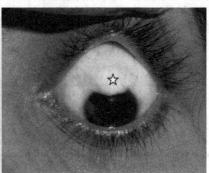

1. Most common (full thickness guarded) filtering surgery for glaucoma is
   (A) Goniotomy
   (B) Trabeculotomy
   (C) Trabeculectomy
   (D) Deep Sclerectomy
2. Trabeculectomy can be modified by the following antifibrotic agents **EXCEPT**
   (A) Mitomycin C
   (B) 5 Fluorouracil (5-FU)
   (C) Corticosteroids
   (D) Bevacizumab
3. The minimum size of fistula (if there is no inflammation or fibrous scaring) sufficient for aqueous to filter (in μ) is
   (A) 15
   (B) 30
   (C) 60
   (D) 120
4. The area marked by star in the figure is
   (A) Trabeculectomy Bleb
   (B) Trabeculotomy bleb

(C) Goniotomy bleb

(D) Deep sclerectomy bleb

5. Test for Leakage of bleb can be determined by

   (A) Seidels

   (B) Schirmer

   (C) Jones

   (D) Tear break up time

Answers:

1. C

   Only trabeculectomy is full thickness guarded filtering surgery for glaucoma

2. C

   Corticosteroids are anti inflammatory while others inhibit fibrosis

3. A

4. A

5. A

   All others are tests for dry eye

References:

1. McEvan WK. Application of Poiseuille's law to aqueous outflow. Arch Ophthalmol. 1958;60:290-294.

2. Sihota R, Tandon R (editors). Parsons' diseases of the eye; Elsevier, New Delhi. 21st edition, 2011, Chapter 19, pages 280 – 300.

3. Allingham RR, Damji KF, Freedman S, Moroi SE, Rhee DJ. Shields textbook of glaucoma. 6th edition. Philadelphia. Wolters Kluwer & Lippincott Williams and Wilkins. 2011

4. Kanski JJ, Bowling B. Clinical Ophthalmology – A systemic approach. 7th edition. New York: Elsevier; 2011.

5. Neema HV, Neema N. Textbook of Ophthalmology; 5th edition, New Delhi, Jaypee brothers medical publishers (P) Ltd; 2008, chapter 15, pages 214 – 249

6. Khurana N. Comprehensive ophthalmology, 6th edition, New Delhi, Jaypee brothers medical publishers (P) Ltd. ; 2015, Chapter 10, pages 219 - 256

PRIMARY OPEN ANGLE GLAUCOMA

Dr. S K Bhasker, Professor, Department of Ophthalmology

A 48 year old female presented with diminution of vision for 2 years. The diminution of vision was gradual in onset, painless and was progressive in nature. There was a history of frequent change of glasses. Patient had attained menopause at the age of 39years of age. Patient had family history for glaucoma (her mother has glaucoma) and by medication the target pressure (IOP) has been achieved.

On examination the visual acuity was 6/12 (OD) and 6/9 (OS). The disc sizes were average with the cup to disc ratio being 0.75 (OD) and 0.8 (OS). On pachymetry central corneal thickness in right and left eyes were 499μ and 501μ respectively. Intra ocular pressure (IOP) at time of examination was 21 and 22 mm of Hg in right and left eyes respectively. Goniscopy showed open angle.

Optical coherence tomography (OCT) showed marked thinning in Arcuate areas in both eyes. Biarcuate visual field defects were present on Humphry perimeter. (vide photo of OCT and Humphry visual field printouts below)Therefore a diagnosis of advanced open angle glaucoma was made and patient was prescribed bimatoprost and dorzolamide. Target IOP (in low teens) was achieved. Treatment was continued with regular follow-up at 2 months interval.

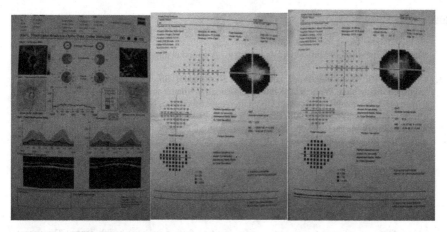

1. Glaucoma is a condition characterised by
   (A) Increased intraocular pressure
   (B) Ocular pain
   (C) Decreased visual acuity
   (D) Optic N Neuropathy
2. Basic patho-physiology in glaucoma is loss of
   (A) Rods and cones by apoptosis
   (B) Rods and cones by necrosis
   (C) Retinal ganglion cells by apoptosis
   (D) Retinal ganglion cells by necrosis
3. Which of the following is **NOT** usually a visual field defect in patients with glaucoma
   (A) Arcuate Bjerrum
   (B) Seidel's
   (C) Central
   (D) Paracentral
4. Clinically the loss of optic nerve fibres at optic disc in glaucoma is characterised by
   (A) Increased cup to disc ratio (CD ratio)
   (B) Decreased cup to disc ratio
   (C) Fullness of cup
   (D) Colobomatous disc
5. The sequence of angle structures from cornea to iris (anterior to posterior) is
   (A) Ciliary body, Scleral spur, Trabecular meshwork, Schwalbe's line
   (B) Scleral spur, Trabecular meshwork, Schwalbe's line, Ciliary body
   (C) Schwalbe's line, Trabecular meshwork, Scleral spur, Ciliary body
   (D) Scleral spur, Schwalbe's line, Trabecular meshwork, ciliary body

Answers:
   1. D
      According to current definition glaucoma is optic nerve neuropathy with characterstic disc changes and corresponding visual field changes.
      Corticosteroids are anti inflammatory while others inhibit fibrosis
   2. C
      Glaucoma is characterised by loss of retinal ganglion cell by apoptosis ie. cells involute and are lost without any inflammation.
   3. C
      Central vision is retained till the end. Due to this patient has tubular vision before he goes blind.
   4. A
      As retinal ganglion cells are lost, the cup size increase. Therefore the cup to disc ration in glaucoma increases
   5. C

References:

1. Sihota R, Tandon R (editors). Parsons' diseases of the eye; Elsevier, New Delhi. 21st edition, 2011, Chapter 19, pages 280 – 300.
2. Kanski JJ, Bowling B. Clinical Ophthalmology – A systemic approach. 7th edition. New York: Elsevier; 2011.
3. Allingham RR, Damji KF, Freedman S, Moroi SE, Rhee DJ. Shields textbook of glaucoma. 6th edition. Philadelphia. Wolters & Kluwer, Lippincott Williams and Wilkins. 2011
4. Neema HV, Neema N. Textbook of Ophthalmology; 5th edition, New Delhi, Jaypee brothers medical publishers (P) Ltd; 2008, chapter 15, pages 214 – 249
5. Khurana N. Comprehensive ophthalmology, 6th edition, New Delhi, Jaypee brothers medical publishers (P) Ltd. ; 2015, Chapter 10, pages 219 - 256

BUPHTHALMOS

Dr. S. K. Bhasker, Professor, Department of Ophthalmology

A 2 month male infant was referred to our tertiary care institute from a primary health centre. The parents complained that the infant had whitish coloration of both eyes since birth. Size of eyeballs is also increasing for last one and half months. They consulted local health centre from where the child was referred here. Antenatal history was non contributory.

On examination no congenital defect was detected except buphthalmos. The corneal diameter was 12mm in both axis in both eyes. Intra ocular pressure was 14mm (OU) by Perkins tonometer. Gonioscopy by Koeppe lens could not be done due to hazy cornea with central corneal opacity . Above examination was conducted under anesthesia. (vide figure below)

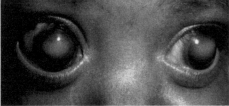

Trabeculectomy with trabeculotomy was done in both eyes at one sitting. Post operative IOP was 10mm in both eyes by rebound tonometer, and the haziness of cornea cleared except for the central opacity.

1. In an infant average normal corneal diameter (in mm) is
   (A) 5
   (B) 10
   (C) 12
   (D) 14
2. Intra ocular pressure measured in an infant with buphthalmos may be
   (A) Normal
   (B) Decreased
   (C) Increased
   (D) Depend on corneal diameter
3. Typical Haab's striae seen in cornea of buphthalmos are
   (A) Single tram track radial
   (B) Single tram track concentric to limbus
   (C) Double tram track radial
   (D) Double tram track concentric to limbus
4. Medication to be avoided in buphthalmic infant due to its crossing the blood brain barrier is
   (A) Pilocarpine
   (B) Timolol
   (C) Brimonidine
   (D) Dorzolamide
5. Definitive management of buphthalmic patient is
   (A) Medical
   (B) Surgical
   (C) Laser

(D) Keratoplasty

Answers:

1. B

   Average corneal diameter in infant is 10mm. Cornea with diameter of 5mm will be micro cornea, while with 12 or 14 mm may be associated with buphthalmos or megalocornea.

2. A

   Sclera in infant is elastic, therefore any increase in IOP is compensated by increase in size of eye ball, leading to buphthalmos with normal IOP. If IOP is decreased, enlargement of globe will not occur. The size of cornea is dependent on IOP and not vice versa.

3. D

4. C

   Brimonidine crosses the blood brain barrier and causes depression of central nervous system.

5. B

   Surgical procedures will divert the aqueous in paediatric glaucomas. Medical treatment is used till surgery is conduced. The effects or side effects of antiglaucoma medication for a very long period, has not been studied. These glaucomas are associated with congenital anomalies (mainly in angle), which may render the antiglaucoma medication ineffective.

References:

1. Sihota R, Tandon R (editors). Parsons' diseases of the eye; Elsevier, New Delhi. 21st edition, 2011, Chapter 19, pages 280 – 300.

2. Kanski JJ, Bowling B. Clinical Ophthalmology – A systemic approach. 7th edition. New York: Elsevier; 2011.

3. Allingham RR, Damji KF, Freedman S, Moroi SE, Rhee DJ. Shields textbook of glaucoma. 6th edition. Philadelphia. Wolters Kluwer & Lippincott Williams and Wilkins. 2011

4. Neema HV, Neema N. Textbook of Ophthalmology; 5th edition, New Delhi, Jaypee brothers medical publishers (P) Ltd; 2008, chapter 15, pages 214 – 249

5. Khurana N. Comprehensive ophthalmology, 6th edition, New Delhi, Jaypee brothers medical publishers (P) Ltd. ; 2015, Chapter 10, pages 219 - 256

PRE PERIMETRIC GLAUCOMA

Dr. S. K. Bhasker, Professor, Department of Ophthalmology

A 44 year old female came to our department with complains of diminution of vision (more for near vision) for 1 year. She was advised refraction.

On refraction patient was mildly hypermetropic. Fundus examination revealed cup to disc ratio of 0.7:1 and 0.75:1 in right and left eye respectively. Retinal nerve fiber wedge defects were also seen. (vide the areas marked by stars in fundus photographs below). She was referred to glaucoma unit for detailed glaucoma evaluation.

Patient's history was non contributory except that her elder sister has glaucoma and is on medication. Intra ocular pressures were 14 mmHg (OD) and 16 mmHg (OS). Central corneal thickness was 583☐☐ for right eye and 588☐☐ for left eye. Goniscopy showed open angle in both eyes.

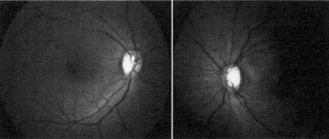

Optical coherrance tomography showed marked thinning in nerve fiber layer in left eye (vide OCT printout below). The visual fields were within normal limits. She was diagnosed to be a case of pre perimetric glaucoma and was kept on regular followup at 3 months interval.

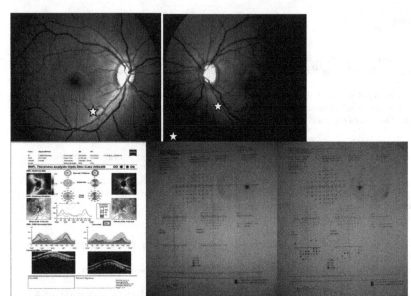

1. Visual field defects on Standard Automated Perimetry (white on white) in glaucoma appear when the loss of ganglion cells is more than
   (A) 13%
   (B) 33%
   (C) 63%
   (D) 93%

2. Well established neuroprotective medication is
   (A) Bimatoprost
   (B) Brimonidine
   (C) Betaxolol
   (D) Brinzolamide

3. Pre perimetric glaucoma can be estabilished by all **EXCEPT**
   (A) 30-2 Short wave automated perimetry (SWAP)
   (B) 30-2 Standard automated perimetry (SAP)
   (C) Optical coherrence tomography
   (D) GDx

4. Short wave automated perimetry (SWAP) detects visual field defects earlier than standard automated perimeter (SAP) is by using
   (A) Blue spot on white background
   (B) Blue spot on yellow background
   (C) White spot on yellow background
   (D) White spot on white background

5. The area marked by stars in the fundus photos above are wedge defects due to loss in
   (A) Retinal nerve fiber layer
   (B) Bipolar cells
   (C) Outer plexiform layer
   (D) Outer nuclear layer

Answers:
1. B
   Initial changes occur when 33% or more retinal ganglion cells are lost.
2. B
3. B
   33% of retinal ganglion cells are lost before field changes can be detected on visual field. But they can be detected by imaging and SWAP
4. B
5. A

The axons of retinal ganglion cells form the innermost nerve fiber layer in retina. Glaucoma is a condition where these cells are lost due to apoptosis, leading to formation of wedge defects in retina.

References:

1. Sihota R, Tandon R (editors). Parsons' diseases of the eye; Elsevier, New Delhi. 21st edition, 2011, Chapter 19, pages 280 – 300.
2. Kanski JJ, Bowling B. Clinical Ophthalmology – A systemic approach. 7th edition. New York: Elsevier; 2011.
3. Allingham RR, Damji KF, Freedman S, Moroi SE, Rhee DJ. Shields textbook of glaucoma. 6th edition. Philadelphia. Wolters Kluwer & Lippincott Williams and Wilkins. 2011
4. Neema HV, Neema N. Textbook of Ophthalmology; 5th edition, New Delhi, Jaypee brothers medical publishers (P) Ltd; 2008, chapter 15, pages 214 – 249
5. Khurana N. Comprehensive ophthalmology, 6th edition, New Delhi, Jaypee brothers medical publishers (P) Ltd. ; 2015, Chapter 10, pages 219 - 256

GLAUCOMATOUS OPTIC DISC ATROPHY

Dr. S K Bhasker, Professor, Department of Ophthalmology

Evaluate the optic disc photograph and answer the questions that follow.

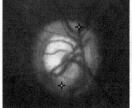

1. The C/D ratio shown is
   (A) 0.4:1
   (B) 0.6:1
   (C) 0.8:1
   (D) 1.0:1
2. Visual field of the patient will show
   (A) Superior Arcuate Scotoma
   (B) Inferior Arcuate Scotoma
   (C) Biarcuate Scotoma
   (D) Nasal Step Scotoma
3. Significant Thinning of Nerve fiber layer at the disc on OCT imaging will be present at the
   (A) Superior pole
   (B) Inferior pole
   (C) Nasal margin
   (D) Temporal margin ..
4. Area marked by star is
   (A) Alfa (☐) zone
   (B) Notch in the neural rim
   (C) Coloboma disc
   (D) Beta (☐) zone
5. The vessel (marked by blue arrows) is showing
   (A) Overpass cupping
   (B) Bayoneting
   (C) Baring
   (D) Proximal constriction

Answers:

1. B
2. A
   Notch (deficiency of nerve fibres) is seen in the inferiorly, therefore visual field defect would be seen in superior Arcuate region

3. B
OCT is a imaging technique for the disc. Therefore inferior pole will show thinning.
4. B
Loss of nerve fibers causes a notch in the neural rim of the disc. Alfa (☐) and beta (☐) zones are areas around the disc, while coloboma is a congenital defect.
5. B

References:
1. Sihota R, Tandon R (editors). Parsons' diseases of the eye; Elsevier, New Delhi. 21st edition, 2011, Chapter 19, pages 280 – 300.
2. Kanski JJ, Bowling B. Clinical Ophthalmology – A systemic approach. 7th edition. New York: Elsevier; 2011.
3. Allingham RR, Damji KF, Freedman S, Moroi SE, Rhee DJ. Shields textbook of glaucoma. 6th edition. Philadelphia. Wolters Kluwer & Lippincott Williams and Wilkins. 2011
4. Neema HV, Neema N. Textbook of Ophthalmology; 5th edition, New Delhi, Jaypee brothers medical publishers (P) Ltd; 2008, chapter 15, pages 214 – 249
5. Khurana N. Comprehensive ophthalmology, 6th edition, New Delhi, Jaypee brothers medical publishers (P) Ltd. ; 2015, Chapter 10, pages 219 - 256

CENTRAL SEROUS CHOROIDOPATHY

Dr. Sandeep Saxena , Professor, Department of Ophthalmology

A 49-year male, with coexistent well-controlled type 2 diabetes mellitus of 8 years duration, presented to our tertiary care center with the complaints of decreased and distorted vision in both the eyes since 1 year. The best corrected logMAR visual acuity was 1 (20/200) in both the eyes. Slit lamp examination results were unremarkable. Fundus examination of both the eyes revealed central serous chorioretinopathy. Spectral domain optical coherence tomography (SD-OCT) of both the eyes showed neurosensory detachment of the macula with retinal pigment epithelial detachment (PED). 3D reconstruction on SD-OCT further enhanced the understanding of the plane of fluid collection. The RPE layer was found to be hyperplastic in the right eye. Single-layer RPE map topography showed surface alterations in both eyes.

The patient was treated with 1.25 mg/0.05 ml of intravitreal bevacizumab in the right eye and 4 weeks later in the left eye. Each eye was reassessed 6 weeks after therapy. The best-corrected logMAR visual acuity was 0.78 (20/120) in the right eye and 0.30 (20/40) in the left eye.

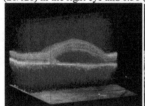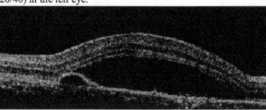

Optical coherence tomography of the right eye showed resolution of subretinal fluid with persistent PED. Foveal contour was restored. Residual granularity at OPL and proliferative RPE cells were visualized. Small cystic spaces were also observed.The ILM-RPE macular thickness reduced. SD-OCT of the left eye showed minimal subretinal fluid in the macula with residual PED. Multiple cystic spaces were also observed temporally. At 1-year follow up, visual acuity was maintained in both the eyes.

1. Differential diagnosis of central serous chorioretinopathy are all except:
   (A) choroidal melanoma
   (B) optic disc pit
   (C) polypoidal choroidalvasculopathy
   (D) macular edema
2. Risk factors for central serous chorioretinopathy:
   (A) Type A personality
   (B) emotional stress
   (C) corticosteroid
   (D) All of the above.
3. False about central serous chorioretinopathy:

(A) Leakage of dye from choroidal vessels through focal RPE defect on fluorescein angiography.

(B) Presence of subretinal fluid and thickening of choroid on optical coherence tomography.

(C) delineation of edge of area of RPE dysfunction on fundus autofluorescence.

(D) pooling within two disc diameter of fovea is found in more than 75% patients.

4. Complication of central serous retinopathy is:

(A) retinal detachment

(B) neovascular glaucoma

(C) choroidal neovascularization

(D) explusivechoroidal haemorrhage

5. Conventional dose of verteporfin may cause all except:

(A) choroidal neovascularization

(B) diffuse retinal atrophy

(C) severe retinal thinning

(D) choiroidal haemorrhage

Answers:

1. A
2. D
3. D
4. C
5. D

References:

1. Schaal KB, Hoeh AE, Scheuerle A, Schuett F, Dithmar S. Intravitreal bevacizumab for treatment of chronic central serous chorioretinopathy. Eur J Ophthalmol. 2009; 19:613–7.

2. Simo R, Villarroel M, Corraliza L, Hernandez C, Garcia-RamirezM. The retinal pigment epithelium: something more than a constituent of the blood-retinal barrier-implications for the pathogenesis of diabetic retinopathy. J Biomed Biotechnol. 2010. doi:10.1155/2010/190724.

3. Piccolino FC, Llongrais RR, Ravera G, et al. The foveal photoreceptor layer and visual acuity loss in central serous chorioretinopathy. Am J Ophthalmol. 2005;139:87–99.

4. Kroll AJ, Machemer R. Experimental retinal detachment in the owl monkey. III. Electron microscopy of retina and pigment epithelium. Am J Ophthalmol. 1968; 66:410–27.

5. Anderson DH, Guerin CJ, Erickson PA, Stern WH, Fisher SK. .Morphological recovery in the reattached retina. Invest OphthalmolVis Sci. 1986; 27:168–83.

6. Cook B, Lewis GP, Fisher SK, Adler R. Apoptotic photoreceptor degeneration in experimental retinal detachment. Invest Ophthalmol Vis Sci. 1995; 36:990–6.

7. Hisatomi T, Sakamoto T, Goto Y, et al. Critical role of photoreceptor apoptosis in functional damage after retinal detachment. Curr Eye Res. 2002;24:161–72.

DIABETIC RETINOPATHY

Dr. Sandeep Saxena, Professor, Department of Ophthalmology

A 56-year male, with type 2 diabetes mellitus of 17 years duration, presented to our tertiary care center with the complaints of decreased vision in both the eyes since 6 months. The best corrected visual acuity (BCVA) was 6/36 in right eyeand 6/24 in the left eye. Slit lamp examination was unremarkable. Fundus examination of both the eyes revealed non proliferative diabetic retinopathy (NPDR): superficial and deep retinal hemorrhages, microaneurysms with clinically significant macular edema (CSME). Blood investigations showed blood sugar level fasting of 98mg/dl and post prandial 150mg/ dl, glycated hemoglobin of 8.35 %.On SD-OCT macular cube analysis using 512×128 feature demonstrated,central sub foveal thickness (CST) of2ßfn in right eye and 259μm in left eye, central average thickness (CAT) of 300μm in right eye and 268μm in left eye, cube volume of 9.5 and 7.8 in right and left eye respectively and grade 1 disruptionof ISel band of both the eyes.The patient was treated with 1.25 mg/0.05 ml of intravitreal bevacizumab in the right eye and 4 weeks later in the left eye. Each eye was reassessed 6 weeks after therapy. The BCVA was 6/12in the right eye and 6/9 in the left eye. SD-OCT showed CST of 221μm in right eye and 214 μm in left eye, CAT of 245 μm and 233 μm in right and left eye respectively, cube volume of 8 mm^3 in right eye and 6.5 mm^3 cube volume in left eye.

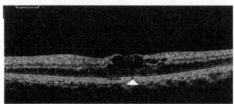

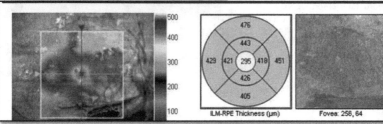

1. Oral hypoglycemic agents of choice in patients with diabetic retinopathy:
   (A) Metformin
   (B) Sulfonylurea
   (C) Pioglitazone
   (D) Statin
2. Optical coherence tomography was developed by:
   (A) Huang
   (B) Rosen
   (C) Gullstrand
   (D) Snellen
3. External limiting membrane is considered to be a part of:
   (A) blood- retinal barrier
   (B) Retinal pigment epithelium
   (C) Bruch's membrane
   (D) Retinal nerve fibre layer.
4. Avastin (Bevacizumab) has an approximate molecular weight of :
   (A) 149 kD
   (B) 178 kD
   (C) 100 kD
   (D) 70 kD
5. Cotton wool spots are found in:
   (A) Nerve fibre layer
   (B) External limiting membrane
   (C) Outer nuclear layer
   (D) Inner nuclear layer

Answers:

1. C
   Pioglitazone
2. A
   Huang
3. A
   Blood- retinal barrier
4. A
   149 kD
5. A
   Nerve fibre layer

References:

1. Jain A, Saxena S, Khanna VK, Shukla RK, Meyer CH. Status of serum VEGF and ICAM-1 and its association with external limiting membrane and inner segment-outer segment junction disruption in type 2 diabetes mellitus. Molecular Vision 2013.19; 1760-68.

2. Browning D, Glassman A, Aiello L. Relationship between optical coherence tomography-measured central retinal thickness and visual acuity in diabetic macular edema. Ophthalmology 2007; 114:525-36.

3. SharmaSR, Saxena S, Mishra N, Akduman L, Meyer CH. The Association of Grades of Photoreceptor Inner Segment-Ellipsoid Band Disruption with Severity of Retinopathy in Type 2 Diabetes Mellitus. Journal of Case Reports and Studies 2014.

4. Saxena S, Srivastav K, Akduman L. Spectral domain optical coherence tomography based alterations in macular thickness and inner segment ellipsoid are associated with severity of diabetic retinopathy. Int J Ophthalmolol Clin Res 2015; 2007.

RETINAL DETACHMENT

Dr. Sanjiv Gupta, Professor, Department of Ophthalmology

A 45 years old lady, resident of Kanpur presented in the KGMU OPD with a 5 months history of sudden painless diminuition of vision in right eye which has been stationary since then. She was prescribed glasses with no improvement in vision. There is no history of ocular trauma or surgery. No history of flashes or floaters. No history of Diabetes or Hypertension. History of valvular heart surgery 3 years back. Vision in right eye was finger counting 1ft PR full with no improvement on pinhole. Direct and consensual pupillary reflexes were present with RAPD right eye. IOP taken using Rebound tonometry was 14 in both eyes. On Slit lamp examination of right eye, Shaffers sign was present with degenerated vitreous behind lens. RE Fundus as seen with indirect ophthalmoscopy with indentation revealed subtotal RD with macula off, corrugated convex surface with tortuous blood vessels with subretinal fluid present extending upto superotemporal and superonasal arcades and multiple atrophic holes with lattice degeneration (snail track degeneration)

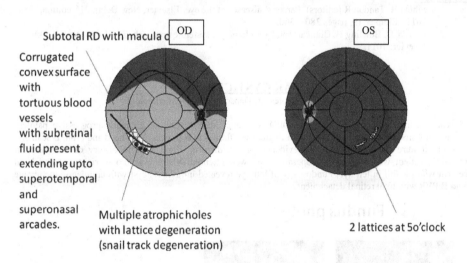

Subtotal RD with macula off | OD | | OS

Corrugated convex surface with tortuous blood vessels with subretinal fluid present extending upto superotemporal and superonasal arcades.

Multiple atrophic holes with lattice degeneration (snail track degeneration)

2 lattices at 5o'clock

1. What is the most likely diagnosis:
   (A) Vitreous hemorrhage
   (B) Retinal Detachment
   (C) CRAO
   (D) BRVO
2. The following retinal findings are associated with rhegmatogenous RD
   (A) Lattice degeneration
   (B) Cystic retinal tuft
   (C) Congenital hypertrophy of RPE
   (D) Meridonal folds
3. RD resulting from break in retina is called
   (A) Rhegmatogenous RD
   (B) Tractional RD

(C) Exudative RD
(D) Retinoschisis
4. Findings consistent with rhegmatogenous RD are all <u>EXCEPT</u>
   (A) Increased IOP
   (B) Shaffer's sign
   (C) Convex surface of detached retina
   (D) Presence of lattice
5. Most common type of RD
   (A) Rhegmatogenous
   (B) Tractional
   (C) Exudative
   (D) None

Answers:
1. B
   RAPD, Shaffer's sign and sub-total RD are indicative of retinal detachment
2. A
   Lattice degeneration can lead to retinal break and subsequent retinal detachment.

3. A
   As per nomenclature and classification of retinal detachment
4. A
   IOP is usually lower or normal
5.   A
   Rhegmatogenous RD is most common type

References:
1. Sihota R, Tandon R (editors). Parsons' diseases of the eye; Elsevier, New Delhi. 21st edition, 2011, Chapter 19, pages 280 – 300.
2. Kanski JJ, Bowling B. Clinical Ophthalmology – A systemic approach. 7th edition. New York: Elsevier; 2011.

OCULAR CYSTICERCOSIS
Dr. Sanjiv Gupta, Professor, Department of Ophthalmology

A 45 years old male presented at KGMU OPD with a 25 days history of gradually progressive painless diminution of vision in left eye associated with floaters and flashes in both eyes. MRI head and orbit, B scan and Fundus photo were done which showed evidence of the disease. There was no history of seizures. On examination, patient was conscious, cooperative and well oriented. Vision was 6/6 in right eye and hand movement with PR full in left eye. Fundoscopy of left eye revealed intravitreal cyst with undulating membrane with gd B PVR with total retinal detachment.

Fundus photo

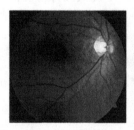 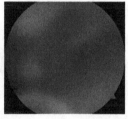

RE   LE

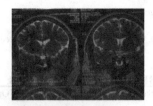

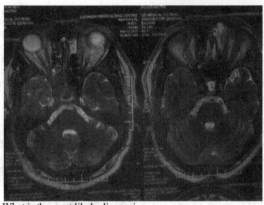

1. What is the most likely diagnosis:
   (A) Brain tumor
   (B) Disseminated cysticercosis
   (C) Tuberculoma
   (D) Brain abcess
2. Most common site of ocular cysticercosis is:
   (A) subretinal and intravitreal
   (B) lids and conjuctiva
   (C) anterior chamber
   (D) extraocular muscle
3. All are true **EXCEPT**
   (A) Antihelminthic should not be started in cases of extraocular musle cysticercous
   (B) Oral antihelminthic may predispose to endophthalmitis in cases of intravitreal cysticercous
   (C) Intravitreal cysticercous causes rhegmatogenous RD
   (D) Intravitreal cyst may lead to uniocular diplopia in early stages
4. Imaging studies used for establishing diagnosis are all except
   (A) B scan
   (B) CT scan
   (C) MRI
   (D) X Ray
5. Treatment of choice for intravitreal cysticercosis is
   (A) Pars Plana Vitrectomy
   (B) Systemic antihelmenthics
   (C) Wait and watch till the Cysticercus undergoes spontaneous death.
   (D) Intravitreal injection of antimicrobial drugs.

Answers:

1. B

   the fundus photo shows the cyst with MRI showing ring enhancing lesion
2. A

   Intravitreal is the most common site followed by sub-retinal
3. A

   The treatment of choice is antihelmintics for extraocular cysts

4. D
    X-ray cannot show cysticercus cyst
5. A
    Removal of cyst by surgery is only treatment.

Reference:
1. Yanoff M, Duker J. Ophthalmology. 4th edition. United States: Elsevier Saunders; 2014

DIABETIC RETINOPATHY & OCT
Dr. Sandeep Saxena, Professor, Department of Ophthalmology

A 56-year male, with type 2diabetes mellitus of 13 years duration, presented to our tertiary care center with the complaints of decreased vision in both the eyes since 2 year. The best corrected visual acuity (BCVA) was 4/60 and 3/60 (Snellen) in right and left eye respectively. The patient had immature senile cataract in both eyes. Rest slit lamp examination was unremarkable. Fundus examination of right eyes revealed proliferative diabetic retinopathy with clinically significant macular edema (PDR with CSME) superficial and deep retinal hemorrhages in all four qaudrants, neovascularization at disc and hard exudates temporal to the foves. Fundus examination of left eye revealed PDR with CSME: neovascularization along the supero-temporal vascular arcade, IRMA in two quadrants, venous beading.

Fasting blood sugar and post prandial blood sugar levels were 98 mg/dl, 135 mg/dl. Glycosylated hemoglobin level was 8.1 %.

SD-OCT for macular thickness analysis using macular cube 512x 128 feature showed centr al subfield thickness of 289 µm, cube average thickness of 300 µm and cube volume of 10.9 mm3of right eye and central subfield thickness(CST) of 372 µm, cube average thickness(CAT) of 328 µm and cube volume of 11.9 mm3 of left eye. Single layer retinal pigment epithelium (RPE) map showed alteration in two quadrants in right eye and three quadrants in left eye . External limiting membrane (ELM) and Inner segment ellipsoid band (ISel) were both disrupted in the two eyes.

The patient was treated with 1.25 mg/0.05 ml of intravitreal bevacizumab in the right eye and 4 weeks later in the left eye. Each eye was reassessed 6 weeks after therapy. The BCVA was 6/36 in the right eye and 6/60 in the left eye. OCT showed resolution of subretinal fluid. Right eye showed a CST and CAT was 260 µm, 258 µm, while left eye documented a CST and CAT of 230 µm, 270 µm.

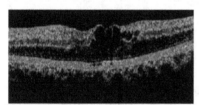

Figure 1: Spectral domain optical coherence tomogrphy showing macular edema (Right eye).

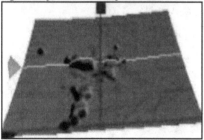

Figure 2: Single layer retinal pigment epithelium topographical map showing alteration in two quadrants (Right eye).

1. True about Inner segment ellipsoid band:
    (A) it is the inner segment-outer segment junction of photoreceptor
    (B) outer highly reflective band next to RPE
    (C) concept given by Spaeth
    (D) ISel disruption is not related with visual prognosis.

2. N-carboxy methyl Lysine is:
   (A) anti-VEGF
   (B) advancedglycated end product
   (C) VEGF
   (D) ICAM
3. Increase in macular central subfield thickness is related with:
   (A) Increased LDL cholesterol
   (B) severity of diabetic retinopathy
   (C) ELM amdISel disruption
   (D) All of the above.
4. Bruch's membrane is a :
   (A) Penta-laminal structure
   (B) Housed most amount of lysozymes
   (C) most prone to age related dysfunction
   (D) highly cellular structure
5. ETDRS definition includes :
   (A) Hard exudates within 500 micron of the fovea
   (B) Retinal thickening of 500 microns or more
   (C) Retinal thickening of 500 microns a part of which lies within 1 DD of the fovea
   (D) Retinal thickening within 1 DD of the disc

Answers:

1. A
   It is the inner segment-outer segment junction of photoreceptor
2. B
   Advanced glycated end product
3. D
   All of the above.
4. A
   Pentalaminal structure
5. D
   Retinal thickening within 1 DD of the disc

References:

1. Sharma SR, SaxenaS, Mishra N, Akduman L, Meyer CH. The association of grades of photoreceptor inner segment-ellipsoid band disruption with severity of retinopathy in type 2 diabetes mellitus. J Case Rep Stud. 2014; 2:205.
2. Jain A, Saxena S, Khanna VK, Shukla RK, Meyer CH. Status of serum VEGF and ICAM-1 and its association with external limiting membrane and inner segment-outer segment junction disruption in type 2 diabetes mellitus. Molecular Vision 2013.19; 1760-68.
3. Saxena S, Mishra N, Khanna V, Jain A, Shukla R, et al. Increased Serum N-CML, VEGF and ICAM-1 is Associated with Photoreceptor Inner Segment Ellipsoid Disruption in Diabetic Retinopathy. JSM Biotechnol Bioeng 2014; 2(2): 1039.
4. Saxena S, Srivastav K, Akduman L. Spectral domain optical coherence tomography based alterations in macular thickness and inner segment ellipsoidare associated with severity of diabetic retinopathy. Int J Ophthalmolol Clin Res 2015; 2007.

Chapter-14

Orthopaedics

MULTIPLE HEREDITARY EXOSTOSIS

Dr. Ashish Kumar and Dr. Vineet Sharma, Professor, Department of Orthopaedics

A 15-year-old boy presents with a painless mass over his right shoulder. It has been slowly growing over the past year. On examination similar swelling was found on right knee. Patient's sibling has similar swelling over shoulder and knee.

1. What is the most likely diagnosis?
   - (A) Lipoma
   - (B) Osteochondroma
   - (C) Osteosarcoma
   - (D) Ewing's sarcoma
2. This patient may have all complications except
   - (A) absence of the thumb
   - (B) ulnar deviation of the wrist
   - (C) valgus deformity of the knee
   - (D) limb-length discrepancy
3. All of the following are true of multiple hereditary exostoses (MHE) EXCEPT
   - (A) The rate of transformation to chondrosarcoma is less than 10% in MHE
   - (B) The most common joint affected is the knee
   - (C) Exostoses grow towards the joint in MHE but away from the joint in solitary osteochondromas
   - (D) Caused by mutation(s) in the EXT1/EXT2/EXT3 genes
4. All of the following statements regarding hereditary multiple exostosis (HME) are correct EXCEPT?
   - (A) Radiographically, the exostoses grow towards the physis
   - (B) Radiographically, the exostoses are in direct connection to the medullary cavity
   - (C) It is caused by mutations in either EXT1, EXT2, or EXT3 genes
   - (D) Mutations in HME affect the prehypertrophic chondrocytes of the growth plate

Answers:

1. B
2. A
3. C
4. A

Reason-The solitary osteochondroma, a common pediatric bone tumor, is a cartilage-capped exostosis. Multiple Hereditary Exostoses is an autosomal dominant inherited disease cause by mutations in the EXT1, EXT2, or EXT3 genes. Like solitary osteochondromas, periarticular lesions grow away from joints. Although exostoses are benign lesions, they are often associated with characteristic progressive skeletal deformities and may cause clinical symptoms. The most common deformities include short stature, limb-length discrepancies, valgus deformities of the knee and ankle, asymmetry of the pectoral and pelvic girdles, bowing of the radius with ulnar deviation of the wrist, and subluxation of the radiocapitellar joint.

References:

1. Schmale GA, Conrad EU III, Raskind WH: The natural history of hereditary multiple exostoses. J Bone Joint Surg Am 1994;76:986-992
2. Stieber JR, Dormans JP: Manifestations of hereditary multiple exostoses. J Am Acad Orthop Surg 2005;13:110-120

EWING'S SARCOMA

Dr. Ashish Kumar and Dr. Vineet Sharma, Professor, Department of Orthopaedics

A 10-year-old male presents with ongoing complaints of left thigh pain after fall during a soccer game. He has tenderness and general warmth over the lateral aspect of his left thigh. His ESR is 82 and his WBC is 15,000. Radiograph shows lytic destructive lesion in mid shaft region.

1. What is most likely diagnosis?
   - (A) Ewing Sarcoma
   - (B) Osteosarcoma
   - (C) Osteochondroma
   - (D) Acute Osteomyelitis

2. Possible management of above condition
   (A) Neoadjuvant chemotherapy and surgical excision
   (B) Neoadjuvant chemotherapy, surgical excision, and radiation therapy
   (C) Neoadjuvant chemotherapy, surgical excision, and adjuvant chemotherapy
   (D) Neoadjuvant radiation therapy and surgical excision
3. All of the following could be a differential for above condition except
   (A) Embryonal rhabdomyosarcoma
   (B) Primitive neuroectodermal tumors (PNET
   (C) Ewing's sarcoma
   (D) Synovial sarcoma
4. What is the most likely translocation associated with this condition?
   (A) t(10;20)
   (B) t(11;22)
   (C) t(X;18)
   (D) t(9;22)

Answers:
1. A
2. C
3. D
4. B

Reason-Ewing's sarcoma primarily occurs in patients that are less than 20 years of age and is the 2nd most common (primary) malignant bone tumor in children. The etiology of Ewing's sarcoma is an 11:22 chromosomal translocation that produces the EWS/FLI1 fusion gene, which can be detected by polymerase chain reaction (PCR). Treatment consistently includes neoadjuvant multiagent chemotherapy followed by either surgical resection or radiation. Neuroblastoma, primitive neuroectodermal tumors (PNET), Ewing's sarcoma, and embryonal rhabdomyosarcoma are tumors having round cell components.

References:
1. Patterson FR, Basra SK. Ewing's sarcoma. In: Schwartz HS, ed. Orthopaedic Knowledge Update: Musculoskeletal Tumors 2. Rosemont, IL: American Academy of Orthopaedic Surgeons; 2007:175-183.
2. Damron T.A. Orthopaedic Surgery Essentials, Oncology and Basic Science. Philadelphia, PA: Lippincott Williams & Wilkins; 2008:187-191.

RECURRENT DISLOCATION OF SHOULDER
Dr. Ashish Kumar and Dr. Vineet Sharma, Professor, Department of Orthopaedics

A 30 year old patient comes to the OPD with history of trauma over shoulder one year back which resulted in dislocation of the shoulder and since then whenever he tries to wear clothes by overhead movements his shoulder pops out in front. MRI shows altered signal intensity in anterior labrum with effusion.
1. What is the likely diagnosis?
   (A) Rotator cuff tear
   (B) Posterior dislocation of shoulder
   (C) Recurrent anterior dislocation of shoulder
   (D) SLAP tear
2. What is the movement called for testing the condition?
   (A) Hamilton test
   (B) Apprehension test
   (C) Pivot shift test
   (D) Hawkins test
3. What is the treatment of the condition?
   (A) Single row cuff repair
   (B) Bankarts repair for anterior instability
   (C) Sub-acromial decompression
   (D) Biceps tenodesis
4. What is the most appropriate investigation?
   (A) X-ray
   (B) USG

(C) MRI Scan
(D) Arthrogram

Answers:

1. C
2. B
3. B
4. C

Reason: Recurrent dislocation of shoulder is one of the most common sports injury encountered in athletes. It is best diagnosed by MRI and clinically by Apprehension test. High demand patient requires arthroscopic repair of labrum to prevent instability.

References:

1. Taylor DC, Arciero RA: Pathologic changes associated with shoulder dislocations: Arthroscopic and physical examination findings in first-time, traumatic anterior dislocations. Am J Sports Med 1997; 25:306-311
2. Hintermann B, Gachter A: Arthroscopic findings after shoulder dislocation. Am J Sports Med 1995; 23:545-551 PMID:8526268 (Link to Abstract)

RECURRENT DISLOCATION OF PATELLA

Dr. Ashish Kumar and Dr. Vineet Sharma, Professor, Department of Orthopaedics

A 24 year old female comes to the OPD with six weeks old history of knee trauma. She is now giving history that whenever she tries to kneel for her prayers her patella moves and comes to lie in lateral side of knee.

1. What is the likely diagnosis?
    (A) Medial Collateral ligament injury
    (B) Recurrent dislocation of Patella
    (C) ACL injury
    (D) PCL injury
2. What is the most appropriate diagnostic test?
    (A) Apprehension test
    (B) Lachman's test
    (C) O'Brien Test
    (D) Hawkins Test
3. What is the most appropriate investigation?
    (A) MRI
    (B) X-ray
    (C) USG
    (D) Arthrogram
4. What is the likely cause of above clinical condition?
    (A) Hypoplasia of medial femoral condyle
    (B) Hypoplasia of lateral femoral condyle
    (C) Medial patella-femoral ligament disruption
    (D) ACL rupture
5. How do you manage the above patient?
    (A) MPFL reconstruction
    (B) Patellar osteotomy
    (C) Plication of patellar tendon
    (D) Quadricepsplasty

Answers:

1. B
2. A
3. A
4. C
5. A

Patellofemoral instability may results from trauma or due anatomic defect in femoral condyles. Patellofemoral instability following trauma results in rupture of medial patellofemoral ligament. Patellofemoral instability can be diagnosed clinically by apprehension test and radiologically by MRI.Management requires arthroscopic reconstruction of medial patellofemoral ligament.

References:

1. Toritsuka Y, Horibe S, Hiro-Oka A, Mitsuoka T, Nakamura N. Medial marginal fracture of the patella following patellar dislocation. Knee. 2007 Dec; 14(6):429-33.
2. Nomura E, Horiuchi Y, Inoue M. Correlation of MR imaging findings and open exploration of medial patellofemoral ligament injuries in acute patellar dislocations. Knee. 2002 May; 9(2):139-43.

NEGLECTED CONGENITAL TALIPES EQUINOVARUS

Dr. Ajai Singh and Dr. Vineet Sharma, Professor, Department of Orthopaedics

A 12 years old female child presented to orthopaedic OPD with club feet. Her parents gave history that the deformity was present since birth but due to poverty she was not subjected to any treatment. Child was walking on deformed feet with callosities on outer aspect of her feet. There was no clinical evidence suggestive of any secondary cause of these club feet.

1. What is the most appropriate diagnosis?
   (A) Relapsed club feet
   (B) Neglected club feet
   (C) Rigid club feet
   (D) Recurrent club feet
2. Which of the following investigations should be commonly required before the management of this child?
   (A) Ultrasound of feet
   (B) Plain radiographs of feet
   (C) CT scan feet
   (D) MRI Feet
3. Which of the following angles will be suggestive of the forefoot adduction?
   (A) Talo-Ist Metatarsal
   (B) Talo-Vth Metatarsal
   (C) Talo- calcaneal
   (D) Foot axis
4. Equinus deformity 'primarily' occurs at
   (A) Ankle joint
   (B) Hind foot
   (C) Talonavicular joint
   (D) Calcaneocuboid joint
5. Which of the following treatment modality will be most appropriate for her?
   (A) Corrective plasters alone
   (B) Soft tissue release alone
   (C) Corrective osteotomies alone
   (D) Arthrodesis alone

Answers:

1. B
   As the patient is walking so she developed callosities, which signifies that no treatment was given in form of plasters or any surgery i.e., it was neglected.
2. B
   As the bones are ossified by this age and it's a relatively common, cheap and informative investigation.
3. A
   Fore foot adduction occurs at intertarsal joints (talo navicular joint on medial and calcaneocuboid joint on lateral side). So, on X-rays talo 1st metatarsal angle is suggestive of foot adduction deformity.
4. A
   Equinus is planter flexed attitude at ankle joint. Plater and dorsiflexion occurs at ankle joint (tibio talar).
5. D
   Soft tissue procedures won't help as the bones are ossified by this age and soft tissues are non compliant to stretch.

References:
1. Sobel E Giorgini R Velez Z. Surgical correction of adult neglected clubfoot: three case histories. J Foot Ankle Surg. 1996;35(1):27-38
2. Bitariho D, Penny JN. Triple arthrodesis in children for severe neglected clubfoot deformity. Presented at the Association of Surgeons of East Africa; December 3–5, 2003
3. C. Radler, H. M. Manner, R. Suda et al., "Radiographic evaluation of idiopathic clubfeet undergoing Ponseti treatment," The Journal of Bone and Joint Surgery, vol. 89, no. 6, pp. 1177–1183, 2007.

CUBITUS VARUS DEFORMITY

Dr. Ajai Singh and Dr. Vineet Sharma, Professor, Department of Orthopaedics

An eight years old child sustained injury around left elbow three months back. He was managed by a local practitioner in an above elbow plaster for three weeks. Child presented in orthopedics OPD after six months with cubitus varus deformity of left elbow.

1. What could be the most appropriate case of cubitus elbow in this child?
   (A) Fracture medial epicondyle humerus
   (B) Fracture supracondylar humerus
   (C) Fracture olecranon
   (D) Fracture lateral epicondyle humerus
2. What will be the relationship of three points of elbow in this case?
   (A) Distance between medial epicondyle and tip olecranon will be altered
   (B) Distance between lateral epicondyle and tip olecranon will be altered
   (C) Intercondylar distance will be altered
   (D) Relationship will remain unaltered
3. Which of the following is a component of cubitus varus
   (A) Internal torsion of distal fragment
   (B) Internal torsion of proximal fragment
   (C) External rotation of distal fragment
   (D) External torsion of distal fragment
4. Cubitus varus is commonly managed by
   (A) Temporary epiphysiodesis
   (B) Permanent epiphysiodesis
   (C) Corrective osteotomy
   (D) Elbow arthrodesis
5. Cubitus varus is defined as decrease of
   (A) Q angle
   (B) Carrying angle
   (C) Kite angle
   (D) Anatomical axis

Answers:
1. B
   Most common long term complication of this fracture also known as gun stock deformity.
2. D
   Three point bony relationship is between the two epicondyles and olecranon tip. As the fracture is at supracondylar level so they are supposed to be maintained
3. A
   Common displacements in fracture supracondylar humerus are:
   Posterior displacement and tilt
   Medial rotation
   Lateral / Medial displacement
4. C
   Provides immediate correction (clinical and radiological) with good results. Step cut osteotomy helps in three directional correction of the deformity.
5. B
   Bauman's angle defines it radiologically and carrying angle clinically. It is the angle between long axis of arm and forearm in anatomic position.

Reference:

1. John Ebnezar. Textbook of Orthopaedics. Jaypee Brothers Medical Publishers Pvt. Ltd; India. 4th edition; 2010; pg. 148-62

CHRONIC OSTEOMYELITIS

Dr. Ajai Singh and Dr. Vineet Sharma, Professor, Department of Orthopaedics

A five years old child presented with discharging sinus over medial side of lower part of right thigh. Sinus was fixed to underlying bone. Plain radiographs of the part showed a lytic lesion over lateral side of lower third of femur with thickening of bone with sclerosis.

1. What can be the diagnosis of the patient?
   (A) Acute osteomyelitis
   (B) Subacute osteomyelitis
   (C) Chronic osteomyelitis
   (D) Chronic osteitis
2. Out of the following complications, which one needs a regular long term follow up?
   (A) Angular deformity of knee
   (B) Pathological fracture of femur
   (C) Septic arthritis of knee
3. The aim to correct the angular deformity of joint is to
   (A) Restore mechanical axis
   (B) Restore the length of the limb
   (C) Improve the appearance of the limb
   (D) None of the above
4. Which of the following treatment modality will be preferred in this patient
   (A) Open wedge osteotomy
   (B) Close wedge osteotomy
   (C) Temporary epiphysiodesis
   (D) Permanent epiphysiodesis
5. To avoid genu recurvatum deformity while managing angular deformity around knee, one should use
   (A) One figure of eight plate
   (B) Two figure of eight plate
   (C) Three figure of eight plate
   (D) Four figure of eight plate

Answers:

1. C
   Thickening of bone and sclerosis indicates its chronic nature and lytic lesion in bone and fixity of sinus to the underlying skin indicates infection of bone and marrow (osteomyelitis)
2. A
   B and C are complications with acute presentation. They don't need regular follow up. Neuro vascular structures are not involved in chronic osteomyelitis. Angular deformity can be there in long term as the patient is of growing age group and distal physes can get involved leading to limb length discrepancies and deformities.
3. A
   It's a rule to maintain mechanical alignment of the appendicular skeleton, especially of weight bearing extremities to avoid complications related to gait and joint pain/ arthritis
4. C
   Because the child is of growing age, so a temporary and reversible procedure is preferable.
5. B
   Two are required to address equally anterior and posterior physes

Reference:

1. Stuart L. Weinstein, Joseph A. Buckwalter: Turek's Orthopaedics: Principles and Their Application; Lippincott, Williams and Wilkins; US; 6th edition; pg., 577-79: 138-48.

CONGENITAL TALIPES EQUINOVARUS

Dr. Ajai Singh and Dr. Vineet Sharma, Professor, Department of Orthopaedics

A newborn female child presented to orthopedics OPD with bilateral club foot

1. Following lesion should be looked for in the above child
   (A) DDH
   (B) Malnutrition
   (C) Sensory involvement
   (D) Congenital inguinal hernia
2. The sequence of correction of club feet by Ponseti technique is
   (A) Cavus, abduction, subcutaneous tenotomy of tendoachilles
   (B) Cavus, supination, abduction, subcutaneous tenotomy of tendoachilles
   (C) Cavus, pronation, abduction, subcutaneous tenotomy of tendoachilles
   (D) Cavus, supination, adduction, subcutaneous tenotomy of tendoachilles
3. In Ponseti technique, the fulcrum of correction is
   (A) Calcaneocuboid joint
   (B) Head of talus
   (C) Lateral malleolus
   (D) Lateral border of foot
4. The conservative treatment of club feet by .... plaster
   (A) Below knee plaster
   (B) Above knee plaster
   (C) Single POP hip spica
   (D) 1 ½ pop Hip spica
5. Most common complication of correction by Ponseti technique is
   (A) Osteoarthritis foot
   (B) Osteonecrosis of tarsals
   (C) Recurrence of deformity
   (D) Contractures

Answers:

1. A

   If one congenital anomaly is present then one should look for other congenital anomalies also and in CTEV patients, DDH is a common association.

2. B

   The forefoot adduction deformity is corrected by abducting the foot and fore foot cavus is first to be corrected by supinating the forefoot as fore foot is in pronation with respect to hindfoot.

3. B

   This was one of the modifications done in Kite's technique while correcting the foot adduction deformity.

4. B

   So that the POP doesn't slips out as socks and the thigh extension of cast helps in maintaining the correction of adduction deformity.

5. C

   One of the reasons for this is a long treatment protocol and the patient/ attendants are noncompliant to such a lengthy treatment schedule.

Reference:

1. Lynn Staheli. Clubfoot: Ponseti Management: Global HELP Organization; 3rd edition; 2009; pg.,1-28

POSTERIOR DISLOCATION OF HIP

Dr. Kumar Shantanu, Assistant Professor and Dr. Vineet Sharma, Professor, Department of Orthopaedics

A 33 years old male is brought to the trauma centre after a high speed motor-vehicle accident. He was the unrestrained passenger in a car that was travelling 80km/hr when it rear-collided a pick-up truck. On arrival to the trauma centre, the patient is writhing in pain, complaining of (L) hip pain. His vitals are within normal limits. His left lower limb is flexed, internally rotated and adducted at hip. He is unable to extend his hip, although he is able to extend his great toe as well as dorsiflex or plantar flex the foot. There are no signs of distal neurovascular deficit.

An Antero-Posterior plain radiograph of the pelvis is shown.

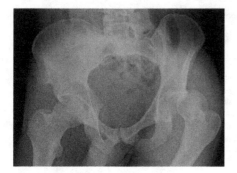

1. What is the most likely diagnosis?
    (A) Fracture pelvis
    (B) Posterior dislocation of hip
    (C) Anterior dislocation of hip
    (D) Central fracture dislocation of hip
2. What is the most likely concomitant injury?
    (A) Lumbar burst fracture
    (B) Right knee meniscus tear
    (C) Left knee Anterior cruciate ligament tear
    (D) Subdural hematoma
3. After a successful attempt at closed reduction in the trauma centre using conscious sedation, what is the next step in management?
    (A) CT scan of the hip and pelvis
    (B) Hip spica cast application
    (C) Further evaluation of hip instability via an exam under anesthesia in the operating room
    (D) Femoral skeletal pin traction
4. The patient is about to be discharged, he asks to review what position he can and cannot place his hip. You explain to him that precautions does not include
    (A) Leg crossing
    (B) Flexing the hip to greater than 90 degrees
    (C) Twisting the hip inward
    (D) Hip extension

Answers:
1. B
   As there is classical limb attitude of flexion, adduction and internal rotation, and is also evident in radiograph
2. C
   Most common mechanism of injury is hit on anterior aspect of knee in a person sitting on a chair, either with legs crossed/ normally sitting, resulting in additional ligamentous injury (ACL).
3. A
   To rule out associated fracture of acetabulum and/ or head of femur.
4. D
   As rest of the other three are the attitude in posterior dislocation of hip.

Reference:
1. Louis Solomon, David J. Warwick, Selvadurai Nayagam. Apley's System of Orthopaedics and Fractures; 9th Edition; Hodder Arnold, an imprint of Hodder Education, an Hachette UK Company, 2010: page 862-865

LIS FRANC INJURY
Dr. Kumar Shantanu, Assistant Professor and Dr. Vineet Sharma, Professor, Department of Orthopaedics

A football player who is lying on the ground after being tackled attempts to stand up. While he is still prone on the ground, another player falls directly on his left heel. He immediately experiences mid-foot pain and is unable to place any weight on his left foot.

1. In this setting, the team physician be most concerned about?
   (A) High ankle sprain
   (B) Achilles tendon rupture
   (C) Lis franc injury
   (D) Ankle fracture
2. Which one X-ray will be required for diagnosing this injury?
   (A) X-ray foot AP and oblique view
   (B) X-ray ankle with leg AP and lateral
   (C) X-ray knee with leg AP and lateral
   (D) X-ray pelvis with both hips AP view
3. An AP radiograph of the foot reveals a 4mm diastasis between the first and 2nd metatarsals, which structure connects the medial cuneiform to the base of the 2nd metatarsal?
   (A) Chopart ligament
   (B) Deltoid ligament
   (C) Lis franc ligament
   (D) Spring ligament
4. What is the most appropriate treatment?
   (A) Open reduction and internal fixation
   (B) Non-weight bearing in a short leg cast
   (C) Protected weight bearing in a cam walker boot
   (D) Chevron osteotomy

Answers:
1. C
   Lis franc injury is tarso metatarsal joint dislocation which is the region of mid foot.
2. A
   For foot and hand we get AP and Oblique views for better delineation of fractured bone
3. C
   Lis franc ligament is attached to the base of second metatarsal, which is avulsed and is the prime culprit in attaining reduction. It needs to be addressed for accurate reduction
4. A
   ORIF is necessary to properly address lisfranc ligament.

Reference:
1. Louis Solomon, David J. Warwick, Selvadurai Nayagam. Apley's System of Orthopaedics and Fractures; 9th Edition; Hodder Arnold, an imprint of Hodder Education, an Hachette UK Company, 2010: page 949 – 951

RADIUS AND ULNA FRACTURES

Dr. Kumar Shantanu, Assistant Professor and Dr. Vineet Sharma, Professor, Department of Orthopaedics

An 8 years old right handed dominant girl presents to the trauma centre with severe left forearm pain. Her mother states that she had been playing on their trampoline with some friends when she fell, landing on her outstretched left hand one hour ago. On examination, the forearm is deformed and she is exquisitely tender to palpation. She is not able to pronate or supinate. The radial pulse is palpable.
1. What is the most likely diagnosis?
   (A) Fracture distal end radius
   (B) Fracture ulnar styloid process
   (C) Fracture both bone forearm
   (D) Fracture supracondylar humerus
2. If radiograph shows a middle third diaphyseal both bone forearm fracture with end to end cortical apposition and 12 degrees dorsal angulation, what is the preferred method of treatment?
   (A) Percutaneous pinning of both radius and ulna
   (B) Closed reduction and long arm cast application in supination
   (C) Closed reduction and long arm cast application in neutral
   (D) Long arm cast application without any manipulation
3. Which of the following is most accurate regarding bone remodeling in children
   (A) The distal radial epiphysis will correct angular deformity at approx 20 degrees per year , independent of age, as long as the physis remains open
   (B) As the bone lengthen through growth, remodeling will also occur and lead to decreased angulation

(C) Intramembranous apposition on the convex side and resorption on the concave side of bone lead to remodeling

(D) Children older than 11 years are more effective at correcting bone angulation than younger ones

4. Which of the following statements is most accurate regarding the radiographic evaluation of anatomic forearm alignment after reduction?

(A) On AP radiograph, the ulnar styloid and the coronoid process are oriented 270 degrees apart.

(B) On lateral radiograph, the ulnar styloid and the coronoid process are oriented 90 degrees apart.

(C) On AP radiograph, the radial styloid and tuberosity are oriented 180 degrees apart

(D) On lateral radiograph, the radial styloid and tuberosity are oriented 90 degrees apart

Answers:

1. C

Site of deformity and pain well denotes towards the site of lesion.

2. C

Immobilization is done in neutral (mid prone) position in fractures of mid both bone forearm in order to neutralize the effect of supinators and pronators at the fracture site.

3. B

Remodeling at the fracture site is an inherent property of fracture healing and is more in children by virtue of their growth potential.

4. C

This is in normal anatomical position of radius bone.

Reference:

1. Louis Solomon, David J. Warwick, Selvadurai Nayagam. Apley's System of Orthopaedics and Fractures; 9th Edition; Hodder Arnold, an imprint of Hodder Education, an Hachette UK Company, 2010: page 786 – 794

FRACTURE CLAVICLE

Dr. Kumar Shantanu, Assistant Professor and Dr. Vineet Sharma, Professor, Department of Orthopaedics

A 5 years old boy falls on the ground during playing and presents with pain and swelling over right shoulder and is unable to lift his right hand overhead. The doctor noticed that the front of his right shoulder appears swollen in comparison with the contra-lateral side. He has a strong radial pulse, and sensation to light touch is intact throughout the whole extremity. The X-ray is shown below

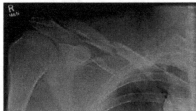

1. What is the most likely diagnosis?

(A) Anterior dislocation of shoulder

(B) Posterior dislocation of shoulder

(C) Fracture clavicle

(D) Fracture scapula

2. Which view is shown in this X-ray?

(A) X-ray shoulder lateral view

(B) X-ray shoulder AP view

(C) X-ray clavicle

(D) X-ray chest PA view

3. What will be the management for this injury?

(A) Shoulder immobilizer application

(B) Figure of four strapping

(C) Figure of eight strapping

(D) Below elbow pop application

4. What is the minimum duration for which splintage will be needed?
   (A) 2 months
   (B) 3 weeks
   (C) 6 months
   (D) 1 week only

Answers:
   1. A
      Fracture clavicle is one of the most common bone to be fractured in children. Mode of injury is fall on an outstretched hand. X-ray confirms the clinical diagnosis.
   2. B
      AP view of shoulder because whole of the shoulder is seen with glenohumeral articulation.
   3. C
      Figure of eight strapping is done in mid clavicular fractures in order to neutralize the effect of pull of sternocleidomastoid muscle.
   4. B
      By this time in children the fracture ends are expected to become sticky enough (union) to do well without splintage.

Reference:
   1. Louis Solomon, David J. Warwick, Selvadurai Nayagam. Apley's System of Orthopaedics and Fractures; 9th Edition; Hodder Arnold, an imprint of Hodder Education, an Hachette UK Company, 2010: page 752 – 755

SPINAL TUBERCULOSIS

Dr. Kumar Shantanu, Assistant Professor and Dr. Vineet Sharma, Professor, Department of Orthopaedics

A 23 year-old male was admitted with low back pain. Pain was present for 3 months and was getting worse. Physical examination was normal except some loss of lumbar lordosis. The x-ray of the spine is shown.

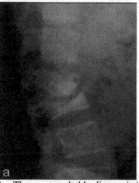

1. The most probable diagnosis is?
   (A) Ganglioma
   (B) Tuberculosis spine
   (C) Scheuermann's disease
   (D) Intervertebral disc prolapse
2. Which of the following is false for following disease
   (A) Multiple levels are commonly involved
   (B) Dorsolumbar vertebra are the commonly affected
   (C) Posterior elements are commonly involved
   (D) Starts in the anteroinferior aspect of vertebrae
3. Which of the following is not a radiological picture in this disease?
   (A) Ivory vertebra
   (B) Vertebra within vertebra
   (C) Picture frame vertebra
   (D) Vertebra plana
4. Which of the following is false for the disease
   (A) This disease rarely involves the neural arch

(B) Effects body of vertebra in 50-60 % of cases

(C) Has a very poor prognosis

(D) Typically erodes the spinous end plate

Answers:

1. B

    Because the end plates of vertebrae are destroyed with loss of disc space.

2. C

    Paradiscal area are most common to get involved because of blood supply as the involvement of vertebral body by tuberculosis is secondary and the spread is commonly hematogenous.

3. C

    Picture frame vertebrae is seen in Paget's disease.

4. B

    Rarely effects body and commonly involves the paradiscal area.

Reference:

1. Louis Solomon, David J. Warwick, Selvadurai Nayagam. Apley's System of Orthopaedics and Fractures; 9th Edition; Hodder Arnold, an imprint of Hodder Education, an Hachette UK Company, 2010: page 503- 507

AVASCULAR NECROSIS OF HIP

Dr. Santosh Kumar and Dr. Vineet Sharma, Professor, Department of Orthopaedics

34 years male presented with right side hip pain for last one and half years, with painful limp, with symptoms aggravated by walking and stair climbing and relieved by rest. On repeated questioning he revealed history of alcohol intake for last 10 years. On examination all movements are terminally painful but with no significant shortening. The other hip is perfectly normal. The clinician advised the x-ray of the part.

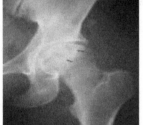

1. Most probable diagnosis is
    (A) Healed TB arthritis
    (B) Ankylosing spondylitis
    (C) Rheumatoid arthritis
    (D) Avascular necrosis of hip
2. What is true about sectoral sign?
    (A) With extended hip internal rotation is almost full.
    (B) With extended hip external rotation is almost full.
    (C) With flexed hip internal rotation is almost full.
    (D) With flexed hip external rotation is almost full.
3. What is the Investigation of choice if this patient would have been presented earlier?
    (A) X ray
    (B) CT Scan
    (C) MRI
    (D) PET scan
4. At this stage which modality of treatment is preferred?
    (A) Medical management
    (B) Core decompression
    (C) Core decompression with fibular graft
    (D) Total hip replacement arthroplasty

Answers:

1. D

No H/O fever and no sign of infection to rule out infective etiology. Mono articular involvement with classical H/O chronic alcoholism in addition to X-ray picture indicates towards AVN. In AS, SI joint is first to be involved followed by spine. RA (Rheumatoid Orthritis) is mostly symmetrical and poly articular.

2. A
3. C
   MRI is the most sensitive means of diagnosing avascular necrosis (AVN).
4. C
   It is a Ficat and Arlet stage 2 AVN and in this stage the recommended surgical treatment is Core decompression and vascularized fibular graft

References:

1. J Beltran, , L J Herman, , J M Burk, , W A Zuelzer, , R N Clark, , J G Lucas, , L D Weiss, and , A Yang. Femoral head avascular necrosis: MR imaging with clinical-pathologic and radionuclide correlation January 1988 Volume 166, Issue 1
2. Castro FP Jr, Barrack RL. Core decompression and conservative treatment for avascular necrosis of the femoral head: a meta-analysis. American Journal of Orthopedics (Belle Mead, N.J.) [2000, 29(3):187-194]

FRACTURE PELVIS

Dr. Santosh Kumar and Dr. Vineet Sharma, Professor, Department of Orthopaedics

22 year old male presented in emergency department with gross swelling and bruise over B/L groin with PR-110/min instead of BP-80/50 mmHg , RR-26/min, cold and clammy limbs, talkative but with irritation, maintaining SpO_2 99% with nasal prongs

1. Which of the following should be performed during primary survey
   (A) Cervical spine x ray
   (B) Per rectal examination
   (C) GCS
   (D) ABG
2. What would be the first stage of management
   (A) 2 L iv crystalloid and 2 unit blood
   (B) 2 L iv crystalloid ,mannitol,iv steroid
   (C) 1 unit albumin and compression stocking
   (D) 2 Lcrystalloid and vasopressor if BP does not respond
3. After hemodynamic stabilization on X-Ray pelvis, bilateral superior and inferior pubic rami fracture was revealed. What was the most likely cause of his condition?
   (A) Cardiac shock
   (B) Neurogenic shock
   (C) Septic shock
   (D) Hemorrhagic shock
4. Which one of following is indication of CT in this patient with minor traumatic brain injury?
   (A) 10 cm isolated scalp laceration
   (B) Fracture mandible
   (C) Haemotympanum
   (D) None of the above

Answers:

1. C
   Primary survey does not require neurological evaluation.
2. D
   Hemorrhage is the predominant cause of preventable post-injury deaths. Hypovolemic shock is caused by significant blood loss. Two large-bore intravenous lines are established and crystalloid solution may be given. If the person does not respond to this, type-specific blood, or O-negative if this is not available, should be given.
3. D
   In fracture pelvis there is an estimated loss of 2-3 litres of fluid (blood)
4. C
   Bleeding through ear is indicative of brain injury

Reference:
1. ATLS student course manual,9th edition, page no 52-63

ANKYLOSING SPONDYLITIS
Dr. Santosh Kumar and Dr. Vineet Sharma, Professor, Department of Orthopaedics

A 28 years old male complains of low back ache with bilateral hip pain and morning stiffness, which improves once he starts walking. His father has similar spinal restriction with stooped back. On examination there is gross limitation of hip movements and limited chest expansion.

1. What will be the most sensitive blood test
   (A) Vit. D3 level
   (B) CRP
   (C) Anti ccp
   (D) HLA B27
2. Drug of choice
   (A) Methotrexate+HCQS
   (B) Indomethacin
   (C) Tramadol
   (D) Colchicine
3. Cardinal sign on x ray pelvis
   (A) Erosion and fuzziness of SI joint
   (B) Periarticular sclerosis on sacral side of SI joint
   (C) Periarticular sclerosis on iliac side of SI joint
   (D) Periarticular cyst in iliac side of SI joint
4. Commonest site of spinal fracture in this case
   (A) C5-C7
   (B) T8-T12
   (C) L2 –L5
   (D) Sacrum

Answers:
1. D
   Most people with ankylosing spondylitis test positive for HLA-B27, but so do some people who don't have the condition. A positive test may point to AS but it won't confirm the diagnosis.
2. B
   NSAIDs (nonsteroidal anti-inflammatory drugs) are still the cornerstone of treatment and the first stage of medication in treating the pain and stiffness associated with spondylitis.
3. A
   Sacroiliitis occurs early in the course of ankylosing spondylitis and is regarded as a hallmark of the disease. Radiographically, the earliest sign of sacroiliitis is indistinctness of the joint. The joints initially widen before they narrow.
4. A
   This region is particularly susceptible to injury because of oblique facet joints, proximity to the weight of the head, and its location at the junction of a fused thoracic area with a more mobile head and neck

References:
1. Braun J, Sieper J. Ankylosing spondylitis. *Lancet.* 2007; 369(9570):1379–1390.
2. Saad ((B) Chaudhary, Heidi Hullinger, and Michael J. Vives. Review Article Management of Acute Spinal Fractures in Ankylosing Spondylitis. Volume 2011, Article ID 150484, 9 pages

FRACTURE DISLOCATION HIP
Dr. Santosh Kumar and Dr. Vineet Sharma, Professor, Department of Orthopaedics

36 years old male following RTA complains of pain over Right hip and inability to move Right lower limb. On examination bruise around Right hip.

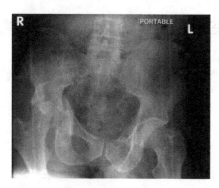

BP 118/80 mmHg
PR 68 /minute
RR 18/ minute
Urine output 50 ml/hour

1. Which nerve is likely to damage?
    (A) Femoral nerve
    (B) Sciatic nerve
    (C) Obturator nerve
    (D) Lateral cutaneous nerve of thigh
2. Which radiological line indicate anterior column fracture
    (A) Ilio- pectineal line
    (B) Ilio- ischial line
    (C) Tear drop
    (D) None of the above
3. Preferred surgical approach
    (A) anterior ilio inguinal
    (B) Kocher Langenbach
    (C) Both A&B
    (D) Stoppas
4. Long term complication in this case are all except:
    (A) Ilio-femoral venous thrombosis
    (B) Heterotopic calcification
    (C) AVN femoral head
    (D) degenerative osteoarthritis

Answers:
1. B
   In Posterior dislocation/ fracture dislocation the most common nerve to get injured is sciatic nerve
2. A
   In pelvis ischial tuberosity is posteriorly and pectineal line and symphysis forms the anterior part of the ring
3. B
   Posterior column and wall are more important to stabilize as weight bearing part of acetabulum is postero superior dome and this is a case of posterior fracture dislocation hip.
4. D
   There is post traumatic arthritis not degenerative

References:
1. S. Terry Canale and James H. Beaty. Campbell's Operative Orthopaedics; Mosby: 12th Edition: vol; 3 page; 2777
2. GA Hunter. Posterior dislocation and fracture-dislocation of the hip. A review of fifty-seven patients. From the Accident Service, Radcliffe Infirmary, Oxford- J Bone Joint Surg Br, 1969; pg.,38-44
3. PENNAL, GEORGE F. M.D, M.CH., F.R.C.S.C; TILE, MARVIN M.D, B.SC (MED),F.R.C.S.C; WADDELL, JAMES P. M.D; GARSIDE, HENRY. Pelvic Disruption: Assessment and Classification.Clinical Orthopaedics & Related Research: September 1980 - Volume 151 - Issue - pg 12-21

OSTEOARTHRITIS KNEE

Dr. Santosh Kumar and Dr. Vineet Sharma, Professor, Department of Orthopaedics

A 67 years old female patient complaining of right knee pain while walking and climbing stairs and experiences stiffness after prolonged period of sitting and joint swelling after extended period of walking. The relevant X-ray is shown.

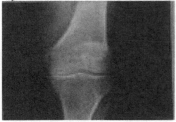

1. Identify the clinical condition?
   (A) Osteoarthritis knee
   (B) Rheumatoid arthritis
   (C) Reiter's disease
   (D) Pseudo gout
2. Which of the following is not a cardinal radiological feature of this clinical condition?
   (A) Asymmetric Reduced joint space
   (B) Subchondral sclerosis
   (C) Subchondral cyst
   (D) Juxta-articular osteopenia
3. Which classification is used for grading this clinical condition?
   (A) Kellgren Lawrence system
   (B) Neer's system
   (C) Tile's system
   (D) Fernandez system
4. What would be the initial management for this clinical condition?
   (A) Analgesics, quadriceps exercise and use of walking stick
   (B) Intra-articular steroids
   (C) Arthroscopic washout
   (D) Realignment osteotomy

Answers:
   1. A
      Demographic features, clinical features and radiological picture classically defines OA knee
   2. D
      Juxta-articular osteopenia is a feature of rheumatoid arthritis not osteoarthritis
   3. A
      Kellgren Lawrence system is used for grading OA knee.
   4. A
      Conservative management is the first line of treatment in OA knee.

References:
   1. Kellgren JH, Lawrence JS, Bier F. Genetic factors in generalized osteoarthrosis. Ann Rheum Dis. 1963 Jul; 22:237-55.
   2. Johnson C. Chapter 12. Approach to the Patient with Knee Pain. CURRENT Rheumatology Diagnosis & Treatment. (2e)

Chapter-15

Otolaryngology

LARYNGOCOELE

Dr. Anupam Mishra, Professor, Department of Otolaryngology

A 40 year old male patient presented with a 3.5 year history of slowly progressive swelling left side of the upper part of neck. There was no history of hoarseness of voice, difficulty in swallowing or cough. The patient was a chronic bidi smoker and farmer by occupation. Past history was not significant.

The General physical examination was normal. Otorhinolaryngological examination revealed a non-tender soft and reducible swelling on left side of upper half of neck that increased in size on Valsalva manoeuvre. Indirect laryngoscopy showed a fullness of left false vocal cord. The patient's haematological examination was normal while X-ray chest was consistent with findings of chronic bronchitis.. Ultrasound of the neck revealed an air filled cavity on the left side of neck. Computed tomography of the neck was done (Fig).

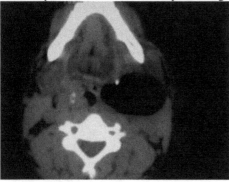

1. The diagnosis is
   (A) Pharyngocele
   (B) Laryngocele
   (C) Gas gangrene due to impacted foreign body
   (D) Zenker's diverticulum
2. The best option of management will be
   (A) Conservative intralaryngeal surgery
   (B) Radical surgery through extra laryngeal approach
   (C) Removal of the obstructive foreign body
   (D) Radiotherapy to induce fibrosis and collapse.
3. The most important associated disease to rule out in such a situation is
   (A) Cancer
   (B) Traumatic impact in past
   (C) Impaction of a radiolucent Foreign body with a ball-valve airway obstruction
   (D) Past history of Kirmer's disease
4. The most feared complication of surgery of choice in this case is
   (A) Dysphagia
   (B) Hoarseness
   (C) Salivary fistula
   (D) Respiratory distress

Answers:

1. A

   A laryngocele is an abnormal dilation or herniation of the saccule of the larynx. If this dilation lies within the limits of the thyroid cartilage, the laryngocele is internal. If it extends beyond the thyroid cartilage in a cephalad direction to protrude through the thyrohyoid membrane, thelaryngocele is external.

2. B

   Surgical excision through an external approach is the management of choice

3. A

   Hoarseness, cough, dyspnea, and dysphagia strongly suggest a laryngocele and these are the common presenting symptoms of carcinoma of larynx.

4. A

Surgical excision through an external approach is the management of choice wherein the most trouble complication is the injury to the laryngeal nerve resulting in long term hoarseness.

Reference:

1. Flint PW, Haughey BH, Lund VJ, Niparko JK, Richardson MA (Eds). Differential diagnosis of Neck Masses. In: Cummings Otolaryngology Head and Neck Surgery, 5th Edition Mosby Elsevier Philadelphia 2010,pp 2817-2818.

NASOPHARYNGEAL ANGIOFIBROMA
Dr. Anupam Mishra, Professor, Department of Otolaryngology

A 13 year old patient presents with progressive right nasal obstruction that has now resulted in complete blockade since 15 days and associated with marked pallor with tachypnoea. There is positive history of recurrent profuse nasal bleed since last 2 months and the family history is positive for heart disease. He happens to be a student and works for his family business with his father who is a blacksmith by occupation (hence exposed to heat). The pulse rate is 90 per minute, regular while his blood pressure is within normal limits. Nasal examination reveals a smooth pinkish mass in the right nostril. The ear and throat examinations are within normal limits. On neck examination a single 1cm size left submandibular lymph gland is palpable that is firm, non-tender and freely mobile. The imaging of his nasal mass is shown in the figure.

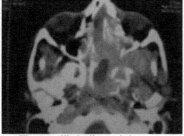

1. The most likely diagnosis is
   (A) Hemangiopericytoma
   (B) Nasal septal hemangioma
   (C) Epidermoid cancer
   (D) None of the above
2. The clinical diagnosis of the above case can be best achieved by
   (A) Imaging
   (B) Nasal examination, palpation and probing
   (C) Endoscopy
   (D) Biopsy in the office.
3. The most important diagnostic radiological sign involves the involvement of
   (A) Nasal cavity and nasopharynx
   (B) Spheno palatine foramina
   (C) Greater palatine foramina
   (D) Lesser palatine foramina
4. The treatment of choice for this case is
   (A) Chemotherapy followed by Surgery
   (B) Surgery followed by Chemotherapy
   (C) Surgery
   (D) Radiotherapy

Answers:
1. D
   Juvenile Nasopharyngeal Angiofibroma is the most common benign nasopharyngeal tumour seen in adolescent males. It is characterized by nasal blockage, profuse recurrent nasal bleeding and reveals a reddish pink nasal mass in one or the both nostrils.
2. A
   The clinical diagnosis is suspected in the presence of reddish nasal mass and history of profuse epistaxis further confirmed by radiologically on the basis of classical signs including widening of sphenopalatine foramina.

3. B
    Widening of sphenopalatine foramen is classical radiological sign of angiofibroma.
4. C
    The treatment of choice is complete surgical excision.

Reference:

1. Flint PW, Haughey BH, Lund VJ, Niparko JK, Richardson MA (Eds). Benign tumours of sinonasal tract. In: Cummings Otolaryngology Head and Neck Surgery, 5th Edition Mosby Elsevier Philadelphia 2010, page 721-722.

RHINOLITH
Dr. Anupam Mishra, Professor, Department of Otolaryngology

A 10 year old girl presented with a history of left sided nasal obstruction with off and on mild epistaxix with pain since 2 years. She was otherwise cheerful and did not remember any foreign body insertion in her nose. Her previous consultations did not give her any relief while she has been on topical decongestants since last 4 months. On anterior rhinoscopy examination a smooth polypoidal obstructive swelling was seen in the left nostril the inside of which was felt a bit hard on probing. Slight amount of bleeding on touch was appreciated but was associated with significant foul smelling debris. Posterior rhinoscopy was within normal limits. Imaging of nose and paranasal sinus is shown in the figure.

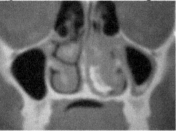

1. The diagnosis is
    (A) Ringertz tumor with calcification
    (B) Radiopaque foreign body
    (C) Rhinoliith
    (D) Fungal rhinusinusitis with heterogenous pattern
2. The most important diagnostic modality affecting the treatment outcome for the above pathology is
    (A) Imaging and nasal examination
    (B) Simple Angiography
    (C) DSA
    (D) Biopsy
3. The treatment of choice for the above disease is
    (A) Intra / Extra – nasal removal
    (B) Biopsy followed by radiotherapy
    (C) Chemotherapy
    (D) Nasal steroids
4. The post treatment prognosis can be best explained by
    (A) High changes of recurrence with involvement of the other side
    (B) Low chances of recurrence with central necrosis
    (C) Malignant conversion
    (D) No chances of recurrence with a possibility of atrophic changes

Answers:

1. C
    A rhinolith usually forms around the nucleus of a small exogenous foreign body, blood clot or secretion by slow deposition of calcium and magnesium salts. Over a period of time, they grow into large irregular masses that fill the nasal cavity. They may cause pressure necrosis of the nasal septum or lateral wall of nose. Rhinoliths present as unilateral nasal obstruction. Foul-smelling, blood-stained discharge is often present. Epistaxis and pain may occur due to the ulceration of surrounding mucosa. It is not uncommon to see hypertrophied inflamed

mucosa overlying the hard stone underlying that can only be appreciated on probing / palpation.
2. A
    Imaging along with clinical examination is hence the most important modalities top arrive at a correct diagnosis.
3. A
    Intranasal extraction is preferred unless the stone is so large as to require a lateral rhinotomy external approach.
4. D
    There are NO chances of recurrence provided nasal hygiene is maintained but chances of atrophic rhinitis prevail in case of a massive stone removal leaving behind a roomy nasal cavity.

Reference:

1. Dhingra PL. Miscellaneous Disorders of Middle Ear. Dhingra PL (Ed.). Diseases of Ear, Nose and throat, 5th Edition. Elsevier, New Delhi 2010, pp 199-200.

BRANCHIAL FISTULA

DrAnupam Mishra, Professor, Department of Otolaryngology

A 10 year old boy presented to outpatient clinic with the main complaint of a cutaneous opening in the middle of the neck lateral to the midline. The patient had been completely asymptomatic in his early childhood days till the age of 5 years after which he has been continuously suffering from recurrent attacks of pus discharge from the opening off and on, only to resolve temporarily with treatment. His otolaryngological examination is otherwise normal and neck is soft on palpation. A radiopaque dye injected through the opening is seen to proceed superiorly through a tract as shown in the figure.

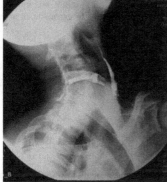

1. The diagnosis of the above case is
    (A) Branchial fistulous track
    (B) Thyroglossal tract remnant
    (C) Bronchial sinus
    (D) Thyroglossal fistula
2. The most likely superior extent / opening is likely to be at
    (A) Base of tongue
    (B) Foramen caecum
    (C) Tonsillar pillar
    (D) Nasopharynx
3. The most likely treatment of choice of this particular case is
    (A) Sistrunk Operation
    (B) Excision of the track with inclusion of tongue base but excluding the body of hyoid
    (C) Excision of the track upwards between the carotid-fork with or without tonsillectomy
    (D) Antibiotics and anti inflammatory drugs at the time of pus discharge with no role of surgery
4. The recurrence after incomplete excision for the above pathology is
    (A) More difficult to deal with surgery.
    (B) More easy to deal with second surgery as the size of the recurrence is usually small.
    (C) No additional difficulty as the primary surgery.

(D) The recurrence always goes unnoticed and does not require any treatment.

Answers:
1. A

   Second Branchial cleft anomalies are the commonest amongst all the branchial cleft anomalies and present as a cyst or sinus / fistula at the anterior boarder of sternomastoid muscle in the lower half of neck.

2. C

   The track usually ascends up to the tonsillar fossa coursing in between the internal and external carotid arteries.

3. C

   The well accepted treatment involves complete excision of the tract upto the tonsillar fossa with or without tonsillectomy.

4. A

   The incomplete resection leaves epithelial residue to recur again and then in that case the surgery becomes more difficult.

Reference:
1. Flint PW, Haughey BH, Lund VJ, Niparko JK, Richardson MA (Eds). Differential diagnosis of Neck Masses. In: Cummings Otolaryngology Head and Neck Surgery, 5th Edition Mosby Elsevier Philadelphia 2010, pp 1636.

PARAGANGLIOMA

Dr Anupam Mishra, Professor, Department of Otolaryngology

A 49 years old female presented with a slow growing lateral neck swelling since past 5.7 years along with dysphagia and hoarseness appearing since 2 years. The indirect laryngoscopy was normal and NO parapharyngeal bulge could be seen on oropharyngeal examination. The cervical swelling was mobile laterally but less mobile in the cranio-caudal direction. Moreover as it was pulsatile but NOT expansile an angiography was undertaken as shown in the figure.

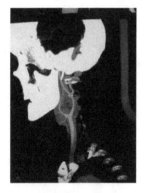

1. The diagnosis is
   (A) Hemangioma
   (B) Hemangiopericytoma
   (C) Paraganglioma
   (D) Schwannoma
2. Positive Fontaine sign refers to
   (A) A cervical swelling that is mobile laterally but less mobile in the cranio-caudal direction
   (B) Pulsatile but non-expansile neck swelling
   (C) Triad of neck mass with dysphagia and hoarseness
   (D) Neck mass in upper part of neck presenting with parapharyngeal bulge
3. The diagnostic radiological sign seen in the above figure is
   (A) Holman's sign
   (B) Millar sign
   (C) Lyre sign

(D) Phelp's sign
4. The treatment of choice in an 85 years old patient with the above disease presenting with dysphagia, odynophagia, hoarseness, and cranial nerve (IX-XII) deficits is
    (A) Surgery followed by radiotherapy
    (B) Surgery alone
    (C) Radiotherapy alone
    (D) Sclerosing agents

Answers:

1. C
    The paraganglioma occurring at the carotid bifurcation is known as carotid body tumour. It is a highly vascular tumour and enhances with contrast imaging.
2. A
    Paraganglioma is attached with the carotid axis and it can be easily moved at right angle to the axis, than along the axis longitudinally. This is Fontaine sign.
3. C
    Radiologically the splaying of carotid fork is known as Lyre's sign.
4. C
    The treatment of choice is surgical excision but in case of advanced/extensive tumour especially in the elderly, it is preferable to opt for non surgical intervention especially radiotherapy.

Reference:

1. Flint PW, Haughey BH, Lund VJ, Niparko JK, Richardson MA (Eds).Neoplasms of the Neck. In: Cummings Otolaryngology Head and Neck Surgery, 5th Edition Mosby Elsevier Philadelphia 2010, pp1659.

BRAIN ABSCESS

Dr. Anupam Mishra, Professor, Department of Otolaryngology

A 70 year old male patient of chronic left ear discharge presented with acute exacerbation of blood tinged discharge, moderate grade headache and dizziness / gait ataxia. Pulse was 90 per minute regular and temperature was NOT raised. The otolaryngological examination showed foul smelling pus discharge in left ear with attic disease along with spontaneous nystagmus. The neck rigidity was absent but the 'heel to shin test' was abnormal. The gait assessment showed marked central sway with tendency to fall on either side (more towards left). A preoperative imaging is shown in the figure.

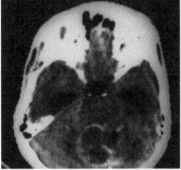

1. The diagnosis of chronic suppurative otitis media is complicated by
    (A) Temporal lobe abscess
    (B) Extradural abscess
    (C) Brain abscess
    (D) Subdural venous thrombosis
2. The most likely cause of truncal ataxia is
    (A) Lesion of Vermis
    (B) Lesion of temporal lobe
    (C) Lesion of the cerebellar hemisphere
    (D) Compression of dura adjoining labyrinth
3. All are the following are localizing signs of temporal lobe SOL (space occupying lesion) except:
    (A) Auditory hallucinations and Tinnitus

(B) Sensory aphasia and Amnesia

(C) Seizures

(D) Dyslexia, dysgraphia and dyscalculia

4. All are the localising sign of intracranial SOL (space occupying lesion) involving cerebellum except:

(A) Disdiadokokinesia

(B) Abnormal finger nose test

(C) Brun's nystagmus

(D) Absent neck rigidity

Answers:

1. C

Diagnosis is CSOM with Cerebellar Abscess involving predominantly the midline.

2. A

Truncal gait ataxia is characteristic of lesions of Vermis.

3. D

Complex partial seizures are well known in temporal lobe epilepsy while Dyslexia, Dysgraphia and Dyscalculia are characteristic of parietal lobe involvement.

4. D

Neck rigidity as a feature whether positive or negative is not anywhere related to cerebellum.

References:

1. Nedzelski JM.Cerebellopontine angle tumors: bilateral flocculus compression as cause of associated oculomotor abnormalities Laryngoscope. 1983 Oct; 93(10):1251-60

2. Dhingra PL. Complications of Suppurative otitis media. Dhingra PL (Ed.). Diseases of Ear, Nose and throat, 5th Edition. Elsevier, New Delhi 2010, 107-109.

BILATERAL PERIPHERAL VESTIBULOPATHY

Dr. Anupam Mishra, Professor, Department of Otolaryngology

A 40 year old male patient presented with the mild vertigo without subjective hearing loss. He showed particular concern about his oscillopsia during head movements and about unsteadiness, especially while walking in the dark. The bedside vestibular test battery revealed a positive head impulse test, reduced dynamic visual acuity and a positive Romberg test on foam rubber.

1. The most likely diagnosis is

(A) Unilateral peripheral vestibular dysfunction

(B) Bilateral peripheral vestibular dysfunction (BVL)

(C) Central vestibular dysfunction

(D) Mixed picture of unilateral vestibular dysfunction and psychogenic vertigo

2. The probability of which of the following disease(s) is likely to result in the above picture:

(A) Vestibulotoxic antibiotics

(B) Autoimmune ear diseases

(C) Menière's disease

(D) All of above

3. Computerised dynamic posturography (CDP) provides information about:

(A) Functional status only

(B) Assessment of Site of lesion only

(C) Both Functional status and anatomical site of lesion

(D) None of the above

4. The most essential requirement of dynamic visual acuity testing (DVA) is

(A) Slit lamp

(B) Snellen's chart

(C) Retinoscope

(D) Fundoscope

Answers:

1. B

Clinical diagnosis of BVL is based on the result of three simple bedside tests: a positive head impulse test, reduced dynamic visual acuity and a positive Romberg test on foam rubber. With these signs, diagnosis of severe BVL is usually straightforward to establish.

2. D

The causes of BVL are vestibulotoxic antibiotics, autoimmune ear diseases, Menière's disease and meningitis.

3. A

    Computerized Dynamic Posturography can identify and differentiate the functional impairments associated with the pathological processes, but by itself, Computerized Dynamic Posturography cannot diagnose the source of the problem.

4. B

    DVA assesses a subject's ability to perceive objects accurately while the head is moved passively. To measure DVA clinically , the examiner oscillates the patient's head horizontally or vertically at 0.5–2 Hz and asks the patient to read optotypes on a visual acuity chart

Reference:

1. Petersen JA, Straumann D, Weber KP. Therapeutic Advances in Neurological Disorders. Ther Adv Neurol Disord. (2013) 6(1) 41–45.

JUGULAR VENOUS PHLEBECTASIA

Dr. Anupam Mishra, Professor, Department of Otolaryngology

A 45 year old male patient presented with an otherwise normal neck until doing strenuous job. He is farmer by occupation and does not reveal any traumatic impact on the neck in past. The physical examination including otolaryngological workup seems to be reasonably fine. The patient on valsalva as shown in the picture presents with a swelling in the lower part of neck that feels like "bag of worms'.

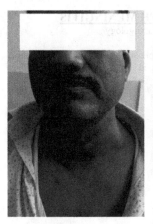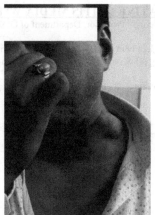

1. The diagnosis is
    (A) Venous phlebectasia
    (B) Arteriovenous malformation
    (C) Lymphangiomatous hemangioma
    (D) Laryngocele
2. Long-Term Complications of the above condition may include
    (A) Hoarseness
    (B) Dysphagia
    (C) Respiratory compromise
    (D) None of the above
3. The treatment of choice for the above condition is
    (A) Immediate total surgical excision for the fear of rapid growth and rupture
    (B) Tight Compression bandage
    (C) Radiotherapy to induce fibrosis and collapse
    (D) Wait and watch policy till size increases sufficiently enough to undertake local excision
4. Swellings increasing on valsalvamanuever include all except
    (A) Laryngocele
    (B) Tumours and cysts of upper mediastinum
    (C) Lymphangioma
    (D) Internal jugular phlebectasia

Answers:
1. A

   External Jugular venous phlebectasia manifests as intermittent neck swelling during lying down or straining (Valsalvamaneuvre)
2. D

   No reports of complications such as include Hoarseness, Dysphagia or Respiratory compromise exist in the literature
3. D

   radical treatment is not indicated unless for cosmetic / emotional reasons or it being symptomatic due to its increased size
4. C

   The differential diagnosis of swellings appearing in the neck on Valsalva maneuvre or on straining, coughing, bending, are laryngoceles, pharyngoceles, venous enlargement of internal jugular vein, tumours and cysts of upper mediastinum and inflation of the cupola of the lung

References:
1. Zohar Y, Ben-Town R, Talmi YP. Phlebectasia of the jugular system. J Craniomaxfac Surg 17: 96-98. 1989
2. Nwako FA, Agugua NE, Udeh CA Osuorji RI. Jugular phlebectasia. J Pediatr Surg 24: 303-305, 1989).

CHRONIC SUPPURATIVE OTITIS MEDIA WITH MENINGITIS
Dr. Veerendra Verma, Professor, Department of Otolaryngology

A 25 yr adult male came to emergency dept with c/o Headache, fever, photophobia, Neck rigidity and vomiting for 2 days. On past history he was having off & on ear discharge since childhood.
1. What is your probable diagnosis-
   - (A) CSOM with Lateral sins thrombosis
   - (B) CSOM with Meningitis
   - (C) CSOM with Brain abscess
   - (D) CSOM with Labyrynthitis
2. All the sign can be elicited in this patient EXCEPT-
   - (A) Neck rigidity
   - (B) Brudzinsky sign
   - (C) Kernig's sign
   - (D) Schwartz sign
3. CSF finding on lumbar puncture shows all EXCEPT-
   - (A) CSF is turbid
   - (B) Cell count is increased
   - (C) Sugar is increased
   - (D) Protein is increased
4. Mode of infection in children -
   - (A) AOM
   - (B) CSOM tubo tympanic type
   - (C) CSOM atticoantral type
   - (D) Blood borne
5. Treatment of choice of this patient-
   - (A) Conservative
   - (B) Surgical
   - (C) Medical & Surgical
   - (D) Hib Vaccination

Answers:
1. B

   Fever, neck rigidity and vomiting are the signs of meningitis.
2. D

   Schwartz sign is seen in otosclerosis while rest seen in meningitis.
3. C

   In CSF finding sugar is reduced in meningitis
4. D

In such cases mode of infection is retrograde thrombophlebitis
5. C
    Treatment is medical for symptom and surgical for underlying Disease CSOM.

Reference:
1. Dhingra PL. Complications of Suppurative Otitis Media. Dhingra PL(Ed.). Diseases of Ear, Nose and throat, 5th edition.Elsevier, New Delhi 2010, pp 92.

PRESBYACUSIS
Dr. Veerendra Verma, Professor, Department of Otolaryngology

A70 yrs old male came to OPD with c/o difficulty in hearing which was gradually progressive. On examination both tympanic membrane was intact. His Audiogram shows B/L Sensory neural hearing loss.

1. What is likely the diagnosis –
    (A) Presbyopia
    (B) Presbylaryngis
    (C) Presbycusis
    (D) Presbystasis
2. How many type of Presbycusis have been identified-
    (A) 3 type
    (B) 4 type
    (C) 2 type
    (D) 5 type
3. Degenertion of organ of corti is seen in which type of Presbycusis-
    (A) Sensory
    (B) Neural
    (C) Strial or Metabolic
    (D) Cochlear conductive
4. Stiffening of basilar membrane is seen in which type of Presbycusis-
    (A) Sensory
    (B) Neural
    (C) Strial or Metabolic
    (D) Cochlear conductive
5. Treatment of above patient is-
    (A) Surgery
    (B) Medicine
    (C) Hearing aids
    (D) No treatment

Answers:
1. C
    Hearing loss associated with physiological aging is called Presbycusis.
2. B
    Four types of presbycusis Sensory, Neural, Strial and cochlear
3. A
    In Sensory type organ of corti is involved.
4. D
    Stiffening of basilar membrane is seen in cochlear conductive type.
5. C
    As cochlea is involved Hearing aids are best options

Reference:
1. Dhingra PL. Hearing Loss. Dhingra PL(Ed.). Diseases of Ear, Nose and throat, 5th edition. Elsevier, New Delhi 2010, pp 41-42.

LABYRINTHITIS
Dr. Veerendra Verma, Professor, Department of Otolaryngology

A 30 yrs male came to OPD with c/o vertigo whenever he tries to clean ear with swab stick. Sometimes even nausea and vomiting occurs. His past history includes off & on ear discharge for 10 yrs.

1. Which test would you like to perform to confirm your diagnosis
   (A) Caloric test
   (B) Modified Kobrak test
   (C) Bithermal caloric test
   (D) Fistula test
2. When positive pressure is applied to ear canal by siegle's speculum the quick Component of nystagmus is towards-
   (A) Towards disease side
   (B) Towards normal side
   (C) No nystagmus
   (D) Vertical nystagmus seen
3. What is your diagnosis
   (A) Meniere's disease
   (B) BPPV
   (C) Labyrinthitis
   (D) Vestibular neuronitis
4. All are types of labyrinthitis EXCEPT-
   (A) Circumscribed labyrinthitis
   (B) Diffuse serous labyrinthitis
   (C) Diffiuse suppurative labyrinthitis
   (D) Vestibular neuronitis
5. Fistula of labyrinth is caused by all EXCEPT
   (A) CSOM with cholesteatoma
   (B) Neoplasm of middle ear
   (C) Surgical or accidental trauma
   (D) Serous otitis media

Answers:
   1. D
      Fistula test is done to check labyrinthine fistula
   2. A
      the quick component of nystagmus would be towards affected Ear due to ampullopetal displacement of cupula.
   3. C
      Labyrinthitis as Vertigo on pressure change mean labyrinthine Fistula.
   4. D
      Vestibular neuronitis is viral infection of 8th nerve.
   5. D
      serous otitis media is non bone eroding disease.

Reference:
   1. Dhingra PL. Complications of suppurative otitis media. Dhingra PL(Ed.). Diseases of Ear, Nose and throat, 5th edition. Elsevier, New Delhi 2010, pp 90.

CANCER LARYNX
Dr. Veerendra Verma, Professor, Department of Otolaryngology

A 50 yrs old male came to the OPD with c/o of change in voice for 3 months which was gradually worsening? He is chronic smoker for past 10 yrs.
1. What is your diagnosis
   (A) Malignancy supraglottic larynx
   (B) Malignancy glottis larynx
   (C) Malignancy sub glottis larynx
   (D) Malignancy hypopharynx
2. Stage **T1b** include
   (A) Tumour limited to one vocal cord with normal mobility
   (B) Tumour limited to one vocal cord with impaired mobility
   (C) Tumour involving both vocal cords with normal mobility
   (D) Tumour involving both vocal cords with impaired mobility
3. Treatment of **T1b** carcinoma of glottis is
   (A) Surgery

(B) Radiotherapy

(C) Laser

(D) Striping of vocal cord

4. Conservative surgery can not be done if

(A) Both vocal cords are involved

(B) Ant commissure is involved

(C) Arytenoids are involved

(D) Preepiglottc space is involved

Answers:

1. B

Change in voice is seen in glottic disease.

2. C

Both vocal cords involve with normal mobility

3. B

Since mobility is normal so Radiotherapy is the treatment of choice

4. D

Pre epiglottic space involvement means extra laryngeal Spread.

Reference:

1. Dhingra PL. Cancer larynx. Dhingra PL (Ed.). Diseases of Ear, Nose and throat, 5th Edition.Elsevier, New Delhi 2010, pp 330.

FOREIGN BODY BRONCHUS

Dr. Veerendra Verma, Professor, Department of Otolaryngology

A 3 yrs old child during playing suddenly developed coughing, dyspnoea and wheezing. After some time child become normal but after few days he develops fever and mild distress.

1. What is your diagnosis

(A) Laryngotracheo bronchitis

(B) Laryngeal diptheria

(C) Foreign body bronchus

(D) Pneumonia

2. Foreign body is common in

(A) Trachea

(B) Rt bronchus

(C) Lt bronchus

(D) Larynx

3. X-ray finding shows all except

(A) Cavity

(B) Emphysema

(C) Atelactasis

(D) Normal

4. Treatment for above patient is

(A) Antibiotics

(B) Bronchoscopy

(C) Oesophagoscopy

(D) Steroid

5. Check valve &ball valve mechanism are seen in

(A) Foreign body Bronchus

(B) Foreign body oesophagus

(C) Foreign body larynx

(D) Foreign body nose

Answers:

1. C

sudden onset symptom is foreign body inhalation.

2. B

Rt bronchus as it is in alignment with trachea and wider than lt bronchus.

3. A

Cavity is seen in infection.

413

4. B

Bronchoscopy and Foreign body removal
5. A

In early stage check valve and in late stage, ball valve Mechanism takes place.

Reference:

1. Dhingra PL. Foreign bodies of air passages. Dhingra PL (Ed.). Diseases of Ear, Nose and throat, 5th Edition.Elsevier, New Delhi 2010, pp 342.

MALIGNANCY MAXILLA

Dr. Veerendra Verma, Professor, Department of Otolaryngology

A 50 yrs old working in furniture industry has developed nasal stuffiness, for 2 months and Blood stained nasal discharge epiphora for 15 days.

1. What is your diagnosis
   (A) Angiofibroma
   (B) Carcinoma maxilla
   (C) Foreign body
   (D) Dacrocystitis
2. Investigation to see extension of disease in above case-
   (A) X-ray PNS
   (B) CT scan
   (C) MRI
   (D) USG
3. Ohngren's line extend from-
   (A) Lateral canthus of eye to midline of mandible
   (B) Medial canthus of eye to angle of mandible
   (C) Lateral canthus of eye to angle of mandible
   (D) Medial canths of eye to midline of mandible
4. Accordiing to which classification para nasal sinuses are divided into Supra ,Meso & Infra structure.
   (A) Ohngren's line classification
   (B) Lederman's classification
   (C) TNM classification
   (D) AJCC classification
5. 5 yrs cure rate of malignancy maxilla is
   (A) 20%
   (B) 25%
   (C) 30%
   (D) 40%

Answers:

1. B

   Carcinoma maxilla is common cause of blood stained nasal discharge in middle age.
2. B

   CT scan as it gives 3D image.
3. B

   One of method of classification of carcinoma maxilla.
4. B

   Lederman classification divides maxilla into supra, meso and infra structure.
5. C

   30% as given in literature.

Reference:

1. Dhingra PL. Neoplasm of Paranasal Sinuses. Dhingra PL (Ed.). Diseases of Ear, Nose and throat, 5th Edition. Elsevier, New Delhi 2010, pp 222.

FRACTURE NASAL BONE
Dr. Veerendra Verma, Professor, Department of Otolaryngology

A boy while playing Football suddenly collided with the other player. He started bleeding from nose, swelling over dorsum of nose and nasal deformity.

1. What is your diagnosis
    (A) Septal hematoma
    (B) Deviated nasal septum
    (C) Angiofibroma
    (D) Fracture nasal bone
2. How many types of fracture nasal bone are seen
    (A) Two types
    (B) Three types
    (C) Four types
    (D) Single types
3. Complication of fracture nasal bone are all except
    (A) Cosmetic deformity
    (B) CSF leak
    (C) Nasal block
    (D) Loss of smell
4. Which is not true about Nasal bone fracture:
    (A) Simple fracture
    (B) Compound fracture
    (C) Incomplete fracture
    (D) Complete fracture
5. All are true regarding management of fracture of nasal bone except
    (A) Manual alignment
    (B) Closed Reduction and setting
    (C) Open reduction and plating
    (D) Bone grafting

Answers:
1. D
    Fracture nasal bone due to trauma.
2. B
    Three type of fractures seen Chevorlet, Jarjaway and Nasoorbitoethmoid.
3. D
    Loss of smell is usually not seen in fracture nasal bone.
4. D
5. D
    Bone grafting is not required.

Reference:
1. Dhingra PL. Trauma to the Face. Dhingra PL (Ed.). Diseases of Ear, Nose and throat, 5th Edition. Elsevier, New Delhi 2010, pp 195.

BENIGN PAROXYSMAL POSITIONAL VERTIGO
Dr. Veerendra Verma, Professor, Department of Otolaryngology

A 50 yrs old male presented to OPD with sudden onset of spinning sensation (it appears that whole world is moving around). This attack lasted for less than 40 sec. The attack occurred in spells specially when turning head to one side.

1. What is your diagnosis
    (A) Meniere's disease
    (B) BPPV
    (C) Vestibular neuronitis
    (D) Epileptic vertigo
2. Dix hallpike test is used to diagnose
    (A) Meniere's disease

(B) BPPV
(C) Vestibular neuronitis
(D) Epileptic vertigo
3. Sensory neural hearing loss is present in
(A) Meniere's disease
(B) Vestibular neuronitis
(C) BPPV
(D) Vertibro basilar insufficiency
4. Treatment of this patient is
(A) Steroids
(B) Anti viral therapy
(C) Anti vertigo
(D) Epley'smaneuver

Answers:
1. B
   Sudden onset and less duration is BPPV.
2. B
   BPPV
3. A
   Sensory neural hearing loss is seen in Meniere's disease.
4. D
   Canalolith repositioning like Epley's maneuver is the treatment of choice.

Reference:
1. Dhingra PL. Disorders of Vestibular System. Dhingra PL (Ed.). Diseases of Ear, Nose and throat, 5th Edition.Elsevier, New Delhi 2010, pp 51.

SERIOUS OTITIS MEDIA
Dr. Veerendra Verma, Professor, Department of Otolaryngology

A 15 yrs old boy comes to OPD with c/o decrease hearing for 3 months Sensation of fluid in right ear. His otoscopic finding is given below.

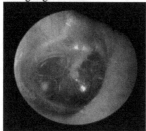

1. What is your likely diagnosis
   (A) Acute otitis media
   (B) Tubercular otitis media
   (C) Serous otitis media
   (D) Chronic otitis media
2. In this patient Impedance audiometry shows which type of curve-
   (A) Type –A
   (B) Type –B
   (C) Type –C
   (D) Type –As
3. Pure tone audiometry of this patient shows
   (A) Normal hearing
   (B) Conductive hearing loss
   (C) Sensory neural hearing loss
   (D) Mixed hearing loss
4. Treatment of choice in above patient
   (A) Antibiotics
   (B) Tympanolsty

(C) Cortical mastoidectomy
(D) Myringotomy with grommet insertion
5. All can be squeals of above disease EXCEPT-
(A) Atelectasis of the tympanic membrane
(B) Adhesive otitis media
(C) Cholesteatoma
(D) Otosclerosis

Answers:
1. C
   Serous otitis media.
2. B
   Type B Flat curve.
3. B
   Conductive Hearing loss due to middle ear pathology.
4. D
   Myringotomy with Grommet insertion.
5. D
   Otosclerosis as it is auto immune disease.

Reference:
1. Dhingra PL. Disorders of Middle Ear.Dhingra PL (Ed.). Diseases of Ear, Nose and throat, 5th Edition. Elsevier, New Delhi 2010, pp 71-73.

CHRONIC SUPPURATIVE OTITIS MEDIA ATTICOANTRAL DISEASE WITH LEFT FACIAL PALSY

Dr H P Singh, Assistant Professor, Department of Otolaryngology

This 35 years gentleman presented to ENT outdoor with one week history of left sided weakness of face with inability to close his left eye. He had history of Left ear discharge since childhood. Discharge was scanty, foul smelling and purulent. On examination of the ear, there was attic perforation with whitish flakes, which could not be removed by ear suctioning. Reddish granulations were also present with greenish-yellow discharge. His routine blood investigations including chest x-ray were normal.

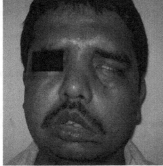 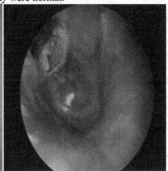

1. What is the most probable diagnosis?
   (A) Serous otitis media
   (B) Acute suppurative otitis media
   (C) Chronic suppurative otitis media unsafe type
   (D) Acute necrotizing otitis media
2. Which of the following is false about the disease?
   (A) Cholesteatoma is usually present
   (B) Attic perforation is present
   (C) Complications are more common
   (D) Usually central perforation is seen
3. In this disease, which of the following is correct-
   (A) Facial nerve palsy is of LMN type
   (B) Facial nerve palsy is of UMN type

(C) Facial nerve functions remain poor in spite of adequate surgical and medical management.

(D) Decompression of facial nerve is not usually preferred.

4. What is the preferred modality among radiological investigation for this condition?

(A) High Resolution CT Scan

(B) X-ray of mastoids

(C) MRI study of tympanomastoid region

(D) None of the above

Answers:

1. C

    Chronic suppurative otitis media Unsafe type usually presents with the off and on ear discherge and hearing impairment. The discharge is typically scanty, foul smelling and purulent.

2. D

    In such type of CSOM attic or marginal perforation is present along with cholesteatoma and granulations.

3. A

    One of the complications of this disease is LMN type facial palsy.

4. A

    Pre-operative high resolution CT scan helps in localization of disease and important anatomical landmarks.

Reference:

1. Flint PW, Haughey BH, Lund VJ, Niparko JK, Richardson MA (Eds). Complications of Temporal Bone Infections. In: Cummings Otolaryngology Head and Neck Surgery, 5th Edition Mosby-Elsevier Philadelphia 2010, pp 1991.

VALLECULAR CYST

Dr. H P Singh, Assistant Professor, Department of Otolaryngology

An otherwise well, normally delivered 4 month old boy was referred to our hospital for progressive difficulty in breathing. He was asymptomatic till 2 months of age when he developed stridor and progressive respiratory distress. A flexible upper airway scopy revealed a cystic lesion in the supraglottic area. He was then referred to our hospital for further management.

Upon examination in our hospital, his vital signs were stable. It was observed that he had inspiratory stridor as well as suprasternal and subcostal recession. The air entry was decreased in both lungs. Other systems were normal.

A diagnostic direct laryngoscopy under GA demonstrated a cystic mass adherent to the base of the tongue and valleculae. The epiglottis was compressed posteriorly and the laryngeal inlet was not well visualized. The aryepiglottic folds were short. The vocal cord and subglottic region were normal. An emergency tracheostomy has to be performed in view of the impending airway obstruction.

1. What is the most probable diagnosis?

(A) Laryngomalacia

(B) Laryngocoel

(C) Vallecular cyst

(D) Saccular cyst

2. What is the most pertinent investigation required to confirm the diagnosis and for planning of management?

(A) X ray of neck

(B) CT Scan of neck

(C) Barium swallow

(D) Angiography

3. What is the definitive management of the disease?

(A) Incision and marsupialization

(B) Micro laryngeal surgery

(C) Laryngofissure

(D) Partial laryngectomy

Answers:

1. C

    Vallecular cysts are typically present at birth in the tongue base of affected infants.

2. B

    These can be well demonstrated on CT scan of neck.

3. B

Treatment of vallecular cyst consists of excision via micolaryngeal surgery.

Reference:

1. Flint PW, Haughey BH, Lund VJ, Niparko JK, Richardson MA (Eds). Aspiration and Swallowing Disorders. In: Cummings Otolaryngology Head and Neck Surgery, 5th Edition Mosby- Elsevier, Philadelphia 2010, pp 2951-2952.

VOCAL CORD NODULES

Dr. H P Singh, Assistant Professor, Department of Otolaryngology

36 year old female, mother of two, with a 4-year history of intermittent hoarseness of voice presented to outdoor of ENT department. She was non smoker, generally very healthy. She was a teacher by occupation. She had gradual deterioration of voice over the past few years. On examination, the patient had moderate dysphonia and a mild strained quality in normal speech. During pitch-range exercises, voicing is intermittent but overall frequency range relatively normal. Videolaryngoscopic examination reveals bilateral vocal cord masses, which impedes normal voicing. However, closure is not complete, due to the bilateral mass lesions.

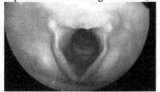

1. What is the probable diagnosis?
   (A) Vocal cord polyp
   (B) Vocal cord nodule
   (C) Leukoplakia of vocal cord
   (D) Granuloma of vocal cord
2. Which one is true about the disease?
   (A) Recurrence is common after surgery
   (B) Regress with the steroids
   (C) Malignant transformation can occur
   (D) Vocal abuse is the most common cause
3. What is the treatment of choice?
   (A) Wait and watch
   (B) Steroid inhalation
   (C) Micro-laryngeal surgery
   (D) Partial laryngectomy

Answers:

1. B
   A **vocal cord nodule** is a mass of tissue that grows on a vocal fold (vocal cord). Typically this mass appears on the junction of the anterior 1/3 and posterior 2/3 of the vocal fold, where contact is most forceful.
2. D
   The cause of these formations is usually strenuous or abusive voice practices such as yelling and coughing. Those who use their voices constantly in a loud environment such as teachers, actors and singers, are susceptible.
3. C
   Treatment of choice of this condition is micro-laryngeal surgery.

Reference:

1. Flint PW, Haughey BH, Lund VJ, Niparko JK, Richardson MA (Eds). Benign Vocal Fold Mucosal Disorders. In: Cummings Otolaryngology Head and Neck Surgery, 5th Edition Mosby- Elsevier, Philadelphia 2010, pp 865-866.

ATROPHIC RHINITIS

Dr. H P Singh, Assistant Professor, Department of Otolaryngology

This 18 year old girl presented to out-patient department of ENT department with the complaints of inability to smell for last 3 years. She also complained of passage of yellowish crusts during forceful clearing of nose and occasional epistaxis. Her father informed us that she had foul smell coming from nose, so much so that her friends do not want to talk to her and yet she is not aware of this fact. On general examination, patient had mild pallor. On external examination of the nose, it was seen that patient had depression of nasal bridge. The nasal cavity were roomy on both the sides and were filled with foul smelling crusts.

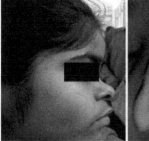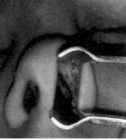

1. What is the most probable diagnosis?
   (A) Allergic rhinitis
   (B) Vasomotor rhinitis
   (C) Atrophic rhinitis
   (D) Hypertrophic rhinitis
2. "She had foul smell coming from nose, so much so that her friends do not want to talk to her and yet she is not aware of this fact." What does this phrase signifies?
   (A) Hopeful anosmia
   (B) Merciful anosmia
   (C) Sensory anosmia
   (D) Conductive anosmia
3. The surgical treatment of this disease is done by
   (A) Septoplasty
   (B) Submucous resection of septum
   (C) Young's operation
   (D) Caldwell-luc's operation

Answers:

1. C
   atrophic rhinitis is a chronic inflammation of nose characterized by atrophy of nasal mucosa, including the glands, turbinate bones and the nerve elements supplying the nose.
2. B
   Microorganisms are known to multiply and produce a foul smell from the nose, though the patients may not be aware of this, because their elements (responsible for the perception of smell) have become atrophied. This is called merciful anosmia.
3. C
   Surgical interventions include:Young's operation; Modified Young's operation; Narrowing of nasal cavities, submucosal injection of Teflon paste, section and medial displacement of the lateral wall of the nose.

Reference:

1. Dhingra PL. Acute and Chronic Rhinitis, In: Dhingra PL (Ed.). Diseases of Ear, Nose and throat, 3rd Edition. Elsevier, New Delhi 2004, pp 190-192.

MENIERE'S DISEASE

Dr. HP Singh, Assistant Professor, Department of Otolaryngology

A 45 year old gentleman presented with episodic dizziness, hard of hearing and tinnitus from right ear for last 6 years. During initial years, all of his complaints used to occur after every 3-4 months and last for about 4-5 days. For the last 2 years, he is experiencing persistent hearing loss and tinnitus from right ear. On examination, his tympanic membrane was normal. There was no nystagmus, either spontaneous or induced. His pure tone audiogram was performed which is given below-

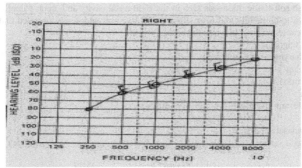

1. What is the most probable diagnosis?
   (A) Meniere's disease
   (B) Otosclerosis
   (C) CSOM
   (D) Acoustic neuroma
2. What major class of pharmacologic agent is used for management of acute phase of this disease?
   (A) Vestibular sedatives
   (B) Vasodilators
   (C) Tranquilizers
   (D) Antibiotics
3. Which is not a variant of this disease
   (A) Cochlear hydrops
   (B) Drop attacks
   (C) Lermoyez syndrome
   (D) Otosclerosis
4. All are the components of this disease except
   (A) Tinnitus
   (B) Hard of hearing
   (C) Vertigo
   (D) Ear discharge

Answers:

1. A

    Meniere's disease is a disorder of the inner ear that causes spontaneous episodes of vertigo along with fluctuating hearing loss, ringing in the ear (tinnitus), and sometimes a feeling of fullness or pressure in ear.

2. A

    Vestibular sedatives forms the mainstay of treatment in acute phase of the disease.

3. D

    Cochlear hydrops, Drop attacks and Lermoyez syndrome are among the many variants of the disease.

4. D

    Patients of meniere's disease do not exhibit ear discharge as a symptoms because of intact tympanic membrane.

Reference:

1. Dhingra PL. Meniere's Disease, In: Dhingra PL (Ed.). Diseases of Ear, Nose and throat, 3rd Edition. Elsevier, New Delhi 2004, pp 129-134.

ANTROCHOANAL POLYP

Dr. H P Singh, Assistant Professor, Department of Otolaryngology

The patient, a 14-year-old girl, complained of a foreign-body sensation in her mouth for approximately 3 months. The sensation was associated with difficulty in breathing from right nostril. Early complaints were unilateral nose blockage, post-nasal drainage and rhinorrhea. The patient reported having previously been healthy and had no history of allergy and nasal bleeding. Examination of the mouth revealed a large polypoid mass hanging from the nasopharynx into the oropharynx. This mass had anteriorly and superiorly displaced the uvula and soft palate. The mass was mobile upon palpation with a tongue depressor. Upon examination with a nasal speculum, a whitish soft-tissue mass was seen in the right nasal cavity and, upon palpation with a suction tube, the mass was found to be mobile and insensitive to touch. Nasal endoscopy revealed that the mass arose from the right middle meatus and extended into the nasopharynx.

1. Name the probable diagnosis-
   (A) Juvenile nasopharyngeal angiofibroma
   (B) Antrocoanal polyp
   (C) Malignancy of maxilla
   (D) Rhinoscleroma
2. What is the most relevant investigation for this condition?
   (A) MRI of nose
   (B) CT scan of paranasal sinuses
   (C) X ray PNS water's view
   (D) Nasal smear
3. What is preferred modality of treatment of this disease?
   (A) Surgical
   (B) Medical
   (C) Radiotherapy
   (D) Streptomycin therapy

Answers:

1. B

   Nasal polyps are polypoidal masses arising mainly from the mucous membranes of the nose and paranasal sinuses. They are overgrowths of the mucosa that frequently accompany allergic rhinitis. They are freely movable and nontender.Nasal polyps are usually classified into antrochoanal polyps and ethmoidal polyps. Antrochoanal polyps arise from the maxillary sinuses and are the much less common, ethmoidal polyps arise from the ethmoidal sinuses. Antrochoanal polyps are usually single and unilateral whereas ethmoidal polyps are multiple and bilateral.

2. B

   CT scan is a preferred method for diagnosis since it is able to give exquisite bony detail of the paranasal sinus anatomy.

3. A

   Surgery is the only feasible treatment. Several surgical techniques have been described in the literature.Functional endoscopic sinus surgery (FESS) is, currently, the gold standard technique.

Reference:

1. Dhingra PL. Nasal Polypi, In: Dhingra PL (Ed.). Diseases of Ear, Nose and throat, 3rd Edition. Elsevier, New Delhi 2004, pp 210-214.

GLOMUS TYMPANICUM

Dr. H P Singh, Assistant Professor, Department of Otolaryngology

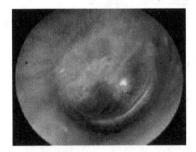

A 46 year old male patient presented to ENT OPD with the complaints of pulsatile tinnitus, hearing loss and heaviness in right ear for 8 months. He denied any history of trauma, ear discharge and vertigo. His otoscopic picture is given below-

1. Name the sign seen in the picture
   (A) Hollman-Millar sign
   (B) Rising Sun sign
   (C) Schwartze sign

(D) Hanneburt sign
2. Name the Probable diagnosis
   (A) Acoustic neuroma
   (B) Otosclerosis
   (C) Endolymphatichydrops
   (D) Glomus tympanicum
3. What is most pertinent investigation?
   (A) CT Scan of tympanomastoid region
   (B) Complete blood counts
   (C) Pure tone audiogram
   (D) X-Ray of mastoid Schuller's view
4. What is the treatment of this condition?
   (A) Wait and watch
   (B) Intratympanic Gentamycin injection
   (C) Surgical excision
   (D) Medical treatment with neurotonics and vasodilators

Answers:
1. B
   Due to the highly vascular nature of the tumor, a reddish mass is typically observed behind the eardrum i.e. **rising sun sign.**
2. D
   Glomustympanicum tumors (also known as paragangliomas of the middle ear) are highly vascular, benign (non-cancerous) tumors that arise from paraganglia in the middle ear. Conductive hearing loss is common due to the tumor occupying space within the middle ear and preventing transmission of sound through the eardrum and ossicular chain. Additionally, pulsatile tinnitus occurs frequently due to the vascular nature of these tumors. Very large glomustympanicumtumors may cause vertigo (feeling that the world around you is spinning when you are not moving), facial paralysis and sensorineural hearing loss.
3. A
   CT scan of tympanomastoid region is the most pertinent investigation as it reveals the complete outline of the tumor and its extension.
4. C
   Complete surgical excision is the treatment of choice.

References:
1. Flint PW, Haughey BH, Lund VJ, Niparko JK, Richardson MA (Eds). Interventional Neuroradiology of the Skull base, Head and Neck. In: Cummings Otolaryngology Head and Neck Surgery, 5th Edition Mosby- Elsevier, Philadelphia 2010, pp 1935.
2. Dhingra PL. Tumours of Middle Ear and Mastoid, In: Dhingra PL (Ed.). Diseases of Ear, Nose and throat, 3rd Edition. Elsevier, New Delhi 2004, pp 139-142.

CHRONIC SUPPURATIVE OTITIS MEDIA
Dr. Sunil Kumar, Assistant Professor, Department Of Otorhinolaryngology

A 20 Years old male presented to the outpatient department with off and on right ear discharge and decreased hearing for 10 years. Discharge was profuse, non-foul smelling and mucopurulent. On routine ENT examination, there was central perforation. He had deviated nasal septum towards tight side. His routine blood investigations including chest x-ray were normal.

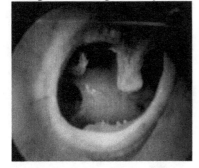

1. What is the most probable diagnosis?
    (A) Serous otitis media
    (B) Acute suppurative otitis media
    (C) Chronic suppurative otitis media
    (D) Acute necrotizing otitis media
2. Which of the following is true about the disease?
    (A) Cholesteatoma is usually present
    (B) Attic perforation is present
    (C) Complications are more common
    (D) Usually central perforation seen
3. What is the most preferred treatment of choice?
    (A) Myringotomy
    (B) Radical mastoidectomy
    (C) Modified radical mastoidectomy
    (D) Tympanoplasty

Answers:
    1. C
       Profuse, mucopurulent and non-foul smelling is found in chronic suppurative otitis media with tubotympanic disease.
    2. D
       Chronic suppurative otitis media with tubotympanic disease is assosciated with central perforation while cholesteatoma, attic perforation are seen in attico-antral disease.
    3. D
       The mainstay of the treatment of chronic suppurative otitis media with tubotympanic disease is tympanoplasty.

Reference:
    1. FlintPW, Haughey BH, Lund VJ, Niparko JK, Richardson MA(Eds). Chronic Otitis Media, Mastoiditis and Petrositis In: Cumming's Otolaryngology Head & Neck Surgery, 5th Edition, Mosby Elsevier Philadelphia 2010, pp 1975-1990.

VOCAL CORD POLYP
Dr. Sunil Kumar, Assistant Professor, Department Of Otorhinolaryngology

A 30 years old male patient presented to OPD with the change in voice for 1 yr. He is student and part time school teacher. Videolaryngoscopy revealed a small smooth pale mass present over right vocal cord at the junction of anterior 1/3 and posterior 2/3. Vocal cord movement was normal. Routine investigation were normal.

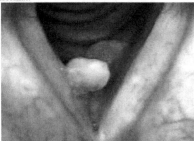

1. What is the most probable diagnosis?
    (A) Vocal nodule
    (B) Vocal polyp
    (C) Malignancy vocal cord
    (D) Papilloma vocal cord
2. Which one is true about the disease?
    (A) Recurrence is common after surgery
    (B) Does not regress with the steroids
    (C) Malignant transformation can occur
    (D) Vocal abuse is the most common cause

3. What is the treatment of choice?
- (A) Wait and watch
- (B) Steroid inhalation
- (C) Micro-laryngeal surgery
- (D) Partial laryngectomy

Answers:
1. B
   Vocal polyp is unilateral and present at the junction of ant 1/3 and post 2/3 of junction.
2. B
   Vocal cord polyp does not regress with the steroid while early vocal nodule may regress with the steroid.
3. C
   Microlaryngeal surgery is the mainstay of the treatment of vocal polyp.

Reference:
1. FlintPW, Haughey BH, Lund VJ, Niparko JK, Richardson MA(Eds). Benign Vocal Fold Mucosal Disorders In: Cumming's Otolaryngology Head & Neck Surgery, 5th Edition, Mosby Elsevier Philadelphia 2010, pp 859-882.

ALLERGIC FUNGAL RHINOSINUSITIS
Dr. Sunil Kumar, Assistant Professor, Department Of Otorhinolaryngology

A 40 years male patient presented the OPD with complaints of off and on nasal obstruction, loss of smell and rhinorrhea for last 5 years. There was no history of nasal bleeding. There was no history of tuberculosis, hypertension, diabetes mellitus or any chronic illness. Patient got relieved with conservative treatment in the form of steroid nasal spray. CT scan was advised after 3 weeks treatment which showed heterogenous mass present in all the paranasal sinuses. Rest of the hematological investigations were normal.

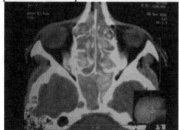

1. What is the most probable diagnosis?
- (A) Invasive fungal sinusitis
- (B) Allergic fungal sinusitis
- (C) Antrohoanal polyp
- (D) Inverted papilloma
2. What is the treatment of choice?
- (A) FESS
- (B) Long term steroid treatment
- (C) Long term antifungal treatment
- (D) Medial Maxillectomy
3. What is true about the disease?
- (A) Commonly occur in immunocompromised patients
- (B) Recurrence never seen after surgery
- (C) Antifungal treatment is the mainstay of the treatment
- (D) Post-operative steroid treatment is given to prevent the recurrence

Answers:
1. B
   Allergic fungal sinusitis presents with nasal obstruction, nasal discharge and loss of smell. It regresses with the steroids.
2. A
   Functional endoscopic sinus surgery is the treatment of choice while steroid is used to prevent the recurrence.

3. D

   After endoscopic sinus surgery steroid is used to prevent the recurrence. Pre-operatively it is used to downgrade the polyposis for better intra-operative field.

Reference:

1. FlintPW, Haughey BH, Lund VJ, Niparko JK, Richardson MA (Eds). Fungal Rhinosinusitis In: Cumming's Otolaryngology Head & Neck Surgery, 5th Edition, Mosby Elsevier Philadelphia, pp 709-716.

THYROGLOSSAL FISTULA

Dr. Sunil Kumar, Assistant Professor, Department Of Otorhinolaryngology

A 20 years old patient presented to OPD with complains of pus discharge from an opening in neck for 1 yr. Patient had previous history of recurrent swelling in midline neck for which he had undergone incision and drainage by a local medical practitioner 1 yr back. Since then he has intermittent watery and purulent discharge from that site. On protrusion of tongue there is puckering at the site of opening

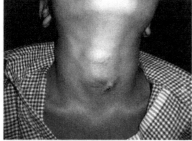

1. What is the most probable diagnosis?
   (A) Thyroglossal fistula
   (B) Branchial fistula
   (C) Branchial sinus
   (D) Thyroglossal cyst
2. What is the most preferred treatment?
   (A) Sistrunk operation
   (B) Medical treatment
   (C) Modified neck dissection
   (D) None of the above
3. Most important step during surgery is to?
   (A) Removal of the body of hyoid bone
   (B) Ligation of major vessels
   (C) Removal of part of thyroid cartilage
   (D) Removal of tonsil

Answers:

1. A

   Thyroglossal fistula occurs after incision and drainage of cyst. There is puckering of surrounding skin on protrusion of tongue.
2. A

   Sistrunk operation is the mainstay of treatment of thyroglossal fistula.
3. A

   Removal of body of hyoid bone is the most important step of sistrunk operation to prevent the recurrence.

Reference:

1. FlintPW, Haughey BH, Lund VJ, Niparko JK, Richardson MA(Eds). Differancial Diagnosis Of Neck MASSES In: Cumming's Otolaryngology Head & Neck Surgery, 5th Edition, Mosby Elsevier Philadelphia 2010, pp 2812-2821.

RHINOSCLEROMA

Dr. Sunil Kumar, Assistant Professor, Department Of Otolaryngology

A 45 years male presented in OPD with the complaints of off and on bleeding from nasal cavity and nasal obstruction for 1 Patient also had purulent fowl smelling discharge from nasal cavity. On clinical examination nasal cavity was filled with rubbery polyps with bluish red nasal mucosa. Rest of the investigation were normal.

1. What is the most probable diagnosis?
   - (A) Antrochoanal polyp
   - (B) Ethmoidal polyp
   - (C) Rhinoscleroma
   - (D) Tuberculosis
2. This disease is a---infection
   - (A) Bacterial
   - (B) Viral
   - (C) Fungal
   - (D) Protozoal
3. Which is the most probable causative organism?
   - (A) Klebsiellarhinoscleromatis
   - (B) Pseudomonas aeruginosa
   - (C) Mybacterium tuberculosis
   - (D) Streptococcus pneumonae

Answers:

1. C

   Rhinoscleroma presents as recurrent nasal bleeding, nasal obstruction, and fowl smelling nasal discharge with rubbery polyp and bluish red nasal mucosa. Biopsy shows the typical Mikulicz cells and Russell bodies.

2. A

   Rhinoscleroma is a bacterial infection. It starts in the nose and nasopharynx, oropharynx, larynx,trachea and bronchi.

3. A

   Rhinoscleroma is caused by gram negative bacillus called Klebsiellarhinoscleromatis or Frisch bacillus.

Reference:

1. Dhingra PL. Granulomatous diseases of nose, In: DhingraPL(ed.) Diseases of Ear Nose And Throat 3rd Edition. Elsevier New Delhi 2004, pp 194-198.

Chapter-16

Pathology

ASK UPMARK KIDNEY

Dr. Atin Singhai, Associate Professor, Department of Pathology

A 3 years old female child presented with hematuria. Urine examination showed presence of 30-40 fresh as well as crenated RBCs, 8-10 pus cell with occasional cluster formation, and 2-3 epithelial cells per high power field. Radiological examination showed segmental contracted kidney with mild hydronephrosis and cortical thinning accompanied by compensatory enlargement of right kidney. Clinically, the child was also found to be mildly hypertensive. Subsequently left nephrectomy was planned and a specimen was received measuring 2.8 x 2 x 1 cms. Cut surface showed contracted areas as well as few dilated cystic areas. Microscopic sections(as shown in the figure) prominently revealed disorganized renal parenchyma with primitive glomeruli and immature tubules surrounded by muscular cuff. In vicinity of these areas, mature looking glomeruli and tubules with focal tubular necrosis and thyroidisation were also evident. Blood vessels were prominent for marked medial hyperplasia. There was no other remarkable pathology evident.

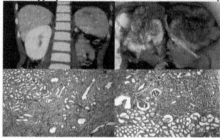

1. What is the most likely diagnosis?
   - (A) Cystic Dysplasia of Kidney
   - (B) Renal Segmental Hypoplasia
   - (C) Polycystic Kidney Disease
   - (D) Renal Aplasia
2. What is the most common clinical presentation?
   - (A) Weakness and fatigue
   - (B) Abdomin lump
   - (C) Hematuria with hypertension
   - (D) Loss of appetite and weight loss
3. What is the proposed aetiology for this entity?
   - (A) Developmental defect
   - (B) Vesicoureteric reflex
   - (C) Both of the above
   - (D) None of the above
4. What is the hallmark microscopic finding?
   - (A) Segments of primitive glomeruli, immature tubules and hyperplastic vessels
   - (B) Areas of immature cartilage and dermal elements including hair follicles
   - (C) Dilated cystic spaces lined by narrow rim of renal cortex
   - (D) Areas of chronic tubulonephritis with prominent thyroidisation of tubules
5. What is the treatment modality of choice?
   - (A) Nephrectomy alone
   - (B) Nephrectomy with adjuvant therapy
   - (C) Conservative treatment
   - (D) Renal artery embolization

Answers:

1. B

   Renal Segmental Hypoplasia or commonly called as Ask Upmark Kidney.
2. C

   Hypertension with or without hematuria is most common clinical presentation.
3. C

   Developmental as well as reflux, both have been described as possible aetiologies.
4. A

   Immature tubules, primitive glomeruli and hyperplastic vessels are confirmatory.
5. A

Nephrectomy alone is the treatment of choice.

Reference:
1. Bostwick DG, Cheng L, MacLennan GT. Non Neoplastic Diseases of the Kidney. In: Urologic Surgical Pathology. Mosby Elseiver. Second Edition 2008. pp 50-51.

DIABETIC NEPHROPATHY

Dr. Atin Singhai, Associate Professor, Department of Pathology

A 55 years old male patient presented to Medicine OPD with chief complaints of fatigue and foot edema since 8 months. The edema was progressively increasing. He also reported of passing foamy urine and was found to be mildly hypertensive on clinical examination (150/100 mm Hg). Investigations revealed: Serum Creatinine 3.5 mg/dl, Blood Urea 105 mg/dl, Serum Protein 3.9 gm/dl, 24 hours Urinary Protein 4.5 gm/day, Microalbuminuria 2.8 gm/ 24 hrs, Fasting Blood Sugar was 156 mg/dl, Hemoglobin 10.6 gm/dl, Total Leucocyte Count 7200/cumm, Polymorphs 70%, Platelets 2.5 lakhs/cumm. Subsequent renal biopsy displayed adequate number of glomeruli with uniform involvement of all glomeruli, depicting prominent nodular glomerulosclerosis. The nodules showed both PAS and JSM (Silver) positivity, but were negative for any deposits on Immunofluorescence. Tubules were moderately degenerated with occasional presence of proteinaceous casts. Vessels were prominent for subintimalhyalinosis.

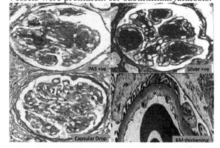

1. What is the most likely diagnosis?
   (A) Focal Segmental Glomerulosclerosis
   (B) Amyloidosis
   (C) Diabetic Nephropathy
   (D) Light Chain Deposition Disease
2. The nodular lesions in Diabetic Nephropathy are commonly referred as?
   (A) Kimmelstiel Wilson Nodules
   (B) Armani Ebstein Nodules
   (C) SpuhlerZollinger Nodules
   (D) Falk Hennigar Nodules
3. The nodules in Diabetic Nephropathy are:
   (A) Both PAS and Silver negative
   (B) PAS positive, Silver negative
   (C) PAS negative, Silver positive
   (D) Both PAS and Silver positive
4. Microalbuminuria cut off value is:
   (A) <30 mg / 24 hrs
   (B) 30 – 100 mg / 24 hrs
   (C) 30 – 200 mg / 24 hrs
   (D) 30 – 300 mg / 24 hrs
5. Which of the following is not a risk factor for progression of nephropathy?
   (A) Poor Glucose control
   (B) Low Blood Pressure
   (C) Higher Urinary Albumin excretion
   (D) Smoking

Answers:
1. C
   Microscopic as well as clinical findings suggest Diabetic Nephropathy.

2. A

Kimmelstiel and Wilson first recognized nodular lesions in Diabetic Nephropathy.
3. D

Nodules in Diabetic Nephropathy are both PAS and JSM positive.
4. D

Microalbuminuria cutoff values range between 30 – 300 mg / 24 hrs.
5. B

High Blood Pressure is a risk factor for progression of Nephropathy.

Reference:
1. Jennette JC, Oslen JL, Schwartz MM, Silva FG. Diabetic Nephropathy In: Pathology of the Kidney. Wolter Kluwer, Lippincott Williams & Wilkins. Sixth Edition 2007. pp 803-52.

PERIPHERAL NEUROECTODERMAL TUMOR OF KIDNEY

Dr. Atin Singhai, Associate Professor, Department of Pathology

A 22 years old female patient, native of Gangetic plains, was admitted to Urology wards for complaints of right flank pain and hematuria for last 4 months. On radiological evaluation, she was found to have a well defined infiltrating mass of 8.8 X 6.7 cm occupying the lower and mid portions of right kidney on lateral aspect and infiltrating the perirenal fascia. Subsequently, she underwent radical nephrectomy under epidural anaesthesia. A gross specimen was received with attached perinephric fat measuring, 11 X 9.5 X 8 cm. Cut section revealed a variegated growth involving two thirds of the renal parenchyma with obvious capsular breach. Microscopy of the sections from growth showed a malignant neoplasm disposed mainly as solid sheets and nests separated by thick fibrovascularseptae. Individual tumor cells were monomorphic small round cells having high nucleo-cytoplasmic ratio, round to oval nuclei with fine chromatin and mild to moderate amount of eosinophillic cytoplasm. Occasional ill formed rosettes were also seen. Capsular breach was evident. Immunohistochemistry was strongly positive for CD99, focally positive for Vimentin and negative for Cytokeratin (CK) and Leucocyte Common Antigen (LCA).

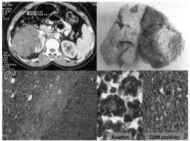

1. What is the most likely diagnosis:
    (A) Rhabdoid Sarcoma of Kidney
    (B) Lymphoma of Kidney
    (C) Peripheral Neuroectodermal Tumor of Kidney
    (D) Adult Wilm's Tumor of Kidney
2. What can be the possible differential diagnosis:
    (A) Rhabdoid Sarcoma of Kidney
    (B) Adult Wilm'sTumor of Kidney
    (C) Lymphoma of Kidney
    (D) All of the above
3. Most common age and gender for presentation of PNET Kidney is:
    (A) Elderly females
    (B) Young to middle aged females
    (C) Young to middle aged males
    (D) Elderly males
4. The most consistent positive Immunohistochemistry markers for PNET kidney are:
    (A) CD 99 and FLI 1
    (B) CD 99 and WT 1

(C) WT 1 and LCA

(D) FLI 1 and LCA

5. The most consistent molecular marker of PNET Kidney is:

    (A) PRCC and TFE 3 fusion

    (B) EWS and FL1 fusion

    (C) Biallelic inactivation of hSNF 5 / INI1 on 22q

    (D) Loss of heterozygosity of the TSC2 gene on 16p13

Answers:

    1.   C

            CD 99 positivity with microscopic and clinical features favours PNET Kidney.

    2.   D

            On the basis of microscopy alone, all can be the possible differential diagnosis.

    3.   C

            Middle aged males, with peak age around 26 years, are predominantly involved.

    4.   A

            IHC positivity for CD 99 and/or FLI1 is confirmatory for PNET Kidney.

    5.   B

            PNET belongs to Ewing Family of Tumors and hence marked by EWS FLI1 fusion.

Reference:

    1.   Bostwick DG, Cheng L, MacLennan GT. Neoplasms of the Kidney. In: Urologic Surgical Pathology. Mosby Elseiver. Second Edition 2008. pp 77-172.

OVARIAN CARCINOMA

Dr. Ajay Kr. Singh, Associate Professor, Department of Pathology

A 58 year-old woman with two healthy children visited a gynecologist with a 2-month history of vague pelvic discomfort and abdominal distension. Pelvic examination revealed a right adnexal mass. There was no previous history of co-morbid illness, or family history of breast or ovarian cancer. On radiology, abdominal-pelvic CT revealed an 8 x 8-cm right adnexal mass and a small volume of ascitic fluid. Chest xray, CBC and biochemical profile were within normal limit. Except CA125 which was elevated to 178 U/mL. The patient underwent total abdominal hysterectomy with bilateral salpingo-oopherectomy, omentectomy and pelvic peritoneal debulking surgery.CA125 decreased to 95 U/mL following surgery.The gross and microscopic findings of the patient were as shown below.

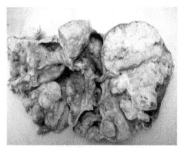 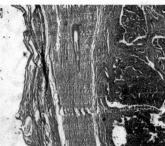

1. Which of the following is not a common symptom of ovarian cancer.

    (A) Distention of abdomen

    (B) Pelvic/abdominal pain

    (C) Urinary symptoms such as urgency or frequency

    (D) Dysfunctional uterine bleeding

2. Which is not a risk factor for ovarian cancer.

    (A) Diabetes mellitus

    (B) Early menarche

    (C) Late age at menopause

    (D) Personal or family history of breast, ovarian, fallopian tube, or colon cancer

3. Which of these markers is most useful in the diagnosis of ovarian cancer

    (A) PSA

    (B) CA-125

(C) CEA

(D) CA-19.9

Answers:

1. **D**

   Dysfunctional uterine bleeding is mainly symptoms of endometrium or cervical cancer.

2. **A**

   Diabetes mellitus is mainly predisposing factor for endometrial carcinoma.

3. **B**

   CA-125 is a tumour marker which is elevated in approximately 85% of patients with stage III/IV ovarian cancer. The endometrial cancer may be sometime elevated CA-125.

References:

1. Mansoor NA, Jezan HS. Spectrum of ovarian tumors: Histopathological study of 218 cases. Gulf J Oncolog. 2015 May;1(18):64-70.

2. Cramer DW, Welch WR. Determinants of ovarian cancer risk:II. Inference regarding pathogenesis . J Natl Cancer Inst.1983;71:717-721.

3. Russell P, Merkur H. Proliferating ovarian "epithelial" a clinicopathological analysis of 144 cases. Aust NZJ ObstetGynaecol 1979;19:45-51.

DERMOID CYST OVARY

Dr Ajay Singh, Associate Professor, Department of Pathology

A 21 year old student presented with left iliac fossa pain since 6 months which gradually increased in frequency and severity. The pain was intermittent withnoparticular pattern,however it generally worsened on exercise.Her menstrual cycle was regular and unremarkeable. The physical examination revealed a palpable mass in left iliac fossa which was firm and mobile. It was moderately tender. Per speculum findings were unremarkeable. Bimanual examination confirmed an 8.0 cm mass in left adnexa which was also confirmed by USG. The uterus was palpable separately, mobile and anteverted. The right adnexa was normal. On the basis of clinicoradiological findings surgery was done for removal of left adnexal mass. The radiological, gross and microscopic findings were as follows:

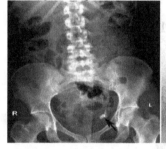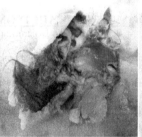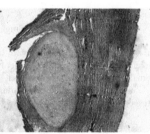

1. Which is not a clinical diagnosis on this given history?
   (A) Dermoid cyst of ovary
   (B) Simple cyst of ovary
   (C) Chocolate cyst of ovary
   (D) Torsion of follicular cyst

2. On opening the cyst, hemorrhagic fluid came out so which is not a differential diagnosis.
   (A) Chocolate cyst of ovary
   (B) Torsion of any cyst
   (C) Luteal hemorrhagic cyst
   (D) Simple cyst

3. Dysfunctional uterine bleeding is not a clinical symptom of?
   (A) Endometrial carcinoma
   (B) Chocolate cyst of ovary
   (C) Complex hyperplasia of endometrial
   (D) Carcinoma cervix

4. Not true about dermoid cyst (mature cystic teratoma).
   (A) Benign tumour

(B) Teeth and hair is found in this cyst

(C) CA-125 is increases in dermoid cyst

(D) They commonly display a classical appearance on x-ray and ultrasound

5. Which is not a differential diagnosis of acute right iliac fossa pain ?

(A) Dermoid cyst

(B) Ovarian cyst torsion

(C) Ectopic pregnancy

(D) Appendicitis

Answers:

1.   D

Torsion of follicular cyst .Torsion of any cyst is emergency and presents with acute abdomen with heavy pain.

2.   D

Except simple cyst on cutting serous fluid came out, all other option cyst on cutting hemorrhage came out.

3.   B

Chocolate cyst of ovary.Because dysfunctional uterine bleeding is a symptoms of endometrial and cervical lesions not an ovarian lesions.

4.   C

CA-125 is increased in dermoid cyst

5.   A

Dermoidcyst. All other problems is acute but dermoid cyst is not acute lesion. If dermoid cyst on torsion then they present acute pain

References:

1.   Ozgur T[1], Atik E, Silfeler DB, Toprak S. Mature cystic teratomas in our series with review of the literature and retrospective analysis. Arch Gynecol Obstet. 2012;285(4):1099-101.

2.   Peterson WF, Prevost EC et.al. Benign cystic teratoma of ovary.A clinicostatistical study of 1007 cases with review of literature. Am J ObstetGynecol 1955; 70:368

3.   Chiang AJ, La V, Peng J, Yu KJ, Teng NN.Squamous cell carcinoma arising from mature cystic teratoma of the ovary. Int J Gynecol Cancer. 2011; 21(3):466-74.

ENDOMETRIAL CARCINOMA

Dr. Ajay Singh, Associate Professor, Department of Pathology

A 50-year-old female presented with history of vaginal spotting. The complaint appeared after two years of menopause. She had two children. Her mother and maternal grandmother died in their 40's of colon cancer and a maternal aunt had endometrial cancer. The non-gynecologic physical examinations were within normal limits. On USG there was mild thickening of endometrium.Sheunderwenttotal hysterectomy. The gross and microscopicphotographs were as shown below:

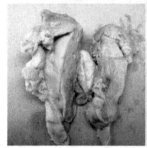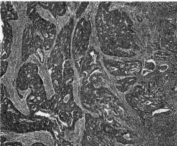

1. Which is LEAST likely to be the differential diagnosis of her complaint?

(A) Ovarian cancer

(B) Cervical cancer

(C) Endometrial cancer

(D) Endometrial hyperplasia

2. Which is not an investigation indicated for this woman at this time?

(A) PAP smear

(B) Transvaginal ultrasound and endometrial biopsy

(C) Colposcopy of the cervix

(D) Hysteroscopy

3. Which is not a risk factor for endometrial carcinoma?

(A) Obesity

(B) History of breast cancer

(C) Grand multiparty

(D) Diabetes mellitus

4. Which tumor marker might be positive in this patient?

(A) CEA

(B) CA 19-9

(C) CA 125

(D) CA 1492

5. Which defines Stage 3 endometrial carcinoma?

(A) Carcinoma confined to the corpus uteri

(B) Cancer involving the corpus and cervix but has not extended outside the uterus

(C) Cancer extending outside the uterus but confined to the true pelvis and/or retroperitoneal lymph nodes

(D) Cancer involving the bladder or bowel mucosa or that has distant metastases

Answers:

1. A

It is rare for ovarian cancer to present with vaginal bleeding. Each of the other choices can cause vaginal bleeding.

2. C

She should have bimanual and rectovaginal examinations. An endometrial biopsy can usually be performed safely in the office setting and approaches the D&C in accuracy. The Pap smear would detect any cervical abnormalities. Hysteroscopy and saline infusion sonography can visualize endometrial lesions and can be useful adjuncts to endometrial biopsy. A colposcopy of the cervix is indicated only if there is evidence for cytological abnormalities on the Pap smear.

3. C

Women who have had many children are thought to have some protection from endometrial carcinoma. Other protective factors are oral contraception for at least one year and cigarette smoking. There are multiple risk factors for endometrial carcinoma including increasing age, obesity, physical inactivity, early menarche, late menopause, low parity or infertility, diabetes mellitus, hypertension, and chronic use of unopposed estrogens.

4. C

The CA 125 can be positive in endometrial cancers, especially papillary serous carcinomas, and should be looked for. Elevated CA 125 may also indicate metastasis or large deeply invasive tumors in women with Type 1 endometrial cancers. However, it is usually associated with ovarian CA. CEA is most often associated with colon, lung, and breast cancer. The CA 19-9 is associated with pancreatic and biliary malignancies. The CA 1492 is fictitious.

5. C

Stages of endometrial cancer the choices are different stages as follows.
a= Stage 1; b= Stage 2; c= Stage 3; and d= Stage 4.

References:

1. Gerli S, Spanò F, Di Renzo GC. Endometrial carcinoma in women 40 year old or younger: a case report and literature review. Eur Rev Med Pharmacol Sci .2014; 18 (14): 1973-8

2. K. Uma Devi. Current status of gynecological cancer care in India.JGynecolOncol2009; 20(2):77-80.

3. Dunton CJ, Balsara G, MC Farland M. Uterine papillary serous carcinoma: a review. ObstetGynecolSurv 1991; 46:97-102.

FOLLICULAR CARCINOMA OF THYROID

Dr. Madhu Kumar, Associate Professor, Department of Pathology

A 60yrs old female presentedwith slowly enlarging painless midline neck mass for 10 yrs. We received a thyroidectomy specimen of the same patient, which measured 8x6x4cm in size and was nodular in appearance. On cutting, dirty white in color,solid to cystic colloid filled follicles with fibrotic & small hemorrhagicareas were identified. On microscopic examination, low power view showed capsular invasion by tumor cells (white arrow-capsule, blue arrow-capsular invasion). On high power, uniformtumour cells forming nests and sheetswere identified, however no colloid was seenwithout colloid. At some places repetitive follicles containing colloid areas were also seen.

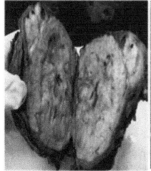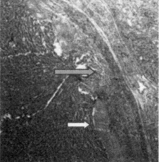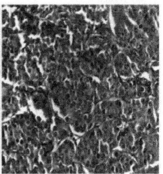

1. Which statement is true about follicular carcinoma?
   (A) It has no relationship to dietary iodine.
   (B) Lymphatic spread is the main route of metastasis.
   (C) Individual malignant nuclei have nuclear groove with fine powdery chromatin.
   (D) Capsular and vascular invasion are the diagnostic feature of invasive follicular carcinoma.
2. Common mode of spread may be associated with follicular carcinoma is
   (A) Vascular spread
   (B) Lymphatic spread
   (C) Direct spread
   (D) all of the above
3. All lesions of thyroid can be diagnosed on fine needle cytology except
   (A) Papillary thyroid carcinoma
   (B) Follicular thyroid carcinoma
   (C) Medullary carcinoma
   (D) Anaplastic carcinoma
4. Nuclear features of follicular carcinoma are usually all except
   (A) Presence of repetitive follicles
   (B) Lined by cuboidal epithelium
   (C) Nuclear overlapping & crowding
   (D) Ground glass appearance/Orphan Annie eye nuclei.

Answers:
   1. D
      Because Capsular and vascular invasion are the important diagnostic feature of invasive follicular carcinoma.[2]
   2. A
      Vascular invasion causes distant metastasis by vascular dissemination.[1,2]
   3. B
      The cytological appearances of follicular carcinoma &adenoma aresimilar. It is difficult to appreciate and we cannot see capsular invasion in the FNAC smears.[3]
   4. D
      The nuclei of papillary carcinoma cells contain fine chromatin, which imparts an optically clear or empty appearance looking like to Ground glass appearance.[4]

References:
   1. Baloch ZW, LiVolsi VA.Prognostic factors in well-differentiated follicular-derived carcinoma and medullary thyroid carcinoma. Thyroid 2001; 11:637
   2. Collini P, Sampietro G, Rosai J, Pilotti S. Minimally invasive (encapsulated) follicular carcinoma of the thyroid gland is the low-risk counterpart of widely invasive follicular carcinoma but not of insular carcinoma. Virchows Arch 2003; 442:71.
   3. Gita Jayaram and Svante R Orell, Thyroid, Svante R Orell and Gregory F. Sterrett,Orell and Sterrett's Fine Needle Aspiration Cytology, 5th Edition,118-155;2012.

4. AnirbanMaitra,The Endocrine System,Thyroidgland.Vinay Kumar, Abul K. Abbas, Jon C. Aster. Robbins &Cotran Pathologic Basis of Disease, 8th Edition,1107-1126;2010.

HASHIMOTO THYROIDITIS
Dr. Madhu Kumar, AssociateProfessor, Department of Pathology

A 40 years old female patient presented with diffuse, painless enlargement of the thyroid for 6months. Her free T4& T3 level were low and TSH waselevated. Grossly, the capsule of resected gland was intact. Microscopic examination revealed dense infiltration of thyroid tissue by a mononuclear infiltrate & well developed germinal centers. Follicles were lined by cuboidal epithelium as well as hurthle cells.

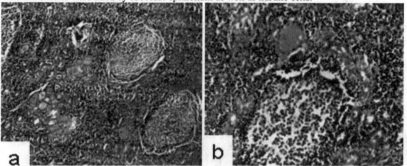

1. Which is the most likely diagnosis seen in the microphotograph.
    (A) Granulomatous thyroiditis.
    (B) Hashimoto thyroiditis.
    (C) Colloid goiter.
    (D) Graves disease.
2. Histopathology of Hashimoto's thyroiditis is   characterized by all except
    (A) Infiltration of the thyroid tissue by lymphocytic infiltrate.
    (B) Infiltration of the thyroid tissue by plasma cells&hurthle cells
    (C) Presenceof well-developed germinal centers
    (D) Presence of multinucleated giant cells.
3. Hashimoto's thyroiditis is at increased risk for development of
    (A) Papillary carcinoma thyroid
    (B) Medullary carcinoma thyroid
    (C) B-cell non-Hodgkin lymphomas
    (D) Follicular carcinoma thyroid
4. Diagnosisof Hashimoto's thyroiditis is usually made by elevated levels of antibodies
    (A) Anti-thyroglobulin antibodies (anti-Tg).
    (B) Anti-thyroid peroxidase antibodies (anti-TPO).
    (C) Anti-microsomal antibodies.
    (D) All of the above.
5. Which of the following is an autoimmune disease:
    (A) Viral thyroiditis.
    (B) Hashimoto's thyroiditis.
    (C) Suppurative Thyroiditis
    (D) Riedel's thyroiditis

Answers:
    1. B
       Thyroid tissue contains with a dense lymphocytic infiltrate with germinal centers.[1]
    2. D
       Multinucleated giant cells are present in the granulomatous thyroiditis.[1]
    3. C
       Oncogenic mutation occur most frequently in germinal center B cell during attempted antibody diversification.[1]
    4. D
       Breakdown of self tolerance to thyroid autoantigens.so presence of autoantibodies

anst the thyroglobin,thyroid peroxidase& microsomal antibodies.[1]

5.   B

Breakdown of peripheral tolerance to thyroid autoantigens,results in progressive autoimmune destruction of thyrocytes by infiltrating cytotoxic T cells or by antibody dependent cytotoxicity.[1]

Reference:

1.   MaitraA,The Endocrine System,Thyroidgland.Vinay Kumar, Abul K. Abbas, Jon C. Aster. Robbins &Cotran Pathologic Basis of Disease, 8th Edition.1097-1164; 2010.

MULTINODULAR COLLOID GOITER
Dr. Madhu Kumar, Associate Professor, Department of Pathology

A 20 yr old female patient presented with slowly enlarging large midline neck swelling for 2 yrs. Other associated symptom was dysphagia. TSH, T3 &T4 were within normal range.On gross examination of hemi-thyroidectomy specimen, size was 4.5x3x1cm.Outer surface was smooth,nodular& covered with fibrous capsule. Cut surface showed lobulated colloid filled thyroid parenchyma.On microscopic examination well capsulated thyroid tissue   was identified which showed variably sized follicles, lined by flattened bland cuboidal epithelium and filled with eosinophilic colloid (as shown in the figures below).

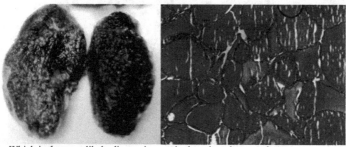

1. Which is the most likely diagnosis seen in the microphotograph.
    (A) Follicular carcinoma
    (B) Follicular adenoma
    (C) Colloid goiter
    (D) Graves disease
2. Multinodular goiter is characterized by all of the following except
    (A) It is most often caused by dietary deficiency of iodine.
    (B) Serum T3 &T4 are usually normal.
    (C) Diffuse hyperplasia, infiltrative ophthalmopathy&dermatopathy.
    (D) Histologically,it shows cystic inactive follicles & areas of follicular hyperplasia.
3. The following statement is true about Multinodular goiter except
    (A) They are more likely to be benign than solitary thyroid nodules.
    (B) Functioning nodules are more likely to be benign.
    (C) They are less likely to be malignant in younger patients.
    (D) All long standing multinodular goiters convert into malignancy.
4. The most precise diagnostic screening procedure for differentiating benign thyroid nodules from malignant ones is:
    (A) Thyroid ultrasonography.
    (B) Thyroid scintiscan.
    (C) Fine-needle-aspiration cytology.
    (D) Thyroid hormone essay.
5. Out of these thyroid function tests, most specific test is/are for hyper/hypo thyroidism
    (A) TSH
    (B) T3
    (C) T4
    (D) All of the above.

Answers:
1.   C

Gross & microscopic findings are consistent with the diagnosis of colloid goiter.[1]

2. C
All clinical findings are associated with Graves disease.[1]
3. D
Not all convert in to malignancy but less than <5% multinodular goiter convert in to malignancy.[1]
4. C
Fine-needle-aspiration cytology helpful in differentiating benign thyroid nodules from malignant nodule.[1]
5. A
It is regulated by ant. Pituitary gland which control the T3& T4 level by negative feedback mechanism.[1]

Reference:

1. Anirban Maitra,The Endocrine System,Thyroidgland.Vinay Kumar, Abul K. Abbas, Jon C. Aster. Robbins &Cotran Pathologic Basis of Disease, 8th Edition, 1097-1164; 2010.

FIBROADENOMA: BREAST

Dr. Malti Kumari Maurya, Associate Professor, Department of Pathology

A 25 year old female presented with complaint of left breast lump since one year, which was gradually increasing in size. There was no associated pain, change during menstrual periods, nipple discharge or fever. On physical examination, the mass was located in the upper outer quadrant of the breast. It was 3.7 x 3.5 cm smooth; non-tender and freely mobile. Overlying skin and nipple areola complex were normal. The lump was excised and sent for histopathological examination.

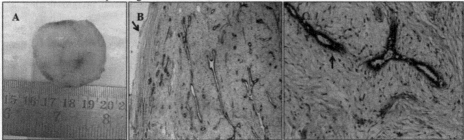

Figure: (A) Cut surface of well encapsulated, homogenous, rubbery white nodular lesion of breast. (B) Biphasic tumor composed of proliferating stroma and epithelial component (arrow: capsule). (C) Myxoid stroma compressing the duct (arrow).

1. What is the most likely clinical diagnosis
   (A) Fibroadenoma
   (B) Fibrocystic changes
   (C) Breast carcinoma
   (D) Fat necrosis
2. Fibroadenomas have all of the following common characteristics except:
   (A) Occur in young women (20-30s)
   (B) Benign biphasic tumor with both epithelial and stromal components
   (C) Very low risk of developing cancer
   (D) Associated with lymph node enlargement
3. Gross appearance of fibroadenoma is characterised by:
   (A) Size varies from1- 5 cm
   (B) Frequently multiple and bilateral
   (C) Rubbery, white well circumscribed mass, often with small slit like spaces
   (D) All of the above
4. Most easy and safe diagnostic technique for fibroadenoma is:
   (A) Fine needle aspiration cytology
   (B) Core biopsy
   (C) Mammography
   (D) Hormone assay
5. The clinical behaviour and outcome of fibroadenoma is not characterised by
   (A) Hormonally responsive, grows during pregnancy and late luteal phase, regresses after menopause

(B) Excellent prognosis after excision

(C) Recurrence is uncommon

(D) High potential for malignancy

6. Fibroadenoma differs from Phyllodes tumor that it has

(A) Typical leaflike architecture

(B) Increase stromal cellularity, over growth and mitotic count

(C) Smooth borders and hypocellularstroma

(B) Increase risk of recurrences

Answers:

1. A

Fibroadenoma is most common benign tumor of female breast, usually presents in young female as a discrete, freely mobile painless nodule.

2. D

Benign breast disease.

3. D

All are the characteristic features of fibroadenoma.

4. A

Fine needle aspiration cytology is safe and coast effective and reliable method.

5. D

Fibroadenoma has very low risk of developing cancer. However the increase risk was associated with cyst larger than 0.3cm, sclerosingadenosis, epithelial calcification, papillary apocrine changes.

6. C

Smooth borders and hypocellularstroma. Phyllodestumor have stromal overgrowth (leaf like pattern) hypercellularstroma and increase mitotic count.

Reference:

1. Kumar V, Abbas AK, Aster JC. Robbins and Cotran Pathologic Basis of Disease.South Asia Edition Vol II. Elsevier, 2014, p. 1068-69.

INFILTRATING DUCTAL CARCINOMA (NOS): BREAST

Dr. Malti Kumari Maurya, AssociateProfessor, Department of Pathology

A 50 year old woman presented with large irregular mass in right breast for last three months. The mass was associated with dirty and bloody discharge from the nipple, off and on. Physical examination revealed a huge mass measuring about 7.0 x 7.0 cm with irregular margins, located in upper and middle compartment.Overlying skin was fixed with retracted nipple. Right axilla had single palpable lymph node of 1.0 cm size. Radical mastectomy was performed.(Fig. A) The cut surface showed an 8.0 x 7.0 cm firm to hard, gray white growth with foci of necrosis, which was irregularly extending into surrounding adipose tissue. Histology showed (fig B) neoplastic epithelial cells having hyperchromatic nuclei with prominent nucleoli and scant amount of cytoplasm. Tumor cells were infiltrating into stroma in the form of tubules, nests and sheets. Lymph node showed infiltration by morphologically similar cells as thegrowth in the breast.

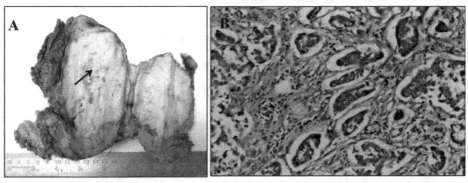

Figure: (A) Cut surface of mastectomy specimen showing large grey white growth with foci of necrosis (arrow). (B) Atypical epithelial cells infiltrating into stroma in form of tubules, nests and sheets.

1. The most likely diagnosis is:
   (A) Lobular carcinoma
   (B) Infiltrating ductal carcinoma
   (C) Papillary carcinoma
   (D) Medullary carcinoma
2. What is the stage of the disease?
   (A) Stage II A
   (B) Stage II B
   (C) Stage III A
   (D) Stage III B
3. Further work-up of this patient should include:
   (A) WBC count
   (B) Bone scan for evidence of metastatic disease
   (C) Lung biopsy
   (D) Study for antibodies to HLA antigens
4. In Bloom Richardson grading system (Nottingham system) the score depends on following criteria *except*:
   (A) Tendency to form tubular structures
   (B) Nuclear size, shape (pleomorphism)
   (C) Comedonecrosis
   (D) Mitotic rate
5. Regardless of histological type, the prognosis of infiltrating ductal carcinoma depends on:
   (A) Tumor size
   (B) <u>Histological grade</u>
   (C) Vascular invasion
   (D) All of the above
6. Each of the following is considered a risk factor in the development of breast carcinoma *except* :
   (A) Early menarche
   (B) Oral contraceptive use
   (C) Nulliparity
   (D) Previous breast cancer
7. Which of the following statements is false regarding treatment of early stage breast cancer?
   (A) Axillary lymph node assessment, Hormone receptors status, and HER-2neu over expression, is important to guide adjuvant therapy.
   (B) Adjuvant hormone therapy in ER/PR positive breast cancer reduces the risk of recurrence.
   (C) Adjuvant chemotherapy benefits both premenopausal and postmenopausal women irrespective of hormone receptors
   (D) Aromatase inhibitors are standard adjuvant hormone therapy in premenopausal women
8. False statement about triple negative (basal like) breast cancers:
   (A) Comprising of about 15% of breast cancers.
   (B) Associated with germline BRCA1 mutations
   (C) Poorly differentiated

(D) Associated with germline BRCA2 mutations

Answers:
1. B
   Infiltrating ductal carcinoma- tubule and sheets of atypical cells
2. C
   Stage III A (T3) tumor>5cm, N1- lymph node positive, M0-no metastasis
3. C
   Bone scan for evidence of metastatic disease –bone metastasis are common.
4. C
   Comedonecrosis.
5. D
   All of the above
6. B
   Oral contraceptive use and breast feeding have protective effect.
7. C
   Adjuvant systemic therapy refers to the administration of hormone therapy, chemotherapy and trastuzumab (a humanized monoclonal antibody directed against HER2) after definitive local therapy for breast cancer. ER and PR negative breast cancers do not respond to hormone therapy. Therefore, adjuvant hormone therapy is not indicated in ER/PR negative breast cancer. In premenopausal women with operable ER/PR positive tumours, tamoxifen reduces the risk of recurrence and breast cancer mortality. In postmenopausal women, third-generation aromatase inhibitors are superior to 5 years of adjuvant tamoxifen therapy. Adjuvant chemotherapy benefits both premenopausal and postmenopausal women irrespective of hormone receptors status,
8. D
   Associated with germline BRCA2 mutations

References:
1. Kumar V, Abbas AK, Aster JC. Robbins and Cotran Pathologic Basis of Disease.South Asia Edition Vol II. Elsevier, 2014, p. 1051-68.
2. Sinn, HP; Kreipe, H (May 2013). "A Brief Overview of the WHO Classification of Breast Tumors, 4th Edition, Focusing on Issues and Updates from the 3rd Edition.".Breast care (Basel, Switzerland)8 (2): 149–154 Rosai, J. (2004).
3. Rosai and Ackerman's Surgical Pathology (9th ed.).
4. Tavassoli, F.A., Devilee, P., ed. (2003). World Health Organization Classification of Tumours: Pathology & Genetics: Tumours of the breast and female genital organs. Lyon: IARC Press

RETINOBLASTOMA: EYE
Dr Malti Kumari Maurya, AssociateProfessor, Department of Pathology

A three year old boy presented to the eye clinic with history of diminished vision in right eye since three months. On clinical examination child had leukocoria. Fundus examination revealed an endophytic nodular creamy white growth with increased vascularisation. There was no family history of blindness or eye tumor. Enucleation was done. Histopathology showed small round cells arranged in clusters, rosettes and pseudorosettes with foci of necrosis and calcification.

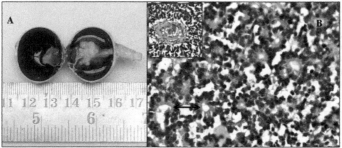

Figure: (A) Cut surface of eye ball with endophytic creamy white growth and attached stump of optic nerve at posterior pole. (B) Small round cell tumour, composed of Flexner-Wintersteiner rosettes (double headed arrow) formed by small round cells surrounding an empty lumen; and Pseudorosette (inset).

1. What is your most likely diagnosis?
   (A) Neuroblastoma
   (B) Coat's disease
   (C) Retinoblastoma
   (D) Meduloblastoma
2. All are true regarding retinoblastoma except:
   (A) Typically affect young children less than 4 years
   (B) 94% of cases are sporadic tumor
   (C) Patients with sporadic retinoblastoma do not pass their genes to their offspring
   (D) 4% cases are bilateral associated with germ line mutation
3. Trilateral retinoblastoma is:
   (A) Germ line disease with bilateral retinoblastoma
   (B) Increase risk of secondary tumor in brain like pinealoblastoma
   (C) Poor prognosis
   (D) All of the above
4. Which is incorrect about retinoblastoma:
   (A) Tumor arises from primitive retinal epithelium,and composed of small blue cells
   (B) Calcification often present, can be detected on ultrasound scan of orbit
   (C) Flexner-Wintersteiner rosettes and fleurettes reflecting photoreceptor differentiation
   (D) Flexner-Wintersteiner rosettes are pseudorosette
5. Which one of the following statements is false regarding treatment and prognosis retinoblastoma :
   (A) 5 year survival in 90% if unilateral, slightly less if bilateral
   (B) Poor prognostic factors are invasion of optic nerve, invasion of uveal tract or sclera, seeding of vitreous, involvement of anterior segment
   (C) Tumor differentiation has good prognostic value
   (D) Reese Ellsworth classification is useful in predicting visual prognosis following radiotherapy

Answers:

1. C
   Retinoblastoma
2. B
   94% of cases are sporadic tumor. 60% sporadic, 40% familial (autosomal dominant). Develops in 80-90% of those with mutant alleles in retinoblastoma (Rb) gene at 13q14.Patients with hereditary retinoblastoma have a germline mutation in one allele; develop tumors after somatic mutation in second allele ("second hit"); in sporadic cases, both alleles have somatic mutations
3. D
   All of the above.Some patients with bilateral tumors also have similar tumor of pineal gland, termed "trilateral" retinoblastoma, associated with poor prognosis
4. D
   Flexner-Wintersteiner rosettes are pseudorosettes. Flexner-Wintersteiner rosettes are true rosette (cells line up around empty lumen delineated by a distinct eosinophilic circle composed of terminal bars analogous to outer limiting membrane of normal retina) Homer-Wright rosettes (nuclei are displaced away from lumen), fluerettes (tumor cells arranged side by side which show differentiation towards photoreceptor.
5. C
   Tumor differentiation have good prognostic value.
   Poor prognostic factors: invasion of optic nerve (report as prelaminar or retrolaminar involvement, with or without resection line involvement), invasion of uveal tract or sclera, seeding of vitreous, involvement of anterior segment; extensive ocular tissue and tumor necrosis is associated with other factors. Tumor differentiation does not appear to have prognostic value.

References:

1. Kumar V, Abbas AK, Aster JC. Robbins and Cotran Pathologic Basis of Disease.South Asia Edition Vol II. Elsevier, 2014, p. 1339.
2. Abramson DH, Schefler AC. Update on retinoblastoma. Retina.2004 Dec; 24:828-48.
3. Lin P, O'Brien JM. Frontiers in the Management of Retinoblastoma. Am J Ophthalmol 2009; 148: 142-8.
4. Shields JA, Shields CL. Ocular tumors. A text and atlas. Philadelphia, PA: Saunders; 1992. p.311-12.

ORAL SQUAMOUS CELL CARCINOMA
Dr Mala Sagar, Associate Professor, Department of Pathology

A 40 years old male presented with complaints of left upper cervical lymphadenopathy, weakness, weight loss & anorexia for 2-3 months. Lymph node was solitary, about 2×3 cm in size, firm to hard, fixed and non-tender. On examination oral hygiene of the patient was poor and an ulcer was noticed in the left bucccal mucosa. Biopsy from buccal mucosa and fine needle aspiration from lymph node was advised. Their findings are shown below:

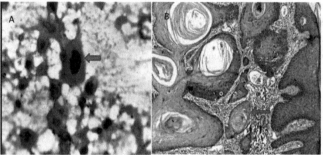

Fig. A. characteristic pleomorphic cells with abundant dense orangeophilic cytoplasm and irregular enlarge nucleus*(arrow)*. Fig. B, malignant squamous cells and keratin pearls*(arrow)*.

1. What is the most likely diagnosis:
   (A) Squamous cell carcinoma
   (B) Basal cell carcinoma
   (C) Melanoma
   (D) Transitional cell carcinoma
2. The most characteristic histological feature of squamous cell carcinoma is:
   (A) Keratin pearl
   (B) Peripheral palisading of cells
   (C) Presence of osteoid
   (D) Herring bone pattern
3. The clinical condition having maximum malignant potential to develop in oral squamous cell carcinoma is:
   (A) Leukoplakia
   (B) Erythroplakia
   (C) Human papilloma virus infection
   (D) Herpes simplex virus infection
4. Virus commonly associated with cutaneous squamous cell carcinoma is:
   (A) HPV TYPE 4
   (B) HPV TYPE 2
   (C) HPV TYPE 36
   (D) HPV TYPE 7

Answers:
1. A
   Figure A, fine needle aspirate of lymph node shows a large keratinized squamous cell with prominent hyperchromatic nucleus. B, section from buccal mucosa shows keratin pearls surrounded by malignant squamous cells, so the most likely diagnosis is squamous cell carcinoma
2. A
   Keratin pearl
3. B
   Leukoplakia and erythroplakia   both are precancerous lesions but erythroplakia   is much less common as well as carry higher risk of malignant transformation .
4. C
   HPV TYPE 1, 2, 4 & 7 are associated with benign squamous papilloma in human beings.

Reference:
1. Kumar et al. Robbins and CotranPATHOLOGIC BASIS OF DISEASE.7/e 2005.324, 778-79,1242.

PAROTID PLEOMORPHIC ADENOMA

Dr Mala Sagar, AssociateProfessor, Department of Pathology

A 30 years old female presenting with history of painless, slowly increasing right parotid swelling. It was about 2×1 cm in size firm and non-tender. There was no history of fever, sore throat, trauma, anorexia and weight loss. Patient sent to pathology lab for fine needle aspiration and later on excisional biopsy was done. The findings were as shown below:

Fig. A. Myoepitelialcells(thick arrow) in the fibrillarychondromyxoid background (thin arrow). Fig. B, Photomicrograph of pleomorphic adenoma showing ducts(thick arrow),myoepithelial cells in the chondroid background (thin arrow).

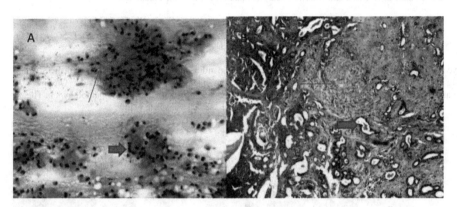

1. What is the most likely diagnosis:
   (A) Basal cell adenoma
   (B) Pleomorphic adenoma
   (C) Squamous cell carcinoma
   (D) Basal cell carcinoma
2. What are the characteristic features of pleomorphic adenoma :
   (A) Ductal cells,myoepithelial cells and chondroid matrix
   (B) Squamouscells,myoepithelial cells and chondroid matrix
   (C) Squamous cells and chondroid matrix
   (D) Ductalcells, myoepithelial cells and osteoid matrix
3. Pleomorphic adenoma is a benign tumor which can:
   (A) Recur and rarely metastasize,
   (B) Never recur and metastasize,
   (C) Recur but never metastasize,
   (D) Usually metastasize
4. PA usually recur after simple enucleation because of:
   (A) Rich blood supply
   (B) Presence of inconcipicuous nodules in the surrounding of main mass
   (C) Because of faulty surgical technique
   (D) chondroid matrix present in the tumor.

Answers:

1. B

   Figure A, fine needle aspirate of parotid swelling showing ductal cells with bland nucleus in the thick chondroidbackground.B,section from biopsy specimen showing ductal and myoepithelial cells disposed in duct formations, tubules and sheets in the background of chondroid matrix. The most likely diagnosis is pleomorphic adenoma.

2. A

   Ductal cells,myoepithelial cells and chondroid matrix are typical findings in pleomorphic adenoma[1].

3. A

    Recurrence rate of pleomorphic adenoma is low about 4% after adequate parotidectomy. Usually benign tumors do not metastasize but under rare circumstances PA can metastasize into lymph nodes, lungs and bones[2].

4. B

    Standard treatment of PA is superficial parotidectomy with preservation of facial nerve. Usually minute protrusions in the surrounding of main mass of pleomorphic adenoma are present, if simple enucleation is done these small masses may left behind and cause tumor recurrence[2].

References:

1. Kumar etal. Robbins and CotranPathologic Basis Of Disease.7/e,2005.791-92.
2. Rosai J et al. Rosai and Akerman'ssurgical pathology, 9/e (vol.1)2004.881.

MUCOEPIDERMOID CARCINOMA

Dr Mala Sagar, AssociateProfessor, Department of Pathology

A 45 years old female presented with complaints of large submandibular swelling on left side and difficulty in opening of mouth for one year. The swelling was about 4×3 cm in size firm, fixed and non-tender. On fine needle aspiration,mucoid fluid was aspirated. Excisional biopsy was done and sent to histopathology lab. The findings of FNA of swelling and histomorphology of biopsy tissue were as given below:

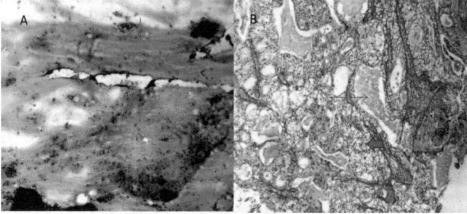

Fig. A: Smears from aspirated fluid showedmucoidbackground *(thin arrow)*, inflammatorycells, macrophages and dense dark cluster at the upper right side probably of intermediate epithelial cells. Fig. B, micrograph showing pale acellularmucoidmaterial (thin arrow), mucus and intermediate cells having clear cytoplasm (thick arrow) and sheets of dark squamous cells on the right side.

1. What is the most likely diagnosis?
    (A) Basal cell adenoma
    (B) Pleomorphic adenoma
    (C) Squamous cell carcinoma
    (D) Mucoepidermoid carcinoma
2 . What are the characteristic features of mucoepidermoidcarcinoma?
    (A) Mucus secreting cells, intermediate cell and squamous cells.
    (B) Squamouscells,myoepithelial cells and chondroid matrix
    (C) Squamouscells,ductal cells and chondroid matrix
    (D) Spindle cells, multinucleated giant cells and osteoid matrix
3. Most common malignant tumor of salivary gland in childhood is:
    (A) Pleomorphic adenoma
    (B) Mucoepidermoid carcinoma
    (C) Adenoid cystic carcinoma
    (D) Warthintumor
4. Themost common gland affected by Mucoepidermoid Carcinoma:
    (A) Lacrimal gland
    (B) Submandibular gland

(C) Sublingual gland
(D) Parotid gland

Answers:

1. D

   Figure A, fine needle aspiration of submandibular swelling shows clusters of clear and intermediate cells in the mucinous background. B, section shows clear cells, intermediate cells and sheets of squamous cells along with pools of mucin (arrow).So most likely diagnosis is mucoepidermoid carcinoma (MEC).

2. A

   The characteristic features of mucoepidermoid carcinoma are mucus secreting cells, intermediate cell and squamous cells[1-2].

3. B

   MEC is most common primary malignancy of salivary gland and it is also the most common malignant tumor of salivary gland in children[2].

4. D

   MEC occurs most commonly (60%-70%) in parotid glands[1-2].

References:

1. Kumar etal.Robbins and CotranPathologic Basis Of DIsease.7/E,2005.793.
2. Juan Rosai et al. Rosai and Akerman'ssurgical pathology, 9/e (vol.1)2004.890-91.

ADENOCARCINOMA GALL BLADDER WITH CHOLELITHIASIS AND XANTHROGRANULOMA

Dr. Preeti Agarwal, Assistant Professor, Department of Pathology

A 45year old lady resident of Lucknow, presented with complaints of off and on pain in left hypochondrium with nausea after heavy meals for six months. On general examination palpebral pallor and bulbar icterus was noted, abdominal examination was unremarkable. Total Serum Bilirubin was 3.2 mg/dl and direct: 2.8mg/dl, SGPT was 34 IU/L; Alkaline phosphatase was 465 mg/dl. Abdominal Sonography revealed enlarged thickened gall bladder with multiple tiny stones. Resected specimen was received as an irregular enlarged gall bladder measuring 13cms in length, mucosa was atrophic and wall thickness was 0.6-0.9cms with intramural yellowish areas. Multiple small greenish-black stones were found in the lumen. H& E stained sections from different areas show a rounded pigmented intramuscular structure with cholesterol clefts (Figure 1). Section form other areas showed intramuscular invasive irregular acini lined by atypical cells (Figure 2) along with intramuscular collection of foamy histiocytes and lymphocytes (Figure 3)
The Histopathological picture shows:

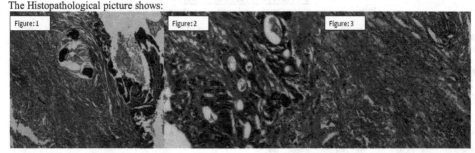

1. What is the most likely clinical diagnosis?
   (A) Acute viral Hepatitis
   (B) Acute Cholecystitis with cholelithiasis
   (C) Chronic cholecystitis with cholelithiasis
   (D) Carcinoma gall bladder
2. What is the most likely morphological diagnosis?
   (A) Acute viral Hepatitis
   (B) Acute Cholecystitis with cholelithiasis
   (C) Chronic cholecystitis with cholelithiasis
   (D) Carcinoma gall bladder

3. Identify the type of stone shows in Figure 1?
   (A) Pigmented
   (B) Cholesterol
   (C) Mixed
   (D) Oxalate
4. Name the premalignant condition associated in the present case?
   (A) Xanthogranuloma
   (B) Gall stones
   (C) Antral metaplasia
   (D) Intestinal metaplasia
5. Which is the most common type of carcinoma seen in gall bladder?
   (A) Adenocarcinoma
   (B) Mucinous carcinoma
   (C) Squamous cell carcinoma
   (D) Adenosquamouscarcinoma

Answers:

1. B
   Direct hyperbilirubinemia with increased ALP and normal SGOT and SGPT are consistent with Obstructive jaundice. Enlarged gall bladder and stones points out towards the probable cause
2. D
   In figure 2 invasive glands are seen and as written in explanation they are lined by atypical cells and are infiltrative
3. C
   Stones are formed by cholesterol clefts along with bile pigment= Mixed stone
4. A
   Sheets of foam cells are seen in figure 3. Though Intestinal metaplasia, gall stones and xanthogranuloma all of them are associated with carcinoma gall bladder; but xanthogranuloma has maximum incidence of carcinoma gall bladder as compared to these options
5. A
   Adenocarcinoma is the most common carcinoma seen in gall bladder followed by mucinous carcinoma. Squamous cells carcinoma and adenosquamous carcinoma may be seen but are rare.

Reference:

1. Thiese ND. Liver and Gall BLadder. In: Kumar V,AbbasAK and AsterJC editors. Robbins and Cotran Pathologic Basis of Disease 9th ed. Canada: Elsevier; 2015.

CHORIOCARCINOMA

Dr. Riddhi Jaiswal, Associate Professor, Department of Pathology

A 25-year-old female presenting with recurrent abortions and off and on vaginal bleeding over the last three years. The previous endometrial biopsies were either inconclusive or showed Arias-Stella reaction. The recent biopsy shows the following histopathological features.

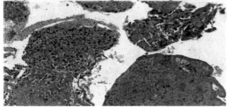

1. What is the diagnosis?
   (A) Choriocarcinoma
   (B) Placental Site trophoblastic tumor
   (C) Complete mole
   (D) Invasive mole
2. Poor prognostic factors include all except
   (A) High human chorionic gonadotrophin levels
   (B) Metastasis to brain and liver

(C) Large interval to diagnosis

(D) Age less than 39 years

3. True about this entity are all except

(A) 50% arise from normal pregnancies

(B) Persistently raised hcg is an important finding

(C) Chemotherapy is associated with 100% survival if tumour is restricted to uterus

(D) It is the most aggressive form of gestational trophoblastic diseases.

4 . The important microscopic findings include

(A) Two cell population comprise of mononuclear trophoblasts and multinucleated   syncytiotrophoblast

(B) Prominent vascular invasion

(C) Absence of villi

(D) high mitotic activity

(E) All of the above

Answers:

1.   A

Choriocarcinoma[1]

2.   D

Age less than 39 years[2]

3.   A

50% arise from normal pregnancies[2]

4.   E

All of the above[1]

References:

1.   Lewis SH, Perrin EV. Pathology of the placenta. New York, 1999, Churchill Livingstone

2.   SanderCH. The surgical pathologist examines the placenta. PatholAnnu 1985, 20(Pt 2): 235-288

HYDATID CYST

Dr. Riddhi Jaiswal, Associate Professor, Department of Pathology

A 40-year-old male presented with chronic cough and mild grade fever with vague discomfort in the right side of abdomen for the last five months. X-ray chest was unremarkable but CT abdomen showed a 12 cm cystic lesion in the liver.

Histopathology of the excised liver lesion is given below.

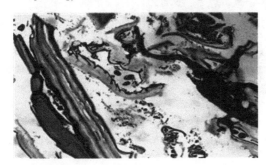

1.   What is the interpretation?

(A) An inflammatory condition

(B) A parasitic infestation (Echinococcusgranulosus showing laminated cyst wall and 2 scolices)

(C) A tumor

(D) A malignant lesion

2.   The infecting stage is

(A) Eggs

(B) Larva

(C) Adult male

(D) Adult female worm.

3.   Which of the following is true.

(A) Echinococcus is a trematode

449

(B) The infection may remain silent for a long time

(C) The cyst wall is opaque black in colour

(D) Removal of the cyst alone may cure the patient

Answers:

1. B

   A parasitic infestation (Echinococcusgranulosus showing laminated cyst wall and 2 scolices)[1]

2. B

   Larva[2]

3. B

   The infection may remain silent for a long time[1]

References:

1. Munzer D.New perspectives in the diagnosis of Echinococcus disease. J ClinGastroenterol 1991,13:415-423.

2. Magistrelli P, Sasetti R, Coppola R, Messia A, Nuzzo G, Picciocchi A. Surgical treatment of hydatid disease of the liver. A 20-year experience. Arch Surg 1991,126:518-523.

RHINOSPORIDIOSIS

Dr. Riddhi Jaiswal, Associate Professor, Department of Pathology

A 31-year-old male with epistaxis and nasal mass. Contrast-enhanced CT PNS **(A)** Axial and **(B)** Coronal sections show an enhancing soft tissue mass lesion in the right inferior nasal cavity (thin black arrow) extending anteriorly into the vestibule and posteriorly into the nasopharynx. Another similar mass lesion is seen arising from the posterior aspect of the left inferior turbinate (thick black arrow).

(C) Axial CT PNS image shows associated rarefaction of the right inferior turbinate (white arrow)

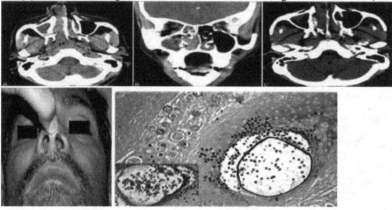

1 What is the diagnosis?

   (A) Rhinosporidiosis

   (B) Mycetoma

   (C) Allergic fungal rhino-sinusitis

   (D) Rhinoscleroma

2. Infecting unit is a

   (A) Spore

   (B) Intermediate sporangium

   (C) Hyphae

   (D) Yeast

3. Malignant rhinosporidiosis is

   (A) Nasal

   (B). Ocular

   (C) Cutaneous

   (D) Genital

4. The drug of choice is
   (A) Fluconazole
   (B) Dapsone
   (C) Penicillin
   (D) Metronidazole

Answers:
   1. A
      Rhinosporidiosis[1]
   2. A
      Spore[2]
   3. C
      Cutaneous[1]
   4. B
      Dapsone[2]

References:
   1. Ahluwalia KB. New interpretations in rhinosporidiosis, enigmatic disease disease of the last nine decades. L Submicroscopic CytolPathol 1992, 24:109-114
   2. Van der Coer JM, Marres HA, Wielinga EW, Wong-Alcala LS. Rhinosporidiosis in Europe. J LaryngolOtol 1992, 106: 440-443

STOMACH ADENOCARCINOMA
Dr. Riddhi Jaiswal, Associate Professor, Department of Pathology

A 45-year-old male smoker presented with abdominal discomfort, nausea and loss of appetite for the last three months. He had two episodes of hematemesis.

He was subjected to endoscopy which showed irregular antral wall mucosa with an old haemorrhagic area. (Fig 1) and microscopy showed 'signet ring cells' infiltrating the muscle layer of the stomach wall. (Fig 2)

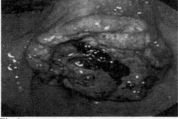

Fig 1

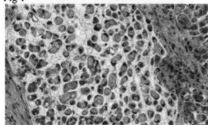

Fig 2.

1. Risk factors for gastric carcinoma include
   (A) Prior partial gastrectomy
   (B) H. pylori infection
   (C) Co-existing pernicious anemia
   (D) All/any of the above
2. Early spread via thoracic duct to the following lymph node is known as the node of Virchow
   (A) Right supra-clavicular lymph node
   (B) Left supra-clavicular lymph node
   (C) Right para-aortic lymph node
   (D) Left sub-mandibular lymph node

3. Which of the following is false about stomach tumors
   (A) Gross appearance varies from superficial, polyloid, fungating, ulcerating to diffuse
   (B) Adenocarcinoma is the most common histological variant
   (C) Majority of priamary lymphomas are MALT lymphomas
   (D) GIST arises from mucosal glands
4. Gross variants of stomach carcinoma may be all escept
   (A) Fungating/exophytic
   (B) Ulcerative
   (C) Linitisplastica
   (D) Nodular

Answers:
1. D
   All/any of the above[1]
2. B
   Left supra-clavicular lymph node[2]
3. D
   GIST arises from mucosal glands[2]
4. D
   Nodular[1]

References:
1. Ming SC. Gastric carcinoma. A pathobiological classification. Cancer 1977,39: 2475-2485
2. World Health Organization. Classification of tumors of the digestive system. Hamilton S, Aaltouen R, (eds). Lyon, IARC Press, 2000, p. 38

WILMS TUMOR

Dr. Suresh Babu, Professor, Department of Pathology

A 9 months old male infant presented with chief complaints of left flank mass with occasional episodes of hematuria as reported by his mother. On CT scan, a heterogeneously enhancing mass with predominantly solid and focal cystic components was present. Subsequently nephrectomy was done. Gross examination showed a grayish brown growth with focal cystic areas, separated from normal renal parenchyma. Histology showed a triphasic pattern comprising of epithelial component in form of abortive tubules, blastemal component as solid sheets of small round cells with scanty cytoplasm, overlapping nuclei with finely dispersed chromatin, and fibroblast like stroma signifying the mesenchymal component. On immunohistochemistry, all the components were diffusely positive for WT1.

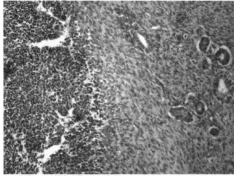

1. What w ll be diagnosis?
   (A) Wilms Tumor
   (B) Neuroblastoma
   (C) MesoblasticNephroma
   (D) RhabdoidTumor
2. What is commonest clinical presentation of Wilms tumor?
   (A) Abdomen mass
   (B) Haemturia
   (C) Abdomen pain

(D) Asymptomatic

3 Above diagnosis associated with which of the following syndrome/s?
   (A) Beckwith Wiedeman syndrome
   (B) WAGR syndrome
   (C) Denys Drash syndrome
   (D) All of the above

4. WT gene is located on which chromosome?
   (A) 11
   (B) X
   (C) Both
   (D) None

5. Which of the following is not a prognostic marker for Wilms Tumor?
   (A) Histology
   (B) Immunohistochemistry expression
   (C) Age at presentation
   (D) Stage of presentation

Answers:

1. A

   A typical triphasic presentation is hallmark of Wilms Tumor.

2. A

   Abdominal mass or lump is the first clinical presentation in most cases.

3. D

   Wilms tumor is known to be associated with all mentioned syndromes.

4. A

   WT gene is located on chromosome 11.

5. B

   Immunohistochemistry is not a prognostic marker for Wilms Tumor.

Reference:

1. Bostwick DG, Cheng L, MacLennan GT. Non Neoplastic Diseases of the Kidney. In: Urologic Surgical Pathology. Mosby Elseiver. Second Edition 2008. . pp 117-21.

IMMEDIATE HAEMOLYTIC TRANSFUSION REACTION

Dr. Mili Jain, Assistant Professorr, Department of Pathology

21 year old male with a road traffic accident was brought to the casuality unit. On examination he was conscious, had multiple fracture in the lower limb and was bleeding profusely. Initial resuscitation was done and 2 units of whole blood were requested. During transfusion the patient developed fever and started complaining of chest discomfort, dyspnoea. On examination he had tachycardia and hypotension.

1 What must be the first step in this situation?
   (A) Stop transfusion immediately
   (B) Start vasopressor drugs
   (C) Start hydration
   (D) Start steroids

2. What is the patient most likely suffering from?
   (A) Immediate haemolytic transfusion reaction (IHTR)
   (B) Transfusion related lung injury (TRALI)
   (C) Anaphylaxis
   (D) Delayed haemolytic transfusion reaction (DHTR)

3. Which investigation is NOT REQUIRED for confirming the diagnosis:
   (A) Direct Coombs Test
   (B) Repeat cross match of patient and donor sample
   (C) Visual inspection of post transfusion sample
   (D) Renal function tests

Answers:

1. A

   Stop transfusionimmediately

Steps of management of suspected haemolytic transfusion reaction include:
Immediate discontinuation of transfusion
Maintain hydration, normal saline infusion to prevent renal failure
Diuretics to maintain urine output
Vasoactive drugs for hypotension

2.   A

Immediate haemolytic transfusion reactions (IHTR)

IHTR occurs soon after incompatible blood transfusion has begun. These are most commonly due to ABO incompatibility.

Fever is the most common manifestation. Other features are anxiety,chest or back pain, flushing, dyspnoea, tachycardia and hypotension. Complications may lead acute renal failure, shock, and intravascular coagulation.

TRALI is acute lung injury within 6 hours of transfusion.

Anaphylactic reaction will be associated with rashes, bronchospasm, angioedema.

DHTR is seen 2-10 days after transfusion.

3.   D

Renal function test is not required for diagnosis of IHTR but for monitoring renal status.

For investigating IHTR:

1.   Check patient identity and donor blood label for clerical errors
2.   A new post transfusion sample and blood bag is returned to the blood bank for blood grouping and cross match
3.   Post transfusion sample must be visually checked for hemolysis (pink plasma after centrifugation)
4.   Direct antiglobulin test (DAT) in the sample submitted at the time of reaction
5.   Also check pre-transfusion sample for blood grouping and cross matching
6.   Antibody identification if DAT is positive

Reference:

1.   Greer JP, Foerster J, Rodgers GM,Paraskevas F, GladerB,Arber DA, *etal.*Wintrobe's clinical hematology. 12thed.Philadelphia: Wolters Kluwer Health; p.697-700.

PAROXYSMAL NOCTURNAL HEMOGLOBINURIA
Dr. Mili Jain, Assistant Professor, Department of Pathology

A 40 year male presented to the medicine outdoor with complaints of weakness, progressively increasing pallor for 3 months. The patient also complained of off and on reddish discoloration of first voided urine which was painless. He had also developed the complaint of abdominal pain for last 1 week. On examination he had pallor++ and icterus +. His systemic examination did not reveal any organomegaly. His hemogram showed an haemoglobin of 7.1gm/dl MCV 108fl,MCH 29.9pg,MCHC 34.4g/dl, TLC 5.9X10^9/L, Platelet count 196x10^9/L, Lymph% 27.7,Gran% 67.6,Mid% 4.7. His total bilirubin was 3.5 mg/dl with conjugated bilirubin accounting for 0.8mg/dl. SGPT was 50IU/L, SGOT was 42IU/L, and SALP was 60 IU/L. His serum creatinine was 1.2 mg/dl. The reticulocyte count was 15%.

1.   What is the most probable diagnosis?
(A) Chronic renal failure
(B) Hemolytic uremic syndrome
(C) Intravascular hemolysis
(D) Extravascular hemolysis
2.   What is the most probable cause of abdominal pain in this patient?
(A) Acute hepatitis
(B) Mesenteric vein thrombosis
(C) Renal stone
(D) Acute appendicitis
3.   The abnormality in PNH cells is seen in:
(A) Red blood cells (RBCs)
(B)   Granulocytes
(C)   RBCs, Platelets
(D)   RBC, Granulocytes, platelets
4.   What is the mechanism of hemolysis in PNH:
(A) Increase sensitivity to complement lysis

(B)   Antibody mediated hemolysis
(C)   Increased activity of Decay accelerating factor(DAF)
(D)   Increased activity of Membrane inhibitor of reactive lysis(MIRL)

Answers:
1.   C
Intravascular hemolysis
Patient is presenting with macrocytic normochromic anemia with reticulocytosis and unconjugated jaundice. Renal function is normal, excluding chronic renal failure and haemolytic uremic syndrome. Also for HUS platelet count is not decreased. As the patient complains of reddish discoloration of urine, it indicates hemoglobinuria and hence intravascular hemolyisis.
2.   B
Mesentric vein thromboses
PNH is associated with striking pre-disposition to vascular thrombosis especially venous thrombosis. Abdominal pain may be a result of mesenteric or portal vein thrombosis, transient intestinal ischemia or infarction, hepatic vein thrombosis (Budd Chiari syndrome).
3.   D
PNH is due to an acquired mutation affecting hemopoietic stem cells (HSC), hence all cell lineages RBC, platelets and granulocytes are abnormal.
4.   A
PIGA gene defect leads to deficiency of GPI-anchored complement regulatory proteins i.e. CD55 (Decay accelerating factor) and CD59 (Membrane inhibitor of reactive lysis). These defects lead to increased susceptibility of PNH cells to complement lysis.No autoantibodies are implicated in hemolysis.

Reference:
1.   Greer JP, Foerster J, Rodgers GM,Paraskevas F, GladerB,Arber DA, *etal.*Wintrobe's clinical hematology. 12thed.Philadelphia: Wolters Kluwer Health; p.998-1101.

ACUTE PROMYELOCYTIC LEUKEMIA (FAB- AML M3)
Dr. Rashmi Kushwaha, Associate Professor, Department of Pathology

A 23 year male presented to hematology clinic with history of on and off fever, progressive pallor, multiple petechial rashes, epistaxis and bleeding PR.
His peripheral smear showed TLC 41500/cu.mm
Differential showed 43% blast cells,
Platelet Count -15000/cu.mm
Bone marrow aspirate – Hypercellular marrow with 90% blasts of large size with kidney shaped nuclei, cytoplasm densely packed with granules.

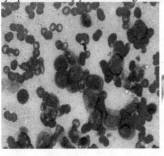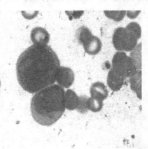

1.   What is probable diagnosis?
(A) Acute PromyelocyticLeukemia
(B)   Immune Thrombocytopenic Purpura
(C)   Acute Lymphoblastic Leukemia
(D)   Metastatic Carcinoma
2.   The genetic abnormality associated with above condition is
(A) RUNX1-RUNX1T1

(B) PML-RARA

(C) CBFβ- MYH11

(D) MLLT3-MLL

3. Patients with which of the following leukemias may go into DIC if given routine chemotherapeutic agents?
   (A) Acute promonocyticleukemia
   (B) Acute promyelocyticleukemia
   (C) Acute lymphoblastic leukemia
   (D) Chronic myeloid leukemia

4. Following is a myeloid marker
   (A) CD 3
   (B) CD 10
   (C) CD 13
   (D) CD 19

5. Myeloid blasts are positive for
   (A) MPO
   (B) Non Specific Esterase
   (C) PAS
   (D) None of the above

Answers:

1. A
   Acute PromyelocyticLeukemia
2. B
   PML-RARA fusion is the associated genetic abnormality
3. B
   This is a medical emergency as the patient can go in to DIC
4. C
   CD13, CD33, CD117 are myeloid markers
5. A
   Myeloid blasts are positive for MPO and SBB

Reference:

1. Swerdlow HS, Campo E, Harris NL, Jaffe ES, Pileri SA, Stein H et al (Eds.). WHO Classification of Tumours of Haematopoetic and Lymphoid Tissues. International agency for research on cancer (IARC), Lyon France. 321-34.

HODGKINS LYMPHOMA

Dr. Rashmi Kushwaha,Associate Professor, Department of Pathology

A22 year old male presented with bilateral cervical lymphadenopathy since one year duration, progressively increasing in size. He also had on and off fever, night sweats and weight loss.
Biopsy from cervical lymphnode was as shown below:

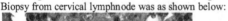

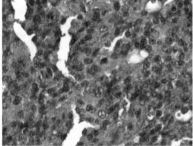

1. What is most the likely diagnosis?
   (A) Tuberculous lymphadenitis
   (B) Hodgkin Lymphoma
   (C) Non Hodgkin Lymphoma
   (D) Metastatic Carcinoma

2. This characteristic cell is known as
   (A) Tuton giant cell
   (B) Reed Sternberg cell
   (C) Langerhans cell
   (D) Langhans giant cell
3. The above mentioned case is (Modified Cotswold Ann Arbour staging)
   (A) Stage I
   (B) Stage II
   (C) Stage III
   (D) Stage IV
4. In classical Hodgkins Lymphoma, RS cells are positive for
   (A) CD15 and CD30
   (B) CD10 and CD15
   (C) ALK and CD30
   (D) CD 45 and CD30
5. HRS cells have origin from
   (A) Dendritic Reticulum cell
   (B) Germinal Center B cell
   (C) Perifolliculr T cell
   (D) Plasma cell

Answers:

1. B
   The figure is showing typical Reed Sternberg cell which is diagnostic of Hodgkins Lymphoma
2. B
   the characteristic cell is known as Reed Sternberg cell/ RS Cell
3. A
4. A
   : RS cells are positive for CD15, CD30 and negative for CD45
5. B
   HRS cells arise from germinal center B cell

Reference:

1. Swerdlow HS, Campo E, Harris NL, Jaffe ES, Pileri SA, Stein H et al (Eds.). WHO Classification of Tumours of Haematopoetic and Lymphoid Tissues. International agency for research on cancer (IARC), Lyon France. 321-34.

GLANZMANNSTHROMBASTHENIA

Dr. Rashmi Kushwaha, AssociateProfessor, Department of Pathology

A 15 year girl presented with history of puberty onset menorrhagia. She also had history of repeated epistaxis since childhood. Her coagulation screening investigations revealed:
BT- 15 min
CR 30% at end of one hour
PT- 12 sec
APTT – 24 sec
Peripheral smear is shown below

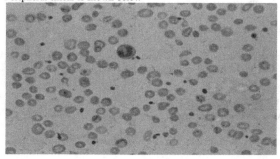

Aggregation studies with 5 µm ADP and 1.25mg/ml Ristocetin shows the following results

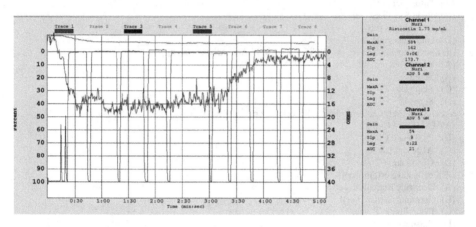

1. What is probable diagnosis?
   (A) Bernard –Soulier disease
   (B) Glanzmann'sThrombasthenia
   (C) HermanskyPudlack syndrome
   (D) Gray platelet syndrome
2. What is the inheritance pattern of above mentioned disorder?
   (A) Autosomal Recessive
   (B) Autosomal Dominant
   (C) X-Linked Recessive
   (D) X- Linked Dominant
3. In above mentioned disorder, Platelets are deficient in
   (A) Glycoprotein Ib/IX
   (B) Glycoprotein IIb/IIIa
   (C) Glycoprotein V
   (D) Dense Granules
4. Inherited platelet defects are
   (A) Bernard –Soulier disease
   (B) Glanzmann'sThrombasthenia
   (C) Gray platelet syndrome
   (D) All of the above

Answers:
1. B
   GlanzmannsThrombasthenia, there are no platelet aggregates seen in peripheral smear
2. A
   GT is autosomal recessive
3. B
   platelets are deficient in Glycoprotein IIb/IIIa
4. D
   All conditions mentioned here are inherited platelet defects.

Reference:
1. Thomas JK, Diane JN. Qualitative disorders of platelet function. In   John PG et al (eds). Wintrobe's Clinical Hematology, 12thedn. Lippincott Williams and Wilkins. 1361.

VON WILLIBRANDS DISEASE
Dr. Rashmi Kushwaha, AssociateProfessor, Department of Pathology

A 16 year female presented with history of unexplained menorrhagia. She also gave history of repeated epistaxis and prolonged wound healing since childhood.
Folllowingwere her lab parameters:

Hemoglobin: 7.5 gm%
BT : 16 minutes
CR: 38% at end of one hour
PT: 12 sec
APTT: 62 sec
Correction studies showed full correction with factor IX deficient plasma
Aggregation studies with 5 μm ADP was normal and absent with 1.25mg/ml Ristocetin.

1. What is probable diagnosis?
    (A) Glanzmann's
    (B) Haemophilia A
    (C) vWD
    (D) Hemophilia B
2. VWF monomer is:
    (A) Factor VIII carrier molecule
    (B) Factor IX carrier molecule
    (C) Factor VII carrier molecule
    (D) Forms fibrin multimeres
3. Most common type of vWD is:
    (A) Type 1
    (B) Type 2A
    (C) Type 2B
    (D) Type 2N
4. Which variant is also called as *Normandy Variant* or *Autosomal Hemophilia?*
    (A) Type 1
    (B) Type 2A
    (C) Type 2B
    (D) Type 2N
5. In what type of vWD is the RIPA test result positive when ristocetinis used at a low concentration of less than 0.5 mg/ml?
    (A) Type 1
    (B) Type 2A
    (C) Type 2B
    (D) Type 2N

Answers:

1. C
    Most likely diagnosis is vWD
2. A
    VWF monomer is a factor VIII carrier molecule
3. A
    Type I is the most common type of vWD
4. D
    Type 2N is also called as Normandy variant or autosomal Hemophilia
5. C
    Type 2B

References:

1. Swerdlow HS, Campo E, Harris NL, Jaffe ES, Pileri SA, Stein H et al (Eds.). WHO Classification of Tumours of Haematopoetic and Lymphoid Tissues. International agency for research on cancer (IARC), Lyon France. 321-34.
2. Thomas JK, Diane JN. Qualitative disorders of platelet function. In John PG et al (eds). Wintrobe's Clinical Hematology, 12thedn. Lippincott Williams and Wilkins. 1361.

Chapter-17

Pediatric Surgery

PSEUDOPANCREATIC CYST

Dr Anand Pandey, Assistant Professor, Dr JD Rawat, Professor, Dr Ashish Wakhlu, Professor, Dr SN Kureel, Professor, Pediatric Surgery

A 6-year-old boy presented with a lump in upper abdomen for duration of 2 months. The lump is painless and is not increasing in size. There is a history of fall from tree about 4 months ago, followed by abdominal pain for 1 week. On examination, the lump is cystic.
1. What is the probable diagnosis?
   (A) Post-traumatic pseudo-pancreatic cyst
   (B) Omental cyst
   (C) Cystic teratoma
   (D) Choledochal cyst
2. How will you confirm your diagnosis?
   (A) CT scan abdomen
   (B) USG abdomen
   (C) Abdominal X-ray
   (D) MRCP
3. What will be the findings on an ultrasonography abdomen?
   (A) Aortic dilatation
   (B) Retroperitoneal hematoma
   (C) Cystic mass in relation to pancreas
   (D) Any of the above
4. The surgical option for treating this entity?
   (A) roux-en-Y choledocho-jejunostomy
   (B) cysto-gastrostomy
   (C) excision
   (D) billroth II operation

Answers:
1.   A
     This history is typical of post-traumatic pseudopancreatic cyst. Trauma is the most common cause of pancreatitis in children.
2.   A
     CT scan abdomen will delineate a cystic structure in relation to the pancreas. Also it can define the relation of the cyst to the surrounding structures.
3.   C
     Cystic mass in relation to pancreas in a patient suspected of having sustained abdominal trauma is highly suggestive of post-traumatic pseudopancreatic cyst.
4.   B
     Cysto-gastrostomy is the most commonly performed operation for this entity.

Reference:
1.   Adzik NS. The Pancreas, In, Coran AG, Krummel TM, Laberge J, Shamberger RC, Caldamone AA (Eds) Pediatric Suregry 7th Ed Elsevier Saunders Philadelphia PA. 2012; 1371-84

NEURAL TUBE DEFECT
Dr Anand Pandey, Assistant Professor, Dr JD Rawat, Professor, Dr Ashish Wakhlu, Professor, Dr SN Kureel, Professor, Pediatric Surgery

A 2-day-old neonate presented with a swelling in his lower back since birth. On examination, the swelling is in lumbosacral region. The size of the swelling is about 5x5 cm. It is cystic in consistency. Translucency test is positive. On Translucency test, there are some black structures are visible inside the swelling. The skin in the central part of the swelling is missing and a parchment like covering is present over it.

1. What is the probable diagnosis?
   (A) Lymphangioma
   (B) Neural tube defect
   (C) Lipoma
   (D) Sacrococcygeal teratoma

2. What additional examinations are **not** needed in this patient?
   - (A) Examination of lower limbs
   - (B) Examination of upper limbs
   - (C) Examination of head
   - (D) All of the above
3. **Single best** test to diagnose it in the antenatal period is-
   - (A) Chorionic villous sampling
   - (B) Maternal MRI
   - (C) Antenatal USG
   - (D) X-ray abdomen
4. On Translucency test, if the black structures are not visible, and the swelling is brilliantly translucent, what would be the probable diagnosis?
   - (A) Meningocele
   - (B) Lipoma of the back
   - (C) Sacrococcygeal teratoma
   - (D) Meningomyelocele
5. What is the investigation of choice to diagnose it?
   - (A) Non contrast CT scan of spine
   - (B) Contrast enhanced CT of spine
   - (C) MRI spine
   - (D) PET scan
6. What is the role of cranial ultrasonography in this patient?
   - (A) Cranial metastasis
   - (B) Hydrocephalus evaluation
   - (C) Cerebral Hemangioma
   - (D) None

Answers:
1. B

   Neural tube defect is the diagnosis associated with this clinical presentation. The central part has missing skin. Sacrococcygeal teratoma has variegated consistency. Lipoma is not transluminant. Lymphagioma does not have any negative shadows.
2. B

   Since NTD may affect nerves distal to the site of involvement, the swelling being lumbo-sacral in this patient, will not affect the upper limbs.
3. C

   Antenatal USG will assess the spine and the defect, if present.
4. A

   The black structures are suggestive of nerve tissue. Absence suggests that the swelling has only CSF, thus making it a meningocele.
5. C

   MRI of the spine is the best modality to delineate the soft tissue structures and tethering of the cord.
6. B

   About 80-90% of patients have coexisting hydrocephalus. This can be evaluated by a cranial USG.

Reference:
1. Smith JL. Management of Neural Tube Defects, Hydrocephalus, Refractory Epilepsy, and Central Nervous System Infections. In, Coran AG, Krummel TM, Laberge J, Shamberger RC, Caldamone AA (Eds) Pediatric Suregry 7th Ed Elsevier Saunders Philadelphia PA. 2012; 1673-97

INTUSSUSCEPTION

Dr Anand Pandey, Assistant Professor, Dr JD Rawat, Professor, Dr Ashish Wakhlu, Professor, Dr SN Kureel, Professor, Pediatric Surgery

A 7-month-old male child presented with vomiting and bleeding per rectum for 1 day. There is presence of severe episodes of pain followed by period of relief. On examination, the right iliac fossa is empty and a mass is present in the epigastric region.

1. What is the likely diagnosis?
   (A) Meckel's diverticulum perforation
   (B) Intussusception
   (C) Hirschsprung disease
   (D) Gastroenteritis
2. What is the name of the stool seen in this condition?
   (A) Black currant jelly stool
   (B) Red currant jelly stool
   (C) Rice water stool
   (D) All of the above
3. What is the sign name when right iliac fossa is empty?
   (A) Sister Mary Joseph nodule
   (B) Cullen sign
   (C) Dance's sign
   (D) Puddle sign
4. What is the shape of the mass present in the epigastric region?
   (A) Globular
   (B) Irregular
   (C) Sausage
   (D) All of the above
5. What is the non-operative management of this condition?
   (A) Pneumatic enema
   (B) Ultrasound guided aspiration
   (C) Oral contrast study
   (D) Abdominal compression
6. What is claw sign in this condition?
   (A) Clumpke's paralysis
   (B) Contrast in large bowel taking shape of claw
   (C) Claw like mass coming out per rectally
   (D) None of the above
7. What is the feature in USG abdomen picture given below called?

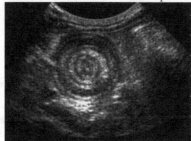

   (A) Pseudo-kidney sign
   (B) Whirlpool sign
   (C) Cork screw sign
   (D) Crescent sign

Answers:
   1. B
      This history is characteristic of intussusception. Hirschsprung disease will present wit constipation since birth. Meckel's perforation presents with pain and persistent distension.
   2. B
      Red currant jelly stool is the characteristic name given to the blood mixed mucoid stool.
   3. C
      It is signe d' dance or dance's sign. Sister Mary Joseph nodule is seen in metastasis at umbilicus. Cullen sign is seen in pancreatitis, and Puddle sign is to test for ascitis.
   4. C
      It is sausage shaped mass.
   5. A

Pneumatic enema or contrast enema under fluoroscopic guidance is the standard treatment for intussusception.

6. B

    Claw sign is seen on contrast enema study.

7. A

    It is a pseudo kidney or target sign. Crescent sign is seen in severe hydronephrosis on IVU. Cork screw is seen in esophageal spasm. Whirlpool sign is seen on USG abdomen in malroation.

Reference:

1. Columbani PL, Scholz S. Intussusceptions. In, Coran AG, Krummel TM, Laberge J, Shamberger RC, aldamone AA (Eds) Pediatric Suregry 7th Ed Elsevier Saunders Philadelphia PA. 2012; 1093-1110.

PURE ESOPHAGEAL ATRESIA

Dr Anand Pandey, Assistant Professor, Dr JD Rawat, Professor, Dr Ashish Wakhlu, Professor, Dr SN Kureel, Professor, Pediatric Surgery

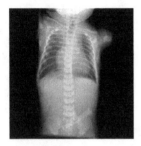

A 2-day-old child presented with drooling of saliva and a gasless abdomen. A red rubber tube could not be passed beyond 8 cm from the oral cavity.

1. What is the likely diagnosis?
    (A) Choanal atresia
    (B) Pharyngeal web
    (C) Esophageal atresia
    (D) Cleft palate
2. What is "R" in VACTERL stand for?
    (A) Radial
    (B) Renal
    (C) Rhomboid
    (D) Rectal
3. Had the child presented with gas in abdomen and drooling of saliva, what would have been the appropriate operation for this condition?
    (A) Thal's operation
    (B) Ligation of fistula with esophageal anastomosis
    (C) Heller's operation
    (D) All of the above
4. In a patient with no native esophagus, all are options for its substitution **except-**
    (A) Stomach
    (B) Jejunum
    (C) Ileum
    (D) Colon
5. What is the **most common** organ for esophageal replacement in such pediatric patients?
    (A) Stomach
    (B) Colon
    (C) Jejunum
    (D) Any of the above
6. What should be the management in this patient?
    (A) Cervical esophagostomy and gastrostomy

(B) Pharyngioplasty
(C) Primary esophageal anastomosis
(D) None
7. Right colon grafts is based on which artery?
    (A) Ileocolic artery
    (B) Right colic artery
    (C) Middle colic artery
    (D) Left colic artery

Answers:

1. A
    It is diagnostic of esophageal atresia. In case of choanal atresia, the tube may not pass through nose but it will pass via mouth.
2. B
    VACTERL is an acronym for **V**ertebral, **A**norectal malformation, **C**ardiac, **T**rachea-**E**sophageal, **R**enal, and **L**imb deformities.
3. B
    It will be a patient of Type C esophageal atresia with trachea-esophageal fistula, for which the standard surgery is ligation of fistula with esophageal anastomosis. Others are operation for gastro-esophageal reflux.
4. C
    Excluding ileum, all others are used for esophageal replacement.
5. B
    It is colon.
6. A
    Since it is type A esophageal atresia, primary anastomosis will not be possible. Cervical esophagostomy with gastrostomy is the appropriate treatment.
7. C
    It is middle colic artery.

Reference:

1. Harmon CM, Coran AG. Congenital anomalies of the esophagus. In, Coran AG, Krummel TM, Laberge J, Shamberger RC, Caldamone AA (Eds) Pediatric Suregry 7th Ed Elsevier Saunders Philadelphia PA. 2012; 893-918

HEMANGIOMA

Dr Anand Pandey, Assistant Professor, Dr JD Rawat, Professor, Dr Ashish Wakhlu, Professor, Dr SN Kureel, Professor, Pediatric Surgery

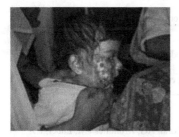

A female infant presented with a reddish swelling over her right cheek. Initially, it appeared as a mosquito bite after about 15 days of birth; however, thereafter the size increased rapidly.

1. What is the likely diagnosis?
    (A) Kaposiform hemangioendothelioma
    (B) Tufted angioma
    (C) Infantile hemangioma
    (D) Port wine stain
2. This condition is common in which sex?
    (A) Male

(B) Female
(C) Both
(D) Intersex
3. All are complication if this lesion becomes very large except-
    (A) Bleeding
    (B) Respiratory distress
    (C) Squint
    (D) Scarring
4. Kasabach-Merritt phenomenon is-
    (A) Thrombocytopenia
    (B) Leucopenia
    (C) Anemia
    (D) Eosinophilia
5. Treatment of this entity includes **all except-**
    (A) Propanolol
    (B) Steroids
    (C) Cyclophosphamide
    (D) Decarbazine
6. As regard to pharmacologic therapy, the **most recent drug** used for its treatment is
    (A) Propanolol
    (B) Steroids
    (C) Cyclophosphamide
    (D) Decarbazine
7. **True about** natural history of this condition is-
    (A) It appears at birth
    (B) It enlarges rapidly during first year of life
    (C) Involution is completed by second year of life.
    (D) All of the above.

Answers:

1. C
   This history and clinical appearance is suggestive of infantile hemangioma.
2. B
   It is common in females in a ratio of 3-5:1.
3. B
   This being a facial lesion may affect patient by all others except respiratory distress. Distress may be present in tracheal or laryngeal hemangioma.
4. A
   It is entrapment thrombocytopenia usually seen in kaposiform hemangioendothelioma.
5. D
   Excluding decarbazine, which is used for malignant melanoma, all others are used for hemangioma treatment.
6. A
   Prapanalol was serendipitously discovered as treatment modality in 2008.
7. B
   Infantile hemangioma appears after about 15 days of birth, enlarges during first year of life. Thereafter involution starts, which is completed by 7-10 years of life, leaving behind scarring in about 50% of patients.

Reference:

1. Kulungowaski AM, Fishman SJ. Vascular anomalies. In, Coran AG, Krummel TM, Laberge J, Shamberger RC, Caldamone AA (Eds) Pediatric Suregry 7th Ed Elsevier Saunders Philadelphia PA. 2012; 1613-45

SACROCOCCYGEAL TERATOMA

Dr Anand Pandey, Assistant Professor, Dr JD Rawat, Professor, Dr Ashish Wakhlu, Professor, Dr SN Kureel, Professor, Pediatric Surgery

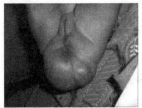

A 1-month-old girl child presents with a swelling in the lower back since birth. The swelling is increasing gradually. On examination, the consistency is variegated. Some areas are cystic and others solid. Cystic areas are translucent. The swelling is painless. Anus is displaced anteriorly. There is no lower limb paresis. X-ray of the swelling shows some areas of radio-opaque shadows.

1. What is the likely diagnosis?
   (A) Sacrococcygeal teratoma
   (B) Meningomyelocele
   (C) Sacral lymphangioma
   (D) lipoma
2. What is the standard classification system of this disease?
   (A) Gross classification
   (B) Altman classification
   (C) Evans classification
   (D) None
3. What is the blood supply of this swelling?
   (A) Inferior vesical artery
   (B) Internal pudendal artery
   (C) Median sacral artery
   (D) Internal iliac artery
4. Which serum marker is especially important to corroborate the diagnosis?
   (A) Alfa feto protein
   (B) Lactate dehydrogenase
   (C) Serum ferritin
   (D) Beta HCG
5. What is the impact of delaying the diagnosis beyond 6 months?
   (A) More fibrosis leading to difficult excision
   (B) More chances of malignancy
   (C) Possibility of mass at other body locations
   (D) No effect
6. During surgery, what special precaution is taken?
   (A) Radical cystectomy is needed.
   (B) Sigmoid colostomy is a must.
   (C) Coccyx needs complete excision
   (D) External iliac vessel needs to be secured.

Answer
   1. A
      None of the abovementioned conditions, excluding Sacrococcygeal teratoma, will displace the anus anteriorly. Also the variegated consistency points towards teratoma. MMC and lymphagioma will have cystic consistency, where as lipoma has soft consistency.
   2. B
      It is the Altman classification. Gross classification is for esophageal atresia and Evan classification is for some malignancy like neuroblastoma.
   3. C
      It is median sacral artery.
   4. A
      AFP is elevated in this condition.
   5. B

Delaying the surgery beyond six months causes increase likelihood of development of malignancy.
6. C

Failure to excise the coccyx carries 37% more chances of recurrence of the mass.

Reference
1. Rescorla FJ. Teratomas and other germ cell tumors. In, Coran AG, Krummel TM, Laberge J, Shamberger RC, Caldamone AA (Eds) Pediatric Suregry 7th Ed Elsevier Saunders Philadelphia PA. 2012; 507-16

EXTRAHEPATIC BILIARY ATRESIA
Dr Sudhir Singh, Assistant Professor, Dr JD Rawat, Professor, Dr Ashish Wakhlu, Professor, Dr SN Kureel, Professor, Paediatric Surgery

A 2 ½ months female child presented with progressive jaundice, acholic stools, darkurine, firm hepatomegaly andspleenomegaly.Blood investigation show direct hyperbilirubinemia> indirect hyperbilirubinemia and raised gammaglutamyltranspeptidase.

1. What is the probable diagnosis?
    (A) Extra hepatic biliary atresia.
    (B) Physiological jaundice
    (C) Choledochal cyst
    (D) Breast milk Jaundice
2. HIDA Scan (24 hours delayed film) of the above patient is below. What is your opinion?

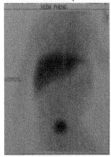

    (A) Hepatocellular function is poor.
    (B) It is non excretory, support the diagnosis of EHBA.
    (C) Shows the radiotracer in gastrointestinal tract.
    (D) Suggest physiological jaundice.
3. An USG finding of above condition support the diagnosis of EHBA?
    (A) Triangular cord sign.
    (B) Gallbladder is normal appearing and distended.
    (C) Bile duct seen clearly.
    (D) Intrahepatic dilated biliary radical may be seen.
4. What is the finding on hepatobiliary scintigraphy that excludes the condition?
    (A) Presence of isotope in the intestine.
    (B) Absence of isotope in intestine after 24 hours.
    (C) Absence of hepatic uptake of isotope.
    (D) Presence of isotope at bladder area.
5. Finding on intraoperative cholangiogram that exclude the diagnosis of Biliary atresia.
    (A) Presence of contrast in gastrointestinal tract.
    (B) Cystic structure seen near porta.
    (C) Normal opacification of branching of intrahepatic biliary redicals.
    (D) Atretic gallbladder.
6. Surgical procedure indicated for above patient?
    (A) Intra operative cholangiogram and Kasai Procedure.
    (B) Hepaticojejunostomy.
    (C) Cystojejunostomy.
    (D) Liver transplantation.

7. Finding of liver biopsy in biliary atresia is?
   (A) Portal tracts inflammation with ductular proliferation.
   (B) Paucity of biliary ductules.
   (C) Bridging necrosis and fibrosis.
   (D) Central necrosis.
8. Which one is NOT a prognostic factor for biliary atresia?
   (A) Age at operation.
   (B) Severity of liver disease.
   (C) Operative technique.
   (D) Operative time.

Answers:
1. A
   Direct hyperbilirubinimea, acholic stool, hepatospleenomegaly and raised gamma GT suggest diagnosis of EHBA.
2. B
   On HIDA scan if radiotracer seen in gastrointestinal tract suggest patency of biliary tree and rule out biliary atresia.
3. A
   USG finding in biliary atresia are gallbladder is either shrunken or normal appearing and the bile ducts are not easily delineated. An abnormal "cord" can be appreciated in the area of the portal plate.
4. A
   Presence of radioisotope in gastrointestinal tract suggest patency of biliary system and exclude biliary atresia.
5. C
   Normal anatomy of intrahepatic and extrahepatic biliary system exclude biliary atresia.
6. A
   The Roux-en-Y hepatic portoenterostomy procedure (Kasai Procedure) is the standard initial operation for treatment of infants with biliary atresia.
7. A
   On histopathological examination of liver in biliary atresia findings are varying degrees of inflammation with ductular proliferation at portal tracts.
8. D
   Prognostic factors are -Age at operation, operative technique, severity of liver disease, gross and microscopic aspects of the biliary tree and portal plate, and the presence of co morbid conditions.

Reference:
1. Cowles R A.The Jaundiced Infant: Biliary Atresia. In: Arnold G. Coran, Pediatric surgery seventh edition, Elsevier Saunders; 2012. P. 1321-30.

CHOLEDOCHAL CYST

Dr Sudhir Singh, Assistant Professor, Dr JD Rawat, Professor, Dr Ashish Wakhlu, Professor, Dr SN Kureel, Professor, Paediatric Surgery

A 4 years male presented with abdominal pain,Jaundice, and a palpable right upper quadrant abdominalmass since 2 months. On blood investigation conjugated hyperbilirubinemia and increased serum alkaline phosphatise was found.

1. What is the probable diagnosis?
   (A) Biliary Atresia.
   (B) Choledochal cyst.
   (C) Right hydro nephrosis
   (D) Pseudo pancreatic cyst.

2. What is your diagnosis on the basis of MRCP shown below?

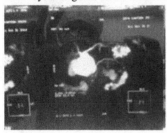

   (A) Choledochal cyst type IV.
   (B) Choledochal cyst type I.
   (C) Pseudo pancreatic cyst
   (D) Choledochoceles.
3. The infantile form of Choledochal cyst occurs before 12 months of age, these patients tend to present with all EXCEPT?
   (A) Obstructive jaundice.
   (B) Acholic stools.
   (C) Hepatomegaly.
   (D) Suprapubic mass.
4. What radiological investigation is now considered gold standard for above case?
   (A) Magnetic resonance cholangiopancreatography (MRCP).
   (B) USG abdomen.
   (C) HIDA scan.
   (D) CECT abdomen.
5. What is the surgical procedure of choice for this condition?
   (A) Cystojejunostomy.
   (B) Cyst excision and Roux-en-Y hepaticojejunostomy.
   (C) External drainage of cyst.
   (D) Cystoduodenostomy.
6. Complications of choledochal cyst are all EXCEPT?
   (A) Cholangitis.
   (B) Malignancy.
   (C) Pancreatitis.
   (D) Renal stone.

Answers:

1. B
   Choledochal cyst can present as Cholangitis (recurrent pain abdomen, abdominal mass, obstructive jaundice, fever) pancreatitis.
2. B
   MRCP suggest fusiform Dilatation of CBD and CHD.
3. D
   Suprapubic mass is not a presentation of Choledochal cyst.
4. A
   Magnetic resonance cholangiopancreatography (MRCP) is now considered the gold standard for imaging choledochal cyst.
5. B
   Treatment of choice for Choledochal cyst is cyst excision and Roux-en-Y hepaticojejunostomy.
6. D
   cholangitis, pancreatitis, intrahepatic stone formation, and malignancy are complications of choledochal cyst.
   Renal stone is not a complication of Choledochal cyst.

Reference:

1. Gonzales K D, Lee H. Choledochal Cyst. In: Arnold G. Coran, Pediatric surgery seventh edition, Elsevier Saunders; 2012. p. 1331-39.

PORTAL HYPERTENSION

Dr Sudhir Singh, Assistant Professor, Dr JD Rawat, Professor, Dr Ashish Wakhlu, Professor, Dr SN Kureel, Professor, Paediatric Surgery

A 4 years male presented in emergency with complains of fresh blood vomiting around 3 -4 times, patient had also history of previous episodes of bleeding 2 months back.On examination tachycardia and pallor was present, jaundice was not present. On examination of abdomen liver and spleen was palpable. On haemograme Hb-6.5 gm%, TLC-2400 and Platelets counts -60000/micro lit.

1. The probable diagnosis of above condition is?
   (A) Duodenal ulcer.
   (B) Portal hypertension with hypersplenism.
   (C) Coagulation disorders.
   (D) Meckel's diverticulum.
2. Initial management of the above condition is?
   (A) Urgent surgical management.
   (B) Medical management and stabilisation of patient.
   (C) Emergency endoscopy.
   (D) Embolisation of bleeding vessel.
3. Investigation needed to confirm the diagnosis is?
   (A) Doppler USG of portal venous system and upper GI endoscopy.
   (B) CECT abdomen.
   (C) Complete blood count and electrolyte levels.
   (D) Liver biopsy.
4. Drug used for control of acute bleeding is?
   (A) Insulin.
   (B) Octreotide.
   (C) Propranolol
   (D) Ciprofloxacin.
5. Drug used for prophylaxis for rebleedingis?
   (A) Insulin.
   (B) Octreotide.
   (C) Propranolol.
   (D) Ciprofloxacin.
6. Indications for surgical intervention of above condition are all EXCEPT?
   (A) Failed medical and endoscopy treatment.
   (B) Sever hypersplenism.
   (C) Patient with a severe liver disease.
   (D) Gastric varices.

Answers:
1. B
   The probable diagnosis is portal hypertension with varices bleeding.
2. B
   Patient should be intense resuscitation with blood and crystalloids, replacement of coagulation factor deficiencies with fresh frozen plasma, and control of the bleeding.
3. A
   Investigations needed are complete blood count and electrolyte levels, renal function tests, liver function test, coagulation profile, abdominal USG with Doppler, Computed tomography (CT) and magnetic resonance (MR) angiography, liver biopsy can be done after correction of coagulation profile. Among above Doppler USG of portal venous system, Computed tomography (CT), magnetic resonance (MR) angiography, and upper GI endoscopy is important to access anatomy.
4. B
   Somatostatin analogues such as vapreotide and Octreotide is used as a continuous infusion in emergency bleeding.
5. C
   Propranolol is used for prophylaxis of variceal bleeding
6. C
   In severe liver disease shunt surgery is not indicated.

Reference:
1. Superina R. Portal Hypertension. In: Arnold G. Coran, Pediatric surgery seventh edition, Elsevier Saunders; 2012. p. 1355-70.

CONGENITAL DIAPHRAGMATIC HERNIA

Dr Sudhir Singh, Assistant Professor, Dr JD Rawat, Professor, Dr Ashish Wakhlu, Professor, Dr SN Kureel, Professor, Paediatric Surgery

A 24 hrs neonate presented with complains of respiratory distress since birth. On examination chest was asymmetric distended and abdomen was scaphoid, heart sounds will be heard best over the right chest. There was antenatal history of Polyhydramnios. X ray chest shown below.

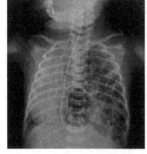

1. Diagnosis of above mentioned condition is?
   (A) Left congenital lobar emphysema.
   (B) Tracheoesophageal fistula.
   (C) Left side congenital diaphragmatic hernia.
   (D) Bronchogenic cyst.
2. Should NOT be done during resuscitation of above baby?
   (A) Nasogastric tube insertion.
   (B) Endotracheal intubation in sever distress.
   (C) Ventilation by mask and Ambu bag.
   (D) Minimal iatrogenic injury.
3. Ventilators strategies used to stabilise the baby is?
   (A) High rates and modest peak airway pressures.
   (B) Low rate and high pressure.
   (C) High rate and high pressure.
   (D) Low rate and low pressure.
4. Surgical intervention should be done?
   (A) Urgently.
   (B) Within 6 hrs of delivery
   (C) After a period of medical stabilization.
   (D) Surgery should not be done.
5. Indication for Extracorporeal membrane oxygenation are all EXCEPT?
   (A) OI (oxygen Index) of 40 or greater.
   (B) Alveolar–arterial oxygen difference AaDO2 of 610 or greater.
   (C) Multiple congenital anomalies.
   (D) Acute severe respiratory or cardiac failure.

Answers:
1. C
   Clinical and radiological finding suggestive of left sided congenital CDH.
2. C
   Ventilation by mask and Ambu bag is contraindicated to avoid distension of the stomach and intestines that may be in the thoracic cavity.
3. A

Most infants can be successfully managed using a combination of high rates (100 breaths per minute) and modest peak airway pressures (18 to 22 cm H2O and no PEEP).
4. C
A period of medical stabilization and delayed surgical repair, in an attempt to improve the overall condition of the infant with CDH, was proposed.
5. C
Multiple congenital anomalies is a contraindication for ECMO.

Reference:

1. Charles J H, Stolar, Dillon P W. Congenital Diaphragmatic Hernia and Eventration. In: Arnold G. Coran, Pediatric surgery seventh edition, Elsevier Saunders; 2012.p. 809-24.

TESTICULAR TUMOR

Dr Sudhir Singh, Assistant Professor, Dr JD Rawat, Professor, Dr Ashish Wakhlu, Professor, Dr SN Kureel, Professor, Paediatric Surgery

A 3 year's male presented with progressive increasing painless scrotal mass since 2 months. On examination, right hard testicular mass was present. No abdominal mass was palpable. AFP (alfa-fetoprotein) is elevated significantly.

1. The probable diagnosis is?
    (A) Testicular torsion
    (B) Congenital hernia
    (C) Benign testicular teratoma.
    (D) Malignant germ cell tumor testis.
2. What is the half-life of alfa-fetoprotein?
    (A) 5 days
    (B) 5 weeks
    (C) 5 months
    (D) 10 months
3. The initial surgical treatment in above condition is?
    (A) Trans-scrotal biopsy
    (B) FNAC
    (C) High inguinal orchidectomy
    (D) Chemotherapy
4. Chemotherapy drug used in above mentioned condition all EXCEPT?
    (A) Cisplatin
    (B) Etoposide
    (C) Bleomycin
    (D) Actinomycine D
5. Follow up of the above mentioned case after completion of treatment should be done with all EXCEPT?
    (A) Clinical examination.
    (B) Alfa fetoprotein.
    (C) USG abdomen.
    (D) Testosterone.

Answers:

1. D
Painless hard scrotal mass with raised alfa protein suggest diagnosis of malignant testicular tumor.
2. A
Half-life of alfa fetoprotein is 5-7 days.
3. C
For malignant testicular mass high inguinal orchidectomy should be done. Scrotal route should not be used.
4. D
BEP-Bleomycin, etoposide, cisplatin used for chemotherapy in testicular germ cell tumor.
5. D
Testosterone not used for follow up.

Reference:

1. Frederick J, Rescorla. Teratomas and Other Germ Cell Tumors. . In: Arnold G. Coran, Pediatric surgery seventh edition, Elsevier Saunders; 2012.p. 507-16.

CYSTIC LUNG LESIONS

Dr Sudhir Singh, Assistant Professor, Dr JD Rawat, Professor, Dr Ashish Wakhlu, Professor, Dr SN Kureel, Professor, Paediatric Surgery

A4 month's child presented with complains of respiratory distress.Patient had history of recurrent respiratory infection since birth.Antenatal USG s/o polyhydromnios. On examination baby has tachycardia,tachypnea, tracheal deviation, mediastinal shift, shifted heart sounds towards left side, and decreased air entry on the right part of chest. Abdominal examination was normal. X Ray chest, and CECT thorax is below.

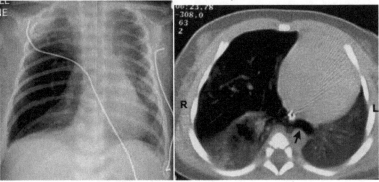

1. What is the probable diagnosis?
   (A) Congenital cystic adenomatoid malformation.
   (B) Congenital lobar emphysema.
   (C) Bronchopulmonary sequestration.
   (D) Cystic Mediastinal Lesions.
2. Most common lobe involved in above condition is?
   (A) Left upper lobe.
   (B) Left lower lobe.
   (C) Right lower lobe.
   (D) Right upper lobe.
3. Air trapping in the emphysematous lobe may be the result of all EXCEPT?
   (A) Dysplastic bronchial cartilages creating a ball-valve effect.
   (B) Endobronchial obstruction from inspissated mucus.
   (C) Extrinsic compression of the bronchi.
   (D) "Adenomatoid" increase of terminal respiratory bronchioles that form cysts of various sizes.
4. What is the treatment option for this child?
   (A) Right lower lobectomy.
   (B) Inter costal tube drainage.
   (C) Medical treatment with antibiotics only
   (D) Right upper lobectomy.
5. Just after birth on chest X ray the affected lobe of the above mentionedconditionis?
   (A) Radio opaque.
   (B) Radiolucence.
   (C) Honey coomb appearance
   (D) Cystic lesion.
6. Finding of a ventilation-perfusion scan in above mentioned patient is?
   (A) Delayed uptake and washout of the radioisotope from the affected lobe.
   (B) Early uptake and washout of the radioisotope from the affected lobe.
   (C) Early uptake and delayed washout of the radioisotope from the affected lobe.
   (D) Delayed uptake and early washout of the radioisotope from the affected lobe.

Answers:

1. B
   Clinical features and Radiology is in favour of CLE.

2. A

The most common site of involvement for CLE is the left upper lobe (40% to 50%), followed by the right middle lobe (30% to 40%), right upper lobe (20%), lower lobes (1%), and multiple sites for the remainder.

3. D

Adenomatoid malformation of terminal bronchioles is a feature of CCAM.

4. A

Symptomatic patient should be treated surgically with resection of involved lobe.

5. A

At the time of birth, the affected lobe may be radiopaque on chest radiography because of delayed clearance of foetal lung fluid.

6. A

Delayed uptake and washout of the radioisotope from the affected lobe.

Reference:

1. Adzick N S, Farmer D L. Cysts of the Lungs and Mediastinum. In: Arnold G. Coran, Pediatric surgery seventh edition, Elsevier Saunders; 2012.p. 825-35.

INFANTILE HYPERTROPHIC PYLORIC SYNDROME

Dr Archika, Assistant Professor, Dr JD Rawat, Professor, Dr Ashish Wakhlu, Professor, Dr SN Kureel, Professor, Pediatric Surgery

A mother comes to Pediatric surgery opd and says that her 2 5-week old boy is vomiting that began 2 days ago and is now occurring after every feeding. The vomiting is nonbilious and projectile. He was a term infant without perinatal problems. He is breast-fed. On examination, baby is dehydrated, visible peristalsis seen in left upper abdomen and on palpation, mobile lump is palpable in epigastrium

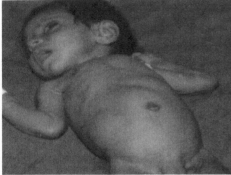 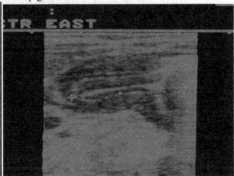

1. What is the most probable clinical diagnosis?
    (A) Infantile Hypertrophic Pyloric Stenosis (IHPS)
    (B) Pylorospasm
    (C) Antral web
    (D) Gastroesophageal reflux
2. All of the following can be clinical manifestation of above condition except
    (A) Presence of bilious vomiting soon after feeding
    (B) visible peristalsis and palpable lump
    (C) Dehydration and electrolyte imbalance
    (D) Hungry child despite vomiting
3. What type of electrolyte abnormality is seen with this condition
    (A) Hypochloremic, hypokalemic metabolic alkalosis and paradoxical aciduria
    (B) Hypochloremic, hyperkalemic metabolic alkalosis and paradoxical aciduria
    (C) Hyperchloremic, hypokalemic metabolic acidosis and aciduria
    (D) Hypochloremic, hypokalemic metabolic alkalosis and alkuluria
4. All of the following can be differential-diagnosis of non-bilious emesis in a neonate except
    (A) Prepyloric diaphragm
    (B) Duplication cysts of antropyloric region

(C) Pyloric atresia

(D) None of the above

5. Which is the gold standard investigation used to confirm your diagnosis?

(A) USG abdomen,

(B) An Upper GI (UGI) contrast study

(C) An Upper GI (UGI) endoscopy

(D) CECT abdomen

6. What is the Procedure of choice to correct the condition?

(A) Fredet-Ramstedt pyloromyotomy

(B) Heineke-Mikulicz Pyloroplasty

(C) Finney Pyloroplasty

(D) Gastroduodenostomy

Answers:

1. A

    Presence of Non-bilious projectile emesis, visible peristalsis and palpable olive are the cardinal features of infantile Hypertrophic Pyloric Stenosis

2. A

    The typical clinical finding IHPS is non bilious projectile vomiting in 3-5 week old fullterm neonate. Infants with IHPS remain hungry after vomiting and is otherwise not illappearing or febrile. A significant delay in diagnosis can lead to severe dehydration. Visible peristaltic waves may be present in the mid to left upper abdomen. The pyloric mass (i.e., "olive") is usually palpable in a relaxed neonate.

3. A

    The hallmark metabolic derangement of hypochloremic, hypokalemic metabolic alkalosis is usually seen in most patients. This was usually associated with paradoxical aciduria.

4. D

    Differential diagnosis of nonbilious emesis emesis in a neonate includes

    A. Medical causes

    Gastroesophageal reflux

    Pylorospasm

    Gastroenteritis

    Increased intracranial pressure

    Metabolic disorders

    B. Surgical causes

    Antral web

    Pyloric atresias

    Duplication cysts of antropyloric region

    Ectopic pancreatic tissue within the pyloric muscle

5. A

    USG abdomen is done to confirm diagnosis of IHPS. It is the gold standard imaging for the diagnosis of IHPS. USG findings of pyloric muscle thickness≥4mm and a pyloric channel length of≥16mm and a pyloric diameter of ≥14mm are considered positive for the diagnosis of IHPS. An Upper GI (UGI) contrast study can also be done, if USG is not available or diagnostic. UGI study shows an elongated pyloric channel and indentation on the antral outline.

6. A

    The operative procedure of choice is the Fredet-Ramstedt pyloromyotomy. It is done both as open procedure and laparoscopic procedure. Myotomy is extended towards antrum while care is taken at duodenal end, few fibres left intact to prevent duodenal perforation.

Reference:

1. Schwartz MZ. Hypertrophic Pyloric Stenosis. In: Coran AG, Adzick NS, Krummel TM, Laberge JM, Shamberger RC, Caldamone AA (eds). Peditric Surgery 7th edn, Elsevier Saunders, Philadelphia p1021-28)

TESTICULAR TORSION

Dr Archika, Assistant Professor, Dr JD Rawat, Professor, Dr Ashish Wakhlu, Professor, Dr SN Kureel, Professor, Pediatric Surgery

A 10 year boy presents in pediatric surgical emergency with sudden onset of pain in right testis, associated with nausea and vomiting and swelling and redness in right scrotum of 12 hour duration. The boy also had previous history of similar type short-lived pains. On examination, right scrotum is swollen, erythematous and tender and pain on palpation of testis, and there is loss of the cremasteric reflex.

1. What is the most probable clinical diagnosis?
   (A) Right Testicular torsion
   (B) Right Testicular appendages torsion
   (C) Right Epididymoorchitis
   (D) Right epididymitis
2. Which of the following clinical feature can be seen with the condition?
   (A) Pain in lower quadrant of abdomen
   (B) Dysuria
   (C) Pyuria
   (D) Fever
3. Blue dot sign is seen with
   (A) Testicular appendages torsion
   (B) Epididymoorchitis
   (C) Fat necrosis of scrotum
   (D) None
4. What will you do to confirm your diagnosis?
   (A) Clinical examination along with Color doppler ultrasound
   (B) Clinical examination alone
   (C) Color doppler ultrasound
   (D) Radionuclide scan
5. What is the treatment of choice?
   (A) Nonoperative
   (B) Immidiate surgical exploration of ipsilateral hemiscrtoum with detorsion of testion and fixation of testis through inguinal incision
   (C) Immidiate surgical exploration of ipsilateral hemiscrtoum hemiscrtoum with detorsion of testion and fixation of testis through scrotal median raphe incision
   (D) Immidiate surgical exploration of ipsilateral hemiscrtoum hemiscrtoum with detorsion of testion and fixation of testis along with contralateral hemiscrotum for fixation of testis through scrotal median raphe incision

Answers:
   1. A
      The presence of acute scrotal pain with swelling and erythema strongly suggest the possibility of Testicular torsion. Strong suspicion should be made in a case of acute scrotum for the possibility of testicular torsion due to risk of permanent ischemic damage to the testis if there is delay in diagnosis
   2. A
      Clinical presentation of testicular torsion is usually heralded by the sudden onset of severe, unilateral pain in the testis, lower thigh, lower abdomen, or groin, associated with nausea and vomiting. A previous history of short-lived, similar pains suggests prior incomplete torsion with spontaneous resolution. Physical examination may reveal the involved testis retracted up toward the inguinal region with a transverse orientation and an anteriorly located epididymis. A horizontal lie of the testis when the boy stands indicates a long mesorchium. The torsed testis is usually enlarged and tender throughout, unless the testis and the epididymis are necrotic. The hemiscrotum rapidly becomes red and edematous, and, if untreated, infarction of the testis may give the hemiscrotum a bluish discoloration. The inflammatory signs usually end abruptly at the edge of the hemiscrotum because this coincides with the limits of the peritoneum, tunica vaginalis. A reactive hydrocele from effusion of edema fluid into the tunica may make the physical signs more difficult to interpret. The cremasteric reflex is often absent with testicular torsion. However, the presence of this reflex does not reliably exclude torsion
   3. A
      Classically called the "blue dot" sign may be seen in Testicular appendages torsion. The inflamed and ischemic appendage may be seen through the skin at the upper pole of the testis as a bluish black spot (blue-dot).

4. A

Often the diagnosis of testicular torsion is clinically apparent, adjunctive high-resolution ultrasonography with color flow Doppler to confirm the presence of testicular blood flow can help in confirmation of diagnosis. If torsion is strongly suspected clinically, further studies will only delay emergent surgical exploration.

5. D

Immidiate surgical exploration of ipsilateral hemiscrtoum hemiscrtoum with detorsion of testion and fixation of testis along with contralateral hemiscrotum for fixation of testis through scrotal median raphe incision is the recoomended treatment for testiculat torsion.

Reference:

1. Hutson JM. Undescended Testes, Torsion, and Varicocele. In: Coran AG, Adzick NS, Krummel TM, Laberge JM, Shamberger RC, Caldamone AA (eds). Peditric Surgery 7th edn, Elsevier Saunders, Philadelphia p1003-19)

CONGENITAL HYDROCELE

Dr Archika, Assistant Professor, Dr JD Rawat, Professor, Dr Ashish Wakhlu, Professor, Dr SN Kureel, Professor, Pediatric Surgery

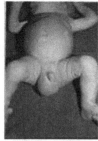

A Mother of 7 month old boy complains that boy is having right sided inguinoscrotal swelling of 1 month duration that increases in size during crying and during the day while the child is upright and decrease in size overnight when the child is supine. On examination, a right sided inguinoscrotal swelling is seen that is cystic, nontender, fluctuant and transilluminant, cry impulse present but it is difficult to reduce the swelling.

1. What is the most probable clinical diagnosis?
    (A) Congenital Hydrocele
    (B) Congenital inguinal hernia
    (C) Epididymoorchitis
    (D) Testicular torsion
2. Which of the following is not part of the differential diagnosis of an inguinal-scrotal swelling in children?
    (A) Varicocele
    (B) Undescended or retracted testis
    (C) Volvulus
    (D) Testicular torsion
3. What is the most appropriate modality of diagnosis?
    (A) Clinical examination
    (B) Inguinoscrotal USG
    (C) Clinical examination + Inguinoscrotal USG
    (D) Color Doppler
4. How will you manage this patient?
    (A) Watchful expectancy with reassurance to parents
    (B) Elective repair
    (C) Emergency repair
    (D) Conservative treatment
5. Which procedure if required is done for the correction of anomaly?
    (A) Herniotomy
    (B) Herniorraphy
    (C) Herniotomy with herniorraphy

(D) Inguinal exploration with detorsion of testis

6. Which of the following statements is false?

(A) A hydrocele can result from incomplete fusion of the processus vaginalis.

(B) A scrotal hydrocele, or simple hydrocele, is a type of non-communicating hydrocele.

(C) Hydroceles are often bilateral and have a higher rate of occurrence on the right side.

(D) None

Answers:

1. A

Clinically, presence of a cystic transilluminant inguinoscrotal swelling in a child with history of reduction in size in morning and increase in size of swelling during the day, points to the diagnosis of congenital hydrocele.

2. C

Possible scrotal masses are:

Hydrocele

Incarcerated hernia

Torsion of the testis

Appendage torsion

Testis tumor

Epididymitis

Epididymal cyst

Epididymal tumor

Paratesticular tumor

Varicocele

Henoch–Schönlein purpura

Idiopathic edema

Cavernous hemangioma

Funiculitis

Lesions that result from a patent process vaginalis.

3. C

Clinically, presence of a cystic transilluminant inguinoscrotal swelling in a child with history of reduction in size in morning and increase in size of swelling during the day, points to the diagnosis of congenital hydrocele. Further confirmation of diagnosis may be done with inguinoscrotal USG that shows patent processus vaginalis and presence of fluid in the sac around testis that is usually used to differentiate congenital hydrocele from reactive hydrocele due to epididymo-orchitis.

4. A

Only wait and watch policy with reassurance to parents is followed and no intervention is required, as the connection with the peritoneal cavity (via the processus vaginalis) may be very small and may have already closed or be in the process of closing. In the majority of children with congenital hydrocele, the processus vaginalis closes behind the hydrocele and the hydrocele typically resolves spontaneously by age 2. If the hydorcoele persists after this observation period, operative repair is indicated and appropriate.

5. A

Herniotomy is the high ligation of the sac or patent processus vaginalis. The distal hydrocele sac is opened and drained. The open sac is left in place and the edges do not require suturing.

6. D

References:

1. Glick PL, Boulanger SC. Inguinal Hernias and Hydroceles. In: Coran AG, Adzick NS, Krummel TM, Laberge JM, Shamberger RC, Caldamone AA (eds). Peditric Surgery 7th edn, Elsevier Saunders, Philadelphia p985-1001)

2. Docimo SG, Canning DA, Khoury AE (eds) The Kelalis–King–Belman Textbook of Clinical Pediatric Urology 5th edn Informa Healthcare, UK p61-102)

GASTROSCHISIS

Dr Archika, Assistant Professor, Dr JD Rawat, Professor, Dr Ashish Wakhlu, Professor, Dr SN Kureel, Professor, Pediatric Surgery

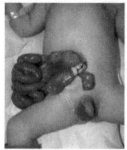

A 1 day-old male baby, born via vaginal delivery at 36 weeks gestation, presented with an abdominal wall defect and prolapsed bowel since birth. On examination, A small defect is seen in abdominal wall with normal appearing umbilical cord attached to left of abdominal wall defect, small bowel is prolapsing through the abdominal wall defect.

1. What is the clinical diagnosis?
   (A) Gastroschisis
   (B) Omphalocele with ruptured sac
   (C) Ruptured Umbilical hernia
   (D) Hernia of umbilical cord
2. In gastroschisis, the abdominal wall defect is
   (A) Right to Umbilical cord
   (B) Left to Umbilical cord
   (C) Above Umbilical cord
   (D) Below Umbilical cord
3. Criteria used to diferentiate Gastroschisis from Omphalocele include all except
   (A) Fascial defect is lateral to umbilicus
   (B) Increased incidence of congenital anomalies
   (C) Urgent surgical intervention required
   (D) All
4. True about Gastroschisis is?
   (A) occurs lateral to the umbilical stump
   (B) can be diagnosed antenatally
   (C) at birth often have edematous matted intestinal loops
   (D) all of the above
5. What are the anomalies associated with gastroschisis?
   (A) prematurity,
   (B) ileal atresia
   (C) undescended testes
   (D) All of the above
6. All are the components of Pentology of Cantrell except?
   (A) thoracoabdominal ectopia cordis.
   (B) Infraumbilical omphalocele,
   (C) cleft sternum, and
   (D) central tendon diaphragmatic and pericardial defects.
7. What are the principles of management of gasroschisis
   (A) protection of the eviscerated bowel and prevention of hypothermia
   (B) provision of appropriate fluid resuscitation
   (C) reduction of bowel into abdominal cavity followed by repair of fascial defect either primarily or with silo
   (D) All of the above
8. All of the following option are used if primary closure of fascial defect is not possible except
   (A) only closure of skin after mobilization of skin flaps,
   (B) creation of a silo by suturing two Dacron reinforced Silastic it all around the medial aspect of the rectus fascia on either side, superiorly, inferiorly and across the top

(C) Use of a prefabricated spring loaded silo that can be placed into the fascial opening,

(D) Painting with escharotics agents

Answers:

1. A

   Gastroschisis is a small congenital abdominal wall defect present almost always to the right of the umbilical cord and has no covering membrane, and usually contains only the midgut with the stomach and possibly a gonad.

   Omphalocele is a congenital midline abdominal wall defect that is covered by a membrane, consisting of amnion externally and peritoneum internally with Wharton's jelly in between two and contains midgut and other abdominal organs including the liver and often the spleen and gonad Umbilical cord is the extension of this covering and present of tip of the defect.

   Hernia of the umbilical cord is a small abdominal wall defect in which there is a defect in the peritoneum, as well as an open fascial defect at the umbilicus. Intestines herniate into the substance of the umbilical cord itself and are covered only by amnion. In fact, hernia of the umbilical cord is a very small omphalocele.

   An umbilical hernia is a full-thickness protrusion of the umbilicus with an associated fascial defect, and may contain peritoneal fluid, pre-peritoneal fat, intestine or omentum. It appears after falling off the umbilical cord.

2. B

   Gastroschisis is a small congenital abdominal wall defect present almost always to the right of the umbilical cord and has no covering membrane, and usually contains only the midgut with the stomach and possibly a gonad.

3. B

   In gastroschisis, defect present almost always to the right of the umbilical cord and has no covering membrane while in omphalocele, defect is in midline and covered with a membrane with umbilical cord attached to tip of the defect. Gastroschisis contains only midgut while omphalocele contains usually midgut and liver. Bowel is usually normal in omphalocele while it is usually thickened, matted, edematous, and covered with fibrinous peel in gastroschisis. There is increased incidence of congenital anomalies in omphalocele as compared to that in gastroschisis. Urgent surgical intervention required in gastroschisis while in omphlaocele there is no such urgency.

4. D

5. D

   In gastroschisis incidence of associated anomalies is low. Associated anomalies include prematurity, ileal atresia (10%) and undescended testes (25%)

6. B

   Pentology of Cantrell is a constellation of anomalies consisting of thoracoabdominal ectopia cordis and other cardiac defects, supraumbilical omphalocele, cleft sternum, and central tendon diaphragmatic and pericardial defects.

7. D

   As neonates with gastroschisis have herniation of bowel that is responsible for increased heat loss and fluid loss, immediate care should be on protecting the eviscerated bowel, preventing hypothermia, and providing appropriate fluid resuscitation. This is done by following measures:

   - Wrapping the eviscerated bowel in warm saline-soaked gauze

   - Position the neonate laterally on the right side with support provided for the prolapsed viscera to prevent kinking of the mesentery and intestine at the fascial level.

   - Placing the neonate in a plastic drawstring bowel bag up to the torso or in clear thermoplastic wrap such as plastic kitchen wrap to further reduce evaporative losses and improve temperature homeostasis.

   -Transport the neonate in heated incubator in a lateral position with bowel contents supported if required.

   -Once in NICU, placing the baby should be under a radiant heater to prevent heat loss.

   -Placing a nasogastric or orogastric tube with continuous drainage for gastric decompression and to prevent undue distention of the stomach and intestine.

   -Intubation should be performed if indicated.

   - Appropriate intravenous access preferably in an upper extremity for substitution of fluid losses and Central venous access (a cuffed Broviac catheter or a peripherally inserted central catheter line) established for providing parenteral nutrition.

   - Appropriate fluid resuscitation is needed to ensure adequate urine output and acid-base balance. An initial normal saline bolus of 20 mL/kg followed by 5% to 10% dextrose one-fourth normal saline at two times the maintenance fluid rate is initiated. In addition, gastric output should be replaced.

- A bladder catheter is placed for monitoring of adequate urine output.

- The neonate is evaluated thoroughly for growth retardation and any other anomalies. In addition, the bowel must be carefully examined assessed for midgut volvulus, segmental bowel ischemia, intestinal atresia, necrosis, or perforation. The degree of serositis and inflammatory peel should be documented. When the inflammatory peel is thick, an atresia may not be seen. No attempt should be made to remove the reactive peel.

- Anal dilatation and rectal irrigation with warm sterile 0.9% NaCl solution in sterile conditions to evacuate meconium resulting in the decrease in size of bowel that may help in reduction of bowel.

- Bacteriological smear from bowel wall is taken and preoperative institution of broad-spectrum antibiotic therapy

- After stabilization and adequate resuscitation, reduction of the bowel loop by loop into the abdominal cavity followed by primary repair of fascial defect without tension in the operation theatre under general anaesthesia and continuous monitoring of intra-abdominal pressure.

8. D

Multiple methods of closure have been described for children in whom primary fascial closure cannot be achieved.

These methods include only closure of skin after mobilization of skin flaps, incorporation of the umbilicus as an allograft, use of prosthetic nonabsorbable mesh or bioprosthetic materials such as dura or porcine small intestinal submucosa, use of amnion-Vicryl net to cover the fascial defect. There occurs formation of massive abdominal wall hernia requiring its repair months to years later after all these procedures.

Another option is to reduce the bowel and place a piece of Silastic sheeting under the abdominal wall to prevent evisceration, removal of Silastic sheet in 4 to 5 days, and closure of the abdominal wall and skin.

One another option is to create a silo by suturing two Dacron reinforced Silastic it all around the medial aspect of the rectus fascia on either side, superiorly, inferiorly and across the top under general anaesthesia followed by bedside gradual reduction of viscera into the peritoneal cavity over the next week.

Use of a prefabricated spring loaded silo that can be placed into the fascial opening, without the need for sutures or general anesthesia, and reduction of the bowel once to twice daily into the abdominal cavity by sequential ligation of the silo is shortened.

Painting with escharotics agents is used in neonates with omphalocele who cannot tolerate operation due to prematurity, pulmonary hypoplasia, congenital heart disease, or other anomalies or with giant omphaloceles

Reference:

1. Klein MD. Congenital Defects of the Abdominal Wall. In: Coran AG, Adzick NS, Krummel TM, Laberge JM, Shamberger RC, Caldamone AA (eds). Peditric Surgery 7th edn, Elsevier Saunders, Philadelphia p973-84)

UMBILICAL HERNIA

Dr Archika, Assistant Professor, Dr JD Rawat, Professor, Dr Ashish Wakhlu, Professor, Dr SN Kureel, Professor, Pediatric Surgery

A Mother of 1month baby comes to OPD and says that her baby has a swelling at umbilicus that increases on crying and reduces when baby is sleeping. On examination, a swelling covered with skin is seen at umbilicus with defect felt at umbilicus. Overlying skin is normal.

1. What is the clinical diagnosis?
   (A) Umbilical hernia.
   (B) Hernia of umbilical cord.
   (C) Small omphalocele.
   (D) Gastroschisis
2. The clinical manifestations of condition include all except
   (A) Asymptomatic
   (B) incarceration of intestine or omentum
   (C) strangulation

(D) None
3. What is the most appropriate treatment in this patient?
    (A) Pressure dressings
    (B) serial follow-up with watchful observation till the age of 2 years
    (C) Surgical repair
    (D) Nothing done
4. With this condition, Surgical treatment is indicated in
    (A) Age <2 years and having incarceration,
    (B) Age <2 years and having strangulation,
    (C) Age < 2 years and size > 4 cm,
    (D) All
5. What are the associated conditions with this condition?
    (A) Down syndrome
    (B) mucopolysaccharidoses
    (C) congenital hypothyroidism
    (D) All of the above.

Answers:

1. A

    Failure of umbilical ring to close at birth results in a fascial defect in linea alba through which a peritoneal sac attached to the overlying skin protrudes resulting in umbilical hernia. Thus, umbilical hernia is a full-thickness protrusion of the umbilicus with an associated fascial defect, and may contain peritoneal fluid, pre-peritoneal fat, intestine or omentum.

    Hernia of the umbilical cord is a defect in the peritoneum, as well as an open fascial defect at the umbilicus. Intestines herniate into the substance of the umbilical cord itself and are covered only by amnion.

2.. D

    Usually umbilical hernias are aymptomatic, however, in rare events it may present with incarceration of intestine or omentum, strangulation, perforation or evisceration.

3. B

    As most of the umbilical hernia are asymptomatic and close spontaneously, these are simply observed until age of first 2 years allowing for spontaneous closure. Parents are convinced that serial follow-up with watchful observation, regarding the occurrence of rare events like incarceration, strangulation, perforation or evisceration, alone will be successful in most cases and an operation is not indicated for their child in first 2 years of life.

    Pressure dressings and other devices to keep the hernia reduced do not speed the resolution and may result in skin irritation and breakdown and are therefore not advisable.

4. D

    Incarceration requiring reduction, strangulation, perforation, and evisceration, though rare presentations of umbilical hernia, are the only absolute indicators for surgical repair. Umbilical hernias that persist at 5 years of age should also be repaired.

5. D

    Increased incidence of Umbilical hernias are seen in infants with prematurity, low birth weight, Down syndrome, trisomy 18, trisomy 13, trisomy 21, mucopolysaccharidoses, congenital hypothyroidism, and the Beckwith-Wiedemann syndrome.

Reference:

1. Cilley RE. Disorders of the Umbilicus. In: Coran AG, Adzick NS, Krummel TM, Laberge JM, Shamberger RC, Caldamone AA (eds). Peditric Surgery 7th edn, Elsevier Saunders, Philadelphia p961-72)

HYPOSPADIAS

Dr Archika, Assistant Professor, Dr JD Rawat, Professor, Dr Ashish Wakhlu, Professor, Dr SN Kureel, Professor, Pediatric Surgery

A 1.5 year old boy presented to pediatric surgery opd with complaints of absence of normal urethral opening at the tip of penis and passing of urine through an abnormal opening on undersurface of penis. On examination, normal meatus is absent, there is ectopic urethral opening on ventral surface of distal penile shaft, and ventral penile curvature.

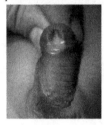

1. What is the clinical diagnosis?
    (A) Distal Penile Hypospadias
    (B) Epispadias
    (C) Congenital Urethral Fistula
    (D) Congenital Hyposplatic Urethra
2. Incidence rate of hypospadias is
    (A) 1 in 250 New borns
    (B) 1 in 500 New borns
    (C) 1 in 150 New borns
    (D) 1 in 50 New borns
3. Chordee occurs due to
    (A) fibrosis or deficiency of skin-dartos complex,
    (B) fibrosis of Bucks fascia,
    (C) fibrosis of urethral plate,
    (D) All of the above
4. Most common site of hypospadias is
    (A) Distal Penile
    (B) Mid Penile
    (C) Scrotal
    (D) Penoscrotal
5. Increased incidence of associated congenital anomalies is seen in
    (A) Distal Penile
    (B) Mid Penile
    (C) Glanular
    (D) Penoscrotal
6. Penis consists of
    (A) Two corpora cavernosa and two corpus spongiosum
    (B) Two corpora cavernosa and one corpus spongiosum
    (C) One corpora cavernosa and two corpus spongiosum
    (D) One corpora cavernosa and one corpus spongiosum
7. Component of hypospadias repair include
    (A) Orthoplasty
    (B) Urethroplasty
    (C) Meatoplasty and glansplasty
    (D) All
8. Optimum age for hypospadias repair is
    (A) 6-18 months
    (B) 12-24 months
    (C) 15-18 months
    (D) 6-12 months
9. What is the most common complications of hypospadias repair is
    (A) Meatal Stenosis
    (B) Urethrocutaneous Fistulas
    (C) Persistent Chordee
    (D) Strictures

Answers:

1. A

    Hypospadias is a developmental anomaly characterized by absence of normal meatus, ectopic urethral meatus opening on ventral surface of penis, anywhere along the shaft of the penis, from the glans to the perineum, chordee, and deficient ventral preputial skin with dorsal preputial hood.

2. A

    Hypospadias is one of the most common congenital anomalies, occurring in approximately 1 in 250 newborns, or roughly 1 in 125 live male births.

3. D

    Chordee occurs due to; (a) fibrosis or deficiency of skin-dartos complex, (b) fibrosis of Bucks fascia, (c) fibrosis of urethral plate, and (d) deficiency of corpora or corporal disproportion on ventral surface of penis

4. A

    Hypospadias is classified on the basis of the location of the urethral meatus into; Anterior hypospadias (65%-70%), Middle hypospadias (10%-15%), and Posterior hypospadias (20%). These types are further subclassified as below;
    Anterior (65%-70% of cases)
    Glanular - meatus on the ventral surface of the glans penis
    Coronal - meatus in the balanopenile furrow
    Distal penile shaft - in the distal third of the penile shaft
    Middle (10%-15% of cases)
    Middle penile shaft - along the middle third of the penile shaft
    Posterior (20% of cases)
    Proximal penile shaft - proximal third of the penile shaft
    Penoscrotal - at the base of the shaft in front of the scrotum
    Scrotal - on the scrotum or between the genital swellings
    Perineal - behind the scrotum or behind the genital swelling

5. D

    Greater incidence of associated anomalies is seen in posterior hypospadias when the meatus is more proximal. Inguinal hernia and undescended testes are the most common anomalies associated with hypospadias, with an incidence of 7%-13%,. An enlarged prostatic utricle also is more common in posterior hypospadias, with an incidence of about 11%.

6. B

    The human penis consists of two corpora cavernosa and one corpus spongiosum encircling the urethra on ventral side, intimately engaged between the two corporal bodies. Corpora cavernosa are covered by a thick, elastic tunica albuginea, with a midline septum. The Buck fascia surrounds the corpora cavernosa and splits to contain the corpus spongiosum in a separate compartment. The Buck fascia also envelops the neurovascular bundle, that, and where the two crural bodies join to form the corporal bodies, the neurovascular bundle completely fans out around the corpora cavernosa, where the two crural bodies join to form the corporal bodies, all the way to the junction of the corpus spongiosum.

7. D

    The components of hypospadias correction include;
    1. Complete straightening of the penis (Orthoplasty)
    2. Locating the meatus at the tip of the glans (Meatoplasty)
    3. Forming a symmetric, conically shaped glans (Glansplasty)
    4. Constructing a neourethra uniform in calibre (Urethroplasty)
    5. Completing a satisfactory cosmetic skin coverage

8. A

    The optimum age for the repair of hypospadias is 6-18 months.

9. B

    Postoperative complications of hypospadias repair include Bleeding, Infection, Devitalized Skin Flaps, Strictures, Fistulas, Diverticulum, Retrusive Meatus, Meatal Stenosis, and Persistent Chordee. Urethrocutaneous Fistula is the most common complication occurring to the tune of 20-60%.

Reference:

1. Baskin LS. Hypospadias. In: Coran AG, Adzick NS, Krummel TM, Laberge JM, Shamberger RC, Caldamone AA (eds). Peditric Surgery 7th edn, Elsevier Saunders, Philadelphia p 1531-53

NEUROBLASTOMA.

Dr.Nitin Pant, Assistant Professor, Dr JD Rawat, Professor, Dr Ashish Wakhlu, Professor, Dr SN Kureel, Professor, Pediatric Surgery

A 4-year-old girl is referred from another hospital. She has been 'unwell' for the past 3 weeks. According to the mother the child is irritable and has a decreased oral intake. She complains of pain in her left thigh. On examination the child is sick looking, pale and uncooperative. Her BP is 140/80 mmHg high for her age group. Per abdomen there is a large, hard tender mass with irregular surface occupying nearly whole of the right upper and central abdomen and crossing the midline towards the left. There are no significant clinically palpable lymph nodes.

1. What is the most likely diagnosis?
   (A) Ovarian tumor
   (B) Neuroblastoma
   (C) Ewings Sarcoma
   (D) Lymphoma
2. What might be the most common site of origin for this mass in this child?
   (A) Kidney
   (B) Gall bladder
   (C) Right Adrenal gland
   (D) Liver
3. Embryologically which type of tissues are these tumors derivative of?
   (A) Intestinal
   (B) Renal
   (C) Neural
   (D) Hematogenous
4. A plain X ray abdomenof the child shows scattered opacities in right paravertebral region as shown in the figure. What might these be?

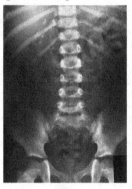

   (A) Renal Calculi
   (B) Gall bladder stones
   (C) Punctate Calcifications in the Adrenal gland
   (D) Extra osseous bone deposition
5. What is the reason of increased BPin this child?
   (A) Brain stem metastases
   (B) Catecholamine metabolites secreted by the tumor
   (C) Bone marrow metastases
   (D) Increased steroid production by tumor
6. What tests should one NOT ORDER to confirm diagnosis and measure the extent of tumor?
   (A) Ultrasonography
   (B) CECT scan abdomen
   (C) Bone marrow biopsy
   (D) MRI spine

1. C
    This is likely to be a child with neuroblastoma.She is a 4 year child presenting with constitutional symptoms of being unwell, decreased oral intake and fever. The child is **sick**looking, pale, **irritable and uncooperative**. She has a **markedly raised BP & Bone pain**. Per abdominally there is a **hard, tender, irregular, mass**which is crossing the midline.
2. C
    Adrenal gland (medulla)
3. C
    The neuroblastoma is derived from primordial neural crest cells of sympathetic origin.
4. C
    Punctate calcifications which are typical of neuroblastoma.
5. B
    Increased level of catecholamine metabolites VMA (vanillylmandelicAcid)/ HVA (homovanillic Acid)/ Metanephrine/ Normetanephrine secreted by the tumor is the cause of increased BP in this child.
6. D
    For Imaging of the primary tumor its origin and loco regional extension one should order USG abdomen, CECT abdomen and chest.
    For confirming the diagnosis a Bilateral posterior iliac crest marrow aspirates and trephine (core) bone marrow biopsies.
    A 24-h urine collection to assess the excretion of catecholamines and their breakdown products vanillylmandelic acid (VMA), homovanillic acid (HVA), dopamine, 3,4-dihydroxyphenylalanine (DOPA), adrenaline and noradrenaline. In the majority of patients these levels are high; metabolites may also serve as markers for follow-up
    MIBG (Metaiodobenzylguanidine) scintigraphy to assess the skeletal and extra-skeletal extent of disease (MIBG is fixed specifically by neuroblasts)

Reference:

1. Rich B.S., La Quagila M.P. Neuroblastoma. In : Coran AG, Adzick NS, Krummel TM, Laberge JM. Pediatric Surgery. 7th Edition. Pheladelphia. 2012.Elsevier Saunders.

TRACHEOESOPHAGEAL FISTULA(TEF)

Dr.Nitin Pant, Assistant Professor, Dr JD Rawat, Professor, Dr Ashish Wakhlu, Professor, Dr SN Kureel, Professor, Pediatric Surgery

A baby boy was born at 38-weeks of gestation, who despite initial suctioning, appears to be salivating excessively. He has mild tachypnoea, but is pink with good cry. Antenatal USG was suggestive of polyhdramnios.

1. What is the most likely diagnosis?
    (A) Choanal Atresia
    (B) Congenital diaphragmatic hernia
    (C) Duodenal atresia
    (D) Esophageal atresia
2. What should be done to confirm the diagnosis?
    (A) Ultrasound thorax
    (B) Ultrasound Abdomen
    (C) CECT Chest
    (D) Gentle passage of a 10 Fr. Red rubber catheter into the oropharynx
3. What should be done to prevent aspiration of saliva in this baby?
    (A) High pressure continuous suction
    (B) High pressure intermittent
    (C) Low pressure continuous suction
    (D) Repeated moping of the oropharynx
4. Which of the following investigations is not necessary in this child?
    (A) Echocardiography
    (B) USG Spine

(C) USG KUB Region

(D) MIBG scan

5. Which is not the appropriate surgical approach in these patients?

    (A) Right Lateral Thoracotomy

    (B) Right posterior lateral Thoracotomy

    (C) Thoracoscopy

    (D) Sternotomy

Answers:

1. D

    Esophageal Atresia

2. D

    One should pass a 10 Fr. red rubber catheter/ tube per orally. If it does not traverse beyond 10 cm. one can suspect an esophageal atresia. Secondly one should get a CXR done with the tube in situ. If CXR shows gas filled bowel loops in the abdomen it indicates accompanying tracheoesophageal fistula. If there is no gas in the abdomen cavity it indicates a pure esophageal atresia.

3. C

    Replogel tube/ small Sump suction tube can be used for low pressure upper pouch suction.

4. D

Associated Anomalies with Esophageal Atresia	Relevant Investigation
Anorectal Anomalies	Clinical Examination/X Ray
Cardiac Anomalies	Echocardiography
Spinal/Skeletal Anomalies	Xray/ USG Spine
Renal Anomalies	USG KUB region
Chromosomal (Trisomy 18, 21)	Clinical examination and if required Chromosomal analysis

5. D

    The condition is managed surgically. The Procedure consists of a Right lateral/ Posterolateral thoracotomy, Ligation and division of the tracheoesophageal fistula with end to end esophageal anastomosis whenever possible. Now days the surgery is also done laparoscopically.

Reference:

1. Harmon CM, Coran AG. Congenital Anomalies of the Esophagus.In : Coran AG, Adzick NS, Krummel TM, Laberge JM. Pediatric Surgery. 7th Edition. Pheladelphia. 2012.Elsevier Saunders.

UNDESCENDED TESTIS (UDT)

Dr.Nitin Pant, Assistant Professor, Dr JD Rawat, Professor, Dr Ashish Wakhlu, Professor, Dr SN Kureel, Professor, Pediatric Surgery

An 11-month-old boy is referred for evaluation of a missing left testicle. According to the parents and the pediatrician, the left testicle has never been in the scrotum since birth. The child has been healthy otherwise.On physical examination, the right testicle is easily found in the scrotal sac and is palpably normal. The left testicle can be palpated using bimanual examination in the inguinal region but cannot be brought down to the scrotum.

1. What is the diagnosis?

    (A) Left Palpable undescended testis

    (B) Absent testis

    (C) Testicular tumor

    (D) Hydrocele

2. How this testis shouldbe managed?

    (A) Watchful waiting till 2 years

    (B) Emergency orchidopexy

    (C) Early elective orchidopexy

    (D) Orchidectomy

A full term male child is born with a single left testicle. Right testis is not palpable. There is no associated hypospadias.

3. Which of the following is true regarding management?

    (A) Orchidopexy in the neonatal period.

(B) Wait for testis to descend till 3 months of age.

(C) Orchidopexy before child goes to school

(D) Orchidopexy once child attains puberty

4. Following statements regarding an undescended testis are trueexcept?

   (A) The degeneration of germ cells starts at 2 years

   (B) The degeneration of germ cells starts at 6 months

   (C) There is impairment of spermatogenesis

   (D) There is an increased chance of torsion

A 1 year old child is brought to the OPD with complaints of an absent Right testis in the scrotum. The opposite testis is normally placed and there is no hypospadias. On examination testis is neither felt in the scrotum nor in the inguinal region.

5. All are the clinical possibilities except?

   (A) The testis is present in the inguinal canal but the examining physician was not able to elicit its presence.

   (B) An intra abdominal testis

   (C) An Absent testis

   (D) It is a case of DSD (Disorder of Sexual Differentiation)

6. In a case of UDT, Orchidopexyis useful in?

   (A) Improving fertility

   (B) Reducing the future tumor potential

   (C) Allow surveillance for the presence of a tumor by physical examination.

   (D) Increasing leydig cell mass

7. Which among the following is not a complication of orchidopexy?

   (A) Seminoma later in life.

   (B) Secondary atrophy of testis due to damage of testicular vessels.

   (C) Injury (occlusion) of vas deferens.

   (D) Hematoma due to poor hemostasis

Answers:

1. A

   Left Palpable Undescended testis

2. C

   In the case of a true palpable undescended testicle, the recommended management is watchful waiting during the first 6 months of life, and surgery (elective orchidopexy) if it persists beyond 6 months of age since degeneration of germ cells starts at 6months.

3. B

   Parents should be told to wait for at least 3 months as in this period the testis might descend spontaneously. They will have to keep child in close follow up. If the testis does not descend within this time then surgery (orchidopexy) should be considered after 6 months.

4. A

   The degeneration of germ cells and somniferous tubules in cases of an Undescended testis starts at 6 months and is nearly complete by 2 years. Also this testis is at an increased risk of impaired spermatogenesis, Torsion and malignant degeneration.

5. D

   One considers DSD (Disorder of Sexual Differentiation) as a possible diagnosis when there is a proximal hypospadias (penoscrotal, scrotal, perineal) associated with an undescended testis and not with a distal hypospadias.

6. C

   The benefits of orchidopexyare.

   It helps in palpation of the testis for any future development of tumor. It gives a sense of psychological well being. Fixation of the testis in the sub dartos pouch prevents torsion.

7. A

   Following are the common complications following orchidopexy. Secondary atrophy of testis due to injury to testicular vessels. Injury/ occlusion of the vas deferens. Hematoma due to poor hemostasis. Wound infection. Malignancy in UDT is due to the malignant transformation of gonocytes in such testis. Malignant potential does not change with orchidopexy.

Reference:

1. Hutson J.M Undescendes Testis, Torsion and Varicocele.In : Coran AG, Adzick NS, Krummel TM, Laberge JM. Pediatric Surgery. 7th Edition. Pheladelphia. 2012.Elsevier Saunders.

HIRSCHSPRUNG'S DISEASE

Dr. Nitin Pant, Assistant Professor, Dr JD Rawat, Professor, Dr Ashish Wakhlu, Professor, Dr SN Kureel, Professor, Pediatric Surgery

A 5 day old, 3 Kg. full term male child is brought in the emergency referred from a private clinic. According to parents he has not passed meconium since birth and has feeding intolerance with occasional bilious emesis. On examination he looks slightly pale but active with a distended, non tender abdomen. The anal opening is normally present. On inserting a no.8 Fr infant feeding tube per rectum a gush of air was passed by the child followed by copious meconium. An infantogram done outside shows multiple dilated bowel loops throughout the abdomen.

1. What is the likely diagnosis?
    (A) Ileal Atresia
    (B) Colonic Atresia
    (C) Anorectal Malformation
    (D) Hirschsprungs disease
2. Which of the following is not true of Hirschsprung`s disease?
    (A) Absence of ganglion cells in the myenteric and submucosal plexuses of the rectum and rectosigmoid.
    (B) Absent peristalsis in the affected bowel.
    (C) Development of a mechanical intestinal obstruction.
    (D) There are no skip lesions.
3. Which is the initial investigation in the diagnostic workup of this case?
    (A) Ultrasonography of abdomen and pelvis
    (B) Water Soluble contrast enema
    (C) Barium enema
    (D) Air contrast enema
4. How will a definitive diagnosis of Hirschsprung's disease be reached in this neonate?
    (A) Contrast enema
    (B) Per operative examination
    (C) Genetic markers
    (D) Histological evaluation

A 1 year old child is brought to the emergency with history of fever, anorexia, severe abdominal distension and passage of foul smelling liquid stools. Parents give a history that child had a recurrent history of abdominal distension and constipation since birth. On examination the child was pale and dehydrated. X ray abdomen showed a massively dilated sigmoid and descending colon containing a large air fluid level.

5. What is the probable diagnosis?
    (A) Sigmoid volvulus
    (B) Intussusception
    (C) Malrotation
    (D) Hirschsprung`s associated enterocolitis
6. The initial management of this child includes by all of the following except?
    (A) Antibiotics
    (B) I/V fluids
    (C) Gentle rectal irrigation
    (D) Colonoscopy

Answers:

1. D
    In a newborn who fails to pass meconium 48 hours after birth one should suspect hirschsprung`s disease. Forceful evacuation of liquid stools along with air following per rectal examination strongly suggests Hirschsprung`s disease.
2. C
    Hirschsprung disease is a developmental disorder of the enteric nervous system that is characterized by the absence of ganglion cells in the myenteric and submucosal plexuses of the distal intestine (most commonly rectum and rectosigmoid). This results in absent peristalsis in the affected bowel and the development of a functional intestinal obstruction. The extent of aganglionosis can vary from an ultra short segment of 1to 2 cm. above the dentate line to that involving the entire colon. There are no intervening segments of normal ganglion innervations (skip lesions).
3. B

One uses a water soluble contrast in neonates since it also acts as a definitive treatment for some of the other conditions in the differential diagnosis, such as meconium ileus and meconium plug syndrome. In older infants a barium enema can be used. The pathognomonic finding of Hirschsprung disease on contrast enema is a transition zone between normal (dilated) and aganglionic (collapsed) bowel, although in 10% cases no transition zone is seen in neonates.

4. D

The definitive diagnosis in Hirschsprung`s disease is made by histological evaluation of rectal biopsy specimen. Depending on the availability & expertise, rectal biopsy can either be a submucosal biopsy using suction gun/ punch biopsy forceps or full thickness open biopsy. The absence of ganglion cells under H&E stain is the hallmark of the disease.

5. D

Many children with hirschsprung`s disease present for the first time during late infancy. There usually is a history of recurrent constipation responding to per rectal suppositories and enemas. Sometimes the presentation is more acute and severe with rapid clinical deterioration and massive abdominal distension. One should always suspect a Hirschsprung`s associated enterocolitis in these cases.

6. D

Such a child should be managed with iv fluids, Broad spectrum antibiotics. He/she should be kept nill per orally. A gentle rectal saline irrigation should be done to decompress the colon. A blood culture should be sent. Once stabilized he should be kept on daily dilatations and or saline enemas till the colon comes to a normal caliber. Following which a contrast enema can be done to confirm the diagnosis. If on the other hand the episode of enterocolitis does not respond to conservative management an emergency decompressing stoma should be performed. Colonoscopy is not recommended and can cause perforation.

Reference:

1. Langer JC. Hirschsprung Disease.In : Coran AG, Adzick NS, Krummel TM, Laberge JM. Pediatric Surgery. 7th Edition. Pheladelphia. 2012.Elsevier Saunders.

NEONATAL BOWEL OBSTRUCTION

Dr. Nitin Pant, Assistant Professor, Dr JD Rawat, Professor, Dr Ashish Wakhlu, Professor, Dr SN Kureel, Professor, Pediatric Surgery

A newborn baby develops abdominal distension with repeated bile-stained vomiting and does not pass meconium.

1. Which of the following is not included in the differential diagnosis in this case?
   (A) Small bowel atresia (ileal)
   (B) Pyloric atresia
   (C) Meconium ileus
   (D) Colonic atresia.
2. Which of the following is not one of the etiological factors responsible for small intestinal atresia?
   (A) Intrauterine intussusceptions
   (B) Maternal use of cocaine
   (C) Intra abdominal hernias
   (D) Intrauterine growth retardation
3. Which is not the findings on a plain X ray in cases of a neonatal small intestinal obstruction?
   (A) Multiple dilated air fluid levels.
   (B) Paucity of gas in pelvis
   (C) Step ladder pattern
   (D) Football sign
4. All of the following are associated problems in neonatal intestinal obstruction except?
   (A) Hyperglycemia
   (B) Fluid loss
   (C) Respiratory distress
   (D) Sepsis

A 1-day-old baby presents with bile-stained vomiting but no abdominal distension.
5. At what level the obstruction is likely?
   (A) Stomach
   (B) Duodenum
   (C) Ileum

(D) Colon

6. X ray of a case of duodenal atresia shows?
    (A) 1 air fluid level
    (B) 2 air fluid levels
    (C) 3 air fluid levels
    (D) Multiple air fluid levels

Answers:

1. B

   The child is a case of distal neonatal intestinal obstruction which is defined by the triad of bile-stained vomiting, abdominal distension and failure to pass meconium. The possible causes could be- Small bowel atresia (ileal), Meconium ileus, Total colonic Hirschsprung disease, colonic atresia. A pyloric atresia will lead to non bilious vomit.

2. D

   The classic etiology considered responsible for intestinal atresiais in utero vascular insufficiency after organogenesis.Possible causes of vascular insult include volvulus, intussusception,embolic or thrombotic events, and incarceration orstrangulation secondary to hernias or abdominal wall defects.Maternal use of cocaine, amphetamines, nicotine, anddecongestants has been implicated in intestinal atresia.

3. D

   Thumb sized Multiple dilated air fluid levels with a step ladder pattern with a paucity of gas in the pelvis indicates a distal bowel obstruction. Foot ball sign is seen in case of neonatal bowel perforation (pneumoperitoneum).

4. A

   Problems associated with neonatal intestinal obstruction are

Problem	Reason
Fluid Loss	Decrease intake Vomiting Sequestration in GUT
Low tissue glucose	Low glucose store in neonates Decrease oral intake Decrease perfusion to tissues
Respiratory distress	Diaphragmatic stenting due to abdominal distension. Aspiration pneumonitis
Sepsis	From gut organisms (due to transmigration of organisms through the ischaemic or perforated gut wall
End result is a child who is Hypothermic and acidotic	

5. B

   It is likely to be a high intestinal obstruction in the duodenum distal to the papilla of vater. Gastro pyloric obstruction will lead to non bilious vomit. Ileal and colonic obstruction will cause distension.

6. B

   Two air fluid levels in X ray (double bubble sign) is suggestive of Duodenal Atresia. Three to four air fluids levels in the upper abdomen with paucity of gas below is suggestive of jejunal atresia. Multiple air fluid level is suggestive of a distal intestinal obstruction.

References:

1. Frischer JS, Azizkhan RG. Jujunoileal Atresia and Stenosis.In : Coran AG, Adzick NS, Krummel TM, Laberge JM. Pediatric Surgery. 7th Edition. Pheladelphia. 2012.Elsevier Saunders.
2. Peterson Al, Olsen L. Intestinal Congenital Malformations In: Zachariou Z. Pediatric Surgery Digest. 1st Edition. Berlin. 2009.Springer

ANTENATAL DIAGNOSIS

Dr. Nitin Pant, Assistant Professor, Dr JD Rawat, Professor, Dr Ashish Wakhlu, Professor, Dr SN Kureel, Professor, Pediatric Surgery

At 32weeks 'of gestation the routine ultrasound findings in a fetus are as follows- Left kidney shows mild hydronephrosis with pelvis AP diameter measuring 7 mm. No calyceal dilatation. Right kidney, bladder, both ureters and amniotic fluid volume are normal.

1. Which of the following statement is true?
   (A) This is a case of antenatal hydronephrosis of the Left kidney
   (B) There is a need to do a chromosomal analysis
   (C) This is a normal finding and the parents need to be reassured
   (D) One should order a fetal MRI for confirmation.

A fetus is diagnosedwith gastroschisis on antenatal USG at 20 weeks of gestation?
2. Which is not a proper statement?
   (A) Gastroschisis is a surgically treatable condition at birth with a good prognosis.
   (B) The mother should be referred to a tertiary care centre for delivery
   (C) The mode of delivery should always be caesarian section.
   (D) All fetuses diagnosed with gastroschisisantenatally are liveborn.

Findings of Fetal USG done at 24 weeks of gestation were as follows- Presence of polyhydramnios with fetal stomach lying in the thorax at thesame cross-sectional level as the heart&presence of the liver in the thorax.
3. What is the likely diagnosis?
   (A) Congenital diaphragmatic hernia.
   (B) Congenital cystic adenomatous malformation
   (C) Congenital short esophagus
   (D) Para esophageal hernia
4. Which of the following is the most widely used index to assess the severity of the lesion on antenatal USG?
   (A) Right lung to Left lung Ratio.
   (B) Lung to Cardiac Ratio
   (C) Lung to Diaphragm Ratio
   (D) The lung-to-head ratio
5. "Key hole sign" on Antenatal Ultrasound is found in case of
   (A) Extrophy Bladder
   (B) Posterior Urethral Valve
   (C) Ureterocoele
   (D) Bladder Diverticulum

Answers:
1. C
   A renal pelvic dilatation of 7 - 10 mm appearing late in the pregnancy is considered normal and is not significant. This is a mild upper tract late third trimester dilatation. The parents need to be reassured that there is nearly an 80% chance that the pelvic dilatation will resolve at birth. One has to confirm this by doing a USG of the baby 3 days after birth. Any significant dilatation at birth will have to be investigated further.
2. D
   Gastroschisis is a surgically treatable condition at birth with a good prognosis. As per available literature about 59% of fetuses with gastroschisisdiagnosed antenatally are live-born. Such mothers should be referred to a tertiary care centre for delivery, with adequate neonatal ICU and pediatric surgical specialties. The mode of delivery is to be decided by the obstetrician on the basis of obstetric indication and not on the basis of presence of this defect.
3. A
   Congenital diaphragmatic hernia.
4. D
   The **lung-to-head ratio (LHR)** is the most widely used index to assess the severity of CDH on antenatal USG . Strength of association with survival is strongest for those fetuses with LHR greater than 1.4(survival 95%) compared with LHR less than 1(75%mortality). These parameters are used as prognostic indicators.
5. B
   The keyhole sign is an ultrasonograhic sign seen in boys with posterior urethral valves. It refers to the appearance of posterior urethra which is dilated, and associated thick walled distended bladder which on ultrasound may resemble a key hole.

Reference:
1. Zachariou Z. Pediatric Surgery Digest. 1st Edition. Berlin. 2009. Springer

POSTERIOR URETHRAL VALVES

Dr Tanvir Roshan Khan, Assistant Professor, Dr JD Rawat, Professor, Dr Ashish Wakhlu, Professor, Dr SN Kureel, Professor, Pediatric Surgery

It is the most common obstructive anomaly of the urethra. The incidence is between 1 in 5000 to 1 in 8000 male births. The etiology is probably a result of the mesonephric ducts entering the cloaca more anteriorly than normal and fusing in the midline.

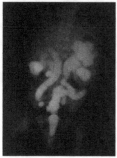

1. What is the condition being discussed above?
    (A) Posterior Urethral Valves(PUV).
    (B) Congenital urethral stricture.
    (C) Persistent urogenital sinus
    (D) Anterior urethral diverticulum
2. The diagnosis can be made precisely by which of the following investigations?
    (A) USG
    (B) CT scan pelvis
    (C) MRI
    (D) Voiding cysto-urethrography (VCUG).
3. Best initial management for the above case would be?
    (A) Vesicostomy
    (B) Cystoscopy
    (C) Bladder catheterization.
    (D) Antibiotics.
4. "Pop off" mechanisms in PUV,s are all except?
    (A) High grade unilateral reflux
    (B) Bladder diverticulum.
    (C) Urinary ascites.
    (D) Dilated posterior urethra.
5. The prognosis of PUV depends on all except?
    (A) Degree of unilateral reflux.
    (B) Degree of renal dysplasia.
    (C) Incidence of UTI with or without VUR.
    (D) Bladder function.

Answers:
    1. A
        Posterior urethral valves are the commonest cause of congenital obstructive uropathy.
    2. D
        Voiding cystourethrographycan only clearly outline the anatomical details of the urethral obstruction as well as the grade of reflux.(Image).
    3. C
        Best initial management is to catheterize the child and relieve the obstruction and wait for the creatinine levels to get normalize.
    4. D
        The pop off mechanisms save the kidney from the deleterious effects of the reflux and preserve the upper tracts unilaterally or bilaterally.
    5. A
        The long term prognosis of PUV depends on all factors that deteriorate the function of upper tracts.

Reference:
1. J. Patrick Murphy, Johan M Gatti. Abnormalities of the urethra, penis and scrotum. Textbook of Pediatric Surgery,7th edn,vol-2.Elsevier saunders;2012: 1555-1557.

DISORDER OF SEXUAL DIFFERENTIATION (XX,DSD)

Dr Tanvir Roshan Khan, Assistant Professor, Dr JD Rawat, Professor, Dr Ashish Wakhlu, Professor, Dr SN Kureel, Professor, Pediatric Surgery

A baby is born with hyperpigmentedlabio-scrotal folds. The gonads are symmetrical and there is evidence of phallus like structure with a single opening below it which on further examination reveals a urogenital sinus. Karyotype is suggestive of 46XX.

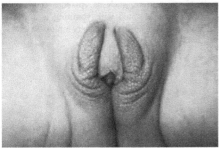

1. What is the probable diagnosis?
   (A) Congenital Adrenal Hyperplasia (CAH).
   (B) Ambigous genitalia.
   (C) Persistent urogenital sinus.
   (D) Mixed gonadal dysgenesis.
2. What is true about these patients.
   (A) Theycan not conceive.
   (B) Ovaries are abnormally placed.
   (C) High androgens and 17 hydroxy progesterone.
   (D) Normal electrolytes.
3. What is the gender assignment in these patients?
   (A) Male
   (B) female.
   (C) Ambiguos.
   (D) Depends upon the social upbringing.
4. True regarding the management of these are all except?
   (A) Corticisteriods and saline rehydration
   (B) Clitoral reduction.
   (C) Vaginoplasty
   (D) Orchiectomy.
5. The clinical finding not true for CAH is?
   (A) Clitoral hypertrophy
   (B) Gonadal asymmetry.
   (C) Enlarged labioscrotum.
   (D) Hyperpigmentation.

Answers:
   1. A
      46 XX DSD(Over androgenized female), Congenital adrenal Hyperplasia(CAH).
   2. B
      The ovaries in these patients are normally placed and they can reproduce as well.
   3. B
      The gender assignment in these patienrs are female as the internal sex organs are normal and the karyotype is XX.
   4. D

All procedures described are needed for the female genitoplasty. No orchiectomy is done as no tetes are there.

5. B

There is always symmetric gonads in CAH.

Reference:
1. Rafael V Pieretti, Patricia K Donahoe, Disorders of sexual differentiation. Textbook of Pediatric Surgery,7th edn,vol-2.Elsevier saunders;2012: 1565-1584.

PELVIURTERIC JUNCTION OBSTRUCTION

Dr Tanvir Roshan Khan, Assistant Professor, Dr JD Rawat, Professor, Dr Ashish Wakhlu, Professor, Dr SN Kureel, Professor, Pediatric Surgery

Although often asymptomatic, these children may have variable symptoms such as episodic flank pain, abdominal pain or less commonly UTI. Cyclic abdominal pain often associated with vomiting is a classic finding. In spite of the most common congenital urinary obstruction its management remains complex.

1. What is the condition being discussed above?
   (A) Posterior urethral valves.
   (B) Ureteroceles.
   (C) PUJO (Pelvi-urteric junction obstruction).
   (D) Congenital urethral stricture.
2. What is the cause of the condition discussed?
   (A) Failure of canalization of the upper ureter.
   (B) Failure of canalization of the renal pelvis.
   (C) Congenital stenosis of upper ureter.
   (D) Adynamic segment of upper ureter or external compression of the pelvi ureteric junction.
3. In how many cases of there is associated (vesicoureteric reflux)VUR?
   (A) 50-75%.
   (B) 25-50%.
   (C) 10-15%.
   (D) 0-5%.
4. The diagnosis of renal function in these patients can be made by?
   (A) DTPA scan.
   (B) DMSA scan.
   (C) IVP.
   (D) Ultrasosnography.
5. The most commonly performed surgery in these patients is.
   (A) Dismemeberedpyeloplasty.
   (B) Nephrostomy.
   (C) D J stent.
   (D) Nephrectomy.

Answers:
1. C
   PUJO (Pelvi-urteric junction obstruction).The incidence is 1:250, most common in males and majority on the left side.
2. D
   There are two types the most common intinsisc type is caused by is due to the adynamic segment of the upper ureter and are typically probe patent but fail to propel the urine. The extrinsic variety is related to the mechanical causes such as crossing vessels or adhesive bands.
3. C
4. A
   The renal scintigraphy studies done by 99m Tc DTPA are preferentially concentrated by the kidney and freely filtered by the glomerulus are used for the renal function studies.
5. A
   The dismembered pyeloplasty also known as Anderson hynespyeloplasty is the most common surgery performed for PUJO with success rate reaching upto 100%.

Reference:
1. Travis W.Groth, M E Mitchell. Ureteropelvic junction obstruction.Textbook of Pediatric Surgery, 7th edn,vol-2.Elsevier saunders;2012. P 1565-1584: 1411-1424.

HEPATOBLASTOMA

Dr Tanvir Roshan Khan, Assistant Professor, Dr JD Rawat, Professor, Dr Ashish Wakhlu, Professor, Dr SN Kureel, Professor, Pediatric Surgery

This is the 10th most common childhood tumor representing 0.5% to 2% of all pediatric tumors. Median age at the time of diagnosis is 1 years and most occur during the first 1.5 years of life. The maternal exposure to metals has high risk for it and congenital anomalies are frequently associated with it. Precocious puberty may arise as this produces beta-HCG.

1. Which tumor of the childhood is being discussed above?
   (A) Neuroblastoma.
   (B) Wilm,s tumor.
   (C) Hepatoblastoma.
   (D) Rhabdomyosarcoma.
2. What is the most common presentation of this tumor?
   (A) Jaundice
   (B) Portal hypertension
   (C) Weight loss, anorexia and weakness.
   (D) Asymptomatic abdominal mass.
3. The most important tumor marker for this condition is?
   (A) Serum ferritin.
   (B) Serum alpha feto protein.
   (C) HCG.
   (D) CA-125.
4. Which classification is used for pre surgical assessment?
   (A) PRETEXT.
   (B) TNM.
   (C) Couinads classification.
   (D) None.
5. Commonest chemotherapeutic agent used for it.
   (A) Vincristine.
   (B) Cisplatin and Doxorubicin.
   (C) Etoposide and vincristine
   (D) Cyclophosphamide.

Answers:

1. C
   Hepatobalstoma is the most common malignant pediatric liver tumor with incidence of around 1 per million.Occurs more in boys and median age at the time of diagnosis is 1 years.
2. D
   The tumor usually presents as an asymptomatic abdominal mass. Systemic symptoms such as weight loss, anorexia and weakness are less common. Severe osteopenia, with back pain, refusal to walk and pathological fractures may be seen at the time of presentation.
3. B
   Serum alpha protein is most valuable laboratory tool for both diagnosing and monitoring of hepatic tumors.
4. A
   PRETEXT(PreTreatment Extent of Disease) is used most commonly in which the liver is divided into four sectors; left lobe of the liver consists of a lateral sector(Segment II and III) and a medial sector(segment IV) and right lobe consists of of an anterior sector(segments V and VIII) and a posterior sector(segments VI and VII).
5. B
   PLADO regimen consisting Cisplatin and Doxorubicin is the widely used chemotherapy for hepatoblastoma.

Reference:

1. Kenneth W Gow, C H Chui, Sani Malagool, B Rao. Malignant Liver Tumors in children and adolescents. Pediatric Oncology. Jaypee 2007: 200-226.

ANO-RECTAL MALFORMATIONS

Dr Tanvir Roshan Khan, Assistant Professor, Dr JD Rawat, Professor, Dr Ashish Wakhlu, Professor, Dr SN Kureel, Professor, Pediatric Surgery

A just born male neonate presented in surgical emergency with parent complains of absence of anal opening. Patient was evaluated and some investigations done and observed for 24 hrs. There after some surgical intervention was done. Now answer the following questions(See image).

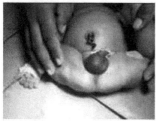

1. What is your diagnosis?
    (A) High type of Ano-rectal malformation.
    (B) Anal membrane.
    (C) Low type of Ano-rectal malformation.
    (D) Anal stenosis.
2. Best preoperative X-ray to make the diagnosis of the above condition is?
    (A) Prone cross table lateral X-ray.
    (B) Invertogram.
    (C) X-ray pelvis.
    (D) X-ray abdomen erect.
3. What is the provisional diagnosis if newborn presented with absence of anal opening, upper abdominal distention and excessive salivation, respiratory distress since birth with inability to put infant feeding tube.
    (A) Meconium aspiration syndrome.
    (B) Esophageal atresia.
    (C) GERD.
    (D) Duodenal atresia.
4. The following syndromes are associated with ano-rectal malformations except?
    (A) Down,s syndrome.
    (B) VACTREL syndrome.
    (C) Currarino,s triad.
    (D) Denys-Drash Syndrome.
5. The type of colostomy usually performed in cases of high ARM?
    (A) Transeverse colostomy.
    (B) Low sigmoid colostomy.
    (C) High sigmoid colostomy.
    (D) Right ascending colostomy.

Answers:

1. A

   High type of ano-recatlmalformations(old terminology-imperforate anus) commonly present with absence of anal opening,flat perineum and or discharge of meconium form the urethra.
2. A

   Prone cross table X-ray is now preferred technique to assess the level of distal rectal pouch as it is more easy and safe to perform and the cahnces of aspiration is also minimized.
3. C

   Esphageal atresia with or without fistula may be associated with these patients leading to salivation/frothing and respiratory distress.
4. D

Denys drash syndrome is associated with pseudohermaphroditism, mesangial renal sclerosis, and Wilms' tumor.

5. C

A high sigmoid diverting colostomy is preferred over other as it provides sufficient length for pullthrough and complications are less.

Reference:
1. Marc A Levitt, A Pena,Ano-Rectal malformations.Textbook of Pediatric Surgery,7th edn,vol-2.Elsevier saunders;2012:1289-1305)

HIRSCHPRUNG'S DISEASE
Dr. J.D. Rawat, Professor Department of Pediatric Surgery

Five months old male infant, born full term normal vaginal delivery, presented to the pediatric surgical emergency with complaint of abdominal distension, fever and bilious vomiting for 2 days along with history of recurrent episodes of constipation, diarrhea and abdominal distension which got relieved on giving enema. In newborn period there is history of delayed passage of meconium.

1. What is the provisional diagnosis?
    (A) Chronic Constipation
    (B) Duodenal Web
    (C) Intestinal Tuberculosis
    (D) Hirschprung's Disease
2. The following anomalies are associated with the diagnosis of above condition except?
    (A) Down's Syndrome
    (B) Currarino's Syndrome
    (C) Waardenberg Shah Syndrome
    (D) Smith LemliOpitz Syndrome
3. Which is not true regarding the radiological investigation in above condition?
    (A) Bird beak sign
    (B) Presence of transition zone in water soluble enema
    (C) Pneumoperitoneum
    (D) Reversed rectosigmoid index
4. Which is the gold standard diagnostic technique in above condition?
    (A) X-ray Abdomen
    (B) Water soluble contrast enema
    (C) Delayed passage of meconium beyond 48 hours
    (D) Rectal biopsy
5. Cause of non-passage of meconium beyond 48 hours are all except?
    (A) Hirscprung's Disease
    (B) Meconium Plug Syndrome
    (C) Hypothyroidism
    (D) Tracheo – esophageal fistula
6. Laparoscopic pull through for the above disease was described by?
    (A) Swenson
    (B) Georgeson
    (C) Duhamel
    (D) Alberto Pena

Answers:
1. D

Hirschprung's Disease is a common cause of delayed passage of meconium, with history of recurrent constipation and abdominal distention.

2. B

Currarino's Syndrome is associated with Anorectal malformations.

3. A

Bird beak sign is not a finding of Hirschprung's Disease.

4. D

Rectal biopsy is gold standard technique in Hirschprung's Disease to see the absence of ganglions cells and hypertrophic nerve bundles.

5. D

In Tracheo-esophageal Fistula there was no delayed passage of meconium.

6. B
    Laparoscopic pull through for the Hirschprung's Disease was first described Georgeson in 1995.

Reference:
1. Langer J. C.Hirschsprung Disease. In: Arnold G. Coran, Pediatric surgery seventh edition, Elsevier Saunders; 2012. P. 1265-75.

MALROTATION
Dr. J.D. Rawat, Professor Department of Pediatric Surgery

20 days neonate presented with sudden onset bilious vomiting with bleeding per rectum with intolerable cry to the emergency department.

1. What is the most likely diagnosis?
    (A) Hirschprung's disease
    (B) Intestinal atresia
    (C) Malrotation with midgut volvulus
    (D) Duodenal web
2. Whirlpool sign is a feature of?
    (A) Color Doppler
    (B) CECT
    (C) Both
    (D) None
3. Ladd's Procedure comprises of all except?
    (A) Normal positioning of bowel
    (B) Lysis of Ladd's band
    (C) Straightening of duodenum
    (D) Appendicectomy
4. Intraoperative finding present in the above condition are all except?
    (A) Abnormal peritoneal bands extending from duodenum and right colon
    (B) Duodenojejunal junction to the right
    (C) Hypermobile caecum
    (D) Wide mesentery base
5. Whirlpool sign is due to?
    (A) SMA and SMV
    (B) Duodenum and SMA
    (C) SMA and Aorta
    (D) A and B

Answers:
1. A
    Malrotation with midgut volvulus presents with bilious vomiting and vitals instability in infants.
2. C
    Whirlpool sign may see in color Doppler or CECT, due to mesenteric vessels rotation.
3. A
    In Malrotation after surgical correction small bowel should be placed in right side and large bowel should be placed in left side.
4. D
    In Malrotation mesentery is narrow.
5. A
    Whirlpool sign occurs due to mesenteric vessels rotations.

Reference:
1. Dassinger M. S. Smith S. D. Disorders of Intestinal Rotation and Fixation. In: Arnold G. Coran, Pediatric surgery seventh edition, Elsevier Saunders; 2012. P. 1111-25.

INFANTILE HYPERTROPHIC PYLORIC STENOSIS
Dr. J.D. Rawat, Professor Department of Pediatric Surgery

A 1.5 month old male infant, born full term with a weight of 3.6 Kg presented with erratic feeding, recurrent, projectile, non-bilious vomiting and failure to weight gain since 2 week of age. He was on exclusive breast feeding initially and tolerated well up to 2 week. Patient attendant noticed visible peristalsis in upper abdomen just after feed. He was usually hungry and keen for feed. A test feed showed a visible peristalsis also.

1. What is your clinical diagnosis?
    (A) Gastroesophagel Reflux disease
    (B) H type Tracheoesophageal fistula
    (C) Infantile hypertrophic pyloric stenosis
    (D) Malrotation of gut
2. What is the initial resuscitation IV fluid in this patient in minimal dehydration?
    (A) NS + I meq KCL/100ml
    (B) N/2 NS in D5% + 1 ml KCL/100ml
    (C) N/4 NS in D5% + I ml KCL/100ml
    (D) N/3 NS in D5% + 1 meq KCL/100ml
3. Metabolic changes occur in this disease?
    (A) Metabolic acidosis,hypokalimia,hyponatremia
    (B) Metabolic alkalosis, hypokalimia,hyponatremia
    (C) Metabolic alkalosis,hypernatremia,hypokaeimia
    (D) Respiratory acidosis, hypokalimia,hyponatremia
4. What we look for in USG abdomen?
    (A) Gastric content movement and gastroesphageal reflux
    (B) Pyloric muscle thickness, pyloric channel length
    (C) Relation of superior mesenteric vessel in relation to Aorta
    (D) Collapsed duodenum and dilated stomach with to and fro movement of gastric content
5. Normal USG Criteria of pyloric channel length and pyloric muscle thickness in neonates,above which it is supposed to be abnormal?
    (A) 14 cm and 4 cm
    (B) 14mm and 4 mm
    (C) 1.4 cm and 4 mm
    (D) 1.4 mm and 4 cm
6. As per Benson and Alpern severity of disease defined by measurement of?
    (A) Serum Co_2
    (B) Serum CO
    (C) Serum O_2
    (D) Vomiting episode per day and electrolyte imbalance
7. Investigation of choice is?
    (A) Endoscopy
    (B) USG abdomen
    (C) Barium swallow in trendelenberg Position
    (D) Manometric evaluation of GE junction.
8. Surgical procedure in this case?
    (A) Nissen fundoplication
    (B) Pyloroplasty
    (C) Pyloromyotomy
    (D) Ladd's procedure

Answers:

1. C
    Clinical features suggests IHPS.
2. B
    In IHPS with mild dehydration high sodium with potassium supplement fluid should be given.
3. B
    In IHPS metabolic abnormalities are hypokalemic, hyponatremic metabolic alkalosis.
4. B
    In USG pyloric muscle thickness should be more than 4 mm and length of pyloric channel should be more than 16 mm for suggestion of IHPS.
5. B
    In USG pyloric muscle thickness should be more than 4 mm and length of pyloric channel should be more than 16 mm for suggestion of IHPS.
6. A
    Level of serum CO2 (HCO3) used for severity of disease.
7. B
    USG is simple and noninvasive diagnostic investigation for IHPS.

8. C
    Ramstedt's pyloromyotomy is the surgical procedure of choice.

Reference:

1. Schwartz M. Z. Hypertrophic Pyloric Stenosis. In: Arnold G. Coran, Pediatric surgery seventh edition, Elsevier Saunders; 2012. P. 1021-28.

Chapter-18

Pediatrics

CONGENITAL HEART DISEASE

Dr. Shally Awasthi, Professor, Department of Pediatrics

Deshraj, 8 years old male was admitted with history of fever for 15 days, headache for 7 days and off and on vomiting for 2 days. There was history of bluish discoloration of lips and nails since the age of 6 months. Developmental milestones were all delayed. On general examination, Glasgow coma scale was 9, pulse was of normal volume and character and rate was 70/minute. Grade III clubbing was present. On examination, left precordial bulge was present and apex was in the 5th intercostal space in mid-clavicular line. On cardiac auscultation, 1st heart sound was normal and 2nd heart sound was soft and single. Pansystolic murmur was present in the left para-sternal border with fan shaped radiation. In addition there was a short ejection systolic murmur at the apex. Fundus examination was normal. Cerebrospinal fluid protein was 20 mg/dL, glucose 100 mg/dL and there were no cells. Simultaneous blood glucose level was 130 mg/dL. EKG strips are pasted below:

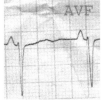
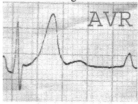
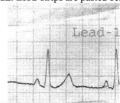
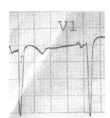
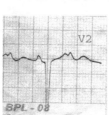
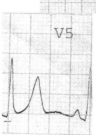

1. EKG findings are suggestive of:
    (A) Left axis deviation with left ventricular hypertrophy
    (B) Normal axis with left ventricular hypertrophy
    (C) Right axis deviation with right ventricular hypertrophy
    (D) Normal axis with right ventricular hypertrophy
2. What is the most likely cause of congenital heart disease?
    (A) Tetrology of Fallot
    (B) Eisenmenger complex
    (C) Ebstein's anomaly
    (D) Tricuspid atresia
3. What is the most likely cause of presenting symptoms of fever with headache?
    (A) Hypertension
    (B) Brain abscess
    (C) Pyogenic meningitis
    (D) Cerebral venous thrombosis
4. EKG findings are suggestive of which electrolyte abnormality?
    (A) Hypocacemia
    (B) Hypokalemia
    (C) Hyperkalemia
    (D) Hypercalcemia

Answers:

1. A
    Since in Lead I, R wave is positive and in Lead $_a$VF it is negative, hence the axis is between 0 and -90^0
2. D
    Since cyanosis began in early infancy and there is Grade III clubbing it is cyanotic heart disease.
    As EKG is showing left axis deviation (leads I and $_a$VF) right precordial leads are showing rS the most likely diagnosis is tricuspid atresia.

3. B

Patients of congenital cyanotic heart disease beyond 2 years of age are more likely to develop brain abscess. Since CSF findings are within normal limits it is not pyogenic meningitis. (2)

4. C

Since there are tall T waves in V5, it is likely to be hyperkalemia. In tricuspid atresia the T wave is flat, biphasic or inverted in left precordial leads. (3)

References:

1. Park MK. Basic tools in routine evaluation of cardiac patients. Electrocardiography in Park's Pediatric cardiology for practitioners. 6th Edition. Elsevier Saunders, Philadelphia, 2014; pages 41-47.

2. Bernstein D. Congenital cyanotic heart lesions: Lesions associated with decreased pulmonary blood flow. In Nelson Textbook of Pediatrics. Kliegman RM, Stanton BF, Geme III, JW, Schor NF, Behrman RE (Eds) 19th Edition, Elsevier Saunders, Philadelphia,2011; pages1573 – 1583.

3. Bernstein D. Evaluation of cardiovascular system. Laboratory evaluation. Electrocariography. In Nelson Textbook of Pediatrics. Kliegman RM, Stanton BF, Geme III, JW, Schor NF, Behrman RE (Eds) 19th Edition, Elsevier Saunders, Philadelphia,2011; pages 1537- 1540.

CONGENITAL HYPOTHYROIDISM

Dr. Durga Prasad, SR, Department of Pediatrics

A 1 year old female child was taken to pediatric OPD with complaints of - not gaining height and dull expression. Child was born through normal vaginal delivery at hospital, birth weight - 2.8 kg and cried soon after birth. Developmental milestones were delayed. On examination she had large tongue &umbilical hernia. Investigations revealed free T_3 – 8 pmol/L (12-33), TSH-12 mIU/L (0.7-6.4).

1. What is the most likely clinical diagnosis?
   (A) Galactosemia
   (B) Congenital hypothyroidism
   (C) Down syndrome
   (D) Hurler disease
2. What is the most common cause of this condition?
   (A) Maternal ingestion of propylthiouracil
   (B) Iodine transport defect
   (C) Thyrotropin deficiency
   (D) Thyroid dysgenesis
3. What investigation would you like to do first?
   (A) Thyroid function test (T3/T4/TSH)
   (B) Thyroid scan
   (C) X- Ray of knee joint
   (D) Ultrasound neck
4. What is the treatment of choice for this condition?
   (A) Levothyroxine
   (B) Propylthiouracil
   (C) Steroid
   (D) Vitamin D_3
5. Best method to detect this condition:
   (A) Amniotic fluid testing
   (B) Antenatal ultrasound
   (C) Newborn screening
   (D) Maternal hormone levels

Answers:

1. B

Newborns with congenital hypothyroidism are usually asymptomatic at birth but may become symptomatic in next 2- 3weeks and present with hypotonia, feeding difficulties, puffy face, large tongue, constipation, macroglossia, letharginess, umbilical hernia and delayed developmental milestone.

2. D

Most common cause of congenital hypothyroidism is defective thyroid gland development (aplasia, hypoplasia, ectopic gland)

3. A

If congenital hypothyroidism is suspected urgent thyroid function test should be done.

4. A

Thyroxine replacement therapy should be started as early as possible to prevent irreversible mental retardation in congenital hypothyroidism.

5. C

Universal newborn screening is the best method for prevention of this condition.

Reference:

1. LeFranchi S. Disorders of thyroid gland.Hypothyroidism.In. Kliegman RM, Stanton BF, St. Jeme JW, Schor NF, Berman RE.Nelson Textbook of Pediatrics. 19th ed. Philadelphia: Sounders Elsevier; 2012, 1895- 99.

FANCONI'S ANEMIA

Dr. Nishant Verma, Assistant Professor, Department of Pediatrics

Six year boy is brought to the out-patient department with complaints of severe pallor. On examination, the child is stunted, has abnormal looking hands (Figure), multiple café-au-lait spots, hyperpigmentation of the trunk, neck, and intertriginous areas, micropenis, undescended testes and severe pallor. There is no jaundice or hepatosplenomegaly.

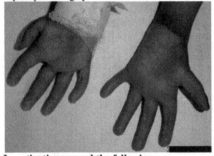

Investigations reveal the following:

Hb-4.5gm/dl, TLC-2000/cu.mm (N20L77E3), Platelet-23000/cu.mm, MCV-101fL, MCH-30pg.
Bone marrow biopsy- Hypoplastic marrow (Bone marrow cellularity < 25%)

1. What is the likely diagnosis in this child?
   (A) Megaloblastic anemia
   (B) Fanconi anemia
   (C) Dyskeratosis congenital
   (D) Shwachman-Diamond syndrome
2. Which of the following is the most is the most common mode of inheritance of this disorder?
   (A) X linked recessive
   (B) X linked dominant
   (C) Autosomal dominant
   (D) Autosomal recessive
3. Which of the following is the most characteristic chromosomal abnormality associated with this condition?
   (A) Increased chromosomal fragility
   (B) Shortening of telomeres
   (C) Trisomies
   (D) Chromosomal deletions
4. Which of the following treatment interventions provides a cure for the hematologic abnormalities in Fanconi's anemia?
   (A) Androgens
   (B) Anti thymocyte globulin + Cyclosporine
   (C) Recombinant growth factors
   (D) Hematopoietic stem cell transplantation

Answers:

1. B

   Presence of pancytopenia, hypoplastic bone marrow and characteristic physical findings like: hypoplastic thumbs, hyperpigmentation, growth failure is characteristic of Fanconi's anemia. The anemia in children with Fanconi's is usually Macrocytic, which explains the MCV of 101fL.

2. D

   The mode of inheritance of Fanconi's anemia is autosomal recessive.

3. A

   All patients with Fanconi's anemia have increased chromosomal fragility. The fragility is further enhanced if diepoxybutane (DEB) is added to the cell culture medium. Telomere shortening is associated with Dyskeratosis congenital.

4. D

   Although androgens can produce a hematological response in 50% of patients with Fanconi's anemia, the only curative therapy for the hematological abnormalities is hematopoietic stem cell transplantation. There is no role of immunosuppression with Anti thymocyte globulin + Cyclosporine in these children, and the role of recombinant growth factors like G-CSF is also not well defined.

References:

1. D'Andrea AD. The Constitutional Pancytopenias. In: Kliegman RM, Stanton BMD, Geme JS, Schor N, Behrman RE, editors, Nelson Textbook of Pediatrics 19th edition vol.2 New Delhi: Elsevier; 2008. Pg 1642-44.

HEMOLYTIC UREMIC SYNDROME
Dr. Akansha Gupta, SR, Department of Pediatrics

A 3 year old girl presents to your office with acute onset of lethargy and pallor. The child's mother reports that the child has bloody diarrhea for 5 days that cleared 1 day before presenting to your office. She also notes acute onset of cola coloured urine along with decreased urine output. On examination, the patient is pale and lethargic. Blood pressure is 120/80 mm Hg. On investigation –Hb 5gm/dL, and schistocytes are seen in peripheral blood smear. Serum Na is 130 mg/dl, K is 5.5 mg/dl, BUN is 100mg/dl, creatinine 4.0 mg/dl and urine analysis reveals hematuria and proteinuria 3+.

1. The most likely diagnosis is:
   - (A) Acute tubular necrosis
   - (B) Hemolytic uremic syndrome
   - (C) Acute glomerulonephritis
   - (D) Prerenal acute renal failure
2. The most appropriate next step in diagnosis would be:
   - (A) Complete blood cell count
   - (B) Urine analysis
   - (C) Urine culture
   - (D) Pro thrombin time
3. What is the most common causative organism for HUS in Asian subcontinent:
   - (A) Salmonella typhi
   - (B) E coli
   - (C) Shigella dysenteriae type 1
   - (D) Campylobacter jejuni
4. All of the following statement about HUS are true Except:
   - (A) HUS is the most common cause of acute renal failure in young children
   - (B) Vero toxin elaborated by E coli 0157:H7 initiates endothelial cell injury in HUS
   - (C) HUS always presents after an episode of enteritis
   - (D) The diagnosis of HUS requires micro-angiopathic haemolytic anemia, thrombocytopenia and acute renal failure.
5. All of the following are accepted treatment for this patient except:
   - (A) Antihypertensive pharmacotherapy to maintain blood pressure below the 90th percentile for age and height
   - (B) Fluid replacement at rate to cover insensible losses plus urine output
   - (C) Institution of antibiotic treatment against E.coli bacteria
   - (D) Early institution of dialysis if required

Answers:
1. B
2. A
   HUS is characterised by triad of microangiopathic hemolytic anemia, thrombocytopenia and renal insufficiency therefore CBC is essential to document thrombocytopenia.
3. C
   In the subcontinent of Asia and southern Africa shiga toxin of shigella dysenteriae type 1,whereas in western countries verotoxin producing Ecoli(VTEC) are the usual causes
4. C
   The various etiologies of HUS allow classification into infection induced,genetic, medication induced, systemic disease characterised by micro vascular injury.
5. C
   Antibiotic therapy to clear the toxigenic organism can result in increased toxin release, potentially exacerbating the disease, and therefore is not recommended.

Reference:
1. Scott K. Van Why and Ellis D. Avner. Hemolytic Uremic Syndrome.Chapter 512 Nephrology. In Nelson Textbook of Pediatrics,19th Edition. Kleigman RM et al, Elsevier Saunders press;1791-1794.

HYPERTROPHIC PYLORIC STENOSIS
Dr. Mala Kumar, Professor, Department of Pediatrics

A 6 weeks old playful full term male infant presented with history of non bilious vomiting for 2 weeks. He vomited in the OPD after a feed. On immediate examination he was found to weigh   3kg, had mild jaundice and an olive shaped lump in the epigastrium. He continued to feed eagerly after the vomit. On investigation his pH was 7.6, potassium 5meq/dl and sodium 128 meq/dl.

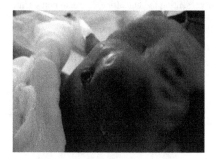

1. What is the most likely diagnosis?
   (A) Gastroesophageal reflux
   (B) Acute cholecystitis
   (C) Hypertrophic pyloric stenosis
   (D) Congenital adrenal hyperplasia
2. What do you think will be the colour of urine be?
   (A) Deep yellow
   (B) Colorless
   (C) Greenish
   (D) Red
3. Which investigation would confirm the diagnosis?
   (A) Plain X ray abdomen
   (B) Ultrasound abdomen
   (C) Barium enema
   (D) Liver function test
4. What is essential in the preoperative management?
   (A) Weight gain
   (B) Domperidon
   (C) Correcting alkalosis

(D) Phototherapy
5. What is the definitive management of the condition?
 (A) Ramstedtpyloromyotomy
 (B) Fontan's procedure
 (C) Fundoplication
 (D) Rex shunt

Answers:

1. C
 Non bilious vomiting with failure to thrive and an olive like mass in the epigastrium indicates gastric obstruction. Progressive loss of hydrogen ion and chloride in vomitus leads to hypochloremic metabolic alkalosis.

2. B
 There is an associated decreased level of glucuronyltransferase in about 5 % of affected infants causing prolonged unconjagated hyperbilirubinemia which does not cause yellow discoloration of urine.

3. B
 Ultrasound abdomen confirms the diagnosis in majority of patients. It has a sensitivity of approximately 95%. Criteria for diagnosis include pyloric thickness more than 4mm or pyloric length greater than 14mm. Upper GI barium studies may show "shoulder sign" or "double tract sign".

4. C
 Fluid resuscitation with dextrose normal saline and correction of metabolic alkalosis are essential to prevent postoperative apnea which may be associated with anesthesia.

5. A
 The incision is usually transverse. The pyloric mass is split without cutting the mucosa and incision is closed.

References:

1. Hunter AK, Liacouras CA. Hypertrophic pyloric stenosis. In: Kliegman, Stanton, ST. Geme, Schor, Behrman editors. Nelson textbook of Pediatrics 19th ed. Philadelphia, PA: Elsevier Saunders; p.1274-1275

LEUKOCYTE ADHESION DEFECT

Dr. Mala Kumar, Professor, Department of Pediatrics

A 2 month old infant was admitted with pneumonia. He was treated with antibiotics which had to be upgraded as he did not respond. His total leukocyte count was 56,000/cu mm with 80 percent neutrophils. There was previous history of omphalitis which needed intravenous antibiotics, required surgical intervention and was accompanied by delayed healing, no formation of pus and reinfection. There was history of falling of the cord at 16 days of life. During treatment for pneumonia his respiratory symptoms improved slowly but he cried incessantly for days, had a distended abdomen but no obvious evidence of inflammation or obstruction. Ultrasound abdomen revealed peritonitis.

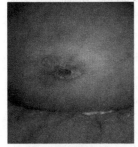

1. What is the likely diagnosis?
 (A) Leukocyte adhesion defect type 1
 (B) T and B cell immunodeficiency
 (C) B cell immunodeficiency
 (D) T cell immunodeficiency

2. What is the cut off for delayed separation of cord?
   (A) 7 days
   (B) 14 days
   (C) 21 days
   (D) 28 days
3. Which of these is NOT a cause for delayed separation of cord?
   (A) Histiocytosis X
   (B) Caesarean delivery
   (C) Neonatal sepsis
   (D) Intrauterine growth retardation
4. The common organisms infecting infants with leukocyte adhesion defects are all EXCEPT
   (A) Staphylococcus aureus
   (B) Escherichia coli
   (C) Candida
   (D) Mycobacterium tuberculosis
5. Management of patients with severe leukocyte adhesion defect includes all EXCEPT
   (A) Antibiotics
   (B) Prophylactic antibiotics
   (C) Bone marrow transplantation
   (D) Corticosteroids

Answers:

1. A

   Leukocyte adhesion defect type 1 is a rare autosomal recessive disorder of leukocyte function in which leukocyte adhesion, chemotaxis and ingestion of C3bi opsonised microbes is impaired owing to mutations in the gene on chromosome 21q22.3 for CD18 β subunit of the β2integrins. The severe variety has less than 0.3% of the normal amount of leukocyte β2 integrin molecules on the cell surface. The diagnosis should be suspected in an infant with unusually severe or recurrent infections with persistently high peripheral neutrophil count, no pus formation and delayed separation of cord.

2. B

   The cord usually falls in the first 14 days of life. In 10% of normal term neonates it may fall by 3 weeks.

3. D

   There is delayed colonisation of the cord in babies born by caesarean section and therefore decreased neutrophils required for falling off the cord.

4. D

   Infection with Staphylococcus aureus, Gram negative organisms, fungi and viruses is common in leukocyte adhesion defect as in neutropenic individuals.

5. D

   Death usually occurs by 2 years of age in children with severe disease. Treatment is broad spectrum antibiotics for acute infection, prophylactic antibiotics and bone marrow transplantation. Corticosteroids decrease neutrophil adhesion.

References:

1. Dinauer MC. The phagocyte system and disorders of granulopoiesis and granulocyte function. In David G. Nathan, Stuart H.Orkin, David Ginsburg and A Thomas Look, editors. Hematology of infancy and childhood, 6th edition. Saunders. Philadelphia Pennsylvania p 964-966
2. Boxer LA, Peter E. Newburger. Disorders of phagocyte function. In: Kliegman, Stanton, ST. Geme, Schor, Behrman editors. Nelson textbook of Pediatrics 19th ed. Philadelphia, PA: Elsevier Saunders; p.741-744.

LOWER RESPIRATORY TRACT INFECTION

Dr. Shally Awasthi, Professor, Department of Pediatrics

A 5 month old is brought to the emergency room with history of fever, cough and breathing difficulty for 3 days. She is also refusing to breastfeed. She has severe lower chest in-drawing and central cyanosis. Her respiratory rate is 72 breaths per minute, and pulse-oximeter shows 87% oxygen saturation in room air. On auscultation, there is diminished air entry on left side. Additional information: unimmunized, birth weight of 2 kg, full term normal vaginal delivery, exclusively breastfed. Investigations: C-reactive protein 60 mg/dL and Chest X-ray is given below:

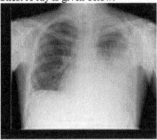

1. What is the most likely clinical diagnosis?
    (A) Acute bronchiolitis
    (B) Pneumonia
    (C) Very severe pneumonia
    (D) Severe pneumonia
2. What therapy would you give this child at first level health care facility?
    (A) Cotrimoxazole
    (B) Amoxycillin
    (C) IV/IM penicillin
    (D) IV penicillin + gentamycin
3. What is the most likely cause of this disease?
    (A) Staphylococcus
    (B) Hemophilus
    (C) Pneumococcus
    (D) E.coli
4. What evidence is NOT against viral etiology?
    (A) Raised C-reactive protein level
    (B) End stage consolidation on chest X-ray
    (C) Pulse oximetry showing 87% oxygen saturation
5. This is a risk factor for pneumonia in the child:
    (A) Low birth weight
    (B) Exclusive breast feeding
    (C) Raised C-reactive protein level
    (D) X-ray showing end stage consolidation

Answers:

1. C
   Very severe Pneumonia, since lower chest in-drawing and cyanosis is present with cough, fast breathing above age specific cutoff.
2. D
   This is the treatment recommended by the World Health Organization at first level care facility
3. C
   Pneumococcus as x-ray chest shows lobar (end stage) consolidation
4. C
   Pulse oxi-metry showing 87% oxygen saturation, since this can be present in acute bronchiolitis and laryngotracheobronchitis, which are predominantly caused by viruses
5. A
   Low birth weight

References:
1. Kabra SK. Lower Respiratory Tract Infections. Chapter 14 Disorders of respiratory system. In Ghai Essential Pediatrics, 8th Ed. Paul VK, Bagga A (Eds) New Delhi, CBS Publishers and Distributers Pvt Ltd 2013; 376-382.
2. WHO recommendations on management of pneumonia in children at first level health facility. WHO/ARI/91.20 Geneva: World Health Organization, 1991

GAUCHER'S DISEASE

Dr. Sarika Gupta, Assistant Professor, Department of Pediatrics

A 4 year boy, product of a consanguineous marriage, presented with regression of milestones and myoclonic seizures for 2 years. Past history was insignificant. There was anemia and hepatosplenomegaly in his younger sibling.On examination he had wasting, stunting, severe splenomegaly and mild hepatomegaly. His investigations showed anemia, thrombocytopenia, leukocyte counts in normal range and a normal blood picture. His liver function tests and k-39 test was normal.

1. What would be the next investigation to confirm the diagnosis:
   (A) Ultrasound abdomen with color doppler
   (B) MRI brain
   (C) Bone marrow examination
   (D) Haemoglobin electrophoresis
2. What is the probable diagnosis:
   (A) Chronic myeloid leukemia
   (B) Chronic malaria
   (C) Storage disorder
   (D) Kala azar
3. Wrinkled paper appearance of the abnormal cell on bone marrow examination is characteristic of:
   (A) Niemann-pick disease
   (B) Tay-sachs disease
   (C) Gaucher disease
   (D) Sandhoff disease
4. Enzyme replacement therapy is not available for:
   (A) Niemann-pick disease
   (B) Gaucher disease
   (C) Fabry disease
   (D) Pompe disease
5. For diseases with autosomal recessive inheritance, what is the recurrence rate in a family With a previously affected child:
   (A) 100%
   (B) 75%
   (C) 50%
   (D) 25%

Answers:
1. C
   Bone marrow examination
2. C
   Storage disorder
3. C
   Gaucher disease
4. A
   Niemann-pick disease
5. D
   25%

References:
1. Scott DA and Lee B. Patterns of genetic transmission. In Nelson Textbook of Pediatrics. Kliegman RM, Stanton BF, Geme III, JW, Schor NF, Behrman RE (Eds) 19th Edition, Elsevier Saunders, Philadelphia,2011; pages385.

2. McGovern MM and Desnick RJ. Lipidoses. In Nelson Textbook of Pediatrics. Kliegman RM, Stanton BF, Geme III, JW, Schor NF, Behrman RE (Eds) 19th Edition, Elsevier Saunders, Philadelphia,2011; pages 487.

MECONIUM ASPIRATION SYNDROME

Dr. Mala Kumar, Professor, Department of Pediatrics

A term neonate weighing 4.0 kg was delivered vaginally 12 hours after rupture of membranes. There was no history of maternal fever or chorioamnionitis however there was evidence of fetal distress. Soon after birth he developed severe respiratory distress. His chest appeared hyper inflated and on auscultation air entry was decreased bilaterally and crepitations were audible. His distress kept on deteriorating and he had to be ventilated using a bag and mask. The condition seemed to improve initially but suddenly deteriorated while still being bagged.

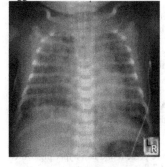

1. The most likely diagnosis is
   (A) Hyaline membrane disease
   (B) Meconium aspiration syndrome
   (C) Tracheo-esophageal fistula
   (D) Diaphragmatic hernia
2. The typical Xray chest in meconium aspiration syndrome has all these, EXCEPT
   (A) Diffuse asymmetric patchy infiltrates
   (B) Areas of consolidation
   (C) Hyperinflation
   (D) Hilar prominence
3. Neonates born through meconium stained liqor need tracheal suctioning if
   (A) Meconium is thick
   (B) Heart rate is < 100/ min
   (C) They are hyperactive
   (D) Respiratory rate is < 60/ min
4. The following are complications of meconium aspiration syndrome, EXCEPT
   (A) Pneumothorax
   (B) Pneumomediastinum
   (C) Persistent pulmonary hypertension
   (D) Left to right shunt
5. The causes of the sudden deterioration could be all, EXCEPT
   (A) Improper seal
   (B) Improper position
   (C) Pneumothorax
   (D) Gram negative sepsis

Answers:

1. B
   Meconium is aspirated into the lungs either in utero or with the 1st breath. The resulting small airway obstruction may produce respiratory distress within the 1st hours, with tachypnea, retractions, grunting, and cyanosis observed in severely affected infants. Overdistention of the chest may be prominent.

2. D

The aspirated meconium obstructs the small airways and causes atelectasis and a ball- valve effect with resultant air trapping and possible air leak. It also causes a chemical pneumonitis.

3. B

Only non vigorous neonates born through meconium stained liqor need tracheal suctioning. Non vigorous babies are those who have a heart rate of < 100/min, poor respiratory effort or poor tone.

4. D

Partial obstruction of some airways may lead to pneumomediastinum and pneumothoraxin 15-30% of patients with meconium aspiration syndromespecially in those who are ventilated. Pneumothorax can be detected by transillumination.Persistent pulmonary hypertension occurs in one third of the cases.

5. D

A poor seal, secretions in the airway, improper position of neck of neonate and inadequate pressure applied to the bag are all causes of ineffective bag and mask ventilation.

References:

1. Amblavanan A and Carlo WA. Meconium aspiration. In: Kliegman, Stanton, ST. Geme, Schor, Behrman editors.Nelson textbook of Pediatrics 19th ed. Philadelphia, PA: Elsevier Saunders; p.590-591.

2. Burris H H. Meconium aspiration. In:John P Cloherty,Eric CEichenwald,Anne R. Hansen,Ann R.Stark editors.Manual of neonatal care7th ed.Philadelphia, PA:Wolters Kluwer Lippincott Williams and Wilkins;p.429-434.

MEGALOBLASTIC ANEMIA
Dr. Shalini Tripathi, Assistant Professor, Pediatrics

A 7 month old infant admitted in pediatric emergency with complaints of tremors, respiratory distress. On examination severe pallor was present, signs of congestive heart failure were present and had hyper pigmented knuckle. Investigations showed Hb- 2.5 gm %, Mean corpuscular volume 107 fl.

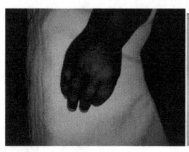 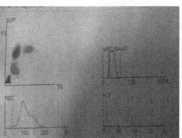

1. The most probable diagnosis is:
   (A) Septicemia
   (B) Congenital heart disease
   (C) Bronchopneumonia
   (D) Megaloblastic anemia
2. The most probable cause of this condition is:
   (A) Iron deficiency
   (B) Zinc deficiency
   (C) Vitamin B6 deficiency
   (D) Vitamin B12 deficiency
3. Dietary deficiency of B12 is seen in:
   (A) People who are strictly vegetarian
   (B) Who do not eat eggs
   (C) Non vegetarians
   (D) Do not eat leafy vegetables
4. A diagnostic feature in peripheral smear in this case would be:
   (A) Reticulocytosis
   (B) Microcytosis

(C) Leukocytosis

(D) Hypersegmented Neutrophils

Answers:

1.   D

Children with Vitamin B12 deficiency often present with pallor, glossitis, vomiting, diarrhea, and icterus. Neurologic symptoms also occur and can include paresthesias, sensory deficits, hypotonia, seizures, developmental delay, developmental regression, and neuropsychiatric changes.

2.   D

Almost all cases of childhood megaloblastic anemia result from folic acid or vitamin B_{12} deficiency; rarely, they may be caused by inborn errors of metabolism.

3.   A

Almost all cases of childhood megaloblastic anemia result from folic acid or vitamin B_{12} deficiency. It does occur in cases of extreme restriction (e.g., strict vegetarians or vegans) wherein no animal products or vitamin B_{12} supplements are consumed

4.   D

The peripheral blood smear is notable for large, often oval, RBCs with increased mean corpuscular volume (MCV). Neutrophils are characteristically hypersegmented, with many having >5 lobes.

Reference:

1. Lerner NB. Megaloblastic Anemias, In Nelson Textbook of Pediatrics. Kliegman RM, Stanton BF, Geme III, JW, Schor NF, Behrman RE (Eds) 19th Edition, Elsevier Saunders, Philadelphia,2011.

CYSTECERCAL ENCEPHALITIS

Dr. Nishant Verma, Assistant Professor, Department of Pediatrics

An eight year old boy presented to the pediatric emergency room with complaints of multiple episodes of generalised tonic clonic seizures for last 1 day. At the time of admission, child was in status epilepticus. He was started on oxygen inhalation, an iv access was immediately obtained and iv Lorazepam was administered @ 0.1mg/kg. The status epilepticus persisted, so a second dose of lorazepam was administered, but the seizures still persisted.

1. Which of the following represents the most appropriate next step for the control of seizures in this child:

(A) Intravenous infusion of midazolam @ 1mcg/kg/min

(B) Loading dose of phenytoin @ 20mg/kg

(C) Intravenous diazepam @ 0.3mg/kg

(D) Loading dose of Levetiracetam @ 20mg/kg

Child remained in altered sensorium even after the control of seizures. His fundus revealed evidence of papilledema in both the eyes. His blood sugar and electrolytes were normal. A contrast enhanced CT scan of the head was obtained, which revealed the following:

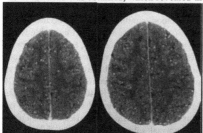

2. What is the most likely diagnosis in this child?

(A) Tubercular meningitis

(B) Cystecercal encephalitis

(C) Herpes simplex encephalitis

(D) Dengue encephalitis

3. Which of the following medications is not indicated in management of a child with cystecercal encephalitis with features of raised intracranial pressure?

(A) Dexamethasone

(B) Mannitol

(C) Albendazole

(D) Antiepileptic drugs

4. Which of the following is the most common mode of acquiring Neurocysticercosis?

    (A) Ingestion of undercooked pork infected with cystecercal larvae

    (B) Ingestion of food contaminated with eggs of *Taenia solium*

    (C) Autoinfection from *Taenia solium* in the gut of humans

    (D) Ingestion of food contaminated with cystecercal larvae

Answers:

1.   B

Benzodiazepines are first line drugs for treatment of status epilepticus in children. After using short-acting benzodiazepines, phenytoin is the preferred second-line anticonvulsant. Midazolam infusion and valproate are reserved for use in refractory status epilepticus (1)

2.   B

The CT scan shows multiple small, contrast enhancing lesions involving the entire brain parenchyma forming the characteristic 'starry-sky' appearance seen in Neurocysticercosis (2)

3.   C

Dexamethasone and Mannitol are indicated for treatment of cerebral edema. Antiepileptics are indicated for control of seizures. Antiparasitic drug, Albendazole should not be used in cystecercal encephalitis because the destruction of numerous live parasites exposes antigens throughout the brain parenchyma and triggers an intense local inflammatory reaction which can be lethal because of sudden increase in intracranial pressure (2,3). Albendazole is also contraindicated in management of intraocular cysticercosis to avoid damage to the eye (2).

4.   B

NCC is caused by infection of the human central nervous system (CNS) with encysted larvae of the tapeworm *Taenia solium*. Humans are the definite hosts and acquire intestinal *T. solium* (taeniasis) from pigs by ingestion of undercooked pork infected with cysticerci. These cysticerci release larvae that develop into adult tapeworms that mature in the intestine, and shed thousands of extremely contagious eggs in the faeces. NCC is acquired by eating food accidently contaminated with these eggs (2).

References:

1.   Mishra D, Sharma S, Sankhyan N, Konanki R, Kamate M, Kanhere S, Aneja S. Consensus guidelines on management of childhood convulsive status epilepticus. Indian Pediatr 2014;51(12):975-90

2.   Singhi P. Neurocysticercosis. Ther Adv Neurol Disord 2011; 4(2):6781

3.   Garcia HH, Gonzalez AE, Gilman RH. Cysticercosis of the central nervous system: how should it be managed? Curr Opin Infect Dis. 2011;24(5):423-7

NEONATAL RESUSCITATION

Dr. Shalini Tripathi, Assistant Professor, Pediatrics

You are asked to attend an emergent caesarean section delivery of a 40 weeks' gestation. Antenatal period was uneventful. Membranes are ruptured at the time of delivery revealing bloody amniotic fluid, but no meconium. At delivery, you receive a floppy, apneic, and blue term male infant. You bring him to the warming table where he is quickly positioned, dried, stimulated and given free-flow oxygen. At 30 seconds of life, he remains apneic and cyanotic. His heart rate is 30 beats per minute. You administer positive pressure ventilation and note good chest wall rise with each positive pressure breath. The infant continues to be apneic and bradycardic with a heart rate of 40 bpm. Chest compressions are begun and positive pressure ventilation is continued. Following 30 seconds of coordinated ventilation and chest compressions, his heart rate is still 40 bpm. Intravenous epinephrine is given. Positive pressure ventilation and chest compressions are continued as you reassess the infant. Good breath sounds are heard bilaterally, but his skin remains pale and mottled and pulses are difficult to palpate. Suspecting hypovolemia, you then administer 10ml/kg of normal saline through the umbilical vein catheter over 5 minutes. The infant's heart rate rises to 150 and his color gradually improves. You check the security of the endotracheal tube and umbilical catheter and prepare for transport to the newborn intensive care unit.

1. What is the most important step in cardiopulmonary resuscitation of the newborn infant:

    (A) Chest compression

    (B) Ventilation

    (C) Hypothermia prevention

    (D) Suction

2. About .... % neonates require assistance to breath.
   (A) 1%
   (B) 5%
   (C) 10%
   (D) 15%
3. The 3 characteristics used to identify newborn infants who do not require resuscitation are
   (A) Gestation, breathing, tone
   (B) Respiration, colour, heart rate
   (C) Respiration, colour, oxygenation
   (D) Tone, heart rate, breathing
4. What is the recommended dose of epinephrine for neonates?
   (A) 0.01-0.03 ml/kg of 1: 10,000 dilution IV
   (B) 0.1-0.3 ml/kg of 1: 10,000 dilution IV
   (C) 0.1-0.3 ml/kg of 1: 1000 dilution IV
   (D) 0.5-1 ml/kg of 1: 1000 dilution IV
5. Target preductal oxygen saturation at 1 minute after birth is-
   (A) 60-65%
   (B) 65-70%
   (C) 70-75%
   (D) 75-80%

Answers:
1. B
   The most important and effective action in neonatal resuscitation is to ventilate the baby's lungs.
2. C
   Approximately 10% of newborns need some assistance at birth to begin breathing at birth.
3. A
   Those newly born infants who do not require resuscitation can generally be identified by a rapid assessment of the following 3 characteristics: Term gestation? Crying or breathing? Good muscle tone?
4. B
   IV administration of 0.01 to 0.03 mg/kg per dose is the preferred. While access is being obtained, administration of a higher dose (0.05 to 0.1 mg/kg) through the endotracheal tube may be considered, but the safety and efficacy of this practice have not been evaluated (Class IIb, LOE C). The concentration of epinephrine for either route should be 1:10,000 (0.1 mg/mL).
5. A
   60-65%

References:
1. Kattwinkel J, Perlman JM,Aziz K, Colby C, Fairchild K, Gallagher Jet al. Special Report—Neonatal Resuscitation: 2010 American Heart Association Guidelines for Cardiopulmonary Resuscitation and Emergency Cardiovascular Care *Pediatrics* published online Oct 18, 2010. DOI: 10.1542/peds.2010-2972E.

NEONATAL SEPSIS
Dr. Mala Kumar, Professor, Department of Pediatrics

A 32 weeks preterm newborn was admitted to the nursery on day one of life with complaints of respiratory distress since birth. Crepitations were audible bilaterally. Mother had received antenatal steroids. There was history of leaking per vaginum for two days. Baby had cried immediately after birth.X ray chest revealed normal volume of lungs and few infiltrates.

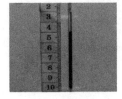

Micro ESR

1. The most likely diagnosis is?
   (A) Early onset neonatal sepsis
   (B) Transient tachypnoea of newborn
   (C) Hyaline membrane disease
   (D) Meconium aspiration syndrome
2. Neonatal sepsis is classified into early and late onset depending on onset of symptoms within or more than how many hours?
   (A) 24
   (B) 36
   (C) 48
   (D) 72
3. Sepsis screen revealed:(a) Total leukocyte count of 18,000/cumm (b) Micro ESR of 20 mm in first hour (c) C- reactive protein of 12 mg/dl (d)Absolute neutrophil count of 6,000/cumm. The positive components are
   (A) a + b
   (B) b + c
   (C) c + d
   (D) d + a
4. Cerebrospinal fluid examination was normal, but CSF culture showed growth of E. coli, the intravenous antibiotics of choice would be
   (A) Vancomycin + Gentamicin
   (B) Ampicillin + Gentamicin
   (C) Meropenem + Vancomycin
   (D) Ampicillin + Gentamicin + Cefotaxim
5. Which are the commonest organisms causing neonatal sepsis in India?
   (A) Group B beta hemolytic streptococcus, E coli, Klebsiella
   (B) Klebsiella, Staphylococcus aureaus, E coli,
   (C) E coli, Enterococcus fecalis,Pseudomonas
   (D) Klebsiella, Pseudomonas, Enterobacter

Answers:

1. A

   Infants with early onset neonatal sepsis usually present with respiratory distress and pneumonia.Meconium aspiration syndrome and transient tachypnoea of newborn occur in term neonates. Ground glass appearance, air bronchogram and low lung volume is seen in Xray chest in hyaline membrane disease.

2. D

   Neonatal sepsis is classified as early- onset if it occurs within 72 hours of birth and as late-onset if it occurs after 72 hours of birth.

3. B

Components of Sepsis screen	Abnormal value
1. Total leukocyte count	<5000/mm3
2. Absolute neutrophil count	Low counts as per Manroe chart for term and Mouzinho's chart for VLBW infants
3. Immature/total neutrophil	>0.2
4. Micro-ESR	>15 mm in 1st hour
5. C reactive protein (CRP)	>1 mg/dl

4. D

   First line antibiotics for neonatal sepsis are Penicillin or Ampicillin + Gentamicin. Cefotaximeis added in cases of meningitis for total duration of 21 days.

5. B

   Commonest organisms for neonatal sepsis in India are, Klebseilla, Staphylococcus aureus and Ecoli

Reference:

1. Neonatal sepsis In: Ramesh Agarwal, Ashok Deorari and Vinod K Paul editors AIIMS Protocols in Neonatology.BS Publishers & Distributers;p163-173

A CHILD WITH ANASARCA
Dr. Chandrakanta, Professor, Department of Pediatrics

A seven years old male child presented with history of generalized swelling and reduced urine output. The child was apparently well eight days before hospitalization when mother noticed some peri-orbital puffiness. Edema progressed over a period of three days and became generalized. After onset of edema, frequency of micturition was reduced from initial 5-6 times per day to 1-2 times per day. There was no history of orthopnoea, jaundice, hematuria, pallor or similar episodes in the past.

On examination HR 90bpm, RR 24/min, BP 100/64 mm/Hg, temp 98.4 deg. F. There was no pallor, clubbing, icterus, cyanosis and lymphadenopathy. General examination revealed facial, periorbital edema, ascites, scrotal edema and pitting edema over legs and feet. Cardiac auscultation revealed normal heart sounds and normal rhythm and no murmur. Chest auscultation showed reduced air entry on right side. Abdomen was distended with flanks full. There was no organomegaly. Shifting dullness was present. There was no thrill and hernia sites were normal. Complete blood counts, renal functions and electrolytes were abnormal. Urine analysis revealed 4+ proteinuria, no RBCs, 15 WBCs per hpf.

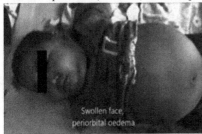

Swollen face, periorbital oedema

1. What is the probable clinical diagnosis?
   A) Nephritic syndrome
   B) Nephrotic syndrome
   C) Acute renal failure
   D) Chronic renal failure
2. All methods are used for assessing proteinuria EXCEPT?
   (A) Sulphosalicylic test
   (B) Spot protein to creatinine ratio
   (C) Dipstick test
   (D) Hay's sulphur test
3. What should be the first step in management of this child?
   (A) Steroids and antibiotics
   (B) Antibiotics and diuretics
   (C) Steroids and diuretics
   (D) Only diuretics
4. All are indications of renal biopsy in a child with nephrotic syndrome EXCEPT?
   (A) Onset at 4 months of age
   (B) 2 relapses over 3 years
   (C) Prior to starting cyclosporine
   (D) A girl with systemic lupus erythematosus
5. Which one of the following complications should be suspected if a child with nephrotic syndrome comes to you with altered sensorium and seizures without fever?
   (A) Cortical vein thrombosis
   (B) Intraventricular hemorrhage
   (C) Subdural hemorrhage
   (D) Acute disseminated encephalomyelitis

1. B
   Acute onset swelling followed by reduced urine output and nephrotic range proteinuria points towards diagnosis of nephrotic syndrome.
2. D
   Sulphosalicylic, urine dipstic andspot protein to creatinine ratiotests are used for detecting proteinuria. Hays's sulphur test is used for detection of bile acids in urine.
3. B
   As child has gross edema and urinary tract infection, so child should be put on diuretics and antibiotics. Steroids can be started after the treatment of infections.
4. B
   Relapses are common in cases of minimal change disease and do not require a biopsy. Other options given point towards a non minimal change disease, so need a biopsy.
5. A
   Thrombosis (venous, arterial) of major blood vessels (eg. Renal veins, cortical venous sinus and mesenteric vein) is a complication of nephrotic syndrome.

Reference:

1. Bagga A, Srivastava RN. Nephrotic syndrome. Bagga A, Srivastava RN. In, Pediatric nephrology, fifth edition, New Delhi: Jaypee Medical limited, 2011: 301-23.

NEUROCYSTICERCOSIS

Dr. Abhinav Sharma, SR and Dr. Rashmi Kumar, Professor, Pediatrics

A seven year old male child presented to pediatric emergency with 2 episodes of generalized tonic clonic convulsions over the last one week – the last one starting half hour back. The child had been previously well till one week prior and there was no preceding history of fever, headache, vomiting, jaundice or any seizure activity in the past. There was no family history of epilepsy. Seizure was treated with i.v. diazepam. After a period of 30 minutes child was fully conscious with Glasgow Coma Score of 15 (E4V5M6), no signs of meningeal irritation, no cranial nerve involvement and no focal neurological deficit. CECT brain showed a 1.5 cm ring enhancing cystic lesion in temporo-parietal region with a small eccentric hyperdensity.

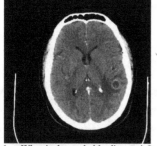

1. What is the probable diagnosis?
   (A) Neurocysticercosis
   (B) Tuberculoma
   (C) Brain abcess
   (D) CNS neoplasm
2. What is the most common presentation of neurocysticercosis ?
   (A) Focal neurological deficit
   (B) Acute onset seizure
   (C) Encephalopathy
   (D) Headache
3. Which organism is responsible for neurocysticercosis?
   (A) Taenia solium
   (B) Strongyloides stecoralis
   (C) Ascaris lumbricoides
   (D) Trichinellaspiralis

4. What is the drug of choice for neurocysticercosis?
   (A) Albendazole
   (B) Ivermectol
   (C) Piperazine
   (D) Mebendazole
5. What does eccentric hyperdensity represent?
   (A) Scolex
   (B) Hemorrhage
   (C) Calcification
   (D) Artifact

Answers:

1. A

   Patient has recent onset seizures with no prior or family history. Recent onset seizures in a well child is often the presentation of neurocysticercosis in the Indian subcontinent, which shows a typical ring or disc like enhancing lesion on imaging. Tuberculoma as compared to neurocysticercosis is usually more than 20 mm in diameter, associated with symptoms of raised intracranial tension, has midline shift, mass effect, presence of a neurodeficit and thick, irregular wall with absent scolex.

2. B

   Acute onset seizures (80%) are the most common manifestation of neurocysticercosis, followed by raised intracranial pressure, focal deficits and rarely meningeal signs.

3. A

   Neurocysticercosis is caused by larval stage of taenia solium. Pigs and humans acquire infections by ingesting food and water contaiminated with parasite eggs.

4. A

   Cysticidal therapy used for neurocysticercosis includes albendazole and praziquantel. Dose of albendazole is 15 mg/kg/day in two divided doses for a duration of seven days. Steroids prednisolone (1-2 mg/kg/day) are started two days prior to inititation of cysticidal therapy. Cysticidal therapy is indicated in viable cysts and ring enchancing lesions. It is contraindicated in cysticercal encephalitis, intraventricular cyst and ocular neurocysticercosis. Anti-epileptic drug therapy is continued for a period of 6 months (till resolution of lesion). Calcified lesion require anti-epileptic drug treatment alone.

5. A

   Neurocysticercosis is the most common cause of cranial ring enhancing lesion. Lesion is disc or ring like with a hypodense center. It may be single or multiple. A scolex is seen within the ring as hyperdense dot. There may be edema surrounding the lesion. There is no midline shift. Cysts are usual in supratentorial areas. MRI is useful in doubtful cases.

References:

1. Dua T, Aneja S. Neurocysticercosis: Management Issues.Indian Pediatrics 2006; 43:227-235.
2. Singhi P. Neurocysticercosis. TherAdvNeurDisord 2011; 4(2): 67-81.

POISONING

Dr. Sarika Gupta, Assistant Professor, Pediatrics

A 8 year boy, living in rural area, presented in pediatric emergency with complaints of multiple episodes of loose stools and vomiting with copious secretions in the mouth with severe respiratory distress followed by altered sensorium. Father told the incident happened 4 hours after they came back from the field. On examinationthe child was in the state of confusion, there were excessive secretions in the mouth and pupils were bilaterally constricted.

1. What is the probable diagnosis:
   (A) Dhaturapoisoning
   (B) Opium poisoning
   (C) Salicylates poisoning
   (D) Organophosphate poisoning
2. Which of the following is the method for decreasing the absorption of poison:
   (A) Administration of antidotes
   (B) Manipulation of urinary pH
   (C) Exchange transfusion
   (D) Use of Cathartics

3. Antidote of choice for salicylate poisoning is
   (A) Atropine
   (B) Physostigmine
   (C) Sodium bicarbonate
   (D) N-acetyl cysteine
4. What is the effect on heart rate in the TOXIDROME of sedative/hypnotic drugs
   (A) No alteration
   (B) Bradycardia
   (C) Tachycardia
   (D) Arrythmia
5. Garlic odour is seen with ingestion of
   (B) Salicylates
   (C) Cyanide
   (C) Organophosphate
   (D) Kerosene

Answers:
1. **D**
   Organophosphate poisoning, as it causes cholinergic toxidrome with constricted pupils, diaphoresis, confusion, fasciculation and increased secretions.
2. **D**
   Use of cathartics
   Various methods to decrease the absorption of toxin are
   - Dilution
   - Emesis, gastric lavage
   - Binding agents-charcoal
   - Cathartics-sorbitol
   - Whole bowel irrigation
   - Endoscopic or surgical removal
3. **C**
   Sodium bicarbonate
4. **D**
   Arrythmia
5. **C**
   Organophosphate

References:
1. O'Donnell and Ewald MB. Poisonings. In Nelson Textbook of Pediatrics. Kliegman RM, Stanton BF, Geme III, JW, Schor NF, Behrman RE (Eds) 19th Edition, Elsevier Saunders, Philadelphia,2011; pages252.
2. Menon PR. Poisonings, injuries and accidents. In Ghai Essential Pediatrics. Paul VK, Bagga A (Eds). Eighth edition, CBS publishers & distributors, 2013; pages 697-701.

PULMONARY HYPERTENSION
Dr. Shalini Tripathi, Assistant Professor, Pediatrics

A 8 years old male child has a history of progressively exercise intolerance and fatigability. On the day of admission she had a chest pain and dizziness. On examination, she has a systolic ejection click and a loud, narrowly split 2nd heart sound. There is a soft systolic murmur. The chest radiograph (fig1) demonstrates prominent pulmonary arteries and an enlarged right ventricle. The peripheral pulmonary vascular markings are greatly decreased.

1. The most likely diagnosis is:
    (A) Tetralogy of Fallot
    (B) Stills murmur
    (C) Rheumatic fever
    (D) Cor pulmonale
    (E) Primary pulmonary hypertension
2. The Electrocardiocadiogram of this patient is suggestive of:

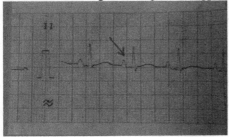

    (A) Broad P wave in lead II
    (B) Tall , narrow, and spiked P waves in lead II
    (C) Normal p wave in lead II
    (D) Bifid P wave in lead II
3. Diseases causing secondary pulmonary hypertension:
    (A) Sickle cell anemia
    (B) Pulmonary venocclusive disease
    (C) Alveolar capillary dysplasia
    (D) All of the above

Answers:
1. E
    The predominant symptoms include exercise intolerance and fatigability; occasionally, precordial chest pain, dizziness, syncope, or headaches are noted. The 2nd heart sound is narrowly split, loud. Chest roentgenograms reveal a prominent pulmonary artery and right ventricle. The pulmonary vascularity in the hilar areas may be prominent, in contrast to the peripheral lung fields in which pulmonary markings are decreased.
2. B
    Tall (>2.5 mm), narrow, and spiked P waves are indicative of right atrial enlargement and are seen in congenital pulmonary stenosis, Ebstein anomaly of the tricuspid valve, tricuspid atresia, and sometimes cor pulmonale.
3. D
    Pulmonary hypertension is a common complication of sickle cell anemia and other hemolytic anemias. In children, pulmonary veno-occlusive disease may account for some cases of primary pulmonary hypertension. Before a diagnosis of primary pulmonary hypertension can be made, other causes of elevated pulmonary arterial pressure must be eliminated.

Reference:
1. Bernstein D. Pulmonary Hypertension. In Nelson text book of Pediatrics, 19th Ed, Chapter 427, pp1600.

RENAL TUBULAR ACIDOSIS
Dr. Abhinav Sharma, SR, Department of Pediatrics

A 5 yrs old male child presented with weakness of all four limbs without any preceding history of diarrhea or other illness. There was a history of two similar episodes of weakness in the past both occurring during evening with spontaneous improvement after sometime. Parents also gave history of polyuria, polydipsia and craving for salty foods. On examination limbs were hypotonic, power grade 1/5 in all four limbs. There was no history of diplopia, dysarthria, respiratory difficulty or bladder and bowel involvement. His weight was 10 kg and height 85 cms were below 3rd percentile for age. He was born of non-consaingenous marriage and third in birth order.
Her serum sodium was 133 meq/l (135-148) and serum potassium 1.4 meq/l (3.5-5). His electrocardiogram (ECG) showed ST depression, flat T waves and appearance of U waves. He was given intravenous followed by

oral potassium supplementation which brought his serum potassium to 3.3 meq/l. Urine output was measured about 5 ml/kg/hr.

His other investigations are given below-

- Blood investigations-
  - o Serum chloride- 105 meq/l
  - o Serum calcium- 8.4 mg/dl
  - o S. phosphorus- 3.1 mg/dl
  - o S. alkaline phosphatase-461 IU/L.
  - o Anion gap on arterial blood gases -14meq/L
  - o Blood sugar, renal and liver function test were normal.
- Urine analysis-
  - o Urine pH- 7.0
  - o Specific gravity- 1.00
  - o 24 hours urinary potassium excretion- 189 meq/L (normal 40-80),
  - o Fractional excretion of potassium- 22%.
  - o 24 hour urinary calcium excretion was 193 mg in 24 hours (> 4mg/Kg/d)
  - o Urinary anion gap was positive (49 mEq/L).
  - o Urine examination did not show any glucose, protein or pus cells
  - o Ammonium chloride acidification (0.1 mg/Kg) after obtaining serum pH caused fall in serum pH from 7.4 to 7.2 but urinary pH was 7.0
- Xray wrist showed changes of rickets
- Ultrasonography of abdomen showed medullary cysts in kidneys.

1. What is probable clinical diagnosis?
   (A) Primary renal tubular acidosis
   (B) Distal renal tubular acidosis
   (C) Type four renal tubular acidosis
   (D) Hyperaldosteronism
2. All are ECG changes of hypokalemia EXCEPT?
   (A) ST depression
   (B) P wave widening
   (C) Elevated T waves
   (D) U waves
3. All of the following are features of distal renal tubular acidosis EXCEPT?
   (A) Increased urinary anion gap
   (B) Urinary potassium wasting
   (C) Nephrocalcinosis
   (D) Urinary pH<5.5
4. Which of the following statement regarding distal renal tubular acidosis is true?
   (A) Hypocalciuria
   (B) Impaired bicarbonate reabsorption
   (C) Obesity
   (D) Failure of urine acidification despite systemic acidosis
5. Which of the following is true regarding proximal renal tubular acidosis?
   (A) There may be global impairment in proximal tubular absorption
   (B) Urine pH>5.5
   (C) Fractional excretion of bicarbonate is reduced
   (D) Hyperkalemia

Answers:

1. B

   Renal potassium wasting with hypercalciuria and failed acidification point towards diagnosis of distal renal tubular acidosis.

2. C

   ECG changes in hypokalemia include:Depression of ST segment, P wave widening, flattening of T waves, and appearance of U waves.

3. D

Name of investigation	Proximal RTA	Distal RTA	Type IV RTA
Plasma K$^+$	Normal/low	Normal/low	High
Urine pH	<5.5	>5.5	<5.5

Urine anion gap	Positive	Positive	Positive
Urine NH$_4^+$	Low	Low	Low
Fraction HCO$_3^-$ excretion	>10-15%	<5%	<5%
Urine calcium	Normal	High	Normal
Bone disease	Common	Often present	Uncommon
Nephrocalcinosis	Absent	Present	Absent
Other tubular defects	Often present	Absent	Absent

4. D

There is hypercalciuria. Bicarbonate reabsorption is impaired in proximal RTA. There is polyuria and failure to thrive. There is failure of urine acidification despite sysytemic acidosis.

5. A

Proximal RTA may be associated with generalized tubular absorption defects. Urine pH is usually less than 5.5 as mechanisms of distal acidification are intact. Fractional excretion of bicarbonate is increased. Serum potassium is normal/low.

References:
1. Bagga A, Srivastava RN. Tubular disorders. In, Pediatric nephrology, fifth edition, New Delhi: Jaypee Medical limited, 2011: 301-23.

VITAMIN D DEFICIENCY
Dr.ShaliniTripathi, Assistant Professor, Pediatrics

A toddler presents to the pediatric outpatient department with short stature. On examination there was wrist widening (figure 2) and X-ray wrist was as shown in the figure1.

(Figure 1.)   (Figure 2.)

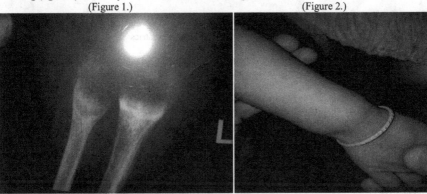

1. The most likely diagnosis is:
   (A) Hypothyroidism
   (B) Vitamin D deficiency
   (C) Skeletal dysplasia
   (D) Chondrodysplasia
2. Rickets can be caused by:
   (A) Nutritional vitamin D deficiency
   (B) Overuse of aluminum antacids
   (C) Prematurity
   (D) Distal renal tubular acidosis
   (E) All of the above
3. Physical features of vitamin D–deficiency rickets include all of the following EXCEPT:
   (A) Craniotabes
   (B) Enlargement of the costochondral junction
   (C) Thickening of the ankles and wrists
   (D) Large anterior fontanel
   (E) Bitot spot
4. The recommended daily allowance of vitamin D in infants and children is
   (A) 100 IU and 200 IU per day
   (B) 200 IU and 400 IU per day

(C) 400 IU and 600 IU per day

(D) 600 IU and 800 IU per day

Answers:

1. B

   Most manifestations of rickets are due to skeletal changes. **Growth plate** widening is also responsible for the enlargement at the wrists and ankles. Rachitic changes are most easily visualized on postero-anterior radiographs of the wrist. Decreased calcification leads to thickening of the growth plate. The edge of the metaphysis loses its sharp border, which is described as *fraying*. The edge of the metaphysis changes from a convex or flat surface to a more concave surface. This change to a concave surface is termed *cupping* and is most easily seen at the distal ends of the radius, ulna, and fibula.

2. E

   There are many causes of rickets including vitamin D disorders, calcium deficiency, phosphorous deficiency, and distal renal tubular acidosis.

3. E

   The classic syndrome of rickets is marked by: craniotabes, rachitic rosary, wrist thickening, and pigeon breast deformity, Harrison groove, flaring epiphyses, and bowing of the legs.

4. B

   The recommended daily allowance in infant is 5 µg (200IU) and children is 10 µg (400IU) per day

References:

1. Gulati A, Bagga A. Micronutrients in health and disease. In Paul VK, Bagga A, Sinha A (Eds).Ghai essential Pediatrics, 8th ed.2013, pp-110-123.

2. Kane AB, Kumar V. Food and Nutrition. In: Cotran RS, et al (Eds). Robbins Pathologic Basis of Disease, 6th edition. 1999, Philadelphia: W.B. Saunders, pp. 436-456.

SEPTIC SHOCK
Dr. Sarika Gupta, Assistant Professor, Pediatrics

A 7 months old child is brought to emergency department with the complaints of fever, 10-12 episodes of watery stool and refusal to feed. On examination he had fever of 101.4°F, heart rate of 180/minutes, Respiratory rate was 64/minutes and blood pressure 50/35 mm of Hg. Skin was mottled, capillary refill time was 6 seconds with weak peripheral pulses. His leukocyte counts were elevated and arterial blood gas analysis showed pH of 7.20. The child was given an intravenous bolus of normal saline 20 ml/kg twice. After the bolus, there was no significant improvement in the clinical sign.

1. What is the cut off systolic BP for a 7 months old infant to label as "**hypotension**":
   (A) <60mm Hg
   (B) <70 mm Hg
   (C) <80mm Hg
   (D) <90 mm Hg
2. All of the following are features of warm shock **except**:
   (A) Decreased cardiac output
   (B) Decreased systemic vascular resistance
   (C) Decreased mean arterial pressure
   (D) Decreased central venous pressure
3. What is the drug of choice for cardiogenic shock:
   (A) Dopamine
   (B) Dobutamine
   (C) Epinephrine
   (D) Norepinephrine
4. The normal anion gap is:
   (A) 4-11mEq/L
   (B) 12-16 mEq/L
   (C) 17-20 mEq/L
   (D) 21-26 mEq/L

Answers:

1. B

   <70 mm Hg

2. A

Decreased cardiac output
3. B
   Dobutamine
4. A
   4-11mEq/L

Reference:
1. Turner DA and Cheifetz IM. Shock.In Nelson Textbook of Pediatrics.Kliegman RM, Stanton BF, Geme III, JW, Schor NF, Behrman RE (Eds) 19th Edition, Elsevier Saunders, Philadelphia, 2011; pages 306-311.

SUBACUTE SCLEROSING PANENCEPHALITIS
Dr. Lalit Takia, SR and Dr.Rashmi Kumar, Professor Pediatrics

A formerly healthy 4.5-year-old boy belonging to a rural background presented with a two-month history of frequent falls during walking.This was followed by frequent sudden, rapid movements of different parts of the body. His condition progressed to a bedridden state, followed by inability to talk and then inability to swallow and respond within 7 weeks after onset of symptoms.

The patient had a prior history suggestive of measles at age of 1.5 years. His developmental milestones prior to onset of illness had been normal.

On physical examination his Glasgow Coma Score was E2V2M4, pupils were normal in size and reaction and fundus examination was normal. Muscle tone was decreased and power was 3/5 in all limbs. No deep tendon reflexes were elicitable but Babinski's sign was positive bilaterally.
CSF analysis showed no cells, protein of 13 mg/dl and sugar of 70 mg/dl. IgG anti measles antibody was present in both cerebrospinal fluid and serum.
EEG showed typical burst suppression pattern.

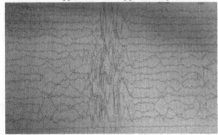

1. The clinical course of this patient is consistent with which of the following?
   (A) Stroke
   (B) Central nervous system infection
   (C) Degenerative brain disorder
   (D) Peripheral neuropathy
2. The following is true about Glasgow Coma Score:
   (A) The highest score is 10
   (B) The lowest score is 3
   (C) There are 4 domains of the score
   (D) Extension to deep painful stimulus gives a motor score of 3
3. Causes of burst suppression on EEG include all of the following EXCEPT:
   (A) Otohara syndrome
   (B) West syndrome
   (C) Severe birth asphyxia
   (D) Absence epilepsy
4. Which of the following is true about subacutesclerosingpanencephalitis ?
   (A) It is caused by modified measles virus persisting in the brain.
   (B) The average age of onset is 4 years
   (C) It is more common in girls
   (D) It never occurs after vaccination.

5. Which of the following features in this patient goes *against* the diagnosis?
    (A) Sudden rapid movements of different parts of his body
    (B) Rapid downhill course
    (C) Positive bilateral Babinski responses
    (D) Inability to swallow

Answers:
1. C
    Degenerative brain disorder
2. B
    The lowest score is 3
3. D
    Burst suppression on EEG is seen in disorders of grave prognosis. Absence epilepsy has a typical 3 per second spike and wave pattern.
4. A
5. B
    This patient has an unusually rapid course for his illness (subacute sclerosing Panencephalitis).

References:
1. Ghai OP Essential PediatricsEds Paul VK, Bagga A. 8thEdn, pp 583 CBS Publishers & Distributors, Delhi 2013
2. Lehman RK, Schor NF in Nelson Textbook of Pediatrics. EdsKliegman RM, Stanton BF, St Geme III, JW, Schor NF, Behrman RE 19th Edition, Elsevier Saunders, Philadelphia,2011; pages 2069-74.

TUBERCULOUS MENINGITIS
Dr. Abhinav Sharma, SR & Dr. Rashmi Kumar, Professor, Pediatrics

A5 year old girl child had been febrile for past one month.According to her parents she was peevish and irritable and her appetite was reduced.After three weeks suddenly child had 6-7 episodes of vomiting followed by 3 episodes of generalized tonic spasms, each lasting for about 10-15 minutes. Along with these she went into altered sensorium. The child had not received any vaccination apart from oral polio vaccine. Child's aunt had a history of pulmonary tuberculosis for which she was on treatment with category one anti-tubercular regimen. On examination Glasgow Coma score was 7 (E2V2M3), signs of meningeal irritation were present, tone was increased in all four limbs, power in all 4 limbs was 3/5, deep tendon reflexes were exaggerated (3+) and plantar responses were extensor bilaterally. Cranial nerve examination was normal. Lumbar puncture was done and CSF examination showed 200 cells/cc with 80% lymphocytes, sugar 60 mg/dl (concomitant blood sugar 110 mg/dl) and protein 210 mg/dl. Fundus examination revealed bilateral papilloedema. Contrast enhanced computed tomography brain showed meningeal enhancement, communicating hydrocephalus, basal exudates and periventricular ooze.

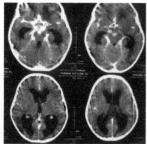

1. What is your diagnosis of the child on the basis of above findings?
    (A) Tubercular meningitis.
    (B) Pyogenic meningitis.
    (C) Acute encephalitis syndrome.
    (D) Brain abscess.
2. Which statement regarding BCG is **false**?
    (A) BCG is a live attenuated vaccine using Danish 1331 strain.

(B) BCG is contraindicated in immune-compromised host.

(C) Efficacy of vaccine varies from 50-80%.

(D) Maternal antibodies interfere against development of effective cellular immune response post-vaccination.

3. Patient's meningitis would fall in which stage?

(A) Stage of prodrome/invasion

(B) Stage of meningeal irritaion

(C) Stage of coma

(D) Stage of neurodeficit

4. The CSF findings in TB meningitis include?

(A) CSF sugar > 2/3 of plasma glucose + raised proteins + lymphocytosis

(B) CSF sugar< 2/3 of plasma glucose + low proteins + lymphocytosis

(C) CSF sugar< 2/3 of plasma glucose + raised proteins + lymphocytosis.

(D) CSF sugar > 2/3 of plasma glucose + raised proteins + lymphopenia.

5. All the following statements regarding tubercular meningitis are true **except**?

(A) Tubercular meningitis isa basal meningitis.

(B) Decerebrate posturing indicates poor prognosis.

(C) Steroids are not indicated in CNS tuberculosis.

(D) Intellectual disability may be a long term complication.

Answers:

1. A

A prodromal phase of three weeks prior to onset of seizures, history of contact and CSF findings suggest a diagnosis of tubercular meningitis rather than an acute process like viral encephalitis or bacterial meningitis.

2. D

BCG is a live attenuated vaccine manufactured using Danish 1331 strain, Pasteur and Glaxo. BCG vaccine is contraindicated in cellular immunodeficiency and symptomatic HIV. Efficacy of BCG vaccine is variable. Against severe forms of tuberculosis (eg. miliary and central nervous system tuberculosis efficacy is 80%) but against less severe forms of tuberculosis it is only 50%. Maternal antibodies do not interfere with development of effective cellular immunity, rather administration at birth ensures compliance and is convenient to implement.

3. B

Stages of CNS tuberculosis can be classified into :

1. Stage of prodrome/invasion: low grade fever, loss of appetite, disturbed sleep, vomiting, head banging and photophobia. Child becomes peevish, irritable and is not interested in play activities.

2. Stage of meningeal irritation: signs of meningeal irritation, increase muscle tone, motor deficits, delirium/stupor and convulsions.

3. Stage of coma: multiple cranial nerve palsies, coma, decerebrate and decorticate rigidity, Cheyne-Stokes or biot's breathing.

4. C

CSF findings in tubercular meningitis include raised CSF pressure 30-40 cm of H_2O, lymphocytic pleocytosis (100-500 cells/cc), elevated protein (more than 40 mg/dl), mild hypoglychorrachia (<2/3of plasma sugar) and low chloride (less than 600 mg/dl).

5. C

Tubercular meningitis is a basal menigitis with a propensity for basal areas of brain, cranial nerves, brain stem and basal ganglia. Decerebrate posturing , younger age and stage 3 disease carry poor prognosis. Steroids are indicated for 4-8 weeks in CNS tuberculosis. Intellectual disability, seizures, motor deficits, cranial nerve deficits, hydrocephalus, optic atrophy are common complications.

References:

1. Ghai OP et al. (2013) *Essentials Of Pediatrics. Tubercular meningitis.* New Delhi: CBS, 566-68.

2. Seth V, Kabra SK. (2011). *Essentials of tuberculosis in children. Neurotuberculosis.* New Delhi: Jaypee, 144-93.

WEST SYNDROME

Dr. Rashmi Kumar, Professor, Department of Pediatrics

A 5 month male infant is brought to the pediatric OPD with history of not smiling, not recognizing mother and not holding head. The baby had a history of full term normal vaginal birth with 'normal' birth weight but did not cry at once. He was revived with difficulty and shifted to newborn intensive care unit and kept there for 9 days on oxygen and intravenous fluids besides other treatment. On specifically asking his mother admitted that he also 'startles' several times a day, without apparent reason, especially on awakening from sleep, with sudden flexion of head and limbs.

On examination, weight was 6 kg; baby had increased tone in all 4 limbs, head circumference of 40 cm and ill sustained ankle clonus bilaterally. Developmental age conformed to about 6 weeks. Other examination was unremarkable.

MRI brain was done and was reported as multicysticencephalomalacia. EEG is shown below.

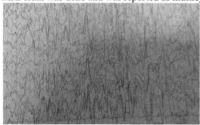

1. What is the EEG diagnosis?
   (A) Generalised seizure
   (B) Hypsarrhythmia
   (C) Myoclonic epilepsy
   (D) Absence seizures
2. What is the clinical diagnosis?
   (A) Lennox Gastaut syndrome
   (B) West syndrome
   (C) Otohara syndrome
   (D) Landau Kleffner syndrome
3. Treatment should include which of the following?
   (A) Phenobarb
   (B) Carbamazepine
   (C) Phenytoin
   (D) ACTH
4. What are the type of seizures?
   (A) Epileptic spasms
   (B) Absence seizures
   (C) Generalised tonic seizures
   (D) Myoclonic seizures
5. At what age should the infant develop social smile?
   (A) 2 weeks
   (B) One month
   (C) 2 – 3 months
   (D) 4 months

Answers:

1. B
   Chaotic record without a proper baseline – hypsarrhythmia
2. B
   Syndrome is West syndrome – a triad of epileptic spasms, developmental delay or regression and hypsarrhythmia on EEG. It is the most common epileptic encephalopathy.
3. D
   ACTH is given
4. A
   Seizures are epileptic spasms
5. C
   Social smile normally develops by about 2 months of age. If not present by 3 months, it is definitely delayed.

References:

1. Fenichel GM Pediatric Neurology : a signs and symptoms approach 6th Edition (South Asia), Saunders 2009 pg 19-20

2. MikatiMA Seizures in childhood in Nelson Textbook of Pediatrics. EdsKleigmanRM, Stanton BF, Schor NF, St Geme JW, Behrman RE 19thEdn Elsevier (Saunders), South Asia, 2011; pp 2013-37.

CYSTIC FIBROSIS

Dr Krishna Kumar Yadav, ICMR Fellow, Department of Pediatrics

A 2year old male child resident of Sitapur district presented with chief complains of recurrent episodes of chest infections and wheezing. Baby was delivered in a government hospital at term gestation with birth weight of 2.8 kg through normal vaginal route. There was history of meconium ileus in neonatal period, otherwise neonatal period was unremarkable. Mile stones were age appropriate and immunized as per age. Current weight is 6.5 kg and height is 65 cm. General examination showed presence of mild grade of pallor, Clubbing grade II in all fingers and features of Vit D deficiency like frontal bossing, rachitic rosary and widening of wrist. There was no icterus, edema, lymphadenopathy. Skin was healthy. In systemic examinations, Cardiovascular, Central Nervous System and Abdominal system were unremarkable. Respiratory system showed normal shape and movement of chest and bilateral coarse crepitations present all over chest fields during all phases of respiration. No other respiratory findings were remarkable. X ray chest showed bilateral central bronchiectatic changes. There is no history of recurrent sinus infections, chronic diarrhoea, rectal prolapse, pancreatitis.

1. What is **false** about cystic fibrosis
   A) CFTR mutation
   B) Screening at neonatal period is possible
   C) Pulmonary function may show combined obstructive and restrictive pattern of disease
   D) W 1282X mutation is least prevalent mutation in cystic fibrosis in Ashkenazi Jews population
2. Inheritance pattern of Cystic Fibrosis
   A) Autosomal Dominance
   B) Autosomal Recessive
   C) X linked Recessive
   D) Mosaic pattern
3. Most common mutation of cystic fibrosis
   A) W1282X
   B) Delta F 508
   C) TGF b1
   D) MBL/IRFD1
4. Which is **false** about Cystic Fibrosis
   A) Occurrence of Liver disease can be predicted by CFTR genotype.
   B) CFTR mutation has resistance (protective) to cholera toxins or infectious dysenteries.
   C) Polymorphism of IRFD1 gene, has been associated with a more serious Cystic fibrosis
   D) Variant allele of Mannose Binding Lectin (MBL) are more associated with more serious lung infections
5. Diagnosis of cystic fibrosis can be established by all **except**
   A) Clinical features with two times sweat chloride more than 60 meq/l
   B) Clinical features with identification of two CF mutations
   C) Clinical features with an abnormal nasal potential difference measurement
   D) Clinical features with history of proven CF in sibling

Answers:
1. D
   W 1282X mutation is most prevalent mutation (>60%) in cystic fibrosis in Ashkenazi Jews population
2. B
   Cystic fibrosis is inherited as autosomal recessive trait.
3. B
   The most prevalent mutation of CFTR is the deletion of a single phenylalanine residue at amino acid 508 (delta F 508)
4. A
   Occurrence of Liver disease can not be predicted by CFTR genotype.
5. D
   Cystic Fibrosis is diagnosed as Clinical features with a-Two times sweat chloride more than 60 meq/l or b- Two CF mutations c- An abnormal nasal potential difference measurement

Reference:
1. Marie Egan. Cystic Fibrosis. In:Kliegman RM, Stanton BF, Geme JW, Schor NF, Behrman RE (Eds.). Nelson Textbook of Pediatrics.19th Edition, Saunders, Philadelphia PA, 2012, pp.1481-97.

PYOTHORAX / EMPEMA
Dr Krishna Kumar Yadav, ICMR Fellow, Department of Pediatrics

A 5 year old boy residence of Faizabad, studying in 1st standard, presented in paediatrics emergency with chief complains of fever since 5 days, continuous, high grade and associated with chills. Taken some oral medicines but not relieved. He also developed respiratory distress since one day. On general examination, oriented to time place and person, lying on couch in left lateral position, febrile, dyspnoeic with head nodding and nasal flaring. Pulse euvolumic, no pulse deficit, no radio-femoral delay, BP 110/64mm Hg, capillary refill time<3 seconds, SpO2 at room air 94%. There is no pallor, icterus, clubbing, edema, lymphadenopathy and cyanosis. Systemic examinations cardiovascular and central nervous system were unremarkable. Respiratory system showed decreased movement left side, mediastinal shift towards right, decreased air entry left side and bilateral crepts. Abdominal system were unremarkable except just palpable spleen. X ray chest done and shown here

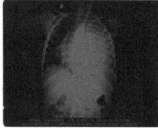

1. Most likely diagnosis is
   A) Congenial heart disease with cardiomegaly
   B) Complicated community acquired pneumonia
   C) Infective endocarditis with congestive heart failure
   D) Complicated malaria/ severe malaria
2. Most common bacteria resulting in empyema
   A) Staphylococcus aureus
   B) Streptococcus pneumonia
   C) Klebsiella pneumonia
   D) Hemophilusinfluenzae B
3. Which is **not** a radiological feature of empyema
   A) Ipsilateral widening of ribs
   B) Contralateral pushed down diaphragm
   C) Ipsilateral homogenous opacity
   D) Contralateral shift of cardiac shadow
4. All **except** are true of pleurocentesis in empyema
   A) pH < 7.20
   B) Polymorphic leucocytosis
   C) Protein>3.5gm/dl
   D) Glucose > 50 mg/dl
5. Treatment of empyema includes all **except**
   A) Systemic Antibiotics
   B) Tube Thoracocentesis
   C) Video assisted thoracoscopic surgery(VATS) before use of fibrinolytic agents
   D) In case, extensive fibrosis open thoracotomy

Answers:
1. B
   Empyema is an accumulation of pus in the pleural space. It is most often associated with pneumonia due to *Streptococcus pneumoniae* and characterised by fever with chills, increased work of breathing and often appears more ill.
2. A

Empyema is most often associated with pneumonia due to *Streptococcus pneumoniae*, although *Staphylococcus aureus* is most often in developing nations and Asia.

3. B
    Radiological findings of empyema includes homogenous opacity, widening of ribs and shifting of diaphragm down on same side and opposite shift of mediastinum.

4. D
    Pleural fluid examinations in empyema is turbid colour, gram staining suggestive of bacteria, pH < 7.20,sugar < 50 mg/dl, Protein more than 3.5 gm/dl, LDH > 2/3 rd of Plasma.

5. C
    Treatment of empyema includes Systemic antibiotics, Tube toracocentesis. If fever persist beyond 72 hrs, then use of fibrinolytic agents are indicated. After use of fibrinolytic agents if fever persist then VATS is indicated and in case of presence of extensive fibrosis open thoracotomy is indicated.

Reference:

1. Winnie GB, LossefSV.Purulent Pleurisy or empyema. In:Kliegman RM, Stanton BF, Geme JW, Schor NF, Behrman RE (Eds.). Nelson Textbook of Pediatrics.19th Edition, Saunders, Philadelphia PA, 2012, pp.1507-09.

Chapter-19

Pharmacology

OPIOID DRUGS
Dr. K. K. Pant, Professor, Department of Pharmacology & Therapeutics

A 70 year-old man is diagnosed with small cell lung cancer with extensive metastasis. The patient is also complaining of excruciating pain all over the chest, vertebral column and pelvis. Along with anticancer drugs, patient is also prescribed analgesic drug to control pain.

1. Use of which pain medication is most suitable in the given situation?
   (A) Acetaminophen
   (B) Ibuprofen
   (C) Ketorolac
   (D) Morphine
2. Which opioid receptor subtype is responsible for most of the dysphoric or negative psychological side effects of opioids such as an *"ill-feeling"* or *"seeing spiders on the wall"*?
   (A) δ
   (B) κ
   (C) μ
   (D) σ
3. Which of the following is **NOT** a sign of morphine overdose?
   (A) Respiratory depression
   (B) Miosis
   (C) Hypertension
   (D) Coma
4. Preferred drug for morphine poisoning is:
   (A) Naltrexone
   (B) Naloxone
   (C) Nalmephene
   (D) Methyl naltrexone
5. Morphine depresses all of the following **EXCEPT**:
   (A) Respiratory centre
   (B) Cough centre
   (C) Temperature regulating centre
   (D) Vagal centre

Answers:
   1.　　D
   　　　In presence of severe pain, the opioids are the preferred drugs.
   2.　　B
   　　　κ-receptor activation is responsible for dysphoric or negative psychological side effects.
   3.　　C
   　　　Respiratory depression, miosis, hypotension, and coma are signs of morphine overdose.
   4.　　B
   　　　Naloxone specificity is such that reversal by this agent is virtually diagnostic for the contribution of an opiate to the depression. It acts rapidly to reverse the respiratory depression associated with high doses of opioids.
   5.　　D
   　　　Opioids suppress cough centre, temperature regulating centre and vasomotor centre; Opioids stimulate Chemoreceptor Trigger Zone, Edinger Westphal nucleus, and vagal centre.

References:
   1. Welch SP, Martin BR. Opioid and nonopioid analgesics. In: Craig CR, Stizel RE, editors. Modern pharmacology with clinical applications. 5th ed. Boston (MA): Little, Brown & Company; 1997. p. 327-9.
   2. Tripathi KD. Essentials of medical pharmacology. 7th ed. New Delhi: Jaypee Brothers Medical Publishers; 2013. p. 470-1.
   3. Yaksh TL, Wallace MS. Opioids, analgesia and pain management. In: Brunton LL, Chabner BA, Knollmann BC, editors. Goodman & Gilman's the pharmacological basis of therapeutics. 12th ed. New York: Mc Graw-Hill; 2011. p. 481-525.

ANTIRETROVIRAL DRUG

Dr. K. K. Pant, Professor, Department of Pharmacology & Therapeutics

Mr X is HIV positive and has been prescribed zidovudine, lamivudine and nevirapine for the past 6 months. Following this treatment, his condition improved and plasma viral load reached to undetectable level (< 50 copies of HIV- RNA/ml). However he was found to have hepatic dysfunction.

1. Which drug amongst the three is responsible for hepatic dysfunction?
   (A) Zidovudine
   (B) Lamivudine
   (C) Nevirapine
   (D) All of the above
2. What is false statement regarding highly active antiretroviral therapy (HAART)?
   (A) The use of combination HAART should be the standard medical care for all patients
   (B) Didanosine and stavudine combination should be avoided owing to an increased risk of pancreatitis and neuropathy
   (C) Zidovudine and stavudine should be used together because these agents are synergistic
   (D) If Protease Inhibitor (PI) based HAART is desired, ritonavir-boosted regimens are preferred
3. The mechanism of action of Nevirapine is:
   (A) Nucleoside reverse transcriptase inhibitor
   (B) Nonnucleoside reverse transcriptase inhibitor
   (C) Protease Inhibitor
   (D) Fusion inhibitor
4. Common adverse effects associated with Nucleoside reverse transcriptase inhibitors (NRTIs) include:
   (A) Bone marrow suppression
   (B) Central fat accumulation and peripheral fat wasting
   (C) Drug interactions involving cytochrome P450 enzymes
   (D) Dyslipidemia and insulin resistance
5. Drugs effective against retrovirus are all **EXCEPT**:
   (A) Raltegravir
   (B) Enfuvertide
   (C) Famciclovir
   (D) Ritonavir

Answers:

1. C
   Elevated hepatic transaminases and severe hepatitis has been associated with nevirapine use.
2. C
   Stavudine and zidovudine exhibit mutual antagonism by competing for the same activation pathway.
3. B
   Nevirapine is nucleoside unrelated compound which directly inhibits HIV reverse transcriptase without the need for intracellular phosphorylation.
4. A
   Myelotoxicity is associated with NRTI. Fat redistribution, drug interactions involving CYP3A4, dyslipidemia, and diabetic symptoms are all side effects commonly associated with protease inhibitors.
5. C
   Famciclovir inhibits H. simplex, H. zoster and some activity against hepatitis B virus (HBV) also has been noted.

References:

1. Dyke KV, Woodfork K. Therapy of human immunodeficiency virus. In: Craig CR, Stizel RE, editors. Modern pharmacology with clinical applications. 5th ed. Boston (MA): Little, Brown & Company; 1997. p. 593-5.
2. Flexner C. Antiretroviral agents and treatment of HIV Infection. In: Brunton LL, Chabner BA, Knollmann BC, editors. Goodman & Gilman's the pharmacological basis of therapeutics. 12th ed. New York: Mc Graw-Hill; 2011. p. 1623-64.
3. Tripathi KD. Essentials of medical pharmacology. 7th ed. New Delhi: Jaypee Brothers Medical Publishers; 2013. p. 798-815.

CORTICOSTEROIDS

Dr. K. K. Pant, Professor, Department of Pharmacology & Therapeutics

A 20 year old female who is a known asthmatic presented to the emergency with the complaint of severe breathlessness which was sudden in onset. She was so breathless that she was not even able to complete her sentences. Intensive bronchodilator therapy was started, but there was no improvement in her condition. 100 mg of hydrocortisone was given intravenously as a bolus followed by 100 mg 8 hourly by i.v. infusion. The patient showed a positive response to this treatment and was later shifted to 50 mg of prednisolone orally.

1. Amongst corticosteroids, why was hydrocortisone chosen for the above condition?
   - (A) Most efficacious
   - (B) Most rapid onset of action
   - (C) Slow rate of elimination
   - (D) More volume of distribution
2. Why are synthetic steroids **NOT** preferred in this condition?
   - (A) Because synthetic steroids have a low volume of distribution
   - (B) Because synthetic steroids have low plasma protein binding capacity
   - (C) Because synthetic steroids must be enzymatically reduced to their biologically active forms
   - (D) Because synthetic steroids have a rapid onset of action
3. Hydrocortisone induces the synthesis of the following protein which in turn inhibits the enzyme phospholipase-A_2:
   - (A) Heat shock protein-90
   - (B) Inhibin
   - (C) Transcortin
   - (D) Annexins
4. Which of the following is the correct statement for hydrocortisone?
   - (A) Glucocorticoid with minimum mineralocorticoid activity
   - (B) Glucocorticoid with maximum mineralocorticoid activity
   - (C) Mineralocorticoid with maximum glucocorticoid activity
   - (D) Mineralocorticoid with minimum glucocorticoid activity
5. Following are the contraindications for corticosteroid therapy **EXCEPT**:
   - (A) Peptic ulcer
   - (B) Psychosis
   - (C) Systemic Lupus Erythematosus
   - (D) Osteoporosis

Answers:
1. B
   Hydrocortisone is the steroid of choice because it has the most rapid onset (5-6 hours after administration), compared with 8 hours of prednisolone.
2. C
   Status asthmaticus is an emergency situation where rapid onset of action is required. Therefore, those steroids should be used which do not require enzymatic activation.
3. D
   Glucocorticoids inhibit Phospholipase A_2 by inducing the synthesis of a group of proteins termed annexins or lipocortins that modulate PLA_2 activity.
4. B
   Hydrocortisone is a glucocorticoid which has got significant mineralocorticoid activity as well.
5. C
   Corticosteroids are needed in collagen diseases such as systemic lupus erythematosus.

References:
1. Barnes PJ. Pulmonary pharmacology. In: Brunton LL, Chabner BA, Knollmann BC, editors. Goodman & Gilman's the pharmacological basis of therapeutics. 12th ed. New York: Mc Graw-Hill; 2011. p. 1031-66.
2. Schimmer BP, Funder JW. ACTH, adrenal steroids, and pharmacology of the adrenal cortex. In: Brunton LL, Chabner BA, Knollmann BC, editors. Goodman & Gilman's the pharmacological basis of therapeutics.12th ed. New York: Mc Graw-Hill; 2011. p. 1209-36.
3. Smyth EM, Grosser T, FitzGerald GA. Lipid-derived autacoids: Eicosanoids and platelet activating factor. In: Brunton LL, Chabner BA, Knollmann BC, editors. Goodman & Gilman's the pharmacological basis of therapeutics. 12th ed. New York: Mc Graw-Hill; 2011. p. 937-58.

ORGANOPHOSPHORUS POISONING

Dr. A. K. Saksena, Professor, Department of Pharmacology & Therapeutics

A 35 year old male, came in medical emergency unit with excessive salivation and sweating. He was also suffering from difficulty in breathing, colic pains, diarrhoea and involuntary urination. History further revealed that the patient was farmer by occupation and his problems started 4-5 hours before, when he came back from his fields after spraying insecticide on his crop. He had taken his meals also in the field itself. Physical examination revealed- miosis, ronchi and coarse crepitations, BP was 80/50 mm of Hg. A probable diagnosis of organophosphorus poisoning was made.

1. The organophosphorus compounds produce poisoning by:
   (A) Acting as agonist on muscarinic cholinergic receptors
   (B) Increasing release of acetylcholine from cholinergic neurones
   (C) Blocking re-uptake of acetylcholine in nerve terminals
   (D) Inhibiting the activity of cholinesterase enzyme
2. The antidote of organophosphorus poisoning is:
   (A) Atropine
   (B) Adrenaline
   (C) Physostigmine
   (D) Neostigmine
3. The long term treatment of organophosphorus poisoning is:
   (A) Pantoprazole
   (B) Propantheline
   (C) Pralidoxime
   (D) Pipanzolate
4. If a patient of organophosphorus poisoning develops seizures, then which of the following drug is given by intravenous route?
   (A) Sod. thiopentone
   (B) Phenobarbitone
   (C) Sod. Valproate
   (D) Diazepam

Answers:
   1. D
      Organophosphorus compounds are irreversible inhibitors of cholinesterase enzyme.
   2. A
      Atropine is a competitive antagonist at muscarinic receptors.
   3. C
      Pralidoxime re-activates the enzyme cholinesterase.
   4. D
      Diazepam is the drug of choice for drug induced convulsions.

References:
   1. Tripathi KD. Essentials of medical pharmacology. 6th ed. New Delhi: Jaypee Brothers Medical Publishers; 2008. p. 104-5.
   2. Osterhoudt KC, Penning TM. Drug toxicity and poisoning. In: Brunton LL, Chabner BA, Knollmann BC, editors. Goodman & Gilman's the pharmacological basis of therapeutics. 12th ed. New York: Mc Graw-Hill; 2011. p. 73-87.

MYASTHENIA GRAVIS

Dr. A. K. Saksena, Professor, Department of Pharmacology & Therapeutics

A 50 year old woman presented in out patient department of ophthalmology with double vision for last 4-5 months, which used to increase in the evening. Her problem was slow in onset but was gradually increasing. She was prescribed correction glasses also but was not relieved. History also revealed that of late she used to get tired early. On examination the pulse was 80/min. and blood pressure was 140/86 mm of Hg. There was no sensory loss however ptosis was found to be present- right eye was affected more than left eye. A probable diagnosis of Myasthenia gravis was made.

1. Which investigation is required to confirm the diagnosis?
   (A) MRI head

(B) CT head
(C) Edrophonium test
(D) d-Tubocurarine test
2. What is the aetiology of myasthenia gravis?
    (A) It is an infective disorder
    (B) It is a degenerative disorder
    (C) It is an auto-immune disorder
    (D) It is an ischaemic disorder
3. What is the preferred drug for myasthenia gravis?
    (A) Physostigmine
    (B) Neostigmine
    (C) Edrophonium
    (D) Rivastigmine
4. Which of the following is used for treatment of myasthenia gravis?
    (A) Gabapentin
    (B) Levodopa
    (C) Methylcobalamine
    (D) Glucocorticoids

Answers:

1. C
    Edrophonium is a very short acting reversible cholinesterase inhibitor. Intravenous injection of edrophonium increases the power of skeletal muscles, thus, improves the symptoms of myasthenia gravis.
2. C
    Myasthenia gravis is an auto-immune disorder in which antibodies are formed against nicotinic cholinergic receptors.
3. B
    Neostigmine is less lipid soluble as compared to physostigmine, hence it is used for treatment of myasthenia gravis.
4. D
    Glucocorticoids act as immunosuppressant and inhibit the formation of auto-antibodies against nicotinic cholinergic receptors.

Reference:

1. KD Tripathi. Essentials of medical pharmacology. 6th ed. New Delhi: Jaypee Brothers Medical Publishers; 2008. p. 102-4.

HYPERTENSIVE CRISIS

Dr. A. K. Saksena, Professor, Department of Pharmacology & Therapeutics

An elderly male aged about 64 years presented in medical emergency with severe headache, vertigo and epistaxis. He was known hypertensive and was taking a Atenolol 100 mg and Hydrochlorthiazide 12.5 mg per day, however, he had stopped taking these medications for last two days. On examination his blood pressure was recorded to be 220/124 mm Hg and papilodema was also present. He was diagnosed as a case of hypertensive crisis.

1. What is the preferred drug for hypertensive crisis?
    (A) Glyceryl trinitrate
    (B) Sodium valproate
    (C) Telmisartan
    (D) Sodium nitroprusside
2. Which of the following route is employed for administration of sodium nitroprusside?
    (A) Sublingual
    (B) Intravenous
    (C) Intraarterial
    (D) Intramuscular
3. What is the onset of action of sodium nitroprusside when given by intravenous route?
    (A) 30 seconds

(B) 60 seconds
(C) 90 seconds
(D) 120 seconds
4. Which of the following is a toxic effect of sodium nitroprusside:
   (A) Bleeding episode
   (B) Cyanide poisoning
   (C) Myocardial infraction
   (D) Cerebrovascular accident

Answers:

1. D
   Sodium nitroprusside dilates both arteries and veins so it produces more fall in blood pressure.
2. B
   To get rapid fall in blood pressure and for controlled administration, sodium nitroprusside is administered by intravenous infusion.
3. A
   The onset of action is approximately 30 seconds.
4. B
   After metabolism, sodium nitroprusside produces cyanide radicals, hence poisoning may be produced in larger doses.

References:

1. Tripathi KD. Essentials of medical pharmacology. 7th ed. New Delhi: Jaypee Brothers Medical Publishers; 2013. p. 572-4.
2. Michel T, Hoffman BB. Treatment of myocardial Ischaemia and Hypertension. In: Brunton LL, Chabner BA, Knollmann BC, editors. Goodman & Gilman's the pharmacological basis of therapeutics. 12th ed. New York: Mc Graw-Hill; 2011. p. 745-88.

ANTIAMOEBIC DRUGS

Dr. R. K. Dixit, Professor, Department of Pharmacology & Therapeutics

A 58 years old alcoholic male develops amoebic dysentery for which he took medicine. After that he developed severe headache, flushing of face. After few days he develops neuropsychiatric disorders and doctor told to attendants that patient has developed hepatic coma (due to long term use of alcohol which caused hepatic cirrhosis). He was prescribed lactulose along with one antimicrobial agent and slowly he recovered.

1. What is the name of clinical condition the patient developed after taking anti-amoebic drug?
   (A) Disulfiram like reaction
   (B) Stevens-Johnson syndrome
   (C) Red man syndrome
   (D) Alcohol withdrawal syndrome
2. Which drug might have caused the flushing, and severe headache?
   (B) Metronidazole
   (C) Diloxinide furoate
   (D) Ivermectine
   (D) Tetracyclin
3. Inhibition of which enzyme was responsible for the patient flushing and headache?
   (A) Alcohol dehydrogenase
   (B) Aldehyde dehydrogenase
   (C) Alcohol synthetase
   (D) Aldehyde polymerase
4. Which antimicrobial was prescribed along with lactulose for managing the hepatic coma?
   (A) Amikacin
   (B) Gentamicin
   (C) Streptomycin
   (D) Neomycin

Answers:

1. A
   Disulfiram like reaction is the name of condition which is produced in alcoholics who take drugs like metronidazole.

2. A

Metronidazole produces disulfiram like reaction.

3. B

Inhibition of aldehyde dehydrognease by disufiram, metronidazole, cefoperazone produced accumulation of acetaldehyde leading to aldehyde syndrome manifesting in form of severe headache & flushing.

4. D

Hepatic coma is due to increased entry of ammonia from blood to the brain. Ammonia is produced mainly in the intestine by action of microbes. Neomycin is an amino- glycoside which is not absorbed in gut but kills the microbes present inside intestine there by reducing the production of ammonia.

References:

1. Rosenthal PJ. Antiprotozoal drugs. In: Katzung BG, Masters SB, Trevor AJ, editors. Basic and clinical pharmacology. 11th ed. New Delhi: Tata Mc Graw-Hill; 2010. p. 899-921.
2. Tripathi KD. Essentials of medical pharmacology. 6th ed. New Delhi: Jaypee Brothers Medical Publishers; 2008. p. 380-7.
3. Tripathi KD. Essentials of medical pharmacology. 6th ed. New Delhi: Jaypee Brothers Medical Publishers; 2008. p. 719-26.

PSEUDOMEMBRANOUS ENTEROCOLITIS
Dr. R. K. Dixit, Professor, Department of Pharmacology & Therapeutics

A 74 years woman developed bloody diarrhoea after three days of treatment with an antibiotic for pneumonia. Her stool was tested positive for clostridium difficile toxin. Her antibiotic was stopped immediately and a new drug was administered for the treatment of bloody diarrhoea.

1. Which of the following is correct regarding diarrhoea of this female?
   (A) She developed amoebic diarrhoea
   (B) She developed fungal diarrhoea
   (C) She developed pseudomembranous colitis
   (D) She developed viral diarrhoea
2. Which of the following drug was prescribed for the treatment of diarrhoea to this female?
   (A) Streptomycin
   (B) Ampicillin
   (C) Neomycin
   (D) Metronidazole
3. Which of the following drug is **NOT** likely to cause the diarrhoea of this female?
   (A) Clindamycin
   (B) Ampicillin
   (C) Lincomycin
   (B) Vancomycin

Answers:
   1. C

   Clostridium difficile produced bloody diarrhoea by causing pseudomembrenous colitis.

   2. D

   Metronidazole, and vancomycin are drugs for the treatment of pseudomembrenous colitis.

   3. D

   Vancomycin is used for treatment of pseudomembrenous colitis.

References:

1. Chambers HF, Deck DH. Beta lactam and other cell wall and membrane active antibiotics. In: Katzung BG, Masters SB, Trevor AJ, editors. Basic and clinical pharmacology. 11th ed. New Delhi: Tata Mc Graw-Hill; 2010. p. 773-93.
2. Tripathi KD. Essentials of medical pharmacology. 6th ed. New Delhi: Jaypee Brothers Medical Publishers; 2008. p. 667-81,732.
3. Tripathi KD. Essentials of medical pharmacology. 6th ed. New Delhi: Jaypee Brothers Medical Publishers; 2008. p. 727-38.

SULPHONAMIDES

Dr. R. K. Dixit, Professor, Department of Pharmacology & Therapeutics

A female with history of nine month pregnancy suffered from urinary tract infection. She was prescribed antimicrobials for one week for this condition. She delivered a baby which was jaundiced. The baby was managed by giving phenobarbitone.

1. Which of the following was responsible for the jaundice in preterm new born baby?
   (A) Ampicillin
   (B) Gentamicin
   (C) Streptomycin
   (D) Sulphamethoxazole
2. In premature new born baby kernicterus can be caused by which of the following?
   (A) Reduced binding site of bilirubin with albumin
   (B) Reduced glomerular filtration of bilirubin
   (C) Reduced conjugation of bilirubin in liver
   (D) Reduced distruction of bilirubin in skin
3. What is the name of condition in which the bilirubin concentration in premature neonate in brain increases?
   (A) Kernicterus
   (B) Icterus
   (C) Cortical degeneration
   (D) Cerebellar degeneration
4. What is the mechanism of action by which phenobarbitone improved the above neonate condition?
   (A) Increased metabolism of bilirubin
   (B) Increased albumin binding of bilirubin
   (C) Decreased albumin binding of bilirubin
   (D) Decreased metabolism of bilirubin

Answers:

1. D
   Sulphonamides cross placental barrier and enter in the foetus. In foetus they bind with albumin and displace the bilirubin from the albumin binding sites. The free albumin becomes more in the blood and leads to development of severe jaundice in the newborn.

2. A
   Kernicterus is caused by binding of albumin with sulphonamides and displacing bilirubin from the binding sites.

3. A
   The name of increased concentration of bilirubin reaching in the brain of newborn is called kernicterus. The bilirubin gets deposited in the basal ganglia of new born.

4. A
   Phenobarbitone is microsomal enzyme inducer and enhances the metabolism of bilirubin leading to reduction in bilirubin concentration of baby.

References:

1. Chambers HF, Deck DH. Sulphonamides, trimethoprim & quinolones. In: Katzung BG, Masters SB, Trevor AJ, editors. Basic and clinical pharmacology. 11th ed. New Delhi: Tata Mc Graw-Hill; 2010. p. 815-7.
2. Tripathi KD. Essentials of medical pharmacology. 6th ed. New Delhi: Jaypee Brothers Medical Publishers; 2008. p. 682-93.

TUBERCULOSIS

Dr. Rajendra Nath, Professor, Department of Pharmacology & Therapeutics

A 37 year old women presenting with cough for 2 months, off and on pyrexia of mild to moderate degree & diminution in appetite . She has multiple cervical lymph nodes & her X- ray chest (PA –view) has shown the following findings:-Bilateral hilar enlargement (right>left)

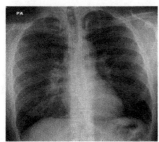

1. Suspecting tuberculosis in the above patient which of the following antitubercular agent has best action against slow multiplying intracellular bacteria ?
   (A) Isoniazid
   (B) Rifampicin
   (C) Pyrazinamide
   (D) Ethambutol
2. Suppose the above patient after 2 months of anti-tuberculosis therapy (ATT) (rifampin + pyrazinzmide + isoniazid + ethambutol) develops numbness & parasthesia (peripheral neuropathy) in the limbs, which of the following drugs may be responsible for this complaint ?
   (A) Rifampicin
   (B) Pyrazinamid
   (C) Isoniazid
   (D) Ethambutol
3. To treat the above patient's complaint of numbness & parasthesia (peripheral neuropathy), which of the following drug is given ?
   (A) Thiamine
   (B) Riboflavin
   (C) Cynocobalamine
   (D) Pyridoxine
4. Suppose the above patient is having 12 weeks pregnancy, which one of the following drug should be avoided?
   (A) Isoniazid
   (B) Ethambutol
   (C) Streptomycin
   (D) Rifampicin
5. Which Antitubercular drug is implicated in transient memory loss?
   (A) Ethambutol
   (B) Isoniazid
   (C) Ethionamide
   (D) Pyrazinamide

Answers:
   1. C
       Suitable drug for slow multiplying intracellular bacteria is Pyrazinamide,isoniazid also as intra as well as extracellular action but in rapidly multiplyingbacteria. Rifampicin is also equally effective on intra as well as extracellularbacteria but more on dormant & in caseous lesions. Ethambutol is bacteristaticdrug.
   2. C
       INH is the only drug in above mentioned alternatives which causes peripheral neuropathy on prolonged use resulting in numbness & paraesthesia.
   3. D
       Pyridoxin (vitamin B6) is administered for the prevention & treatment of isoniazid induced peripheral neuropathy.
   4. C
       Streptomycin is absolutely contra-indicated in pregnant female as it can cause deafness in the new born.
   5. B
       Mental abnormalities such as euphoria, transient impairment of memory and florid psychosis may appear during the use of isoniazid.

References:
1. Gumbo T. Chemotherapy of tuberculosis, mycobacterium avium complex disease, and leprosy. In: Brunton LL, Chabner BA, Knollmann BC, editors. Goodman & Gilman's the pharmacological basis of therapeutics. 12th ed. New York: Mc Graw-Hill; 2011. p. 1549-70.
2. Tripathi KD. Essentials of medical pharmacology. 7th ed. New Delhi: Jaypee Brothers Medical Publishers; 2013. p. 765-79.

ANGINA

Dr. Anuradha Nischal, Professor, Department of Pharmacology & Therapeutics

A 55 year old man presented with complaints of tightness and discomfort over middle part of chest felt episodically, particularly after walking briskly or climbing stairs. This is relieved within 5-10 minutes of rest. One or two episodes occur daily. He was a chronic smoker. Four years ago he was diagnosed to be suffering from chronic obstructive pulmonary disease (COPD) subsequent to which he quit smoking. He has been prescribed ipratropium and salbutamol inhalations twice daily which he is taking regularly. On examination pulse was 90/min, BP 120/80 mm Hg. Resting ECG was normal, but stress test was positive. It was diagnosed as a case of exertional angina.

1. What therapy would you give this patient on SOS basis?
    (A) Nicorandil
    (B) Glyceryltrinitrate
    (C) Clopidogrel
    (D) Atorvastatin
2. Should he be prescribed another drug on regular basis to prevent episodes of angina? If so which drug can be given?
    (A) Nicorandil
    (B) Glyceryltrinitrate
    (C) Clopidogrel
    (D) Amlodipine
3. What is the preferred route of administration of glyceryltrinitrate in the above patient?
    (A) Subcutaneous
    (B) Sublingual
    (C) Transdermal
    (D) Intranasal
4. Which of the following phenomenon is **NOT** seen with nitrates when used in angina?
    (A) Tolerance
    (B) Cross tolerance
    (C) Cumulation
    (D) Dependence

Answers:
1. B
    Glyceryltrinitrate is effective in angina for terminating an acute attack where it is taken on 'as and when required basis'.
2. C
    Clopidogrel is an anti-platelet drug which is very helpful in preventing ischaemic episodes and is utilized for checking restenosis of stented coronaries, thus effectively preventing the episodes of angina.
3. B
    The sublingual route is used when termination of an attack of angina is the aim. It acts within 1-2 minutes because of direct absorption into systemic circulation.
4. C
    Tolerance, cross tolerance and dependence are commonly observed with nitrates when used in angina.

References:
1. Michel T, Hoffman BB. Treatment of myocardial ischemia and hypertension. In: Brunton LL, Chabner BA, Knollmann BC, editors. Goodman & Gilman's the pharmacological basis of therapeutics. 12th ed. New York: Mc Graw-Hill; 2011. p. 745-88.

2.   Tripathi KD. Essentials of medical pharmacology. 7th ed. New Delhi: Jaypee Brothers Medical Publishers; 2013. p. 539-57.
3.   Tripathi KD. Essentials of medical pharmacology. 7th ed. New Delhi: Jaypee Brothers Medical Publishers; 2013. p. 613-33.

ORGANOPHOSPHATE POISONING
Dr. Anuradha Nischal, Professor, Department of Pharmacology & Therapeutics

A farmer 35 years of age was admitted in the emergency in comatose state. He had history of profuse sweating, lacrimation, diarrhoea and urination. On examination, the pupil was pin point, heart rate was 102/min, blood pressure was 174/110 mmHg. He developed this condition while working in the field.

1. What is the preferred drug for this condition?
    (A) Oximes
    (B) Atropine
    (C) Acetylcholine
    (D) Adrenaline
2. Which enzyme is deactivated in this condition?
    (A) Pseudocholinesterase
    (B) Butylcholinesterase
    (C) Acetylcholinesterase
    (D) Plasma cholinesterase
3. Which of the following drugs cause constriction of pupil?
    (A) Acetylcholine
    (B) Adrenaline
    (C) Noradrenaline
    (D) Atropine
4. Pin point pupil is characteristic of:-
    (A) Belladona poisoning
    (B) Methanol poisoning
    (C) Digoxin poisoning
    (D) Organophosphate Poisoning

Answers:
1. B
    Atropine, in sufficient dosage, crosses the blood brain barrier and effectively antagonizes the actions at muscarinic receptor sites. Saving the life of the patient is most important. Therefore, atropine is the preferred drug for organophosphorus poisoning.
2. C
    Organophosphates irreversibly inhibit the enzyme acetylcholinesterase at neuromuscular junctions.
3. A
    Acetylcholine produces miosis by contracting the pupillary sphincter muscle which is mediated by M_3 muscarinic receptors. All the other three drugs produce mydriasis.
4. D
    Anticholinesterase agents cause constriction of the pupillary sphincter muscle around the pupillary margin of the iris, resulting in *pin point pupil*. Belladona poisoning results in dilated pupil.

References:
1.   Osterhoudt KC, Penning TM. Drug toxicity and poisoning. In: Brunton LL, Chabner BA, Knollmann BC, editors. Goodman & Gilman's the pharmacological basis of therapeutics. 12th ed. New York: Mc Graw-Hill; 2011. p. 73-87.
2.   Taylor P. Anticholinesterase agents. In: Brunton LL, Chabner BA, Knollmann BC, editors. Goodman & Gilman's the pharmacological basis of therapeutics. 12th ed. New York: Mc Graw-Hill; 2011. p. 239-54.
3.   Brown JH, Laiken N. Muscarinic receptor agonists and antagonists. In: Brunton LL, Chabner BA, Knollmann BC, editors. Goodman & Gilman's the pharmacological basis of therapeutics. 12th ed. New York: Mc Graw-Hill; 2011. p. 219-38.

TUBERCULOSIS

Dr. Anuradha Nischal, Professor, Department of Pharmacology & Therapeutics

A 40 year old male presents with cough for more than 3 weeks, haemoptysis, low grade fever, loss of appetite, weight loss and production of sputum. His chest X ray revealed the presence of cavities in the left upper lobe. He was prescribed a combination of four drugs for a period of 2 months, after which the patient started complaining of tingling and numbness in the left lower limb.

1. Which drug is responsible for the tingling and numbness in the patient?
   (A) Isoniazid
   (B) Rifampicin
   (C) Ethambutol
   (D) Pyrazinamide
2. Which of the following drug should be prescribed to the patient to correct tingling and numbness?
   (A) Folic acid
   (B) Pyridoxine
   (C) Biotin
   (D) Niacin
3. Which of the following anti tubercular drugs is **NOT** hepatotoxic?
   (A) Isoniazid
   (B) Rifampicin
   (C) Ethambutol
   (D) Pyrazinamde
4. Which of the following drugs is bacteriostatic?
   (A) Rifampicin
   (B) Pyrazinamide
   (C) Isoniazid
   (D) Ethambutol
5. The primary reason for the use of multidrug therapy in the treatment of tuberculosis is to:
   (A) Ensure patient compliance
   (B) Decrease incidence of adverse effects
   (C) Provide prophylaxis against other bacterial infections
   (D) Prevent the emergence of resistance

Answers:

1. A
   Treatment with isoniazid results in peripheral neuritis (most commonly paresthesias of feet and hands) in approximately 2% of patients.
2. B
   Pyridoxine should be given concurrently with isoniazid to prevent peripheral neuritis.
3. C
   Hepatotoxicity is commonly observed with isoniazid, rifampicin as well as pyrazinamide. The most important side effect of ethambutol is optic neuritis, resulting in decreased visual acuity and loss of the ability to differentiate red from green.
4. D
   Isoniazid, rifampicin, pyrazinamide and streptomycin have tuberculocidal effect on Mycobacteria. Only ethambutol is selectively tuberculostatic.
5. D
   Use of any single drug in tuberculosis reults in the emergence of resistant organisms and relapse in almost 3/4th patients. Therefore, a combination of two or more drugs may be used.

References:

1. Gumbo T. Chemotherapy of tuberculosis, mycobacterium avium complex disease, and leprosy. In: Brunton LL, Chabner BA, Knollmann BC, editors. Goodman & Gilman's the pharmacological basis of therapeutics. 12th ed. New York: Mc Graw-Hill; 2011. p. 1549-70.
2. Tripathi KD. Essentials of medical pharmacology. 7th ed. New Delhi: Jaypee Brothers Medical Publishers; 2013. p. 765-79.

LEAD POISONING

Dr. Rishi Pal, Assistant Professor, Department of Pharmacology & Therapeutics

A painter of 32 years presented with a two weeks history of lethargy, malaise, headaches, nausea, cramping abdominal pain and weakness in hands. His serum lead level was 4.09 μmol l^{-1} (85.2 μg 100 ml^{-1}). On examination anaemia was noted but he was otherwise well and exhibited no neurological or intellectual impairment. Investigation showed: Hb 9.7 g 100 ml^{-1} with moderate polychromasia and basophilic stippling of the red cells. His blood count was otherwise within normal limits as were his electrolytes and liver function tests. The case was diagnosed with lead toxicity. He received calcium disodium edetate (Ca Na_2 EDTA). When reviewed 4 weeks later his symptoms had resolved and his Hb was 11.3 g 100 ml^{-1}.

1. What is the mechanism of lead neurotoxicity?
   (A) Interferes with neurotransmitter release
   (B) Affecting intracellular messenger cGMP
   (C) Interferes with synthesis of neurotransmitters
   (D) Affecting neuronal cell death
2. What is the main route of lead exposure?
   (A) Oral
   (B) Sublingual
   (C) Inhalational
   (D) Dermal
3. Which of the following analytical technique used for lead detection in blood?
   (A) UV-Vis spectrophotometer
   (B) Mass-spectrophotometer
   (C) Photoactometer
   (D) Atomic absorbtion spectrophotometer
4. What is the main organ of lead storage?
   (A) Liver
   (B) Bone
   (C) Lung
   (D) Brain
5. Which of the following reflects over 3 months lead exposure in blood?
   (A) Zinc protoporphyrin (ZPP) concentration
   (B) Low level of Zinc
   (C) Low level of Calcium
   (D) Low level of zinc and calcium

Answers:

1. A
    At the neurosynaptic junction, it appears that lead interferes with transmitter release and signal transduction. In adults the classical picture of severe lead toxicity includes bilateral wrist drop. The histology shows segmental axonal demyelination and degeneration, and decreased nerve conduction velocities have been demonstrated in lead workers with blood lead concentrations of 1.9 μmol l^{-1} (40 μg 100 ml^{-1}). The underlying mechanism may be substitution of calcium and zinc by lead at the synapse, affecting intracellular messengers such as cAMP and protein kinase.

2. C
    The main route of lead exposure is through inhalational route. The setting of the exposure, removing leaded paint, represents an established source of danger. The main route of absorption in adults is the respiratory tract where 30–70% of inhaled lead finds its way into the circulation. Particle size is the most important determinant of absorption. Gastrointestinal absorption in adults is generally less complete and averages approximately 10% of the ingested load.

3. D
    Atomic absorption spectrophotometer (AAS) is the analytical technique used for the analysis of heavy metals, like lead, arsenic, mercury in biological sample/fluids.

4. B
    Bone is the main organ of lead storage and over the period of time redistribution of lead from bone into the blood takes place.

5. A
    Inhibition of mitochondrial ferrochelatase results in accumulation of erythrocyte precursors including protoporphyrin, which binds to available zinc in blood. Therefore ZPP (zinc

protoporphyrin) remains in the blood for the life-time of erythrocyte and reflects lead exposure over the prior three months lead exposure.

Reference:

1. Gordon JN, Taylor A, Bennett PN. Lead poisoning: case studies. Br J Clin Pharmacol. 2002 May; 53(5): 451-58.

VITAMIN B$_{12}$ DEFICIENCY
Dr. Rishi Pal, Assistant Professor, Department of Pharmacology & Therapeutics

A 58 year old woman comes with complaint of increasing symptoms of painful paresthesia in both legs for past 18 months. Physical examination reveals impaired position sense and vibration sense. The serum vitamin B$_{12}$ level was found 195 pg/ml, haematocrit was 42% with MCV of 96 fl. The serum methylmalonic acid level was 3600 nm/L (Normal level, <400) and serum homocysteine level 49.1 μm/L (normal level, <14).

1. What is the normal range of vitamin B$_{12}$ levels in blood?
   (A) 400-800 pg/ml
   (B) 300-600 pg/ml
   (C) 200-900 pg/ml
   (D) 250-500 pg/ml
2. What is the cause of painful paresthesia?
   (A) Loss of neurotransmitters
   (B) Demyelination of nerves
   (C) Excessive release of neurotransmitters
   (D) Loss of neurons
3. Causes of vitamin B$_{12}$ deficiency include all **EXCEPT**:
   (A) Pernicious anemia
   (B) Celiac disease and Crohn disease
   (C) Lack of intrinsic factor
   (D) Hyperthyroidism
4. Treatment for vitamin B$_{12}$ deficiency **DOES NOT** include:
   (A) Parenteral high-dose of vitamin B$_{12}$
   (B) Advice to take food of animal origin
   (C) Folic acid, iron and ascorbic acid supplements
   (D) Over growth of gut bacteria

Answers:
1. C
   Normal laboratory reference range of vitamin B$_{12}$ lies between 200 to 900 picogram/ml. This range may vary with the age. In the older adults it lies between 200-500 picogram/ml. Values of less than 200 pg/ml are a sign of a vitamin B$_{12}$ deficiency. People with this deficiency are likely to have or develop symptoms.
2. B
   Vitmin B$_{12}$ is necessary for the development of initial myelination of central nervous system as well for the maintenance of its normal function. Vitamin B$_{12}$ deficiency leads to demyelination of cervical, thoracic dorsal and lateral column of the spinal cord as well as demyelination of cranial & peripheral nerve and demyelination of white matter in the brain.
3. A
   Vitamin B$_{12}$ deficiency leads to pernicious anemia not pernicious anemia lead to vitamin B$_{12}$ deficiency.
4. D
   Some people develop vitamin B$_{12}$ deficiency as a result of conditions that slow the movement of food through the intestines (diabetes, scleroderma, strictures, diverticula), allowing intestinal bacteria to multiply and overgrow in the upper part of the small intestine. These bacteria steal B$_{12}$ for their own use, rather than allowing it to be absorbed by the body.

References:

1. Stabler SP. Vitamin B$_{12}$ Deficiency. N Engl J Med 2013; 368:149-160.
2. Mason JB. Vitamins, trace minerals, and other micronutrients. In: Goldman L, Schafer AI, editors. Goldman's Cecil Medicine. 24th ed. Philadelphia (PA): Elsevier Saunders; 2011.

3. Salwen MJ. Vitamins and trace elements. In: McPherson RA, Pincus MR, editors. Henry's clinical diagnosis and management by laboratory methods. 22nd ed. Philadelphia (PA): Elsevier Saunders; 2011.

IMMUNOSUPPRESSION WITH ACTINIC KEROTOSIS

Dr. Rishi Pal, Assistant Professor, Department of Pharmacology & Therapeutics

A 60 year old white man had renal transplantation seven years ago for polycystic kidney disease and receiving immunosuppressive therapy with cyclosporine and prednisolone to protect against organ rejection. 3 years after kidney transplantation, several verrucae and actinic keratosis (AK) developed in sun exposed areas, including face, neck and hands and 10-20 new AK appearing every month. In addition patients experienced considerable pain and blistering. It was diagnosed as a case of Non-melanoma skin cancer.

1. What could be the possible treatment regimen?
    (A) Immunosuppressive drugs
    (B) Photodynamic therapy (PDT) alone
    (C) Anti-neoplastic agents and photodynamic therapy (PDT)
    (D)I mmunostimulants drugs
2. What is the preffered drug for treatment?
    (A) 5-Fluorouracil (5-FU)
    (B) Cyclophosphamide
    (C) Cyclosporine
    (D) Levamisole
3. What is the cause of actin keratosis (AK)?
    (A) Increased activity of immune system
    (B) Not related with immune system
    (C) Activation of proto-oncogene
    (D) Suppressed immune surveillance system
4. What is the mechanism of action of cyclosporine?
    (A) False nucleotide incorporation
    (B) IL-2 receptor blocker
    (C) Calcineurin inhibitor
    (D) mTOR inhibitor

Answers:

1. C
    Since it is skin cancer in immune-compromised patient photodymanic therapy (PDT) with anti-neoplastic chemotherapeutic agents can be used particularly anti-metabolite like 5-fluorouracil (5-FU).
2. A
    Preferred drug for the treatment of non-melanoma skin cancer is 5- fluorouracil (5-FU).
3. D
    Since, the patient has been taking immunosuppressant for long time immune system is compromised and the activity of immunesurveillance system of the body becomes inadequate. So the defense system in the body/skin against UV radiation becomes poor, as result skin cancer developed.
4. C
    Cyclosporine acts by inhibiting calcineurin (phosphatase enzyme inhibitor). Calcineurin catalysed dephosphorylation which is required for the movement of a component of the nuclear factor of activated T-lymphocytes (NFAT) into the nucleus. NFAT, in turn is required to induce signal transduction of a number of cytokine genes, including IL-2.

References:

1. Krensky AM, Bennett WM, Vincenti F. Immunosuppressants, tolerogens, and immunostimulants. In: Brunton LL, Chabner BA, Knollmann BC, editors. Goodman & Gilman's the pharmacological basis of therapeutics. 12th ed. New York: Mc Graw-Hill; 2011. p. 1008-9.
2. Chabner BA, Amrein PC, Druker BJ, Michaelson MD, Mitsiades CS, Goss PE, et al. Anti-neoplastic agents. In: Bruton LL, Lazo JS, Parker KL, editors. Goodman and Gillman's the pharmacological basis of therapeutics, 11th ed. New York: Mc Graw-Hill; 2011. p. 1342-43.

DIARRHOEA

Dr. Sarvesh Singh, Assistant Professor, Department of Pharmacology & Therapeutics

A 3-year-old child was suffering from watery diarrhea lacking blood. He had mild fever also. The child was given one tablet three times a day to control loose motions. The diarrhoea stopped but next day the child was brought in a toxic condition with abdominal distention and vomiting. He had paralytic ileus, mild dehydration, low blood pressure and sluggish reflexes.

1. Which anti-diarrheal drug could have caused this condition?
   (A) Iodochlorhydroxyquinoline
   (B) Furazolidone
   (C) Metronidazole
   (D) Loperamide
2. First line management for watery diarrhea in this child should be:
   (A) Norfloxacin
   (B) Norfloxacin and Tinidazole combination
   (C) Norfloxacin and oral rehydration solution (ORS)
   (D) Only oral rehydration solution (ORS)
3. Which of the following statement is true regarding the loperamide?
   (A) It is not an opioid analogue
   (B) It is indicated in noninfective diarrhea
   (C) CNS side effects are common
   (D) It does not increase anal sphincter tone

Answers:

1. D
   Loperamide is a synthetic opioid analogue. It is contraindicated in children < 4 year because complications like paralytic ileus, toxic megacolon with abdominal distension may occur in young children.
2. D
   Most common causes of watery diarrhea lacking blood with little or no fever in children are by rota virus and other viruses. These organisms stimulate massive secretion by activating cAMP in intestinal mucosal cell. ORS and not anti-microbials are the main therapy.
3. B
   Loperamide is an opioid analogue with major peripheral μ opioid receptor action. Entry into brain is negligible so CNS effects are rare. Antimotility agents like loperamide may be given to control non-infective diarrhea and mild traveller's diarrhea. These drugs are contraindicated in acute infective diarrhea because they delay clearance of the pathogen from the intestine. It also increases anal sphincter tone so may be useful in some patients who suffer from anal incontinence.

References:

1. Sharkey KA, Wallace JL. Treatment of disorders of bowel motility and water flux; anti – emetics; agents used in biliary and pancreatic disease. In: Brunton LL, Chabner BA, Knollmann BC, editors. Goodman & Gilman's the pharmacological basis of therapeutics. 12 th ed. New York: Mc Graw-Hill; 2011. p. 1323-50.
2. Tripathi KD. Essentials of medical pharmacology. 7th ed. New Delhi: Jaypee Brothers Medical Publishers; 2013. p. 672-87.

DEPRESSION

Dr. Rahul Kumar, Assistant Professor, Department of Pharmacology & Therapeutics

A 30 year old female attended the outpatient department (OPD) with the complaints of difficulty in sleeping, early morning awakening, diminished interest in normal activities, poor appetite and weight loss. It was diagnosed as a case of depression and she was prescribed amitriptyline 50 mg. Three weeks later, she again visited OPD with no improvement in condition and with two new complaints of dry mouth and constipation.

1. The prescribed drug amitriptyline belongs to which drug class?
   (A) SSRIs (selective serotonin reuptake inhibitors)
   (B) TCAs (tricyclic antidepressants)
   (C) Phenothiazines
   (D) RIMAs (reversible inhibitors of MAO-A)
2. There was no improvement in symptoms even after three weeks. This may be due to:
   (A)Inappropriate dose
   (B)Inappropriate frequency
   (C)Wrong diagnosis
   (D)Therapeutic lag of 3-4 weeks
3. The new symptoms of dry mouth and constipation were due to:
   (A)Worsening of the disease itself
   (B)Anti-muscarinic effect of amitriptyline
   (C)Serotonin reuptake inhibiting effect of amitriptyline
   (D)Noradrenaline reuptake inhibiting effect of amitriptyline
4. Which one of the following drugs can be prescribed as an alternative of amitriptyline to
   avoid adverse effects like dry mouth and constipation?
   (A)Sertraline
   (B)Imipramine
   (C)Clomipramine
   (D)Nortriptyline

Answers:
1. B
   Amitriptyline belongs to tricyclic antidepressants group. It is nor-adrenaline and serotonin reuptake inhibitor.
2. D
   Antidepressant drugs have a therapeutic lag period of 3-4 weeks before a measureable t herapeutic response is evident.
3. B
   TCAs like amitriptyline have potent anti-muscarinic effects. Some tolerance may occur for these anti-muscarinic effects.
4. A
   SSRIs like sertraline are free of anti-muscarinic side effects.

Reference:
1. O'Donnell JM, Shelton RC. Drug therapy of depression and anxiety disorders. In: Brunton LL, Chabner BA, Knollmann BC, editors. Goodman & Gilman's the pharmacological basis of therapeutics. 12th ed. New York: Mc Graw-Hill; 2011. p. 397-415.

ALCOHOLISM
Dr. Rahul Kumar, Assistant Professor, Department of Pharmacology & Therapeutics

A 40 year old chronic alcoholic decided to abstain from alcohol. But shortly thereafter he felt anxiety, sweating, tremor, hallucinations and impairment of sleep. He has no apparent liver disease.

1. Which one of the following drug can be used to avoid above stated symptoms?
   (A)Disulfiram
   (B)Phenytoin
   (C)Diazepam
   (D)Triazolam
2. If the above alcoholic person had some liver disease which one of the following drug will be preferred to control withdrawal phenomenon?
   (A)Diazepam
   (B)Triazolam
   (C)Flurazepam
   (D)Disulfiram
3. To avoid alcohol consumption in future the above alcoholic was prescribed a drug. Name that drug:
   (A)Phenobarbital
   (B)Phenytoin
   (C)Diazepam

(D)Disulfiram

Answers:
1. C

    Long acting benzodiazepines like diazepam are preferred in alcohol withdrawl. Diazepam can be gradually withdrawn later.
2. B

    In presence of liver disease a benzodiazepine of shorter duration of action is preferred like triazolam.
3. D

    Disulfiram is used in controlling alcohol consumption.

Reference:
1. Schuckit MA. Ethanol and Methanol. In: Brunton LL, Chabner BA, Knollmann BC, editors. Goodman & Gilman's the pharmacological basis of therapeutics. 12th ed. New York: Mc Graw-Hill; 2011. p. 629-47.

PSYCHOSIS
Dr. Rahul Kumar, Assistant Professor, Department of Pharmacology & Therapeutics

A 50 year old female was brought to the psychiatry department because of a recent history of spontaneously removing cloths outside her house and claiming that she can talk to souls. There was no history of diabetes or hypertension. But on starting the antipsychotic drug she had syncope. This was found to be a condition of orthostatic hypotension.

1. Which drug was most likely prescribed to her?
    (A) Olanzapine
    (B) Sertindole
    (C) Haloperidol
    (D) Chlorpromazine
2. Orthostatic hypotension is caused by some of the antipsychotic drugs. This is due to:
    (A) α_1 receptor blockade
    (B) α_2 receptor blockade
    (C) β_1 receptor blockade
    (D) β_2 receptor blockade
3. If patient's psychotic symptoms are well controlled with a particular drug and patient has few other antipsychotic options, orthostatic hypotension as a side effect can be controlled by:
    (A) Triamcinolone
    (B) Fludrocortisone
    (C) Betamethasone
    (D)Deflazacort

Answers:
1. D

    Among antipsychotics, chlorpromazine is the most likely drug to cause orthostatic hypotension.
2. A

    Antagonism of α_1 adrenergic receptors is associated with the risk of orthostatic hypotension and can be particularly problematic for elderly patients who have poor vasomotor tone.
3. B

    If patients have few other antipsychotic options, the potent mineralocorticoid fludrocortisone is sometimes tried at the dose of 0.1 mg/day as a volume expander to minimize the chance of orthostatic hypotension.

Reference:
1. Meyer JM. Pharmacotherapy of psychosis and mania. In: Brunton LL, Chabner BA, Knollmann BC, editors. Goodman & Gilman's the pharmacological basis of therapeutics. 12th ed. New York: Mc Graw-Hill; 2011. p. 417-55.

GENERAL PHARMACOLOGY
Dr. Narendra Kumar, Assistant Professor, Department of Pharmacology & Therapeutics

A 25 year old male presented with the complaint of irregular episodes of high fever since the last 3 days. The fever was preceded by chills and accompanied by headache, nausea and weakness. The fever lasted 4-6 hours and subsided after sweating. The doctor advised peripheral blood smear to be done. Reports were positive for malaria parasite Plasmodium vivax. He was prescribed chloroquine 600mg stat followed by 300 mg after 8 hours and then for the next two days along with 15mg of primaquine to be taken once daily for 14 days, after he was tested negative for G-6-PD deficiency.

1. Why is a higher dose of chloroquine prescribed initially?
   (A) Because chloroquine has a low volume of distribution
   (B) Because chloroquine has a large volume of distribution
   (C) Because chloroquine undergoes metabolism quickly
   (D) Because chloroquine gets excreted quickly
2. Why is the patient tested for G-6-PD deficiency before advising primaquine?
   (A) Because primaquine is well absorbed orally in G-6-PD deficient state
   (B) Because primaquine is not bound extensively to the tissues in G-6-PD deficient state
   (C) Because primaquine can cause fatal haemolytic anaemia in G-6-PD deficient state
   (D) Because primaquine is rapidly metabolized by the liver in G-6-PD deficient state
3. Why is oral administration preferred over parenteral administration for chloroquine?
   (A) Because rapid entry into the bloodstream together with slow exit from this compartment can result in toxicity
   (B) Because chloroquine undergoes extensive first pass metabolism
   (C) Because chloroquine is extensively protein bound
   (D) Because chloroquine is rapidly hydrolysed

Answers:
1. B
   If a drug is having large volume of distribution and its effect is required soon than it is given in loading dose.
2. C
   G-6-PD deficiency is responsible for hemolysis with oxidising drugs, e.g. Primaquine, Chloroquine.
3. A
   Intravenous injection can cause hypotension, cardiac depression arrhythmias and CNS toxicity including seizures.

References:
1. Vinetz JM, Clain J, Bounkeua V, Eastman RT, Fidock D. Chemotherapy of malaria. In: Brunton LL, Chabner BA, Knollmann BC, editors. Goodman and Gilman's the pharmacological basis of therapeutics. 12th ed. New York: McGraw-Hill; 2011. p. 1383-418.
2. Sharma KK. Principles of Pharmacology. 2nd ed. Hyderabad: Paras Medical Publishers; 2011. p. 53,807-18.
3. Tripathi KD. Essentials of medical pharmacology. 7th ed. New Delhi: Jaypee Brothers Medical Publishers; 2013. p. 65-6.

ANTI-HYPERTENSIVE AGENTS
Dr. Pradeep Dwivedi, Senior Resident, Department of Pharmacology & Therapeutics

Ram Kumar is a 44-year-old man who presents to Medicine OPD (KGMU) concerned about high blood pressure (BP). At health screening camp last month he was told he had stage 1 hypertension. He has family history of diabetes mellitus and hypertension. He smokes one pack per day of cigarettes and thinks his BP is high because of job-related stress. He does not engage in any regular exercise and does not restrict his diet. Physical examination shows his body mass index (BMI) 35.2 kg/m2, BP is 148/88 mm Hg (left arm) and 146/86 mm Hg (right arm) while sitting, heart rate is 80 beats/minute. Fundoscopic examination reveals mild arterial narrowing and arteriovenous nicking, with no exudates or hemorrhages. The other physical examination findings are essentially normal. His fasting laboratory serum values are within normal limits. An electrocardiogram (ECG) is normal except for left ventricular hypertrophy.

1. Which antihypertensive agents are appropriate first-line treatments for Ram Kumar?
   (A) Angiotensin converting enzyme inhibitors/angiotensin receptor blockers
   (B) Calcium channel blockers
   (C) Thiazide diuretics
   (D) All of the above

2. When using a standard dose monotherapy of first-line antihypertensive agents, the average reduction in systolic blood pressure /diastolic blood pressure is only:
   (A) 10/5 mmHg
   (B) 20/10 mmHg
   (C) 30/15 mmHg
   (D) 40/20 mmHg
3. If chlorothiazide is used then which of the ion will **NOT** be increased in the urine of Ram Kumar?
   (A) K^+
   (B) Mg^{++}
   (C) Na^+
   (D) Ca^{++}
4. If Ram Kumar is also taking Insulin for diabetes then which antihypertensive drug should be cautiously used?
   (A) Prazosin
   (B) Guanethidine
   (C) Methyldopa
   (D) Propanolol
5. Which is **NOT** a contraindication for ACE inhibitors?
   (A) Pregnancy
   (B) Bilateral renal stenosis
   (C) Hypernatremia
   (D) Hypovolumia

Answers:
   1. D
       Angiotensin converting enzyme inhibitors/angiotensin receptor blockers, calcium channel blockers, thiazide diuretics are the first line druge for the management of Hypertension.
   2. A
       With standard dose monotherapy of first-line antihypertensive agents, the average reduction in systolic blood pressure /diastolic blood pressure is only 10/5mmHg.
   3. D
       Thiazide therapy decreases Ca++ excretion.
   4. D
       Propranolol slows the recovery from hypoglycemia caused by Insulin.
   5. C
       Hyponatremia is a contraindication.

Reference:
   1. Saseen JJ. Essential hypertension. In: Alldredge BK, Corelli RL, Ernst ME, Guglielmo BJ, Jacobson PA, Kradjan WA, et al, editors. Koda-Kimle & Young's Applied Therapeutics: The clinical use of drugs. 10th ed. Philadelphia (PA): Wolter Kluwer Health Lippincott Williams & Wilkins; 2013. p. 291-331.

ANTI-ANGINAL DRUGS
Dr. Pradeep Dwivedi, Senior Resident, Department of Pharmacology & Therapeutics

Shashi Kant, a 68 year old weighing 80 kg man was being admitted to the emergency department after experiencing an episode of sustained chest pain while brisk walking. Heart rate and rhythm were regular, and S3 or S4 sounds were absent. Vital signs included blood pressure 150/90 mm Hg, heart rate 95 beats/minute, and respiratory rate 28 breaths/minute. The pain radiated to his left arm and jaw. His pain responded to sublingual (SL) nitroglycerin (NTG) tablets at home. His ECG revealed slight ST segment elevation.

1. Which of the following hemodynamic effects of nitroglycerin are primarily responsible for the beneficial results observed in patients with angina?
   (A) Reduction in the force of myocardial contraction
   (B) Reduction in systemic vascular resistance (afterload)
   (C) Reduction in venous capacitance (preload)
   (D) Increased blood flow to the subepicardium
2. The therapeutic action of propanolol in angina pectoris is believed to be due to:
   (A) Reduced production of catecholamines
   (B) Dilation of Coronary vasculature

(C) Decreased requirement of myocardial oxygen

(D) Increased peripheral resistance

3. Which of the following is considered most effective in relieving and preventing episode in variant angina?

    (A) Propranolol

    (B) Nitroglycerin

    (C) Sodium Nitroprusside

    (D) Nifedipine

4. Six month later the above patient suffers acute MI and was treated with alteplase. What is the mechanism of action?

    (A) Inhibition of platelet thromboxane production

    (B) Antagonism of ADP receptor

    (C) Antagonism of Glycoprotein IIb/IIIa

    (D) Activation of plasminogen from plasmin.

Answers:
1. C

    Nitroglycerin can reduce preload, which in turn reduces wall tension and increases subendocardial blood flow. Nitroglycerin also reduces afterload, but this is a small effect compared to the reduction in preload. Its effects on heart rate and contractility are minimal, and if anything reflex tachycardia and increase in contractility would be detrimental effects of too much nitroglycerin.

2. C

    Beta Blockers decrease heart rate, contraction and BP result in decreased oxygen demand.

3. D

    Coronary vasospasm is antagonized by slow Ca^{++} Channel blocker.

4. D

    Alteplase, a recombinant tissue plasma activator, is FDA-approved for treatment of MI with ST-elevation (STEMI), acute ischaemic stroke (AIS), acute massive pulmonary embolism, and central venous access devices (CVAD).

Reference:
1. Page RL, Nappi JM. Acute coronary syndrome. In: Alldredge BK, Corelli RL, Ernst, ME, Guglielmo BJ, Jacobson PA, Kradjan WA, Williams BR, editors. Koda-Kimle & Young's applied therapeutics: the clinical use of drugs. 10th ed. Philadelphia (PA): Wolter Kluwer Health Lippincott Williams & Wilkins; 2013. p. 407-36.

HEART FAILURE MANAGEMENT

Dr. Pradeep Dwivedi, Senior Resident, Department of Pharmacology & Therapeutics

Jugal Kishore, a 66 year old man, presents for a routine checkup in the clinic. His medical history includes type 2 diabetes mellitus, systolic heart failure, hypertension, and gout for the last 5 years. There is no history of rhematic heart disease, myocardial infarction, pulmonary embolism or thyroid disease. Medications include glyburide 5 mg twice daily, lisinopril 40 mg every day, furosemide 40 mg twice daily, metoprolol 50 mg twice daily and allopurinol 300 mg/day. He does not smoke or drink alcohol. Physical examination reveals a blood pressure (BP) of 136/84 mm Hg, pulse of 70 beats/minute in normal sinus rhythm, respiratory rate of 12 breaths/minute, and temperature of 98.2°F. His body mass index (BMI) is 32 kg/m^2.

1. What is the primary mechanism of action of furosemide?

    (A) Inhibition of $Na^+ K^+$ ATPase

    (B) Inhibition of $Na^+ K^+ Cl^-$ co-transport

    (C) Inhibition of $Na^+ Cl^-$ co-transport

    (D) Inhibition of Cl^- transport

2. Digitalis functions to improve congestive heart failure by:

    (A) Activation of β-adrenergic receptors

    (B) Improving survival in patients of heart failure

    (C) Binding to and inhibiting the Na–K ATPase enzyme in cardiac myocytes

    (D) Deactivation of the angiotensin receptor

3. Beta-Blockers have been effective in the treatment of heart failure. They primarily exert their effect by:

    (A) Binding to the receptor that binds norepinephrine

    (B) Inducing a prominent diuretic effect

    (C) Increasing contractility

(D) Increasing heart rate to meet the additional demands placed upon the heart in CHF
4. Which of the following drug has beneficial effects on "cardiac remodelling"?
    (A) Hydrochlorothiazide
    (B) Enalapril
    (C) Furosemide
    (D) Carvedilol
5. The following statement concerning drugs in heart failure is correct:
    (A) The combination of furosemide (loop diuretic) and ramipril (ACE inhibitor) should be avoided
    (B) Candesartan (angiotensin-II receptor antagonist) is generally better tolerated than captopril (ACE inhibitor)
    (C) Beta blockers are contraindicated in heart failure
    (D) The combination of loop diuretic, ACE inhibitor and spironolactone must always be avoided because of the risk of hyperkalaemia

Answers:
1. B
    Furosemide causes Inhibition of $Na^+ K^+ Cl^-$ co-transport in the thick ascending loop of henle.
2. C
    Digoxin inhibits $Na^+ K^+$ ATPase (Na^+ pump) in the myocytes.
3. A
    Beta Blockers bind to the receptor that binds norepinephrine and inhibit sympathetic activation of the heart.
4. B
    Angiotensin converting enzyme inhibitors (ACE inhibitors) have beneficial effect on cardiac remodelling.
5. B
    Angiotensin receptor blockers (ARBs) are better tolerated than ACE inhibitors.

Reference:
1. Singh H, Marrs JC. Heart failure. In: Alldredge BK, Corelli RL, Ernst ME, Guglielmo BJ, Jacobson PA, Kradjan WA, et al, editors. Koda-Kimle & Young's applied therapeutics: the clinical use of drugs. 10th ed. Philadelphia (PA): Wolter Kluwer Health Lippincott Williams & Wilkins; 2013. p. 407-89.

TYPE 1 DIABETES MELLITUS
Dr. Arpit Jain, JR III, Department of Pharmacology & Therapeutics

Parents of a 10 year-old child have noted that his thirst and appetite have increased over the past 2 months, but he has lost 5 kg. He is urinating more frequently. On physical examination there are no abnormal findings. Urine dipstick analysis shows specific gravity 1.011, pH 6, glucose 4+, ketones 4+, no blood, no protein, and no urobilinogen. Urine microscopic analysis shows a few oxalate crystals but no RBCs or WBCs. Laboratory findings show serum creatinine 2.0 mg/dL and random blood glucose 500 mg/dL. It was diagnosed as a case of Type I Diabetes Mellitus.

1. Which of the following pathologic abnormalities most likely led to this disease?
    (A) Chronic pyelonephritis
    (B) Decreased islet cell mass
    (C) Insulin resistance
    (D) Nodular glomerulosclerosis
2. What is the treatment of choice for the given condition?
    (A) Sulfonylureas
    (B) Insulin
    (C) Metformin
    (D) Hydrocortisone
3. Which of the following is a common long term complication of the given condition?
    (A) Metabolic alkalosis
    (B) Hypoglycemia
    (C) Acute tubular necrosis
    (D) Kimmelstiel Wilson Syndrome
4. Which of the following drug is most appropriate for hypertension associated with the concerned disease?
    (A) Amlodipine

(B) ACE inhibitors
(C) Furosemide
(D) Clonidine

Answers:

1. C

   Decreased islet cell mass due to antibody mediated destruction is the prime cause of Type I Diabets mellitus.

2. B

   Insulin is the treatment of choice due significant loss of pancreatic β islet cell mass which leads to absolute insulin deficiency. Oral hypoglycaemic drugs offer no benefit in such patients.

3. D

   Kimmelstiel Wilson syndrome refers to the diabetic nodular glomerulosclerosis which is a long term complication of diabetes mellitus.

4. B

   Enalapril has a renoprotective effect in diabetic nephropathy and is preferred in hypertension associated with it.

Reference:

1. Powers AC, Alessio DD. Endocrine pancreas and pharmacotherapy of diabetes mellitus and hypoglycemia. In: Brunton LL, Chabner BA, Knollmann BC, editors. Goodman and Gilman's the pharmacological basis of therapeutics. 12th ed. New York: McGraw-Hill; 2011. p. 1237-73.

HYPERPROLACTINEMIA
Dr. Arpit Jain, JR III, Department of Pharmacology & Therapeutics

A 22 year old female presented to you with complains of headache and vomiting for last two months. She is having amenorrhoea but urine pregnancy test is negative. She also complained of secretion of milk from the breasts. A brain MRI scan was performed which reported the presence of a large pituitary tumour, suggesting of prolactinoma.

1. What is the cause of galactorrhoea and amenorrhoea in the given case?
   (A) Decreased production of prolactin
   (B) Increased production of prolactin
   (C) Increased production of LH
   (D) Increased production of FSH

2. Which of the following medications is most likely to be prescribed?
   (A) Sumatriptan
   (B) Cabergoline
   (C) Ergotamine
   (D) Lanreotide

3. Which of the following drugs may lead to similar symptoms?
   (A) Bromocriptine
   (B) Haloperidol
   (C) Levodopa
   (D) Pegvisomant

4. Which of the following drugs is preferred more in pregnancy associated with the given disease?
   (A) Quinagolide
   (B) Cabergoline
   (C) Bromocriptine
   (D) Pergolide

Answers:

1. B

   Increased production of prolactin from the pituatary adenoma will lead to excess production of milk from mammary glands and amennorhoea due to feedback inhibition.

2. B

   Cabergoline, an ergot derivative with agonistic activity at dopamine receptor, is used in the cases of prolactinomas. Dopamine is analogous to prolactin inhibitory hormone derived from hypothalamus and reduces the secretion of prolactin from pitutary. Treatment with cabergoline may decrease the size of the tumour to an extent that the drug can be discontinued without recurrence.

3. B
Haloperidol has a dopamine D_2 receptor antagonistic action and may thus cause hyperprolactinemia.

4. C
Both bromocriptine and cabergoline have been found to be relatively safe in pregnancy but because of its greater track record, bromocriptine is more preferable. Quinagolide has been associated with some fetal abnormalities so is not used in pregnancy.

Reference:
1. Parker KL, Schimmer BP. Introduction to endocrinology: the hypothalamic-pituitary axis. In: Brunton LL, Chabner BA, Knollmann BC, editors. Goodman and Gilman's the pharmacological basis of therapeutics. 12th ed. New York: McGraw-Hill; 2011. p. 1129-61.

HYPERTHYROIDISM
Dr. Arpit Jain, JR III, Department of Pharmacology & Therapeutics

A 30-year-old female complains of palpitations, fatigue, insomnia and loss of weight. On physical exam, her extremities are warm and she has tachycardia. There is diffuse thyroid gland enlargement and proptosis. There is a thickening of the skin in the pretibial area. Her thyroid profile results are free triiodothyronine (FT3) - 865 pg/dl, free thyroxine (FT4)- 2.5 ng/dl, thyroid stimulating hormone (TSH)- 0.01 µU/dl. The condition was diagnosed as a case of Grave's disease.

1. The cause of this patient's thyrotoxicosis is:
   (A) Autoimmune disease
   (B) Benign tumor
   (C) Malignancy
   (D) Viral infection of the thyroid
2. The treatment of choice in this patient, with which remission from Graves' disease is possible, is:
   (A) Methimazole
   (B) Radioactive iodine
   (C) Thyroid surgery
   (D) Oral corticosteroids
3. What is the mechanism of action of propylthiouracil that may be prescribed in such a case?
   (A) Inhibit incorporation of iodine into tyrosyl residues of thyroglobin
   (B) Inhibit reuptake of iodine
   (C) Inhibit release of thyroid hormone from the gland
   (D) Inhibit interaction of hormone with the receptors
4. What is the role of β-blockers in management of thyrotoxicosis?
   (A) Inhibit reuptake of iodine
   (B) Inhibit release of thyroid hormone from the gland
   (C) Reduces symptoms associated with sympathetic activity
   (D) Inhibits incorporation of iodine into tyrosyl residues of thyroglobin

Answers:
1. A
Grave's disease is an autoimmune phenomenon. The extra thyroidal manifestations of the disease are due to immunologically activated fibroblasts in extraocular muscles and skin.

2. A
Antithyroid drugs are considered by most to be the treatment of choice in a patient with Grave's disease when the underlying illness may remit. Those with large goitres or severe disease usually require definitive therapy with either surgery or radioactive iodine. These are, however, associated with a substantial risk of developing hypothyroidism.

3. A
Propylthiouracil inhibits the formation of hormone by interfering with the incorporation of iodine into tyrosyl residues of thyroglobin and also the coupling of these residues. It also partially inhibits peripheral conversion of T_4 to T_3.

4. C

β adrenergic blockers are effective in antagonizing the sympathetic/adrenergic effects of thyrotoxicosis, thereby reducing the tachycardia, tremor and stare and relieving palpitations, anxiety and tension.

Reference:
1. Brent GA, Koenig RJ. Thyroid and anti-thyroid drugs. In: Brunton LL, Chabner BA, Knollmann BC, editors. Goodman and Gilman's the pharmacological basis of therapeutics. 12th ed. New York: McGraw-Hill; 2011. p. 1129-61.

GASTROESOPHAGEAL REFLUX DISEASE
Dr. Anjula Sachan, JR III, Department of Pharmacology & Therapeutics

A 42-year-old morbidly obese woman complains of a non-productive cough for 8 months. She denies abdominal discomfort after eating and has never "suffered" from heartburn. Rarely, she has regurgitation, and when she does it has a sour taste to it. Abdominal examination is normal. Rectal examination is FOBT (fecal occult blood test) negative. The condition was diagnosed as a case of Gastroesophageal reflux disease (GERD).

1. Which of the following drug**DOES NOT** improve lower esophageal sphincter tone or prevent gastroesophageal reflux but used as the first line treatment of gastrophageal reflux disease?
   (A) Sodium alginate + aluminium hydroxide
   (B) Omeprazole
   (C) Mosapride
   (D) Metoclopramide
2. Which of the following is **NOT** an anti-helicobacter Pylori drug?
   (A) Metronidazole
   (B) Omeprazole
   (C) Mosapride
   (D) Amoxicillin
3. Choose the antiulcer drug that inhibits gastric acid secretion, stimulates gastric mucus and bicarbonate secretion and has cytoprotective action on gastric mucosa:
   (A) Misoprostol
   (B) Sucralfate
   (C) Carbenoxolone sodium
   (D) Colloidal bismuth subcitrate
4. Most specific drug for the treatment of peptic ulcer disease due to chronic use of aspirin is:
   (A) Omeprazole
   (B) Misoprostol
   (C) Pirenzepine
   (D) Ranitidine

Answers:
1. B
   GERD is usually due to relaxation of lower esophageal sphincter (LES) in the absence of swallowing. Treatment of GERD can be accomplished by decreasing gastric acid secretion with PPIs (PPIs do not improve LES tone) and by increasing gastrointestinal motility and LES tone with prokinetic drugs.
2. C
   Mosapride is a 5-HT$_4$ agonist used for GERD. It has no role in H. pylori.
3. A
   Misoprostol acts by increasing the release of mucus and bicarbonate and by increasing the mucosal blood flow.
4. B
   Misoprostol (PGE$_1$ analogue) is the most specific for treatment and prevention of NSAID induced peptic ulcer.

Reference:
1. Wallace JL, Sharkey KA. Pharmacotherapy of gastric acidity, peptic ulcers, and gastroesophageal reflux disease. In: Brunton LL, Chabner BA, Knollmann BC, editors. Goodman and Gilman's the pharmacological basis of therapeutics. 12th ed. New York: McGraw-Hill; 2011. p. 1309-22.

PEPTIC ULCER DISEASE

Dr. Anjula Sachan, JR III, Department of Pharmacology & Therapeutics

A 38 year old man arrives at the emergency room with the chief complaint of hematemesis for 1 h. He does not drink alcohol and has previous history of epigastric pain. He spent the previous night with severe epigastric pain after eating some "bad chicken." He is afebrile with a heart rate of 120/min and a blood pressure of 90/60 mm Hg. Abdominal exam is positive for diffuse tenderness, but the patient has no rigidity, guarding, or rebound tenderness. There is no hepatosplenomegaly. Rectal exam is negative for occult blood. A nasogastric tube is inserted and reveals coffee ground emesis. The condition was diagnosed as a case of peptic ulcer disease.

1. On chronic use which of the following drug may cause reversible gynaecomastia?
    (A) Cimetidine
    (B) Omeprazole
    (C) Pirenzepine
    (D) Sucralfate
2. Antacid drug that typically cause diarrhoea is:
    (A) Sodium bicarbonate
    (B) Magnesium hydroxide
    (C) Calcium bicarbonate
    (D) Aluminium hydroxide
3. Carbenoxolone sodium is used in peptic ulcer as:
    (A) Systemic antacid
    (B) Orally used antacid
    (C) Promoter of ulcer healing
    (D) Defoaming agent
4. Which of the following 5-HT receptors play an important role in causing emesis?
    (A) 5-HT$_1$
    (B) 5-HT$_{1B/1D}$
    (C) 5-HT$_3$
    (D) 5-HT$_4$

Answers:
1. A
   Cimetidine inhibits degradation of estradiol by liver. High dose given for prolonged period produces gynacoemastia.
2. B
   Magnesium hydroxide causes diarrhoea
3. C
   Carbenoxolone promotes healing of gastric ulcer by increasing mucus production, prolongation of lifespan of gastric epithelial cells, prevention of bile reflux and slowing of prostaglandin degradation in gastric mucosa.
4. C
   5 HT$_3$ receptors cause emetogenic impulse of central origin by stimulation of CTZ.

Reference:
1. Wallace JL, Sharkey KA. Pharmacotherapy of gastric acidity, peptic ulcers, and gastroesophageal reflux disease. In: Brunton LL, Chabner BA, Knollmann BC, editors. Goodman and Gilman's the pharmacological basis of therapeutics. 12th ed. New York: McGraw-Hill; 2011. p. 1309-22.

BRONCHIAL ASTHMA

Dr. Anjula Sachan, JR III, Department of Pharmacology & Therapeutics

A 45-year-old woman asthmatic presents with acute attack of non-productive cough with dyspnoea. The cough is associated with environmental exposure. She has never smoked cigarettes. She has no nasal discharge, heartburn, or cardiac symptoms. She denies fever and chest pain. Wheezing is present. Chest radiograph shows hyperinflation in bilateral lung field.

1. Which of the following drug is the fastest acting inhaled bronchodilator?
    (A) Ipratropium bromide
    (B) Formoterol

(C)Salmeterol
(D)Salbutamol
2. Which of the following drug is contraindicated in bronchial asthma?
(A)Propranolol
(B)Ipratropium bromide
(C)Theophylline
(D)Ketotifen
3. The following drug is **NOT** useful during acute attack of bronchial asthma:
(A)Salbutamol
(B)Hydrocortisone
(C)Cromolyn sodium
(D)Theophylline
4. Which of the following drug **CANNOT** precipitate acute attack of asthma?
(A)Phenylbutazone
(B)Naproxen
(C)Glucocorticoid
(D)Aspirin

Answers:

1. D
    Salbutamol and terbutaline are the fastest acting bronchodilators
2. A
    Beta blockers are contraindicated in bronchial asthma
3. C
    Cromolyn sodium prevents the degranulation of mast cells. It is indicated only for prophylaxis of bronchial asthma.
4. C
    COX inhibitors inhibit the formation of PGs from arachidonic acid. Large excess of LTs are produced with the use of NSAIDs. These drugs therefore can result in precipitation of acute attack of asthma.

Reference:

1. Barnes PJ. Pulmonary pharmacology. In: Brunton LL, Chabner BA, Knollmann BC, editors. Goodman and Gilman's the pharmacological basis of therapeutics.12 th ed. New York: McGraw-Hill; 2011.p. 1031-60.

MALARIA

Dr. Hiten Saresa JR II, Department of Pharmacology & Therapeutics

A 20-year old girl reported to the district hospital OPD with irregular episodes of high fever for the past 3 days. The fever is preceded by chills and shivering and attended by headache, body ache, pain in abdomen, nausea and weakness. The fever lasts 4-6 hours and subsides after sweating. On enquiry she informed that she belongs to a village in the tribal area of Madhya Pradesh. About a month back she had returned from her home after 3 weeks vacation and she works as a house maid in the city. Blood smear examination showed presence of intraerythrocytic P. vivax parasites. She was treated with the standard 1.5 g chloroquine(base) course over 3 days, and was given primaquine 15 mg tab to be taken once daily for 14 days, after she tested negative for G-6PD deficiency. She was afebrile on the 4th day, but returned back 7 days later with similar episode of chills and fever. Finger prick blood smear was positive for P. vivax. She confirmed continuing to take daily primaquine medication.

1. Preferred drug for treatment of malaria due to P. vivax in a 25 year old pregnant female is:
(A)Chloroquine
(B)Primaquine
(C)Sulfadoxine-pyrimethamine
(D)Quinine
2. Drawback of artesunate is:
(A)Poor bioavailability
(B)Rapid recrudescence of malaria
(C)Hypoglycaemia
(D)Hemolysis

3. Preferred drug for treatment of chloroquine resistant falciparum malaria is:
   (A)Artesunate
   (B)Chloroquine
   (C)Pyrimethamine
   (D)Primaquine
4. Tissue schizontocide which prevents relapse of vivax malaria is:
   (A)Quinine
   (B)Primaquine
   (C)Pyrimethamine
   (D)Chloroquine
5. Volume of distribution for chloroquine is:
   (A)5-8 L
   (B)9-15 L
   (C)100-650 L
   (D)Above 1300 L

Answers:
1. A
   Chloroquine is safe during pregnancy.
2. B
   Because of short duration of action, recrudescence rates are high. For this reason, they must be used in combination with long-acting schizontocide which acts by a different mechanism.
3. A
   Artesunate is preferred drug for chloroquine resistant falciparum malaria.
4. B
   Primaquine 15 mg daily for 14 days is drug of choice for radical cure of vivax malaria.
5. D
   It is the drug possessing largest volume of distribution (>1300 L).

Reference:
1. Vinetz JM, Clain J, Bounkeua V, Eastman RT, Fidock D. Chemotherapy of malaria. In: Brunton LL, Chabner BA, Knollmann BC, editors. Goodman and Gilman's the pharmacological basis of therapeutics. 12th ed. New York: Mc Graw-Hill; 2011. p. 1383-418.

ANTI-PROTOZOAL DRUGS
Dr. Hiten Saresa JR II, Department of Pharmacology & Therapeutics

A 50-year old gardener weighing 58 kg was admitted to the hospital with fever for 4 days, severe pain in right upper part of abdomen, loss of appetite, vomiting and marked weakness. He was not well for the past 2-3 weeks and had lost weight. There was no history of chronic diarrhoea. Palpation of abdomen revealed soft tender enlargement of liver 2 cm below costal margin. Marked tenderness was noted in the lower right intercostal region. Ultrasound showed a solitary 2.5 cm diameter abscess with sharp margins in the right lobe of liver. Stool examination was negative for any kind of ova and cysts. A clinical diagnosis of amoebic liver abscess was made and he was treated with metronidazole 500 mg i.v. over 1 hour every 8 hours for 5 days along with infusion of glucose-saline and vitamins. The fever and vomiting subsided and he started eating food. The injections were substituted by oral metronidazole 800 mg 3 times a day for another 5 days, and the patient became well, except weakness and mild tenderness in the right lower chest. Repeat ultrasound showed abscess cavity size to decrease to 1.5 cm. The patient was discharged with advice for vitamins and food.

1. Which of the following drugs is least effective luminal amoebicide?
   (A) Metronidazole
   (B) Diloxanidefuroate
   (C) Iodoquinol
   (D) Paromomycin
2. Which of the following drug causes disulfiram like reaction if used in patient taking alcohol?
   (A) Iodoquinol
   (B) Paromomycin
   (C) Metronidazole
   (D) Emetine
3. Tetracycline is indicated in the following form(s) of amoebic infection:
   (A) Acute amoebic dysentery
   (B) Chronic intestinal amoebiasis

(C) Amoebic liver abscess

(D) All of the above

4. The following antiamoebic drug should **NOT** be used in children because of risk of causing blindness:

(A) Quiniodochlor

(B) Diloxanidefuroate

(C) Tinidazole

(D) Secnidazole

5. The following drug is effective in hepatic amoebiasis but **NOT** in intestinal amoebiasis:

(A) Chloroquine

(B) Emetine

(C) Tetracycline

(D) Diloxanidefuroate

Answers:

1. A

Metronidazole is almost completely absorbed in the proximal intestine and very little amount reaches the colon.

2. C

Metronidazole causes disulfiram like reaction if used in patient taking alcohol.

3. B

Tetracycline reduce proliferation of entamoebae in the colon and are valuable in chronic, difficult to treat cases who have only the luminal cycle with little mucosal invasion.

4. A

Prolonged/repeated use of relatively high doses of quiniodochlor causes a neuropathic syndrome called 'subacutemyelo-optic neuropathy'. Its use in pediatric population is prohibited.

5. A

Chloroquine kills trophozoites of E. histolytica and is highly concentrated in liver. Therefore it is used in hepatic amoebiasis only.

Reference:

1. Phillips MA, Stanley SL Jr. Chemotherapy of protozoal infections: amebiasis, giardiasis, trichomoniasis, trypanosomiasis, leishmaniasis, and other protozoal infections. In: Brunton LL, Chabner BA, Knollmann BC, editors. Goodman and Gilman's the pharmacological basis of therapeutics. 12th ed. New York: Mc Graw-Hill; 2011. p. 1419-42.

ANTIVIRAL DRUGS

Dr. Hiten Saresa JR II, Department of Pharmacology & Therapeutics

A 58-year-old man presents for the evaluation of a painful rash. He says that for 3 or 4 days he had a sharp, burning pain radiating from his midback around to his left side. He thought that he was having a kidney stone. Yesterday he noticed a rash which spread in a distribution *"like a line"* in the same area in which he had the pain. He is on glyburide for type II diabetes, simvastatin for high cholesterol, and lisinopril for hypertension, all of which he has been taking for several years. He does have a history of having chickenpox as a child. On examination he has a low-grade fever and otherwise normal vital signs. His skin examination is remarkable for a rash in a belt-like distribution from his spine around his left flank to the midline of the abdomen. The rash consists of erythematous patches with clusters of vesicles. The remainder of his examination is normal. Diagnosis of herpes zoster was made and he was prescribed a course of acyclovir (ACV).

1. Which of the following viruses is most susceptible to acyclovir?

(A) Herpes simplex type I virus

(B) Herpes simplex type II virus

(C) Varicella-zoster virus

(D) Epstein-Barr virus

2. Ganciclovir is preferred over acyclovir in the following condition:

(A) Herpes simplex keratitis

(B) Herpes zoster

(C) Chickenpox

(D) Cytomegalovirus retinitis in AIDS patients

3. Choose the correct statement about famciclovir:

(A) It is active against acyclovir resistant strains of herpes simplex virus

(B) It does not need conversion to an active metabolite

(C)It is used orally to treat genital herpes simplex

(D)It is the drug of choice for cytomegalovirus retinitis

4. What is true of acyclovir treatment of genital herpes simplex?

(A)Topical treatment affords symptomatic relief in primary as well as recurrent disease

(B)Oral therapy for 10 days affords symptomatic relief as well as prevents recurrences

(C)Oral therapy for 10 days affords symptomatic relief but does not prevent recurrences

(D)Continuous long-term topical therapy is recommended to prevent recurrences

5. Iodoxuridine is indicated in:

(A)Herpes simplex keratitis

(B)Herpes zoster

(C)Chickenpox

(D)All of the above

Answers:

1. A

HSV-1 is most sensitive followed by HSV-2> VZV=EBV, while CMV is practically not affected.

2. D

Ganciclovir's active metabolite attains much higher concentration inside CMV infected cells.

3. C

Famciclovir is ester prodrug of penciclovir which inhibits H. simplex but not acyclovir-resistant strains.

4. C

Both local and oral therapies afford symptomatic relief and rapid healing of lesions but do not prevent recurrences.

5. A

Idoxuridine is effective only against DNA viruses and clinical utility is limited to topical treatment of H. simplex keratitis.

Reference:

1. Acosta EP, Flexner C. Antiviral agents (nonretroviral). In: Brunton LL, Chabner BA, Knollmann BC, editors. Goodman and Gillman's the pharmacological basis of therapeutics. 12th ed. New York: Mc Graw-Hill; 2011. p. 1593-622.

CARCINOMA BREAST

Dr. Shweta Singh JR II, Department of Pharmacology & Therapeutics

A 60 year old female was diagnosed with breast cancer. She was given chemotherapy with doxorubicin and cyclophosphamide. Few days after the start of the therapy, she developed swelling of the lower extremities and febrile neutropenia. Amphotericin B and imipenem were administered. She now complains of muscle weakness, palpitations, blood in urine and burning sensation during micturition. Her ECG was done which showed prominent U waves indicative of hypokalemia along with signs of left ventricular hypertrophy, which pointed towards dilated cardiomyopathy.

1. Which drug is responsible for hypokalemia in this patient?

(A) Doxorubicin

(B) Cyclophosphamide

(C) Amphotericin B

(D) Imipenem

2. Which drug is responsible for blood in urine?

(A) Doxorubicin

(B) Cyclophosphamide

(C) Amphotericin B

(D) Imipenem

3. Which of the following is used to treat haematuria in the above patient?

(A) Folic acid

(B) Daunorubicin

(C) Methotrexate

(D) Mesna

4. Which of the following drugs is responsible for dilated cardiomyopathy?

(A) Doxorubicin

(B) Cyclophosphamide
(C) Amphotericin B
(D) Imipinem

5. Which of the following is administered to reduce dilated cardiomyopathy?
   (A) Desferrioxamine
   (B) Deferiprone
   (C) Dexrazoxane
   (D) D-penicillamine

Answers:
   1. C
      Renal wasting of K^+ is seen during and for several weeks after therapy with amphotericin B.
   2. B
      Therapy with cyclophosphamide generates 2 metabolites phosphoramide mustard and acrolein. Acrolein is responsible for haemrrhagic cystitis.
   3. D
      Haemorrrhagic cystitis caused by cyclophosphamide can be reduced in intensity or prevented by parenteral coadministration of mesna which conjugates acrolein in urine. Mesna does not negate the systemic antitumor activity of the drug.
   4. A
      Cardiomyopathy is the most important long term toxicity of doxorubicin.
   5. C
      Dexrazoxane is a cardioprotective iron chelating agent which reduces troponin T elevations and averts cardiotoxicity.

References:
   1. Chabner BA, Bertino J, Cleary J, Ortiz T, Lane A, Supko JG, et al. Cytotoxic agents. In: Brunton LL, Chabner BA, Knollmann BC, editors. Goodman & Gilman's the pharmacological basis of therapeutics. 12th ed. New York: Mc Graw-Hill; 2011. p. 1677-730.
   2. Bennett JE. Antifungal agents. In: Brunton LL, Chabner BA, Knollmann BC, editors. Goodman & Gilman's the pharmacological basis of therapeutics. 12th ed. New York: Mc Graw-Hill; 2011. p. 1571-92.

DEEP VEIN THROMBOSIS
Dr. Shweta Singh JR II, Department of Pharmacology & Therapeutics

A 30 year old obese female presented with the complaints of pain and swelling in her left lower limb for past 1 month. She was already taking isoniazid and rifampicin for tuberculosis. Venography was done and she was diagnosed as a case of deep vein thrombosis. Warfarin was started but her prothrombin time was not raised.

1. Prolongation of only prothrombin time indicates defect in:
   (A) Extrinsic coagulation pathway
   (B) Intrinsic coagulation pathway
   (C) Both extrinsic and intrinsic coagulation pathways
   (D) Common pathway

2. Prothrombin time was **NOT** raised due to which drug interaction?
   (A) Isoniazid + warfarin
   (B) Rifampicin + warfarin
   (C) Heparin + warfarin
   (D) Isoniazid + rifampicin

3. What should be the next step in the manangement?
   (A) Increase the dose of warfarin
   (B) Replace warfarin with acenocoumarin
   (C) Switch ethambutol for rifampicin
   (D) Use LMWH

4. Which of the following drugs follows zero order kinetics?
   (A) Warfarin
   (B) Heparin
   (C) Isoniazid
   (D) Rifampicin

5. What is the antidote for warfarin?
   (A) Protamine sulfate

(B) Vitamin K
(C) Naloxone
(D) Disulfiram

Answers:

1. A

   A patient with a prolonged PT and a normal aPTT has a defect in the extrinsic coagulation pathway because thromboplastin is extrinsic to the plasma.

2. B

   Warfarin is metabolized principally by CYP2C9. Rifampicin potently induces CYP2C9, so its administration results in a decreased $t_{1/2}$ of warfarin.

3. D

   Rifampicin is the most effective drug for tuberculosis, hence should not be replaced.

   Warfarin follows zero order kinetics and increase in its dose can result in saturation of metabolism and thus toxicity. Therefore, increasing the dose of warfarin is not advisable.

   Acenocoumarin 's metabolism is also subjected to induction by rifampicin.

4. A

   The elimination of warfarin approaches saturation over the therapeutic range.

5. B

   Warfarin acts as competitive antagonists of vitamin K and interferes with the synthesis of vitamin k dependent clotting factors. Therefore, excess vitamin K can reverse the effects of warfarin.

References:

1. Weitz JI. Blood coagulation and anticoagulant, fibrinolytic, and antiplatelet drugs. In: Brunton LL, Chabner BA, Knollmann BC, editors. Goodman & Gilman's the pharmacological basis of therapeutics. 12th ed. New York: Mc Graw-Hill; 2011. p. 849-76.
2. Gumbo T. Chemotherapy of tuberculosis, mycobacterium avium complex disease, and leprosy. In: Brunton LL, Chabner BA, Knollmann BC, editors. Goodman & Gilman's the pharmacological basis of therapeutics. 12th ed. New York: Mc Graw-Hill; 2011. p. 1549-70.
3. Tripathi KD. Essentials of medical pharmacology. 7th ed. New Delhi: Jaypee Brothers Medical Publishers; 2013. p. 22-36.

DYSLIPIDEMIA

Dr. Shweta Singh JR II, Department of Pharmacology & Therapeutics

A 52 year old diabetic male patient presented with a hard yellow patch over the inside corner of his left eyelid. The doctor explained to him that this hard yellow patch is known as xanthelasma which occurs due to deposition of fat under the skin and is associated with an increased risk of ischaemic heart disease. The doctor gave him the necessary treatment and advised him to get his lipid profile checked. The lipid profile report showed that HDL levels were markedly lowered and LDL levels were raised. He was advised a combination of atorvastatin and nicotinic acid.

1. Which of the following drugs is mainly responsible for raising HDL?
   (A) Statins
   (B) Nicotinic Acid
   (C) Fibrates
   (D) Ezetimibe

2. Risk of which of the following is increased in the above patient?
   (A) Ototoxicity
   (B) Nephrotoxicity
   (C) Neurotoxicity
   (D) Myopathy

3. Which of the following is responsible for lowering of lipoprotein (a)?
   (A) Nicotinic Acid
   (B) Fibrates
   (C) Statins
   (D) Ezetimibe

4. Which of the following statins can be taken anytime during the day?
   (A) Pravastatin
   (B) Simvastatin
   (C) Atorvastatin
   (D) Lovastatin

5. Which enzyme is inhibited by atorvastatin?
   (A) HMGCoA synthetase
   (B) HMGCoA reductase
   (C) HMGCoA dehydrogenase
   (D) HMGCoA hydroxylase

Answers:
   1. B
      Niacin is the best agent available for increasing HDL cholesterol.
   2. D
      Concomitant administration of niacin increases the risk of statin induced myopathy.
   3. A
      Niacin decreases VLDL and LDL levels, and Lp(a) in most patients.
   4. C
      Atorvastatin has a long $t_{1/2}$ which allows administration of this statin at any time of the day.
   5. B
      Statins exert their effect by competitively inhibiting HMG CoA reductase.

References:

   1. Bersot TP. Drug Therapy for hypercholesterolemia and dyslipidemia. In: Brunton LL, Chabner BA, Knollmann BC, editors. Goodman & Gilman's the pharmacological basis of therapeutics. 12th ed. New York: Mc Graw-Hill; 2011. p. 877-908.
   2. Malloy MJ, Kane JP. Agents used in dyslipidemia. In: Katzung BG, Masters SB, Trevor AJ, editors. Basic and clinical pharmacology. 11th ed. New Delhi: Tata McGraw-Hill; 2010. p. 605-20.

ARRHYTHMIA
Dr. Dheeraj Kumar Singh JR I, Department of Pharmacology & Therapeutics

A 55 years old male presented with palpitation felt off and on, both during activity as well as at rest for last 1 month. He also complained of tiredness and anxiety. The pulse was irregular in volume and frequency with average rate of 104/min, respiration 20/min, BP 130/84mmhg, apex beat was irregular, with an average rate 120/min. heart sounds were irregular, but there was no murmur. The ECG showed atrial fibrillation (AF) with no sign of ischemia. A diagnosis of persistent AF was made, and it was decided to electrically cardiovert him. He was put on warfarin 5mg once daily and dose to be adjusted to an international normalized ratio (INR) between 2-2.5. This was to be maintained for 1 month before attempting cardioversion.

1. The purpose of putting patient on warfarin therapy before attempting cardioversion is:
   (A) To prevent thromboembolism
   (B) To convert atrial fibrillation into atrial flutter
   (C) To decrease the dose of other drugs required
   (D) To prevent the development of other arrhythmias.
2. Which of the following drug can be given during meantime to control and regularize his heart rate?
   (A) Lidocaine
   (B) Mexilitine
   (C) Quinidine
   (D) Verapamil
3. After cardioversion which of the following drug can be given to maintain sinus rhythm and prevent recurrence of atrial fibrillation (AF)?
   (A) Sotalol
   (B) Lidocaine
   (C) Verapamil
   (D) Diltiazem
4. In case of unsuccessful cardioversion which of the following drug should be given to revert him to sinus rhythm?
   (A) Lidocaine
   (B) Amiodarone
   (C) Dofetilide
   (D) Propranolol
5. During AF which of the following drug can be given for urgent ventricular rate control?
   (A) Lidocaine I.V.
   (B) Verapamil

(C) Esmolol I.V.

(D) Digoxin

Answers:

1. A

   Current guideline is to give warfarin to a target INR of 2-3 in AF patients with high for stroke.

2. D

   Verapamil may be used to control ventricular rate in AF (atrial fibrillation) or AFl (atrial flutter).

3. A

   Sotalol is effective in polymorphic VT (ventricular tachycardia) and for maintaining sinus rhythm in AF (atrial fibrillation) /AFl (atrial flutter).

4. B

   Amiodarone is used to maintain sinus rhythm in AF (atrial fibrillation) when other drugs have failed. Resistant VT (ventricular tachycardia) and recurrent VF (ventricular fibrillation) are most important indication.

5. C

   Esmolol is quick and short acting beta blocker administered i.v and is very useful for emergency control of ventricular rate in AF (atrial fibrillation)/AFl (atrial flutter).

Reference:

1. Tripathi KD. Essentials of medical pharmacology. 6th ed. New Delhi: Jaypee Brothers Medical Publishers; 2008. p. 508-20.

CONGESTIVE HEART FAILURE

Dr. Dheeraj Kumar Singh JR I, Department of Pharmacology & Therapeutics

A 72 year old man presents with swelling over ankle and feet, also noticeable over face in the morning, shortness of breath and palpitation on walking around 100m, weakness, fatigue and cough at night. The pulse is 110/min, BP 114/78, there is pitting edema over feet, liver is enlarged 2cm below costal margin, neck veins are filled upto 3 cm above clavicle, crepitations are heard at the base of lungs, apex beat is in the 6th intercostals space and heart sounds are muffled. Chest X-Ray and echocardiography shows enlarged cardiac shadow and ejection fraction of 28%. A diagnosis of moderate grade congestive heart failure due to dilated cardiomyopathy is made. The doctor prescribed bed rest, salt restriction, tab. enalapril 5mg twice a day and tab. furosemide 40mg in the morning.

1. Enalapril differs from captopril in that:
   (A) It blocks angiotensin II receptors
   (B) It does not produce cough as a side effect
   (C) It is less liable to cause abrupt first dose hypotension
   (D) It has a shorter duration of action

2. The following drug increases cardiac output in congestive heart failure without having any direct myocardial action:
   (A) Captopril
   (B) Digoxin
   (C) Amrinone
   (D) Dobutamine

3. Select the drug that can help restore cardiac performance as well as prolong survival in CHF patients:
   (A) Spironolactone
   (B) Furosemide
   (C) Dobutamine
   (D) Metoprolol

4. Which of the following drugs can afford both haemodynamic improvement as well as disease modifying benefits in CHF?
   (A) Furosemide
   (B) Milrinone
   (C) Losartan
   (D) Digoxin

5. The preferred diuretic for mobilizing edema fluid in CHF is:
   (A) Hydrochlorothiazide
   (B) Furosemide
   (C) Metolazone
   (D) Amiloride

Answers:

1. **C**

   Onset of action of enalapril is slower due to need for conversion to active metabolite, therefore it is less liable to cause abrupt first dose hypotension.

2. **A**

   ACE inhibitors have no direct action on myocardium though stroke volume and cardiac output are increased, while heart rate is reduced.

3. **D**

   Beta blockers cause antagonism of ventricular wall enhancing, apoptosis promoting and pathological remodelling effects of excess sympathetic activity in CHF as well as due to prevention of arrhythmias.

4. **C**

   ARBs improve hemodynamic as well as cardiac status by reversing ventricular/ vascular hypertrophy/remodelling.

5. **B**

   Furosemide (I.V.) causes prompt increase in systemic venous capacitance and decreases left ventricular filling pressure. This action is responsible for quick relief in CHF patients.

Reference:

1. Tripathi KD. Essentials of medical pharmacology. 6th ed. New Delhi: Jaypee Brothers Medical Publishers; 2008. p. 493-507.

ANGINA

Dr. Dheeraj Kumar Singh, JR I, Department of Pharmacology & Therapeutics

A 60 year old man comes to emergency with pain, tightness and discomfort over middle part of the chest. According to patient, one or two such episodes occur every day, episodic in nature and usually occur during climbing stairs or moderate exercise. Pain is relieved after 5-10 min of rest. He has quit smoking 4 years back when he was diagnosed with COPD for which he regularly takes 2 inhalations of ipratropium bromide 3 times a day and 2 puffs of salbutamol whenever he feels out of breath. Pulse was 88/min and BP 128/84 mm hg. Resting ECG was normal but stress test was positive. The diagnosis of exertional angina was made and he was prescribed tab. glyceryl trinitrate 0.5 mg to be put under the tongue as soon as he begins to feel the chest discomfort as well as before taking any physical exertion.

1. Choose the correct statement about the action of nitrates on coronary vessels:
   (A) They mitigate angina pectoris by increasing total coronary flow
   (B) They preferentially dilate conducting arteries without affecting resistance arterioles
   (C) They preferentially dilate autoregulatory arterioles without affecting the larger arteries
   (D) They increase subepicardial blood flow without affecting subendocardial blood flow
2. Select the organic nitrate which undergoes minimal first-pass metabolism in the liver:
   (A) Glyceryl trinitrate
   (B) Isosorbide dinitrate
   (C) Isosorbide mononitrate
   (D) Erythrityl tetranitrate
3. The following anti-anginal drug is most likely to produce tachycardia as a side effect:
   (A) Amlodipine
   (B) Nifedipine
   (C) Diltiazem
   (D) Verapamil
4. Propranolol should **NOT** be prescribed for a patient of angina pectoris who is already receiving:
   (A) Nifedipine
   (B) Felodipine
   (C) Verapamil
   (D) Isosorbide mononitrate
5. Though nitrates and calcium channel blockers are both vasodilators, they are used concurrently in angina pectoris, because:
   (A) They antagonise each other's side effects
   (B) Nitrates primarily reduce preload while calcium channel blockers primarily reduce afterload
   (C) Nitrates increase coronary flow while calcium channel blockers reduce cardiac work

(D) Both 'B' and 'C' are correct

Answers:
1. B
   Nitrates preferentially dilate conducting coronary arteries than resistance arterioles. This may cause favourable redistribution of blood flow to ischaemic ares while in non ischaemic areas resistance vessels maintain their tone.
2. C
   All nitrates except isosorbide mononitrate undergo extensive and variable first pass metabolism.
3. B
   Nifedipine does not depress SA node or A-V conductance. Reflex sympathetic stimulation of heart predominates. There is tachycardia, increased contractility and cardiac output.
4. D
   Propranolol may counteract the effect of nitrates.
5. B
   Nitrates primarily reduce preload while calcium channel blockers primarily reduce afterload. Both lead to beneficial action in angina.

Reference:
1. Tripathi KD. Essentials of medical pharmacology. 6th ed. New Delhi: Jaypee Brothers Medical Publishers; 2008. p. 521-38.

MIGRAINE
Dr. Sartaj Hussain, JR I, Department of Pharmacology & Therapeutics

A 25-year-old medical student routinely develops headaches on the weekend. The headaches are almost always limited to the right side of her head and centered about the right temple. She knows that a headache is coming because of changes in her vision that precede the headache by 20 to 30 min. She sees scintillating lights just to the left of her center of vision. This visual aberration then expands and interferes with her vision. The blind spot that it creates appears to have a scintillating margin. As the blind spot clears, the headache starts. It rarely lasts more than 1 hour, but is usually associated by nausea and vomiting. The condition was diagnosed as a case of classical migraine.

1. Appropriate therapy for this patient's presented with headache in emergency department might include which of the following drug?
   (A) Sumatriptan
   (B) Ergotamine
   (C) Verapamil
   (D) Amitriptyline hydrochloride
2. Appropriate long-term management might include a prescription for daily use of which of the following medications?
   (A) Ergotamine tartrate
   (B) Sumatriptan
   (C) Oral contraceptives
   (D) Amitriptyline hydrochloride
3. Sumatriptan is:
   (A) $5HT_{1D}$ antagonist
   (B) $5HT_{1A}$ agonist
   (C) $5HT_{1D}$ agonist
   (D) $5HT_{1A}$ antagonist
4. Drug used in migraine prophylaxis are all **EXCEPT**:
   (A) Flunarizine
   (B) Propanolol
   (C) Cyproheptadine
   (D) Sumatriptan

Answers:
1. A
   Sumatriptan (subcutaneous) is the drug of choice for aborting acute attack of migraine.
2. D

Several medications are effective as prophylactic agents in the treatment of migraine. These include amitriptyline hydrochloride, propranolol, verapamil, and valproate. Most experts recommend initiating prophylactic therapy only when headaches occur at least one to two times per month. Metoclopramide hydrochloride, sumatriptan, and ergotamine tartrate are appropriately used to treat an acute attack of migraine, and should not be prescribed on a daily basis.

3. C

Sumatriptan acts as a selective agonist at $5HT_{1B/1D}$ receptors.

4. D

Metoclopramide, sumatriptan, and ergotamine tartrate are used to treat an acute attack of migraine. Several medications are effective as prophylactic agents in the treatment of migraine. These include amitriptyline hydrochloride, propranolol, verapamil, valproate, flunarizine and topiramate.

References:

1. Sanders-Bush E, Hazelwood L. 5-Hydroxytryptamine (serotonin) and dopamine. In:Brunton LL, Chabner BA, Knollmann BC, editors. Goodman & Gilman's the pharmacological basis of therapeutics. 12th ed. New York: Mc Graw-Hill; 2011. p. 335-62.
2. Katzung BG. Histamine, serotonin, & the ergot alkaloids. In: Katzung BG, Masters SB, Trevor AJ, editors. Basic and clinical pharmacology. 11th ed. New Delhi: Tata McGraw-Hill; 2010. p. 271-92.

RHEUMATOID ARTHRITIS

Dr. Sartaj Hussain, JR I, Department of Pharmacology & Therapeutics

A 42-year-old female complains of 8 weeks of pain and swelling in both wrists and knees. The patient complained of fatigue and lethargy several weeks before noticing the joint pain. The patient notes that after a period of rest, resistance to movement is more striking. On examination, the metacarpophalangeal joints and wrists are warm and tender, tenderness and effusion has occurred in both the knee joints. The rheumatoid factor is positive and subcutaneous nodules are noted on the extensor surfaces of the forearm. There are no other joint abnormalities. The clinical picture is suggestive of rheumatoid arthritis. There is no alopecia, photosensitivity, kidney disease or rash.

1. The following are rheumatoid disease modifying drugs **EXCEPT**:
   (A) Chloroquine
   (B) Gold
   (C) Penicillamine
   (D) BAL
2. Which of the following disease modifying anti-rheumatic drugs (DMARDs) is drug of first choice?
   (A) Penicillamine
   (B) Methotrexate
   (C) Gold
   (D) Anakinra
3. What is the most likely mechanism by which etanercept suppresses the signs, symptoms, or underlying pathophysiology of rheumatoid arthritis?
   (A) Inhibits eicosanoid synthesis by inhibiting phospholipaseA_2
   (B) Inhibits leukocyte migration by blocking microtubular formation
   (C) Neutralizes circulating tumor necrosis factor (TNF-α)
   (D) Selectively and effectively inhibits COX-2
4. In case of Hemophilia with Rheumatoid arthritis, the analgesic of choice is:
   (A) Ibuprofen
   (B) Aspirin
   (C) Acetaminophen
   (D) Phenylbutazone

Answers:

1. D

   Disease modifying anti-rheumatic drugs (DMARDs) are methotrexate, gold compounds, d-penicillamine, chloroquine and sulfasalazine.

2. B

   Methotrexate is first choice DMARD.

3. C

   TNF-α plays major role in joint destruction in patients with rheumatoid arthritis. Three drugs etanercept, adalimumab, and infliximab act as DMARDs by blocking the action of TNF-α.

4. C

   Acetaminophen does not inhibit platelet aggregation, therefore it is analgesic of choice when bleeding tendencies are an issue. Acetaminophen is particular useful for those with bleeding disorders such as bleeding ulcers or hemophilia and has been used for pain control in rheumatoid arthritis.

References:

1. Smyth EM, Grosser T, FitGerald GA. Lipid derived autacoids: eicosanoids and platelet activating factor. In: Brunton LL, Chabner BA, Knollmann BC, editors. Goodman & Gilman's the pharmacological basis of therapeutics. 12th ed. New York: Mc Graw-Hill; 2011. p. 937-58.
2. Smyth EM, FitzGerald GA. The eicosanoids: prostaglandins, thromboxanes, leukotrienes, & related compunds. In: Katzung BG, Masters SB, Trevor AJ, editors. Basic and clinical pharmacology. 11th ed. New Delhi: Tata McGraw-Hill; 2010. p. 313-30.
3. Tripathi KD. Essentials of medical pharmacology. 6th ed. New Delhi: Jaypee Brothers Medical Publishers; 2008. p. 202-12.

GOUT

Dr. Sartaj Hussain, JR I, Department of Pharmacology & Therapeutics

A 49-year-old man presents with painful, recurring episodes of swelling in his left great toe. He takes 25 mg of hydrochlorothiazide daily for blood pressure control but otherwise is in good health. On physical examination, the patient is afebrile but his great toe is warm, swollen, erythematous, and exquisitely tender to palpation. He has several subcutaneous nodules in his pinna and monosodium urate crystals were found in synovial fluid.

1. All of the following drugs can produce hyperuricemia **EXCEPT**:
   (A) Sulfinpyrazone
   (B) Pyrazinamide
   (C) Ethambutol
   (D) Hydrochlorthiazide
2. Preferred drug for acute gout is:
   (A) Colchicine
   (B) Indomethacin
   (C) Allopurinol
   (D) Dexamethasone
3. Select the drug which is used in chronic gout but is **NOT**uricosuric:
   (A) Probenecid
   (B) Phenylbutazone
   (C) Sulfinpyrazone
   (D) Allopurinol
4. Allopurinol has a therapeutic effect in the following conditions **EXCEPT**:
   (A) Radiotherapy induced hyperuricaemia
   (B) Hydrochlorothiazide induced hyperuricaemia
   (C) Acute gouty arthritis
   (D) Kala-azar

Answers:

1. A

    Drugs causing hyperuricemia are aspirin, chlorthalidone, cyclosporine, cytotoxics, ethacrynic acid, fructose (IV), furosemide, pyrazinamide and thiazides. Sulfinpyrazone is a uricosuric agent and is used in the treatment of hyperuricemia.

2. B

    NSAIDs except aspirin are the agent of choice for treatment of gout.

3. D

    Allopurinol inhibits the formation of uric acid from hypoxanthine and xanthine by inhibiting the enzyme xanthine oxidase.

4. C

    Allopurinol is contraindicated in acute gout because may precipitate an acute attack of gouty arthritis. Allopurinol is indicated in chronic gout, in secondary hyperuricemia (due to chemotherapy, radiotherapy or thiazide diuretics), recurrent renal urate stone and kala-azar.

References:

1. Grosser T, Smyth EM, FitzGerald GA. Anti-inflammatory, antipyretic, and analgesic agents; pharmacotherapy of gout. In: Brunton LL, Chabner BA, Knollmann BC, editors. Goodman & Gilman's the pharmacological basis of therapeutics. 12th ed. New York: Mc Graw-Hill; 2011. p. 959-1004.
2. Furst DE, Ulrich RW, Varkey AC. Nonsteroidal anti-inflammatory drugs, disease-modifying antirheumatic drugs, nonopioid analgesics, & drugs used in gout. In: Katzung BG, Masters SB, Trevor AJ, editors. Basic and clinical pharmacology. 11th ed. New Delhi: Tata McGraw-Hill; 2010. p. 621-42.

Chapter-20

Physical Medicine & Rehabilitation

SPINAL CORD INJURY

Dr. Anil Kumar Gupta, Associate Professor & Dr. Arvind Kumar Sharma, Junior Resident-3, Physical Medicine & Rehabilitation

A 29 year old man who was a rear passenger in a motor vehicle accident presented to trauma emergency with severe mid-back pain. His airway was clear and vitals were stable. On neurological examination, AIS was A. There was tenderness present at the thoracolumbar region in the back and there was a suspicion about posterior ligamentous complex disruption on local examination of spine. There was no visceral injury. There was no prior history of spinal complaints. X-ray (AP and lateral) demonstrated a flexion compression injury of T12.

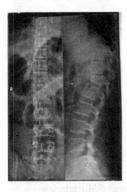

X-ray Dorsolumbar Spine

1. Most appropriate method for determining stability of the spine
    (A) Modified Denis 3 column classification
    (B) CT spine
    (C) MRI spine
    (D) TLICS score
2. What is the TLICS score for the above case
    (A) 3
    (B) 5
    (C) 7
    (D) 9
3. Management for this case would be
    (A) Surgical stabilization
    (B) Spinal bracing
    (C) Complete bed rest only
    (D) Surgical or conservative
4. Which of the following is not a component of TLICS score
    (A) Injury morphology
    (B) Posterior ligamentous complex integrity
    (C) Dynamic X ray of spine
    (D) Neurological status

5. Find the correct match for TLICS scoring

	Neurologically intact	Nerve root injury	Spinal cord (complete injury)	Spinal cord (incomplete injury)
a.	3	2	3	2
b.	0	2	2	3
c.	0	1	3	2
d.	1	3	2	4

Answers:

1. **D**

   Dennis anatomic divisions of columns are easily visualized on CT images but Dennis classification system is unclear on how ligamentous injuries can be identified. With the advent of MRI, occult ligamentous injuries may be easier to define. Yet, there is no classification system to date that incorporates this new technology in its scheme. TLICS scoring was conceptualized based on a survey given to Spine Trauma Study Group, which consists of worldwide experts in the field of spinal trauma. The goal of this survey was to identify similarities in treatment algorithms for common thoracolumbar injuries as well as to identify characteristics of injury that played a key role in decision making process.

2. **B**

   TLICSS is summation of points on 3 categories: fracture morphology, neurological status, and integrity of the posterior ligamentous complex.

   Fracture morphology
   Compression Injuries (1pt)
   Burst (2pts)
   Translational/Rotational Injuries (3pts)
   Distraction Injuries (4pts)
   Neurologic status
   Intact (0)
   Root Injury (2pts)
   Complete injury (2pts)
   Incomplete injury (3pts)
   Cauda Equina injury (3pts)
   Integrity of posterior ligamentous complex (PLC) - Supraspinous ligament (SSL), interspinous ligament (ISL), capsular ligaments and ligamentum flavum
   Intact (0)
   Injury suspected (2pts)
   Injured (3pts)
   In this patients it is 1 point for morphology + 2 points for complete neurological injury(AIS score A) + 2 points for suspected PLC injury . Total TLICS= 5.

3. **A**

   Management according to summation of point values from each category
   3 or less - nonoperative
   4 - either operative or nonoperative manaagement
   5 or more - surgical candidate

4. **C**

   Explanation same as 2

5. **B**

   Explanation same as 2

References:

1. Patel AA, Vaccaro AR, Albert TJ et al. The adaptation of a new classification system: time dependent variation in interobserver reliability of the thoracolumbar injury severity score classification system. The Spine J. Feb 1 2007; 32 (3) : E105-10.
2. Lee JY, Vaccaro AR, Lim MR, et al. Thoracolumbar injury classification and severity score: a new paradigm for the treatment of thoracolumbar spine trauma. J Orthop Sci. Nov 2005; 10(6):671-5.
3. AR Vaccaro, RA Lehman, RJ Hurlbert et al. A new classification of thoracolumbar injuries. The Spine J. 2005; 30 (20): 2325-33.

DVT IN SCI

Dr. Anil Kumar Gupta, Associate Professor & Dr. Arvind Kumar Sharma, Junior Resident-3, Physical Medicine & Rehabilitation

A patient of traumatic spinal cord injury was referred to the Dept of PMR from Dept of Orthopedics after spinal fixation for rehabilitation. On the day 15th of surgery, he developed swelling of right lower limb. On local examination, the temperature was raised; there was presence of swelling and erythema in right lower limb from calf downwards. Fever was absent. All the peripheral pulses were normal. Routine blood examination was normal. On special investigation, D- dimer level was 430 microgram/litre.

1. What is the provisional diagnosis?
   - (A) Cellulitis
   - (B) DVT
   - (C) Drug allergy
   - (D) Dependent edema
2. What will be the next investigation?
   - (A) X ray right Lower Limb
   - (B) Duplex venous USG
   - (C) Arteriography
   - (D) Venography
3. Gold standard for the diagnosis of this condition:
   - (A) Duplex venous USG
   - (B) Arteriogram
   - (C) Venogram
   - (D) MRI
4. Immediate management of this patient includes:
   - (A) Promote mobilization
   - (B) LMWH/UFH
   - (C) Warfarin only
   - (D) Active exercises
5. Prophylaxis for prevention of DVT in a SCI patient includes all except
   - (A) LMWH.
   - (B) Elastic stockings.
   - (C) Pneumatic compression device.
   - (D) Complete bed rest.

Answers:

1. B
   Unilateral involvement of lower limb excludes dependent edema and drug allergy. Absence of fever excludes cellulitis.
2. B
   Duplex venous USG(B-mode.i.e. two dimensional, imaging, and pulse-wave Doppler interrogation).The noninvasive test used most often to diagnose DVT. The sensitivity approaches 95% for proximal DVT and 75% for symptomatic calf vein thrombosis.
3. C
   Venogram is gold standard. Contrast medium is injected in to superficial vein of the foot and directed to deep system by using a tourniquets. The presence of a filling defect or absence of filling of the deep veins is required to make the diagnosis
4. B
   Immediately anticoagulation is initiated with a parentral drug, UFH or LMWH. Long term anticoagulation is given with a vit K antagonist (warfarin). Warfarin requires 5-7 days to achieve a therapeutic level, during that time one should overlap the the parentral and oral drugs.
5. D
   Early ambulation is the simplest method of prophylaxis. It acts by activating the calf pump mechanism.

References:
1. Dan L Longo, Dennis L Kasper, J Larry Jameson (eds) Harrison's principles of internal medicine. 18th edition USA: McGraw Hill companies 2012.p2175-76.
2. Randall L Braddom.(ed) *Physical Medicine and Rehabilitation*. 3rd edition.Elsivier Saunders Philadelphia 2011 p. 1323.
3. Denise I. Campagnolo(ed.), Geno J. Merli. Autonomic and cardiovascular complication of spinal cord injury. Steven Kirshblum, M.D.,Denise I. Campagnolo, Joel A. Delisa, M.D.(eds.).*Spinal Cord Medicine,* Philadelphia: Lippincott Williams & Wilkins2002.p128-132
4. Powell M, Kirshblum S, O'Connor KC. Duplex ultrasound screening for deep vein thrombosis in spinal cord injured patients at rehabilitation admission. *Arch Phys Med Rehabil.* Sep 1999;80(9):1044-6
5. Consortium for Spinal Cord Medicine Clinical Practice Guidelines. *Prevention of Thromboembolism in Spinal Cord Injury.* 2nd ed. Washington, DC: Paralyzed Veterans of America; 1999.

CHARCOT JOINT

Dr. Anil Kumar Gupta, Associate Professor & Dr. Arvind Kumar Sharma, Junior Resident-3, Physical Medicine & Rehabilitation

A 35 year old female presented with gradual increasing swelling of right knee joint since last 6 months. Initially there was no pain, but since last 2 months she complains of pain in right knee. Further enquiry revealed a past history of spinal anesthesia given for caesarean section. There was no previous history of joint pains, joint swellings, or trauma. In the CNS examination higher mental functions, cranial nerves and speech were normal. The right knee had a warm swelling and a circumference of 46cm (left knee girth being 37 cm) with no tenderness or crepitus. There was laxity of knee joint on medial and lateral movements. Anterior and posterior drawer test were positive. Radiograph of her right knee showed fracture dislocation of the tibia with destruction of lateral condyle of femur and medial condyle of tibia and grossly disorganized knee joint. Synovial fluid analysis from the knee showed clear fluid, protein of 3 g/dl, an total cells 0.153×10^9/L (all lymphocytes); culture for bacterial, mycobacterial and fungal elements was negative and polarized light microscopy did not reveal any crystals. Fasting blood sugar was 98 mg%, blood VDRL was non reactive and the X-ray chest normal. MRI spine revealed syrinx at distal cord and conus region.

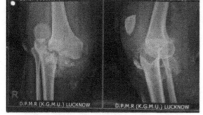

1. The most likely diagnosis is:
   (A) Charcot knee joint
   (B) Tuberculous arthritis
   (C) Septic arthritis
   (D) Osteoarthritis knee
2. How will you differentiate neuropathic knee joint from osteoarthritis knee?
   (A) Soft tissue swelling
   (B) Osteophytes
   (C) Joint effusion
   (D) Bony fragments
3. What would be the cause of neuropathic joint in this patient?
   (A) Tabes dorsalis
   (B) DM
   (C) Leprosy
   (D) Syringomyelia
4. All of the following are pathological findings of neuropathic knee except .
   (A) Increased vascularity

(B) Decreased osteoclast function

(C) Joint effusion

(D) Thickening of synovial membrane

5. The following are treatment of this condition except

(A) Analgesics for pain

(B) Splints & calipers

(C) Arthrodesis

(D) Replacement arthroplasty

Answers:

1. A

   Destructive arthropathy with normal chest X- ray, and normal synovial fulid examination and presence of bony fragments suggests charcot knee joint

2. D

   Presence of bony fragments, subluxation and periarticular debris occur only in charcot knee while the soft tissue swelling, osteophytes and joint effusion occur in both

3. D

   Charcot knee is a rare complication of the lumbar cord syringomyelia due to spinal anaesthesia. Generally syringomyelia produces bilateral involvement. However, a thin, strategically placed syrinx cavity as seen in the right hemicord may give ipsilateral presentation.

4. B

   Neuropathic knee shows rapid destruction with increased osteoclast activity and increased vascularity.

5. D

   Some patients complain of pain and may need analgesics. Treatment is usually conservative and consists of splintage. Arthrodesis may be attempted. Replacement arthroplasty is not indicated.

References:

1. Sara J. Cuccurullo, *Physical medicine & rehabilitation board review* 3rd edition, Demos Medical USA 2010, p.561

2. Louis Solomon, *Apley's system of orthopaedics and fractures*, 9th edition. Oxford University Press NewYork 2001 p.201

3. Paliwal VK, Singh P, Rahi SK, Agarwal V, Gupta RK Journal of Clinical Rheumatology: practical reports on rheumatic & musculoskeletal diseases 18:4 2012 Jun pg 2078.

CHRONIC WOUND SINUS

Dr. Anil Kumar Gupta, Associate Professor, Dr. Javed Ahmad, Junior Resident,
Physical Medicine & Rehabilitaion

A 20 year old male, admitted to trauma center with crush injury of left lower limb with neurovascular deficit following an agricultural machinery accident. He was managed by left transfemoral amputation, and discharged after 3 weeks. After 6 weeks, he visited PMR OPD with a discharging sinus at posterior aspect of end of the residual limb. Pus culture showed moderate Enterobacter spp, sensitive to Levofloxacin and moderate sensitive to Pipera cillin and Imipenem. Oral levofloxacin was given for two weeks given but could not get relief. On subsequent visit, patient admitted and sinogram done as shown below in photograph.

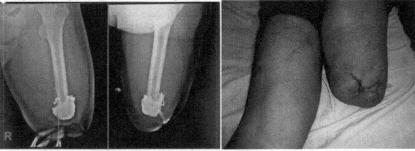

1. Which of the following is not true for above condition

   (A) This condition is known as chronic wound sinus

579

(B) Low grade, localized osteomyelitis may be present

(C) A sinus is best managed surgically during a benign, non acute interval

(D) A sinogram followed by excisional surgery can be curative

(E) All are correct

2. All of the following are correct except

(A) Active adduction, extension exercises should be instituted as early as possible in transfemoral amputation

(B) Diminished sensation in residual limb is common especially in diabetic patients

(C) Socket looseness can cause decreased friction and/or pressures over tibia and fibula

(D) Myodesis or myoplasty are the two techniques available to both providing distal padding and prevent adherence of incisional scar to underlying bones.

3. Most likely developing deformity in transfemoral amputation level is

(A) Flexion, adduction

(B) Flexion, abduction

(C) Extension, abduction

(D) Extension, adduction

4. False statement regarding delayed wound healing

(A) Occurs due to several factors like inappropriate level selection, sub-optimal operative technique, inadequate postoperative management and infection.

(B) If infection is sole cause of dehiscence, the wound should be widely opened for drainage and appropriate antibiotics should be given.

(C) If skin separation is minor, the residual limb may be allowed to heal by secondary intention following conservative debridement under adequate antibiotic coverage.

(D) In the presence of gross necrosis or failure of the wound to produce adequate granulation tissue, the choice is limited to debridement and adequate antibiotics.

5. True statement related to late musculoskeletal complication in amputation is

(A) In transfemoral amputation, if dynamically balanced myodesis has not been performed, the femur may drift anteromedialy.

(B) Transfemoral amputees may complain of burning sensation in ischial weight bearing area, while using a quadrilateral socket.

(C) With ischial containment socket and the advent of flexible socket material has increased pressure discomfort over ischium.

(D) All are correct.

Answers:

1. E

All are correct.

2. C

Socket looseness can cause increased friction and/or pressures over tibia and fibula, fibular head, tibial tubercle, distal end of the patella as the residual limb enters the socket deeply.

3. B

At the transfemoral level a flexion abduction contracture may develop which can be prevented by adduction and extension exercises as early as possible.

4. D

In the presence of gross necrosis or failure of the wound to produce adequate granulation tissue, the choice is limited to revision of residual limb.

5. B

In transfemoral amputation, if dynamically balanced myodesis has not been performed, the femur may drift anterolateraly. With ischial containment socket and the advent of flexible socket material, pressure discomfort over ischium is less common.

References :

1. Dawn M. Ehde, Douglas G Smith. Chronic pain management; Atlas of amputations and limb deficiencies: surgical, prosthetic, and rehabilitation principles 2004; 56: 711-716

2. Matos LA: Enhancement of healing in selected problem wounds, 1989, pp 37- 44

PHANTOM LIMB PAIN

Dr. Anil Kumar Gupta, Associate Professor, Dr. Javed Ahmad, Junior Resident,
Physical Medicine & Rehabilitaion

A 27 year old male, admitted to trauma center with crush injury of right leg with neurovascular deficit following a road traffic accident. He was managed by right transtibial amputation, and transferred to Dept of PM&R for rehabilitation. Three weeks post operatively, he complained of shooting/cramping pain located in the distal part of amputated limb not responding to NSAID's. He also complained that he can feel the amputated part with itching and tingling sensation. He cannot sleep properly in nights due to these complaints.

1. Perception of pain in amputated limb is called as
    (A) Residual limb pain
    (B) Phantom sensation
    (C) Phantom pain
    (D) None
2. Which of the following is correct regarding Phantom pain
    (A) Occurs in around 50% of patients after amputation
    (B) Increases in incidence with time
    (C) Is usually a constant pain
    (D) Is commonly experienced by people with congenitally absent limb
    (E) Is more common in patients with persistent pain
3. Etiology of phantom pain includes
    (A) Severing of nerve axons and the formation of neuroma, which are enlarged, disorganized endings of C-fibers and demyelinated A fibers
    (B) Increase in excitability of spinal cord neurons characterized by abnormal spontaneous activity and exaggerated response to mechanical and thermal stimuli
    (C) Reorganization of primary somatosensory and motor cortices and sub cortical structures
    (D) All of the above
4. Pharmacological treatment includes all except
    (A) NSAID's
    (B) NMDA antagonists
    (C) Sodium channel blockers
    (D) Tricyclic antidepressants
5. Non medical treatment includes all except
    (A) Mirror box/Mental imagery
    (B) Acupuncture and TENS
    (C) Electrical stimulation to the residual limb
    (D) Immediate fitting of prosthesis
    (E) Psychology

Answers:

1. C
    Any sensation in the absent part of body except pain is called Phantom sensation. Painful sensation referred to absent part of body is known as Phantom pain.
2. E
    Around 60-80% amputees will experience phantom pain which is commonly intermittent unlike other neuropathic pains and with time incidence decreases. The incidence of phantom limb pain is however lower in pediatric amputees and it does not occur in children with congenitally absent limbs.
3. D
    All are correct and known as peripheral, spinal, and cerebral mechanism.
4. A
    Phantom limb pain did not respond well to NSAID's.
    Tricyclic antidepressants such as amitriptyline and nortriptyline act by inhibiting the reuptake of noradrenaline and serotonin, thereby potentiating the action of two important central anti-nociceptive pathways.
    Sodium channel blockers like Gabapentin and pregablin bind to voltage gated calcium channels and have been shown to be effective.

NMDA receptor antagonists like Tramadol are also effective, tolerance and dependance is uncommon.

5. C

Electrical stimulation of spinal cord, deep brain structures and motor cortex is effective in refractory cases. Rests are useful nonmedical modalities.

References:

1. Nikolajsen L, Jensen TS. Phantom limb pain. Br. J. Anaesth. 2001; 87 (1): 107-116.
2. Nathanson M. Phantom Limbs as reported by S.Weir Mitchell. Neurology 1988; 38:504-505
3. Spiegel DR et al. A presumed case of phantom limb pain treated successfully with duloxetine and pregabalin. Gen Hosp Psychiatry. 2010; 32(2):228
4. Dworkin RH et al. Pharmacologic management of neuropathic pain: Evidence-based recommendations. Pain 2007; 132 (3): 237-251
5. Jaeger H, Maier C. Calcitonin in phantom limb pain: a double-blind study. Pain 1992; 48: 21–27
6. Diers M et al. Mirrored, imagined and executed movements differentially activate sensorimotor cortex in amputees with and without phantom limb pain. Pain 2010; 149: 296-304.
7. Dawn M. Ehde, Douglas G Smith. Chronic pain management; Atlas of amputations and limb deficiencies: surgical, prosthetic, and rehabilitation principles 2004; 56: 711-716.

ERB'S PALSY

Dr. Anil Kumar Gupta, Associate Professor, Dr. Javed Ahmad, Junior Resident,
Physical Medicine & Rehabilitaion

A two month old male child preterm, appropriate for gestational age with breech presentation delivered by normal vaginal delivery came to OPD of Dept of PMR by their parents with complaint of no movement of his left upper limb. On examination, his left arm was adducted with forearm pronated and extended as seen in picture. X ray of Left shoulder joint was normal.

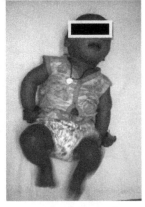

1. What is the diagnosis?
    (A) Klumpke's palsy
    (B) Shoulder dislocation
    (C) Erb–Duchenne palsy
    (D) None
2. Which of the following is incorrect regarding management?
    (A) Nerve transplants from the opposite arm or limb
    (B) Supraspinatous releases
    (C) Latissimus Dorsi Tendon Transfer
    (D) All of the above are correct
3. All of the following are helpful in Erb's palsy except
    (A) Exercises
    (B) Massage
    (C) Electrical stimulation

(D) All
4. Involved nerve root is
   (A) C5-C6
   (B) C7
   (C) C8- T1
   (D) All
5. The deformity in this condition is known as
   (A) Ape thumb deformity
   (B) Waiter's tip hand
   (C) Gun stock deformity
   (D) None

Answers:

References:

1.   Warwick, R., & Williams, P.L, ed. (1973). *Gray's Anatomy* (35th ed.). London: Longman. pp.1037–1047
2.   Tortora, G.J., & Anagnostakos, N.P. (1990). *Principles of Anatomy and Physiology* (6th ed.). New York: Harper & Row. pp.370–374
3.   Abrahams, P (2002). *The Atlas of the Human Body: A Complete Guide to How the Body Works.* Leicester, U.K.: Silverdale Books. pp.76–77

POST POLIO RESIDUAL PARALYSIS REHABILITATION

Dr. Dileep Kumar, Assistant Professor & Dr. Javed Ahmad, Junior Resident,
Physical Medicine & Rehabilitaion

A 30 year old male with Post Polio residual paralysis of left lower limb presented to PMR OPD with hand on knee gait, seeking rehabilitation. On enquiry, no intervention has been done till now. On examination, left lower limb power is- hip flexors 4/5, hip extensors 3/5, hip abductors 4/5, hip adductors 4/5, knee flexors 2/5, knee extensors 0/5, ankle DF 3/5, ankle PF 4/5, evertors 4/5, invertors 3/5, while right lower limb have normal power. There is flexion deformity at left hip and knee 15 degree and 40 degree respectively.

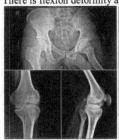 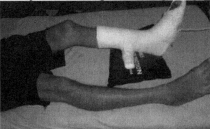

1.   False statement is
     (A) Poliomyelitis is an acute infectious disease caused by a group of neurotropic viruses (type I, II and III)
     (B) Spinal paralysis is due to affection of anterior horn cells of the spinal cord and may involve limb and trunk muscles while bulbar paralysis affects motor cells in brainstem causing difficulty in swallowing, respiration and speech.
     (C) In its natural course, the disease has four major stages: Acute illness, Proliferating stage, Recovery stage, and Residual stage.

(D) In three clinical forms, Bulbar paralysis has high mortality rate.
2. The paralysis of polio virus infection, all are true except
    (A) is upper motor neuron type
    (B) is asymmetrical
    (C) usually affects the lower limbs more severely than the upper limbs
    (D) is more severe if strenuous physical exercise occurred in the incubation period
    (E) may be caused by polio vaccination
3. Functional consequence of paralysis in poliomyelitis are
    (A) Impairment or loss of specific movements like active extension of knee
    (B) Impairment of stability of a joint
    (C) Impairment of general motor performance
    (D) Development of deformities like contractures, valgus, varus, and recurvatum.
    (E) All are correct.
4. False regarding muscle power
    (A) Grade 1- a flicker of contraction, does not bring any movement
    (B) Grade 2- sufficient muscle contraction to move the joint
    (C) Grade 3- sufficient muscle contraction to move the joint against gravity
    (D) Grade 4- sufficient muscle strength to move the joint against gravity and some resistance.
5. Surgical procedure not done in poliomyelitis
    (A) Yount's procedure
    (B) Modified Campbell's procedure
    (C) Modified Huckstep's procedure
    (D) Percutaneous Tenotomy of adductor muscles

Answers:
1. C
    In its natural course the disease has three major stages: Acute illness, Recovery stage, and Residual stage.
2. A
    Paralysis in poliomyelitis is lower motor neuron type, affecting anterior horn cells.
3. E
    All are the functional consequence in poliomyelitis.
4. B
    Grade 2- sufficient muscle contraction to move the joint eliminating gravity.
5. D
    Percutaneous tenotomy done in adductor contracture of hip present in Cerebral palsy patients.

References:
1. J. Krol , Rehabilitation Surgery for deformities due to poliomyelitis Technique for the district hospital, Delhi, World Health Organization, Jaypee First Indian edition 1994.
2. A.H.Crenshaw, Cerebral palsy, Campbell's Operative Orthopedics. Mosby, Seventh Edition 1987, Volume 4, Page 2864-65

SPASTICITY IN SPINAL INJURY
Dr. Anil Kumar Gupta, Associate Professor & Dr. Javed Ahmad, Junior Resident,
Physical Medicine & Rehabilitaion

A 26 year old male presented to Department of PMR with 8 weeks old traumatic paraplegia with bladder bowel involvement with 10x7 cm sacral pressure ulcer. He complained of fever with chills and rigor since 4 days. On examination, LEMS was 0/50, AIS B, Neurological level T12. There was considerable increase in muscle tone and difficulty in passive movement of bilateral lower limb. Pus culture showed moderate E. coli sensitive to Imipenum and Nitrofurantoin, while urine culture showed Significant E. coli sensitive to Levofloxacin.
1. What is the grade of spasticity grading of the patient according to modified Ashworth scale?
    (A) 1
    (B) 1+
    (C) 2
    (D) 3
2. Factor(s)that may increase spasticity
    (A) Ingrown toe nails
    (B) Pressure ulcers
    (C) Poor fit in a brace or wheelchair

(D) Constipation

(E) All of the above

3. All of the following is correct regarding spasticity except

(A) May assist in activities of daily living

(B) May interfere with activities of daily living

(C) Decreases risk of heterotopic ossification (HO)

(D) Maintains muscle tone/bulk

(E) Can be used as "diagnostic tool"

4. Not a negative sign of Upper motor neuron lesion

(A) Lack of strength

(B) Lack of Primitive reflexes

(C) Lack of motor control

(D) Lack of coordination

5. Traditional Step-Ladder Approach to Management of Spasticity

(A) Remove noxious stimuli→ Oral medications → Rehabilitation Therapy→ Neurolysis → Orthopedic→ Neurosurgical

(B) Remove noxious stimuli →Rehabilitation Therapy→ Oral medications → Neurolysis→ Orthopedic→ Neurosurgical

(C) Remove noxious stimuli→ Oral medications → Rehabilitation Therapy→ Neurolysis → Neurosurgical→ Orthopedic

(D) Remove noxious stimuli →Rehabilitation Therapy→ Oral medications → Neurolysis→ Orthopedic→ Neurosurgical

Answers:

1. D 3

Modified Ashworth scale

0 No increase in muscle tone

1 Slight increase in muscle tone, manifested by a catch and release or by minimal resistance at the end of range of motion

1+ Slight increase in muscle tone, manifested by a catch, followed by minimal resistance throughout the remainder (less than half) of the range of motion

2 More marked increase in muscle tone through most of the range of motion, but the affected part is easily moved

3 Considerable increase in muscle tone, passive movement is difficult

4 Affected part is rigid in flexion or extension (abduction or adduction, etc.)

2. E

All of the above

Factors that can increase spasticity

• Urinary tract infections

• Constipation

• Ingrown toe nails

• Pressure ulcers

• Poor fit in a brace or wheelchair

3. C

Decreases risk of heterotopic ossification (HO)

Possible Advantages of Spasticity

• Maintains muscle tone/bulk

• Helps support circulatory function

• May prevent formation of deep vein blood thrombosis

• May assist in activities of daily living

• May assist with postural control

• Can be used as "diagnostic tool" (spasticity can be a sign of exposure to a noxious stimuli-infection, bowel impaction, urinary retention, etc)

Consequences of Spasticity

• May interfere with mobility, exercise, joint range of motion

• May interfere with activities of daily living

• May cause pain and sleep disturbance

• Can make patient care more difficult

• Contractures

- ↑ risk of heterotopic ossification (HO)
- Joint subluxation / dislocation

4. B
   Lack of Primitive reflexes
   Positive Signs
   (Excessive normal resting state)
   - Spasticity
   - Rigidity
   - Hyperreflexia
   - Primitive reflexes
   - Clonus
     Negative Signs
     (Less than normal resting state)
   - Lack of strength
   - Lack of motor control
   - Lack of coordination

5. B
   Remove noxious stimuli →Rehabilitation Therapy→ Oral medications → Neurolysis→ Orthopedic→ Neurosurgical

References:

1. Journal of Neurology, Neurosurgery, and Psychiatry 1994;57:773-77
2. Lance JW. Symposium synopsis. In: Feldman RG, Young RR, Koella WP, editors. Spasticity: disordered motor control. Chicago: Year Book Medical Pubs; 1980. p. 487–9.
3. Young RR. Spasticity: a review. Neurology1994;44(Suppl):S12-20.
4. Rymer W, Katz RT. Mechanisms of spastic hypertonia. In: Katz RT, editor. Spasticity: state of the art review. Vol. 8. Philadelphia: Hanley & Belfus; 1994. p. 441-54.

LEPROSY

Dr. Anil Kumar Gupta, Associate Professor & Dr. Javed Ahmad, Junior Resident,
Physical Medicine & Rehabilitation

A 30 year old man came to PMR OPD with hypopigmented anaesthetic patches over back over last 2 months. On examination there were 3 patches as described above size ranging from 1x1 cm to 3x4 cm. On palpation ulnar nerve of left side was thickened behind medial epicondyle. Split skin smear and nerve biopsy showed acid fast, rod shaped bacillus.

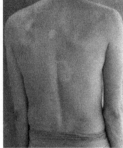

1. What is the diagnosis?
   - (A) Tuberculoid leprosy
   - (B) Borderline leprosy
   - (C) Lepromatous leprosy
   - (D) None of the above
2. False regarding leprosy
   - (A) The goal of the WHO by the end of 2015 is to reduce the rate of new cases with grade-2 disabilities worldwide by at least 35%.
   - (B) Elimination, as defined by the WHO, was defined as a reduction of patients with leprosy requiring multidrug therapy to fewer than 1 per 1,000 population.

(C) Leprosy is a chronic infection caused by the acid-fast, rod-shaped bacillus mycobacterium leprae.

(D) Initially, a mycobacterial infection causes a wide array of cellular immune responses which lead to peripheral neuropathy with potentially long-term consequences.

3. All of the following are true except

(A) Leprosy is generally more common in males than in females, with a male-to-female ratio of 1.5:1.

(B) Leprosy can occur at any age, but, in developing countries, it peaks in children younger than 10 years.

(C) Mode of spread of mycobacterium leprae is by droplets.

(D) Ridley-Jopling classified leprosy in Paucibacillary and multibacillary category.

4. According to WHO pharmacotherapy of multibacillary leprosy includes

(A) Rifampicin -600 mg monthly

(B) Dapsone -100mg daily

(C) Clofazamine -300mg once monthly and 50 mg daily

(D) All of the above

5. False statement regarding care in leprosy patients is

(A) Daily inspection of hands and feet.

(B) Soaking the hand and feet in warm water followed by scraping hard skin.

(C) Active and passive exercise of deformed joints.

(D) Offloading of feet.

Answers:

1. A

   a. WHO system: The WHO recommends classifying leprosy according to the number of lesions and the presence of bacilli on a skin smear. This method is useful in countries where biopsy analysis in unavailable.

   b. Paucibacillary leprosy is characterized by 5 or fewer lesions with absence of organisms on smear. Paucibacillary leprosy generally includes the tuberculoid and borderline lepromatous categories from the Ridley-Jopling system.

   c. Multibacillary leprosy is marked by 6 or more lesions with possible visualization of bacilli on smear. Lepromatous leprosy, borderline lepromatous leprosy, and midborderline leprosy on the Ridley-Jopling scale are included in the multibacillary leprosy category.

2. B.

   In the 1990s, the World Health Organization (WHO) launched a campaign to eliminate leprosy as a public health problem by 2000. Elimination, as defined by the WHO, was defined as a reduction of patients with leprosy requiring multidrug therapy to fewer than 1 per 10,000 population. This goal was achieved in terms of global prevalence by 2002, but 15 of the 122 countries where leprosy was endemic in 1985 still have prevalence rates of greater than 1 per 10,000 population

   The goal of the WHO by the end of 2015 is to reduce the rate of new cases with grade-2 disabilities worldwide by at least 35%. This will be carried out by enforcing activities to decrease the delay in diagnosing the disease and actuate treatment with multidrug therapy. This will also have the impact of reducing transmission of the disease in the community.

   Leprosy is a **chronic granulomatous disease** caused by *Mycobacterium leprae*, an acid and alcohol fast bacillus.

3. D.

   Leprosy is generally more common in males than in females, with a male-to-female ratio of 1.5:1. In some areas in Africa, the prevalence of leprosy among females is equal to or greater than that in males.

   Leprosy can occur at any age, but, in developing countries, the age-specific incidence of leprosy peaks in children younger than 10 years, who account for 20% of leprosy cases. Leprosy is very rare in infants; however, they are at a relatively high risk of acquiring leprosy from the mother, especially in cases of lepromatous leprosy or midborderline leprosy.

   Classification of leprosy: Leprosy has 2 classification schemas: the 5-category Ridley-Jopling system and the simpler and more commonly used WHO standard.

   Ridley-Jopling: Depending on the host response to the organism, leprosy can manifest clinically along a spectrum bounded by the tuberculoid and lepromatous forms of the disease. Most patients fall into the intermediate classifications, which include borderline tuberculoid leprosy, midborderline leprosy, and borderline lepromatous leprosy. The classification of the disease typically changes as it evolves during its progression or management. The Ridley-Jopling system is used globally and forms the basis of clinical studies of leprosy.

The most important mode of spread of Mycobacterium leprae is by **droplets** from the sneeze of leprosy patients, whose nasal mucosa is heavily infected. It is not certain whether the organism enters by inhalation or through the skin. The incubation period is between 2-5 years.

4. D

Who recommended chemotherapy:

Multibacillary- Rifampicin-600 mg monthly, dapsone-100mg daily, Clofazimine 300mg once monthly and 50 mg daily

Paucibacillary-Rifampicin-600mg once monthly, Dapsone-100 mg daily

5. B

Sensory loss leads to loss of perception of pain and heat deprives the hand of its protective mechanism. Motor activities become clumsy and difficult. Because muscle action is not fine tuned, frequent injuries results in anesthetic deformities(shortening of digits). Lack of sweating leads to dryness of palmer skin and cracks at digital creases.

Skin care practice includes daily soaking hands in water for 15 minutes, rubbing palms vigorously and applying liquid paraffin or vegetable oil. Injury care practice includes precaution against burns while cooking, using utensils with insulated handle. Daily inspection of hands, using bulky bandages in case injury occurs.

References:

1. World Health Organisation. Action programme for elimination of leprosy-status report. WHO/LEP/98.2, 1998.
2. Vijayakumaran, P., Prabhakar Rao, T. and Krishnamurthy, P. Pace of leprosy elimination and support teams in Bihar state, India. Lepr. Rev, 1999; 70:452-458
3. Mandal, M.G., Pal, D., Majundar, V., Biswas, P.C., Biswas, S. and Saha, B. Recent trends in leprosy in a large district of West Bengal, India, revealed by a modified leprosy campaign (MLEC). Lepr. Rev. 2000; 71:71-76.

MORQUIO SYNDROME

Prof. V. P. Sharma, Professor & Dr. Arvind Kumar Sharma, JR3, Department of Physical Medicine & Rehabilitaion

A 28 years old male patient presented to PMR OPD with the presenting complain of delayed physical growth and bilateral knee joint deformity since the age of 2 years. The knee joint appeared swollen and medially deviated; according to the patient. Since the age of 5 years, he also noticed chest wall deformity wherein there is forward bulge of the chest wall. The deformities are progressively increasing since then. Gradually he developed joints stiffness and pain all over body with difficulty in walking. Physical examination showed a height of 3 feet 10 inches with muscular weakness, pectus carinatum, stubby neck, kyphoscoliosis of dorsolumbar spine, bilateral genu valgum, equinovarus deformity in right ankle & he has right sided squint. The neurological examination revealed muscular weakness in bilateral lower limb and upper limbs & paresthesias. There was no mental retardation.

The AP radiographic view of the spine showed a mild thoraco-lumbar right scoliosis; the lateral view demonstrated a slight thoraco-lumbar kyphosis with irregular, flat and antero-posteriorly enlarged vertebral bodies particularly in mid-thoracic region, thoraco-lumbar junction and distal lumbar spine. The cervical x-ray showed wedge shape of the vertebral bodies and an hypoplasia of the odontoid process.

Roentgenographic findings of the chest included a relatively small size of his chest with oar-shaped ribs (widening ribs anteriorly and narrowing posteriorly). The iliac wings of the pelvis were flared, with short femoral necks, flattered femoral epiphysis, and marked degenerative changes of the hip joints . In the lower extremity, the lower ends of the femur and the upper ends of the tibia were large with an evident genu valgus deformity. Severe degenerative changes of the knee joints were present.

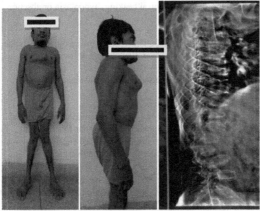

1. What is the most probable diagnosis?
    (A) Achondroplasia
    (B) Morquio's syndrome
    (C) Hurler's syndrome
    (D) Klinefelter's syndrome
2. Not seen in morquio's syndrome
    (A) Pectus excavatum
    (B) Genu valgum
    (C) Coxa valgum
    (D) Dysostosis multiplex
3. Which of the following is not a X ray finding of spine in Morquio syndrome
    (A) Platyspondyly
    (B) Hypoplasia of odontoid process
    (C) Kyphosis
    (D) Hyperplasia of odontoid process
4. The characteristics of Morquio's disease include
    (A) Subnormal/normal intelligence
    (B) Excessive excretion of keratosulphate in urine
    (C) Dwarfism
    (D) All of the above
5. Gold standard for diagnosis of Morquio's disease is
    (A) X ray joints, chest & vertebra
    (B) MRI spine
    (C) Bone biopsy
    (D) Decreased enzyme activity in plasma, leukocytes or fibroblasts.
6. Management of Morquio's syndrome includes all except
    (A) Enzyme replacement therapy
    (B) Orthopedic correction of skeletal changes
    (C) Stretching exercises
    (D) None of the above

Answers:
1.   B
      Skeletal changes of Morquio's syndrome include thoracolumbar kyphosis, flat vertebral bodies (platyspondyly), growth failure, genu valgus, generalized joint stiffness, absent mental retardation and usually no hepatosplenomegaly.
2.   A
      The Morquio syndrome in its variants, is characterized by severe skeletal changes, which include hypoplasia of the odontoid process, short neck, barrel chest with pectus carinatum. Some of X-rays features of Morquio's disease include wide flaring of the ilium, shallow acetabula, flattening of femoral heads, coxa and genua valga, and dysostosis multiplex.
3.   D

Skeletal abnormalities of the spine are platyspondyly with central beaking, hypoplasia or absence of the odontoid process and kyphosis

4. D

Stature in Morquio's syndrome is markedly short (< 4 feet). There is absent mental retardation. The first step in diagnosis is the assessment of urinary GAG excretion, collected over 24 hours.

5. D

The gold standard for diagnosis is the demonstration of decreased enzyme activity in plasma, leukocytes or fibroblasts.

6. D

The efficacy and safety of ERT with recombinant human enzyme is well accepted and confirmed by many clinical trials. Patient disease progression should be observed by regular follow up, at least annually. In addition to pain management, typical comorbidities often need surgical intervention like orthopedic surgeries (correction of skeletal changes) and neurosurgical procedures.

References:

1. Louis Solomon, *Apley's system of orthopaedics and fractures*, 8th edition.Oxford University Press NewYork 2001 p.138-142.
2. L. O. Langer and L. S. Carey, "The roentgenographic features of the KS mucopolysaccharidosis of Morquio (Morquio- Brailsford's disease)," *The American Journal of Roentgenology,Radium Therapy, and Nuclear Medicine*, vol. 97, no. 1, pp. 1– 20, 1966.
3. Jonathan Ray, clinical review articles. *Rhematic rarities*: May 2013; volume 39-2, page 432-445.
4. D. Resnick, "Osteochondrodysplasias, dysostoses, chromosomal aberration mucopolysaccharidoses, mucolipidoses and other skeletal dysplasias," in *Diagnosis of Bone and Joint Disorders*, vol. 5, pp. 3501–3507, WB Saunders, Philadelphia, Pa, USA, 1988.

ADHESIVE CAPSULITIS SHOULDER

Dr. Dileep Kumar, Assistant Professor & Dr. Ashish Srivastava, Junior Resident, Department of Physical Medicine & Rehabilitation

A 52 year old male suffering from type 2 Diabetes Mellitus came to PMR OPD with complaint of pain over right shoulder for last 3 months. The pain was specially felt on overhead activities and increases at night when lying on same side. The patient also felt too much pain while trying to pick out purse from the back pocket. There was no history of any trauma or too much weight lifting by same arm. On examination, abduction of shoulder was found limited at 90^0, internal and external rotation painful and restricted. Patient was on oral hypoglycemic drugs and his RBS was marginally elevated. X-ray of his right shoulder was done but came out normal.

1. What is the provisional diagnosis in this case?

   (A) Rotator cuff tear

   (B) Adhesive capsulitis

   (C) Diabetic neuropathy

   (D) Biceps tendonitis

2. Which of the following statement about this condition is not true?

   (A) More common in women over the age of 40 years

   (B) Synovial tissue of the capsule and bursa become adherent

   (C) Pain, with significant reduction in range of motion both actively and passively

   (D) Arthrography will demonstrate increased volume in the joint

3. Provocative test used for adhesive capsulitis shoulder?

   (A) Yergason's test

   (B) Neer's walsh impingement test

   (C) Speed's test

   (D) None

4. Correct sequence of stages of this disease is?

   (A) freezing - thawing – frozen

   (B) thawing – freezing – frozen

   (C) freezing – frozen – thawing

   (D) can be seen in any sequence

5. Definitive treatment of the condition is?

(A) Suprascapular nerve block
(B) Intraarticular corticosteroid injection
(C) Surgical manipulation under anesthesia
(D) Basically a self resolving disease

Answers:

1. **B**

   Adhesive capsulitis:
   Defined as inflammation of the shoulder joint (glenohumeral) causing painful shoulder with restricted glenohumeral motion. Etiology is unknown, may be related to autoimmune condition, trauma or inflammatory condition.

2. **D**

   It is more common in women over the age of 40 years. Synovial tissue of the capsule and bursa become adherent.

   Associated with a variety of conditions: – Intracranial lesions: CVA, hemorrhage, and brain tumor – Clinical depression – Shoulder-hand syndrome – Parkinson's disease – Iatrogenic disorders – Cervical disc disease – Insulin dependent diabetes mellitus – Hypothyroidism.

   Clinically patient presents with pain and significant reduction in range of motion both actively and passively.
   Plain films (AP) is indicated to rule out underlying tumor or calcium deposit, otherwise normal plain films are indicated in patients whose pain and motion do not improve after 3 months of treatment. Arthrography will demonstrate a decreased volume in the joint, which can be realized by the small amount of contrast (less than 5 ml) that can be injected.

3. **D**

   None
   Yergason's test for bicipital tendinitis.
   Neer-walsh test for rotator cuff tendinitis.
   Speed's test for biceps tendinitis.

4. **C**

   Freezing – frozen – thawing stage
   Painful stage(Freezing): Progressive vague pain lasting roughly 8 months.
   Stiffening stage(Frozen): Decreasing range of motion lasting roughly 8 months.
   Thawing stage: An increase of range of motion with decrease of shoulder pain.

5. **D**

   Basically a self resolving disease
   Treatment: Adhesive capsulitis is basically a self limiting disease. Following options are used for symptomatic treatment.
   Rehabilitation - Restoring passive and active range of motion, Corticosteroid injection: Subacromial and glenohumeral will decrease pain to maximize therapy, Modalities: Ultrasound and electrical stimulation.
   Surgical – Manipulation under anesthesia (MUA) may be indicated if there is no substantial progress after 12 weeks of conservative treatment. Arthroscopic lysis of adhesions—usually reserved for patients with IDDM who do not respond to manipulation.

References:

1. Kelley MJ, McClure PW, Leggin BG. Frozen Shoulder: Evidence and a Proposed Model Guiding Rehabilitation. Journal of Orthopaedic and Sports Physical Therapy. February 2009;39(2):135-136-148.
2. Pearsall AI, MD. Adhesive Capsulitis. eMedicine. 2008. Accessed 06/01/09.
3. Saidoff DC, McDonough AL. Critical Pathways in Therapeutic Intervention: Extremities and Spine. St. Louis: Mosby; 2002:134-144.
4. Rookmoneea M et al. The effectiveness of interventions in the management of patients with primary frozen shoulder. The Journal of Bone $ Joint Surgery (Br). 2010;92-B(9):1267—1272

TRAUMATIC PARAPLEGIA WITH PRESSURE ULCER

Dr. Dileep Kumar, Assistant Professor, Dr. Javed Ahmad, Junior Resident, Department
of Physical Medicine & Rehabilitaion

A 28 year old man admitted to Department of PMR as two month old elsewhere operated case of traumatic paraplegia with bladder bowel involvement with 10x7cm sacral and about 2x2 cm grade 3 pressure ulcers on bilateral heel. Pus culture showed E.coli sensitive to Leuoflokacin and Nitrofurantoin. Oral Nitrofurantoin started and care of bladder, bowel and skin were taught.

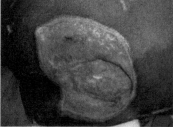

1. All of the following are true regarding pressure ulcer except?
   (A) 25%–40% of SCI patients develop pressure ulcers at some time during their life.
   (B) During the acute period after SCI the most common locations of ulcer is sacrum.
   (C) Patient should be turned and positioned every 4 hours for prevention of pressure ulcers
   (D) Risk factors include immobility, incontinence, lack of sensation and altered level on consciousness.
2. What is the classification of a pressure ulcer with full thickness skin loss involving subcutaneous tissue and extending into but not through fascia?
   (A) Stage I
   (B) Stage II
   (C) Stage III
   (D) Stage IV
3. Pressure Ulcer Complication include(s)?
   (A) Osteomyelitis
   (B) Dehydration
   (C) Endocarditis
   (D) All of the above
4. Not true for development of pressure ulcer?
   (A) Decreases in total protein (< 6.4 g/dL) and albumin (< 3.5 g/dL) (78) have similarly been found to be associated with pressure ulcer development.
   (B) Maintaining the head of the bed slightly elevated decreases risk.
   (C) Minimizing environmental factors leading to skin drying decreases risk.
   (D) Braden scale and Norton scale are used for risk assessment of ulcer development.
5. True statement is
   (A) In chronic SCI patients the most common location of ulcer is greater trochanter.
   (B) Pressure relief every 2 hour when sitting reduces pressure ulcer.
   (C) Prevention of pressure ulcers should always be the first line of defense.
   (D) None

Answers:

1. C
   Patient should be turned and positioned every 2 hours for prevention of pressure ulcers. rest options are true.

2. B

Staging of pressure ulcers

Stage	Description
I	Nonblanchable erythema of intact skin not resolved within 30 minutes; epidermis intact
II	Partial-thickness loss of skin involving epidermis, possibly into dermis; may appear as blisters with erythema
III	Full-thickness destruction through dermis into subcutaneous tissue
IV	Deep-tissue destruction through subcutaneous tissue to fascia, muscle, bone, or joint

3. D

Pressure ulcers have been associated with many complications, including osteomyelitis, endocarditis, heterotopic bone formation, maggot infestation, septic arthritis, sinus tract or abscess, squamous cell carcinoma in the ulcer and dehydration.

4. B

Maintain the head of the bed at the lowest degree of elevation possible. Rest options are true.

5. C

Common Locations of Pressure Ulcers

During the acute period after SCI the most common locations of ulcers are due to the patient lying supine: #1 Sacrum #2 Heels.

In chronic SCI patients the locations of ulcers are as follows: Ischial decubitus (30 %) Greater trochanter (20%) Sacrum (15%) Heels (10%)

Risk Factors • Immobility • Incontinence • Lack of sensation • Altered level on consciousness

Prevention of Pressure Ulcers

1) Minimize extrinsic factors—pressure, maceration, and friction
2) Decrease pressure forces, the patient should be turned and positioned every 2 hours
3) Pressure relief every 30 minutes when sitting
4) Proper cushioning and wheelchair seating (see wheelchairs)
5) Wheelchair pushups

References:

1. Glover D. Let's own up to the real cost of pressure ulcers. Journal of Wound Care 2003; 12: 43.
2. Copeland-Fields LD, Hoshiko BR. Clinical validation of Braden and Bergstrom's conceptual schema of pressure sore risk factors. Rehabilitation Nursing 1987; 14: 257-260.
3. National Pressure Ulcer Advisory Panel. Pressure ulcers prevalence, cost and risk assessment: consensus development conference statement. Decubitus 1989; 2: 24-28.

HETEROTOPIC OSSIFICATION

Dr. Dileep Kumar, Assistant Professor & Dr. Sanjai Singh, Junior Resident, Department of Physical Medicine & Rehabilitaion

A man aged 32 years with 5 year old traumatic paraplegia with spasticity of biltareral lower limb. Patient admitted with the complaint of swelling over his left knee joint with flexion deformity. On examination, local swelling with raised temperature over left knee joint was present and decreased range of motion. Serum Alkaline phosphatase level is 609 IU and X-ray of left knee joint shows some radio-opaque shadow around knee joint.

1. What is the diagnosis?
   (A) Thrombophlebitis
   (B) Cellulitis
   (C) Heterotopic Ossification
   (D) Osteomyelitis
2. Which is the most sensitive test used to identify early heterotopic ossification (HO)?
   (A) X-ray
   (B) Serum alkaline phosphatase
   (C) Computed tomography (CT) scan
   (D) Bone scan
3. What is considered the most effective method for the prevention of heterotopic ossification (HO)?
   (A) Radiation of bone tissue
   (B) Range of motion

(C) Nonsteroidal anti-inflammatory drugs (NSAIDs)

(D) Diphosphonates

4. What is the most common location of heterotopic ossification (HO) in spinal cord injury (SCI) patients?

(A) Hip

(B) Knee

(C) Shoulder

(D) Elbow

5. Which of the following is a risk factor for the development of heterotopic ossification (HO) in spinal cord injury (SCI)?

(A) Gender

(B) Level of lesion

(C) Spasticity

(D) Race

Answers:

1. C

    HO is the formation of true bone in ectopic sites that restricts range of motion. HO can present with swelling, fever, limited mobility, or pain. Ninety percentage of the time, in spinal cord injured patients, it occurs around hip joint. Serum alkaline phosphatase will be elevated, but it is not a specific measure and levels gradually diminish with maturation. HO may not be visible on plain films in the acute phase, but will be seen on bone scan. In chronic phase it is visible in X-ray also in the form of radio-opaque shadow.

2. D

    Phase 1 and 2 of a bone scan can help detect HO within 2 to 4 weeks. To detect HO on x-ray requires bone maturation, which can take as long as 4 weeks. CT scan is not indicated for HO identification, and serum alkaline phosphatase is a nonspecific/ non-sensitive test.

3. B

    Range of motion is the best prophylaxis and treatment of HO. Radiation would have to be given to the whole body because HO development can not be predicted. NSAIDs and diphosphonates have a role in treatment, but not significantly in prevention.

4. A

5. C

    The risk of HO is greater in complete spinal cord injuries, older individuals, in the presence of spasticity, and in patients with pressure ulcers. No relationship has been shown with gender, race, level, or cause of injury.

References:

1. Cuccurullo SJ, ed. Physical Medicine and Rehabilitation Board Review. New York, NY: Demos Medical Publishing; 2004.

2. Schneck CD, Goldberg G, Munin M, Chu A. Imaging techniques relative to rehabilitation. In: DeLisa JA, Gans BM, Bockenek WL, Frontera WR, Gerber LH, Geiringer SR, Pease WS, Robinson LR, Smith J, Stitik TD, Zafonte RD, eds. Physical Medicine & Rehabilitation: Principles and Practice. 4th ed. Philadelphia, PA: Lippincott Williams & Wilkins; 2005: 179–228.

MUSCULAR DYSTROPHY

Dr. Anil Kumar Gupta, Associate Professor, Dr. Sanjai Singh, Junior Resident,
Department of Physical Medicine & Rehabilitation

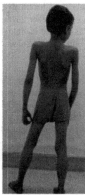

A 8-year-old boy presented in the OPD with mild difficulty in getting up from a seated position on the floor. On examination, we found increased gastrocnemius & calf circumference bilaterally, lordosis, and a waddling gait. His HLA B-27 report is positive.

1. The manoeuvre child performs to assist him in standing is caused by-
   (A) Proximal leg weakness
   (B) Distal leg weakness
   (C) Proximal arm weakness
   (D) Distal arm weakness

2. Which myopathy is characterized by a steadily progressive, X-linked muscular dystrophy that is characterized by absent dystrophin or less than 3% that is normal?
   (A) Becker's muscular dystrophy (BMD)
   (B) Duchenne muscular dystrophy (DMD)
   (C) Limb-girdle muscular dystrophy (LGMD)
   (D) Facioscapulohumeral

3. Which of the following myopathies is not associated with cardiac abnormalities?
   (A) Becker's muscular dystrophy (BMD)
   (B) Duchenne muscular dystrophy (DMD)
   (C) Facioscapulohumeral dystrophy (FSHD)
   (D) Limb-girdle muscular dystrophy (LGMD)

4. Cognition may be impaired in which of the following myopathies?
   (A) Becker's muscular dystrophy (BMD)
   (B) Duchenne muscular dystrophy (DMD)
   (C) Facioscapulohumeral dystrophy (FSHD)
   (D) Limb-girdle muscular dystrophy (LGMD)

5. A patient with Duchenne muscular dystrophy (DMD) is at risk to have which of the following as his or her disease progresses?
   (A) Sudden cardiac death
   (B) Contractures
   (C) Scoliosis
   (D) All of the above

Answers:

1. A

   The manoeuvre noted here is **Gower's sign**, which is the inability to rise from a seated position on the floor. The patient has to use his hands and knees for assistance in a four-point stance. He will bridge the knees into extension and leans the upper extremity forward. This will substitute hip extensior weakness (proximal leg weakness) and lean the upper extremities forward. The patient then moves the upper extremities up the thigh, and a full hip extension is achieved in an upright stance. The Gower's sign indicates proximal muscle weakness. Also, this patient has pseudo hypertrophy, which is seen in patients with either Duchenne or Becker's muscular dystrophy. The enlargement in the calf is not due to increased muscle. It is a result of increased fat and connective tissue.

2. B

DMD is an X-linked disorder with an abnormality in the Xp21 gene locus. There is dystrophin deficiency that disrupts the membrane cytoskeleton and leads to membrane instability. Chronically, this will lead to fibrotic replacement of muscle and failure of regeneration, with muscle fiber death. Absent dystrophin or less than 3% of normal is diagnostic of DMD. Becker's is also an X-linked disorder, but quantitative dystrophin analysis shows either 20% to 80% dystrophin levels. Answer choice C and D are not X-linked disorders.

3. C

The presence of cardiac abnormalities in FSHD is rare. It is important to note that cardiomyopathy is seen prominently in Becker's and Duchenne muscular dystrophy. These patients have abnormalities in the dystrophin protein that is also present in myocardium and Purkinje fibers. ECG abnormalities can be seen, such as Q waves in lateral leads, elevated ST segments, poor R wave progression, and resting tachycardia. Cardiomyopathy is seen in nearly all patients older than 18 years in Duchenne. Cardiomyopathy may also be seen in Limb-girdle dystrophy.

4. B

The dystrophin isomer is present in the brain. Since there is an absence of this dystrophin protein in DMD, there have been lower intelligence quotients seen in affected children. Mean IQ scores have been 1 to 1.5 standard deviations below the normal population. An increase in autism and obsessive-compulsive disorder is also seen in DMD patients.

5. D

Patients with DMD often have contractures by 13 years of age. Contractures may mostly affect ankle plantar flexors, knee flexors, hip flexors, iliotibial band, elbow flexors, and wrist flexors. Scoliosis is prevalent in 33% to 100% in DMD patients and is strongly related to age. 50% will acquire scoliosis by the age of 12 to 15 years. There is no causal relationship between wheelchair use and scoliosis. Cardiac abnormalities happen in DMD patients because of absence of dystrophin, which is also present in myocardium and Purkinje fibres. ECG abnormalities can be seen, such as Q waves in lateral leads, elevated ST segments, poor R wave progression, and resting tachycardia. Cardiomyopathy is seen in nearly all DMD patients older than 18 years.

References:

1. Brooke MH. Muscular dystrophy. In: A Clinician's View of Neuromuscular Diseases. Baltimore, MD: William & Wilkins; 1977: 95– 124.
2. Amato AA, Russell JA. Muscular dystrophies. In: Neuromuscular Disorders. 1st ed. McGraw-Hill Companies; 2008: 529– 577.

OSTEOARTHRITIS

Dr. Dileep Kumar, Assistant Professor & Dr. Ashish Srivastava, Junior Resident,
Physical Medicine & Rehabilitaion

A 50 years old overweight female, came to PMR OPD with complain of dull aching pain over both knee joints which increases with activity and relieves with rest. The patient has special difficulty in sitting and getting up. This was associated with joint stiffness which lasts about 10 min and become worse as the day goes on. The stiffness lasts for short period and decreases after initial range of motion. On examination, there was crepitus on whole range of motion with localised tenderness. There was also mild enlargement of the joint. On X-ray, asymmetrical narrowing of knee joint spaces was found on both sides with some loose bodies.

1. What is the most probable diagnosis:-
   (A) Rheumatoid arthritis
   (B) Osteoarthritis
   (C) Gouty arthritis
   (D) None
2. All of the following statements are correct regarding the given condition except:-
   (A) An inflammatory condition of the joint leading to deterioration of articular cartilage
   (B) Initially it is a disease of cartilage not bone
   (C) Most common form of arthritis seen worldwide
   (D) After 55years it is more common in women
3. Primary form of this disease is seen in all except-
   (A) Knee joint

(B) Carpometacarpal joint

(C) Elbow joint

(D) Distal interphalangeal joint

4. Radiographic findings of this condition are as follows except;-

(A) Asymmetrical narrowing of the joint spaces

(B) Subchondral bony sclerosis

(C) Osteoporosis/ osteopenia with erosive changes

(D) Loose bodies with osteophyte formation

5. True about pathology of this condition is all except:-

(A) In early stages, hypocellularity of chondrocytes with cartilage breakdown is seen

(B) In later stages, hypocellularity of chondrocytes with cartilage fissuring is seen

(C) Water content of cartilage is increased leading to damage of collagen network

(D) Loss of proteoglycans is seen

Answers:

1. B

Osteoarthritis- Because rheumatoid arthritis is associated with stiffness of >30 min duration and gouty arthritis mainly involves 1st metatarsophalangeal joint along with some systemic features like fever or cutaneous erythema etc.

2. A

Osteoarthritis is basically a non inflammatory progressive disorder of the joint leading to deterioration of articular cartilage and new bone formation and joint surfaces and margins.

Male female ratio is equal between ages of 45-55 years and after that it becomes more common in women.

3. C

Classification of Osteoarthritis:-

A. **Primary Osteoarthritis** - it is idiopathic and mainly seen in knees, metatarsophalangeal joint, distal interphalangeal joint, Carpometacarpal joint and hips and spine.

B. **Secondary Osteoarthritis** - follows a recognisable underlying cause. Involves joints like elbow and shoulder. Secondary to chronic trauma, connective tissue disorders, endocrine or metabolic causes, infections, neuropathic and crystal deposition or bony dysplasia's.

C. **Erosive inflammatory Osteoarthritis**

D. **DISH- Diffuse idiopathic skeletal hyperostosis**

4. C

Radiographic findings of Osteoarthritis:-

a. Asymmetrical narrowing of the joint spaces like

In knee- medial joint space narrowing

In hip- superolateral joint space narrowing

b. Subchondral bony sclerosis- new bone formation (white appearance, eburnation)

c. Loose bodies with osteophytes formation

d. Osseous cysts- micro fractures may cause bony collapse

e. No osteoporosis/osteopenia or bony erosions

f. Luschka joint- uncinate process on the superior or lateral aspect of cervical vertebral bodies making them concave

5. A

Microscopic Pathological changes ofOsteoarthritis:-

A. **Early** -hyper cellularity of chondrocytes

-Cartilage breakdown

-Minimal inflammation

B. **Later** -Hypo cellularity of chondrocytes

-Cartilage fissuring, pitting or erosions

-Inflammation causing 2^{0} synovitis

-Osteophytes spur formation seen at joint margins

-Subchondral bony sclerosis

-Cyst formation in juxtra articular bone

C. Increased water content of cartilage causing damage of collagen network.

D. Loss of proteoglycans

References:

1. Altman R, Hochberg M, Moskowitz R, et al. Recommendations for the medical management of osteoarthritis of the hip and knee: 2000 update. Arthritis Rheum 2000;43(9):1905-1915.

2. Felson DT. Epidemiology of osteoarthritis. In: Brandt KD, Doherty M, Lohmander LS, eds. Osteoarthritis. New York: Oxford University Press, 1998.
3. Brandt KD. Osteoarthritis. In: Diagnostic and nonsurgical management of osteoarthritis, 1st ed. 1996:13-25.
4. Erlich MG, Amstrong AL, Treadwell BV, et al. The role of proteases in the pathogenesis of osteoarthritis. J Rheumatol 1987;14:30-32.
5. Bollet AJ, Nance JL. Biochemical findings in normal and osteoarthritic articular cartilage. II. Chondroitin sulfate concentration and chain length, water and ash contents. J Clin Invest 1966; 45:1170.

LEGG– CALVE– PERTHES' DISEASE

Dr. Dileep Kumar, Assistant Professor & Dr. Sanjai Singh, Junior Resident,
Department of Physical Medicine & Rehabilitation

A 9 year old male presented with complaint of pain in Right hip and walking with a limp. He did not have any history of trauma, fever and weight loss.

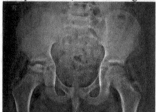

On examination, affected hip has limited range of motion particularly abduction and internal rotation. AP view of X-ray pelvis shows developing fragmentation of the right femoral head with loss of epiphyseal height.

1. What is the diagnosis?
   (A) Tuberculosis of hip joint
   (B) Legg-Calf Perthes' disease
   (C) Transient synovitis
   (D) Juvenile Arthritis
2. Which of the fallowing is not a phase of LCP-
   (A) Synovitis in hip joint
   (B) Fragmentation and reabsorption of bone;
   (C) Reossification when new bone has regrown
   (D) Healing, when new bone reshapes.
3. Orthosis used for the management of LCP-
   (A) Ischial Weight Bearing Orthosis
   (B) Knee Ankle Foot Orthosis
   (C) Ankle Foot Orthosis
   (D) PTB Orthosis
4. How is the hip placed in an orthosis for someone with Legg– Calve– Perthes (LCP) disease?
   (A) Abduction and external rotation
   (B) Adduction and internal rotation
   (C) Abduction and internal rotation
   (D) Adduction and external rotation
5. What is the most common cause of limping and pain in the hip of children?
   (A) Slipped capital femoral epiphysis (SCFE)
   (B) Trochanteric bursitis
   (C) Legg– Calve– Perthes disease
   (D) Transient toxic synovitis

Answers:
1. B

Legg–Calvé–Perthes Disease is a childhood hip disorder initiated by a disruption of blood flow to the ball of the femur called the femoral head. Due to the lack of blood flow, the bone dies (osteonecrosis or avascular necrosis) and stops growing. Common symptoms include hip, knee (hip pathology can refer pain to a normal knee), or groin pain, exacerbated by hip/leg movement, especially internal hip rotation (twisting the leg toward the centre of the body). There is reduced range of motion, particularly in abduction and internal rotation, and the patient presents with a limp. Pain is usually mild.

2. A
    Four stages of LCPD are-
    1. Femoral head becomes more dense with possible fracture of supporting bone;
    2. Fragmentation and reabsorption of bone;
    3. Reossification when new bone has regrown; and
    4. Healing, when new bone reshapes.

3. A
    In Ischial Weight Bearing calipre the body weight is transmitted from the ischial tuberosity to a padded rind or moulded lather (bucket) top, through metal side bars to the shoes and hence the ground. It can be used in Perthes, disease to prevent head femur distruction.

4. C
    The goal of bracing in LCP is to maintain the femoral head completely within the acetabulum to maintain its sphere shape. This is achieved by positioning the hip in hyperabduction and internal rotation.

5. D
    Transient synovitis of the hip (also called toxic synovitis; is a self-limiting condition in which there is an inflammation of the inner lining (the synovium) of the capsule of the hip joint. The term irritable hiprefers to the syndrome of acute hip pain, joint stiffness, limp or non-weight bearing, indicative of an underlying condition such as transient synovitis or orthopaedic infections (like septic arthritis or osteomyelitis). Transient synovitis (TS) is the most common cause of acute hip pain in children aged 3-10 years. The disease causes arthralgia and arthritis secondary to a transient inflammation of the synovium of the hip.SCFE is commonly seen in preadolescent-adolescent obese boys and is a separation of the proximal femoral epiphysis through the growth plate. Trochanteric bursitis is not commonly seen in children. In Legg– Calve–Calve– Perthes disease, there is avascular necrosis at the femoral head. It is seen in children age 4 to 10 who have pain in the groin that radiates to the anterior/ medial thigh toward the knee.

References:

1. American Academy of Paediatrics Committee on Children with Disabilities. Counseling families who choose complementary and alternative medicine for their child with chronic illness and disability. Paediatrics. 2001;107: 598– 601.
2. Rossi R, Alexander M, Cuccurullo SJ. Paediatric rehabilitation. In: Cuccurullo SJ, ed. Physical Medicine and Rehabilitation Board Review. 2nd ed. New York, NY: Demos Medical; 2010: 713– 808.
3. Hart JJ (Oct 1996). "Transient synovitis of the hip in children". Am Fam Physician 54 (5): 1587– 91, 1595–6. PMID 8857781

SPINA BIFIDA(MENINGOMYELOCELE)

Dr. Anil Kumar Gupta, Associate Professor & Dr. Ashish Srivastava, Junior Resident, Department of Physical Medicine & Rehabilitaion

A 7 years old male child came to PMR OPD with complaints of multiple non healing ulcers over both foot, unable to pass urine with self control, unable to walk properly and no sensations below knee on both sides from last 5 years. On elaborating history, patient's parents told that patient had swelling on lower part of back with some hairs on it at the time of birth which was operated after few days. Also there was no significant prenatal or natal history. Patient was born as a result of full term normal vaginal delivery at hospital and cried immediately after birth. On examination ,the ulcers were accompanied with foul smelling discharge, power of both lower limbs below knee was decreased and a scar mark was present on lower part of back. Patient was walking on medial border of both feet with foot drop.

1. What is your provisional diagnosis:-
    (A) Extradural tumour
    (B) Meningomyelocele

(C) Trauma during delivery

(D) None

2. All of the following may be associated causal factors of the disease except:-

    (A) Low socioeconomic status

    (B) Mother taking valproic acid during pregnancy

    (C) Maternal alcohol use

    (D) Vitamin D deficiency in mother antenataly

3. All of the following are associated complications with this condition except:-

    (A) Arnold chiari malformation type 2 and hydrocephalus

    (B) Charcots joint with osteoporosis

    (C) Rib fractures with type 2 respiratory failure

    (D) Malformations of forebrain with tethered cord

4. Which of the following is not true about types of this condition:-

    (A) Occulta type- cystic sac present

    (B) Meningocele- sac contains spinal fluid and meninges

    (C) Meningomyelocele- sac contains spinal fluid, meninges and spinal cord

    (D) Myelocele- central cord remains unfused and exposed

5. All are true about antenatal diagnosis of this condition except:-

    (A) Maternal serum AFP between 13-15 weeks

    (B) Acetylcholinesterases in maternal serum only is confirmatory

    (C) Amniocentesis between 16-18 weeks is nearly 100% accurate

    (D) Fetal USG between 16-24 weeks has >90% reliability

Answers:

1. B

    Extradural tumours will not present with neurosensory deficits. Any trauma during delivery will present immediately after birth.

2. D

    Risk factors associated with etiology of this spina bifida are:-

    Low socioeconomic status

    Maternal obesity

    Maternal febrile illness

    Maternal alcohol use

    Maternal vitamin A and folic acid deficiency

    Familial

3. C

    Associated conditions with spina bifida:-

    Arnold chiari malformation type 2

    Hydrocephalus

    Vasomotor changes over involved area

    Charcots joint

    Osteoporosis

    Malformations of forebrain and hindbrain

    Tethered cord

    Benign lumbosacral tumours

    Diastematomyelia and syringomyelia

    Scoliosis/kyphosis

    Central respiratory dysfunction

    Impaired fine hand co ordination, visual function and ataxia

    Renal malformations like renal hypoplasia, horse shoe kidney, solitary kidney, uretral or lower tract anomalies.

4. A

    Types of spina bifida:-

    a. Spina bifida occulta- failure of fusion of posterior elements of vertebrae. There is no cystic sac formation.50% cases are associated with a pigmented nevus, angioma, hirsute patch or a dimple or dermal sinus overlying the skin.

    b. Spina bifida cystica- divided in three types-

    1.Meningocele- protusion of meninges

    2. Meningomyelocifele- protrusion of meninges and cord

    3. Myelocele- central cord remainunfused and exposed.

5.   B
      Antenatal diagnosis of spina bifida is done by:-
      Maternal serum AFP
      Acetycholinesterases in maternal serum and amniotic fluid
      Fetal USG between 16 – 24 weeks
      Amniocentesis done between 16-18 weeks is nearly 100% accurate for elevated amniotic fluid
      AFP. It does not detect closed NTDs without leakage of fetal CSF.

References:
1.   Ghatan S (2006). Myelomeningocele. In FD Burg et al., eds., Current Pediatric Therapy, 18th ed.,
      pp. 377–380. Philadelphia: Saunders Elsevier.
2.   Liptak GS (2013). Neural tube defects. In ML Batshaw et al., eds., Children with Disabilities, 7th
      ed., pp. 451–472. Baltimore, MD: Paul H. Brookes Publishing.
3.   Liptak GS, Dosa NP (2010). Myelomeningocele. Pediatrics in Review, 30(31): 443–450.
4.   Sandler AD (2010). Children with spina bifida: Key clinical issues. Pediatric Clinics of North
      America, 57(4): 879–892.

STROKE

Dr. Anil Kumar Gupta, Associate Professor & Dr. Sanjai Singh, Junior Resident,
Department of Physical Medicine & Rehabilitation

A 75-year-old man presents to OPD 3 months after sustaining a stroke, with resulting right-sided weakness. He complains of pain over his right shoulder and decreased range of motion. Scarf sign is positive. The patient is noted to have decreased range of motion in all planes.

1.   Techniques to prevent aspiration while eating in a patient with a stroke would include:
      (B) Chin tuck
      (C) Head rotation
      (D) Mendelsohn maneuver
      (E) All of the above
2.   Which of the following is a nonmodifiable risk factor for stroke?
      (A) Hypertension
      (B) Atrial fibrillation
      (C) Age
      (D) Smoking
3.   Shoulder subluxation after stroke:
      (A) Occurs late in the recovery phase
      (B) Is always associated with pain
      (C) Is associated with flaccid hemiplegia
      (D) Will need radiological studies for diagnosis
4.   What is the greatest predictor of community ambulation after a stroke?
      (A) Use of an assistive device
      (B) Walking speed
      (C) Degree of lower extremity motor strength
      (D) Type of stroke
5.   Good prognosis of recovery after stroke is associated with:
      (A) Complete arm paralysis
      (B) Prolonged flaccidity
      (C) Severe proximal spasticity
      (D) Some motor recovery of the hand by 4 weeks

Answers:
1.   D
      All of the above mentioned maneuvers prevent aspiration by providing airway protection. Tucking the chin helps prevent liquid from entering the larynx. Head rotation (turning the head toward the paretic side) helps force the bolus of food into the contralateral pharynx. The Mendelsohn maneuver involves having the patient voluntarily hold the larynx at its maximal height to increase the duration of the cricopharyngeal opening.
2.   C
      Age is a nonmodifiable risk factor for stroke, rest options are modifiable.

3. C
    Shoulder subluxation tends to occur early after a stroke in patients with flaccid hemiplegia. Although shoulder subluxation is listed as a common cause of shoulder pain, the relationship between the two remains controversial. The clinical diagnosis of shoulder subluxation can be made without imaging studies.
4. B
    The greatest predictor of community ambulation after a stroke is walking speed according to a study conducted by Perry et al.
5. D
    If there is some motor recovery of the hand by 4 weeks, there is up to a 70% chance of making a complete or almost complete recovery.

References:

1. Aghalar MR, Araim RJ, Weiss LD. NIH Stroke Scale. In: Weiss LD, ed. Neuromuscular Quick Pocket Reference. New York, NY: Demos Medical Publishing; 2012: 87– 89
2. Harvey R, Macko R, Stein J, Zorowitz R, Winstein C. Stroke Recovery and Rehabilitation. New York, NY. Demos Medical Publishing; 2008.
3. Stein J, Silver JK, Rizzo TD, et al. Stroke. In: Frontera WR, ed. Essentials of Physical Medicine and Rehabilitation. 2nd ed. Philadelphia, PA: Saunders; 2008: 627: Chapter 114. Stein J, Silver JK, Rizzo TD, et al.
4. Stroke. In: Frontera WR, ed. Essentials of Physical Medicine and Rehabilitation. 2nd ed. Philadelphia, PA: Saunders; 2008: 887– 891

Chapter-21
Physiology

EXERCISE PHYSIOLOGY
Dr Sunita Tiwari, Professor& Head, Department of Physiology

A 38 year old adult male during treadmill test showed diminished exercise tolerance. The following data was obtained during catheterization procedure to evaluate the pressures in the cardiovascular system:-

Peak left ventricular pressure:	192mm Hg
Mean left atrial pressure:	16mm Hg
Peak aortic pressure:	119 mm Hg
Peak right ventricular pressure:	30mm Hg
Mean right aortic pressure:	6mm Hg
CO:	4.2 L/min
Arterial O_2 content:	19.3ml/dL
Venous O_2 content:	14.6ml/dL

1. Diminished exercise tolerance in this patient could be due to:
   (A) A decrease in the number of cardiac β receptors
   (B) An elevation in the left ventricular end diastolic pressure
   (C) Stenosis of the aortic valve
   (D) Poor cardiac muscle function after a myocardial infarction (MI)
2. The patient would respond favorably by following one of the following intervention?
   (A) Administration of an α-blocking agent
   (B) Administration of an β-blocking agent
   (C) Administration of supplemental oxygen (O_2)
   (D) Replacement of the aortic valve

Answers:
1.   C
     The large difference between peak left ventricular pressure and peak aortic pressure indicates stenosis of the aortic valve. This prevents adequate amounts of blood from being pumped out of the left ventricle into the aorta.
2.   D
     The stenosed aortic valve needs replacement.

Reference:
1. Roger Tanner Thies. Physiology An Illustrated Review International. 6th ed. New York: Thieme Medical and scientific publishers Pvt. Ltd; 2012. p. 97-9.

PHEOCHROMOCYTOMA
Dr Sunita Tiwari, Professor& Head, Department of Physiology

A 45 year old woman had complaint of recurrent headache episodes, sweating & thumping in her chest. On examination her blood pressure was 190/120mm Hg and heart rate was 136/min. Urine analysis showed elevated levels of epinephrine metabolites (metanephrine). She was diagnosed with a tumor in adrenal medullary tissue and it was postulated that uncontrolled, episodic release of catecholamines and metanephrines are the cause of elevated heart rate and mean arterial pressure.

1. Probable cause of elevated heart rate and BP in this patient could be:
   (A) Action of androgenic steroids
   (B) Action of epinephrine and norepinephrine
   (C) Action of aldosterone
   (D) Action of corticosteroids
2. Increase in the heart rate is due to:
   (A) Alpha adrenergic blocking drug
   (B) Beta adrenergic blocking drug
   (C) Cholinergic blocking drug
   (D) Cholinergic stimulating drug
3. Intravenous (IV) infusion of epinephrine causes:
   (A) A decrease in TPR
   (B) An increase in venous volume
   (C) An increase in cardiac contractility
   (D) A reflexively mediated increase in heart rate

Answers:

1. B

   The patient's tachycardia was due to the increased rate of depolarization of pacemaker cells in the SA node stimulated by the excess catecholamine epinephrine and nor-epinephrine. Epinephrine and nor-epinephrine also increases peripheral resistance by vasoconstriction and stimulate increased contractility, so blood pressure increases.

2. C

   Tonic vagal never activity slows the SA nodal rate of depolarization via activation of muscarinic receptors. Blocking cholinergic muscarinic receptors would increase heart rate.

3. C

   Norepinephrine increase cardiac contractility via cardiac β receptors.

Reference:

1. Roger Tanner Thies. Physiology An Illustrated Review International. 6th ed. New York: Thieme Medical and scientific publishers Pvt. Ltd; 2012. p. 106-8.

GLYCOSURIA

Dr Shraddha Singh, Professor, Department of Physiology

A 11 year old male is having frequent episodes of night bed wetting. He remains constantly thirsty (drinking a total of 5 to 6 litres of liquids daily), urinating every 30 to 40 min. and despite a voracious appetite, he is losing weight. He is diagnosed as a case of diabetes mellitus.

The findings on physical examination and the results of laboratory testsare:

Height	5 feet, 4 inches
Weight	40kg (43 kg at his annual checkup 2 months earlier)
Blood pressure	90/56 mm Hg (lying) 76/45 mm Hg (standing)
Fasting plasma glucose	320 mg/dL (normal 70–110 mg/dL)
Plasma	Na^+ 143 mEq/L (normal, 140 mEq/L)
Urine glucose	4+ (normal, nil)
Urine ketones	2+ (normal, nil)
Urine Na^+ Increased	

1. Transport maximum (Tmax) for glucose is approximately:
   - (A) 125 mg/min
   - (B) 80 mg/min
   - (C) 375 mg/min
   - (D) 480 mg/min
2. In a normal individual glucose should **NOT** appear in urine, if plasma glucose level (approximately) is below:
   - (A) 180 mg/min
   - (B) 240 mg/min
   - (C) 300 mg/min
   - (D) 360 mg/min
3. Glucose is reabsorbed maximally in which part of nephron:
   - (A) First part of the Proximal convoluted tubule
   - (B) Loop of Henle
   - (C) Distal convoluted tubule
   - (D) Second part of the Proximal convoluted tubule
4. Glucose is reabsorbed from the lumen of nephron by which process:
   - (A) Active transport
   - (B) Secondary active transport
   - (C) Facilitated diffusion
   - (D) Carrier mediated
5. In a normal individual glucose concentration of glomerular filtrate is:
   - (A) One third of plasma glucose concentration
   - (B) Half of plasma glucose concentration
   - (C) Two third of plasma glucose concentration
   - (D) Equal to plasma glucose concentration

Answers:

1. C

   For most substances that are actively reabsorbed or secreted, there is a limit to the rate at which the solute can be transported, often referred to as the *transport maximum.*In the adult human, the transport maximum for glucose averages about 375 mg/min.

2. A

   When the plasma concentration of glucose rises above about 200 mg/100 ml, increasing the filtered load to about 250 mg/min, a small amount of glucose begins to appear in the urine. This point is termed the *threshold* for glucose. *Note that this appearance ofglucose in the urine (at the threshold) occurs before thetransport maximum is reached.*

3. A

   In the first half of the proximal tubule, sodium is reabsorbed by co-transport along with glucose, amino acids, and other solutes. But in the second half of the proximal tubule, little glucose and amino acids remain to be reabsorbed.

4. B

   Reabsorption of glucose is referred to as "secondary active transport" because glucose itself is reabsorbed uphill against a chemical gradient, but it is "secondary" to primary active transport of sodium.

5. D

   Glucose is freely filtered across glomerular capillary membrane and therefore glucose concentration of glomerular filtrate is same as that of plasma.

Reference:

1. Hall JE. Guyton and Hall text book of medical physiology. 12th ed. Philadelphia: Saunders Elsevier; 2011. p. 314-15,326-27,329.

DIABETIC NEPHROPATHY

Dr Shraddha Singh, Professor, Department of Physiology

A 42-year-old woman who had proteinuria for past 5 years develops renal failure with hypertension. She also had several bacterial and vaginal yeast infections over the last 10 years. She required cesarean for her past 2 deliveries because oflarge babies (4 kg and 4.5 kg). A kidney biopsy reveals increased mesangialmatrix and acellular periodic acid-Schiff (PAS)-positive nodules. She was diagnosed as case of diabetic nephropathy.

1. Structure forming glomerular membrane (filtration membrane) is:
   - (A) Endothelium of the capillaries, Basement membrane, Bowman's epithelium
   - (B) Epithelium of the capillaries, Basement membrane and Bowman's endothelium
   - (C) Endothelium of the capillaries, Basement membrane, podocytes
   - (D) Both (a) and (c)
2. The diameter of the glomerular membrane pores, is about :
   - (A) 6 nm
   - (B) 6 µm
   - (C) 8 nm
   - (D) 8 µm
3. In normal individual, albumin is not filtered in glomerulus, because of :
   - (A) Small size of the glomerular membrane pore
   - (B) Electrostatic charge
   - (C) High molecular weight of albumin
   - (D) Both (a) and (c)
4. This patient had large babies, because of the actions of:
   - (A) insulin hormone
   - (B) growth hormone
   - (C) cortisols
   - (D) thyroid hormone
5. Glucose is reabsorbed in first part of lumen of PCT via:
   - (A) SGLT 2
   - (B) GLUT 2
   - (C) SGLT 4
   - (D) GLUT 4

Answers:

1. D

   The glomerular capillary membrane is similar to that of other capillaries, except that it has three (instead of theusual two major layers: (1) the endothelium of the capillary, (2) a basement membrane, and (3) a layer ofepithelial cells (podocytes) surrounding the outer surface of the capillary basement membrane.

2. C

   Pores of the glomerular membrane are thought to be about 8 nanometers (80 angstroms).

3. C

   The molecular diameter of the plasma protein albumin is only about 6 nanometers, whereas thepores of the glomerular membrane are thought to be about 8 nanometers (80 angstroms). Albumin is restricted fromfiltrationbecause of theelectrostatic repulsion exerted by negative charges of theglomerular capillary wall proteoglycans.

4. A

   Insulin promotes protein formation and prevents the degradation of proteins. Because of the anabolic action of insulin hormone released in response to hyperglycemia (in mother's blood), growth of fetus accelerates resulting in large baby.

5. A

   Glucose and Na^+ bind to the sodium-dependent glucose transporter (SGLT-2) in the apical membrane, and glucose is carried into the cell asNa^+ moves down its electrical and chemical gradient.

Reference:

1. Hall JE. Guyton and Hall text book of medical physiology. 12th ed. Philadelphia: Saunders Elsevier; 2011. p. 312,316,683,944.

DIARRHEA

Dr. Vani Gupta, Professor, Department of Physiology

A 28 year old male was brought to emergency with high grade fever, slurred speech and confused mental state. He also had severe watery diarrhea since last two days.He is a salesman in a company and his job requires frequent travelling. He was diagnosed as a case of "traveler's diarrhea".

Relevant physical examination and laboratory findings:

Oral mucosa and skin was dry.

Temperature:	103.1^0 F (39.5°C)	
Pulse rate:	120/min	
Respiratory rate :	24/min, deep and rapid respiration	
Blood pressure:	94/ 64 mm Hg in lying position	
	68/56 mm Hg in standing position	
WBC count:	15000/mm³.	
Serum Na^+:	131.5 mEq/L	(normal 140 mEq/L)
Serum Cl^-:	112 mEq/L	(normal 105 mEq/L)
Serum HCO_3^-:	10 mEq/L	(normal 24 mEq/L)
Serum K^+:	2.5 mEq/L	(normal 4.5 mEq/L)
Arterial pCO_2:	25 mm Hg	(normal 40 mm Hg).
Arterial pH:	7.25	(normal 7.4)

1. Acid-base disorder in above patient is:
   (A) Metabolic acidosis
   (B) Respiratory acidosis
   (C) Metabolic alkalosis
   (D) Respiratory alkalosis
2. Orthostatic hypotension is defined as
   (A) Fall in systolic blood pressure of at least 20 mm Hg or diastolic blood pressure of at least 10 mm Hg when a person assumes a standing position.
   (B) Raise in systolic blood pressure of at least 20 mm Hg or diastolic blood pressure of at least 10 mm Hg when a person assumes a lying position.

(C) Fall in systolic blood pressure of at least 20 mm Hg or diastolic blood pressure of at least 10 mm Hg when a person assumes a sitting position.

(D) Fall in diastolic blood pressure of at least 10 mm Hg when a person assumes a sitting position.

3. Anion gap in above case is:
   (A) 8 mEq/L
   (B) 10 mEq/L
   (C) 12 mEq/L
   (D) None of the above

Answers:

1. A

Since pH is less than normal hence its acidosis. In metabolic acidosis there is a decrease in HCO_3^- concentration; this decrease can be caused either by a gain of fixed acid (fixed acid is buffered by extracellular HCO_3^-, leading to a decreased HCO_3^- concentration) or by loss of HCO_3^- from the body.

2. A

Orthostatic hypotension also known as postural hypotension, orthostatic is a form of low blood pressure in which a person's blood pressure falls when suddenly standing up or stretching. It is defined as a fall in systolic blood pressure of at least 20 mm Hg or diastolic blood pressure of atleast 10 mm Hg when a person assumes a standing position. The symptom is caused by blood pooling in the lower extremities upon a change in body position.

3. C

Anion gap = $(Na^+ + K^+)$-$(HCO_3^- + Cl^-)$

References:

1. Hall JE. Guyton and Hall text book of medical physiology. 13th ed. Philadelphia: Saunders Elsevier; 2015. p. 409-426
2. Beitzke M, Pfister P, Fortin J, Skrabal F. Autonomic dysfunction and hemodynamic in vitamin B12 deficiency. Autonomic Neuroscience; 2002; 97(1).p.45-54.

PULMONARY TUBERCULOSIS

Dr Archana Ghildiyal, Associate Professor, Department of Physiology

A 25 years old women, working as a health care worker in a village, presented with complaints of evening fever, night sweats, fatigue, shortness of breath on exertion, anterior chest pain, loss of appetite, weight loss and productive cough with blood for last 1 month. Doctor did her Physical examination and investigated for Hb%, TLC, DLC, sputum smears and cultures. X-ray chest shows an extensive infiltrate in the upper lobe of right lung with air space consolidation and formation of cavities.

1. Ventilation-Perfusion ratio is maximum at which part of the lung?
   (A) Apex
   (B) Base
   (C) Middle
   (D) Equal (at all the places)
2. What is the possible etiology for evening rise of temperature?
   (A) Cytokines
   (B) Thyroxine
   (C) Progesterone
   (D) Testosterone
3. What will happen if the lungs develop areas of fibrosis?
   (A) Decreased thickness of respiratory membrane
   (B) Increased Vital capacity
   (C) Increased breathing capacity
   (D) Decreased pulmonary diffusing capacity

1. A

Ventilation as well as perfusion in the upright position (Normal V/P Ratio is 0.8; 4.2 L per min ventilation/5.5 L per min blood flow) declines in a linear fashion from the base to the apex of the lungs. But ventilation is significantly higher than perfusion at the apex..

2. A

In Tuberculosis, fever produced by cytokines (IL-1, IL-6, -IFN, -IFN, and TNF-alfa) is probably due to local release of prostaglandins in the hypothalamus.

3. D

In Fibrosis, reduced total respiratory membrane surface area and increased thickness of the respiratory membrane result in progressively diminished pulmonary diffusing capacity.

References:
1. Tortora GJ, Derrickson BH. Principles of Anatomy and Physiology 12th ed. Asia: John Wiley &Sons, (Asia) Pte Ltd; 2012. p. 913. (International student edition; vo 2).
2. Hall JE. Guyton and Hall text book of medical physiology. 12th ed. Philadelphia: Saunders Elsevier; 2011. p. 520.

HAEMOPHILIA
Dr Dileep Verma, Associate Professor, Department of Physiology

A 7-year-old boy is brought to the emergency department with injured knee. He was accompanied by a college employee who told that the boy collided with a classmate while running across the schoolyard and fell on the pavement. Upon examination, the patient is extremely uncomfortable, his knee is warm and tender, and there is a large hematoma on the anterior aspect of the knee. The patient also has cuts on both elbows that continue to bleed even after applying pressure to the wound, as well as a number of contusions elsewhere on his arms and legs. Laboratory studies reveal a normal CBC, platelet count, prothrombin time and a markedly elevated partial thromboplastin time. X-rays of the legs are negative for fractures in the femur, tibia, and fibula.

1. Haemophilia can result from deficiency of which clotting factor?
(A) Factor IX
(B) Factor X
(C) Factor XI
(D) Both (a) and (c)
2. Inheritance of Haemophilia is:
(A) Autosomal recessive
(B) Sex linked dominant
(C) Autosomal dominant
(D) Sex linked recessive
3. Partial thromboplastin time is primarily a test for evaluation of the:
(A) Extrinsic pathway of coagulation
(B) Intrinsic pathway of coagulation
(C) Common pathway of coagulation
(D) None

Answers:
1. D

Haemophilia A: deficiency of Factor VIII
Haemophilia B/ Christmas disease: deficiency of factor IX
Haemophilia C: deficiency of factor XI.

2. D

The abnormality is located on the sex chromosome X and is a recessive character. Therefore the females generally do not suffer, being protected by the second X chromosome which is usually normal.

3. B

Thromboplastin generation test (TGT) is primarily a test for evaluation of the intrinsic system of clotting. The various factors required for the generation of thromboplastin by the intrinsic system are factors XII, XI, IX, VIII, PF-3, X and V.

References:

1. Hall JE. Guyton and Hall text book of medical physiology. 12th ed. Philadelphia: Saunders Elsevier; 2011. p. 452,458.
2. Bijlani RL, Manjunatha S. Understanding medical physiology a textbook for medical students. 4th ed. New Delhi (India): Jaypee Brothers Medical Publishers (P) Ltd; 2011. p. 97,98.

IRON DEFICIENCY ANEMIA

Dr Dileep Verma, Associate Professor,Department of Physiology

A 21-year-old woman presents to gynecologistwith history of dysmenorrhea and menorrhagia for past 1 year. She recalls having seven or eight periods over the past 12 months, all of which were heavier than normal. She has been feeling tired for the past 3 months and has trouble waking up each morning because she feels exhausted. She is not taking any medications and denies substance abuse. Her coagulation studies are normal. Her vital signs include a heart rate of 92/min, blood pressure of 135/80 mm Hg, and respiratory rate of 20/min. Relevant laboratory results are as follows:

WBC count:	5600/mm^3
Haemoglobin:	9.2 g/dL
Platelet count:	2,25,000/mm^3
Mean corpuscular haemoglobin:	21 pg
Mean corpuscular haemoglobin concentration:	29%
Mean corpuscular volume:	72 fl (femtolitre)

1. Most common cause of nutritional deficiency anemia in females is:
   (A) Iron deficiency
   (B) Vitamin B12 deficiency
   (C) Folic acid deficiency
   (D) Zinc
2. Maximum absorption of iron from intestine occurs in form of:
   (A) Fe^{++} (ferrous)
   (B) Fe^{+++} (ferric)
   (C) Haem iron
   (D) Nonhaem iron
3. Effect of anemia on circulatory system is/are:
   (A) Increased cardiac output
   (B) Decreased peripheral vascular resistance
   (C) Increased workload of heart
   (D) All of the above
4. What should be serum ferritin level and iron binding capacity in this case:
   (A) Decreased and decreased respectively
   (B) Increased and decreased respectively
   (C) Decreased and increased respectively
   (D) Increased and increased respectively

Answers:

1. A
   Deficiency of iron is the most common nutritional disorder in the world and results in a clinical signs and symptoms that are mostly related to inadequate hemoglobinsynthesis.
2. C
   The intestinal absorption of haem iron is much better(up to 30% may be absorbed) than that of non-haem iron. Non-haem iron is converted into ferrous form before it can enter the enterocyte by a carrier-mediated active process.
3. D
   In severe anemia, the blood viscosity decreases, moreover, hypoxia resulting from diminished transport of oxygen by the blood causes the peripheral tissue blood vessels to dilate. Thus, one of the major effects ofanemiais greatly *increased cardiac output,* as well as *increasedpumping workload on the heart.*

4. C
   Measurements of marrow iron stores, serum ferritin, and total iron-binding capacity (TIBC) are sensitive to early iron-store depletion.

Test	Iron deficiency	Inflammation	Thalassemia	Sideroblastic anemia
TIBC	>360	<300	Normal	Normal
Ferritin(µg/L)	<15	30-200	50-300	50-300

References:
1. Bijlani RL, Manjunatha S. Understanding medical physiology a textbook for medical students. 4th ed. New Delhi (India): Jaypee Brothers Medical Publishers (P) Ltd; 2011. p. 62,407.
2. Hall JE. Guyton and Hall text book of medical physiology. 12th ed. Philadelphia: Saunders Elsevier; 2011. p. 420-21.
3. Longo DL, Fauci AS, Kasper DL, Hauser SL, Jameson JL, Loscalzo J. Harrison's hematology and oncology. 2nd ed. NewYork: McGraw-Hill Education; 2011. p. 75.

CUSHING'S SYNDROME
Dr Jagdish Narayan, Assistant Professor, Department of Physiology

A 46 year old male had gained 14 kg over 2 years, mostly around his trunk, face, and shoulders, although his arms and legs had become very thin. He has purple stretch marks on his abdomen. His appetite has significantly increased in the past 2 years. He is having trouble doing the heavy lifting that is required in his job. His blood pressure was significantly elevated at 170/110 mm Hg.

Table summarizes the laboratory results obtained in the fasting state:

Serum Na^+	140 mEq/L (normal, 140 mEq/L)
Serum K^+	3.0 mEq/L (normal, 4.5 mEq/L)
Fasting glucose	155 mg/dL (normal, 70–110 mg/dL)
Serum cortisol	Increased
Serum ACTH (adrenocorticotropic hormone)	Undetectable

His serum cortisol level remained elevatedeven after administration of low dose dexamethasone. CT scan showed a 7-cm mass on the right adrenal gland.

1. The most common cause of Cushing's syndrome is:
   (A) high plasma levels of ACTH and cortisol
   (B) high plasma levels of cortisol and low levels of ACTH
   (C) high plasma levels of ACTH and low levels of cortisol
   (D) low plasma levels of ACTH and cortisol
2. Major portion of cortisol is secreted from:
   (A) zona reticularis
   (B) zona fasciculata
   (C) zona glomerulosa
   (D) adrenal medulla
3. Fasting glucose level is elevated in this case, because of :
   (A) increased rate of glycogenolysis
   (B) decreased glucose uptake and utilization
   (C) insulin resistance
   (D) both (b) and (c)
4. Patient washaving trouble doing the heavy lifting, because of:
   (A) protein stores of hepatic tissues are utilized in gluconeogenesis
   (B) decreased amino acid transport into hepatic tissues
   (C) both (A) and (B)
   (D) none
5. Cortisol's glucocorticoid activity is:
   (D) equal to mineralocorticoid activity
   (E) 10 times as that of mineralocorticoid activity
   (F) $^1/_{10}$ th of mineralocorticoid activity
   (G) None

Answers:

1. **A**

   Excess ACTH secretion is the most common cause of Cushing's syndrome and is characterized by high plasma levels of cortisol.

2. **B**

   The zona fasciculata, the middle and widest layer, constitutes about 75 percent of the adrenal cortex and secretes the glucocorticoids cortisol and corticosterone, as well as small amounts of adrenal androgens and estrogens.

3. **D**

   Both the increased rate of gluconeogenesis and the moderate reduction in the rate of glucose utilization by the cells cause the blood glucose concentrations to rise. High levels of fatty acids, caused by the effect of glucocorticoids to mobilize lipids from fat depots,impairs insulin actions on the tissues.

4. **D**

   Cortisol causes mobilization of amino acids from theextrahepatic tissues mainly from muscle. As a result, more amino acids become available in the plasma to enter into the gluconeogenesis process of the liver and thereby to promote the formation of glucose.

5. **A**

   Cortisol has equal glucocorticoid and mineralocorticoid activity.

Reference:

1. Hall JE. Guyton and Hall text book of medical physiology. 12th ed. Philadelphia: Saunders Elsevier; 2011. p. 922,924,928-29,935.

HYPERTHYROIDISM

Dr Jagdish Narayan, Assistant Professor, Department of Physiology

A20 year old female presented with weight loss of almost 7 kg in the past 3 monthsdespite of a good appetite. She complains of nervousness, sleeplessness, palpitations, irregular menstrual periods and intolerance to warm weather. On physical examination, she was restless and had a noticeable tremor in her hands. At 5 feet 8 inches tall, she weighed only 44 kg. Her BP was 160/85 mm Hg, and her heart rate was 110 beats/min. She had a wide-eyed stare, and her lower neck appeared full; these characteristics were not present in photographs taken 1 year earlier. Based on her symptoms, the physician suspected that she had thyrotoxicosis.

1. Patient had intolerance to heatbecause of:
   (A) Increase in the number and activity of mitochondria
   (B) Increase cellular metabolic activity
   (C) Increased activity of sodium-potassium ATPase pump
   (D) All of the above

2. The enzyme primarily responsible for the conversion of T_4 to T_3 in the periphery is
   (A)D1 thyroid deiodinase
   (B)D2 thyroid deiodinase
   (C)D3 thyroid deiodinase
   (D)Thyroid peroxidase

3. Thyroid hormone receptors binds to DNA in which of the following form?
   (A)A heterodimer with the prolactin receptor
   (B)A heterodimer with the growth hormone receptor
   (C)A heterodimer with the retinoid X receptor
   (D)A heterodimer with the insulin receptor

4. Thyroid hormone increases heart rate by:
   (A)Sensitizing myocardium to circulating catecholamines
   (B)Directly stimulation
   (C)Both (a) and (b)
   (D)None

5. Tremor in hyperthyroidism is:
   (A) Coarse tremor caused by increased reactivity of the neuronal synapses in the areas of the spinal cord
   (B) Fine tremor caused by increased reactivity of the neuronal synapses in the areas of the spinal cord
   (C) Coarse tremor caused by increased sensitivity of the musclesto circulating catecholamines
   (D)Fine tremor caused by increased sensitivity of the muscles to circulating catecholamines

1. D

   One of the principal functions of thyroxine is to increase the number and activity of mitochondria, which in turn increases the rate of formation of adenosine triphosphate (ATP).

   Activity of *Na-K-ATPase* pump increases in response to thyroid hormone which in turn increases the rate of transport of both Na^+ and K^+ through the cell membrane. This process uses energy and increases the amount of heat produced in the body.

2. A

   Three different deiodinases act on thyroid hormones: D1, D2, and D3. D1 is primarily responsible for maintaining the formation of T3 from T4 in the periphery.

3. C

   The thyroid hormone receptors are either attached to the DNA genetic strands or located in proximity to them. The thyroid hormone receptor usually forms a heterodimer with *retinoid X receptor* (RXR) at specific *thyroid hormone response elements* on the DNA.

4. B

   Thyroid hormone have a direct effect on the excitability of the heart, which in turn increases the heart rate.

5. B

   One of the most characteristic signs of hyperthyroidism is a fine muscle tremor occuring at the rapid frequency of 10 to 15 times per second. This tremor is believed to be caused by increased reactivity of the neuronal synapses in the areas of the spinal cord that control muscle tone.

References:

1. Hall JE. Guyton and Hall text book of medical physiology. 12th ed. Philadelphia: Saunders Elsevier; 2011. p. 910-13.
2. Barret KE, Barman SM, Boitano S, Brooks HL. Ganong's review of medical physiology. 24th ed. NewYork: The McGraw-Hill Companies; 2012. p. 344.

NEPHROTIC SYNDROME

Mayank Agarwal, JR2, Department of Physiology

A 5 year old boy is brought to pediatrician after his mother notices that his limbs seem swollen and stomach distended. She says that the boy received an influenza vaccine 1 week ago. Physical examination reveals generalized pitting edema and shifting dullness of the abdomen suggestive of ascites. Urine analysis reveals 4+ proteinuria, and laboratory findings show decreased serum albumin, hypertriglyceridemia, and normal serum ionized calcium. Blood pressure, blood urea nitrogen (BUN), and serum creatinine values are within normal limits.

1. Cause of pitting edema is:
   - (A) Decreased plasma colloidal oncotic pressure
   - (B) Decreased water filtration from glomerulus
   - (C) Decreased plasma protein
   - (D) Both a and c

2. What is the classical presentation of this condition:
   - (A) Edema, massive proteinuria, hypertension, gross hematuria
   - (B) Edema, mild proteinuria, hypoalbuminemia, hypertriglyceridemia
   - (C) Edema, massive proteinuria, hypertension, hypoalbuminemia
   - (D) Edema, massive proteinuria, hypoalbuminemia, hypertriglyceridemia

3. What is the normal value of plasma colloid oncotic pressure?
   - (A) 8 mm Hg
   - (B) 18 mm Hg
   - (C) 28 mm Hg
   - (D) None

4. What is the range of microalbuminuria?
   - (A) 8-10 mg in 24 hours
   - (B) 30-300 mg per hour
   - (C) 30-300 mg in 24 hour
   - (D) >300 mg per hour

Answers:

1. **D**

   The glomerular basement membrane contains heparin sulfate, which acts as a negative charge barrier that keeps small and negatively charged proteins such as albumin from crossing the membrane. Minimal change disease can be preceded by a recent infection or vaccination. It is believed that T cells release cytokines that injure glomerular epithelial cells. Consequently, the negative charge barrier is lost.

2. **D**

	NEPHROTIC SYNDROME	NEPHRITIC SYNDROME
CLINICAL FINDINGS	Edema (often periorbital) Minimal hematuria	Hypertension Gross hematuria Decreased urine output
LABORATORY FINDINGS	Hypoalbuminemia Hypercholesterolemia Massive Proteinuria	Red cell casts in urine Elevated creatinine Mild proteinuria

3. **C**

   Normal plasma oncotic value is 28 mm Hg.

4. **C**

   Microalbuminuria is excretion of protein in range of 30-300mg/24 hours.

References:

1. Hall JE. Guyton and Hall text book of medical physiology. 12th ed. Philadelphia: Saunders Elsevier; 2011. p. 185,404.
2. Jameson JL, Loscalzo J. Harrison's nephrology and acid base disorders. 2nd ed. New York: McGraw-Hill Education; 2013. p.25,166.

Chapter-22

Plastic Surgery

HEMANGIOMA

Prof. Arun K. Singh, Head, Dr. Divya Narain Upadhyaya, Assistant Professor,
Dr. Veerendra Prasad, Associate Professor, Department of Plastic Surgery

A 3-month-old male child presents with a rapidly growing swelling on the forehead. The parents inform that the swelling was not present at birth and appeared 2 weeks later. It has been growing rapidly ever since and has changed color from a pale pink spot to dark red. The swelling is red in color, warm, non-tender, soft, compressible but not reducible and exhibits no thrill or bruit. It does not trans-illuminate.

1. The most likely diagnosis is –
    (A) Arachnoid cyst
    (B) Branchial cyst
    (C) Venous malformation
    (D) Hemangioma
    (E) Cystic hygroma
2. The most likely next step in the management of the above condition will be –
    (A) Surgical excision
    (B) Laser therapy
    (C) Intra-lesional sclerosant
    (D) Systemic steroids
    (E) Observation only
3. Pharmacotherapy for the above condition consists of all of the following except –
    (A) Systemic corticosteroids
    (B) Intra-lesional steroids
    (C) Systemic propanolol
    (D) Interferon Alpha
    (E) Proton pump inhibitors
4. All of the following are true for the above condition except –
    (A) Greater incidence in white races
    (B) Greater incidence in males than females
    (C) Greater incidence in females than males
    (D) Characterized by endothelial proliferation
    (E) Majority resolve by themselves and do not need treatment
5. All of the following are useful in establishing a diagnosis except –
    (A) Serum levels of angiogenic proteins
    (B) Tissue biopsy
    (C) Ultrasonography
    (D) MRI
    (E) Lymphoscintigraphy

Answers:
1.   D
      A vascular anomaly, which appears after birth and shows rapid growth thereafter, is a hemangioma.
2.   E
      Most hemangiomas will resolve on their own beginning at the age of one year. Those that do not, will require some form of intervention.
3.   E
      Proton pump inhibitors are used to treat gastric ulcers. The others are used in some or other forms for pharmacologic treatment of hemangiomas.
4.   B
      Hemangiomas are seen more in females than in males.
5.   E
      Lymphoscintigraphy is used in the evaluation of diseases of the lymphatic pathways and not for diagnosing hemangiomas.

References:
1.   Morris SF, Mulliken J B. Vascular Anomalies. In: Neligan P C, Chang J (Eds) Plastic Surgery 3rd Edition. Elsevier Saunders, 2005, Vol 1, pp 676-706.
2.   Mulliken J B, Fishman SJ, Burrows P E. Vascular Anomalies. Current Problems in Surgery 2000; 37(8): 517-584

UPPER LIMB TRAUMA

Prof. Arun K. Singh, Head, Dr. Divya Narain Upadhyaya, Assistant Professor,
Dr. Veerendra Prasad, Associate Professor, Department of Plastic Surgery

A 20-year-old male patient is brought to the emergency department at night with a laceration to the volar aspect of his right forearm, which he sustained in a drunken brawl inside a pub. He gives a history of profuse bleed, which was controlled on pressure, and inability to flex his fingers. On examination the radial artery is palpable at the wrist, he is unable to make a fist and has no sensation in the medial one and half fingers of his hand. He has a hurriedly tied cloth on his forearm, which serves as temporary dressing.

1. The first response of the emergency team should be –
   (A) Order a CT angiography
   (B) Order blood transfusion
   (C) CTake consent for surgery
   (D) Apply a sterile dressing over the previous dressing
   (E) Apply a tourniquet and examine the wound
2. Which of the following investigations are you least likely to order
   (A) Radiograph of the forearm and hand
   (B) Color doppler
   (C) CT Angiography
   (D) 2D Echo cardiography
   (E) Hemogram
3. Which of the following structures is most likely to have been injured
   (A) Extensors of the wrist
   (B) Posterior Interosseous Nerve
   (C) Long Flexors of the hand
   (D) Brachial artery
   (E) Biceps tendon
4. What course of treatment will you advise for the patient
   (A) Splintage and limb elevation
   (B) Pressure dressing to arrest bleeding
   (C) Blood transfusion and elective surgery next day
   (D) Emergency exploration under infiltration anesthesia
   (E) Emergency exploration under upper limb block and tourniquet control
5. During exploration which structures are you unlikely to find damaged
   (A) Long flexors of the hand
   (B) Flexors of the wrist
   (C) Ulnar artery
   (D) Posterior Interosseous Artery
   (E) Ulnar Nerve

Answers:

1. E
   The patient has a vascular injury. Attempting to examine him without proximal control can lead to further blood loss and exsanguination of the patient.
2. D
   A young healthy patient is unlikely to have a cardiac condition especially if he has been vigorous enough to be in a fight. Hence a 2D Echocardiography is hardly necessary for evaluating his surgical fitness.
3. C
   Long flexors of the hand are injured, as the patient is unable to make a fist
4. E
   All vascular injuries must undergo emergent exploration under tourniquet control unless contraindicated by the patient's general condition.
5. D
   Posterior Interosseous artery supplies the extensor compartment of the forearm and branches off at the cubital fossa, hence is the least likely to have been injured.

References:

1. Tang J B. Flexor Tendon Injury and Reconstruction. In: Neligan P C, Chang J (Eds) Plastic Surgery 3rd Edition. Elsevier Saunders, 2005, Vol 6, pp 178-209

2. Chang J, Valero-Cuevas F, Hentz V R, Chase R A. Anatomy and biomechanics of the Hand. In: Neligan P C, Chang J (Eds) Plastic Surgery 3rd Edition. Elsevier Saunders, 2005, Vol 6, pp 1-46.

CLEFT LIP AND PALATE

Prof. Arun K. Singh, Head, Dr. Divya Narain Upadhyaya, Assistant Professor,
Dr. Veerendra Prasad, Associate Professor, Department of Plastic Surgery

A one-week-old male child with a cleft of the lip is brought to the hospital by his anguished parents. The child is unable to suckle and keeps regurgitating fluids from his nose. On examination there is a cleft of the alveolus and the palate too. The child is underweight and is crying incessantly.

1. How will you evaluate the child
    (A) Get a hemogram done
    (B) Order a radiograph of the face
    (C) Order a genetic profile of the child and the parents
    (D) Clinically examine the child for other congenital anomalies
    (E) No need to evaluate the child at present, call him back after three months
2. While counseling the parents regarding the care of the child which advice are you unlikely to give
    (A) Feed him with a bottle with a wide hole
    (B) Only breast feed him
    (C) Feed him expressed milk with a spoon
    (D) Frequently burp the child
    (E) Feed him with his head elevated
3. At what age are you likely to recommend a lip repair to the child
    (A) Five years
    (B) One year
    (C) Three months
    (D) Three weeks
    (E) After adolescence
4. At what age are you likely to recommend palate surgery to the child
    (A) Two years
    (B) Five years
    (C) Three months
    (D) At adolescence
    (E) One year
5. All of the following are methods of lip repair except
    (A) Tennison
    (B) Millard
    (C) Zancolli
    (D) Veau
    (E) Blair

Answers:

1. D
    The first visit should be utilised to scan the child for other congenital anomalies clinically and for counseling the parents and educating them about the care of the child.
2. B
    The child has a cleft of the lip and the palate and hence will not be able to suckle. The child should be fed by either a wide hole bottle or a spoon.
3. C
    Most cleft centers around the world will recommend undertaking the cleft lip repair at around three months of age.
4. E
    Most cleft centers around the world will recommend palate surgery around one year of age.
5. C
    Zancolli's operation is recommended for Ulnar claw hand.

References:

1. Chen P K T, Noordoff M S, Kane A. Repair of the unilateral cleft lip. In: Neligan P C, Chang J (Eds) Plastic Surgery 3rd Edition. Elsevier Saunders, 2005, Vol 3, pp 517-549.

2.   Hoffman W Y. Cleft Palate. In: Neligan P C, Chang J (Eds) Plastic Surgery 3rd Edition. Elsevier Saunders, 2005, Vol 3, pp 569-583.

FACIAL TRAUMA

Prof. Arun K. Singh, Head, Dr. Divya Narain Upadhyaya, Assistant Professor,
Dr. Veerendra Prasad, Associate Professor, Department of Plastic Surgery

A forty-year-old male patient is brought to the emergency with facial injuries, which he sustained in an assault. He is conscious, well oriented to time, place and person and able to stand and walk without support. There is no history of loss of consciousness, ear or nasal bleed or seizures. He has a bruised left cheek, a red eye and has sensory loss in his left upper lip. He has not lost any teeth but complains of his teeth not 'sitting together'.

1. The most likely investigation that you should order is
    (A) Hemogram
    (B) ECG
    (C) CT Scan of the face
    (D) 2D Echocardiography
    (E) CT Scan of the brain
2. The patient complains of decreased sensation in his left cheek which is likely due to trauma to the following nerve
    (A) Inferior alveolar nerve
    (B) Infraorbital nerve
    (C) Supraorbital nerve
    (D) Supratrochlear nerve
    (E) Facial nerve
3. All of the following are indicative of fracture of the mandible except
    (A) Malocclusion
    (B) Bony crepitus
    (C) Decreased sensation in lower lip
    (D) Decreased sensation in cheek
    (E) Gingival laceration
4. All of the following are suggestive of a fracture of the zygoma except
    (A) Enopthalmos
    (B) Decreased sensation in cheek
    (C) Conjunctival ecchymosis
    (D) Diplopia
    (E) Malocclusion
5. The following test is used to look for extra-ocular muscle entrapment in cases of fracture of the floor of the orbit.
    (A)Paget's test
    (B)Pointing index test
    (C)Forced duction test
    (D)Valsalva test
    (E)Fegan's test

Answers:
1. C
    The CT Scan of the face is the standard investigation that should be ordered in cases of facial injury where one suspects facial fractures.
2. B
    The infra-orbital nerve supplies sensation to the left cheek and the left upper alveolus. It is often involved in a fracture of the zygomatico-maxillary complex
3. D
    A decreased sensation in the cheek indicates injury to the infra-orbital nerve and thus fractures of the bones of the mid-face
4. E
    The zygoma does not bear teeth hence a pure fracture of the zygoma will not affect the occlusion.
5. C
    The forced duction test is used to look for entrapment of the extra-ocular muscles in fractures of the orbital floor.

Reference:
1. Rodriguez E D, Dorafshar A H, Manson P N. Facial Fractures. In: Neligan P C, Chang J (Eds) Plastic Surgery 3rd Edition. Elsevier Saunders, 2005, Vol 3, pp 49-88.

VENOUS ULCER

Prof. Arun K. Singh, Head, Dr. Divya Narain Upadhyaya, Assistant Professor,
Dr. Veerendra Prasad, Associate Professor, Department of Plastic Surgery

A forty year old male patient walks into the out patient department with complains of an ulcer over the medial malleolar are of his right leg since two years. The ulcer is painless but refuses to heal. On examination his lower limb shows several dilated veins and the skin around the ulcer is thickened and pigmented and appears shiny. The ulcer has red granulation tissue in its floor and sloping edges. It appears to sit right on the medial malleolus and is not mobile over its bed. The peripheral pulses of that limb are palpable.

1. The most likely clinical diagnosis is
    (A) Marjolin's ulcer
    (B) Venous ulcer
    (C) Trophic ulcer
    (D) Syphlitic ulcer
    (E) Decubitus ulcer
2. How should you proceed with examining the patient
    (A) Examine the peripheral arterial system
    (B) Examine the heel and back for other decubitus ulcers
    (C) Examine the nose and genitalia for signs of syphilis
    (D) Examine the nervous system for signs of loss of sensation
    (E) Examine the peripheral venous system for incompetent veins
3. Which investigation are you likely to order for this patient's evaluation
    (A) 2D Echocardiography
    (B) Venous color doppler of the lower limb
    (C) CT Angiography of the lower limb
    (D) Wound culture
    (E) Slit skin smear
4. All except one of the following tests will be used to examine the patient
    (A) Trendelenburg test
    (B) Schwartz test
    (C) Pratt's test
    (D) Fegan's test
    (E) Cottle's test
5. All except one of the following may be offered to the patient as a treatment modality
    (A) Cauterization of wound
    (B) Ligation of perforators
    (C) Ligation sapheno-femoral junction
    (D) Skin grafting
    (E) Venous stripping

Answers:
1. B
    A non-healing ulcer over the medial malleolar area in a patient with varicose veins is most likely a venous ulcer.
2. E
    Examination of the peripheral venous system is the way forward in a patient presenting with a venous ulcer
3. B
    A venous color doppler is likely to reveal the competence of perforators, S-F and S-P valves and also the status of the deep veins.
4. E
    Cottle's test is used to examine airway patency
5. A
    Cauterization of the wound is unlikely to help him as it is not an acute wound and there is no active bleeding

References:
1. Sen C K, Roy S. Wound Healing. In: Neligan P C, Chang J (Eds) Plastic Surgery 3rd Edition. Elsevier Saunders, 2005, Vol 1, pp 240-266.
2. Scurr J H, Coleridge-Smith P D. Venous Disorders. In: Russell R C G, Williams N S, Bulstrode C J K (Eds). Bailey and Love's Short Practice of Surgery. 23rd Edition. Arnold, London. 2000. pp 235-255.

SYNDACTYLY

Prof. Arun K. Singh, Head, Dr. Divya Narain Upadhyaya, Assistant Professor,
Dr. Veerendra Prasad, Associate Professor, Department of Plastic Surgery

A five year old child is brought to the out patient clinic with complains of non-separation of the 3rd and 4th digit of both hands since birth. On examination both the upper limbs are well formed with no digits missing. The child can form a grip with both his hands. The 3rd and 4th digits share a single nail but otherwise the skin covering them is supple and lax. The digits appear normal in length and have well formed PIP and DIP joints.

1. The most likely clinical diagnosis is
   (A) Camptodactyly
   (B) Syndactyly
   (C) Symbrachydactyly
   (D) Acrosyndactyly
   (E) Clinodactyly

2. What investigation are you most likely to order next
   (A) Color doppler examination of both upper limbs
   (B) Radiograph of both hands
   (C) Radiograph of the whole upper limb
   (D) Radiograph of hands and feet
   (E) CT Scan of both hands

3. What advice are you likely to give to the parents regarding the management of the condition
   (A) The condition cannot be corrected by surgery
   (B) Surgery should not be done till skeletal maturity
   (C) Surgery should be done as soon as possible
   (D) Surgery should be done after proper genetic profiling of the family
   (E) Surgery is contraindicated

4. All of the following conditions denote an anomaly of the hand except
   (A) Floating thumb
   (B) Trigger thumb
   (C) Simonart's band
   (D) Syndactyly
   (E) Camptodactyly

Answers:
1. B
   Syndactyly is one of the most common congenital hand anomalies presenting with fingers, which may be variably attached to each other
2. B
   A radiograph is ordered to rule out any osseous union
3. C
   The condition should be rectified as soon as the child is robust enough to with stand surgery to preempt growth disturbances in the fingers
4. C
   Simonart's band is found in the cleft of the lip and palate

References:
1. Tonkin M, Oberg K. Congenital Hand I: Embryology, classification and principles. In: Neligan P C, Chang J (Eds) Plastic Surgery 3rd Edition. Elsevier Saunders, 2005, Vol 6,pp 526-547.
2. Hovius S E R. Congenital hand IV: Disorders of differentiation and duplication. In: Neligan P C, Chang J (Eds) Plastic Surgery 3rd Edition. Elsevier Saunders, 2005, Vol 6, pp 603-633.

NON HEALING ULCERS

Prof. Arun K. Singh, Head, Dr. Divya Narain Upadhyaya, Assistant Professor,
Dr. Veerendra Prasad, Associate Professor, Department of Plastic Surgery

A wound usually heals in a reasonable time depending on its size and location, by contraction of the bed and centripetal growth of the epithelium from the margins. However, sometimes the healing process gets arrested, the granulation tissue either fails to appear due to avascular bed, or is pale, unhealthy and unable to support the growing epithelium. The epithelial margins too may become fibrotic and scarred. Such wounds are called chronic wounds. Local and systemic factors have been implicated in preventing the wound from healing , which if corrected may allow the wound heal.

1. A diabetic patient has a non healing ulcer over the big toe. This is because
   (A) Diabetes is a systemic disorder
   (B) Local factors at wound site are responsible
   (C) Both of the above may be correct
   (D) Medications for diabetes retards wound healing
2. A wound over the scalp with exposed calveria may refuse to heal on its own, because
   (A) The scalp skin is thick
   (B) The wound bed cannot contract
   (C) Oxygen tension at scalp is low
   (D) Infection invariably occurs
3. One of the features differentiating an acute wound from a chronic wound is the epithelium/margins surrounding the wound. In chronic wounds:
   (A) Margins are thick and whitish in colour
   (B) Margin is thin and sloping
   (C) Margins are discharging pus
   (D) It is irregular and their is no demarcated margin.
4. Chronic osteomylitis is often associated with a non healing wound/ sinus. Which of the following statements is correct
   (A) Systemic bacteremia prevents the wound from healing
   (B) Neuropathic changes prevent healing
   (C) Bone is an avascular structure
   (D) Sequestrum acts like a foreign body
5. The most common reason for development of pressure sore in a paraplegic is:
   (A) Sensory loss
   (B) Sudden increase in pressure on the local site
   (C) Atrophy of muscles
   (D) Nutritional deficiency.

Answers:
1. C
    Most chronic wounds are prevented from healing by a combination of local and systemic factors.
2. B
    The wound bed over the calvarium consists of bare bone and thus refuses to heal due to contraction.
3. A
    The margins of a chronic wound usually show scarring and tissue hypoxia and appear thickened and pale.
4. D
    The sequestrum in the bed of a chronic wound acts as a foreign body causing persistent inflammation and reluctance to heal.
5. A
    Loss of sensation at a pressure site in a paraplegic does not allow change in posture thus causing skin breakdown and formation of wound

Reference:
1. Sen C K, Roy S. Wound Healing. In: Neligan P C, Chang J (Eds) Plastic Surgery 3rd Edition. Elsevier Saunders, 2005, Vol 1, pp 240-266.

SECONDARY ALVEOLAR BONE GRAFTING (SABG)

Prof. Arun K. Singh, Head, Dr. Divya Narain Upadhyaya, Assistant Professor,
Dr. Veerendra Prasad, Associate Professor, Department of Plastic Surgery

A 16 years old boy approaches the out patient clinic for the treatment of his malaligned teeth. He complains of an unaesthetic appearance of his upper teeth and his wide nose. He has undergone lip repair at the age of 4 months, palate repair at the age of 18 months and Secondary Alveolar Bone Grafting (SABG) to his alveolus when he was 8 years of age. The patient has a concave facial profile with a small oro-nasal fistula in anterior part of hard palate.

1. Right age for secondary bone grafting is
    (A) After eruption of all permanent teeth in the oral cavity
    (B) After eruption of all permanent canine in the oral cavity
    (C) When root of permanent maxillary canine is formed approximately one-fourth to two Dthirds of its length
    (D) At any age after 6 years
2. The most preferred donor site for SABG is
    (A) Vertebra
    (B) Iliac crest
    (C) Calvarium
    (D) Mandible
3. The best time of closure of fistula in anterior part of hard palate in the above patient is
    (A) As early as possible
    (B) After age of maturity
    (C) Once orthodontic alignment and leveling of teeth are achieved
    (D) None of above
4. The objectives of the orthodontic treatment of a malocclusion in a cleft patient are
    (A) To achieve functional efficiency
    (B) To achieve structural equilibrium
    (C) To achieve aesthetic harmony
    (D) All of above
5. The ideal age for nose deformity correction
    (A) After eruption of all permanent teeth in oral cavity
    (B) Can done at the time of secondary bone grafting
    (C) After passing age of maturity or nasal growth
    (D) At any age

Answers:
1. C
    The right time to bone graft the alveolus is when the canine is just about erupting and its root can be seen on an X-ray.
2. B
    The Iliac crest is the most commonly used donor site for SABG due to the quality of its bone, ease of harvest and relatively less risk
3. C
    The anterior palatal fistula should be closed before any other skeletal corrective surgery is undertaken, preferably after the teeth have been treated by orthodontia to relieve crowding and ease the access to the fistula
4. D
    Orthodontic treatment in a cleft patient helps in planning skeletal surgery as well as giving the finishing touches to the final facial appearance. It also helps in preventing abnormal articulation by proper alignment of the teeth.
5. C
    The ideal age for a definitive rhinoplasty is after the age of skeletal maturity has been achieved and skeletal corrections have been done. Any procedure done before this is likely to require a revision later on.

Reference:
1. Figueroa A A, Poley J W. Orthodontics in cleft lip and palate. In: Sen C K, Roy S. Wound Healing. In: Neligan P C, Chang J (Eds) Plastic Surgery 3rd Edition. Elsevier Saunders, 2005, Vol 3, Part 2. pp 614-630.

Chapter-23

Psychiatry

ELIMINATION DISORDERS

Dr. Amit Arya, Assistant Professor & Dr. Rashmi Tiwari, Senior Resident,
Department of Psychiatry

A 6 years old boy presented with complaints of recurrent abdominal pain, constipation, passing urine and feces in clothes, at inappropriate places, along with attempts to hide the fecal matter in the house. He lived with his adoptive parents, having been removed from his biological parents at age 3 years because of neglect and physical abuse. He had always been enuretic at night, and until this year, he had a history of daytime enuresis as well. Despite experiencing physical abuse, he has never experienced flashbacks or other symptoms. His physical examination revealed tenderness in lower abdomen. Laboratory investigations have been done to rule out organic causes. Family had objectioned to this behaviour and attributed it to his laziness leading to interpersonal stress. The child was diagnosed as a case of encopresis with enuresis. The treatment programme involved use of laxatives and a bladder and bowel training for patient.

1. Which is the correct order of achieving continence?
   (A) Nocturnal fecal continence, diurnal bladder control, diurnal fecal continence, nocturnal bladder control
   (B) Diurnal bladder control, nocturnal fecal continence, diurnal fecal continence, nocturnal bladder control
   (C) Nocturnal fecal continence, diurnal fecal continence, diurnal bladder control, nocturnal bladder control
   (D) Diurnal fecal continence, nocturnal bladder control, diurnal bladder control, nocturnal fecal continence
2. According to DSM-5 what is the minimum age in years to diagnose encopresis and enuresis respectively?
   (A) 3, 5
   (B) 4, 5
   (C) 5, 6
   (D) 5, 5
3. Which one of the following is correct?
   (A) Upto 80% of the children with fecal incontinence have associated constipation.
   (B) Females are more likely to have encopresis than males.
   (C) As the age increases chances of spontaneous remission decreases.
   (D) Surgical intervention is the most effective treatment for enuresis and encopresis.
4. Most effective treatment strategy for enuresis is?
   (A) Behavioral therapy
   (B) Desmopressin
   (C) Reboxetine
   (D) Only psychotherapy
5. Etiology of enuresis could be?
   (A) Maladaptive behavioral habits
   (B) Genetic
   (C) Psychosocial stressors
   (D) All of the above

Answers:
1. C
   nocturnal fecal continence, diurnal fecal continence, diurnal bladder control, nocturnal bladder control
2. B
   4, 5
3. A
   Upto 80% of the children with fecal incontinence have associated constipation
4. A
   Behavioral therapy (bell and pad method, bladder training)
5. D
   All of the above could be associated.

Reference:
1. Sadock J M., Sadock A V., Ruiz P 2009. Comprehensive Textbook of Psychiatry, 9th ed. Wolters Kluwer Health, Lippincott Williams & Wilkins.

SELECTIVE MUTISM

Dr. Amit Arya, Assistant Professor & Dr. Rashmi Tiwari, Senior Resident,
Department of Psychiatry

A first-grade teacher is concerned about a 6-year-old girl in her class who has not spoken a single word since school started. The little girl participates appropriately in the class activities and uses gestures and drawings and nods and shakes her head to communicate. The parents report that the little girl talks only in the home and only in the presence of her closest relatives.

1. Which of the following is the most likely diagnosis?
   (A) Autism
   (B) Expressive language disorder
   (C)School phobia
   (D) Selective mutism
2. Possible etiologies for this presentation could be?
   (A) Maternal anxiety, depression
   (B) Delayed onset of speech and hearing abnormalities
   (C) Early emotional or physical trauma
   (D) All of the above
3. All of the following are correct except?
   (A) Prevalence of selective mutism range between 0.03-1%
   (B) More common in girls than boys
   (C) One half of children with selective mutism improve within 5-10 years
   (D) SSRI's are the treatment of choice
4. Which of the following is not a feature of selective mutism?
   (A) Lack of speaking in certain specific situations like school
   (B) Commonly begins before the age of 5 years
   (C) Difficulty in nonverbal communication through gestures
   (D) Social anxiety can be present
5. Which one of the following is the first line treatment for selective mutism?
   (A) Individual CBT
   (B) SSRI's
   (C) Both
   (D) None

Answers:
1.   D
     In selective mutism, a child voluntarily abstains from talking in particular situations (usually at school) while remaining appropriately verbal at home
2.   D
     All can lead to genesis of selective mutism in a child
3.   D
     A multimodal approach using psychoeducation for the family, CBT, and SSRI's as needed is recommended
4.   C
     Children with selective mutism will communicate with eye contact and nonverbal gestures
5.   A
     Individual CBT is recommended as a first line treatment for selective mutism

Reference:
1.   Sadock J M., Sadock A V., Ruiz P 2009. Comprehensive Textbook of Psychiatry, 9th ed. Wolters Kluwer Health, Lippincott Williams & Wilkins.

SEPARATION ANXIETY DISORDER

Dr.Amit Arya, Assistant Professor & Dr. Rashmi Tiwari, Senior Resident,
Department of Psychiatry

Every morning on school days, an 8-year-old girl becomes tearful and distressed and claims she feels sick. Once in school, she often goes to the nurse, complaining of headaches and stomach pains. At least once a week, she misses school or is picked up early by her mother due to her complaints. Her paediatrician has ruled out organic causes for the physical symptoms. The child is usually symptom free on weekends, unless her parents go out and leave her with a babysitter.

1. Which of the following is the most likely diagnosis?
    (A) Separation anxiety disorder
    (B) Somatization disorder
    (C) Generalized anxiety disorder
    (D) Attachment disorder

2. Normative separation anxiety peaks between which age group?
    (A) 12- 24 months
    (B) 9 -18 months
    (C) 2- 3 years
    (D) 3- 4 years

3. All of the following physiological characteristics are exhibited by behaviorally inhibited children except?
    (A) Higher than average resting heart rate
    (B) Low heart rate variability
    (C) Lower morning cortisol level
    (D) Increased heart rate variability

4. All of the following are correct except?
    (A) Separation anxiety diminishes by about 2.5 years of age
    (B) Separation anxiety is a universal human developmental phenomenon
    (C) Transient separation anxiety is always pathological
    (D) Behaviourally inhibited children are at risk for development of anxiety disorder

5. Best treatment strategy to treat childhood anxiety disorder includes?
    (A) SSRI alone
    (B) Cognitive behaviour therapy and SSRI
    (C) Cognitive behaviour therapy alone
    (D) No treatment is required as anxiety resolves on its own.

Answers:
    1. A
        Separation anxiety disorder is characterized by manifestations of distress when the child has to be separated from loved ones. The distress often leads to school refusal, refusal to sleep alone, multiple somatic symptoms, and complaints
    2. B
        Normative separation anxiety peaks between 9 -18 months.
    3. C
        Morning cortisol level is increased in behaviourally inhibited children.
    4. C
        Transient separation anxiety is a normal phenomenon.
    5. B
        The comparative efficacy of CBT and SSRI was investigated in National Institute of Mental Health which found response rate of 80.7% in comparison to either CBT alone (59.7%) or SSRI alone (54.9%)

Reference:
    1. Sadock J M., Sadock A V., Ruiz P 2009. Comprehensive Textbook of Psychiatry, 9th ed. Wolters Kluwer Health, Lippincott Williams & Wilkins.

AUTISM
Dr. Amit Arya, Assistant Professor, Dr. Rashmi Tiwari, Senior Resident Department of Psychiatry

A 6 year old boy, born to middle class parents both in their early 40's was brought for consultation to a psychiatrist. As an infant the child was undemanding and relatively placid. His motor development proceeded appropriately but language development was delayed. Parents became concerned about his development when he was not able to speak even at the age of 18 months. Parents also complained of his sensitivity to odd noises. He used to get extremely upset when his usual routine was disrupted and played with toys in repetitive and idiosyncratic way. His psychological assessment revealed Intelligence Quotient (IQ) of 60. CT scan of head and EEG were within normal limits. He was diagnosed with Autism spectrum disorder and was enrolled in special education program. At the age of 8 years child began to have serious behavioral problems in the form of screaming loudly, getting markedly upset and throw all of his belongings off his desk, hitting others and difficulty in sleeping.

627

1. Who gave the term "Early Infantile Autism"?
   (A) Leo Kanner
   (B) Eugen Bleuler
   (C) Emil Kraepelin
   (D) Karl Jasper
2. Which one of the following is not included under the term of Autism spectrum disorder in (A)DSM-5?
   (A) Asperger's syndrome
   (B) Rett's syndrome
   (C) Autism
   (D) Childhood disintegrative disorder
3. All of the following are correct except?
   (A) Core feature of autistic disorder include deficits in social communication and restrictive repetitive behaviour
   (B) In Asperger's syndrome marked deficit in language development is present
   (C) About one third of children with autism exhibit intellectual disability
   (D) Prevalence of autism spectrum disorder is about 1%
4. Which of the following is the appropriate strategy to manage these children's behavioral problems?
   (A) Risperidone (0.5 mg-1.5mg) alone
   (B) Parent training and participation
   (C) Both 1 and 2
   (D) Leave the child alone, he will be calm down on his own
5. Following are the core symptoms of autism except?
   (A) Deficit in social interaction
   (B) Restricted repetitive behaviour, interests and activities
   (C) Normal language development
   (D) None of the above.

Answers:
1. A
   "Early Infantile Autism" was described by Leo Canner in 1943.
2. B
   Rett's syndrome
3. B
   Aspergers syndrome does not include language impairment as diagnostic criteria
4. C
   Both Risperidone (0.5 mg-1.5mg) and Parent training and participation
5. C
   Aberrant language development and usage is no longer considered a core feature of autism. However language development is never normal.

Reference:
1. Sadock J M., Sadock A V., Ruiz P 2009. Comprehensive Textbook of Psychiatry, 9th ed. Wolters Kluwer Health,Lippincott Williams & Wilkins.

SPECIFIC LEARNING DISORDER
Dr.Amit Arya, Assistant Professor, Dr. Rashmi Tiwari, Senior Resident, Department of Psychiatry

A 10 year old boy presented with complaints of failing to complete class assignments and homework, and failing tests in reading, spelling, and arithmetic. Parents reported history of language delay. In preschool, the child had more difficulty learning to read than other boys in his class and continued to have problems pronouncing multisyllabic words. Parents showed concern about his declining performance at school. His detailed psychological evaluation revealed above average performance IQ, poor comprehension, poor spelling, weak comprehension of oral language. He was diagnosed as a case of Specific Learning Disorder (SLD), with deficits in reading and written expression.

1. Which of the following is included in specific learning disorder as per DSM-5?
   (A) Difficulty in learning and reading
   (B) Difficulty in written expression
   (C) Difficulty with mathematical reasoning
   (D) All of the above
2. All of the following are correct except?

(A) Increased risk of four to eight times in first degree relatives for reading deficits

(B) Two to three times more common in females than in males

(C) Dyslexia is defined as leaning difficulties including deficits in accurate or fluent word recognition

(D) IQ is no longer a diagnostic criteria for specific learning disorder

3. Which of the following comorbidities are associated with SLD?

(A) Language disorder

(B) ADHD

(C) Depressive disorder

(D) All of the above

4. Which of the following is the characteristic of SLD with Reading impairment?

(A) Difficulty in recognizing words

(B) Slow and inaccurate reading

(C) Poor comprehension and difficulty with spelling

(D) All of the above

5.Which of the following is the appropriate treatment for SLD?

(A) Exposure and response prevention

(B) Remediation strategies

(C) Systemic desensitization

(D) Memory enhancers

Answers:

1. D

DSM-5 combines the diagnosis of reading disorder, mathematics disorder, disorders of written expression and learning disorder not otherwise specified

2. B

SLD is more common in males (Two to three times)

3. D

Comorbid psychiatric disorder associated with SLD are ADHD, ODD, CD, depressive disorders

4. D

All of the above are characteristic of SLD with Reading impairment

5. B

Remediation strategies focus on direct instruction that leads a child's attention to the connections between speech sounds and spellings.

Reference:

1. Sadock J M., Sadock A V., Ruiz P 2009. Comprehensive Textbook of Psychiatry, 9th ed. Wolters Kluwer Health, Lippincott Williams & Wilkins.

ATTENTION DEFICIT HYPERKINETIC DISORDER

Dr. Pawan Kumar Gupta, Assistant Professor, Department of Psychiatry

Master D, 8 years old male child from a middle class, urban Hindu family was brought to the psychiatry OPD with chief complaints of difficult behavior. At home, he prefers to roam around the room, picking up toys here and there but doesn't really get interested in any one activity. During story time with parents he doesn't become involved in the story, but keeps repeating the same questions in a loud tone of voice. He also has the habit of constantly running around in the household, climbing and scaling furniture, even hurting himself on multiple occasions. D's mother states that she avoids family gatherings and celebrations because he gets overly excited and then she can't control him. He has also started to avoid school. His teacher reports that he squirms around in his seat, stands up unexpectedly and seldom finishes his work. The kids sitting near him in class say he's always interrupting and shouting out the answers (generally wrong). His desk is in disarray; papers are on the floor and his work is disorganized. He's often not picked for games during the sports period and then tries to spoil the game for the others.

1. What is the diagnosis?

(A) Intellectual disability

(B) ADHD

(C) ASD

(D) PDD

2. Which of the medications given below is NOT found useful in management of ADHD

(A) Methylphenidate

(B) Atomoxetine

(C) Second generation antipsychotics

(D) Tricyclic antidepressants

3. Methylphenidate and amphetamines belong to which class of medications

(A) Stimulants

(B) Selective monoamine reuptake inhibitors

(A) Second generation antipsychotics

(D) Alpha adrenergic agonist

4. Which of the following is NOT a side effect of stimulant medications

(A) Motor tics

(B) Increased risk for substance abuse in later life.

(C) Reductions in rate of height and weight gain.

(D) Increased irritability and crying

5. Which of the following is NOT a non pharmacological treatment modality in ADHD

(A) Direct contingency management

(B) Intensive behavioral management

(C) Community based management

(D) First line of treatment for the symptoms.

Answers:

1. B

The characteristic of children with ADHD are hyperactivity, attention deficit (short attention span, distractibility, perseveration, failure to finish tasks, inattention, poor concentration), impulsivity, memory and thinking deficit, specific learning disabilities and speech and hearing deficit.

2. C

Methylphenidate, Atomoxetine, TCA are found useful in pharmacotherapy of ADHD but not antipsychotic.

3. A

Amphetamine, dextroamphetamine, methylphenidate belongs to the stimulant group of drugs.

4. B

Side effects associated with stimulant drugs are stomach pain , anxiety, irritability, insomnia, tachycardia, decreased appetite, dysphoria, and less commonly induction of movement disorder such as tics, Tourette's disorder like symptoms.

5. D

Treatment of symptoms with stimulant drug is pharmacological treatment for ADHD.

References:

1. Sadock, B. J., Sadock, V. A., Ruiz, P., & Kaplan, H. I. (2009). Kaplan & Sadock's Comprehensive Textbook of Psychiatry. Philadelphia: Wolters Kluwer Health/Lippincott Williams & Wilkins

2. Jahad A, Boyle M, Cunningham C, Kim M, Schachar R: *Treatment of Attention-Deficit/Hyperactivity Disorder* (AHRQ Publication No. 00-E005). Rockville, MD: Agency for Healthcare Research and Quality, U.S. Department of Health and Human Services; 1999.

3. Newcorn JH, Sharma V, Schulz K, Halperin JM: Childhood disorders: Attention-deficit/hyperactivity and disruptive behavior disorders. In: Tasman A, Kay J, Lieberman JA, First MB, Maj M, eds: *Psychiatry*. 3rd ed. Chichester, UK: Wiley; 2008:804.

ASPERGER'S SYNDROME

Dr. Pawan Kumar Gupta, Assistant Professor, Department of Psychiatry

Master T was an only child from an affluent urban Hindu family. Birth, medical, and family histories were unremarkable. His motor development was somewhat delayed, but communicative milestones were within normal limits. His parents became concerned about him at age 4 when he was enrolled in a nursery school and was noted to have marked difficulties in peer interaction that were so pronounced that he could not continue in the school. In another school, he was enrolled in special education classes and was noted to have some learning problems. His greatest difficulties arose in peer interaction—he was viewed as markedly eccentric and had no friends. His preferred activity, watching the weather channel on television, was pursued with great interest and intensity. On examination at age 13, he had markedly circumscribed interests and exhibited pedantic and odd patterns of communication with a monotonic voice quality. Psychological testing revealed an IQ within the normal range, with marked scatter evident. Formal communication examination revealed age-appropriate skills in receptive and expressive language but marked impairment in pragmatic language skills.

1. What is the most likely diagnosis?
   (A) Rett disorder
   (B) Childhood disintegrative disorder
   (C) Autism
   (D) Asperger disorder
2. The following are characteristic of autism except:
   (A) Onset after 6 years of age
   (B) Repetitive behavior
   (C) Delayed language development
   (D) Severe deficit in social interaction
3. Which of the following regarding Autism is WRONG
   (A) Has 3 core deficiencies: language, social interaction and behaviour (restricted, repetitive interests and behaviours)
   (B) Comorbidities are common
   (C) Risperidone is used for aggression and irritability
   (D) SSRI can be used to improve communication skills in patients with autism
4. Regarding 'irritability' in ASD, which of the following is FALSE?
   (A) Includes: aggression, self injurious behaviour
   (B) Anti-epileptic mood stabilizers are used
   (C) Risperidone is licensed to be used
   (D) Mood stabilizers are more efficacious than SGAs
5. The screening checklist for autism in children aged 16-48 months is
   (A) CHAT
   (B) MCHAT
   (C) GADS
   (D) CAST

Answers:

1. D
   Asperger's disorder is characterized by impairment and oddity of social interaction and restricted interest and behavior. In Asperger's disorder there is no significant delay in language or cognitive delay.
2. A
   The disorder usually manifests early in the developmental period usually before the child enters in the school (<3 year)
3. D
   SSRI are not useful in improving communication skill in children with autism spectrum disorder.
4. D
   Two second generation antipsychotics, risperidone and aripiprazole, have been approved by the FDA for treatment of irritability in children with autism spectrum disorder.
5. B
   MCHAT is a screening checklist to assess the risk of autism.

References:

1. Volkmar F: Autism and the pervasive developmental disorders. In: Lewis M, ed. *Child and Adolescent Psychiatry: A Comprehensive Approach.* 2nd ed. Baltimore: Williams and Wilkins; 2002:489.
2. Sadock, B. J., Sadock, V. A., Ruiz, P., & Kaplan, H. I. (2009). *Kaplan & Sadock's comprehensive textbook of psychiatry.* Philadelphia: Wolters Kluwer Health/Lippincott Williams & Wilkins.

CONDUCT DISORDER

Dr. Pawan Kumar Gupta, Assistant Professor, Department of Psychiatry

Master M is a nine-year-old boy who lives with his biological mother, and his three siblings. At the initial assessment, he presented with unruly behavior. He refused to comply with his mother's requests, blamed others for his mistakes and broke family rules. His mother reported that he often engaged in physical fights with his siblings, and his teachers described him as an angry and spiteful child who often bullied other children and initiated fights with peers, he was in-fact called "terrorist of the 9-year-olds" by his teachers. He punches or bites children and pushes them off the swings in the playground without provocation. He would swing the puppies by the tail in spite of being told how it hurt the animals. His mother reported that he has been difficult to manage since he was an infant. He was also found to be in possession of some cigarettes by his mother, who when confronted him about this, the boy initially refused but later on started using foul language for his mother, threatening her and snatched the cigarettes from her hand, and stormed out of the house, only to return 3 days later.

1. What is the diagnosis?
   (A) ODD
   (B) ADHD
   (C) CD
   (D) ASD

2. According to neurobiological studies of the disorder described in above mentioned case. Following have been found to exhibit except
   (A) Neurological defect
   (B) Genetic history of antisocial behavior amongst first degree relatives
   (C) Higher level of adrenaline
   (D) Difficult temperament as infants

3. Which if the following is NOT a protective factor for Conduct Disorder
   (A) Easy temperament
   (B) Susceptible genes
   (C) Internal locus of control
   (D) Higher IQ

4. Which of the following is NOT a developmental pathway in Conduct Disorder
   (A) Overt pathway
   (B) Covert pathway
   (C) Authority conflict pathway
   (D) Generalized aggression pathway

5. Which of the following is not true regarding management of the child with conduct disorder?
   (A) Monitoring, positive reinforcement along with harsh discipline is needed
   (B) Long, intensive intervention programs are used
   (C) Individual case management
   (D) Intensive collaboration amongst community

Answers:

1. C
   Conduct disorder is an enduring set of behaviors in a child or adolescent usually characterized by aggression, violation of rights of the others, destruction of property, theft or act of deceit, and frequent violation of age appropriate rules.

2. C
   In conduct disorder studies suggest low level of plasma dopamine beta hydroxylase leading to decreased noradrenaline functioning.

3. B
   Susceptible genes are linked to antisocial behavior in conduct disorder.

4. D
   Generalized aggression is not a developmental pathway in Conduct Disorder

5. A
   Positive reinforcement and avoiding punishment is one of the behavioural intervention advised in management of conduct disorder.

References:

1. Volkmar F: Autism and the pervasive developmental disorders. In: Lewis M, ed. *Child and Adolescent Psychiatry: A Comprehensive Approach.* 2nd ed. Baltimore: Williams and Wilkins; 2002:489.
2. Sadock, B. J., Sadock, V. A., Ruiz, P., & Kaplan, H. I. (2009). *Kaplan & Sadock's comprehensive textbook of psychiatry.* Philadelphia: Wolters Kluwer Health/Lippincott Williams & Wilkins.

MENTAL RETARDATION

Dr. Pawan Kumar Gupta, Assistant Professor, Department of Psychiatry

Miss N is 7 years old girl, who was presented to a psychiatric outpatient service with the chief complaints of lagging behind in daily activities since birth. Her mother recalled that she was a difficult delivery as there was history suggestive of a prolonged labor, followed by meconium aspiration and failure to cry soon after birth. The neonate had to be kept under intensive care for 4 days after which she was handed over to her parents.

Since early infancy, she lagged behind her siblings and peers, her mother recalls that it was not before an age of approx. 14 months that the child could sit without support and started walking only by an age of 3 years. The child also vocalized late, at an age of 5 years, and currently could use 10-15 words only and no complete sentences.

She was described as a jolly child, who would keep on smiling most of the time and generally playful. She could maintain eye gaze while being talked to and doted on her mother. She was capable of playing with other children, although they tended to avoid including her in their games, as she would not be able to keep up with the rules. She needed assistance with her daily activities including bathing, and dressing and undressing and had achieved toilet training only an year earlier.

1. What is the diagnosis?
    (A) Mental Retardation
    (B) Rett disorder
    (C) Childhood disintegrative disorder
    (D) ADHD
2. Current understanding of the concept of mental retardation in psychiatry does not include
    (A) Etiological understanding of intelligence and its impairment,
    (B) Assessment methods and management of for associated comorbidity
    (C) Not clinically recognized as a developmental disorder
    (D) Needs to meet criteria of impairment and dysfunction to be called disorder
3. The co-occurrence of psychiatric illness with mental retardation
    (A) Has not been well established
    (B) People with mental retardation are more unlikely to suffer from mental disorders
    (C) The change in prevalence of neuropsychiatric disorders is non specific
    (D) Only prevalence of behavioural disorders, personality disorders, autistic-spectrum disorders and attention- deficit hyperactivity disorder is affected.
4. Masking in people with learning disability refers to
    (A) Unemotional facial expression
    (B) Presence of Autistic symptoms in severe learning disability
    (C) Clinical characteristics of a mental disorder masked by a cognitive, language or speech deficit.
    (D) People with learning disability share many mental health needs with the general population.
5. Which of the following IQ is the ICD-10 defined level for moderate Mental Retardation
    (A) 50-69
    (B) 35-49
    (C) 20-34
    (D) <20

Answers:
1. A
    Mental retardation is characterized by significant limitation in both intellectual functioning and in adaptive behavior that emerges before the age of 18 years.
2. C
    Intellectual disability (MR) is clinically classified under developmental disorder.
3. C
    Epidemiological surveys indicate that children and adults with intellectual disability have comorbid psychiatric disorder several times higher than without intellectual disability.
4. C
    Masking in learning disability refers to clinical feature of a mental disorder masked by a cognitive, language or speech deficit.
5. B
    35-49 I.Q. refers to moderate mental retardation

References:
1. Volkmar F: Autism and the pervasive developmental disorders. In: Lewis M, ed. *Child and Adolescent Psychiatry: A Comprehensive Approach.* 2nd ed. Baltimore: Williams and Wilkins; 2002:489,
2. Jaffe, JH. "Mental Retardation." In: Sadock, B.J. and Sadock, V.A (Eds), Comprehensive Textbook of Psychiatry, 7th edition, Philadelphia, PA: Lippincott Williams and Wilkins; 2000
3. World Health Organization.International statistical classification of diseases and related health problems. 10th revision. Geneva: WHO; 1992.
4. Royal College of Psychiatrists. Diagnostic Criteria for Psychiatric Disorders for Use with Adults with Learning Disabilities (DC-LD): London: Royal College of Psychiatrists; 2001

OPPOSITIONAL DEFIANT DISORDER

Dr. Pawan Kumar Gupta, Assistant Professor, Department of Psychiatry

Master F, A 10-year-old boy belonging to a middle class, urban family is brought to the psychiatrist because his mother says the boy is driving her "nuts." She reports that he constantly argues with her and his father, does not follow any of the house rules, and incessantly teases his sister. She says that he is spiteful and vindictive and loses his temper easily. Once he is mad, he stays that way for long periods of time. The mother notes that the boy started this behavior only about 2 years previously. While she states that this behavior started at home, it has now spread to school, where complaints of aggressiveness, disobedience, stealing, lying, truancy, frequent school fights, and deteriorating school grades were becoming all the more common. The patient maintains that none of this is his fault his parents are simply being unreasonable. He denies feeling depressed and notes that he sleeps well through the night. Recently for last 6 months he had become irritable, throwing tantrums on minor issues, spending long hours in cyber cafes and self-refreshing along with like-minded peers in restaurants. He refused to attend school and often failed to complete the task assigned by the teachers for which there were repeated complaints from the school authorities.

1. What is the diagnosis?
   (A) Conduct Disorder
   (B) Oppositional Defiant Disorder
   (C) ADHD
   (D) Intellectual Disability
2. Which of the following is NOT a predictor of worse outcome in the above case in terms of progression to conduct disorder
   (A) Co-morbid ADHD
   (B) Severe baseline oppositional symptoms.
   (C) Male gender
   (D) Early age of onset
3. Which of the following is FALSE regarding ODD
   (A) Not recognized if symptoms occur during presence of any other psychiatric illness
   (B) Initially, symptoms are less marked in the household, and more pronounced outside.
   (C) Diagnosis of oppositional defiant disorder is not given if symptoms occur within the context of conduct disorder
   (D) It can not be diagnosed in individuals over the age of 18 years
4. Which of the following statements is FALSE regarding treatment of ODD
   (A) Fundamental aspects are primary and secondary prevention
   (B) Key element is intervention in early life
   (C) Medications are important way to control the symptoms
   (D) Intensive treatments, multiple times a week, over long durations are advocated
5. What percent of ODD children eventually develop conduct disorder
   (A) 5-10
   (B) 10-20
   (C) upto 30
   (D) upto 50

Answers:

1. B
   Children with ODD often argue with adults, lose their temper, and are angry, resentful, and easily annoyed by others at a level and frequency that is outside the expected range for their age and developmental level.
2. C
   The prognosis for ODD in a child depends somewhat on family functioning and the development of comorbid psychopathology.
3. B
   Manifestation of the disorder are almost invariably present in the home, but they may not be present at school or with other adults or peers.
4. C
   The primary treatment of ODD is family intervention using both direct training of the parents in child management skills and careful assessment of family interaction.
5. C
   In children who have long history of aggression and ODD there is a greater risk upto 30% of development of conduct disorder.

References:

1. Volkmar F: Autism and the pervasive developmental disorders. In: Lewis M, ed. *Child and Adolescent Psychiatry: A Comprehensive Approach.* 2nd ed. Baltimore: Williams and Wilkins; 2002:489,
2. Sadock, B. J., Sadock, V. A., Ruiz, P., & Kaplan, H. I. (2009). *Kaplan & Sadock's comprehensive textbook of psychiatry.* Philadelphia: Wolters Kluwer Health/Lippincott Williams & Wilkins

ALCOHOL DEPENDENCE
Dr. Haseeb Khan, Senior Resident, Department of Psychiatry

A 41 year old software engineer presented with the desire to stop alcohol intake. He had been drinking approx. 1 bottle of vodka daily for last 1 year, and had never been abstinent in last 2 years. More recently, he had begun to feel "shaky" every morning and would sometimes treat that sensation with a drink, followed by more alcohol during the day. He had started to experience a number of problems related to this behaviour of alcohol intake. His wife threatens him for divorce. He had diminished ability to concentrate at his work. He was spending more time in either recovering from the effect of alcohol or in planning to procure the same. He first tried alcohol in high school and said that he had always been able to hold his liquor. In college his frequency and amount of alcohol intake increased. Through his 30s, he gradually increased the frequency of his drinking from primarily on weekend to daily. Over the prior year he had switched from being exclusively a beer drinker to drinking vodka. There is no history of any other substance use. He has no history of seizure or any medical problems. Family history was significant for alcohol abuse by his father and grandfather. He entered the alcohol treatment program with symptoms of tremor in hand, anxiety, restlessness, irritability, nausea and recent insomnia. Clinical evaluation revealed, he was alert and oriented. No other evident psychopathology was found. Notable features of his physical examination were marked diaphoresis, blood pressure 156/96 mm Hg, heart rate of 104 beats /minute, severe tremor in upper extremity and hyperactive deep tendon reflex. Laboratory tests were within normal limit except aspartate amino-transferase and alanine amino-transferase, which were approx 3 times normal.

1. Drug of choice in alcohol withdrawal
    (A) Haloperidol
    (B) Lithium
    (C) Benzodiazepine
    (D) SSRI(selective serotonin reuptake inhibitor)
2. Wernicke's encephalopathy associated with use of alcohol is characterized by all except
    (A) Ataxia (affecting primarily the gait),
    (B) Seizure
    (C) Ophthalmoplegia
    (D) Confusion
3. All but which are symptoms of a hangover?
    (A) Autonomic hyperactivity
    (B) Insomnia
    (C) Loss of hearing
    (D) Anxiety
4. Disulfiram, a drug used as deterrent in management of alcohol dependency acts by
    (A) Inhibiting alcohol dehydrogenase
    (B) Inhibiting aldehyde dehydrogenase
    (C) Both of the above
    (D) None of the above.
5. All of the following are characteristics of substance dependence except:
    (A)Withdrawal
    (B)Loss of Control
    (C)Denial
    (D)Negative consequences

Answers:

1.   C
      Benzodiazepine is considered to be the primary drug used in patients of alcohol dependency.
2.   B
      Wernicke's encephalopathy is characterized by the triad ophthalmoplegia, ataxia, and confusion
3.   C

Symptoms of a hangover includes tremors, anxiety, nausea and/or vomiting, headache, autonomic hyperactivity, sweating, irritability, confusion, insomnia, nightmares

4.   C

Disulfiram acts by inhibiting both alcohol dehydrogenase and aldehyde dehydrogenase

5.   C

Denial is a defense mechanism usually found in substance use disorder and not as symptoms of dependence.

References:

1. Amato L1, Minozzi S, Vecchi S, Davoli M: Benzodiazepines for alcohol withdrawal. Cochrane Database Syst Rev. 2010 Mar 17;(3):CD005063.
2. Amato L1, Minozzi S, Davoli M: Efficacy and safety of pharmacological interventions for the treatment of the Alcohol Withdrawal Syndrome. Cochrane Database Syst Rev. 2011 Jun 15;(6):CD008537.
3. Sadock BJ, Sadock VA, eds. Kaplan and Sadock's Synopsis of Psychiatry 10th edition. Baltimore: Lippincott Williams & Wilkins; 2015. P391-407.

CANNABIS USE DISORDER

Dr.Haseeb Khan, Senior Resident, Department of Psychiatry

A 19-year-old man is brought to the emergency department by a friend because of strange behavior during the past 2 hours at a party. The patient has seemed confused and has been insisting that someone is following him. On arrival, he is alert but confused. He says that he is angry because his friend had promised that the ride to the hospital would only take 5 minutes, but it seemed to take several hours. He states that he has been hungry all evening, and he asks if there is anywhere he can get something to eat. He is dressed casually in baggy pants and a T-shirt. His temperature is 37.2°C (99°F), pulse is 107/min, respiration is 12/min, and blood pressure is 120/85 mm Hg. Examination shows injected conjunctivae. Deep tendon reflexes are decreased. There is ataxia on finger-nose testing. On mental status examination, he has a mildly anxious affect. His speech is slow, and his thought process is disorganized.

1. Patient is most likely having withdrawal of which substance?
   (A) Alcohol
   (B) Heroin
   (C) LSD
   (D) Marijuana
2. Which of the following is not derived from cannabis sativus?
   (A) Hashish
   (B) Ganja
   (C) Heroin
   (D) Bhang
3. Psychoactive substance present in cannabis sativus is
   (A) Di-hydro-cannabinol
   (B) Tetra-hydro-cannabinol
   (C) Tri-hydro-cannabinol
   (D) Penta-hydro-cannabinol
4. "Flashback" and "amotivation syndrome" is seen with
   (A) LSD
   (B) Amphetamine
   (C) Bhang
   (D) Heroin
5. Cannabis intoxication includes all except;
   (A)Conjunctival injection
   (B)Increased appetite
   (C)Hypersalivation
   (D)Tachycardia

Answers:

1.   D

Marijuana

2.   C

Heroin (diacetylmorphine or morphine diacetate) is an opioid analgesic originally synthesized by adding two acetyl groups to the molecule morphine, which is found naturally in the opium poppy

3.   B
Tetrahydrocannabinol

4.   C
Flashback" and "amotivation syndrome" are usually found in subjects with cannabis (bhang) dependence.

5.   C
Dry mouth rather than hypersalivation occurs in cannabis intoxication.

References:

1. Sadock BJ, Sadock VA, eds. Kaplan and Sadock's Synopsis of Psychiatry 10th edition. Baltimore: Lippincott Williams & Wilkins; 2015:p418-421

2. Huizink AC, Mulder EJ. Maternal smoking, drinking or cannabis use during pregnancy and neurobehavioral and cognitive functioning in human offspring. Neurosci Biobehav Rev 2006;30:24-41.

OPIOID DEPENDENCE

Dr. Haseeb Khan, Senior Resident, Department of Psychiatry

A 42-year-old executive in a public relations firm was referred for psychiatric consultation by his surgeon, who discovered him sneaking large quantities of a codeine-containing cough medicine into the hospital. The patient had been a heavy cigarette smoker for 20 years and had a chronic, hacking cough. He had come into the hospital for a hernia repair and found the pain for the incision unbearable when he coughed.

An operation on his back 5 years previously had led his doctors to prescribe codeine to help relieve the incisional pain at that time. Over the intervening 5 years, however, the patient had continued to use codeine-containing tablets and had increased his intake to 60-90 mg tablets daily. He stated that he often just took them by the handful not to 'feel good' rather just to get by. He spent considerable time and effort developing a circle of physicians and pharmacists to whom he would make the rounds at least three times a week to obtain new supplies of pills. He had tried several times to stop using codeine, but had failed. During this period he lost two jobs because of lax work habits and was divorced by his wife of 11 years.

1. All are signs/symptoms of opioid withdrawal except.
    (A) Muscle aches
    (B) Lacrimation or rhinorrhea
    (C) Pupillary dilatation
    (D) Papillary constriction
2. Which is not the action of "μ-type" opioid receptor
    (A) Diuresis
    (B) Analgesia,
    (C) Aespiratory depression,
    (D) Aonstipation
3. All of the following are opiates except
    (A) Morphine
    (B) Aeroin,
    (C) Codeine
    (D) Methylphenidate
4. Factors responsible for drug/substance dependence:
    (A) Peer pressure
    (B) Social acceptability
    (C) Reinforcement effect of drug
    (D) All of the above
5. Opiate withdrawal is treated with
    (A) Chlorpromazine
    (B) Methadone
    (C) Carbamazepine
    (D) Methylphenidate

Answers:

1.   D
Pupillary constriction is seen in intoxication of opioid not in withdrawal

2. A

Analgesia, sedation, slightly reduced blood pressure, itching, nausea, euphoria, decreased respiration, miosis (constricted pupils) and decreased bowel motility often leading to constipation are the effects of μ-type" opioid receptor.

3. D

Methylphenidate in not an opioid but a CNS stimulant use in patients of ADHD.

4. D

Numerous factors are responsible for substance dependence important ones are as follows.

Peer pressure

As a way to deal with stress

Substance abuse as part of a personality disorder

To promote relaxation

Social acceptability

Reinforcement effect of drug

5. B

Methadone is used for detoxification and maintenance treatment of opioid addiction (heroin or other morphine-like drugs).

References:

1. Sadock BJ, Sadock VA, eds. Kaplan and Sadock's Synopsis of Psychiatry 11[th]edition . Baltimore: Lippincott Williams & Wilkins; 2015:p659-p666
2. Bhatti K. Dinesh Companion to Biology. S. Dinesh & Co. New Delhi, 2009.
3. William T. O'Donohue ,Jane E. Fisher and hayes SC. Cognitive Behavior Therapy: Applying Empirically Supported Techniques in Your Practice, John Wiley &sons 2003, p252.

DEFENSE MECHANISMS IN ADJUSTMENT DISORDERS

Dr. Shweta Singh, Assistant Professor, Department of Psychiatry

A young adult, 18 years old female studying in class XIIth, resident of Lucknow came to the adult psychiatry OPD with the chief complaints of episodes of falling and unresponsiveness, 4-5 times in a week, from past 2 months. These episodes did not have any organic cause and had a direct correlation with the stressor related to her academic poor performance. Mental status examination revealed no abnormal perceptions or formal thought disorder.

1. What could be the most plausible disorder the patient appears to have
   - (A) Depression
   - (B) Bipolar affective disorder
   - (C) Dissociative disorder
   - (D) Obsessive compulsive disorder
2. What kind of defense mechanism is usually used by patients with this disorder
   - (A) Displacement
   - (B) Isolation
   - (C) Dissociation
   - (D) Undoing
3. This defense mechanism is used as an
   - (A) Neurotic defense mechanism
   - (B) Mature defense mechanism
   - (C) Primary defense mechanism
   - (D) Narcissistic defense mechanism
4. Sublimation is a
   - (A) Immature defense mechanism
   - (B) Primary defense mechanism
   - (C) Mature defense mechanism
   - (D) Neurotic defense mechanism
5. Most commonly found comorbid disorder of this condition is
   - (A) Schizophrenia
   - (B) Depression
   - (C) OCD
   - (D) Mania

1. C

   The patient has Dissociative disorder.

   The clinical feature of dissociative disorder is disturbance in the normally integrated functions of consciousness, identity and/ or memory without any organic basis.

2. C

   Dissociation is usually used by people of this disorder.

   Dissociation refers to involuntary splitting or suppression of a mental function from rest of the personality in a manner that allows expression of forbidden unconscious impulses without having any sense of responsibility for actions.

3. A

   Neurotic defense mechanism is used.

   Conversion, dissociation, displacement, isolation, reaction formation, undoing, rationalization, intellectualization, acting out, introjection and inhibition are all neurotic defense mechanism.

4. C

   Sublimation is a mature defense mechanism

   It refers to unconscious gradual channelization of unacceptable infantile impulses into personally satisfying and socially valuable behaviour patterns.

5. B

   Most commonly found comorbid disorder is depression.

   The affective states like depression are usually associated with dissociative disorder.

Reference:

1. Ahuja.N. A short textbook of psychiatry. 4th edition

DEPRESSION

Dr. Shweta Singh, Assistant Professor, Department of Psychiatry

An adult, 23 years old male graduate, resident of Shahjahanpur came to the adult psychiatry OPD with the chief complaints of low mood, decreased sociability and reduced sleep from 2 months. In history of present of present illness it is seen that the low mood is throughout the day. There is anhedonia, decreased concentration, decreased sociability, hopelessness, suicidal ideas, and pessimistic views about future, feeling of emptiness, reduced sleep and appetite. Mental status examination revealed subjective feeling of easy fatigability, pessimistic view about future and hopelessness.

1. What disorder does the patient seem to have-
   - (A) Schizophrenia
   - (B) Generalized anxiety disorder
   - (C) Obsessive compulsive disorder
   - (D) Depressive disorder

2. Which rating scale is most useful with this patient-
   - (A) Beck's depression inventory
   - (B) Hamilton anxiety scale
   - (C) MMSC
   - (D) Y-BOCS

3. What kind of defense mechanism is usually used with this disorder-
   - (A) Introjection
   - (B) Denial
   - (C) Distortion
   - (D) Anticipation

4. What is the category of defense mechanism usually used in this disorder-
   - (A) Immature
   - (B) Mature
   - (C) Narcissistic
   - (D) Repression

5. Which kind of therapy is not useful for this disorder-
   - (A) Pharmacological Treatment
   - (B) Cognitive Behaviour Therapy
   - (C) Exposure response prevention
   - (D) Supportive therapy

Answers:

1. D

   The patient has depressive disorder. Low mood, loss of interest and enjoyment are common symptoms of depression.

2. A

   Beck's depression inventory is most useful with this patient. It tells about the severity of depression more in terms of cognitive symptoms.

3. A

   Introjection is used as defense mechanism in this disorder. It refers to unconscious internalization of the qualities of an object or person.

4. A

   Immature defense mechanism is used in this disorder, which includes conversion, dissociation, displacement, isolation, reaction formation, undoing, rationalization, intellectualization, acting out, introjection and inhibition.

5. C

   Exposure response prevention is not useful in this disorder. It is useful in the treatment of OCD.

Reference:

1. Kaplan & Shadock, Comprehensive Textbook of Psychiatry, 9th edition

OBSESSIVE COMPULSIVE DISORDER-DEFENSE MECHANISMS

Dr. Shweta Singh, Assistant Professor, Department of Psychiatry

An adult, 37 years old married female patient, with an educational qualification of B.Ed., working as a science teacher in a school, resident of Lucknow, came to the adult psychiatry OPD with chief complaints of repetitive checking behaviour, and restlessness which had started four years back. The history of her present illness revealed that these are recurrent, intrusive, distressing to the patient and causes anxiety, as she is unable to control her thoughts as well as her urge of checking and is not able to complete her targets in time, thus causing impairment in her professional life.

Mental status examination revealed the patient has repetitive thought of being jailed, which she identifies as being her own, irrelevant act of checking not under her control, is a cause of distress to her. She is unable to stop it even if she tries to. She realizes that her behaviour is irrational; however it helps her realize her anxiety.

1. What kind of disorder the patient seem to suffer from-
   (A) Depression
   (B) Phobia
   (C) Obsessive compulsive disorder
   (D) Generalized anxiety disorder

2. Which defense mechanism is common in this disorder-
   (A) Regression
   (B) Denial
   (C) Undoing
   (D) Distortion

3. This defense mechanism comes in the category of-
   (A) Immature defense mechanism
   (B) Primary defense mechanism
   (C) Undoing
   (D) Distortion

4. Therapy useful for this condition-
   (A) Interpersonal
   (B) Supportive
   (C) Social
   (D) Exposure response prevention

5. Which tool is useful in determining the severity of this condition-
   (A) SCT
   (B) Rorschach
   (C) TAT
   (D) Y-BOCS

Answers:
1. A

   The patient is suffering from Obsessive compulsive disorder.

   The essential feature of this disorder is recurrent obsessional thoughts or compulsive acts.
2. C

   Undoing is the defense mechanism used in this disorder. It refers to unconsciously motivated acts which magically/ symbolically counteract unacceptable thoughts, impulses or acts.
3. A

   This defense mechanism comes in the category of immature defense mechanism.
4. D

   Exposure response prevention is useful in this condition. It is a form of Cognitive Behavior Therapy
5. D

   Y-BOCS is the tool useful to determine the severity of this condition.

Reference:
1. Kaplan &Shadock, Comprehensive Textbook of Psychiatry, 9th edition

GENERALIZED ANXIETY DISORDER
Dr. Shweta Singh, Assistant Professor, Department of Psychiatry

An adult male 33 years old came to adult psychiatry OPD with chief complaints of apprehensiveness, worrying over simple things and inability to sleep and work for the last 17 years. History revealed that the course of symptoms was fluctuating and their severity would increase prior to a stressor or after it followed.

Mental status revealed rate tone and volume of speech was normal, psychomotor activity was within normal limits, thought content was preoccupied with worries about future and negative views about self. Judgment was intact.

1.What disorder the patient appears to be having
   - (A) Depression
   - (B) Schizophrenia
   - (C) Obsessive compulsive disorder
   - (D) Generalized anxiety disorder
2.What scale is useful in this study
   - (A) HAM-A
   - (B) HAM-D
   - (C) BDI
   - (D) MADRS
3.The evidence of this disorder is usually not present in
   - (A) Antisocial personality disorder
   - (B) Anxious avoidant personality disorder
   - (C) Phobia
   - (D) Obsessive compulsive disorder
4.Which kind of defense mechanism is not used in this condition
   - (A) Humor
   - (B) Repression
   - (C) Regression
   - (D) Projection
5.Which therapy is most useful in this disorder
   - (A) Psychoanalytic therapy
   - (B) Interpersonal therapy
   - (C) Supportive therapy
   - (D) Relaxation techniques

Answers:
1. D

   The patient appears to be having Generalized anxiety disorder (GAD). The symptoms of anxiety should last for at least a period of 6 months for diagnosis of GAD.
2. B

   HAM-D is useful in this condition. It measures the severity level of depression.

3. A
   Evidence of this disorder is not present in Antisocial personality disorder. The traits of Antisocial personality disorder includes callous concern for the feelings of others, gross and persistent attitude of irresponsibility and disregard for social norms, rules and obligations etc.
4. A
   Humor is not used in this condition. It is a mature defense mechanism.
5. B
   The most useful therapy in this disorder is relaxation therapy. Relaxation brings down the anxiety level.

Reference:
1. Kaplan & Shadock, Comprehensive Textbook of Psychiatry. 9th edition

ADJUSTMENT DISORDER
Dr. Shweta Singh, Assistant Professor, Department of psychiatry

An adult female of 27 years of age came to the adult psychiatry OPD on 6/8/14 with the chief complaints of headache and decreased sleep from four months. The onset was acute, course was progressive, second episode of psychiatric illness, precipitating factor is the environmental change after marriage.

History reveals restlessness, anxiousness, headache and decreased sleep and difficulty in doing the daily chores of the day. Past history was suggestive of dissociative episode. Family history reveals strained relations with father, now with brother, husband and in laws. Personal history reveals shy nature of the patient. It also tells that as a child she was very bright and intelligent child. Pre-morbidly she had warm temperament.

MSE findings reveals affect to be anxious and distressed both subjectively and objectively.

1. The patient seems to have a disorder of-
   (A) Psychosis
   (B) Autism
   (C) Adjustment disorder
   (D) Major depression
2. The features of following can't be found with this disorder-
   (A) Depression
   (B) Dissociative disorder
   (C) Anxiety
   (D) Psychosis
3. The assessment tool useful in exploring interpersonal difficulties are-
   (A) Rorschach
   (B) BDI
   (C) TAT
   (D) HAM-D
4. The above test is a-
   (A) Projective test
   (B) Objective test
   (C) Paper pencil test
   (D) Questionnaire
5. The following disorder could be a part of this category-
   (A) Paranoia
   (B) BPAD
   (C) PTSD
   (D) Histrionic personality disorder

Answers:
1. C
   The patient seems to have Adjustment disorder.
   This disorder usually occurs in those individuals who are vulnerable due to poor coping skills or personality factors.
2. D
   Psychosis cannot be found with this disorder.
   The reality contact is impaired in psychotic disorder.
3. C
   TAT is useful in exploring interpersonal difficulties.
   It is also useful in exploring needs, conflict and emotion.

4. A

The above test is a projective test.

Projective tests are used to know the unconscious element of the mind.

5. B

The disorder could be PTSD.

PTSD is delayed and/or protected response to a stressful event or situation.

Reference:
1. Kaplan &Sadock, Synopsis of psychiatry. 9th edition

MAJOR DEPRESSIVE DISORDER

Dr. Eesha Sharma & Dr. Manu Agarwal, Assistant Professors, Department of Psychiatry

43 years old lady had complaints of low mood and lack of interest in work, for the last 2 months. Her appetite and sleep are reduced and at times she feels that she would be better off dead. Her family is unable to cheer her up no matter how hard they try. When she came to see a psychiatrist she reported that she had no hope of getting back to her usual life again and that she only wanted medication to help her sleep at night. She had no medical history and no major psychosocial stressors ongoing.

1. Which of the following is true about depression?
   (A) It is almost always a result of stress
   (B) It is commoner in the 2nd-3rd decade
   (C) Females have a bimodal peak in the age at onset
   (D) The large majority of people who suffer depression tend to have a chronic illness over many years
2. Somatic symptoms of depression include:
   (A) Increased appetite
   (B) Bodily pains
   (C) Gastric symptoms
   (D) Early morning awakening
3. Depression can be treated with all of the following except:
   (A) Serotonin reuptake inhibitors
   (B) Carbamazepine
   (C) Lithium
   (D) Antipsychotics
4. Which of the following is associated with relapse in depression?
   (A) Personality disorders
   (B) Incomplete remission of symptoms in index episode
   (C) Treatment resistance
   (D) All of the above
5. Which of the following has the largest evidence base in treatment resistant depression?
   (A) Electroconvulsive therapy
   (B) Lithium
   (C) Cognitive behavior therapy
   (D) Atypical antipsychotics

Answers:
1. C

Incidence of depression in women occurs in two peaks – in middle age, and post-menopausal age.

2. D

The 'somatic syndrome' of depression includes – early morning awakening, reduced appetite and weight loss, decreased libido, psychomotor retardation, anhedonia.

3. B

Carbamazepine has been used as a mood stabilizer and has some efficacy as an anti-manic agent, however, anti-depressant effects are negligible.

4. D

Personality disorders, resistance to treatment and persistence of sub-syndromal depressive symptoms have all been associated with greater likelihood of relapse.

5. A

ECT is the first line treatment, with the highest reported efficacy, in the management of treatment resistant depression.

Reference:

1. Kaplan &Saddock's Comprehensive Textbook of Psychiatry, 9th edition, Wolters Kluwer/Lippincott Williams & Wilkins

MANIC EPISODE

Dr. Eesha Sharma & Dr. Manu Agarwal, Assistant Professors, Department of Psychiatry

A 14-year-old girl is brought for a psychiatric consultation with complaints of excessive talking, reduced sleep and irritability. These symptoms are reportedly present for the last 15 days and have been progressively increasing. Her father and paternal uncle suffered from 'mood swings' that required treatment for several years. The girl is otherwise well behaved and good at academics; she had no major difficulties growing up. On examination she is cheerful, questioning the doctor in several things, reports wanting 'to fly like a bird', and becomes angry easily if her ideas are challenged. She has no other medical history.

1. Factors associated with a higher likelihood of bipolar disorder include:
   (A) Having an episode of depression in the 4th decade
   (B) Family history of bipolar disorder
   (C) Substance use disorder
   (D) Having an extroverted temperament
2. Which of the following has the largest evidence base for treating bipolar disorder?
   (A) Carbamazepine
   (B) Valproate
   (C) Lithium
   (D) Olanzapine
3. Common side effects of Lithium include all the following except:
   (A) Gastric intolerance
   (B) Tremors
   (C) Increased thirst
   (D) Seizures
4. Role of antipsychotics in the treatment of bipolar disorder lies in their efficacy as
   (A) Anti-manic agents
   (B) Anti-depressive agents
   (C) Prophylactic agents
   (D) All of the above
5. An index depressive episode with the following features is more likely to turn into a bipolar illness later in life:
   (A) Pediatric age of patient
   (B) Presence of psychotic symptoms
   (C) Reversal of vegetative signs
   (D) All of the above

Answers:

1. B

   Bipolar disorder has a high genetic underpinning, and a family history of bipolar disorder is frequently seen in patients.

2. C

   Lithium has the largest evidence base for management of bipolar disorder – including anti-manic, anti-depressive and prophylactic effects.

3. D

   Seizures are a rare side effect, only seen at very high serum levels, or in the presence of other risk factors for seizures.

4. D

   Antipsychotics like olanzapine, quetiapine, aripiprazole, have shown efficacy in all phases of bipolar disorder.

5. D

   An index depressive episode in childhood, with atypical features and psychotic symptoms is more likely to turn into bipolar disorder in follow-up.

Reference:

1. Kaplan &Saddock's Comprehensive Textbook of Psychiatry, 9th edition, Wolters Kluwer/Lippincott Williams & Wilkins

BIPOLAR AFFECTIVE DISORDER

Dr. Sujit Kumar Kar & Dr.Manu Agarwal, Assistant Professor, Department of Psychiatry

A 31 year old man with history of two manic episodes in past (first episode being five years back and 2nd being 3 years ago) presented with complaints of sadness of mood, decreased energy, hopelessness, decreased interest in work and disturbed sleep for last 2 months. The patient had received lithium as mood stabilizer during the last episode along with olanzapine and benzodiazepines but was non-adherent to medications for last one year. His father had history of bipolar affective disorder, who was well maintained on lithium 600mg/day for last 3 years. On mental status examination, the patient had depressed mood. He had pessimistic views about future and subjectively decreased interest in recreational activities. He was diagnosed as "Bipolar affective disorder, current episode moderate depression".

1. Bipolar depression differs from unipolar depression in having all of the following features, except –
   (A) More slow in onset
   (B) Relatively shorter episodes
   (C) More in severity
   (D) Hypersomnia is more common
2. Which of the following statement regarding bipolar depression is incorrect?
   (A) Around 2% people with bipolar depression commit suicide
   (B) Bipolar depression results in more socio-economic burden than mania
   (C) Hyperphagia is more common in bipolar depression than unipolar depression
   (D) All the above
3. The above mentioned patient belongs to which subtype of bipolar affective disorder?
   (A) Type I Bipolar affective disorder
   (B) Type II Bipolar affective disorder
   (C) Type III Bipolar affective disorder
   (D) Type IV Bipolar affective disorder
4. Recent biological researches suggest alteration in the Brain Derived Neurotrophic Factor level is associated with –
   (A) Episodes of mania & depression
   (B) Psychosocial stressor
   (C) Substance abuse
   (D) All the above
5. Which of the following antipsychotic agent is recommended as monotherapy in bipolar depression?
   (A) Olanzapine
   (B) Risperidone
   (C) Haloperidol
   (D) Quetiapine

Answers:

1. A
   Episodes of bipolar depression are, compared with unipolar depression, more rapid in onset, more frequent, more severe, shorter and more likely to involve reverse neurovegetative symptoms such as hyperphagia and hypersomnia.
2. A
   Around 15% people with bipolar depression commit suicide.
3. A
   Patients with manic episodes, interspersed with depressive episodes come under Bipolar I disorder
4. D
   BDNF level is found to be altered in Bipolar disorder, Depression, Substance use disorder, Stress related disorder
5. D
   Quetiapine is recommended as monotherapy in Bipolar depression.

References:

1. Sadock B J, Sadock VA, Ruiz P. Kaplan &Sadock's Comprehensive Textbook of Psychiatry, 9th Edition; Lippincott Williams & Wilkins; 2009, Vol.1:
2. Taylor D, Paton C, Kapur S. The Maudsley Prescribing Guidelines in psychiatry. 11th Edition.Wiley-Blackwell. 2012.

POSTPARTUM DEPRESSION

Dr. Sujit Kumar Kar& Dr.Manu Agarwal, Assistant Professor, Department of Psychiatry

A 27 year old lady with no past history of psychiatric illness was brought for psychiatric consultation with complaints of sadness of mood, anxiety, hopelessness, suicidal ideations and disturbed sleep for 20 days. She had delivered a male child 25 days prior to psychiatric consultation by elective caesarian section. She also had recurrent thoughts to kill her baby which was quite distressing for her. In last two weeks, her self-care had been declined significantly.

This was the first pregnancy of the patient. She had regular antenatal follow ups and had received iron-folic acid as well as calcium supplementation. There was no family history of psychiatric illness. There was no psychosocial stressor. She was diagnosed to be suffering from "Postpartum depression".

1. The risk of having a major depressive episode during the perinatal period is approximately –
   (A) < 5 %
   (B) 10 – 15%
   (C) 20 – 30%
   (D) Approximately 50%
2. Which of the following statement regarding post partum blues is incorrect?
   (A) Nearly 50 – 80% of postpartum women experience postpartum blues
   (B) It is a mood disturbance of transient in nature
   (C) Symptoms usually start by 3rd day postpartum, peak by 5th day and usually resolve by 10th day
   (D) Nearly 50% patient with postpartum blues goes to postpartum depression
3. Which of the following is a risk factor development of postpartum depression?
   (A) Past history of depression in postpartum period
   (B) Past history of depression independent of postpartum period
   (C) Family history of depression
   (D) All of the above
4. Following general principles need to be followed during prescribing psychotropic medications in a lactating mother, except –
   (A) Benefits of breast feeding to the mother and infant must be weighed against the risk of drug exposure in the infant.
   (B) Premature infants are at a greater risk from exposure to drugs
   (C) Infants with renal, hepatic, cardiac impairment are at a greater risk from exposure to drugs
   (D) Breast feeding is to be withheld strictly in mothers who are on psychotropic medications
5. Which of the following antidepressant is not excreted in breast milk?
   (A) Sertraline
   (B) Imipramine
   (C) Bupropion
   (D) None of the above

Answers:

1. B
    10 to 15 percent of postpartum women experience a major depressive episode during perinatal period.
2. D
    Nearly 20 to 25 percent women may go on to experience major postpartum depression
3. D
    Past history of depression, family h/o depression as well as h/o postpartum depression are risk factor for development of postpartum depression.
4. D
    Where a mother has taken a particular psychotropic drug during pregnancy and until delivery, continuation with the drug while breast feeding may be appropriate as this may minimise withdrawal symptoms in the infant.
5. D
    SSRIs, TCAs and Bupripion are secreted in breast milk

References:

1.   Sadock B J, Sadock VA, Ruiz P. Kaplan &Sadock's Comprehensive Textbook of Psychiatry, 9th Edition; Lippincott Williams & Wilkins; 2009, Vol.2:2539 -2561.
2.   Taylor D, Paton C, Kapur S. The Maudsley Prescribing Guidelines in psychiatry. 11th Edition.Wiley-Blackwell. 2012.

OBSESSIVE COMPULSIVE DISORDERS
Dr. Eesha Sharma, Assistant Professor, Department of Psychiatry

A mother brought her 12-year-old son to a psychiatrist. She complained that the boy took excessively long while writing class work or homework. She said that he kept going over the same line again and again, sometimes asking her to check if he had written it correctly. Further exploration also revealed that the boy took a long time to arrange his school bag, wash, bathe, dress-up and for other daily routine activities. This had been going on for the last 1 year and his school grades were going down. On speaking to the boy, he said that he kept getting doubts about everything he did. He could never be sure if he had done things correctly. The psychiatrist also noted that the boy repeatedly blinked his eyes and shrugged his shoulders for no apparent reason. On asking, the mother reported that the boy had had these movements for at least the last 4-5 years. A diagnosis of Obsessive-compulsive disorder (mixed subtype) along with Tic disorder was made.

1. Which of the following statements about OCD is untrue?
   (A) It is a chronic illness with a waxing and waning course
   (B) It is much more common in females than in males
   (C) Serotonin-reuptake inhibitors are the first line of treatment
   (D) Compulsions may not always be present in all patients
2. Which of the following are common co-morbidities with OCD?
   (A) Tic disorder
   (B) Depression
   (C) Obsessive-compulsive spectrum disorders
   (D) All of the above
3. What is the importance of age at onset of symptoms in OCD?
   (A) Psychotherapy is not a mode of treatment in children
   (B) Childhood onset generally implies a poor prognosis for the disorder
   (C) Co-morbidities are not found in adults with OCD
   (D) Age at onset does not matter in OCD
4. Which of the following is the most common type of symptom in OCD?
   (A) Pathological doubts
   (B) Obsessions of contamination
   (C) Sexual obsessions
   (D) Aggressive obsessions
5. The neurotransmitter most commonly implicated in OCD is:
   (A) Dopamine
   (B) Serotonin
   (C) Nor-epinephrine
   (D) Acetylcholine

Answers:
1. B
   The prevalence of OCD has been reported equal across genders, although males tend to have a comparatively early onset with a poorer prognosis.
2. D
   Depression is perhaps the commonest comorbid disorder with OCD. Several other disorders, now called 'obsessive compulsive spectrum disorders' are also seen to be commonly comorbid.
3. B
   A childhood onset of illness is seen to predict a longer duration of illness with a severe course of symptoms.
4. B
   Obsessions of contamination and consequent washing compulsions are the commonest symptoms reported across studies.
5. B
   Serotonergic dysfunction appears to be central to OCD; the most effective currently available treatments increase in levels of serotonin in the brain leading to symptom relief.

Reference:
1. Kaplan &Saddock's Comprehensive Textbook of Psychiatry, 9th edition, Wolters Kluwer/Lippincott Williams & Wilkins

SOMATOFORM DISORDER

Dr. Eesha Sharma, Assistant Professor, Department of Psychiatry

43 years old married lady has visited at least 10 doctors in the last 2-3 years and has a large bundle of prescriptions. She complains of persistent headache, pain in several joints, gastric upset with belching and bloating sensations, off and on complaints of burning in the genital area and frequency of micturition, palpitations, and vague chest discomfort. Her symptoms have been present the last 6-7 years and have shown fluctuations in severity and type. Numerous investigations, several of them repeated 2-3 times, have revealed no abnormality. During her consultations with specialists, she has many a times been told that her symptoms are 'all in the mind'. She has been taking various medications – analgesics, antacids, antibiotics, sleeping pills, etc – none of which seem to have helped her. She denies depressed or anxious mood, however, remains preoccupied with her physical symptoms. She has two sons who live with her and are currently in their final years at school. Her husband, employed with the railways, has a history of alcohol use for the last 25 years. The family has had severe financial difficulties because of her husband's alcohol use.

1. Which of the following describes the clinical presentation given above?
    (A) Medically unexplained somatic symptoms
    (B) Briquet syndrome
    (C) Somatization
    (D) All of the above
2. Which of the following is untrue about somatization disorder?
    (A) It is commoner in females
    (B) There is usually a psychosocial stressor involved
    (C) Dysfunctional personality traits are generally present in patients with this disorder
    (D) Patients should be encouraged to continue taking medicines for symptomatic relief
3. Functional somatic syndromes in medicine include all the following except:
    (A) Globus syndrome
    (B) Tension headache
    (C) Blepharospasm
    (D) Irritable bowel syndrome
4. Somatoform disorders include:
    (A) Undifferentiated somatoform disorder
    (B) Persistent somatoform pain disorder
    (C) Conversion disorder
    (D) All of the above
5. The following should be considered in the differential diagnosis of somatoform disorders:
    (A) Bipolar disorder
    (B) Hypochondriasis
    (C) Depression
    (D) Both b and c

Answers:

1. D
    A presentation with multiple physical symptoms, without medical or psychological symptoms has been called by various names – Medically unexplained somatic symptoms, Briquet syndrome, Somatization disorder, etc.
2. D
    Medication prescription for 'symptom relief' is best avoided in somatization disorder. Adequate psychoeducation should be done and withdrawal of medications negotiated with the patient.
3. C
    Globus syndrome, tension headache and irritable bowel syndrome are considered functional somatic syndromes, due to lack of sufficient medical cause, however blepharospasm is a focal neurological dystonia.
4. D
    Somatoform disorders are a group of disorders that have been classified based on the type of somatic symptoms and sites of involvement.
5. D
    Depression, which can also present with multiple somatic complaints, should always be ruled out before diagnosing somatoform disorders. Hypochondriasis involves preoccupation about having an illness, whereas in somatoform disorders the focus is on physical symptoms.

Reference:
1. Kaplan &Saddock's Comprehensive Textbook of Psychiatry, 9th edition, Wolters Kluwer/Lippincott Williams & Wilkins

PANIC ATTACK
Dr. Eesha Sharma, Assistant Professor, Department of Psychiatry

A 25 years old lady working as a bank clerk presented to the emergency room with palpitations, sweating, trembling limbs, choking sensation and 'light-headedness'. She has no past history of any major medical disorder and the current symptoms started abruptly as she was sitting at her office desk typing out an official letter. The symptoms surged within minutes and stayed for almost half an hour. She reported such 'attacks' having happened to her 2 times in the last two months. While she remained asymptomatic between the attacks, she reported the episodes to be extremely frightening and worried about their recurrence. The emergency room evaluation did not find any abnormalities in her ECG or blood work.

1. What is the most likely explanation for her symptoms?
   (A) Paroxysmal supraventricular tachycardia
   (B) Thyroid storm
   (C) Panic attack
   (D) Episodic hypoglycemia
2. The most common comorbidity with panic disorder is:
   (A) Generalized anxiety disorder
   (B) Depression
   (C) Social phobia
   (D) Agoraphobia
3. Which of the following is a typical cognition in panic disorder?
   (A) A feeling of impending doom
   (B) Persistent concern about having additional attacks
   (C) Fear of losing control/going crazy
   (D) All of the above
4. Which of the following is a mainstay of treatment in panic disorder?
   (A) Benzodiazepines
   (B) Cognitive behavior therapy
   (C) Psychoanalysis
   (D) Electroconvulsive therapy
5. Which of the following is involved in the 'fear circuitry'?
   (A) Frontal lobes
   (B) Thalamus
   (C) Amygdala
   (D) Olfactory bulb

Answers:
1. C
   Episodes of sudden surge in anxiety without accompanying physiological abnormalities, e.g. on ECG, are seen in a panic attack
2. D
   The occurrence of panic attacks induces a fear of being alone in a place, especially from where escape could be difficult, a phenomenon called agoraphobia.
3. D
   People who experience panic attacks commonly report all three thoughts mentioned here.
4. B
   Cognitive behavior therapy is the treatment with best supportive evidence for panic disorder.
5. C
   Amygdala has been shown on fMRI studies to be involved in processing of fear related information and memories.

Reference:
1. Kaplan & Saddock's Comprehensive Textbook of Psychiatry, 9th edition, Wolters Kluwer/Lippincott Williams & Wilkins

SPECIFIC PHOBIA

Dr. Eesha Sharma, Assistant Professor, Department of Psychiatry

A 36 years old lawyer reports anxiety over the last one year. On enquiry it turns out that he becomes very uncomfortable when he sees blood. His 60 years old mother was diagnosed with diabetes 4 years ago. Whenever he has to take her for a blood test and has to stand beside her as they draw her sample, he starts to shiver, sweat and feel anxious that something disastrous could happen. He acknowledges that his fear might be illogical but is not able to overcome it. He cannot recall any initiating event that might have triggered his fear, but it has been becoming an increasing problem in the last few years. Recently he has consciously avoided visiting hospitals, labs, or any other place he might see blood.

1. Specific phobias could be of the following types:
    (A) Animal type
    (B) Natural environment type
    (C) None of the above
    (D) Both of the above
2. Following has the largest evidence base for treatment of phobic disorders:
    (A) Serotonin-dopamine antagonists
    (B) Exposure therapy
    (C) Mindfulness meditation
    (D) Relaxation therapy
3. In the above case what form of exposure therapy would be appropriate?
    (A) Interoceptive exposure
    (B) In vivo exposure
    (C) Imaginal exposure
    (D) Exposure with relaxation
4. Which of the following is untrue for specific phobia?
    (A) There is a bimodal peak for age at onset
    (B) Females are more commonly diagnosed with phobias
    (C) It follows a fluctuating course
    (D) Avoidance of the phobic stimulus is advisable to decrease distress
5. Differential diagnosis for social phobia includes:
    (A)Anxious-avoidant personality disorder
    (B)Agoraphobia
    (C)Depression
    (D)All of the above

Answers:

1. D

    These are the two broad categories of stimuli seen in patients with specific phobia.

2. B

    Exposure that leads to habituation and gradually reduction in anxiety has the best evidence for treatment of phobia.

3. B

    In vivo exposure involves real time exposure to the feared stimulus. Interoceptive exposure is done in panic disorder whereas imaginal exposure is used where it is not feasible to expose in real time, e.g. a person with fear of travelling in aeroplanes.

4. D

    Avoidance results in increasing discomfort with the feared stimulus since habituation of anxiety cannot occur.

5. D

    Any situation that could result in discomfort in social situations could mimic social phobia.

Reference:

1. Kaplan &Saddock's Comprehensive Textbook of Psychiatry, 9th edition, Wolters Kluwer/Lippincott Williams & Wilkins

POST TRAUMATIC STRESS DISORDER

Dr. Eesha Sharma, Assistant Professor, Department of Psychiatry

A 50 year old male was involved in a road traffic accident about a year ago. He was travelling with his family in a car that his 25 years old son was driving. A truck collided with the car leaving his wife and son seriously injured. His son was in the ICU for almost a month and had for a short while been put on a ventilator. Although now they were all healthy and not suffering from any serious residual disabilities, the patient reported being 'permanently affected' by the event. He reported frequently waking up in the night from a nightmare about the accident. He avoided crossing the road where the accident had occurred. He frequently felt as though the events of the accident were happening with him again. His family reported that he had in general become quite dull after the event. Although he participated in all activities of the family and took care of all his daily routines, he just could not forget the accident.

1. The clinical presentation above could be indicative of:
   (A) Chronic depression
   (B) Generalized anxiety disorder
   (C) Post-traumatic stress disorder
   (D) Both a and c
2. Likelihood of developing PTSD increases with:
   (A) Minor accidents
   (B) Long-time after the accident
   (C) Witnessing unrelated persons in an accident
   (D) A high degree of avoidance of stimuli that recall the accident
3. The following appears to be most effective in the treatment of PTSD:
   (A) Cognitive behavior therapy
   (B) Stress inoculation training
   (C) Eye movement desensitization and reprocessing
   (D) All of the above
4. Acute PTSD refers to symptoms lasting:
   (A) Less than 1 month
   (B) Less than 3 months
   (C) Less than 6 months
   (D) Less than 1 year
5. The following features indicate a state of 'increased arousal':
   (A) Hypervigilance
   (B) Difficulty falling or staying asleep
   (C) Flashbacks
   (D) Both a and b

Answers:

1. C
   Nightmares, avoidance of all trauma-related memories, and flashbacks are symptoms of post-traumatic disorder; features such as pervasive sadness, anhedonia, and other features of depression are not present.
2. D
   Avoidance of stimuli associated with the trauma, in a way, hinder processing of trauma related memories and has been seen to be associated with development of PTSD.
3. D
   While no treatment has a very large evidence base for PTSD, and at best moderate effect sizes, cognitive behavior therapy, stress inoculation therapy and eye movement desensitization have been used successfully.
4. B
   Usually, acute PTSD symptoms resolve within 3 months, persistence beyond that could be a harbinger of chronic PTSD.
5. D
   Increased arousal is a feature of PTSD that presents as hypervigilance and difficulty falling asleep.

Reference:

1. Kaplan &Saddock's Comprehensive Textbook of Psychiatry, 9th edition, Wolters Kluwer/Lippincott Williams & Wilkins

ALZHEIMER'S DEMENTIA WITH BEHAVIORAL AND PSYCHOLOGICAL SYMPTOMS

Dr. Diwakar Sharma, Senior Resident, Department of Psychiatry

A 76-year-old woman from urban background was brought to Psychiatry OPD by her son with complaints of forgetfulness since 3 years and suspiciousness with disturbed sleep since last 6 months. She is reported to have gradually progressive worsening in her memory functions related to daily household activities such as leaving tap open, forgetting to lock doors, difficulty in finding objects of limited utility. Of late, she has had difficulty in remembering her last meal on frequent occasions which had resulted in loss of 8 kg weight over last 10-12 months. For a year now she had more than often failed to recall having met a family member or relative who actually visited the house in recent times. Recently she would often lose her way back to her own room within the house. Now for last 6 months, she had begun to suspect all her family members of conspiring against her. She would even get irritable and verbally abusive shouting at times when she is not able to find her things. She does not sleep properly and gets up prematurely in the middle of night to get ready. Upon consultation with a general physician, she had normal laboratory tests for metabolic, haematological, and thyroid function. Her physical examination was within normal parameters. Her mental status examination revealed disorientation to time and day, irritable affect with paranoid delusions. Her recent and immediate memory was impaired. No hallucinations were reported. Her Mini-Mental State Examination (MMSE) score was 12/30.

She was provisionally diagnosed to be suffering from Alzheimer's Dementia with Behavioral and Psychological symptoms.

1. Most common cause of dementia is?
   - (A) Parkinson's Disease
   - (B) Alzheimer's Disease
   - (C) Pick's Disease
   - (D) HIV related

2. Which of the following structures is affected in Alzheimer's disease?
   - (A) Predominantly cerebellum
   - (B) Parieto temporal cortex
   - (C) Predominantly fronto temporal cortex
   - (D) Occipital cortex

3. In what order do the following symptoms generally present in progression of Alzheimer's Disease?
   - (A) Mood changes, behavioural symptoms, cognitive impairment
   - (B) Behavioural symptoms, motor symptoms, decline in functional independence
   - (C) Mood changes, cognitive impairment, decline in functional independence
   - (D) Behavioural symptoms, mood changes, motor symptoms

4. Which of the following is the first line of treatment for behavioural and psychological symptoms of dementia (BPSD)?
   - (A) Atypical antipsychotics
   - (B) Selective serotonin reuptake inhibitor
   - (D) Anti-epileptic drugs
   - (D) Behavioral management

5. Who devised Mini Mental Status examination ?
   - (A) AM Clarfield & DJ Thurman
   - (B) MR Folstein, SE Folstein & PR McHugh
   - (C) CA Luis, AP Keegan & V Bedirian
   - (D) DJ Thurman, JK Rao & JA Stevens

Answers:

1. B
   Of all patients with dementia, 50 to 60 percent have the most common type of dementia, dementia of the Alzheimer's type (Alzheimer's disease).

2. B
   Alzheimer's disease has parietal-temporal distribution of pathological findings. In contrast Pick's disease is characterized by a preponderance of atrophy in the frontotemporal regions.

3. C
   Mood changes, cognitive impairment, decline in functional independence followed by behavioural and motor symptoms

4. D
   Behavioral management is the first line of management. Behavioral treatments that identify antecedents and consequences of problem behaviors and then effect changes in the environment to alter the behaviors have been shown to be beneficial in reducing disruptive behaviors

5. B
    The mini–mental state examination (MMSE) or Folstein test is a sensitive, valid and reliable 30-point questionnaire that is used extensively in clinical and research settings to measure cognitive impairment.

References:

1. Kauffman DM, Milstein MJ. Clinical neorology for psychiatrists. 7th ed. Portland: Elsevier Saunders; 2013 (ch. 7)
2. Folstein MF, Folstein SE, McHugh PR. "Mini-mental state".A practical method for grading the cognitive state of patients for the clinician. J Psychiatr Res.1975 Nov;12(3):189-98.
3. Ballard CG, Gauthier S, Cummings JL, Brodaty H, Grossberg GT, Robert P, Lyketsos CG. Management of agitation and aggression associated with Alzheimer disease. Nat Rev Neurol. 2009 May;5(5):245-55.
4. Stahl SM. Stahl's essential psychopharmacology, 3[rd]ed. New York, NY: Cambridge University Press;2008 (ch. 18)

MILD COGNITIVE IMPAIRMENT (MCI)

Dr. Diwakar Sharma, Senior Resident, Department of Psychiatry

A 70 year old man presented himself in Psychiatry OPD with complaints of memory problems since 1 year. He reports having frequent difficulty in remembering things related to activities of daily living such as misplacing objects, missing doses of medications or keeping appointments. He also finds difficulty in naming objects of household routine more than often. Recently, he had started to put in greater effort in the form of sticking notes in the house, keeping a log of task at hand. There is no history of any anxiety, sadness of mood, disturbance of sleep, trauma or any significant substance use during this period. He has history of hypertension for last 6 months and is currently under treatment. Physical examination was within normal limits. Mental status examination revealed normal orientation to time, place and person. Concentration was intact but he had difficulty in recalling immediate and recent events in clear detail. His MMSE Score was 24/30. CT scan head revealed only age related diffuse cortical atrophy.

He was diagnosed with Mild Cognitive Disorder (or Mild Cognitive Impairment)

1. All of the following are true except
   (A)MCI represents a precursor to Alzheimer's disease
   (B)Acetylcholine esterase inhibitors do not slow deterioration of MCI to dementia
   (C)Cognitive impairment in MCI reverts to normal in many cases
   (D)MCI spares memory and involves executive ability or language function.
2. Which of the following is NOT a risk factor for mild cognitive impairment?
   (A)Hypertension
   (B)Diabetes insipidus
   (C)H/o TIA
   (D)Down's syndrome
3. Which of the following medications are approved for use in MCD (or MCI) ?
   (A)Rivastigmine
   (B)Memantine
   (C)Piracetam
   (D)None of the above
4. Following agents are responsible for memory impairment except
   (A)Antipsychotics
   (B)Benzodiazepines
   (C)Statins
   (D)Piracetam
5. Which of the following is true about pseudo-dementia ?
   (A)Symptoms usually of long duration before medical help is sought
   (B)Patients' complaints of cognitive dysfunction usually detailed
   (C)Nocturnal accentuation of dysfunction common
   (D)Near-miss answers frequent

Answers:
   1. D

The term mild cognitive impairment has been suggested as a diagnostic category designed to fill the gap between cognitive changes associated with aging and cognitive impairment suggestive of dementia. The criteria proposed by the Mayo Clinic Alzheimer's Disease Research Center (MCADRC) are (1) memory complaint, preferably qualified by an informant; (2) objective memory impairment for age and education; (3) preserved general cognitive function; (4) intact activities of daily living; and (5) not demented

2. B
   Diabetes insipidus
3. D
   Currently, there is no evidence for long-term efficacy of pharmacotherapies in reversing MCI.
4. D
   Piracetam has not been reported to cause memory impairment.
5. B
   Some patients with depression have symptoms of cognitive impairment difficult to distinguish from symptoms of dementia. The clinical picture is sometimes referred to as pseudodementia. Patients' complaints of cognitive dysfunction that are usually detailed, emphasize disability, highlight failures, and make little effort to perform even simple tasks.

Refrences:

1. Kauffman DM, Milstein MJ. Dementia. In: Clinical neurology for psychiatrists. 7th ed. Portland: Elsevier Saunders; 2013
2. Grossman H. Amnestic Disorders. In: Sadock BJ, Sadock VA, eds. Kaplan &Sadock's Comprehensive Textbook of Psychiatry. 8th ed. Vol. 1. Baltimore: Lippincott Williams & Wilkins; 2005:1093.
3. Neugroschl JA, Kolevzon A, Samuels SC, Marin DB. Dementia. In: Sadock BJ, Sadock VA, eds. Kaplan &Sadock's Comprehensive Textbook of Psychiatry. 8th ed. Vol. 1. Baltimore: Lippincott Williams & Wilkins; 2005:1068.

DEMENTIA WITH LEWY BODIES (DLW)
Dr. Diwakar Sharma, Senior Resident, Department of Psychiatry

A 75-year-old male farmer was healthy and did not have any significant family psychiatric history. One year ago, he began to suffer from memory loss and insomnia, and sought medical treatment at Neurology department. Laboratory data included normal serum chemistry levels, electroencephalography (EEG) study with steady and generalized theta wave, and brain computed tomography (CT) scan with mild brain atrophy. He was treated with donepezil but did not return regularly for follow-up visits. Six months later, he began to have persecutory delusions, visual hallucinations (appeared obviously frightened from seeing non-existent snakes), incidents of delusional misidentification with television characters and her family members, and physical aggression. He was brought to the Psychiatry OPD for evaluation and was prescribed with low dose antipsychotic agents, including risperidone (0.5 mg/day), which was later changed to haloperidol (0.5mg/day). However, the psychosis did not improve and he exhibited evidence of acute dystonia, akathisia, bradykinesia, syncope and repeated falls. The patient was therefore admitted to the hospital for further treatment. Upon admission, mental status examination revealed that he had limited speech and was not well oriented. Neurological exam only revealed signs of apparent Parkinsonism but no other neurological signs. Biochemical blood tests were within normal limits, and EEG, brain CT results were unchanged. He was treated with amantadine (200mg/day), and switched to another antipsychotic drug olanzapine (5 mg/day later raised to 10 mg/day). However, his psychosis and Parkinsonian symptoms persisted. It was not until olanzapine was replaced with quetiapine (25mg /day) that he showed some improvement in parkinsonian features, activity level, and orientation. Even after discharge from hospital, he still experienced apparent visual hallucinations and had a tendency to fall spontaneously. Several weeks later, he exhibited severe Parkinsonian symptoms with difficulty in feeding or take care of himself, and was thus readmitted.

Clinical course in this case pointed towards a diagnosis of Dementia with Lewy Bodies (DLB).

1. The core features of dementia with Lewy bodies include :
   (A) Fluctuating cognition
   (B) Recurrent detailed visual hallucinations
   (C) Spastic paresis
   (D) Progressive language dysfunction
2. Gradual changes in personality and progressive language dysfunction are the hallmarks of which of the following ?
   (A) Alzheimer's disease

(B) Pick's disease

(C) DLB

(D) HIV related dementia

3. Pathological features associated with dementia with Lewy bodies include all except :

(A) Prominent neurofibrillary tangles

(B) Weakly eosinophilic, spherical, cytoplasmic inclusions

(C) Abundant neuritic plaques

(D) Microvacuolation and synapse loss

4. Which of the following is false ?

(A) Cortical Lewy bodies are exclusively seen in in Parkinson's disease

(B) Parkinson's disease is commonly associated with dementia

(C) Alzheimer's disease is the most common cause of dementia

(D) Lewy body core is composed of aggregates of a protein α-synuclein

5. Features of DLB includes all except.

(A) Increased thyroid levels

(B) Syncope

(C) Sensitivity to neuroleptics

(D) Systematized delusions

Answers:

1. C

The core features of dementia with Lewy bodies include (1) fluctuating cognition with pronounced variations in attention and alertness, (2) recurrent visual hallucinations, which are typically well formed and detailed, and (3) spontaneous motor features of parkinsonism.

2. B

The prototypic clinical presentation of Pick's disease is disturbance of personality and behavior or impairments of language (primary progressive aphasia or semantic dementia).

3. A

Lewy bodies are spherical intracytoplasmic eosinophilic neuronal inclusion bodies. "Classic" Lewy bodies are inclusions with a hyaline core and pale halo and are typically seen in the brainstem nuclei, substantia nigra, and locus coeruleus. Cortical Lewy bodies are less-well-defined spherical inclusions. Lewy bodies are composed predominantly of fibrillar deposits of α-synuclein, and can also include neurofilament proteins and ubiquitin.The presence of cortical neurofibrillary tangles indicates that dementia with Lewy bodies is less likely.

4. A

Cortical Lewy bodies may be present even in individuals with familial early-onset Alzheimer's disease due to mutations in amyloid precursor protein, presenilin 1, and presenilin 2.

5. A

Increased thyroid levels

References:

1. Neugroschl JA, Kolevzon A, Samuels SC, Marin DB. Dementia. In: Sadock BJ, Sadock VA, eds. Kaplan &Sadock's Comprehensive Textbook of Psychiatry. 8th ed. Vol. 1. Baltimore: Lippincott Williams & Wilkins; 2005:1068.

2. Hashimoto, M., Kawahara, K., Bar-On, P., Rockenstein, E., Crews, L. &Masliah, E. (2004) The role of alpha-synuclein assembly and metabolism in the pathogenesis of Lewy body disease. Journal of Molecular Neuroscience 24, 343–352.

3. Haan, M.N., Jagust, W.J., Galasko, D. & Kaye, J. (2002) Effect of extrapyramidal signs and lewy bodies on survival in patients with Alzheimer disease. Archives of Neurology 59, 588–593.

4. McKeith LG, Galasko D, Kosaka K. Consensus guidelines for the clinical and pathologic diagnosis of dementia with Lewy bodies (DLB): Report of the consortium on DLB international workshop. Neurology. 1996;47:1113-1124.

PARANOID SCHIZOPHRENIA

Dr. Kamlendra Kishor, Senior Resident, Department of Psychiatry

A 46 years old man was brought in Psychiatry OPD by his wife and son with 4 years of history that he suspects his neighbors and he feels that whenever he passes by they sneeze and talk about him because of which he abuses his neighbors and at many occasions he tried to fight with them. He also feels that his wife has been replaced by a double and has once called police for help. His son also complains about his weird behavior like keeping shoes in the fridge and wearing vest over shirt. He states that he noticed that the patient stopped going to social activities and spent most of his time in his room. He also states that the patient sometimes makes odd comments and remains self-absorbed. He has stopped going to his duties and has lost interest in his work.It was also observed that he talk to himself saying that he hears voices who comment on his actions.

1. What is most likely diagnosis
    (A)Persistent delusional disorder
    (B)Other nonorganic psychotic disorder
    (C)Hebephrenic schizophrenia
    (D)Paranoid schizophrenia
2. What is a bad prognostic indicator in this patient
    (A)Late onset
    (B)Negative symptoms
    (C)No treatment so far
    (D)Absence of family history
3. Which of the following is least likely to be directly involved in schizophrenia
    (A)Dopamine
    (B)Serotonin
    (C)Noradrenaline
    (D)Endorphins
4. Which of the neuropathology is not found in schizophrenia
    (A)Reduced volume of cortical grey matter
    (B)Increased symmetry of the brain
    (C)Enlarged ventricles
    (D)Atrophy of thalamus
5. Which of the following is not included in management of schizophrenia
    (A)Cognitive behavior therapy
    (B)Social skill training
    (C)Hypnosis
    (D)Art therapy

Answers:

1. D
    In paranoid schizophrenia, delusions or hallucinations must be prominent such as delusions of persecution, reference, exalted birth, special mission, bodily change, or jealousy; threatening or commanding voices, hallucinations of smell or taste, sexual or other bodily sensations.
2. B
    Negative symptoms involve symptoms like marked apathy, paucity of speech, and blunting or incongruity of emotional responses. But these should not occur due to depression or to neuroleptic medication.
3. D
    Dopamine, serotonin, norepinephrine, GABA, neuropeptides, glutamate, aetylcholine and nicotine are involved in pathogenesis of schizophrenia. Endorphins are least likely to be directly involved
4. B
    Reduced symmetry not increased symmetry, in several areas like temporal, frontal and occipital lobe is found in schizophrenia.
5. C
    Cognitive behavior therapy, social skill training, family therapy, case management, group therapy, assertive community therapy, art therapy are non-pharmacological therapies used in management of schizophrenia while hypnosis is used in management of anxiety disorder.

Reference:

1. Kaplan &Saddock's Comprehensive Textbook of Psychiatry, 9th edition, Wolters Kluwer/Lippincott Williams & Wilkins

CATATONIC SCHIZOPHRENIA
Dr. Kamlendra Kishor, Senior Resident, Department of Psychiatry

A 36 year old male was brought in Psychiatry emergency with history that he was suspicious that his family members and neighbors are planning against him and he used to mutter for two months with markedly reduced sleep. For last one month his speech output has gradually reduced and is not giving verbal response for last two week with occasional transient excitement without any specific reason. On examination his vital were stable he had blank facial expression, mutism, negativism and rigidity was also present.

1. What is the diagnosis of the patient?
   (A)Other nonorganic psychotic disorder
   (B)Catatonic schizophrenia
   (C)Undifferentiated schizophrenia
   (D)Persistent delusional disorder with catatonia
2. What is most appropriate treatment for this patient?
   (A)Olanzapine
   (B)Fluoxetine
   (C)Electroconvulsive therapy
   (D)Sodium valproate
3. Which of the following is not a sign of catatonia?
   (A)Selective mutism
   (B)Negativism
   (C)Posturing
   (D)Automatic obedience
4. Which of the following is not a secondary complication of catatonia?
   (A)Pulmonary emboli
   (B)Systemic infection
   (C)Bed sore
   (D)Hyperglycemia
5. Catatonia can be found in all except
   (A)Schizophrenia
   (B)Depression
   (C)Panic disorder
   (D)Mania

Answers:

1. B
   For diagnosis of catatonic schizophrenia symptoms like excitement, posturing or waxy flexibility, negativism, mutism, automatic obedience and stupor should be prominent for period of at least two weeks.
2. C
   Electroconvulsive therapy is treatment of choice if there is no contraindication to it.
3. A
   Mutism is a symptom of catatonia while selective mutism is a disorder in children characterized by persistent lack of speaking in one or more specific social situation.
4. D
   Secondary complications of catatonia include, pulmonary emboli, systemic infection, bed sore, deep vein thrombosis, nutritional deficiencies.
5. C
   Catatonia can be present in psychotic disorder, depression, mania and various neurological disorder but not in anxiety disorder like panic disorder.

Reference:

1. Kaplan &Saddock's Comprehensive Textbook of Psychiatry, 9th edition, Wolters Kluwer/Lippincott Williams & Wilkins

ACUTE AND TRANSIENT PSYCHOTIC DISORDER

Dr. Kamlendra Kishor, Senior Resident, Department of Psychiatry

Mr. A, 25 years old married male was brought by his family members in emergency of Psychiatry department with complaints of suspiciousness, fearfulness, increased physical activity and markedly reduced sleep for 2 weeks. He also used to smile and laugh and would start suddenly crying without any apparent reason. According to family members he also used to say that his wife is not the same and has been replaced by double due to which patient also assaulted his wife once. There is no history of recent substance use. Vitals were within normal limit, detailed physical examination was not possible. On MSE patient's psychomotor activity was markedly increased. He was uncooperative and was muttering and laughing inappropriately.

1. What is the diagnosis?
    (A)Persistent delusional disorder
    (B)Acute and transient psychotic disorder
    (C)Other non-organic psychotic disorder
    (D)Mania
2. As per patient, his wife has been replaced by a double, what is this phenomenology called?
    (A)Fregoli syndrome
    (B)Capgras syndrome
    (C)Erotomanic delusion
    (D)None
3. Which of the following drugs can be used for treatment of this patient?
    (A)Venlafaxine
    (B)Mirtazapine
    (C)Aripiprazole
    (D)Milnacipram
4. What should be appropriate place for management of patient?
    (A)At home
    (B)In hospital
    (C)Day-care setting
    (D)Any of the above
5. Which of the following is not an adverse effect of antipsychotic drugs?
    (A)Dystonia
    (B)Tardive dyskinesia
    (C)Chorea
    (D)Akathisia

Answers:
1. B
    Acute and transient psychotic disorder is diagnosed when psychotic symptoms like delusion and hallucination, have acute onset (within two weeks).
2. B
    Capgras syndrome is a syndrome in which the patient believes that a person to whom they are close, usually family member, has been replaced by an exact double.
3. C
    Antipsychotics like aripiprazole, olanzapine, risperidone, haloperidol etc. are mainstay of treatment for psychotic disorder.
4. B
    When there is risk of homicide or suicide, patient should be ideally hospitalized.
5. C
    Movement disorders due to antipsychotics are caused by D2 blocking property. Chorea is not caused by antipsychotic drugs.

Reference:
1. Kaplan & Saddock's Comprehensive Textbook of Psychiatry, 9th edition, Wolters Kluwer/Lippincott Williams & Wilkins

DHAT SYNDROME
Dr. S. K. Kar, Assistant Professor, Department of Psychiatry

A 17 year old orthodox, Hindu boy from a small city of Uttar Pradesh, India sought psychiatric consultation with complaints of easy fatigability, lethargy, burning urination, poor concentration in studies, anxiety since one year. For these complaints he had consulted many general practitioners and traditional healers. His hematological and urine analysis were within normal limits. He was prescribed with analgesics, multivitamins, nutritional supplements as well as benzodiazepines with insignificant response at different points of time. There is no past or family history of psychiatric illness. The patient reports about his scholastic decline in last year due to inattention. On mental status examination, his predominant mood was anxious. When taken into confidentiality, with initial reluctance, he expressed his concern about loss of semen in the form of nightfall. He attributed his symptoms with loss of semen. He was diagnosed to be suffering from "Dhat syndrome".

1. Who coined the term "Dhat Syndrome"?
   (A) Prof.B. B. Sethi
   (B) Prof. V. K. Verma
   (C) Prof.N. N. Wig
   (D) Prof. J. S. Neki
2. All the following statements regarding "Dhat syndrome" are correct except?
   (A) Dhat syndrome is commonly seen in males of rural background.
   (B) Commonly seen in newly married males.
   (C) It is a disorder commonly seen in higher socio-economic strata.
   (D) Dhat syndrome can also be seen in females.
3. Dhat syndrome is a culture bound syndrome commonly seen in –
   (A) Central Asia
   (B) South East Asia
   (C) Exclusively in India
   (D) South Africa
4. Dhat syndrome is known by different names in different countries. Which of the following combination of "country- name of the illness entity" is correct?
   (A) In Sri Lanka – Prameha
   (B) In China –Latah
   (C) In Malayesia & Indonesia – Imu
   (D) In Japan - ShenK'uei
5. Which of the following treatment strategy is mainstay of management of Dhat syndrome?
   (A) Benzodiazepines
   (B) Addressing the culturally colored sexual myths
   (C) SSRIs
   (D) Family focused therapy

Answers:
1. C
    Prof. N. N. Wig has coined the term "Dhat Syndrome".
2. C
    Dhat syndrome is commonly seen in young males of lower socio-economic status of rural background.
3. B
    Dhat syndrome is commonly seen in South East Asian countries. Cases has also been reported from other parts of the world.
4. A
    In Sri Lanka, the entity Dhat syndrome is known as "Prameha"
5. B
    Pharmcological treatment treatment is of little significance. Addressing the sexual myths is the main focus of management.

References:
1. Prakash O, Kar SK, SathyanarayanaRao TS. Indian story on semen loss and related Dhat syndrome. Indian J Psychiatry 2014;56:377-82.
2. Mehta V, De A, Balachandran C. Dhat Syndrome: A Reappraisal. Indian J Dermatol. 2009 Jan-Mar; 54(1): 89–90.
3. Simons RC, Hughes CC. Dordrecht: D Reidel; 1985. The Culture-bound Syndromes: Folk Illnesses of Psychiatric and Anthropological Interest.

ANOREXIA NERVOSA
Dr. S. K. Kar, Assistant Professor, Department of Psychiatry

A 26 year old fashion designer from a affluent family had been referred by gastroenterologist for psychiatric evaluation. The patient had consulted the gastroenterologist for ulcerations in her mouth and episodes of vomiting for past 4 years. During hospitalization under care of the gastroenterologist, no episode of vomiting was reported, even the patient was without any antiemetic medications. Later on she revealed that she used to induce vomiting, every time she eats, in order to maintain her slimness. General physical examination revealed body mass index of 11.72 (body weight of 30 kg and height 160cms). Family member of the patient had reported that four years back, her weight was 58 kg. She also had amenorrhoea for past one year. Every day she used to spend three hours in rigorous physical exercises in a gym.

She was investigated for systemic causes of weight loss and vomiting. Her endocrinological profile revealed normal thyroid profile, however her estrogen, progesterone as well as FSH level were found to be below normal range. Other hematological examinations had revealed, hemoglobin – 10.8gm% and serum potassium 3.3 mEq/lit. Rest of the hematological parameters was within normal limits. On mental status examination she was anxious. She had expressed her apprehension of becoming fat. She was diagnosed with "Anorexia Nervosa".

1. All the following are the criteria for diagnosis of Anorexia Nervosa as per ICD-10, diagnostic criteria, except –
   (A)Loss of body weight, at least 30% below the normal expected weight for age and height.
   (B)Weight loss is self induced
   (C)Self perception of being fat
   (D)Disturbance in the hypothalamo-pituitary gondal axis
2. Among the following psychiatric disorders, which is the commonest co-morbidity with Anorexia Nervosa?
   (A)Obsessive compulsive disorder
   (B)Generalized anxiety disorder
   (C)Major depression
   (D)Alcohol dependence
3. Which of following endocrinological abnormality is not common in anorexia nervosa?
   (A)Low estrogen & low progesterone
   (B)Low FSH
   (C)Low LH
   (D)Increased level of serum leptin
4. Which of the following statement regarding Anorexia Nervosa is false?
   (A)It occurs more commonly in females than males
   (B)Peaks occur in 3rd decade
   (C)Cluster C personality traits are commonly seen
   (D)Monozygotic to dizygotic ratio: 3:1
5. Which of the following statement regarding management of Anorexia Nervosa is correct?
   (A)SSRIs are highly effective in Anorexia Nervosa
   (B)Atypical antipsychotics are effective in typical Anorexia Nervosa
   (C)Cyproheptadine is helpful in some cases
   (D)Zinc helps in rapid restoration of weight in Anorexia Nervosa

Answers:
1. A
   In Anorexia Nervosa, loss of body weight, is at least 15% below the normal expected weight for age and height
2. C
   Major depression is the commonest psychiatric co-morbidity in Anorexia Nervosa
3. D
   Serum Leptin level is found to be low in Anorexia Nervosa
4. B
   The peak of Anorexia Nervosa is seen in early to late teen years.
5. D
   Zinc (50 to 100mg elemental Zinc) helps in rapid restoration of weight in Anorexia Nervosa

Reference:
1. Sadock B J, Sadock VA, Ruiz P. Kaplan &Sadock's Comprehensive Textbook of Psychiatry, 9th Edition; Lippincott Williams & Wilkins; 2009, Vol.1: 2128 – 2150.

ELECTROCONVULSIVE THERAPY
Dr. S. K. Kar, Assistant Professor, Department of Psychiatry

A 25 year old female with severe depressive episode with psychotic symptoms with poor oral intake leading to compromised general condition was hospitalized for inpatient psychiatric management. Family members had also reported that during this depressive episode, she had two suicidal attempts. She expressed her feelings of hopelessness, helplessness, worthlessness as well as had delusion of guilt during the interview.

She had a similar depressive episode three years back, which was improved after eight sessions of electroconvulsive therapy (ECT). She was diagnosed to be suffering from recurrent depressive disorder, current episode severe depression with psychotic symptoms. She had shown significant improvement in after six sessions of ECT along with antidepressant treatment.

1. Who had first used ECT for therapeutic purpose?
   (A)Von Meduna
   (B)Cerletti and Bini
   (C)Ottosson
   (D)Paracelsus
2. The generation of electrical stimulus in ECT is conceptualized on the basis of –
   (A)Faradey's law
   (B)Ampere's law
   (C)Ohm's law
   (D)Newton's law
3. ECT causes all of the following structural changes in brain, except –
   (A)Increased synaptic plasticity in hippocampus
   (B)Increased cortical connectivity
   (C)Increased neurogenesis
   (D)Increased neuronal apoptosis
4. Presence of following factors attribute to higher risk of development of neurocognitive side effects following ECT, except-
   (A)MRI Brain abnormalities
   (B)Old age
   (C)Male gender
   (D)Base line neurological disorder
5. Which of the following is an absolute contraindication for ECT?
   (A)Pregnancy
   (B)Presence of cardiac pacemaker
   (C)Intracranial space occupying lesion
   (D)None of the above

Answers:
1. B
   Cerletti and Bini first used ECT for therapeutic purpose.
2. C
   Fundamentally, the generation and behavior of the electrical stimulus can be conceptualized in terms of Ohm's law: V (voltage) = I (current) × R (resistance).
3. D
   Synaptic plasticity in hippocampus, including mossy fiber sprouting, alterations in cytoskeletal structure, increased connectivity in perforant pathways, the promotion of neurogenesis, and the suppression of apoptosis have been observed following ECT
4. B
   Those with baseline neurological disease, magnetic resonance imaging abnormalities, and baseline impairments in global cognitive functioning are more vulnerable to developing cognitive deficits, as are older and female patients.
5. D
   There is no absolute contraindication for ECT.

Reference:
1. Sadock B J, Sadock VA, Ruiz P. Kaplan &Sadock's Comprehensive Textbook of Psychiatry, 9th Edition; Lippincott Williams & Wilkins; 2009, Vol.2: 3285 – 3301.

ADVERSE EFFECT OF SSRIs
Dr. S. K. Kar, Assistant Professor, Department of Psychiatry

A 34 year old, married male of urban background was suffering from Generalized Anxiety Disorder since eight years for which he was on escitalopram 20 mg per day for last 2 years with adequate control of his anxiety symptoms. The patient had reported his libido was low for past one year and he was not able to experience pleasure as he used to before. Due to these problems, there was significant marital distress. There were no depressive symptoms, any other medical illness or psychosocial issues attributing to his current complaints. In follow up, the dose of escitalopram was reduced and sessions of cognitive behavior therapy were taken.

Relaxation breathing exercise and Jacobson's progressive muscular relaxation were taught. Over a period of two months, patient's symptoms had been improved significantly.

1. Which of the following selective serotonin reuptake inhibitor (SSRI) is the first SSRI to be introduced?
   (A) Paroxetine
   (B) Dapoxetine
   (C) Fluoxetine
   (D) Fluvoxamine
2. Which of the following SSRI is having highest efficacy?
   (A) Paroxetine
   (B) Fluvoxamine
   (C) Sertraline
   (D) All are equally effective
3. Which of the following SSRI is most effective in premature ejaculation?
   (A) Paroxetine
   (B) Sertraline
   (C) Escitalopram
   (D) Fluoxetine
4. Which of the following SSRI is having maximum anticholinergic side effect?
   (A) Paroxetine
   (B) Escitalopram
   (C) Fluvoxamine
   (D) Citalopram
5. All the following medications are effective in SSRI induced sexual dysfunction, except-
   (A) Amantadine
   (B) Buspirone
   (C) Propranolol
   (D) Cyproheptidine

Answers:

   1. C
      Fluoxetine is the first SSRI to be introduced.
   2. D
      All of the SSRIs, starting with fluoxetine and followed by sertraline, paroxetine, fluvoxamine, citalopram, and escitalopram, are equally effective.
   3. A
      In premature ejaculation, paroxetine may be the most useful of these drugs.
   4. A
      Paroxetine has the greatest affinity for muscarinic cholinergic receptors of the available SSRIs and therefore produces, in a small percentage of patients, dry mouth, constipation, blurred vision, or urinary hesitancy.
   5. C
      There have been a number of strategies suggested to deal with this important adverse effect, including decreased dose, drug holidays for shorter half-life SSRIs, or addition of buspirone, amantadine, yohimbine, cyproheptadine, stimulants, or bupropion.

Reference:
   1. Sadock B J, Sadock VA, Ruiz P. Kaplan &Sadock's Comprehensive Textbook of Psychiatry, 9th Edition; Lippincott Williams & Wilkins; 2009, Vol.2: 3190 – 3205.

ADVERSE EFFECTS OF ANTIPSYCHOTICS
Dr. S. K. Kar, Assistant Professor, Department of Psychiatry

A 42 year old non-diabetic, non-hypertensive, male was suffering from paranoid schizophrenia for last 10 years. He had complaints of hearing voices threatening him to kill, suspiciousness against family members, episodes of aggression and disturbed sleep. He was treated with risperidone (up to 8mg per day) for six months with partial control of symptoms, hence shifted to haloperidol. He was on haloperidol 20mg per day initial few months of initiation of treatment. Subsequently the dose of haloperidol was lowered down to 10 mg per day and for last seven years his symptoms were well controlled on this medication. However, the patient had grinding movement of jaw, abnormal darting movement of the tongue for last 2 years, which causes a lot of distress to the individuals. Patient's symptoms are suggestive of tardive dyskinesia.

1. Which of the following statement regarding tardive dyskinesia (TD) is incorrect?
   (A)Commonly involves the oro-facial musculature
   (B)Choreo-athetoid like limb and trunk movements may be seen
   (C)Hypoparathyroidism sometimes present with TD
   (D)It is mostly seen as an acute side effect of antipsychotic treatment
2. Which of the following factor is attributed to worsening of symptoms of TD?
   (A)Addition of atypical antipsychotic to the ongoing typical antipsychotic treatment.
   (B)Increase in the dose of antipsychotic medication
   (C)Withdrawl or stoppage of antiparkinsonian medication
   (D)Sudden stoppage of the antipsychotic medication
3. All the following statements regarding TD are incorrect except:
   (A)TD is due to decreased sensitivity of dopamine receptors at basal ganglia
   (B)TD does not appear to be a progressive disorder for most patients
   (C)Most patients improve in the severity of TD when FGAs are discontinued
   (D)All the above
4. Which of the following research tool is capable of picking the TD symptoms?
   (A)Simpson Angus Rating Scale (SARS)
   (B)Abnormal Involuntary Movement Scale (AIMS)
   (C)Barne'sAkathesia Rating Scale (BARS)
   (D)All of the above
5. Which of the following medication is effective in reducing the symptoms of TD?
   (A)Trihexyphenidyl
   (B)Propranolol
   (C)Clozapine
   (D)Procyclidine

Answers:
   1. D
      TD is mostly seen as a chronic side effect of antipsychotic treatment.
   2. D
      Decreasing the dose or Sudden stoppage of the antipsychotic medication worsens the symptoms of TD
   3. B
      TD does not appear to be a progressive disorder for most patients
   4. B
      Abnormal Involuntary Movement Scale (AIMS) is capable of picking symptoms of TD.
   5. C
      A trial of clozapine may be effective in TD.

Reference:
   1. Sadock B J, Sadock VA, Ruiz P. Kaplan &Sadock's Comprehensive Textbook of Psychiatry, 9th Edition; Lippincott Williams & Wilkins; 2009, Vol.2: 3105 – 3127.

GENDER DYSPHORIA
Dr. Adarsh Tripathi, Assistant Professor, Department Of Psychiatry

The parents of a 17 year old boy presented to the Psychiatry OPD with patient with the complaints that their boy behaves in a girlish way. They observed child's interest in female clothes, toys and play since early childhood. He would like to wear her sister's clothes and would often like to take female roles during play. He would also like company of girls more. Parents thought it to be a childish phenomenon and thought it to be a passing phase. However, behavior remained persistent and now this behaviour leads to frequent altercation with the boy. On interview, patient reported his desire to be a female and reported that its nature's mistake that he is a boy.

1. Clinical condition is best described as
   (A)Cross dressing disorder
   (B)Gender dysphoria
   (C)Intersex disorder
   (D)Paraphilia

2. All sentences are true about trans-genders except
   (A)It refers to those who identify with a gender different from the one they are born with
   (B)These are people diverse from those with genders dysphoria
   (C)Gender-queer feel that they are between genders, of both gender or of neither gender
   (D)Trans-genders are homosexuals i.e gay or lesbians
3. All of these syndromes can be related to intersex conditions except
   (A)Congenital adrenal hyperplasia
   (BAndrogen insensitivity syndrome
   (C)5-α-reductase deficiency
   (D)Angelman syndrome
4. True about transvestic disorders are all except
   (A)It is recurrent and intense sexual arousal from cross-dressing
   (B)Cross-dressing is pathognomonic of gender dysphoria
   (C)Gender dysphoria and transvestic disorders can be diagnosed together
   (D)It is more common in males
5. Girls with gender identity disorder in childhood, all are true except
   (A) Regularly has male companions
   (B) Usually avoids sports and rough-and-tumble play
   (C) Mmay assert that she has or will grow a penis
   (D) May give up masculine behavior by adolescence

Answers:
   1. B
      Gender dysphoria refers to those with a marked incongruence between their experienced or expressed gender and the one they were assigned at birth.
   2. D
      Transgenders may identify as homosexuals, straight, or bisexual.
   3. D
      There is normal sexual development in patients with Angelman syndrome.
   4. B
      Cross- dressing does not imply gender dysphoria. Many people who cross dress do so while retaining a gender identity that matches their assigned gender.
   5. B
      Girls with gender identity disorder (GID) in childhood regularly have male companions and an avid interest in sports and rough-and-tumble play.

Reference:
   1. Synopsis of Psychiatry, 11th edition, Chapter 18.

BORDERLINE PERSONALITY DISORDER
Dr. Adarsh Tripathi, Assistant Professor, Department of Psychiatry

An unmarried 28 years old unemployed female belonging to an upper middle class family was brought to the medical emergency by the family. She had attempted suicide by taking overdose of lorazepam. The patient was managed symptomatically and transferred to the Psychiatry department. On further evaluation she had history of frequent anger outbursts since early childhood. She left school after graduation and attempted few jobs but quickly left them because "people were idiots" there. She would quickly make relationships with people but often had fights with them as they would not be able to appreciate her abilities and were unable to understand her. She also had history of multiple superficial cuts and had frequent thoughts that she may be better off dead after a fight with somebody. She had few short lasting love affairs which she left after some time of their own. On interview, she was relaxed, comfortable and free from guilt over her act. She said that her life is like a roller coaster. She said that she is there to do something special. Another time she said it's no point in living like a failure. Family said that though she was the same from childhood, difficulties have increased for last few years.

1. What is the diagnosis of the case?
   (A)Bipolar affective disorder
   (B)Borderline personality disorder
   (C)Histrionic personality disorder
   (D)Major depressive disorder
2. Superficial cuts reported in the case are commonly called

(A)Dermatitis artifacta

(B)Self-induced skin lesions

(C)Hesitation cuts

(D)Plica polonica

3. All of the above are true for borderline personality disorder except

(A)Chronic feelings of emptiness

(B)Markedly and persistently unstable self-image or sense of self

(C)Comorbidity with mood disorder is rare

(D)May have micro-psychotic episodes in response to stress

4. All are true for the treatment of the personality disorders except

(A)Positive/negative counter-transference is common

(B)Personality disorders cannot be treated

(C)Direct advice on personal and social problems is often counterproductive

(D)Medications may be useful for treatment

5. Treatment of choice in patients with borderline personality disorder is

(A) Psychotherapy

(B) Anticonvulsants

(C) Antipsychotics

(D) Antidepressants

Answers:

1. B

Patients with borderline personality disorder are characterized by extraordinarily unstable affect, mood, behavior, object relations, and self-image.

2. D

The painful nature of lives of patients with borderline personality disorder is reflected in repetitive self-destructive acts. Such patients may slash their wrists and perform other self-mutilations to elicit help from others, to express anger, or to numb themselves to overwhelming affect.

3. C

Major depression is commonly comorbid with borderline personality disorder..

4. B

Personality disorders can be treated utilizing psychotherapy and pharmacotherapy.

5. B

Psychotherapy for patients with borderline personality disorder is an area of intensive investigation and has been the treatment of choice.

Reference:

1. Synopsis of psychiatry, 11th edition, page no. 742

VAGINISMUS

Dr. Adarsh Tripathi, Assistant Professor, Department Of Psychiatry

A 32 years old recently married female educated upto MBA and sales manager in a multinational brand store presented to the psychosexual OPD with her husband with complaints of inability to have intercourse since marriage. Detailed interview with the couple together and both of them separately revealed that couple is having mutually satisfying relationship and there are no conflicts in the family. Both the partners have adequate sexual desire. Husband is able to achieve satisfactory erection but he fails if he tries vaginal penetration. Wife reported that she has a fear of penetration. Though she enjoys sexual intimacy with her husband and was able to achieve orgasm on manual and oral stimulation. She denied history of premarital sexual relationship and possibility of sexual abuse. She has been raised by a religious and highly organised and strict disciplinarian father. She has earlier visited a gynaecologist who reassured that there is no local vaginal pathology. The couple is getting increasingly frustrated over their inability to have successful intercourse.

1. What is the diagnosis of this case

(A) Hypoactive sexual desire disorder

(B)Dyspareunia

(C)Vaginismus

(D)Orgasmic dysfunction

2. Following about the situation is correct except

(A)Results due to involuntary and persistent constriction of the outer one third of the vagina

665

(B)Medical/surgical factors are often the cause

(C)It most often afflicts highly educated women and those in the higher socioeconomic groups

(D)Many have problems in the dyadic relationship

3. Most common female sexual dysfunction is

    (A)Orgasmic dysfunction

    (B)Dyspareunia

    (C)Vaginismus .

    (D)Post coital headache

4. Medication which can commonly cause sexual dysfunction is

    (A)Clonazepam

    (B)Mirtazepine

    (C)Bupropion

    (D)Sertraline

5. Most appropriate treatment for the above case is

    (A)SSRI

    (B)Progressive muscular relaxation

    (C)Gradual exposure

    (D)Interpersonal therapy

Answers:

1. C

   Vaginismus is an involuntary muscle constriction of the outer third of the vagina that interferes with penile insertion and intercourse. Women with vaginismus may consciously wish to have coitus, but unconsciously wish to keep a penis from entering their bodies.

2. B

   The diagnosis is not made when the dysfunction is caused exclusively by organic factors.

3. A

   Orgasmic dysfunction, sometimes called inhibited female orgasm or anorgasmia.

4. D

   All the SSRIs cause sexual dysfunction, and it is one of the most common adverse effect of SSRIs associated with long-term treatment.

5. C

   In cases of vaginismus, a woman is advised to dilate her vaginal opening with her fingers or with size graduated dilators. Dilators are also used to treat cases of dyspareunia.

Reference:

1. Synopsis of Psychiatry, 11th edition, page no. 580

INSOMNIA

Dr. Adarsh Tripathi, Assistant Professor, Department of Psychiatry

A 42 years old female nurse presented to the Psychiatry OPD with complaints of having problems with sleep. She reported difficulty in initiating sleep and feeling of non-restorative sleep in the morning. She would report difficulty in concentrating on the work and increased irritability in the morning. She would deny pervasive sadness and excessive worry except that of sleep. She would frequently feel increased anxiety before the night which often increased once she would lie down to sleep in her bedroom. Her problems started with her posting in an ICU with irregular working shifts 4 year back. Now she is working in another department with relatively less work and stable day time shift. She had unsuccessfully tried using benzodiazepine of her own which made her condition even worse with day time drowsiness.

1. What is the diagnosis of this case?

    (A)Adjustment disorder

    (B)Insomnia

    (C)Parasomnia

    (D)Pathological worry

2. All of the sentences about normal sleep are true except

    (A)NREM sleep is divided in 4 phases

    (B)Brain activity in REM sleep is low

    (C)Normal REM latency is 90 minutes in adult

    (D)REM sleep is also known as "Paradoxical Sleep"

3. True about insomnia is
   (A)It is a rare disorder
   (B)Excessive worry about sleep is uncommon
   (C)Often involve a conditioned associative response
   (D)Decreased muscle tension while trying to sleep is common
4. Treatment of insomnia involves all except
   (A)Ramelteon has been approved for sleep onset insomnia
   (B)Inadequate sleep hygiene needs to be targeted in every case
   (C)Cognitive behaviour therapy has no definite role in treatment
   (D)Melatonin is used in self-administered food additives to help sleep
5. Stimulus control therapy involves all the steps except
   (A)Go to bed only feeling sleepy
   (B)Leave bed if unable to sleep for few minutes and do something non stimulating till one feels sleepy again
   (C)Awaken at the same time every morning
   (D)Persons are allowed to do activities like watching TV, talking on phone while on the bed

Answers:
1. B
   Insomnia is difficulty initiating or maintaining sleep.
2. B
   Polygraphic measures during REM sleep show irregular patterns, sometimes close to aroused waking patterns. Brain oxygen use increases during REM sleep.
3. D
   Insomnia may have features including increased muscle tension when attempting to sleep, trying too hard to sleep, excessive worry about not being able to sleep and inability to clear one's mind while trying to sleep
4. C
   Studies repeatedly show significant, sustained improvement in sleep symptoms, including number and duration of awakenings and sleep latency from CBT.
5. D
   The bed should be used only for sleeping. Do not watch television in bed, do not read, do not eat, and do not talk on the telephone while in bed.

Reference:
1. Synopsis of Psychiatry, 11th edition, Chapter 16

±

FACTITIOUS DISORDER
Dr. Bandna Gupta, Assistant Professor, Department of Psychiatry

A 25-year-old, married man presented in medical OPD with complaints of square-shaped burns on his left forearm. Two weeks earlier, the patient had been admitted for necrotizing fasciitis of the right forearm as per the discharge summary he had presented. He reported a past medical history of juvenile-onset diabetes from age 1 year, asthma, and accidental hot water burns to his left forearm and left lateral thigh at 10 years of age. He reported allergies to 13 medications.

He described his childhood as "good," and he denied a history of physical or sexual abuse. He said his father died of a fall when he was 10 years of age. He proudly stated that even though he was diabetic, he was admitted to the Air Force at age 18 years, where he worked as a mechanic. Subsequently, he worked at commercial airlines. He stated that he was currently married for the second time. While he was married to his first wife, he said, he lost a son, a daughter, and his marriage all in one day: His 4-year-old daughter was in the hospital dying of a blood cancer; on his way to visit her, his 7-year-old son was killed in a road traffic mishappening; and under the stress of losing both children, his first wife left him that same day.

He remarried, and his second wife was a chain smoker. The records of one hospital, when traced, stated that he had claimed to have been a fighter pilot in navy. Two days after discharge from that hospital, he had to be readmitted and treated for necrosis of a skin graft.

One month later, when he was readmitted for worsening necrotizing fasciitis, he requested amputation of his arm, citing his long treatment course and the wish to be rid of the pain. It was noted that his arm healed whenever it was placed in a tight cast that prevented tampering with the lesions but worsened when it was placed in looser casts. During hospital stay, he received no insulin, and his blood glucose remained within normal range.

Upon psychiatric consultation, he was diagnosed to be suffering from factitious disorder.

The week after discharge, the patient presented with eagerness to seek treatment for his wife, whom he reported to be suffering from lung cancer.

Subsequently, he presented several times to the psychiatric emergency services complaining of urges to be violent toward his wife. For the next 4 months, he was admitted to various hospitals in town and everywhere he continued to deny that his wounds were self-inflicted.

1. Factitious disorder
   (A)Occurs more frequently in women than in men
   (B)Is not associated with economic gain
   (C)May result in death due to needless medical interventions
   (D)All of the above
2. Ganser's syndrome
   (A)Is a factitious disorder
   (B)Is associated with a severe personality disorder
   (C)Has a chronic remitting and relapsing course
   (D)Is motivated by involuntary phenomena
3. Which of the following symptoms would a patient with Munchausen syndrome most likely present with?
   (A)Depression
   (B)Amnesia
   (C)Hemoptysis
   (D)Psychosis
4. Which of the following is the gold standard for diagnosis of factitious disorder by proxy?
   (A)Discovery of illness-inducing agents in the caregiver's possession
   (B)Finding inconsistencies in the medical records
   (C)Improvement when the child is removed from the caretaker
   (D)Direct observation of the caretaker doing harm
5. Management of Factitious Disorder includes all except
   (A)Avoid unnecessary tests and procedures
   (B)Facilitating healing by using the double-bind technique
   (C)Appoint a care provider as a gatekeeper for all kind of treatments pursued
   (D)Prefer aggressive direct confrontation

Answers:

1. D

   It occurs more frequently in women than in men, and the severe syndromes are more frequent in women. The motivation for the behavior is to assume the sick role, and external incentives, such as economic gain, avoiding legal responsibility, or improving physical well-being, as in malingering, are absent.

2. B

   It was previously classified as a factitious disorder but is commonly associated with dissociative phenomena such as amnesia, fugue, perceptual disturbances, and conversion symptoms and is thus classified as a dissociative disorder.

3. C

   Munchausen syndrome is another name for factitious disorder with predominantly physical signs and symptoms. The other choices listed-depression, amnesia, and psychosis-are common presentations of patients with factitious disorder with predominantly psychological signs and symptoms.

4. D

   Direct observation of the caretaker doing harm is the gold standard for diagnosis of factitious disorder by proxy.

5. D

   Steer the patient toward psychiatric treatment in an empathic, nonconfrontational, face-saving manner.

Reference:

1. Dora L.Wang etal Factitious disorder in Kaplan and Sadock's Comprehensive Textbook of Psychiatry, 9th ed., vol. 1, pp. 1949–11964. Philadelphia: Lippincott Williams and Wilkins.

SLEEP DISORDER

Dr. Bandna Gupta,Assistant Professor, Department of Psychiatry

A 25-year-old female was referred with symptoms of muttering, talking and crying out during sleep. She screamed in her sleep at least two to three times in a week. She was often bothered by excessive sleepiness and falling asleep inappropriately, such as during a meeting. When inactive, she was tired and sleepy, even after a full 8-hour night of sleep. However, she did not have any depressive symptoms. Once, she awakened outside her house in the street and the lock had to be broken because she had locked herself out. She could not recall the events preceding her awakening. She also remembered that occasionally she was told by her mother that she yelled loudly in sleep calling out people by their names. From the history, crying seemed to occur in light sleep, but she rarely recalled any sleep-related thoughts or dreams. However, there was a history of occasions when she would get up from her sleep after having a 'bad' dream which she could recall. Leg kicking and mild snoring without gasping or choking were noted. The patient also complained of leg kicking during sleep. Her sleep–wake schedule was irregular, and she averaged between 4 and 8 hours of sleep per night. Irrespective of sleep duration, she occasionally awakened with a headache in the morning.

Previous health history included a hospitalization for febrile convulsions during infancy. There was no history of any other major medical or surgical illness. The patient did not smoke tobacco or drink alcohol. Polysomnography with clinical EEG was done to rule out unrecognized nocturnal seizure disorder or other organic factors. She was diagnosed to be suffering from Parasomnias which included somnambulism, nightmares and somniloquy.

1. Which of the following is a component of good sleep hygiene?
   (A) Arise at the same time daily
   (B) Eat larger meals near bedtime
   (C) Take daytime naps as needed
   (D) Establish physical fitness with exercise in the evening
2. A dysfunction in the hypocretin system plays a critical role in which of the following disorders?
   (A) Insomnia
   (B) Sleepwalking
   (C) Restless legs syndrome
   (D) Narcolepsy
3. Anatomical sites implicated in the generation of NREM sleep include
   (A) The medulla
   (B) The dorsal raphe nucleus
   (C) The basal forebrain area
   (D) All of the above
4. Which of the following features is not typical of REM sleep?
   (A) Dreams are typically concrete and realistic.
   (B) Polygraph measures show irregular patterns.
   (C) The resting muscle potential is lower in REM sleep than in a waking state.
   (D) Near-total paralysis of the postural muscles is present.
5. Sleep latency is defined as
   (A) The period of time from the onset of sleep until the first sleep spindle
   (B) The period of time from the onset of sleep until the first REM period of the night
   (C) The period of time from turning out the lights until the appearance of stage 2 sleep
   (D) The time of being continuously awake from the last stage of sleep until the end of the sleep record

Answers:

1. A
   Maintain regular hours of bedtime and arising.
2. D
   Patients with narcolepsy are deficient in the neurotransmitter hypocretin.
3. D
   All of the above
4. A
   Dreams during REM sleep are typically abstract and surreal.
5. C
   Common polysomnographic measures are used to diagnose and describe sleep disorders. Sleep latency is the period of time from turning out the lights until the appearance of stage 2 sleep.

References:

1. Max Harshkowitetal .Sleep Disorder. Kaplan and Sadock's Comprehensive Textbook of Psychiatry, 9th ed., vol. 1, pp. 2150–2177. Philadelphia: Lippincott Williams and Wilkins.
2. Kaplan BJ, Kaplan VA. Kaplan and Sadock's Synopsis of Psychiatry: Behavioral Sciences/Clinical Psychiatry. 11th ed. Philadelphia, Pa: Lippincott Williams & Wilkins;

Chapter-24

Radiodiagnosis

CHRONIC LIVER DISEASE
Dr. Anit Parihar and Prof. Neera Kohli Department of Radiodiagnosis

A 42 year old chronic alcoholic came to the casualty with vomiting of dark red blood along with clots and loss of appetite for threemonths. There was yellowish discoloration of eyes with presence of ascites and splenomegaly. Hisserum bilirub in was raised and serum albumin was decreased. On nasogastric intubation 200ml of dark blood was aspirated. His ultrasound abdomen showed

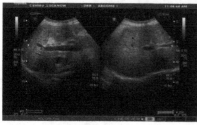 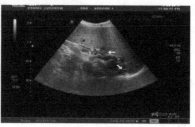

1. What is clinical diagnosis?
    (A) Peptic ulcer
    (B) Chronic liver disease with portal hypertension.
    (C) Erosive gastritis
    (D) Mallory Weis tear
2. Criteria to assess the scenario mentioned above:-
    (A) Ransons criteria
    (B) Modified CT severity scoring
    (C) Child pug scoring system
    (D) Alvardo scoring
3. All are true about the scenario mentioned above except:-
    (A) Increased resistance to blood flow in portal vein
    (B) Portal vein pressure > 12 mm hg
    (C) Most common cause is usually chronic liver disease
    (D) Rarely associated with splenomegaly &hyperdynamic circulation
4. All are true about treatment options of the scenario mentioned above except:-
    (A) Sclerotheraphy and band legation in acute variceal blooding
    (B) Vasopressor along with ongoing endoscopic therapy
    (C) Propranalol in acute variceal bleed
    (D) Sometimes portal vein shunting
5. Absolute Contra indication of liver transplantation in the scenario mentioned above are all except :-
    (A) Multisystem organ failure
    (B) Advanced cardiac / pulmonary disease
    (C) Extrabiliary malignancy
    (D) Hemochromatosis

Answers:
1. B
    History of alchohol; malena, jaundice, decreased S. bilirubin- on usg finding coarse liver with dilated portal vein with Splenomegaly with multiple collaterals along splenic hila s/o CLD with portal hypertension.
2. C
    Ransons criteria and modeified CT severity scoring – acute pancreatitis. Alvardo scoring – Acute appendicitis.
    Child pug scoring – Liver disease.
3. D
    Very commonly associated with Splenomegaly and hperdynamic circulation.
4. C
    Propranalol is used in chronic variceal bleed, not in acute cases.
5. D
    Hemochromatosis – Is a relative contraindication.

Reference:

1. Wilson S R , Withers CE . The Liver.In :Rumack CM, Wilson SR , Charboneau JW, Levine D, Editors. Diagnostic ultrasound . 4th ed. Vol 1, 2005 p. 78 -141

CARCINOMA GALLBLADDER

Dr. Anit Parihar and Prof Neera Kohli Department of Radiodiagnosis

A 40 years old female presented with lump in abdomen, on and off vomiting, jaundice and loss of appetite for last one month. On examination a lump was present in right upper abdomen along with icterus. On investigation his hemoglobin was decreased & serum bilirubin was raised.

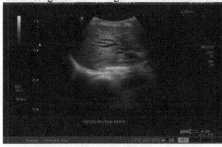
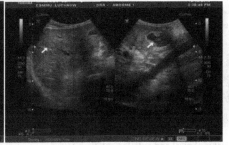

1.What is clinical and radiological Diagnosis:
   (A) Carcinoma gall bladder
   (B) Cholecystitis with cholelithiasis
   (C) Periampullary carcinoma
   (D) Choledocholithiasis

2. Ultrasonography finding in the scenario mentioned above are all except:-
   (A) Diffuse gall bladder wall thickening with increased vascularity
   (B) Gall stone are very rarely associated with Carcinoma Gall bladder.
   (C) Carcinoma gall bladder neck can leads to intra hepatic biliary radical dilatation.
   (D) Carcinoma Gall bladder is associated with retroperitoneal lymphadenopathy

3. Most common site of metastases in the scenario mentioned above is:-
   (A) Liver
   (B) Lung
   (C) Bone
   (D) Brain

4. Which of the following is true about liver metastases:-
   (A) LFT & Ultrasonography used for definitive diagnosis
   (B) 5 yr. survival rate for liver cancer is 15 -20 %
   (C) Primary cancer of liver are much more common than secondary
   (D) Beta HCG& CEA are better predictor than AFP.

5. Best chemotherapeutic agent in the condition mentioned above is :-
   (A) Pacletaxel
   (B) 5 –F U
   (C) Gemcitabine
   (D) Bleomycin.

Answers:

1. A
   Lump in abdomen with jaundice with loss of apetite, on usg finding hypoechoiec lesion noted in gall bladder with multiple mets in liver with gross bilobar IHBRD s/o carcinoma gall bladder.
2. B
   gall stone are very commonly associated with carcinoma gall bladder (80 to 90 % cases).
3. A
4. B
   Definite diagnosis is made by biopsy.Secondaries are much more common than primary cancer of liver
5. C

Reference:

1. Khalili K , Wilson S .The biliary tree and gall bladder. In: Rumack CM, Wilson SR , Charboneau JW, Levine D, Editors. Diagnostic ultrasound .4thedtionVol 1, 2005 p. 172 – 215

PYOGENIC LIVER ABSCESS

Dr. Anit Parihar and Prof. Neera Kohli Department of Radiodiagnosis

A 40 years old alcoholic male presented with chief complaints of right upper abdominal pain, high grade fever and on & off vomiting. On examination mild tender hepatomegaly was present. His total leucocyte count and serum alkaline phosphatase were raised. His Ultrasound showed

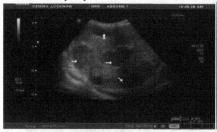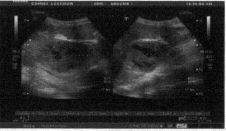

1. What is clinical and radiological diagnosis:-
   (A) Hydatid cyst
   (B) Amoebic liver abscess
   (C) Metastasis with necrotic changes
   (D) Pyogenic liver abscess
2. Most common causative organism related to the lesion showed above is :-
   (A) Staphylococus
   (B) Gram – ve bacilli
   (C) Anerobes
   (D) Echinococcus
3. Pyogenic liver abscess can be differentiated from amoebic liver abscess by:-
   (A)Multiple lesions, jaundice less common , Normal ALP & bilirubin
   (B) Single lesion, Normal ALP and bilirubin, resolves by antibiotics only
   (C) Single lesion, Normal ALP & bilirubin.
   (D) Multiple lesions jaundice more common, increased ALP.
4. Best combination of antibiotic in the lesion showed above is:-
   (A) IIIrd generation cephalosporin + metronidazole
   (B) Azithromycin + metronidazole
   (C) Penicillin + metronidazole
   (D) Linezolid + metronidazole
5. Treatment of choice in the lesion showed above is:-
   (A)Conservative with oral antibiotics
   (B)Open surgery
   (C)IV antibiotics
   (D)Ultrasonography guided p/c neddle aspiration / drainage + IV antibiotics

Answers:
1. D
    History of alcohol, high grade fever, pain, tenderness in right hypochondrium on usg finding multiple hypoechoic lesion with anechoic component noted in liver s/o pyogenic liver abscess. (Amebic liver abscess are generally single instead of being multiple.
2. B
3. D
    Pyogenic liver abscess – multiple, jaundice more common, increased ALP. Amoebic liver abscess – single, jaundice less common, normal / increased ALP.
4. A
5. D

Reference:
1. Wilson S R , Withers CE .The Liver .In : Rumack CM, Wilson SR , Charboneau JW, Levine D, editors.Diagnostic ultrasound . 4th edtion.Vol 1, 2005 p. 78 -141

FATTY LIVER

Dr. Anit Parihar and Prof. Neera Kohli Department of Radiodiagnosis

A 45 yr old obese female presented with right upper abdominal discomfort for 3 months. She had been a diabetic for 5 years. Her ultrasound abdomen showed enlarged liver with diffuse hyperechoic echotexture. On examination hepatomegaly was present. On investigation her Low Density Lipoprotein was increased and High Density Lipoprotein was decreased.

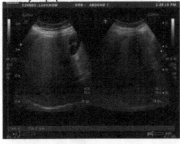

1. What is clinical and radiological diagnosis:-
    (A) Hepatitis
    (B) Chronic liver diseases
    (C) Alcoholic liver diseases
    (D) Nonalcoholic fatty liver
2. All are true in the condition mentioned above except:-
    (A) Frequently associated with obesity, type II DM
    (B) Patient are generally asymptomatic
    (C) AST / ALT > 2
    (D) Hyperbilirubinemia, prologation of PT &hypoalbuminea are uncommon.
3. All drugs can cause the condition mentioned above except:-
    (A) Corticosteroids
    (B) Metformin
    (C) Methotrexate.
    (D) Amiodarone
4. Definitive diagnosis of the condition mentioned above is made by:-
    (A) Raised liver enzymes
    (B) Ultrasonography
    (C) CECT & MRI
    (D) Liver biopsy
5. All are treatment options in the condition mentioned above except-
    (A) Diet & weight controll
    (B) Insulin sensitiser (Metformin)
    (C) Vitamin E &ursodeoxycholic acid
    (D) Trans fat along with corticosteroid

Answers:
1. D
    History of obesity, diabetes, fatigue, discomfort, lipid profile – decreased HDL, increased LDL, on usg finding mild hepatomegaly with increased echogenicity of liver s/o non alcoholic fatty liver.
2. C
    AST / ALT > 2 – s/o alcoholic liver disease
    AST / ALT < 1 – NASH
3. B
    Metformin is used as insulin senstizer it decreases obesity so it is used in treatment of NASH .while other drugs can cause fatty liver

4. D
5. D

Trans fat & corticosteroids can cause fatty liver.

References:

1. Wilson S R , Withers CE .The Liver .In : Rumack CM, Wilson SR , Charboneau JW, Levine D,editorsDiagnostic ultrasound. 4thedtion.Vol 1, 2005 p. 78 -141

HYDATID CYST

Dr. Anit Parihar and Prof. Neera Kohli Department of Radiodiagnosis

A 35 years old female presented with dull abdominal pain, & palpable mass in umblical region. No history of fever was present. His ultrasound showed

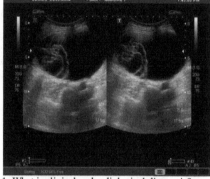

1. What is clinical and radiological diagnosis?
   (A) Pseudopancreatic cyst.
   (B) Mesenteric hydatid cyst.
   (C) Mesenteric abscess.
   (D) Loculated ascites (Tubercular)
2. Most common site of the lesion showed above is
   (A) Liver
   (B) Lung
   (C) Mesentry
   (D) Spleen
3. All are the layers of the lesion showed above except ?
   (A)Pericyst
   (B)Exocyst
   (C)Epicyst
   (D)Endocyst
4. Which test is used for the lesion mentioned above is?
   (A)Frei test
   (B)Casoni skin test
   (C)Weil Felix test
   (D)Patch test
5. Water lily sign is present in :
   (A)Mesenteric cyst
   (B)Hydatid cyst
   (C)Pancreatic pseudocyst
   (D)Splenic pseudocyst.

Answers:
1. B

   History of abdominal pain with compressible mass in umbilical region, on usg finding – thick walled cystic lesion with multiple infolded membrane s/o mesenteric hydatid cyst
2. A
3. C

   Epicyst is not a layer of hydatid cyst
4. B

Frei test – LGV

Explanation: Patch test – contact dermatitis , Weil felix test – Rickettsia
5. B

Reference:
1. Wilson S R , Withers CE .The Liver .In : Rumack CM, Wilson SR , Charboneau JW, Levine D,editors.Diagnostic ultrasound. 4[th]edtion.Vol 1, 2005 p. 78 -141

LEIOMYOMA UTERUS
Dr. Anit Parihar and Prof. Neera Kohli Department of Radiodiagnosis

A 35 Years old married woman presented with chief complaint of menorrhagia and dysmenorrhea. On Ultrasonography, uterus was noted to be bulky with distorted contour. A heterogenous and predominantly hypoechoic lesion was noted in the myometrium with peripheral vascularity

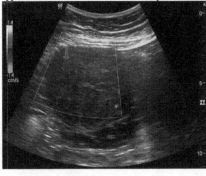

1. What is the most likely diagnosis?
   (A) Leiomyoma
   (B) Polyp
   (C) Adenomyoma
   (D) Myometrial Cyst

   Fibroid is the most common neoplasm of uterus. They occur in 20 to 30% of females over age of 30 yrs. Although frequent ltasymptomatic woman with leiomyomas can experience excessibe bleeding and pain.Typical USG findings—Hypoechoic or heterogeneous mass,distortion of uterine contour, attenuation or shadowing without discrete mass,calcification,degeneration or necrosisOn Doppler peripheral vascularity of the lesion.In the above case we have clinical features as most of USG findings present indicating the most probable diagnosis as Fibroid

2. What is the most common form of above showed lesion :-
   (A) Submucosal
   (B) Intramural
   (C) Subserosal
   (D) Intraligamentous

3. Which of the following drug can result in the growth of above showed lesion:-
   (A) Tamoxifen
   (B) Daunorubicin
   (C) (Methotrexate)
   (D) Iminatib

4. What is best modality for better differentiation between submucosal and intramural lesion and its relationship to endometrial cavity:-
   (A) TVS
   (B) Trans Abdominal Ultrasound
   (C) HSG
   (D) CT

5. Treatment of choice is of above showed lesion :-
   (A) Myomectomy
   (B) Hysterectomy
   (C) Hormonal therapy
   (D) Uterus artery ligation

BICORNUATE UTERUS

Dr. Anit Parihar and Prof. Neera Kohli Department of Radiodiagnosis

A 25 Years old woman presented with chief complaint of repeated abortions. On ultrasonography, 2 endometrial cavities were seen. The endometrial cavities were widely separated and there was a deep indention on fundal contour.

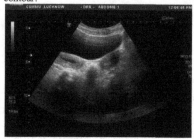

1. What is the probable diagnosis :-
   (A) Arcuate uterus
   (B) Bicornuate Uterus
   (C) Unicornuate Uterus
   (D) Septate uterus
2. What is the current imaging modality of choice for the above condition:-
   (A) Abdominal Ultrasonography
   (B) HSG
   (C) CT
   (D) MRI
3. Additional test should be done because of the woman increased risk of congenital anomalies in which system:-
   (A) Skeletal
   (B) Haematopoietic
   (C) Urinary
   (D) CNS
4. It belongs to which class of Mullerian duct anomaly
   (A) I
   (B) II
   (C) III
   (D) IV

5. What is the treatment of choice for the above condition
   (A) Laprotomy
   (B) Laproscopic assisted transvaginalmetroplasty
   (C) Medical
   (D) None of the above

Answers:
   1. B
   2. D
   3. C
   4. D
   5. B

References:
   1. Salem S .Gynecology. In :: Rumack CM, Wilson SR , Charboneau JW, Levine D,editors Diagnostic ultrasound. 4thedtion.Vol 1, 2005 p. 547 to 612
   2. Chandler TM, Machan LS et al.Mullerian duct anomalies : from diagnosis to intervention. Br J Radiol.2009 dec; 82(984): p.1034-1042

POLYCYSTIC OVARIAN DISEASE
Dr. Anit Parihar and Prof. Neera Kohli Department of Radiodiagnosis

A 20 Years old female presented with oligomenorrhea and increased growth of facial hair. on Ultrasonography bilateral ovaries were found to be enlarged with multiple peripherally arranged follicles (>12) and echogenic stroma.

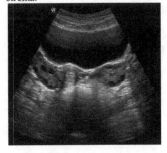

1. What is the most likely diagnosis:-
   (A) Hyperthyroidism
   (B) Hirsutism
   (C) Ovarian hyperthecosis
   (D) PCOD

   PCOD is a common cause of infertility.Clinical manifestations of PCOS range mild sign of hyperandrogenism in thin,normally menstruating women to classic stein-Leventhal syndrome(oligomenorrhea or amenorrhea,hirsutism and obesity) The typical sonographic finding are bilaterally enlarged ovaries containing multiple small follicles and increased stromal echogenicity.Also diagnosis of polycystic ovaries should have either 12 or more follicles measuring 2 to 9 mm in diameter or increased ovarian vol greater than 10 cc.12 or more than 12 follicles is the best diagnostic criterion.

   In above case we see most of these

2. For the above condition which of the following statement is correct:-
   (A) LH/FSH ratio increased
   (B) LH/FSH ratio Decreased
   (C) Both increased
   (D) LH/FSH remains unchanged

3. What further test would you advise :-
   (A) Hormone analysis
   (B) MRI
   (C) TVS
   (D) None of the alone

4. Long term follow up is recommended in patients with above condition because unopposed high estrogen level appears to be associated with increased risk of :-
   (A) Endometrial and Breast CA
   (B) Cervical CA
   (C) Ovarian carcinoma
   (D) None of the above
5. Classical stein Leventhal syndrome includes:-
   (A) Oligomenorrhea or amenorrhea,hirsutism and obesity
   (B) Polymenorrhea, hirsutism and cachexia'
   (C) Convulsion,obesity and dysmenorrheal
   (D) None of the above

Answers:
   1. D
   2. A
   3. A
   4. A
   5. A

Reference:
   1. Salem S .Gynecology. In :Rumack CM, Wilson SR , Charboneau JW, Levine D,editors. Diagnostic ultrasound. 4[th]edtion.Vol 1, 2005 p. 547 to 612

ENDOMETRIOSIS

Dr. Anit Parihar and Prof. Neera Kohli Department of Radiodiagnosis

28 year old woman presented with chief complaint of dysmenorrhea and dyspareunia. She also complained that she was unable to conceive. On Ultrasonography well defined unilocular, predominantly cystic mass containing diffuse low level internal echoes noted in right ovary.

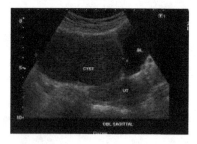

1. What is the likely diagnosis?
   (A)Ovarian malignancy.
   (B)Parovarian cyst
   (C)PCOD
   (D)Endometriosis
2. Most common site for above condition is:-
   (A)Ovary
   (B)Uterus
   (C)Broad ligament
   (D)Peritoneal cavity
3. Above mentioned condition commonly affects women in:-
   (A) Reproductive age
   (B) Post menopausal
   (C) Below 15 years
   (D) Between 5th and 7th decade
4. Localised form of above mentioned condition is known as:-
   (A)Dermoid cyst
   (B)Chocolate cyst
   (C)Parovarian cyst

(D)None of the above
5. Medical management of the above condition is:-
    (A) Combination oral contraceptive pill
    (B) Danazol
    (C) Progestational agents
    (D) All the above

Answers:
    1. D

        PCOD is a common cause of infertility.Clinical manifestations of PCOS range mild sign of hyperandrogenism in thin,normally menstruating women to classic stein-Leventhal syndrome(oligomenorrhea or amenorrhea,hirsutism and obesity) The typical sonographic finding are bilaterally enlarged ovaries containing multiple small follicles and increased stromal echogenicity.Also diagnosis of polycystic ovaries should have either 12 or more follicles measuring 2 to 9 mm in diameter or increased ovarian vol greater than 10 cc.12 or more than 12 follicles is the best diagnostic criterion.

    2. A
    3. A
    4. B
    5. D

Reference:
    1. Salem S .Gynecology. In: Rumack CM, Wilson SR , Charboneau JW, Levine D,editorsDiagnostic ultrasound. 4[th]edtion.Vol 1, 2005 p. 547 to 612

PLACENTA PRAEVIA
Dr. Anit Parihar and Prof. Neera Kohli Department of Radiodiagnosis

A pregnant patient G2P1L1 with a history of LSCS in previous pregnancy present with complaints of sudden onset painless vaginal bleeding. Her ultrasound showed

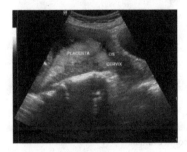

1. What is your diagnosis on the basis on history and Ultrasonography examination
    (A)Placenta praevia
    (B)Abruptio placenta
    (C)Vasa praevia
    (D)Cervical erosion
2. Which test you use to distinguish between maternal and fetal blood?
    (A)APT test
    (B)Kleihauerbetke test
    (C)Bubbin test
    (D)Coomb"s test
3. False statement regarding above mention condition
    (A)Associated with toxemia
    (B)Painless recurrent bleeding
    (C)Maternal blood loss
    (D)Severe bleeding may occur
4. Stallworthy's sign is suggestive of
    (A)Low lying placenta
    (B)Abruptio placenta

(C)Vasa praevia

(D)Cervical erosion

5. In above mention scenario, the regimen use for expectant management is

    (A)Macafee and Johnson regimen

    (B)Page regimen

    (C)McDonald"s regimen

    (D)Brandt Andrew method

Answers:

    1. A

    2. A

    3. A

    4. A

    5. A

Reference:

    1. DUTTA DC. Text book of obstetrics 7[th]edition 2011. Antepartum hemorrhage ,p. 241 -260

TWIN PREGNANCY

Dr. Anit Parihar and Prof. Neera Kohli Department of Radiodiagnosis

A 27 year old female G3P2L2, came for routine antenatal check up. On physical examination uterine fundal height was not corresponding with gestational age. Patient ultrasonography was done which showed a large for date uterus with two sacs with fetal parts separated by intervening membrane.

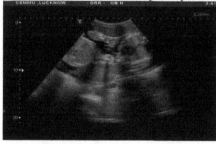

1. What is your diagnosis on the basis of patient history and ultrasonography.

    (A) Wrong date

    (B) Polyhydromnios

    (C)Twin pregnancy

    (D)Red degeneration in fibroid

2. For establishing the diagnosis of monochorionicity which sign we should evaluate

    (A) Twin peak sign

    (B) T sign

    (C) Lambda sign

    (D) None is helpful

3. One yolk sac with two embryos in early gestation signifies

    (A) Monoamniotic twin

    (B) Diamniotic twin

    (C) Dichorionic twin

    (D) Fetal demise

4. Most common type of conjoint twin

    (A) Thoracopagus

    (B) Ischiopagus

    (C) Craniopagus

    (D) Omphalopagus

5. If division of fertilized egg occur at 4TH to 8TH day ,what kind of monozygotic twin pregnancy will it give rise to

    (A) Diamnioticdichorionic

    (B) Diamnioticmonochorionic

(C) Monoamnioticmonochorionic

(D) Conjoint twin

Answers:
1. C
2. B
   Twin peak sign/lambda sign indicate dichorionicity
   T sign indicate monochorionicity
3. A
4. A
   Thoracophagus is most common type of conjoint twin followed by omphalopagus
5. B
   Before 4 days zygote cleave result in dichorionicdiamniotic twin
   Between 4 – 8 th day inner cell mass ckeaves result in monochorionicdiamniotic twin 8-12 day
   embryonic disc cleaves result in monochorionicmonoamniotic twin.

References:
1. Mehta TS , Multifetal pregnancy.In :Rumack CM, Wilson SR , Charboneau JW, Levine D,editors.
   Diagnostic ultrasound. 4th edtion.Vol 2, 2005 . p. 1145 to 1165

OLIGOHYDRAMNIOS
Dr. Anit Parihar and Prof. Neera Kohli Department of Radiodiagnosis

A 27 year old patient come for routine antenatal check up, on examination uterine size is noted to be smaller
than period of amenorrhea. Obstetrician advice Ultrasonography for assessment of fetal well being and
amniotic fluid index showed largest pocket<2 cm in diameter.

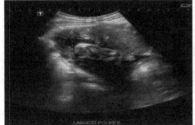

1. On the basis of clinical examination and Ultrasonography what is your diagnosis
   (A) IUGR
   (B) Oligohydramnias
   (C) Wrong date
   (D) Polyhydramnias
2. For defining above mention condition sonograhically vertical pocket of liquor and amniotic fluid index is
   less than
   (A) 2 and 5
   (B) 4 and 6
   (C) 3 and 10
   (D) 1 and 5
3. On the basis of amount of liquor oligohydromnias and polyhydroamnias is defined as
   (A) < 200 and > 2000 ml
   (B) < 500 and > 2000 ml
   (C) < 200 and > 1500 ml
   (D) < 100 and > 1000 ml
4. What is the major source of amniotic fluid in late 2nd and 3rd trimester
   (A) Transudation of fluid from maternal serum
   (B) Transudation of fluid from fetal plasma
   (C) Fetal urine
   (D) Secretion from amniotic epithelium
5 Above mention condition can be associated with all except
   (A) Renal agenesis
   (B) Obstructive uropathy

(C) Post maturity

(D) Chorangioma of placenta

Answers:

1. B

Largest pocket seen on ultrasound is 1.73cm (is less than 2 cm)

2. A

3. A

4. C

5. D

Reference:

1. DUTTA DC. Multiple fetal pregnancy, hydramnias and abnormalities of placenta and cord In: Text book of obstetrics 7thedition 2011. p 200-218

NEUROCYSTICERCUS

Dr. Anit Parihar and Prof. Neera Kohli Department of Radiodiagnosis

A young male patient presented with complaints of recurrent seizure for last 6 months with headache. MRI Brain scan showed multiple ring enhancing lesions as showed in the figure.

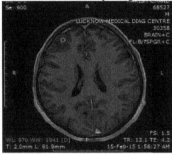

1. This appearance can be found in:-

(A) Neurocysticercosis

(B) Cavernous angioma

(C) Both

(D) None

2. Not true regarding the lesion described above:-

(A) It has 5 stages

(B) Absence of enhancement in typical of nodular calcified stage

(C) Cyst with dot inside

(D) None

Most sensitive tool for tuberculoma :-

(A) NCCT

(B) CECT

(C) MRI

(D) MRA

4. Differential of Ring enhancing lesion can be all except:

(A) Metastasis

(B) Abscess

(C) Inflammatory granuloma

(D) Meningioma

5. All are the stages of above mentioned lesion except:

(A) Vesicular

(B) Nodular calcified

(C) colloidal vesicular

(D) villous

Answers:

1. A

2. A
   4 stages of NCC:
   Vesicular stage
   Colloidal vesicular stage
   Granular nodular stage
   Nodular calcified stage
3. C
4. D
5. D

Reference:

1. Osborn AG.Tuberculosis ,fungal,parasitic and other infections. In:Renlund AR et al.editor Osborn's Brain imaging, pathology and anatomy. edition 1ˢᵗ 2013 p. 337-374

MENINGIOMA

Dr. Anit Parihar and Prof. Neera Kohli Department of Radiodiagnosis

A 38 year old female patient presented with severe headache for 2 months for which CT and MRI scans were done. MRI shows a homogenously enhancing extraxial mass lesion as shown below-

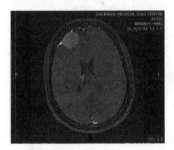

1. Dural tail sign is
   (A) Infolding of dura into the mass
   (B) Thickened and contrast enhancing dura at the periphery of mass.
   (C) CSF trapped between layers of dura adjacent to mass
   (D) De novo neoplasm developing in dura near the primary mass
2. Which of the following is not a sign of these lesions:-
   (A) CSF left around the lesion
   (B) Displacement of gray white matter interface
   (C) Lesion surrounded by brain parenchyma all sides
   (D) Enlargement of the ipsilateral cisterns
3. Most common non- glial primary brain tumor is:-
   (A) Meningioma
   (B) Astrocytoma
   (C) Medulloblastoma
   (D) Ependymoma
4. False about above mentioned lesion-
   (A) Part of NF -2 syndrome
   (B) Part of NF -1 syndrome
   (C) Benign meningioma can metastasis.
   (D) Malignant meningioma can metastases
5. Mother in law sign in seen in:-
   (A) Prolactinoma
   (B) Pituitary fossa tumor
   (C) Meningioma
   (D) Medulloblastoma

Answers:

1. B
2. C
3. A

4. B
5. C
   Mother in law sign – comes early; stays late very dense tumour blush

Reference:
1. Osborn AG.Tumors of meninges. In:Renlund AR et al.editor Osborn's Brain imaging, pathology and anatomy. edition 1st 2013, p. 583-611

SUBDURAL HEMATOMA
Dr. Anit Parihar and Prof. Neera Kohli Department of Radiodiagnosis

A forty years old patient had a history of seizure disorder. She fell down during one such episode and lost consciousness. She was taken to hospital & her MRI scan was done which showed a crescentric collection in left frontoparietal region:-

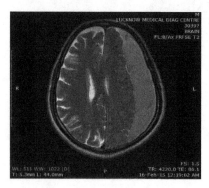

1. It is the classical appearance of:-
   (A) SDH
   (B) EDH
   (C) IVH
   (D) SAH
2. Most Common cause of extraaxial collection in post traumatic patient is:-
   (A) SDH
   (B) EDH
   (C) Both
   (D) None
3. Investigation of choice for head injury patient is:-
   (A) NCCT
   (B) CECT
   (C) MRI with MRA
   (D) CSF examination
4. Classical CT appearance of acute EDH is:-
   (A) Lentiformhyperdense collection
   (B) Lentiform hypodense collection
   (C) Crescentichyperdense collection
   (D) Crescentic hypodense collection
5. What is not indicated in management of Head Trauma
   (A) Hyperventilation
   (B) Intravenous Mannitol
   (C) Head end elevation
   (D) Glucocorticosteroids

Answers:
1. A
   collection noted crossing the suture line suggestive of subdural hemorrhage
2. A
3. A
4. A

5. A

References:
1. Gentry LR , Knoop EA .Head trauma. In: Scott W.Atlaseditor.Magnetic resonance imaging of the brain and spine. 4th edition 2009. vol 1, p.894-928
2. Gerard C, Busl KM. Treatment of acute subdural hematoma. *Curr Treat Options Neurol*. 2014 Jan. 16(1):275.

PITUITARY ADENOMA
Dr. Anit Parihar and Prof. Neera Kohli Department of Radiodiagnosis

A 33yrs old female was referred with decreased visual equity and loss of visual field for 3 years and menstrual irregularities. MRI brain imaging of patient was done which showed a homogenously enhancing mass lesion in sella.

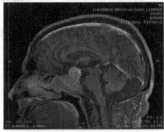

1. What is the most probable diagnosis:-
   (A) Craniopharyngioma
   (B) Optic nerve glioma
   (C) Pituitary adenoma
   (D) Astrocytoma
2. True about craniopharyngioma all except :-
   (A) Suprasellar
   (B) Occurs only in adults
   (C) Cystic
   (D) None
3. True about prolactin microadenoma:-
   (A) Causes galoctorrhoea
   (B) Causes polymenorrhoea
   (C) Hyperdense on CECT
   (D) None
4. Most common posterior fossa tumor in children :-
   (A) Cerebellar astrocytoma
   (B) Medulloblastoma
   (C) Ependymoma
   (D) Glioma
5. McCune-Albright Syndrome has all except
   (A) Endocrinopathy, Precocious Puberty
   (B) Polyostotic Fibrous Dysplasia
   (C) Café-au-lait spots
   (D) Macroglossia

Answer:
1. C
   extraaxial lesion noted in sellaregion,pituitary not visualisedseperately from the lesion with clinical features as described above s/o pituitary adenoma
2. B
3. A
4. A
5. D

References:
1. Zimmerman RA, Bilaniuk T .Pediatric brain tumour. In: Scott W.Atlas editor. Magnetic resonance imaging of the brain and spine. 4[th]edition 2009. vol 1, p.591-643
2. Sympons SP, Montanera WJ, Aviv RI , Kucharczyk W. The sellaturcica and parasellar region. In: Scott W.Atlas editor.Magnetic resonance imaging of the brain and spine. 4[th]edition 2009. Vol2 , p. 1120-1192
3. Fitzpatrick KA, Taljanovic MS, Speer DP et-al. Imaging findings of fibrous dysplasia with histopathologic and intraoperative correlation. AJR Am J Roentgenol. 2004;182 (6): 1389-98

TUBEROUS SCLEROSIS

Dr. Anit Parihar and Prof. Neera Kohli Department of Radiodiagnosis

A child presented with complaints of recurrent seizure and mental impairment on clinical examination Pigmented patches are noted. NCCT head was done which showed multiple calcified nodules lining the lateral ventricle.

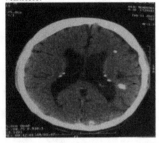

1. What is your diagnosis:-
   (A) Tuberous sclerosis
   (B) Sturge weber syndrome
   (C) Both
   (D) None
2. Cavernous hemangioma of the globe are Most commonly associated with :-
   (A) Von hippellindau disease
   (B) Tuberous sclerosis
   (C) Sturge weber syndrome
   (D) cronkhitecanada syndrome
3. Scenario mentioned above is characterized by all except
   (A) Hamartoma
   (B) Cortical tuber
   (C) Giant cell astrocytoma
   (D) Sphenoid wing dysplasia
4. Tramline calcification seen in: -
   (A) Tuberous sclerosis
   (B) Sturge weber syndrome
   (C) Neurofibromatosis I
   (D) Both a &; b
5. All are true about condition showed above except:-
   (A) Presence of calcified subependymal nodule
   (B) Renal angiomyolipoma
   (C) Intellectual impairement
   (D) Bare orbit sign

Answers:

1. A
    Multiple calcified subependymal nodules noted along with significant clinical history suggestive of tuberous sclerosis
2. A
3. D
4. B

5. D

References:
1. Osborn AG.neurocutaneous syndrome. In:Renlundar et al. editor. osborn's brain imaging, pathology and anatomy. ed 1st 2013 ,p. 1131-1170
2. Blaser SI ,Smirniotopoulos JG and Mmurphy FM . Central nervous system manifestation of phakomatosesphakomatoses In: Scott W.Atlas editor.Magnetic resonance imaging of the brain and spine. 4th edition 2009. Vol1,P. 272-306

CRANIOPHARYNGIOMA

Dr. Anit Parihar and Prof. Neera Kohli Department of Radiodiagnosis

A 12 years old child presented with complain of headache and reduced vision MRI was done to evaluate the cause which showed a cystic mass lesion in suprasellar region. Calcification was seen on CT scan in the lesion (images not shown)-

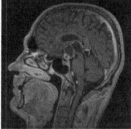

1. Most probable diagnosis is:
    (A) Pituitary macroadenoma
    (B) Craniopharyngioma
    (C) Parasellar meningioma
    (D) Arachnoid cyst
2. Most common non- glial primary brain tumor of children.
    (A) Craniopharyngioma
    (B) Meningioma
    (C) Medulloblastoma
    (D) Pinealoma
3. False about the lesion mentioned above
    (A) Usually both suprasellar and infrasellar
    (B) Usually infrasellar
    (C) cystic
    (D) shows calcification
4. Least common suprasellar lesions is.
    (A) Craniopharyngioma
    (B) Meningioma
    (C) Hypothalamic glioma
    (D) Metastases
5. Treatment of choice for craniopharyngioma
    (A) Gross total resection
    (B) Intracavity Bleomycin
    (C) Brachytherapy
    (D) Chemotherapy

Answer:
1. B
    An enhancing cystic lesion with solid nodule with calcification noted in suprasellar region , pituitary gland visualisedseperately from the lesion , along with significant clinical history suggestive of craniopharyngioma
2. A
3. B
4. D
5. D

References:
1. Osborn AG.Sellar neoplasm and tumor-like lesions. In:Renlund AR et al.editor Osborn's Brain imaging, pathology and anatomy. edition 1st 2013 p. 681-726

CT SCAN-HORSE SHOE KIDNEY
Dr. Anit Parihar and Prof. Neera Kohli Department of Radiodiagnosis

A CT scan of a 24 year old male was performed for pain abdomen. Contrast scan showed an enhancing soft tissue lying across and in front of L2 vertebra

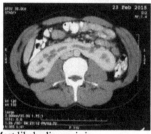

1. Most likely diagnosis is:
   (A) Cross fused ectopic kidney
   (B) Ectopic kidney
   (C) Horseshoe kidney
   (D) Duplex kidney
2. True about the condition mentioned above
   (A) Fusion is usually at lower pole.
   (B) Usually both kidney found on same side.
   (C) Occur due abscess of metanephrogenicblastoma.
   (D) Most common congenital anomaly of urinary tract.
3. All are true about condition mentioned above except
   (A) Kidney are usually lower down in position than normal
   (B) Lower pole project medially usually
   (C) Lower pole of kidney project laterally usually
   (D) May be associated with other anomalies like anorectal malformation.
4. All are true except
   (A) Failure of kidney to ascend during embryonic development result in pelvic kidney.
   (B) If kidney ascends higher it can become thoracic kidney
   (C) Pelvic kidney always have decrease function.
   (D) None
5. Which of the following is not true about PUJ anamoly
   (A) Ureteropelvic junction obstruction is common anomaly
   (B) More common on male.
   (C) Associated with increase incidence of renal agenesis and multi cystic dysplastic kidney in contralateral kidney
   (D) Hematuria in the most common symptom.

Answers:
1. C
   Lower pole of both kideny noted fused in midline and located more medially s/o horse shoe kidney
2. A
   Horse shoe kidney longitudinal axis of the kidney is abnormal, with lower pole located more medially than usual and fusing in the midline anterior to spine
3. C
4. C
5. D

Reference:
1. Babcock DS ,Patriquin HB. The pediatric kidney and adrenal glands .In :Rumack CM, Wilson SR, Charboneau JW, Levine D, editors. Diagnostic ultrasound. 4thedtion.Vol 2, 2005 .p.1845 to 1890

ACOUSTIC SCHWANOMA

Dr. Anit Parihar and Prof. Neera Kohli Department of Radiodiagnosis

A40 year old male patient comes to E N T department with complaints of hearing loss for last 2 month . On examination sensori-neural hearing loss was found . Patient was further sent for MRI to find out the cause. MRI images of the patient given here show an enhancing nodule in right Cerebellopontine angle

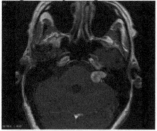

1 Most likely diagnosis is:
   (A) Acoustic schwanoma
   (B) Glomusjugulare
   (C) Vestibular schwanoma
   (D) Both a & c
2 True about the lesion
   (A) Most common tumour of cerebellar pontine angle
   (B) Most common symptom is tinnitus
   (C) Usually occur in children.
   (D) CT is best imaging tool.
3. All are true about the lesion except
   (A) It is benign tumor.
   (B) Most common symptom is symptom unilateral sensorineural hearing loss.
   (C) Can show metastases in upto 20 % cases
   (D) Arises from the schwann cell that wrapvestibulococuler nerve.
4. Ice cream on cone on MRI is diagnostic of-
   (A) Optic nerve glioma.
   (B) Glomusjugulare.
   (C) Vestibular schwanoma
   (D) Meningioma
5. Morphological appearance of vestibular schwannomas are all except-
   (A) When small &intracanalicular, looks like ovoid to cylindrical.
   (B) Larger lesions look like "ice cream (CPA) on cone.
   (C) Calcification are often present.
   (D) CSF-vascular "cleft" between mass & brain may be found.

Answers:
   1. D
   2. A
   3. C
   4. C
   5. C

Reference:
   1. Casselman JW, Mark A and Butman J A, Anatomy and diseases of the temporal bone In: Scott W.Atlas editor. Magnetic resonance imaging of the brain and spine. 4th edition 2009. vol2 p.1193-1257

PSEUDOPANCREATIC CYST

Dr. Anit Parihar and Prof. Neera Kohli Department of Radiodiagnosis

A 45 yr old chronic alcoholic patient was admitted with complain of severe pain in abdomen. On clinical history/examination pain was radiating towards back and patient has some previous episode of such type of pain. Tachycardia and tachypnea noted with raised serum amylase & lipase level. CT imaging of patient were done image is shows bellow.

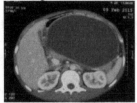

1. Most likely diagnosis based on clinical and radiological findings is:
   (A)Hydatid cyst
   (B)Mesenteric cyst
   (C)Pseudocyst of pancreas
   (D)Ovarian cyst
2. All are true **except**.
   (A)Pseudocyst are more common in chronic pancreatitis than acute pancreatitis
   (B)Trauma in most common cause of pseudocyst.
   (C)Conservative management of pseudo cyst is appropriate unless complication occur.
   (D)Pseudo cyst may resolve spontaneously.
3. All are true about the lesion showed above except
   (A)Well known complication of chronic pancreatitis.
   (B) Comprise 75 – 90 % of an cystic lesion of pancreas.
   (C) Wall consists of fibrosis and granulation tissue
   (D) USG in investigation of choice.
4. All are true except acute pancreatitis
   (A) Enlargement of pancreas is almost universal in acute pancreatitis.
   (B) Abdominal sonography& CECT are useful imaging modality.
   (C)MRCP is investigation of choice
   (D) All.
5. All are true about pancreas except
   (A)Vascular landmark for Pancreatic head is IVC dorsally.
   (B)Alcoholism & trauma most common cause of acute pancreatitis..
   (C)Atlanta scoring is used for carcinoma pancreas
   (D)All

Answers:
   1. C
      correlation with site of lesion and history
   2. B
   3. D
   4. C
      Contrast enhanced CT scan is investigation of choice
   5. C
      The Revised Atlanta Classification: Its importance for the radiologist and its effect on treatment.Radiology 2012;262: p. 751-764

Reference:
   1   Ruedi F. Thoeni . The Revised Atlanta Classification: Its importance for the radiologist and its effect on treatment.Radiology2012; 262: p. 751-764

CHOLELITHIASIS
Dr. Anit Parihar and Prof. Neera Kohli Department of Radiodiagnosis

An 18 yrs. male presented with complaints of acute pain abdomen in right hypochondrium. His NCCT was done. His investigation showed Liver Function and Renal function tests.

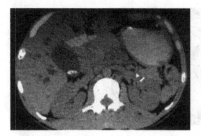

1. Most likely diagnosis is :-
   (A) Cholelithiasis
   (B) Cholelithiasis with choledocholithiasis
   (C) Carcinoma gall bladder
   (D) None

2. Investigation of choice for the above showed pathology is :-
   (A) USG
   (B) CT
   (C) MRI
   (D) MRCP

3. It's commonest complication is :-
   (A) Pancreatitis
   (B) Choledocholithiasis
   (C) Carcinoma Gall bladder.
   (D) Cholangiocarcinoma

4. Sludge induced pancreatitis is known as:
   (A) Microlithiasis phenomenon
   (B) Sludge phenomenon
   (C) Milk of magnesium
   (D) None of above

5. Brown Pigment stones are more common in
   (A) Obesity
   (B) Pregnancy
   (C) Cirrhosis
   (D) Choledochal cyst

Answers:
   1. A
   2. A
   3. A
   4. A
   5. D

References:
   1. Khalili K , Wilson S .The biliary tree and gall bladder. In :Rumack CM, Wilson SR , Charboneau JW, Levine D, editors. Diagnostic ultrasound .4thedtion.Vol 1, 2005 p. 172 – 215)
   2. Heuman DM, Moore EL, Vlahcevic ZR. Pathogenesis and dissolution of gallstones. Zakim D, Boyer TD, eds. *Hepatology: A Textbook of Liver Disease*. 3rd ed. Philadelphia, Pa: WB Saunders; 1996. 1996: 376-417.

HYDATID CYST OF LUNG

Dr. Anit Parihar and Prof. Neera Kohli Department of Radiodiagnosis

A 20 yrs. young male presented to pulmonary medicine department with complaint of cough and chest pain and shortness of breath. No history of fever with chills and rigor. No nausea, no vomiting. His chest CT was done.

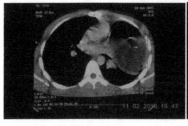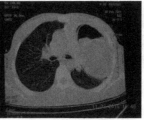

1. Most likely diagnosis is:-
   (A) Complicated Hydatid cyst
   (B) Bronchogenic cyst
   (C) Loculated pleural effusion
   (D) Bronchogenic carcinoma.
2. What other blood investigation you would like to-do
   (A) S. Antibody for echinococcus
   (B) Fluid aspiration and analysis
   (C) CT
   (D) USG
3. Treatment is :-
   (A) Antibiotics
   (B) Surgery
   (C) Follow up with repeat ct
   (D) Both a and b
4. It is caused by:
   (A) Ecchinococcus
   (B) Tinea
   (C) Schistosomiasis
   (D) Any one of above
5. Not an indication for PAIR technique in Hydatid Cyst
   (A) Type II Gharbi cyst
   (B) Size less than 5 cm
   (C) Bone cyst
   (D) Kidney Cyst

Answers:

1. A
   Thick walled cystic lesion with thick fluid attenuation noted in left lung suggestive of complicated hydatid cyst
2. A
3. D
4. A
5. B
   Size more than 5 cm and Type I, II are indications

Reference:

1. Wilson S R , Withers CE . The Liver.In :Rumack CM, Wilson SR , Charboneau JW, Levine D, Editors. Diagnostic ultrasound . 4th ed. Vol 1, 2005 p. 78 -141

EMPHYSEMATOUS PYELONEPHRITIS WITH STAGHORN CALCULUS

Dr. Anit Parihar and Prof. Neera Kohli Department of Radiodiagnosis

A 45 year old diabetic male presented to emergency with complaints of left flank pain, fever, nausea, vomiting, and altered sensorium. The patient was having history of acute colicky pain in recurrent left flank His NCCT abdomen was done. His Total Leucocyte Count was elevated and his renal function tests were markedly deranged

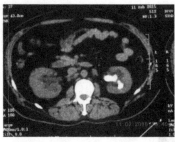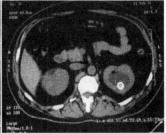

1. What is radiological diagnosis of patient?
   (A) Renal mass
   (B) Staghorn calculus
   (C) Staghorn calculus with pyelonephritis
   (D) Staghorn calculus with pyelonephritis and emphysematous pyonephrosis.
2. What is the clue in the CT scan image which best explains the serious condition of the patient
   (A) No contrast in bowel loops
   (B) Air in the left Renal Pelvis
   (C) Size of Calculus
   (D) Size of Kidneys
3. Contraindication for contrast CT is -
   (A)Renal calculus
   (B)Anaphylaxis
   (C)Cost
   (D)Contrast has no role in diagnosis
4. Commonest type of renal calculus:.
   (A)Oxalate
   (B)Triple phosphate
   (C)Uric acid
   (D)Xanthine
5. Apart from S creatinine what other investigation is needed in all patients of Ureteric colic
   (A) Urinary Sediment/Dipstick test
   (B) 24 Hour Urine Profile
   (C) CBC
   (D) S Electrolyte

Answers:
1. D
   An ill defined hypodensity noted in left renal parenchyma with air specks in upper pole and calculus in pelvis extending into calyces suggestive of staghorn calculus with pyelonehritis and emphysematous pyonephrosis
2. B
3. B
4. A
5. A

References:
1.   Tublin M, Thurston W, and Wilson S.The kidney and urinary tract.In:Rumack CM, Wilson SR , Charboneau JW, Levine D, editors. Diagnostic ultrasound .4[th]edtion.Vol 1, 2005 p. 338-407.
2.   Evan AP, Coe FL, Lingeman JE, Shao Y, Sommer AJ, Bledsoe SB, et al. Mechanism of formation of human calcium oxalate renal stones on Randall's plaque. *Anat Rec (Hoboken).* 2007 Oct. 290(10):1315-23.
3.   European Association of Urology. Guidelines on urolithiasis. National Guideline Clearinghouse. Available http://www.guidelines.gov/content.aspx?id=12528

CARCINOMA GALL BLADDER

Dr. Anit Parihar and Prof. Neera Kohli Department of Radiodiagnosis

A 40 yrs female presented to gastrosurgery department with complaints of pain in upper abdomen & jaundice for 2 months ,itching all over the body x 1 month . No history of fever, pain, vomiting. On investigation his bilirubin was raised and liver function was mildly deranged. His CECT abdomen was done.

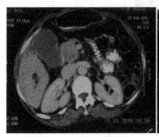 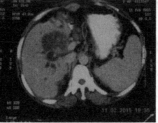

1. What other investigation are needed in the patient:
   (A)USG
   (B) MRCP
   (C) ERCP
   (D) Barium Swallow

2. What is most likely radiological diagnosis of the patient:
   (A) Carcinoma gall bladder
   (B) Cholelithiasis
   (C) Cholecystitis
   (D) Diagnosis cannot be made

3. What is the most common etiological factor for your most likely diagnosis in this patient
   (A) Calculus
   (B) Obesity
   (C) High animal fat diet
   (D) High fibre diet

4.Double duct sign is seen in:
   (A) Carcinoma head of pancreas
   (B) Periampullary carcinoma
   (C) Chronic pancreatitis
   (D) All of the above

5.When a palpable nontender mass is seen in Right upper quadrant with mild jaundice. What is least likely to be the cause
   (A) Carcinoma Gallbladder
   (B) Gall bladder stone
   (C) Carcinoma Pancreas
   (D) Cystic duct stone

Answers:

1. B
   MRCP is done to assess the hepatobiliary system
   ERCP not done as it is an invasive procedure
2. A
   Diagnosis is ca gall bladder made because there is loss of interface between gall bladder and liver parenchyma.
3. A
4. B
5. B
   Courvoisier's Law

References:

1. Khalili K , Wilson S .The biliary tree and gall bladder. In :Rumack CM, Wilson SR , Charboneau JW, Levine D, editors. Diagnostic ultrasound .4thedtion.Vol 1, 2005 p. 172 – 215
2. Schottenfeld D and Fraumeni J. *Cancer. Epidemiology and Prevention.* 3rd. Oxford University Press; 2006. 787-800.

3. Ralls P. The pancreas.In :Rumack CM, Wilson SR , Charboneau JW, Levine D, editors. Diagnostic ultrasound .4thedtion.Vol 1, 2005 p. 216 to 260)

PNEUMOTHORAX

Dr. Anit Parihar and Prof. Neera Kohli Department of Radiodiagnosis

A 36 year man presented with history of breathlessness in emergency department. His chest x ray was done.

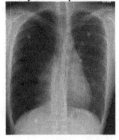

1.What is the diagnosis?
   (A)Pneumothorax
   (B)Pleural effusion
   (C)Hydropneumothorax
   (D)Pneumonia
2.The above mentioned condition causes shift to mediatinum towards
   (A)Contralateral side
   (B)Ipsilateral side
   (C)No shift of mediastinum
   (D)None of the above
3.Treatment of choice in the above mentioned scenario is
   (A)Spontaneous resolutoion
   (B)ICD tube
   (C)Surgery
   (D)Antibiotics
4.Causes of the above mentioned condion:
   (A)Spontaneous
   (B)Traumatic
   (C)Iatrogenic
   (D)All of the above
5.Which is most life threatening condition
   (A)Pleural effusion
   (B)Tension pneumothorax
   (C)Hydropneumothorax
   (D)Pyothorax

Answers:
   1. A
   2. A
      Shift of mediastinum away from the side of pneumothorax may be seen in large pneumothorax
   3. B
   4. D
   5. B
      Tension pneumothorax is life threatening emergency

References:
   1. Prakash A. Pleura and diaphragm.In:Chowdhary V, Gupta AK, Khandelwal N, editors.Diagnostic radiology :chest and cardiovascular imaging ,3rd edition p. 272-300
   2. Kalra N, Kang M, Lal M. Diagnostic and therapeutic interventions in chest. In:Chowdhary V, Gupta AK, Khandelwal N, editors.Diagnostic radiology :chest and cardiovascular imaging ,3rd edition p. 328-340

PLEURAL EFFUSION

Dr. Anit Parihar and Prof. Neera Kohli Department of Radiodiagnosis

A 30 year man presented with history of breathlessness in Pulmonary department . His chest x ray was done.

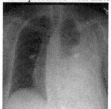

1.What is the diagnosis?
  (A) Pleural effusion
  (B) Pneumothorax
  (C) Pneumonia
  (D) Diaphragmatic hernia
2. What finding is noted in X ray PA view
  (A) Blunting of costophrenic angle initially and a meniscus, on frontal films seen laterally and gently sloping medially
  (B) Lack of pulmonary vessel
  (C) Air under diaphragm
  (D) None of the above
3. The above mentioned condition causes shift to mediastinum towards
  (A) Contralateral side
  (B) Ipsilateral side
  (C) No shift of mediastinum
  (D) None of the above
4. The above mentioned condition is seen in
  (A) Cardiac failure
  (B) Nephrotic syndrome
  (C) Bronchogenic carcinoma
  (D) All of the above
5. Stony dullness is present in which condition
  (A) Emphysema
  (B) Pleural effusion
  (C) Chronic bronchitis
  (D) Pneumothorax

Answers:
  1. A
      Homogenous opacification of lower chest with obliteration of left costophrenic angle and left hemidiaphragm ,upper margin of opacity concave to the lung and is higher laterally than medially
  2. A
  3. A
      Massive pleural effusion causes contralateral mediastinal shift
  4. D
  5. B

Reference:
  1. Prakash A. Pleura and diaphragm. In:Chowdhary V, Gupta AK, Khandelwal N, editors.Diagnostic radiology :chest and cardiovascular imaging ,3rd edition p. 272-300)

EXTRADURAL HEMORRHAGE

Dr. Anit Parihar and Prof. Neera Kohli Department of Radiodiagnosis

A 30 year male patient with history of RTA showed loss of consciousness. For this NCCT was done

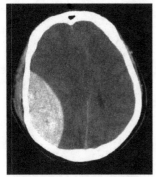

1. The above mentioned condition is
   (A) Extra dural hemorrhage
   (B) Sub dural hemorrhage
   (C) Sub arachnoid hemorrhage
   (D) None of the above
2. Most common source is
   (A) Middle meningeal artery
   (B) Tearing of Bridging veins
   (C) Both of the above
   (D) None of the above
3. The above shown pathology can
   (A) Cross the midline
   (B) Does not cross the midline
   (C) Both of the above
   (D) None of the above
4. The above shown pathology may present with
   (A) Skull fracture
   (B) Abducent nerve palsy
   (C) Lucid interval
   (D) All of the above
5. EDH is seen on CT scan as
   (A) Lenticular
   (B) Concavo-convex
   (C) Biconcave
   (D) None of the above

Answer:

1. A
   Lenticular /biconvex shape hetrogenous predominantly hyperdense lesion noted in right side s/o epidural /extradural hemorrhage
2. A
3. B
4. D
5. A

References:

1. Wasenko JJ, Hocssauserl.Central nervous system trauma . In: Hagga JR, Lanzieri CF, Gilkeson, editors. CTand MR imaging of whole body ,4th edition 2003, vol 1 p. 317 -350)

MIDGUT VOLVULUS

Dr. Anit Parihar and Prof. Neera Kohli Department of Radiodiagnosis

A 24 year old female presented with history of abdominal distension and recurrent vomiting since 2 days. She also has similar episodes of vomiting in the past for which CECT abdomen was done.

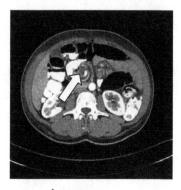

1. What radiological sign is visualized in the above shown picuture.
   (A) Whirlpool sign
   (B) Comet tail sign
   (C) Colon cut off sign
   (D) Chain of lake appearance
2. This sign is seen in
   (A) Midgut volvulus
   (B) Intestinal perforation
   (C) Carcinoma stomach
   (D) Liver abscess
3. Other associated radiological features with the same pathology are:
   (A) Tapering of beaking of the bowel in complete obstruction
   (B) Malrotated bowel configuration
   (C) Both of the above
   (D) None of the above
4. Which other sign is seen in radiograph in the above mentioned condition
   (A) Corkscrew appearance
   (B) Mercedes benz sign
   (C) Signet ring sign
   (D) Double duct sign
5. What is the finding seen on Color Doppler
   (A) Blooming artifact
   (B) Color spill
   (C) Inversion of SMA SMV relationship
   (D) Thrombosis of SMA

Answer:
1. A
   Twisting of the superior mesentric vein and mesentery around the artery is very specific sign of midgut volvulus (whirlpool sign)
2. A
3. C
4. A
5. A

Reference:
1. Thomas KE, Owens CM. The pediatric abdomen .In: Sutton D, Robbinson PJ ,Jenkins JP, editors.Text book of radiology and imaging , 7th edition,2003 volume 1 p. 849 -884

GLIOBLASTOMA MULTIFORME
Dr. Anit Parihar and Prof. Neera Kohli Department of Radiodiagnosis

A 40 year old male presented with history of severe headache and seizures for last 4 months.

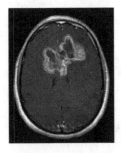

1. Most common adult malignant primary brain tumor.
   (A) Glioblasotomamultiforme
   (B) Medulloblastoma
   (C) Epenymoma
   (D) Lymphoma
2. They have a preferential spreading along
   (A) Corpus callosum.
   (B) Ventricles
   (C) Pituatary gland
   (D) Pineal gland
3. High grade Glioblastoma multiforme is also known as
   (A) Butterfly glioma
   (B) Figure of 8 lesion
   (C) Both of the above
   (D) None of the above
4. Markers of the above mentioned condition
   (A) GFAP+ (intermediate filament)
   (B) Alfa feto protein
   (C) HCG
   (D) None of the above
5. The above shown lesion has all except
   (A) Surrounding edema
   (B) Necrosis
   (C) Well defined margins
   (D) Hemorrhage

Answers:
   1. A
   2. A
   3. C
   4. A
   5. C

References:
   1. Jayaraman MV ,Boxerman JL. Adult brain tumours . In: Scott W.Atlas editor.Magnetic resonance imaging of the brain and spine. 4thedition 2009. vol 1 p. 445-590

Chapter-25

Radiotherapy

BREAST CARCINOMA

Dr. M. L. B. Bhatt, Professor & Head, Department of Radiotherapy

A 50 year old woman presented with lump in right breast .Physical examination revealed 3 cm x 5 cm hard lump with irregular margin in upper outer quadrant of breast with single right sided axillary lymphnode. Histopathology report show infiltrating ductal carcinoma.

1.Genes associated with Ca Breast are all except
- (A) BRCA1
- (B) BRCA2
- (C) P 53
- (D) APC

2.Risk factors for Breast Cancer are all except
- (A) Early age marriage
- (B) Early menarche
- (C) Late menopause
- (D) Oral contraceptive pills

3.True about staging of Ca Breast are all except
- (A) Supraclavicular lymphadenopathy in N3c
- (B) Peau d' Orange in T4b
- (C) Pectoralis major involvement in T4a
- (D) Infraclavicular lymphadenopathy in N3a

4.One of these has the most important prognostic value in ca breast
- (A) size of tumor
- (B) age of the patient
- (C) presence of pain
- (D) Involvement of lymph nodes

5.True about mammography for Ca Breast are all except
- (A) Microcalcification
- (B) Macrocalcification
- (C) Multiple punctuate calcification
- (D) BIRADS classification systems

Answers:

1. D
   APC is associated with colorectal cancer
2. D
   Oral contraceptive pills use does not show increase in risk of Breast cancer
3. C
   T4a is involvement of chest wall; chest wall does not include pectoral muscles
4. D
   Nodal status is the strongest predictor for disease free and overall survival
5. B
   Microcalcification is suggestive of intraducatal disease

Reference:

1. Halperin Edward C, Brady Luther W, Perez Carlos A, Wazer David E. Principles and Practice of Radiation Oncology, 6th ed. USA: Lippincott Williams & Wilkins;2013. Chapter 56, Breast Cancer: Early stage, p.1047,1050, 1058,1062-1065.

CARCINOMA LUNG
Dr. M. L. B. Bhatt, Professor & Head, Department of Radiotherapy

A 45 year old male presented with a 2 months history of fever, productive cough and hemoptysis. He had been a smoker for the last 20 years. On examination, bronchial breath sounds were heard in right infra-axillary area. No neck nodes were palpable. A chest radiograph showed a well defined, round opacity in the right middle zone. Sputum examination for malignant cells was negative. CECT scan showed a 5 cm well-defined, homogenous, contrast-enhancing lesion in the right middle lobe with multiple enlarged (largest 1.8 x 1.5 cm) right peribronchial and hilar lymph nodes. A subsequent fibreoptic bronchoscopy revealed an exophytic growth in the right main bronchus 4 cm from the carina and a biopsy was taken which showed squamous cell carcinoma.

1. What is the TNM stage of lung carcinoma in this case?
   (A) T2N1M0
   (B) T3N1M0
   (C) T2N2M0
   (D) T3N2M0
2. What is the most appropriate treatment for this stage?
   (A) Concurrent chemoradiotherapy
   (B) Sequential chemotherapy and radiotherapy
   (C) Lobectomy with mediastinal node dissection
   (D) Segmentectomy with mediastinal node dissection
3. All of the following are risk factors for lung cancer except
   (A) Asbestos exposure
   (B) Radon exposure
   (C) Smoking
   (D) Obesity
4. Which paraneoplastic syndrome is commonly seen in squamous cell lung carcinoma?
   (A) Cushing syndrome
   (B) SIADH
   (C) Hypercalcemia
   (D) HPO
5. All of the following are prognostic factors for lung cancer except
   (A) High fat diet
   (B) ERCC-1 positivity
   (C) Performance status
   (D) XRCC-1 positivity

Answers:
   1. A
      T2N1M0 tumor >3cm in greatest dimension but <7cm with invasion of main bronchus proximal extent at least 2 cm from carina, involves visceral pleura.
      N1 involvement of ipsilateral intrapulmonary, peribronchial, hilar nodes
   2. C
      The standard treatment for stage I and stage II tumor is surgical resection including lobectomy or pneumonectomy with mediastinal lymphnode dissection
   3. D
      Smoking and environmental carcinogen such as asbestos, arsenic polycyclic aromatic hydrocarbon are risk factor
   4. C
      Squmous cell carcinomas are more commonly associated with hypercalcemia than other lung cancers.
   5. D
      Patient related prognostic factors are –performance status, weight loss, age, gender and marital status Tumor related prognostic factor is - ERCC-1 (excision repair cross-complementation on group 1

Reference:
   1. Halperin Edward C, Brady Luther W, Perez Carlos A, Wazer David E. Principles and Practice of Radiation Oncology, 6th ed. USA: Lippincott Williams & Wilkins;2013. Chapter 51, Lung cancer, p.938, 941-947.

CARCINOMA UTERINE CERVIX
Dr. Kirti Srivastava, Professor, Department of Radiotherapy

A 44-year-old woman presented with post-coital bleeding. On examination, there was a 3 cm growth present replacing the whole cervix and extending to upper third vagina. Left parametrium was involved but not up to the pelvic wall. A punch biopsy from the growth revealed squamous cell carcinoma. She has completed her family.

1. What is the stage of cervical carcinoma?
   (A) II A
   (B) II B
   (C) III A
   (D) III B
2. What is the most appropriate treatment?
   (A) Radical hysterectomy
   (B) External beam radiotherapy with brachytherapy
   (C) Concurrent chemoradiotherapy alone
   (D) Concurrent chemoradiotherapy with brachytherapy
3. Virus associated with cancer cervix is:
   (A) HPV
   (B) HIV
   (C) EBV
   (D) HTLV

Answers:
   1. B
      Parametrium involved but not up to pelvic wall
   2. D
      Treatment for advanced stage is concurrent chemoradiotherapy along with intracavitary Brachytherapy
   3. A
      HPV 16, 18 mainly cause cervical cancer, many strains of HPV are responsible for cervical cancer. HPV is also associated with oropharyngeal malignancy.

Reference:
   1. Halperin Edward C, Brady Luther W, Perez Carlos A, Wazer David E. Principles and Practice of Radiation Oncology, 6th ed. USA: Lippincott Williams & Wilkins;2013. Chapter 69, Uterine Cervix, p.1364,1387-1398, 1423.

NEUROBLASTOMA
Dr. Kirti Srivastava, Professor, Department of Radiotherapy

An eighteen months old infant presented in paediatric OPD with complaints of lump in abdomen associated with anorexia, weight loss and fever. Urinary VMA was found to be elevated, bone marrow revealed formation of clumps and pseudorosettes.

1. The infant is most likely suffering with
   (A) Wilms tumor
   (B) Neuroblastoma
   (C) Rhabdomyosarcoma
   (D) Hypernephroma
2. Most specific investigation to rule out metastasis would be
   (A) Bone scan
   (B) MIBG tagged bone scan
   (C) MRI
   (D) CT Scan
3. Which of the following is not true for Neuroblastoma
   (A) It has the highest rate of spontaneous regression
   (B) Most of the time presents with metastatic disease
   (C) Blue berry muffin sign is a presentation of liver metastasis
   (D) Presence of opsoclonus and myoclonus syndrome indicates favourable prognosis

Answers:
   1. B

Neuroblastomas are most common in infants. Urinary excretion of chatecholamines includes VMA and HMV which is present in more than 95% cases. Bone marrow involvement is a common feature and absence of pseudorosette does not rule out neuroblastoma.

2. B

Meta-iodobenzyleguanidine(MIBG) is concentrated by neurosecretory granules of both normal and metastatic tissues of neural crest origin.It has 85-90% sensitivity and 95% specificity.

3. C

Blue berry muffin sign is a presentation of skin metastasis. The metastasis has a blue tinge, when pressed the release of chatecholamines produces transient blanching.

Reference:
1. Halperin Edward C, Brady Luther W, Perez Carlos A, Wazer David E. Principles and Practice of Radiation Oncology, 6th ed. USA: Lippincott Williams & Wilkins;2013. Chapter 86, Neuroblastoma, p.1665.

CARCINOMA OVARY
Dr. Kirti Srivastava, Professor, Department of Radiotherapy

A 15 years old young female presented with pain in right iliac fossa. USG pelvis revealed unilateral heterogenous ovarian mass of approx 6 x 8 cm. There were no signs and symptoms of hormonal disbalance. None of the serum marker was found to be raised.

1. The most probable diagnosis would be
   (A) Dysgerminoma
   (B) Endodermal sinus tumor
   (C) Granulosa cell tumor
   (D) Mucinous cystadenocarcinoma ovary

2. Which of the tumor marker could be found raised in dysgerminoma
   (A) Alfa feto protein
   (B) Total Inhibin
   (C) Ca-125
   (D) Beta HCG

3. Treatment of choice would be
   (A) Surgery
   (B) Chemotherapy
   (C) Radiotherapy
   (D) Combined approach

Answers:
1. A

In young age dysgerminoma is the commonest ovarian malignancy. Other options are associated with elevated tumor markers.

2. D

Dysgerminomas can present with slight rise in beta HCG however no other marker is found to be elevated.

3. B

Treatment of Dysgerminomas includes conservative management to keep the fertility intact. It has a high incidence of bilaterality however due to availability of effective salvage treatment bilateral oophorectomy is not considered. Patients with advanced stage (>stage I) need chemotherapy 3-4 cycles. Although being radiosensitive, radiation is kept in reserve considering its toxicity in young age.

Reference:
1. Halperin Edward C, Brady Luther W, Perez Carlos A, Wazer David E. Principles and Practice of Radiation Oncology, 6th ed. USA: Lippincott Williams & Wilkins;2013. Chapter 71, Ovarian and Fallopian Tube cancer, p.1462-1463.

CARCINOMA ENDOMETRIUM

Dr. Kirti Srivastava, Professor, Department of Radiotherapy

A 60 years old post menopausal female presented with per vaginal bleeding in Gynaecology OPD, P/v examination was normal. MRI pelvis revealed a heterogeneous growth involving >50% of the myometrium but not reaching up to the serosa or cervix. There is no h/o estrogenic stimulation.

1. The most probable diagnosis would be
   - (A) Fibroid uterus
   - (B) Sarcoma uterus
   - (C) Endometrial cancer type I
   - (D) Endometrial cancer type II
2. According to FIGO staging (2009) tumor is
   - (A) Stage IA
   - (B) Stage IB
   - (C) Stage IC
   - (D) Stage II
3. Which of the following parameters affect the staging
   - (A) Involvement of endocervical glands
   - (B) Involvement of paraaortic lymphnodes
   - (C) Positive peritoneal cytology
   - (D) All of the above

Answers:
1. C
   Type I cancers have strong correlation with estrogen stimulation and occur in pre or perimenopausal age group.
2. B
   Stage I is divided into A &B <50% myometrium invasion means stage IA &>50% myometrium invasion means stage IB. Involvement of cervix is stage II.
3. B
   In the revised FIGO staging endocervical gland involvement & positive peritoneal cytology do not affect the staging as was stated in the earlier staging guidelines.

Reference:
1. Halperin Edward C, Brady Luther W, Perez Carlos A, Wazer David E. Principles and Practice of Radiation Oncology, 6th ed. USA: Lippincott Williams & Wilkins;2013. Chapter 70, Endometrial Cancer, p.1430-1431.

LYMPHOMA

Dr. Rajeev Gupta, Professor, Department of Radiotherapy

A 15 year old male presented with bilateral neck swelling with fever and weight loss. Examination of neck swelling shows multiple bilateral firm non-matted lymph nodes. PET- CT Scan shows FDG uptake in cervical Lymphnode.

1. Most probable diagnosis is,
   - (A) Lymphoma
   - (B) Tuberculosis
   - (C) Secondary Neck
   - (D) Sarcoidosis
2. B symptoms include all except
   - (A) Weight loss
   - (B) High grade fever
   - (C) Night Sweat
   - (D) Pruritis
3. True about Hodgkins lymphoma are all except
   - (A) Bimodal age pattern
   - (B) R-S cells
   - (C) Associated with HPV
   - (D) Associated with EBV

4. CD markers associated with Hodgkins disease
   (A) CD 20 & CD 30
   (B) CD 15 & CD 30
   (C) CD 15 & CD 20
   (D) CD 3 & CD 20
5. Which monoclonal antibody is used in the treatment of non Hodgkins Lymphoma
   (A) Rituximab
   (B) Cituximab
   (C) Bevacizumab
   (D) Bortizumib

Answers:
1. A
   lymphnode involvement in lymphoma are non matted, and show uptake on PET Scan.
2. D
   B symptoms include weight loss, fever, and night sweats
3. C
   Hodgkins lymphoma is associated with Ebstein Bar Virus and not HPV
4. B
   CD15, CD30 these markers are for Reedsternberg cell which are found in Hodgkins disease
5. A
   Rituximab is anti CD 20 antibody and is used in Non- Hodgkins lymphoma

Reference:
1. Halperin Edward C, Brady Luther W, Perez Carlos A, Wazer David E. Principles and Practice of Radiation Oncology, 6th ed. USA: Lippincott Williams & Wilkins;2013. Chapter 66, Intermediate and High risk Prostate Cancer, p.1331-1332,1531-1533, 1559.

CARCINOMA HEAD & NECK
Dr. Sudhir Singh, Department Of Radiotherapy

A 46-year old female presented with a painful mass in the base of the tongue (BOT); the physical examination revealed a ~2 × 2.5-cm palpable lesion in the right base of the tongue that did not extend to the midline, tonsil, or vallecula; there is a right neck palpable level 2 node of ~ 2 × 2 cm. The MRI report noted a right BOT 24 × 28 × 15-mm lesion invading the superior longitudinal muscle not invading the midline, genioglossus muscle, or the floor of the mouth; bilateral level II nodes present (right 22 × 14-mm and left 14 × 9-mm LN). Patient had no distant metastases. Ultrasound- guided biopsy from the right neck node was positive for squamous cell carcinoma.

1. Which of the following could NOT be a risk factor for cancer development in this patient?
   (A) Smoking
   (B) Alcohol
   (C) Chronic irritation
   (D) Tonsillitis
   (E) HPV infection
2. Which of the following diagnostic method is used in the staging of the patient's cancer?
   (A) Indirect laryngoscopy
   (B) MRI
   (C) CT
   (D) Bimanual palpation
   (E) All of the above
3. The patient most likely has which of the following TNM stage of cancer?
   (A) T2 N1 M0
   (B) T4aN2cM0
   (C) T2 N2c M0
   (D) T4a N2bM0
4. The treatment of choice would be
   (A) RT alone

(B) Surgery alone

(C) Concurrent Chemo-RT

(D) Neo-adjuvant chemotherapy with Surgery

Answers:

1. D

Etiology of oropharyngeal cancer: Cigarette smoking, alcohol, chronic irritation, and HPV 16.

2. E

Indirect laryngoscopy with a mirror should be performed to see the base of the tongue and the vallecula. Tumor in this region can easily invade the surrounding soft tissues and present in more advanced stages. However, the actual size of the tumor is determined by bimanual palpation and advanced imaging modalities (MRI, CT). Mandibular invasion is also detected with radiological techniques. The risk of distant metastasis is a bit more than in the case of the oral cavity. Furthermore, the presence of a secondary malignancy or development at a later time in the upper or lower airways are also higher. Thus, the patient should be evaluated and followed for this possibility. The final and exact diagnosis is made via biopsy.

3. C

T2 is tumor larger than 2 cm but no larger than 4 cm in the greatest dimension and N2c is metastasis in bilateral or contralateral lymph nodes, 6 cm or smaller in the greatest dimension.

4. C

Concurrent chemoradiotherapy is standard according to GORTEC 94-01 and Head and Neck Intergroup Data (1, 2):70 Gy at 2 Gy/fraction/day with concurrent bolus CDDP (100 mg/m 2)given on days 1, 22, and 43 or weekly (40 mg/m 2)

Reference:

1. Halperin Edward C, Brady Luther W, Perez Carlos A, Wazer David E. Principles and Practice of Radiation Oncology, 6th ed. USA: Lippincott Williams & Wilkins;2013. Chapter 45, Oropharynx, p.817, 821-822.

CARCINOMA HEAD & NECK

Dr. Sudhir Singh, Department Of Radiotherapy

A 45 yrs old male tobacco chewer presented with 4x4 cm size ulcero-proliferative growth on left buccal mucosa involving lower alveolus with multiple mobile ipsilateral neck nodes less than 6 cm.

1. The most likely TNM stage of this patient is?

(A) T4a N1M0

(B) T4a N2bM0

(C) T2 N1M0

(D) T2 N2bM0

2. Which of the following investigation is least likely needed in this patient is?

(A) CT/MRI of head & neck

(B) OPG (Orthopantomogram)

(C) Chest X-ray PA view

(D) PET-CT scan

3. What is the most appropriate treatment strategy for this patient?

(A) Surgery → Radiotherapy

(B) Radiotherapy alone

(C) Chemoradiotherapy

(D) Surgery alone

4. If this patient underwent surgery, all of the following are indications of post-op radiotherapy except?

(A) Surgical margin positive

(B) Multiple neck nodes positive

(C) Lymphovascular invasion present

(D) High grade tumor

Answers:

1. B
    Involvement of adjacent structures (e.g. skin, deep muscles of tounge, maxillary sinus, through cortical bone) is T4a. Multiple mobile neck node <6 cm is N2b.

2. D
    The actual size of the tumor is determined by bimanual palpation and advanced imaging modalities (MRI, CT). Mandibular invasion is detected with radiological techniques like OPG and CT. Chest X-ray is done to detect lung metastasis. PET scans are optional and may be informative in advanced cases.

3. A
    The treatment of T1-2N0M0 oral cancers is either surgery or radiotherapy alone, whereas the treatment for T3, T4a, N1, N2 oral cancer is Surgery + Postoperative RT.

4. D
    Surgical margin positive and incomplete surgery (i.e. no neck dissection when indicated) are the universal indications for postop RT. Grade is the single most important prognostic factor in sarcomas and in adenocarcinomas also grade is an important prognostic factor treatment planning, but in squamous cell carcinomas grade is not used for treatment planning.

Reference:

1. Halperin Edward C, Brady Luther W, Perez Carlos A, Wazer David E. Principles and Practice of Radiation Oncology, 6th ed. USA: Lippincott Williams & Wilkins;2013. Chapter 44, Oral Cavity, p.803-805.

EWING SARCOMA
Dr. Sudhir Singh, Department Of Radiotherapy

A 15 yrs old boy presented with pain and swelling on lower thigh. X-ray showing lytic lesion with multi-layered subperiosteal reaction on the diaphysis of femur. Biopsy of the lesion shows poorly differentiated nest of small round, PAS positive, blue cells.

1. What is the most likely diagnosis?
    (A) Osteosarcoma
    (B) Ewing's sarcoma
    (C) Osteomylitis
    (D) Eosinophilic granuloma
2. Which would be the most likely cytogenetic abnormality associated?
    (A) t [11:22]
    (B) t [1:16]
    (C) RB1 & p53 gene mutation
    (D) t [9:22]
3. Which of the following diagnostic test should be done in this patient except?
    (A) CT Thorax
    (B) Bone marrow
    (C) CT Abdomen
    (D) Bone scan
    (E) Immunohistochemistry
4. The treatment of choice would be
    (A) Surgery → chemotherapy
    (B) Radiotherapy
    (C) Chemotherapy → surgery / radiotherapy → chemotherapy
    (D) Surgery → Radiotherapy

Answers:

1. **B**

   Ewing's sarcoma is the 2nd most common bone tumor in children and age of presentation between 10-25 yrs. It occurs most commonly in diaphysis of long bone. X-ray features include Lytic, destructive lesion and onion skin effect.

2. **A**

   95% cases of Ewings sarcoma have (t 11,22) & few have (t21,22).

3. **C**

   Ewing's sarcoma is least likely to metastasize in abdomen. The systemic workup should include blood studies, a chest roentgenogram, a CT scan of the chest, a bone scan, and a bone marrow biopsy.

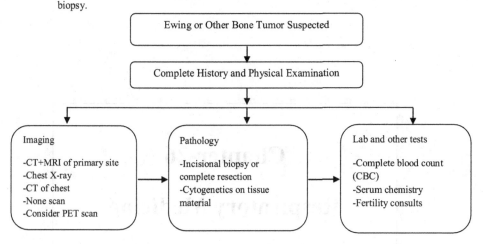

Fig: An algorithm for diagnosis and staging of Ewing tumor

4. **C**

   Effective local and systemic therapy is necessary for the cure of Ewing sarcoma family tumor. Induction chemotherapy is preferred over starting the local therapy and systemic therapy.

Reference:

1. Halperin Edward C, Brady Luther W, Perez Carlos A, Wazer David E. Principles and Practice of Radiation Oncology, 6th ed. USA: Lippincott Williams & Wilkins;2013. Chapter 88, Ewing Tumor, p.1689.

Chapter-26

Respiratory Medicine

ASTHMA

Dr. Surya Kant, Dr. Ajay Kumar Verma, Dr. Anand Srivastava, Dr. Ashwini Kumar Mishra, Dr. Ambarish Joshi
Department of Respiratory Medicine

A 11-year-old boy is referred by his primary care physician for nasal congestion and runny nose for years. His symptoms were getting worse day by day and were persistent. He was taking off and on medications in the past with history of noncompliance and felt that the medications didn't help him significantly. Approximately six months ago, he started to complain of shortness of breath, dyspnea on exertion and cough. The symptoms become worse in the evening and night. He has symptoms throughout the year with worsening of nasal congestion in August and September. He was not exposed to tobacco or pets. Mother and father have allergic rhinitis and his siblings also have allergic rhinitis and atopic eczema.

Physical examination: Thin boy in little distress. Vital signs stable. Temperature 98.8 F, heart rate 80 bpm, respiratory rate 20, blood pressure 110/60 mm/Hg. No Skin rashes. Nose: Pale, boggy turbinate's. Throat: Normal. Respiratory system: On auscultation bilateral wheezing and rhonchi present. Cardiovascular system: Clear S1, S2. Abdomen: Soft, non-tender, non-distended. Extremities: No cyanosis, clubbing, or edema.

1. What is the most likely diagnosis?
   (A) Allergic Rhinitis
   (B) Pulmonary tuberculosis
   (C) Allergic Rhinitis with bronchial asthma
   (D) Bronchiectasis
2. What investigations would you suggest next?
   (A) Skin prick test
   (B) Spirometry
   (C) Differential blood count
   (D) Both b and c
3. You are considering omalizumab therapy for a patient with severe persistent asthma who is requiring oral prednisone at 5-10 mg daily in addition to high-dose inhaled corticosteroids, long-acting bronchodilators, and montelukast to control symptoms. Which of the following is necessary prior to initiating omalizumab?
   (A) Discontinuation of oral prednisone
   (B) Demonstrated elevation in immunoglobulin E levels to greater than 1000 IU/L
   (C) Normalization of FEV_1 or peak expiratory flow rates
   (D) Presence of sensitivity to a perennial aeroallergen
4. What are the characteristic spirometric findings of bronchial asthma
   (A) FEV1/FVC of less than 0.7
   (B) Post bronchodilator improvement in FEV1 of more than 12% and 200ml
   (C) Both a and b
   (D) Normal FEV1/FVC with decreased FVC and FEF25-75%
5. You are considering a diagnosis of allergic bronchopulmonary aspergillosis (ABPA) in a patient of uncontrolled asthma. All the following clinical features are consistent with allergic bronchopulmonary aspergillosis EXCEPT:
   (A) Bilateral peripheral cavitary lung infiltrates
   (B) High-resolution CT thorax S/o bilateral cystic bronchiectasis
   (C) Pulmonary function tests
   (D) Decreased Serum IgE level
6. The mainstay of treatment of bronchial asthma is
   (A) Montelukast and levocetrizine
   (B) Inhaled corticosteroids
   (C) Oral corticosteroids
   (D) Theophyllins

Answers:

1. C
   Asthma is the most common chronic allergic respiratory disease, affecting up to 10% of adults and 30% of children Most patients with asthma have rhinitis suggesting the concept of 'one airway one disease' or 'united airways'.
2. B
   Spirometry is required to confirm asthma.
3. D
   There is no role of anti IGE therapy in a patient of asthma without increased IGE levels and Presence of sensitivity to a perennial aeroallergen

4. C

Hallmark of bronchial asthma on spirometry is obstruction with reversibility of more than 12% and 200ml

5. D

ABPA is considered in a patient of uncontrolled asthma with increased IgE levels usually more than 1000 IU/L

6. B

Inhaled corticosteroids are the first line of therapy for treatment of asthma. Montelukast, Levocetrizine, theophyllins are add on drugs.

References:

1. Global Strategy for Asthma Management and Prevention, Global Initiative for Asthma (GINA) 2014. Available from: http://www.ginasthma.org/.
2. Agarwal R. Allergic bronchopulmonary aspergillosis. Chest 2009;135: 805–826.

LUNG CANCER

Dr. Surya Kant, Dr. Ved Prakash, Dr. Ajay Kumar Verma, Dr. Anand Srivastava, Dr. Ambarish Joshi,
Department of Respiratory Medicine

A 56-year-old male with history of alcohol abuse and smoking is admitted to the hospital with a chief complaint of shortness of breath (SOB) for 2 months. SOB is so severe that he is not able to do his routine activities. Chest pain was also there on right hemithorax. He reports 18-kg weight loss during the last 6 months. The patient says that he has seen blood in his sputum. Tuberculin test (PPD) was negative 2 years ago and he has a 60 pack-years history of smoking. A chest X-Ray was done for work up which prompted the clinician to have a CT thorax. *Physical examination* revealed markedly decreased air entry on the right, with an area of dullness over right infraclavicular and mammary regions.

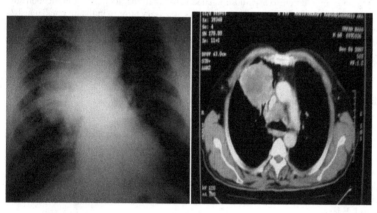

1. What is the diagnosis
   (A)Pleural effusion
   (B)Intrathoracic mass cause?bronchogenic carcinoma
   (C)Pulmonary tuberculosis
   (D)Community acquired pneumonia
2. As an oncologist you are considering treatment options for your patient with lung cancer including small molecule therapy targeting the epidermal growth factor receptor (EGFR). Which of the following patients is most likely to have an EGFR mutation?
   (A)A 23-year-old man with a hamartoma.
   (B)A 33-year-old woman with a carcinoid tumor.
   (C)A 45-year-old woman who has never smoked with an adenocarcinoma
   (D)A 56-year-old man with a 100 pack-year history of tobacco with small cell lung carcinoma
3. Which type of lung cancer is assosciated most commonly with pleural effusion
   (A) Adenocarcinoma
   (B) Small cell carcinoma
   (C) Squamous cell carcinoma

    (D) Large cell carcinoma
4. What is the first line chemotherapy for a patient of lung cancer with EGFR mutation
    (A) Geftinib
    (B) Crizotinib
    (C) Docetaxel
    (D) Bevacizumab
5. Which type of carcinoma lung is commonly associated with paraneoplastic syndrome:
    (A) Squamous cell CA
    (B) Large cell CA
    (C) Small cell cancer
    (D) Adenocarcinoma

Answers:

1. B
   Intrathoracic mass cause? bronchogenic carcinoma.
   Heterogeneously enhancing mass on CT thorax abutting the great vessels with history of weight loss, chest pain and hemoptysis complements the diagnosis of lung cancer.
2. C
   EGFR mutation is most common in non smoker Asian women with histology of adenocarcinoma.
3. B
   Adenocarcinoma is most commonly associated with pleural effusion and pleural dissemination
4. A
   Geftinib is the recommended first line chemotherapy for a patient of lung adenocarcinoma harboring EGFR mutation
5. C
   Small cell carcinoma is associated most commonly with distant metastasis and paraneoplastic syndromes

Reference:

1. Rolf A Stahel. First-line therapy of advanced non small cell lung cancer with activating EGFR mutations.In: Lung Cancer Therapy Annual 7.CRC Press,London2012,pp 75-78.

TUBERCULOSIS

Dr. Surya Kant, Dr. Ajay Kumar Verma, Dr. Anand Srivastava, Dr. Ved Prakash, Dr. Anubhuti
Department of Respiratory Medicine

A 45 year old alcoholic male presented with one month history of low grade fever and productive cough. He was prescribed antibiotics for 7 days by a local practitioner, but did not respond. On physical examination, patient had coarse crepts in left suprascapular region. Chest radiograph revealed infiltrates in left upper zone. Mantoux test showed an induration of 18 mm. Sputum smear examination revealed abundant acid fast bacilli.

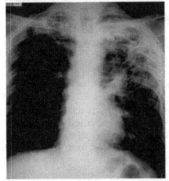

1. What is the most probable diagnosis?
    (A) Bronchiectasis.
    (B) Community acquired pneumonia.
    (C) Pulmonary tuberculosis.

(D) Lung cancer.
2. The highest TB burden country in the world is:
   (A) China.
   (B) India.
   (C) Ethiopia.
   (D) Peru.
3. The most common site of involvement in extra-pulmonary tuberculosis:
   (A) Spine/Musculoskeletal System.
   (B) Genito-urinary system.
   (C) Lymph nodes.
   (D) Pleura.
4. Which of the following drugs is not used in the treatment of multi-drug resistant pulmonary tuberculosis.
   (A) Kanamycin.
   (B) Cyclosporine.
   (C) Levofloxacin.
   (D) Ethambutol.
5. Most common adverse effect experienced by patients on ATT is
   (A) Rash.
   (B) Hepatitis.
   (C) Renal impairment.
   (D) Gastritis and nausea vomiting

Answers:

1. C
   Pulmonary Tuberculosis.
   Cough with expectoration for more than 15 days with fever not responding to antibiotics suggests diagnosis of pulmonary tuberculosis which is confirmed by sputum smear examination which reveals acid fast bacilli.

2. B
   India is the highest TB burden country with prevalence of approximately 9.6 million.

3. C
   Lymph node TB is the most common EPTB which is followed by GUTB.

4. B
   Cyclosporine is not used for MDR TB treatment. The drugs used are Kanamycin, Pyrizinamide, Ethambutol, Ethionamide, Cycloserineand Levofloxacin.

5. D
   Gastritis and nausea vomiting.
   Most common adverse event patients on ATT experience is a mild degree of gastritis in form of nausea, vomiting.

References:

1. WHO Library Cataloguing-in-Publication Data: Treatment of tuberculosis: guidelines – 4th ed. WHO/HTM/TB/2009.420
2. WHO global tuberculosis report 2014. http://www.who.int/tb/publications/global_report/en/

INTERSTITIAL LUNG DISEASE/ IPF

Dr. Surya Kant, Dr. Ved Prakash, Dr. Ajay Kumar Verma, Dr. Anand Srivastava, Dr. Karthik Nagaraju
Department of Respiratory Medicine

A 62 year old male, farmer by occupation, presented with a 7 months history of dry cough and exertional dyspnea. He is smoker for 20 years and smoked nearly 20 cigarettes per day. He was prescribed anti tubercular treatment (ATT) for his illness but got no relief on ATT. His physical examination revealed use of accessory muscles of respiration. RR of 24/min, PR of 126/min, BP 136/84 mm of Hg, SpO291 % on room air, pandigital clubbing of grade 3 was also noted. Auscultation revealed fine inspiratory crepts of Velcro character at the lung bases.

ABG was: pH- 7.32,pO2-54,pCO2-32,HCO3⁻-20.3,SPO2-90.6.Diffusion capacity of lung <50%

SPIROMETRY	PRE		POST	%PREDICTED
FEV1	1.65		1.67	52%
FVC	1.82		1.84	40%
FEV1/FVC	90.6		90.785%	

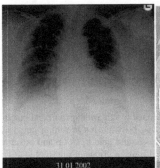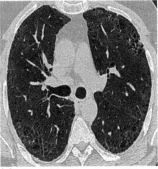

31.01.2002

1. What is the most probable diagnosis?
   (A) COPD.
   (B) Bronchial asthma.
   (C) Interstitial lung disease.
   (D) Bronchiectasis.
2. Which of the following ILD has an association with smoking?
   (A) IPF
   (B) Hypersensitivity pneumonitis
   (C) Sarcoidosis
   (D) Bronchial asthma
3. Which of the following investigations is most helpful in establishing diagnosis?
   (A) Spirometry with DLCO
   (B) HRCT Thorax
   (C) 6 Minute walk test
   (D) 2 D Echocardiography
4. What is the treatment of IPF
   (A) Oxygen therapy and supportive care
   (B) Inhaled corticosteroids
   (C) Inhaled beta 2 agonists
   (D) Systemic corticosteroids
5. Which is not a characteristic feature of IPF on HRCT
   (A) Honeycoomb appearance
   (B) Tractional bronchiectasis
   (C) Ground glassing
   (D) Basal predominance .

Answers:

1. C
   An old aged smoker man with pandigital clubbing and bilateral Velcro crepts with features of restrictive lung disease and decreased DLCO suggest ILD.
   The smoking history and age with clubbing suggest Idiopathic Pulmonary Fibrosis (IPF). HRCT confirms the diagnosis with bibasilar reticular pattern and fibrosis with honey-combing.

2. A
   IPF is the type of ILD most commonly associated with smoking.

3. B
   HRCT is the most useful investigation for confirmation of ILD. It demonstrates fibrosis, reticulation, ground glassing and honeycombing which are specific features of ILD. HRCT is also able to differentiate in between different types of ILD.

4. A
   No drug treatment is effective in IPF including corticosteroids, azathioprine, N-Acetyl Cystine or their combination.

5. C
   Ground glassing is not a feature of IPF. It goes against the suspicion of IPF. Rest three are characteristic features of UIP pattern on HRCT suggesting IPF.

Reference:
1. Raghu G, Collard HR, Egan JJ, Martinez FJ, et al. An official ATS/ERS/JRS/ALAT statement: idiopathic pulmonary fibrosis: evidence-based guidelines for diagnosis and management. Am J Respir Crit Care Med. 2011;183(6):788-824.

PNEUMONIA

Dr. Surya Kant, Dr. Ajay Kumar Verma, Dr. Anand Srivastava, Dr. Ved Prakash, Dr. Prachi Saxena
Department of Respiratory Medicine

A 21-year-old male with a previously unremarkable medical history, developed cough with sputum and blood-stained sputum since 1 week. His temperature was 37.3 °C, his pulse was 114/min, his breathing rate was 32/min and his blood pressure was 105/70 mmHg. The patient was conscious, and able to sit up and breathe. However, he displayed an anemic appearance, with crackles in the mid and lower sections of the right lung on auscultation. Blood test results upon admission were: WBC count = 23.1×10^9/l, 86.3% neutrophils, RBC count = 3.68×10^{12}/l, hemoglobin concentration = 10.1 g/l and platelet count = 2.95×10^9/l. Blood-gas analysis results showed a blood pH of 7.49, a $PaCO_2$ of 36.0 mmHg, a PaO_2 of 50.0 mmHg, a Base Excess of 4.2 mmol/l and a $HCO3-$ concentration of 27.9 mmol/l. Chest X ray is displayed.

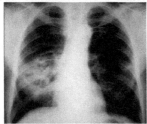

1. What is the most common organism responsible for this kind of presentation?
   (A) Staphylococcus aureus
   (B) Streptococcus pneumoniae
   (C) Haemophilus influenzae
   (D) Escherichia coli
2. What is the most common age group affected by this condition?
   (A) School going children
   (B) Infants
   (C) Adults
   (D) Elderly
3. Which of the following conditions can't present with a similar radiological appearance?
   (A) Cavitating lung cancer
   (B) Loculated pneumothorax
   (C) Congenital cystic adenomatoid malformation (CCAM)
   (D) Empyema necessitans
4. All of the following features make the diagnosis of a pneumatocele more likely than abscess EXCEPT
   (A) Smooth inner margins
   (B) Contains little fluid
   (C) Wall (if visible) is thick and irregular
   (D) Persist despite absence of symptoms
5. The approved antibiotic for community acquired MRSA pneumonia is
   (A) Cephalosporins
   (B) Linezolid
   (C) Carbapenems
   (D) Fluoroquinolones

Answers:
   1. A
       Staphylococcus aureus is the most common organism causing pneumatocele in lung.
   2. B
       Although pneumatoceles are seen in all age groups, they are most frequently encountered in infancy. In premature infants with respiratory distress syndrome, pneumatoceles result mostly from ventilator-induced lung injury.

3. D

The differential diagnosis for a cavitating lung lesion includes:
cavitating lung cancer.
cavitating pulmonary metastasis.
hydatid cyst.
loculated pneumothorax.
large emphysematous bullae.

4. C

pulmonary abscess can be difficult to distinguish but it has thicker irregular walls and should resolve as symptoms resolve.

5. A

For community-acquired methicillin-resistant Staphylococcus aureus infection, add vancomycin or linezolid.

References:

1. Flaherty RA, Keegan JM, Sturtevant HN. Post-pneumonic pulmonary pneumatoceles. Radiology. 1960;74 : 50-3.
2. Mandell, Lionel A, et al. "Infectious Diseases Society of America/American Thoracic Society consensus guidelines on the management of community-acquired pneumonia in adults." *Clinical infectious diseases* 44.Supplement 2 (2007): S27-S72.

Chapter-27

Surgery

DISORDERS OF SUBMANDIBULAR GLAND

Dr. Abhinav Arun Sonkar, Professor and Head, Department of Surgery

A 28 years old male presents to surgical OPD with history of recurrent h/o swelling in right submandibular region specially on eating food, which is painful. The swelling resolves spontaneously with time (2-3 hours). Clinical examination reveals an enlarged firm submandibular gland, tender on bimanual examination.

1. Which of the following statement regarding the submandibular gland is FALSE?
   (A) The deep part of the gland lies on the hyoglossus muscle closely related to the lingual nerve and inferior to the hypoglossal nerve.
   (B) Stafne bone cyst is an ectopic salivary tissue.
   (C) Important anatomical relations include the anterior facial vein running over the surface of the gland and the facial artery.
   (D) They consist of a smaller superficial and a larger deep lobe that are continuous around the posterior border of the stylohoid muscle.

2. Which of the following statement is TRUE regarding Sialolithiasis?
   (A) Fifty per cent of all salivary stones occur in the submandibular glands.
   (B) Eighty per cent of submandibular stones are radio-opaque and can be identified on plain radiography.
   (C) Secretions of submandibular glands are low in viscosity.
   (D) Partial duct obstruction leads to less symptoms and signs, only confined to meals.

3. Regarding management of sialolithiasis which of the following statement is FALSE?
   (A) If the stone is lying within the submandibular duct in the floor of the mouth anterior to the point at which the duct crosses the lingual nerve, the stone can be removed by incising longitudinally over the duct.
   (B) Where the stone is proximal to the second molar, i.e. at the hilum of the gland, stone retrieval via an intraoral approach should be avoided.
   (C) If the stone is lying within the submandibular duct in the floor of the mouth posterior to the second molar, the stone should be removed by total excision of submandibular gland with ligation of the duct.
   (D) Once the stone has been delivered, the wall of the duct should be stitched to avoid free drainage of saliva.

Answers:

1.   D.

   The submandibular glands consist of a larger superficial and a smaller deep lobe that are continuous around the posterior border of the mylohyoid muscle. Important anatomical relations include the anterior facial vein running over the surface of the gland and the facial artery. The deep part of the gland lies on the hyoglossus muscle closely related to the lingual nerve and inferior to the hypoglossal nerve.

   The most common ectopic salivary tissue is the Stafne bone cyst. It is formed by invagination into the bone on the lingual aspect of the mandible of an ectopic lobe of the juxtaposed submandibular gland.

2.   B.

   Eighty per cent of all salivary stones occur in the submandibular glands because their secretions are highly viscous. Eighty per cent of submandibular stones are radio-opaque and can be identified on plain radiography.

   More frequently, the stone causes only partial obstruction when it lies within the hilum of the gland or within the duct in the floor of the mouth. In such circumstances, symptoms are more infrequent, producing minimal discomfort and swelling, not confined to mealtimes.

3.   D.

   If the stone is lying within the submandibular duct in the floor of the mouth anterior to the point at which the duct crosses the lingual nerve (second molar region), the stone can be removed by incising longitudinally over the duct. Once the stone has been delivered, the wall of the duct should be left open to promote free drainage of saliva. Suturing the duct will lead to stricture formation and the recurrence of obstructive symptoms.

Reference:

1.   Smith WP. Disorders of the salivary glands. In: Williams NS, Bulstrode CJK, O'Connell PR (Eds) Bailey and Love's Short Practice of Surgery, 26th edition. CRC Press: Boca Raton 2013,pp 723-728.

ORAL CANCER (CA TONGUE)
Dr. Abhinav Arun Sonkar, Professor and Head, Department of Surgery

A 52 yrs old man chronic tobacco chewer comes to surgical OPD with complaints of a non-healing ulcer over left lateral border of tongue for past 6 months.

On oral examination the ulcer is 3*3 cm in size with a hard base and proliferative margins and pus at floor. On cervical examination patient has left level I and II cervical lymphadenopathy. Patient has no trismus. Incisional biopsy from ulcer margins shows well-differentiated squamous cell carcinoma.

1. Which of the following is TRUE of Ca tongue?
   - (A) OPD examination under anesthesia is rarely required
   - (B) T1 (<2 cm diameter) tumour has no chances of occult metastasis at presentation
   - (C) When performing surgical excision of the primary tumour, a 1-cm margin in all planes should be achieved to ensure a wide, complete excision
   - (D) Lingual Lymph nodes may be a cause for recurrence
2. What effect does the presence of cervical lymph nodal metastasis has on prognosis in head and neck cancer?
   - (A) 10% decrease in survival
   - (B) 30% decrease in survival
   - (C) 50% decrease in survival
   - (D) no effect on overall survival
3. Which of the following factors should NOT be considered in tailoring treatment for a patient of head and neck cancer?
   - (A) Site of the disease
   - (B) Stage of the disease
   - (C) Social factors
   - (D) All of the above

Answers:
1. D.

   When a patient undergoes simultaneous neck dissection, the resection of the primary tumour should preferably be in continuity with the neck node specimen. This eliminates 'lingual' lymph nodes (lying between the primary tumour and submandibular (level I_B) nodes); these nodes may contain micro-deposits of tumour, which may lead to local recurrence.

2. C

   Cervical node metastasis, particularly with extracapsular spread, is the most significant factor in determining prognosis for oropharyngeal cancer.

3. D

   The two principal treatment modalities of oropharyngeal cancer are surgery and radiotherapy. Small tumours can be managed either by primary radiotherapy or surgery. Large-volume disease, i.e. advanced tumour, usually requires a combination of surgery and radiotherapy.

Factors that need to be taken into consideration include:
- the site of disease
- the stage
- histology
- concomitant medical disease
- social factors.

Reference:
1. Smith WP. Oropharyngeal cancer. In: Williams NS, Bulstrode CJK, O'Connell PR (Eds) Bailey and Love's Short Practice of Surgery, 26th edition. CRC Press: Boca Raton 2013,pp 706-722.

PREMALIGNANT ORAL CONDITIONS (LEUKOPLAKIA)
Dr. Abhinav Arun Sonkar, Professor and Head, Department of Surgery

A 36 yrs young male comes to surgical OPD with complaints of a whitish discoloration over left lateral border of tongue for past 3 months. Patient has a history of smoking for past 8 years.

On examination, a whitish area of size 3*3 cm in size is present over lateral border of tongue.There is no cervical lymphadenopathy detected and no trismus.

1. Premalignant lesion with highest rate of malignant transformation is?
   (A) Leukoplakia
   (B) Speckled Leukoplakia
   (C) Erythroplakia
   (D) Erythroplasia
2. The term 'field change' in relation to oral cancer refers to?
   (A) Wide field radiotherapy techniques, which must be, applied to the oral mucosa in head and neck cancer patients.
   (B) Demarcated mucosal changes seen in patients with oral cancer, which resembles the appearance of agricultural fields.
   (C) Effect upon the surrounding oral mucosa conferred by long-standing dental caries.
   (D) Wide spread damage of epithelium leading to mucosal changes and a high incidence of separate tumors.
3. Management of premalignant lesions should NOT include?
   (A) Smoking cessation
   (B) Photographic recording
   (C) Biopsy from more than one site
   (D) Radiotherapy

Answers:

1. B.
   Speckled leukoplakia: This is a variation of leukoplakia arising on an erythematous base. It has the highest rate of malignant transformation.

2. D.
   The diffuse and chronic exposure of the mucosa of the upper aero-digestive tract to carcinogenic substances, e.g. tobacco and alcohol, causes widespread adverse changes in the mucosal epithelium. The consequence of the diffuse exposure is the development of separate tumors at different anatomical sites.

3. D.
   Cessation of smoking, elimination of the areca nut/pan habit and reduction in alcohol consumption should be encouraged in all patients with premalignant lesions. A photographic record of the lesion is useful, particularly for long-term follow up. Biopsy from more than one site provides a better representation of histological changes within a lesion.
   Small lesions may be managed with surgical excision and primary closure by undermining the adjacent mucosa.

Reference:

1. Smith WP. Oropharyngeal cancer. In: Williams NS, Bulstrode CJK, O'Connell PR (Eds). Bailey and Love's Short Practice of Surgery, 26th edition. CRC Press: Boca Raton 2013,pp 706-722.

URINARY BLADDER CARCINOMA

Dr. Harvinder Singh Pahwa, Professor, Department of Surgery

A 50 years male farmer, resident of Barabanki, no concurrent history of hypertension, chronic smoker, without any preceding history of trauma or LUTS, presented in OPD with four episodes of gross painless hematuria each lasting for about 3 to 5 days in past one and half years. Physical examination is normal except pallor. Renal function and liver function tests are normal. Hematuria is confirmed by urine microscopic examination.

1. The most likely diagnosis is?
   (A) Cystolithiasis
   (B) Carcinoma prostate
   (C) Benign prostatic hyperplasia
   (D) Carcinoma urinary bladder
2. Next investigation to be advised for diagnosis?
   (A) USG KUB
   (B) Plain X ray KUB
   (C) CT abdomen
   (D) Cystoscopy and transurethral resection
3. On U/S he had a superficial papillary growth on right posterolateral wall of urinary bladder about size of 2cm. Next step in the management is?
   (A) CT Abdomen
   (B) MRI Abdomen
   (C) Cystoscopy and TURBT

(D) IVU
4. Most likely histopathology report in this case is?
   (A) Adenocarcinoma
   (B) Squamous cell carcinoma
   (C) Transitional cell carcinoma
   (D) Rhabdomyosarcoma

Answers:
1.   D.
   Most common symptom of carcinoma urinary bladder is painless hematuria which is intermittent rather than constant.
2.   A.
   Initial investigation for diagnosis and screening is U/S abdomen or KUB region.
3.   C.
   For superficial bladder cancer, cystoscopy and TURBT is procedure of choice for treatment and staging.
4.   C.
   More than 90% of bladder carcinoma is Transitional Cell Carcinoma.

Reference:
1. Hamdy F. The urinary bladder. In: Williams NS, Bulstrode CJK, O'Connell PR (Eds) Bailey and Love's Short Practice of Surgery, 26th edition. CRC Press: Boca Raton 2013, pp 1329-1338.

SEMINOMA TESTIS
Dr. Harvinder Singh Pahwa, Professor, Department of Surgery

A 28 Years male, resident of Lucknow, bank executive presents in OPD with a painless progressively increasing left scrotal swelling for last six months. On physical examination he had left painless testicular mass, no lymphadenopathy or organomegaly. There is no h/o trauma, fever, jaundice, cough, hemoptysis and respiratory distress.

1. In the evaluation of this patient following is NOT indicated:?
   (A) Chest X ray
   (B) Testicular biopsy
   (C) CT Abdomen
   (D) Tumor markers
2. On further work up and staging it was diagnosed as Stage I Seminoma Testis with normal markers (Beta HCG , ALP and AFP) , treatment of choice is ?
   (A) Radiotherapy and chemothearapy
   (B) High Inguinal Orchidectomy
   (C) Trans scrotal orchidectomy
   (D) High Inguinal Orchidectomy and Radiotherapy
3. Which of the following is TRUE about seminoma testis?
   (A) AFP is raised
   (B) Cured only by Surgery
   (C) It arises only in undescended testis
   (D) It is radiosensitive
4. The first Echelon group of lymph nodes to receive lymphatic metastasis in carcinoma testis is ?
   (A) Internal Iliac
   (B) Deep Inguinal lymph nodes
   (C) Para aortic LN
   (D) Superficial Inguinal LN

Answers:
1.   A.
   FNAC and testicular biopsy is contraindicated (Scrotal seedlings may result in inguinal Lymph node metastasis).
2.   B.
   Histopathological diagnosis is made by high inguinal orchidectomy (the cord is ligated at deep inguinal ring).

3. D

Seminoma is most radiosensitive testicular tumour.

4. C

The primary landing site for the Right testis is the inter aortocaval area and Lt. testis is para-aortic area at the level of renal hilum.

References:

1. Andrew J. Stephenson, Timothy D. Gilligan. Neoplasms of the testis In: Alan J. Wein et al (Eds). Campbell-Walsh Urology. 10th ed. Saunders Elsevier; Philadelphia 2012. pp 3725-3729.
2. Ian Eardley. Testis and Scrotum In: Williams NS, Bulstrode CJK, O'Connell PR. (Eds). Bailey & Love's Short Practice of Surgery. 26th ed. CRC Press: Boca Raton 2013. pp 1384-1387.

URETHRAL INJURY
Dr. Harvindrer S. Pahwa, Professor, Department of Surgery

A 35 Years young male with H/O road traffic accident few hours back was brought in Surgical Emergency. Patient was conscious, BP was 110/80, RR was 32/min, PR was 100/min. On examination blood at urethral meatus was present and pelvic # was suspected. Patient was not able to pass urine and his bladder is palpable on per abdomen examination.

1. The most probable diagnosis is?
   (A) Rupture bladder
   (B) Anuria due to hypovolumia
   (C) Urethral injury
   (D) Kidney Laceration
2. The first investigation to be advised for confirmation of diagnosis?
   (A) U/S Abdomen – KUB
   (B) CT Abdomen
   (C) Retrograde Urethogram
   (D) Intra Venous Urogram
3. Immediate most safe procedure to be done in this patient?
   (A) Urinary catheterization
   (B) Suprapubic Cystostomy
   (C) Observation
   (D) Referral to urologist
4. On the basis of Anatomy of pelvis and perineum, TRUE statement regarding collection of urine in urethral rupture above deep perineal pouch is?
   (A) Medial aspect of thigh
   (B) Anterior abdominal wall
   (C) Scrotum
   (D) True pelvis only
5. Which of the following is NOT a feature of membranous urethral injury ?
   (A) Retention of urine
   (B) Blood at meatus
   (C) pelvic #
   (D) Scrotal Injury

Answers:

1. C

Pelvic # with blood at meatus is suggestive of urethral (membranous) injury.

2. B

For urethral injury first investigation to be done for confirmation of diagnosis is Retrograde urethrogram (RGU).

3. B

First, most safe procedure in urethral injury to be done is suprapubic cystostomy.

4. B

In posterior urethral rupture, there is deep extravasation of urine.

5. D

Membranous urethral injury is associated with blunt pelvic trauma with # pelvis and not with scrotal injury, which may be associated with bulbar urethral injury.

References:
1. Surgery of Penis and Urethra. In: Alan J Weinet al. (Eds)Campbell-Walsh Urology. 10th ed. Saunders Elsevier; Philadelphia 2012. pp 983-984.
2. David S. Sharp, Kenneth W. Angermeier. Urethra and Penis. In: Emil A Tanagho, Jack W McAninch (Eds). Smith's General Urology. 17th ed. McGraw Hill; New Delhi 2008,pp 291-295.
3. Ian Eardley. Urethra and Penis. In: Williams NS Bulstrode CJK, O'Connell PR (Eds). Bailey and Love's Short Practice of Surgery. 26th ed. CRC Press: Boca Raton 2013. pp 1361-1363.

CARCINOMA BREAST
Dr. Sandeep Tiwari, Professor, Department of Surgery

60 year old lady presented with right breast lump of size 12x 10 cm in upper and outer quadrant, which is hard, irregular, fixed to chest wall with peau d' orange and ipsilateral matted fixed nodes in axilla. There is no history of bone pain, hemoptysis or abdominal lump. Histopathology is infiltrating ductal carcinoma, and IHC is ER-ve PR-ve and Herzneu-ve

1. T staging of this patient is?
   (A) T3
   (B) T4a
   (C) T4b
   (D) T4c
2. Triple assessment includes?
   (A) Clinical examination, imaging of breast and histopathology
   (B) Breast Imaging, histology and CBC
   (C) CBC, Breast imaging and CT scan head
   (D) Bone scan, CT scan thorax and Clinical examination to
3. According to molecular classification she belongs to which category?
   (A)Luminal A
   (B)Luminal B
   (C)Luminal C
   (D)Basal like
4. In present scenario best sequence of treatment will be?
   (A) MRM followed by adjuvant therapy
   (B) MRM only
   (C) Neoadjuvant therapy followed by MRM followed by adjuvant therapy
   (D) Hormone therapy only

Answers:
1. D
   According to TNM staging (AJCC 7th edition) T4c is involvement of both skin and chest wall.
2. A
   Triple assessment includes clinical examination, imaging of breast ie. Mammography for > 35 years of age and HR USG for less 35 years, and histopathology.
3. D
   Molecular classification is considered better in terms of management and prognosis and triple negative is classified as basal type and is associated with poor prognosis.
4. C
   It is locally advance disease (stage 3b) therefore neoadjuvant treatment has to be given to downstage the disease followed by MRM and adjuvant treatment.

Reference:
1. Sainsbury R. The Breast. In: Williams NS, Bulstrode CJK, O'Connell PR (Eds) Bailey and Love's Short Practice of Surgery, 26th edition. CRC Press: Boca Raton 2013, pp 798-822.

PHYLLODES TUMOR
Dr. Sandeep Tiwari, Professor, Department of Surgery

40-year-old lady is having 10x10 cm lobulated recurrent lump in her left breast, which is firm in consistency and not fixed to breast tissue or underlying muscle, axillary lymph nodes are not palpable.

1. What could be the most probable provisional diagnosis?
   (A)Simple fibroadenoma
   (B)Phyllodes Tumor
   (C)Traumatic fat necrosis
   (D)Sclerosing Fibroadenosis
2. How will you confirm your diagnosis?
   (A)Trucut biopsy
   (B)Mammography
   (C)CT scan of breast
   (D)HR USG of breast
3. What treatment you will offer to this patient?
   (A)Radical mastectomy
   (B)Simple mastectomy
   (C)Chemoradiation
   (D)Lumpectomy with 1 cm of margin

Answers:
1. B.
   Phyllodes tumor is disease of young adult female and presents as huge bosselated lump in breast notorious for recurrence if not excised properly.
2. A.
   Histopathological confirmation is best way to confirm the diagnosis.
3. B.
   Recurrent, massive or malignant phyllodes tumor require mastectomy.

Reference:
1. Sainsbury R. The Breast. In: Williams NS, Bulstrode CJK, O'Connell PR (Eds) Bailey and Love's Short Practice of Surgery, 26th edition. CRC Press: Boca Raton 2013, pp 798-822.

GRAVE'S DISEASE
Dr. Sandeep Tiwari, Professor, Department of Surgery

35-year-old male presented with anterior neck swelling for 3 months, with history of weight loss, palpitation, tremors and double vision. On examination thyroid is diffusely enlarged and firm in consistency. Pulse rate is 140 beats per minute, palms are moist and exophthalmos is present.

1. What is clinical diagnosis of this patient?
   (A) Plummer's disease
   (B) Graves' disease
   (C) Hashimoto's thyroiditis
   (D) Toxic adenoma
2. What biochemical abnormality do you expect in above patient?
   (A) $\downarrow$ TSH, $\downarrow$ T4, $\downarrow$ T3
   (B) $\uparrow$ TSH, $\downarrow$ T4, $\downarrow$ T3
   (C) $\uparrow$ TSH, $\uparrow$ T4, $\uparrow$ T3
   (D) $\downarrow$TSH, $\uparrow$T4, $\uparrow$ T3
3. The patient can be treated by?
   (A) ATD, RAI, Surgery
   (B) ATD only
   (C) RAI only
   (D) Surgery only
4. If the patient opts for surgical therapy what would be best surgery for him?
   (A) Lobectomy
   (B) Total thyroidectomy
   (C) Subtotal thyroidectomy
   (D) Hemithyroidectomy

Answers:
1. B.
   Diffuse enlargement of thyroid with toxic symptoms and exophthalmos are sufficient to diagnose Grave's disease clinically.
2. B.

In diffuse toxic goiter serum TSH is decreased while Serum T3 and serum T4 are increased.
3. C.
All three modalities of treatment may be given depending upon patient age, pregnancy, patients will and general condition of the patient.
4. B.
For diffuse toxic goiter choice of treatment is total or near total thyroidectomy.

Reference:
1. Krukowski ZH. The Thyroid and parathyroid. In: Williams NS, Bulstrode CJK, O'Connell PR (Eds) Bailey and Love's Short Practice of Surgery, 26th edition. CRC Press: Boca Raton 2013, pp 741-777.

BLUNT ABDOMINAL AND PELVIC TRAUMA
Dr. Vinod Jain, Professor, Department of Surgery

60-year-old male car driver restrained by abdominal belt at umbilicus had high-speed motor vehicle collision. On arrival to hospital his vitals were blood pressure 100/70 mmHg, Heart rate 100/min and respiratory rate 18/min. His GCS score is 15. Patient was complaining of pain in lower chest, abdomen and pelvis. FAST examination showed collection of fluid in hepato-renal, spleno-renal and pelvic cavity. Aspiration of peritoneal cavity revealed 10 ml of frank blood. AMPLE history revealed that patient is taking antihypertensive drugs with beta blockers.

1. Letter "M" in AMPLE history stands for –
   (A)Medical conditions
   (B)Medications
   (C)Middle age
   (D)Motor Vehicle
2. Which x-ray study is done during primary survey of injured patient?
   (A)X-ray chest and x-ray pelvis
   (B)X-ray chest and x-ray cervical spine
   (C)X-ray cervical spine and x-ray long bones
   (D)CT scan of abdomen
3. On laparotomy patient's spleen is lacerated. Which management will be most appropriate and safer?
   (A)Watchful waiting without dislodging haematoma
   (B)Splenorrhaphy
   (C)Splenectomy
   (D)Packing the laceration and apply hemostatic materials
4. Pringle's maneuver is done to minimize bleeding from ?
   (A)Liver
   (B)Spleen
   (C)Mesentery
   (D)Uterine arteries
5. Which of the following is NOT correct?
   (A)Patient is in hemorrhagic shock
   (B)Patient may have Chance fracture of lumbar spine
   (C)Diagnostic peritoneal lavage is also indicated in this patient
   (D)Use of Beta Blockers does not affect the assessment of this patient

Answers:
   1. B.
   AMPLE is mnemonic of history taking
   A – Allergy
   M – Medications
   P – Past Medical history
   L – Last meal
   E – Events of the incident
   2. A.
   As per ATLS protocol
   3. C.
   Splenectomy is the safer option in multiple injury and or patient with age more than 55 year to prevent re bleeding
   4. A.

Pringles maneuver is direct compression of portal triad to reduce the inflow of blood to liver
5. D.
Beta-blocker reduces the heart rate and therefore masks the tachycardia response of hemorrhagic shock. Despite beta-blocker use, patient is having pulse rate 100/min, therefore he is in shock.

Reference :

1. American College Surgeons Committee on trauma, Advanced Trauma Life support for Doctors, ATLS student course manual, 9th edition 2012.

BLUNT CHEST INJURY WITH HYPOTHERMIA
Dr. Vinod Jain, Professor, Department of Surgery

35-year-old male labor was injured due to collapse of roof at construction site. He was pinned under iron girder for more than two hours, which has fallen on his chest. Outside temperature was 14^0 C. He could be rescued from the site and brought to the casualty room of level three-trauma center. At the time of admission his B.P. was 80/40 mm Hg, heart rate 110/min. Respiration rate 12 breath / min smooth. He was having plethora and petechial patches above nipple line. He was non responsive to verbal commands, opened eyes in response to pain and flexed his extremities when pinched. Core body temperature was 32.5^0 C.

1. Patient is suffering from ?
    (A) Cardiac tamponade with hypothermia
    (B) Pneumothorax with hypothermia
    (C) Blunt cardiac injury with hypothermia
    (D) Traumatic asphyxia with hypothermia
2. GCS score of patient is ?
    (A) 6
    (B) 7
    (C) 8
    (D) 9
3. Level 3 - trauma center means a center capable of ?
    (A) Providing assessment, resuscitation and emergency surgery
    (B) 24 hour physician coverage, resuscitation and stabilization of injured patient with no facility for emergency surgery
    (C) Multispecialty services to injured patient under one roof
    (D) Only day care to injured patients
4. Temperature of intravenous fluid to be infused should be ?
    (A) Room temperature
    (B) 37.4^0 C
    (C) 39^0 C
    (D) 41.2^0 C
5. Which of the following statement is NOT correct?
    (A) The patient may have cerebral edema
    (B) Patient needs warmed humidified oxygen
    (C) Patient needs endotracheal intubation
    (D) Patient is in having traumatic pneumothorax

Answers:
1. D
    Because of chest compression due to iron girder, there is compression on superior vena cava causing plethora and petichae above nipple line. This is typical feature of traumatic asphyxia. Patient is having hypothermia as well. Any patient having body temperature below 36^0 C is labelled as hypothermic
2. B.
    Based on factual data –
    No response to verbal commands – 1
    Opening of eye is response to pain – 2
    Flex or response on pinching – 4
    GCS 1+2+4 = 7
3. A.
    Levels of trauma centers are defined as level 1, 2, 3 and 4. Level three trauma center has got emergency surgical facilities

4. C.
    To prevent for and treat hypothermia we need to infuse warm intra-venous fluids. Temperature should be more than body temperature but should not damage the cells.
5. D.
    None of physical finding mentioned supports pneumothorax. No presumptions.

Reference:

1. American College Surgeons Committee on trauma, Advanced Trauma Life support for Doctors, ATLS student course manual, 9th edition 2012.

CHEST TRAUMA
Dr. Vinod Jain, Professor, Department of Surgery

28-year-old male is brought to the casualty of small community hospital. He is having history of stab injury in left fourth intercostal space, anterior to the mid axillary line caused by a long knife. His blood pressure is 70/40 mm Hg. Heart rate 140/min. and respiration rate 34/min. On examination he is having cool and diaphoretic skin, sucking stab wound of 2.5 cm in length in left fourth intercostal space at the site of injury with subcutaneous emphysema, distended neck veins, alert and responds to painful stimuli. He is being given oxygen at 6 liters/minute via mask.

1. First priority of treatment in this patient will be ?
   (A) To cover the chest wound
   (B) To give intravenous fluid rapidly
   (C) To secure airway and cervical spine
   (D) To get a chest x ray
2. Sucking chest wound on left side is due to?
   (A) Simple pneumothorax
   (B) Open pneumothorax
   (C) Flail chest
   (D) Broncho-pleural fistula
3. Distended neck veins is this patient are most likely due to?
   (A) Tension pneumothorax
   (B) Injury to myocardium
   (C) Injury to superior vena cava
   (D) Hemorrhagic shock
4. Preferred flow rate of oxygen (in liter / minute) via a tight fitting mask in trauma patient should be at least?
   (A) 6
   (B) 8
   (C) 11
   (D) 18
5. Arterial blood gas determination of this patient shows pH=7.21, $PaCO_2$ = 39 mm Hg, PaO_2= 58 mm Hg, SaO_2 =83%, HCO_3 = 24. The patient is having?
   (A) Alkalosis with Hypoxemia
   (B) Alkalosis with Hypercarbia
   (C) Acidosis with Hypercarbia
   (D) Acidosis with Hypoxemia

Answers:

1. C.
    As per ATLS protocol, we always follow ABCDE pattern for managing the trauma patient. 'A' stands for airway with cervical spine protection.
2. B
    Air follows the path of least resistance. Whenever the chest wound is more than $2/3^{rd}$ the diameter of trachea, air enters through the wound thus having communication between atmosphere and pleural cavity.
3. B
    Distended neck veins in trauma are due to obstructive shock which is due to poor venous return. This can happen in tension pneumothorax and / or cardiac tamponade. In this patient, there is open pneumothorax. Due to penetrating injury in the myocardium, blood collected in pericardial sac is causing cardiac tamponade.

4. C
5. D
   In ABG analysis pH and saturation of oxygen are low. Carbon dioxide is normal. Therefore patient is having acidosis with hypoxemia.

Reference:

1. American College Surgeons Committee on trauma, Advanced Trauma Life support for Doctors, ATLS student course manual, 9th edition 2012.

PRIMARY HYPERALDOSTERONISM

Dr. Anand Mishra, Associate Professor, Department of Surgery; Arpit Agarwal, MBBS (Stud.),

A 50 years old man presents with headache, generalized muscle weakness, tiredness, polydipsia and polyuria of 7 months duration. He has resistant hypertension. Lab reports show serum potassium is 2.3 mmol/l with metabolic alkalosis.

1. Which of the following is the most likely diagnosis?
   (A) Myasthenia gravis
   (B) Conn's syndrome
   (C) Addison's disease
   (D) Electrolyte imbalance
2. Which of the following is the most appropriate next step in diagnosis?
   (A) Plasma aldosterone and plasma renin ratio
   (B) Serum potassium and serum sodium estimation
   (C) Serum calcium and serum phosphorus estimation
   (D) Urinary aldosterone
3. Which of the following is most likely to confirm the diagnosis EXCEPT?
   (A) Plasma aldosterone to plasma renin ratio more than 30
   (B) Plasma aldosterone concentration more than or equal to 15 mg/L
   (C) Plasma renin activity less than or equal to 1 mg/L
   (D) Low urinary and high plasma aldosterone levels
4. Which of the following is most appropriate pharmacotherapy before surgery after biochemical confirmation of diagnosis of primary hyperaldosteronism?
   (A) Spironolactone
   (B) Alpha blocker
   (C) Centrally acting antihypertensive
   (D) Saline infusion
5. Which of the following radiological investigation is most appropriate after biochemical diagnosis?
   (A) PET CT
   (B) MIBG Scan
   (C) MRI or CECT abdomen
   (D) Ultrasound KUB region
6. Which of the following is the most effective management of Primary hyperaldosteronism?
   (A) Bilateral adrenalectomy
   (B) Medulla sparing adrenalectomy
   (C) Laparoscopic adrenalectomy
   (D) Pharmacotherapy with spirolactone
7. Which of the following is the most common cause of primary hyperaldosteronism?
   (A) Adreno-cortical carcinoma
   (B) Solitary adrenal adenoma
   (C) Bilateral adrenal hyperplasia
   (D) Pituitary neoplasm
8. Which of the following test can differentiate primary hyperaldosteronism from secondary hyperaldosteronism?
   (A) Plasma Aldosterone
   (B) Plasma Renin
   (C) Saline suppression test
   (D) NP-59 scan

Answers:

1. **B**

   Conn's Syndrome or primary hyperaldosteronism is defined by hypertension as a result of hypersecretion of aldosterone hormone. The mean age at presentation ranges from 30 to 50 years, and it is twice as common in women. Patients come to medical attention because of symptoms of hypokalemia or detection of previously unsuspected hypertension. Most complaints are nonspecific symptoms like tiredness, weakness, polydipsia, polyuria, headaches, muscle weakness, cramping and periodic paralytic episodes due to potassium depletion. Blood pressure in patients with primary hyperaldosteronism can range from borderline to severe hypertensive levels. The hypertension is generally indistinguishable from that seen in the population with essential hypertension.

2. **A**

   There are three major steps in the evaluation of patients who are likely to have primary hyperaldosteronism:

   Screen the individual and establish a clear diagnosis of primary hyperaldosteronism by Plasma aldosterone and plasma renin ratio.

   Discriminate between the different causes of primary hyperaldosteronism

   Localize the site of an aldosterone producing adrenocortical adenoma if present.

3. **D**

4. **A**

   All patients planned for surgical treatment adrenalectomy for primary hyperaldosteronism require preoperative medical optimization. Correction of hypokalemia and other electrolyte abnormalities is essential before surgery. Spironolactone is the drug of choice and should be started one to two weeks prior to surgery to minimize potassium wasting and to help achieve adequate control of hypertension.

5. **C**

   Once the biochemical diagnosis is confirmed, MRI or CT should be performed to distinguish unilateral from bilateral disease. Conn's adenoma usually measures between 1 - 2 cm and is detected by CT with a sensitivity of 80-90%.

6. **C**

   Laparoscopic adrenalectomy is the procedure of choice for aldosteronoma. The traditional surgical treatment has required a unilateral total adrenalectomy. Recently, aldosteronoma enucleation or subtotal adrenalectomy has been suggested as an equally effective technique.

7. **B**

   There are six causes of primary hyperaldosteronism that are following:

   Adrenocortical adenoma (APA) (65%)

   Bilateral adrenocortical hyperplasia (25%)

   Primary adrenal hyperplasia (5%)

   Renin-responsive aldosterone-producing adenoma (5%)

   Aldosterone producing adenocarcinoma (Rare)

   Glucocorticoid remediable hyperaldosteronism (Rare)

8. **B**

   It is also known as hyperreninemic hyperaldosteronism, typified by renal artery stenosis, characterized by a decreased renal artery perfusion pressure and flow, which stimulates renin hypersecretion by juxtaglomerular apparatus and leads to increased angiotensin and ultimately high aldosterone.

References:

1. Lennard TWJ. The adrenal glands and other abdominal endocrine disorders. In: Williams NS, Bulstrode CJK, O'Connell PR (Eds) Bailey and Love's Short Practice of Surgery, 26th edition. CRC Press: Boca Raton 2013, pp 778-783.
2. Proye CAG, Carnaille BM, Wemeau JL. Conn's Syndrome: Surgical Primary Hyperaldosteronism. In: Doherty GM, Skogseid B (Eds) Surgical Endocrinology. Lippincott Williams & Wilkins: New York 2001, pp 221-234.

PHEOCHROMOCYTOMA

Dr. Anand Mishra, Associate Professor, Department of Surgery; Arpit Agarwal, MBBS (Stud.)

A 30 years old man presents with complaints of paroxysmal headache, palpitations and sweating for 4 months duration. He also has complaints of feeling generally unwell and weak. The consulting doctor referred him to higher center with recording of intermittent episodes of labile hypertension. There is no family history of goiter and unexplained deaths, bone disease or recurrent fractures.

1. Which of the following is the most likely diagnosis?
   (A)Essential hypertension
   (B)Conn's syndrome
   (C)Pheochromocytoma
   (D)Multiple endocrine neoplasia
2. Which of the following is the most appropriate next step in diagnosis?
   (A)Biochemical testing
   (B)Abdominal CECT scan
   (C)Ultrasound whole abdomen
   (D)MIBG scan
3. Which of the following is most likely to confirm the diagnosis EXCEPT?
   (A)Plasma free metanephrine levels
   (B)Urinary total metanephrine levels
   (C)Urinary fractionated catecholamine levels
   (D)MIBG scan
4. Which of the following radiological investigation is most appropriate after biochemical diagnosis?
   (A)PET CT
   (B)MIBG Scan
   (C)MRI or CECT abdomen
   (D)Ultrasound KUB region
5. Which of the following is most appropriate pre-operative preparation before surgery after biochemical confirmation of diagnosis of pheochromocytoma?
   (A)Alpha and beta blocker simultaneously
   (B)Alpha blocker then beta blocker
   (C)Spironolactone
   (D)Centrally acting antihypertensive
6. Which of the following is the most effective management after biochemical diagnosis and localization of adrenal pheochromocytoma?
   (A)Adrenalectomy
   (B)Medulla sparing adrenalectomy
   (C)Pharmacotherapy with alpha blocker and calcium channel blocker
   (D)Pharmacotherapy with alpha blocker
7. Which of the following is the classic triad of symptoms of pheochromocytoma in adults?
   (A)Hypertension, sweating, palpitation
   (B)Hypertension, breathlessness, sweating
   (C)Headache, sweating, palpitation
   (D)Hypertension, headache, sweating
8. Which of the following is the classic triad of symptoms of pheochromocytoma in pediatric patients?
   (A)Hypertension, sweating, palpitation
   (B)Hypertension, breathlessness, sweating
   (C)Headache, sweating, palpitation
   (D)Headache, sweating, Nausea
9. Pheochromocytoma may be associated with which of the following EXCEPT?
   (A)Von Hippel Lindau disease
   (B)Von Recklinghausen's disease
   (C)Multiple Endocrine Neoplasia type I (MEN I)
   (D)MEN II A

Answers:
1. C
   Pheochromocytoma is a rare tumor of chromaffin cells arising from the adrenal medulla. It is commonly seen in the third to fifth decades of life. Due to the production and release of catecholamines, pheochromocytoma causes hypertension. Pheochromocytoma is the single most important cause of secondary hypertension in young. About half the patients show paroxysmal hypertension with symptom free intervals between attacks (episodic hypertension). Pounding headaches, palpitations, excessive perspiration and less commonly anxiety and tremors are seen. They are sometimes discovered due to severe hypertension noticed during incidental surgery, following trauma, or micturition (bladder pheochromocytoma). It should also be suspected in patients with malignant hypertension not responding to more than 3 different groups of antihypertensive drugs.
2. A

Screening is done by biochemical testing. There are 10 clinical situations in which it is appropriate to screen for a pheochromocytoma and are following:

Symptomatic episodes, especially when paroxysmal and accompanied by hypertension

Refractory hypertension

Accelerated hypertension

Paradoxical hypertensive response to beta-blockers

Hypertensive paroxysms during anesthesia, surgery, parturition, or angiography

Family screening in recognized families

Hypertension coexistent with associated conditions (neurofibromatosis, von Hippel-Lindau disease, Cushing's syndrome)

Marked labile hypertension

Orthostatic hypotension in the absence of antihypertension therapy

Incidentally discovered adrenal tumor

3. D

Measurement of free urinary catecholamines (norepinephrine and epinephrine) or other metabolites, vanillylmandelic acid (VMA) and metanephrines/normetanephrines should be employed first in all patients when pheochromocytoma is suspected. The measurement of plasma catecholamines can also be of value in the diagnosis of pheochromocytoma though availability and cost may be an issue of concern and its limited use.

4. C

Once a pheochromocytoma has been diagnosed by biochemical tests, the anatomic location of the tumor or tumors must be determined. Most often the disease is localized in the abdomen (97%), the thorax (2-3%), and in the neck (1%). A plain CT scan can be performed but does not give adequate information. A contrast enhanced CT scan carries the risk of precipitating a hypertensive crisis but is a very sensitive tool to localize the lesion and for treatment planning. MRI is better as it can distinguish between various types of adrenal tumors without risk of radiation and can be performed in pregnancy.

5. B

All patients of pheochromocytoma are in a state of volume contraction and initially require a slow volume expansion with alpha-adrenergic blocking agent. When orthostatic hypotension is present, intravenous fluids and plasma are administered as the dosage of alpha-blockers is stepped up. Prazosin (1-5 mg) is started at 6 hourly intervals and is gradually increased. Phenoxybenzamine is also used as it is a long-acting non-competitive alpha blocker. Calcium channel blockers may also be added. The duration of preparation is for two weeks prior to surgery. Beta-blockade is useful when tachycardia is present and it also controls perioperative or intraoperative arrhythmias. Beta-blockers should not be started before alpha-blockers otherwise the hypertension may be worsened due to vasoconstriction.

6. A

7. C

8. D

9. C

References:

1. Lennard TWJ. The adrenal glands and other abdominal endocrine disorders. In: Williams NS, Bulstrode CJK, O'Connell PR (Eds) Bailey and Love's Short Practice of Surgery, 26th edition. CRC Press: Boca Raton 2013,pp 778-783.
2. Thompson NW, Gray DK. Pheochromocytoma. In: Doherty GM, Skogseid B (Eds) Surgical Endocrinology. Lippincott Williams & Wilkins: New York 2001, pp 247-262.

CUSHING'S SYNDROME

Dr. Anand Mishra, Associate Professor, Department of Surgery; Arpit Agarwal, MBBS (Stud.)

A 39 years old man presents with recent weight gain of 12 kgs in last 2 months more on the abdomen, chest and face. He also complains of impotence. On examination his blood pressure is 180/90 mm Hg, protuberant belly, purple striae on lower abdomen and inner aspect of thigh, moon facies, buffalo hump and proximal muscle wasting.

1. Which of the following is the most likely diagnosis?

(A) Exogenous obesity

(B) Conn's syndrome

(C) Cushing's Syndrome

(D) Multiple endocrine neoplasia
2. Which of the following is the most common cause of hypercortisolism?
    (A) Adreno-cortical carcinoma
    (B) Solitary adrenal adenoma
    (C) Bilateral adrenal hyperplasia
    (D) Exogenous steroid intake
3. Which of the following is the most common cause of endogenous hypercortisolism?
    (A) Adreno-cortical carcinoma
    (B) Solitary adrenal adenoma
    (C) Bilateral adrenal hyperplasia
    (D) Pituitary hypersecretion of ACTH
4. Which of the following is the most appropriate next step in diagnosis?
    (A) Biochemical testing
    (B) Abdominal CECT scan
    (C) Ultrasound whole abdomen
    (D) MIBG scan
5. Which of the following test are used to confirm the diagnosis of hypercortisolism EXCEPT?
    (A) 24 hour urine cortisol and creatinine
    (B) Low dose dexamethasone suppression test
    (C) Overnight low dose dexamethasone suppression test
    (D) Serum ACTH
6. Which of the following test are used for differential diagnosis of ACTH dependent hypercortisolism EXCEPT?
    (A) CRH test
    (B) High dose dexamethasone test
    (C) Inferior petrosal sinus sampling
    (D) Serum ACTH
7. Which of the following is the most effective management after biochemical diagnosis and localization of adrenal tumor causing Cushing's syndrome?
    (A) Adrenalectomy
    (B) Medulla sparing adrenalectomy
    (C) Bilateral adrenalectomy
    (D) Pharmacotherapy with Ketoconozole, Metyrapone.

Answers:
    1. C
        Cushing's Syndrome commonly presents insidiously in the 3rd or the 4th decade in women with excessive weight gain and truncal obesity. Progressive obesity is usually central involving face (moon facies), neck (buffalo hump), trunk and abdomen, with the extremities spared or even wasted. A facial plethora is seen over the cheeks, and anterior neck. There is profound muscle wasting and the patient complains of fatigue. Weakness is usually associated with proximal muscle wasting. In extreme disease, hypokalemia may aggravate the weakness. Women may have amenorrhea with hirsutism and acne. Oligomenorrhea in women, impotence in men and decreased libido in both sexes are frequent. Androgen excess is manifested by oily facial skin, acne and mild hirsutism in women. Skinbecomes fragile; shows poor wound healing and may peel off. Loss of connective tissue results in striae and easy bruisability. The classical striae are dehiscent, more than 1 cm in width and present in atypical sites. Cutaneous fungal infections, especially, tinea versicolor and fungal infections of the nail are occasionally observed. Emotional instability, agitation, depression, loss of energy and libido, irritability, anxiety, panic attacks and mild paranoia are most common. Most patients have increased appetite and weight gain but some may have anorexia. Occasionally, patients may be suicidal. Insomnia is often an early symptom and is presumably caused by increased levels of cortisol during sleep. Moderate hypertension may be observed in these patients. Cardiovascular complications are a major cause of morbidity and mortality in untreated Cushing's syndrome. Overt or latent diabetes mellitus may occur. Glucose intolerance and hyperinsulinemia are common because of cortisol effects on gluconeogenesis. Vertebral compression fractures, pathological rib fractures and sometimes long bone fractures results from osteoporosis. Polydipsia and polyuria are usually seen in patients with hypercalciuria and glycosuria.
    2. D
        The most common cause of hypercortisolism is exogenous steroid intake prescribed for several illnesses. The most common endogenous cause is pituitary hypersecretion of ACTH (70%). This results in bilateral adrenal hyperplasia with widening of the zona reticularis. Adrenal adenomas are responsible for

the development of Cushing's syndrome in about 10 percent of cases. These tumors affect women more commonly than men. Adrenal carcinoma is a more common cause of Cushing's syndrome in children.

3. D

4. A

The most important first step in the management of patients with suspected Cushing's syndrome is to establish the biochemical confirmation of hypercortisolism after excluding exogenous glucocorticoid use. Diagnosis can be considered if the results of several tests are consistently suggestive of hypercortisolism. So initial step is to perform screening test and then confirmatory test for hypercortisolism. In an established case of Cushing's syndrome serum ACTH helps in differential diagnosis of ACTH dependent and ACTH independent cortisol excess.

5. D

6. D

7. A

Overt Cushing's is associated with poor prognosis if left untreated. In ACTH independent disease, treatment consists of surgical removal of adrenal tumor. In Cushing's disease, the treatment of choice is selective removal of pituitary corticotroph tumor, usually via trans-sphenoidal approach. In recurrent pituitary disease options are second surgery, radiotherapy, stereotactic radiosurgery and bilateral adrenalectomy.

References:

1. Lennard TWJ. The adrenal glands and other abdominal endocrine disorders. In: Williams NS, Bulstrode CJK, O'Connell PR (Eds) Bailey and Love's Short Practice of Surgery, 26th edition. CRC Press: Boca Raton 2013,pp 778-783.
2. Clutter WE. Cushing's Syndrome: Hypercortisolism. In: Doherty GM, Skogseid B (Eds) Surgical Endocrinology. Lippincott Williams & Wilkins: New York 2001, pp 235-246.

BILIARY INJURIES

Dr. Samir Misra, Associate Professor, Department of Surgery

A 30 years female underwent laparoscopic cholecystectomy for symptomatic gall/stone disease. Surgery was uneventful. She was not feeling well on POD 1. She was discharged on POD 2 on painkillers after reassurance. The patient returned on POD 5 with complaints of respiratory distress, abdominal distension, pedal edema, jaundice. The patient remained afebrile. On examination, vitals are stable. Pulse – 92 beats/minute. Blood pressure – 112/70 mmHg. On clinical examination abdomen was distended but soft with no obvious lump palpable. Shifting dullness was positive. Bowel sounds were decreased.

1. What is the most likely diagnosis?
   (A) Biliary ascites following biliary injury
   (B) Decompensated liver cirrhosis
   (C) Acute intestinal obstruction
   (D) Biliary peritonitis following biliary injury
2. Most appropriate next step is?
   (A) Ultrasound abdomen
   (B) Contrast enhanced CT scan
   (C) X ray abdomen
   (D) Ultrasound abdomen with paracentesis
3. What should be the initial management?
   (A) Resuscitation, pig tail drainage and antibiotics
   (B) Resuscitation, pig tail drainage and ERCP with stenting
   (C) Resuscitation, paracentesis, biliary refeeding and monitoring
   (D) Resuscitation and immediate exploration with an attempt to repair the injury
4. External biliary fistula was established (500mL/day for last 7 days). Which investigation will give the correct diagnosis?
   (A) Magnetic resonance cholangiography
   (B) Endoscopic retrograde cholangiography
   (C) Percutaneous transhepatic cholangiography
   (D) Fistulography
5. Surgical reconstruction should be done at?
   (A) 6 weeks after index surgery

(B) 8 weeks after the closure of the fistula
(C) 8 weeks after the establishment of external biliary fistula
(D) 6 months after the establishment of external biliary fistula

Answers:

1. D

   The patient did not have fever and abdomen was soft on examination. So the patient most likely has biliary peritonitis. Jaundice cannot be explained by intestinal obstruction. Liver decompensation without previous history of liver disease and without major liver resection is unlikely.

2. D

   Most appropriate step will be ultrasound and guided paracentesis to establish the diagnosis of bilioma.

3. A

   Best initial management of bilioma is control of sepsis. This can be easily achieved by resuscitation, pigtail drainage and antibiotics.

4. D

   ERCP as the first step is not a good option. Biliary refeeding in a case of bilioma is not indicated. Exploration and repair is not indicated after 24 to 48 hours of injury. Fistulography is the cheapest and most informative initial investigation.

5. C

   Optimum time of repair – 8 weeks of establishment of controlled external biliary fistula.

References:

1. Corvera CU, Alemi F, Jarnagin WR. Benign biliary strictures. In: Blumgart LH, Jarnagin WR, Belghiti J, Buchler MW, Chapman WC, D'Angelica MI, DeMatteo RP, Hann LE (Eds). Blumgart's Surgery of the Liver, Biliary Tract and Pancreas, 5th ed. Philadelphia; Saunders Elsevier: 2012. pp 615-643.

2. Corvera CU, Jarnagin WR, Blumgart LH. Biliary Fistulae. In: Blumgart LH, Jarnagin WR, Belghiti J, Buchler MW, Chapman WC, D'Angelica MI, DeMatteo RP, Hann LE (Eds). Blumgart's Surgery of the Liver, Biliary Tract and Pancreas, 5th ed. Philadelphia; Saunders Elsevier: 2012. pp 615-643.

PERIAMPULLARY CARCINOMA

Dr. Samir Misra, Associate Professor, Department of Surgery

A 50 years male patient presented with painless progressive jaundice with intense itching for last one month. On examination, icterus was present. Per abdomen examination revealed palpable cystic gallbladder. DRE normal. No ascites was present. CECT abdomen of the patient revealed the following picture:

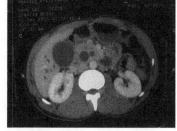

1. What is the most likely diagnosis?
   (A) Gallbladder carcinoma
   (B) Periampullary carcinoma
   (C) Benign biliary stricture
   (D) Choledocholithiasis

2. Definitive treatment for the patient?
   (A) Radical cholecystectomy
   (B) Roux en Y Hepaticojejunostomy
   (C) Whipple's procedure
   (D) ERCP stenting

3. The same patient is planned for definitive surgery. On the morning of surgery, the patient develops high grade fever. What should be done next?
   (A) Go for the definitive procedure as per plan
   (B) ERCP stenting and plan for surgery within 48 hours
   (C) Drainage procedure by surgery and definitive procedure to be done later
   (D) ERCP stenting and wait for the patient to stabilize

Answers:
1.   B
   CECT abdomen shows double duct sign which is classical in periampullary carcinoma.
2.   C
   Definite treatment for periampullary carcinoma will be Whipple's pancreaticoduodenectomy if resectable.
3.   D
   The patient appears to develop cholangitis on the day of surgery. Best option will be ERCP stenting and treat the patient with antibiotic and wait for the fever to subside before taking for surgery.

Reference:
1. Schulick RD, Cameron JL. Pancreatic and periampullary cancer. In: Yeo CJ, Dempsey DT, Klein AS, Pemberton JH, Peters JH (Eds) Shackelford's Surgery of the Alimentary Tract. 7th ed. Philadelphia: Elsevier Saunders; 2013. p. 1187-1205.

PRIMARY SCLEROSING CHOLANGITIS
Dr. Samir Misra, Associate professor, Department of Surgery

A 50-year-old male presents with pain in right upper abdomen, pruritus, jaundice & weight loss with elevated Anti-nuclear antibodies.

1. The likely diagnosis is?
   (A) Primary sclerosing cholangitis
   (B) Klatskin tumour
   (C) Secondary sclerosing cholangitis
   (D) Choledocholithiasis
2. Earliest finding in case of primary sclerosing cholangitis?
   (A) Asymptomatic elevation of GGT
   (B) ALP
   (C) AST
   (D) Serum bilirubin
3. Confirmatory investigation of choice in diagnosis of PSC?
   (A) Cholangiography
   (B) ERCP
   (C) MRCP
   (D) CT Scan

Answers:
    1. A
    2. A
    3. A

Reference:
1. Lazaridis KN, Gores GJ. Primary Sclerosing Cholangitis. In: Yeo CJ, Dempsey DT, Klein AS, Pemberton JH, Peters JH (Eds) Shackelford's Surgery of the Alimentary Tract. 7th ed. Philadelphia: Elsevier Saunders; 2013. p. 1560-1572.

INGUINAL HERNIA
Dr. Jitendra Kumar Kushwaha, Associate Professor, Department of Surgery

A 40 yrs. old male patient has history of left sided inguinal swelling which reduces spontaneously on lying down since last one year. On examination expansile impulse on coughing is present. Abdomen is not distended, bowel sound is normal . No tenderness or rigidity found. Pulse rate is 76/min. TLC-7000.

1. What is most likely diagnosis?
    (A) Irreducible Inguinal hernia
    (B) Obstructed inguinal hernia
    (C) Strangulated inguinal hernia
    (D) Reducible inguinal hernia
2. During surgery it was found that sac of hernia contains a diverticulum of size 2 cm x 2 cm, having wide mouth on antimesenteric border of ileum about 2 feet proximal to Ileocaecal junction , wall of diverticulum is not thickened. Which type of hernia is this?
    (A) Amyand hernia
    (B) Littre's hernia
    (C) Richter's hernia
    (D) Sliding hernia
3. Treatment of above patient will be?
    (A) Wedge resection of diverticulum with hernioplasty
    (B) Hernioplasty only
    (C) Resection and anastomosis of bowel containing divertculum with herniorrhaphy
    (D) Resection and anastomosis of bowel containing divertculum with hernioplasty

Answers:
  1. D
    Expansile impulse on coughing is characteristic finding for hernia. Reducible inguinal hernia reduces spontaneously or manually. In obstructive inguinal hernia abdomen will be distended. Vomiting may present. Patient will not pass feces. In Gangrenous hernia tenderness, rigidity will be present .Patient will have tahychardia, elevated temperature, leucocytosis
  2. B
    If content of hernia is appendix then it is called Amyand hernia. In Littre hernia content of sac is meckel diverticulum which is found 2 feet proximal to ileocaecal junction on antimesenteric border of ileum.
  3. B
    If meckel diverticulum is found incidentally and mouth is wide, not very longer then it is left as such. If length is more or mouth is narrow, features of diverticultis or perforation is present then it needs to be resected.

Reference:
  1. SJ Nixon and Tulloh B. Abdominal wall ,hernia and umbilicus. In: Williams NS, Bulstrode CKJ, O'connell PR (Eds). Bailey and Love's Short Practice of Surgery. 26th ed. CRC Press: Boca Raton 2013. pp 958.

VARICOSE VEIN
Dr. Jitendra Kumar Kushwaha, Associate Professor, Department of Surgery

A 45 yrs. female patient has pain in left leg, which become severe on prolonged standing. On examination dilated and tortuous veins are present on thigh and leg. Skin of lower leg is thick and ankle flare is present.

1. Gold standard Investigation for diagnosis is?
    (A) Doppler Duplex scan
    (B) Venography
    (C) Magnetic resonance angiography
    (D) Varicography
2. If on above investigation saphenofemoral junction is incompetent and few incompetent perforators are found below knee on medial aspect of leg. Saphenopopliteal junction is competent. How will you treat this-

(A) Endovenous laser/Endovenous radiofrequency ablation for main trunk and linton procedure for perforators
(B) Stripping of long saphenous vein from groin to ankle joint with perforators ligation
(C) Endovenous thermal ablation/ High ligation and stripping for main trunk and Subfascial Endoscopic Perforator surgery for perforators
(D) Stripping of Great saphenous vein and short saphenous vein and modified linton procedure

3. Which one is not TRUE regarding complication of varicose veins surgery?
(A) Most common complication is wound infection
(B) Incidence of saphenous nerve neuralgia is 7 % following LSV stripping to knee
(C) Incidence of sural nerve neuroprexia and common peroneal nerve injury may be as high as 20 and 4 % respectively following short saphenous nerve injury.
(D) Incidence of venous thromboembolic complications is approximately 15 % following varicose vein surgery.

Answers:
1. A
   Duplex USG scan is gold standard investigation for varicose vein. Other investigation like Varicography, venography ,magnetic resonance venography is required only in special circumstances.
2. C
   Treatment of Main trunk of GSV varicosity is by endovenous thermal(RF/Laser) ablation or by high ligation and stripping (Trendelenberg procedure). Treatment of below knee perforators are modified linton procedure or SEPS. SEPS is preferred.
3. D
   Incidence of thromboembolism is less than 1 %

Reference:
1. McCollum P and Chetter I. Venous Disorders. In: Williams NS, Bulstrode CJK, O'Connell PR (Eds). Bailey and Love's Short Practice of Surgery. 26th ed. CRC Press: Boca Raton 2013. pp 906-12

RECURRENT INGUINAL HERNIA
Dr. Jitendra Kumar Kushwaha, Associate Professor, Department of Surgery

A 40 yrs. old male patient was operated for inguinal hernia. Open suture repair was done. Hernia recurs after one year. Now Lichtenstein hernioplasty was done. He is known case of COPD. Subsequently pt. again had a recurrence after one year. He is unfit for general anaesthesia.

1. Now most likely this should be treated by
   (A) TAPP
   (B) TEP
   (C) Stoppa's repair
   (D) Shouldice repair

Answer:
1. C
   First time in this case herniorrhaphy was done. Second time Lchtenstein hernioplasty was done. In Lichtenstein hernioplasty mesh is placed anterior to Fascia transversalis. Recurrence after anterior hernioplasty is treated by posterior hernioplasty (TAPP/TEP/Stoppa/Nyhus) TEP and TAPP is performed under general Anaesthesia. In Stoppa's repair mesh is placed behind fascia transversalis under spinal anaesthesia. As patient is unfit for general anaesthesia, TEP and TAPP are not possible in this patient.

Reference:
1. J Nixon SJ and Tulloh B. Abdominal wall ,hernia and umbilicus. In: Williams NS, Bulstrode CJK, O'Connell PR (Eds). Bailey and Love's Short practice of Surgery. 26th ed. CRC Press: Boca Raton 2013. pp 958.

CARCINOMA RECTUM
Dr. Arshad Ahmad, Associate Professor, Department of Surgery

A sixty-five years old male patient presented in surgical OPD with history of bleeding per rectum associated with the act of defecation. Patient had also noticed a change in bowel habits with an increase in frequency. There was no family history of GI diseases. On abdominal examination nothing abnormal was found. Per-rectal examination revealed an irregular, friable mass in rectum about 5 cm from anal verge.

1. The next step in diagnostic evaluation of the patient should be?
    (A) Double contrast barium enema
    (B) USG abdomen
    (C) CT scan
    (D) Proctosigmoidoscopy and biopsy
2. Patients with proven rectal cancer should undergo following investigations EXCEPT.
    (A) Colonoscopy to exclude synchronus tumor
    (B) Capsule endoscopy
    (C) Imaging of the liver and chest
    (D) Pelvic imaging by CT or MRI
3. All are TRUE regarding treatment of rectal cancers EXCEPT?
    (A) In locally advanced disease neoadjuvent chemoradiation makes curative resection possible.
    (B) In resectable cancer preoperative short course radiotherapy reduces local recurrence.
    (C) A sphincter saving operation is not possible for tumors less than 6 cm from pectinate line.
    (D) The presence of liver metastasis does not necessarily rule out the feasibility of cure.
4. Total Meso-rectal Excision (TME) for rectal cancers includes all EXCEPT.
    (A) Suitable for tumors in the middle and lower third of the rectum.
    (B) Radical excision of the rectum together with mesorectum and lymph nodes.
    (C) Low ligation of the inferior mesenteric artery.
    (D) A temporary protecting stoma may be formed.

Answers:
    1. D
        Proctosigmoidoscopy will always show a carcinoma provided the rectum is emptied of feces beforehand. A colonoscopy is required to exclude a synchronous tumor.
    2. B
        All patients with proven rectal cancer require staging by imaging of the liver and chest, local pelvic imaging and colonoscopy to exclude a synchronous tumor.
    3. C
        With the introduction of the stapling gun, sphincter preserving operation is possible for tumors whose lower margin is 2cm above the anal canal.
    4. C
        The principle of the TME involves radical excision of the neoplasm, removal of the mesorectum that surrounds it and high proximal ligation of the inferior mesenteric lymphovascular pedicle.

Reference:
    1. Clark S. The Rectum. In: Williams NS, Bulstrode CJK, O'Connelll PR (Eds). Bailey and Love's Short Practice of Surgery. 26th ed. CRC Press: Boca Raton 2013. pp 1228-29.

ECTAL PROLAPSE
Dr. Arshad Ahmad, Associate Professor, Department of Surgery

A young male patient from a psychiatric ward presented with protrusion during defecation and partial fecal incontinence. On per-rectal examination the resting anal tone was poor. When patient was examined in squatting position and asked to strain, concentric rings of rectal mucosa were seen prolapsing.
1. Routine diagnostic evaluation of the patient may include all EXCEPT.
    (A) Colonoscopy
    (B) Defecography
    (C) Anal manometry
    (D) CT scan abdomen and pelvis
2. All are TRUE regarding rectal prolapse EXCEPT?
    (A) Commences as full thickness rectal intussusception.
    (B) Fecal incontinence is present in approximately 50% of patients with rectal prolapse.

(C) Full thickness prolapse is more common than partial (mucosal) prolapse.

(D) A neoplasm may form the lead point for the rectal prolapse.

3. All are TRUE regarding perineal procedures for rectal prolapse EXCEPT?

(A) Altemeier's procedure involves perineal proctosigmoidectomy.

(B) In Delorme's procedure circumferential rectal mucosectomy is done.

(C)Thiersch operation is reserved for patients with high surgical risk.

(D) Endoluminal stapling technique is suitable for complete rectal prolapse.

Answers:

    1.   D

A neoplasm may form the lead point for rectal intussusceptions. For this reason, colonoscopy should precede an operation. Anal manometry is done to evaluate the symptoms of incontinence. If the prolapse is elusive during clinical evaluation, defecography may reveal the problem.

    2.   C

Full thickness prolapse is less common than the mucosal variety.

    3.   D

The redundant mucosa in partial mucosal prolapse can be excised by endoluminal stapling technique.

Reference:

1.   Robert D. Fry, Najjia N. Mahmoud, David J. Maron, and Joshua I.S. Bleier. Colon and Rectum. In: Townsend CM, Beuchamp RD, Evers BM, Mattox KL(Eds). Sabiston Textbook of Surgery: The Biological Basis of Modern Surgical Practice. 19th ed. Elsevier, Philadelphia 2012: pp 1367-68.

FISTULA -IN-ANO

Dr. Arshad Ahmad, Associate Professor, Department of Surgery

A middle aged male patient presents with history of recurrent perianal abscess drained several times earlier. On examination a discharging sinus is present over the skin about 4 cm posterolaterally from anal verge. On per-rectal examination tender induration is present posteriorly. Proctoscopic examination does not reveal any abnormality.

1. The most likely diagnosis is?

(A) Anal fissure

(B) Pilonidal sinus

(C) Perianal fistula

(D) Hidradenitis suppurativa

2. A trans-sphincteric anal fistula is?

(A) The fistula track is confined to the intersphincteric plane.

(B) The track passes from the rectum to perianal skin external to sphincter complex.

(C) The track loops over the external sphincter and perforates the levator ani.

(D) The track perforates the external sphincter and opens on the skin over the ischiorectal fossa.

3. All are true regarding the management of perianal fistula except.

(A) The aim of treatment is to cure the fistula, prevent recurrence and preserve continence.

(B) Fistulotomy is safe for intersphincteric and low transsphincteric fistulas.

(C) Seton and fibrin glue are alternative methods for complex and deep fistula.

(D) Suprasphincteric fistulas can be laid open without risk of incontinence.

Answers:

    1.   C

Most perianal fistulas are caused by infection originating in the anal glands. The path of spread of infection determines the type of fistula. A fistula may first present as acute abcess or as a draining sinus that may irritate the perianal skin.

    2.   D

In transsphincteric fistula the tract connects the intersphincteric plane with the ischiorectal fossa by perforating the external sphincter.

    3.   D

Because the trajectory of suprasphincteric fistula is above all the muscles of importance to continence, division of all external sphincter muscles results in incontinence.

Reference:

1. Heidi Nelson. The Anus In: Townsend CM, Beuchamp RD, Evers BM, Mattox KL(Eds). Sabiston Textbook of Surgery: The Biological Basis of Modern Surgical Practice. 19th ed. Elsevier; Philadelphia 2012. pp 1394-1398.

PAPILLARY CARCINOMA THYROID

Dr. Kul Ranjan Singh, Assistant Professor, Department of Surgery; Arpit Agarwal, MBBS Std

A 44-year-old female presented with a 3x2 cm right solitary thyroid nodule. On evaluation, TSH – 2.5 mIU/L and HRUSG showed a complex cyst of size 3x2.5 cm in right lobe. The rest of thyroid appeared normal and there was no evidence of enlarged cervical lymph nodes. Guided FNAC was suggestive of colloid nodule. Patient undergoes total thyroidectomy as desired. HPE showed pale empty Orphan Annie eyed nuclei and psammoma bodies. The nodule is surrounded by normal thyroid tissue.

1. Which is the most likely histopathological diagnosis
    (A) Follicular adenoma
    (B) Follicular Thyroid carcinoma
    (C)Papillary thyroid carcinoma
    (D) Colloid adenoma
2. Subsequent Whole body radioactive Iodine scan shows multiple foci of uptake in vertebral column. The patient would be staged as
    (A) Stage 1
    (B) Stage 2
    (C) Stage 3
    (D) Stage 4
3. Which of the following statements are true regarding further management of this patient.
    a. Patient requires maintenance doses of Thyroxine
    b. Patient requires ablative doses of Radioactive Iodine
    c. P atient requires periodical follow up with clinical examination, serum thyroglobulin, S. TSH, +/- Whole body RAI scan and therapy
    d. Patient requires periodical follow up with clinical examination, serum Thyroglobulin, S. anti Thyroglobulin, S. TSH, +/- Whole body RAI scan and therapy
    (A) a,b,c,d are true
    (B) a and c are false , b and d are true
    (C) a,b,d are true and c is false
    (D) a,b,c are true and d is false

Answers:
1. C
    Diagnosis of PTC is made on presence of papillae with a fibro vascular core, overlapping nuclei with finely dispersed optically clear chromatin (ground glass/ Orphan Annie nuclei). Psammoma bodies may also be present.
2. B
    Non metastatic PTC in < 45 years of age fall in Stage 1 and metastatic disease in stage 2.
3. B
    Patient requires suppressive doses of Thyroixine to keep the TSH below the normal range. 20-30 % of the population has anti Thyrogobulin antibodies which interferes with Tg assays and hence should be measured along with Tg

Reference:
1. ZH Krukowski. The Thyroid and Parathyroid glands. In: Williams NS, Bulstrode CJK, O'Connell PR (Eds) Bailey and Love's Short Practice of Surgery. 26th ed. CRC Press: Boca Raton 2013. pp 765-768.

MEDULLARY CARCINOMA THYROID

Dr. Kul Ranjan Singh, Assistant Professor, Department of Surgery; Dr. Devina Singh, MBBS Std

A 60 year old male with slowly progressing 6x4 cm right solitary thyroid nodule and a 2x1 cm right level 3 lymph node. Patient is clinically euthyroid but for history of diarhhoea for last 6 months. No compressive features. Investigations reveal; S. TSH – 0.75 mIu/L, HRUSG shows Rt dominant nodule with multiple Rt level

2,3,4,5 LN, largest 2x2 cm. Serum Calcitonin is in the range of thousands. FNAC resulted in unsatisfactory aspirates on multiple occasions.

1. What is the probable diagnosis?
    (A) Papillary Thyroid carcinoma
    (B) Medullary Thyroid carcinoma
    (C) Follicular Thyroid carcinoma
    (D) MNG with sub clinical Hyperthyroidism
2. Further imaging reveals metastatic disease. What would be the ideal management?
    (A) Surgery with intention of cure followed by Radioactive Iodine ablation
    (B) Surgery with intention of palliation in case patient is fit for surgery
    (C) Radioactive Iodine ablation
    (D) External beam radiotherapy
3. Which of the following is true regarding the probable diagnosis ?
    (1) These are TSH dependent tumors
    (2) Radioactive Iodine is an effective adjuvant treatment
    (3) Blood borne metastasis is uncommon
    (4) Surgery performed after lymph nodal spread has high chances of cure
    (A) 1 & 2 are true and 3 & 4 are false
    (B) 1,2,3 are true and 4 is false
    (C) 1,2, 4 are false and 4 is true
    (D) 1,2,3 and 4 are false

Answers:
   1. B
      Diarrhoea may be one of the presenting symptoms in a patient with advanced medullary thyroid carcinoma. Serum Calcitonin is useful in diagnosis, estimating tumor burden and follow up in cases of MTC.
   2. B
      These are not TSH dependent hence Radioactive Iodine has no role. Surgery is the only effective treatment modality in MTC. Surgery may be performed for metastatic MTC with palliative intent for symptom control and airway control.
   3. D
      Surgery performed after lymph nodal spread may not be curative with high chances of recurrence.

Reference:
   1. ZH Krukowski. The thyroid and parathyroid In: Williams NS, Bulstrode CJK, O'Connell (Eds) Bailey and Love's Short Practice of Surgery. 26th ed. CRC Press: Boca Raton 2013. pp 768-769.

FOLLICULAR CARCINOMA THYROID
Dr. Kul Ranjan Singh, Assistant Professor, Department of Surgery; Dr. Anshuman Singh, MS Std

A 50-year-old woman presents with gradually progressive swelling in anterior aspect of her neck for 20 years with a recent change in voice. TSH – 2.0 mIU/l. HR USG reveals an otherwise unremarkable multi nodular goiter. FNAC is suggestive of Follicular neoplasm. Patient undergoes Total Thyroidectomy. HPE is suggestive of Follicular Thyroid Carcinoma.

1. Which of the following cannot be differentiated on basis of FNAC?
    1) Follicular adenoma from Follicular thyroid carcinoma
    2) Hurthle cell adenoma from Hurthle cell carcinoma
    3) Florid Lymphocytic Thyroiditis from low grade lymphoma
    4) Hyperplastic colloid nodule from papillary thyroid carcinoma
    (A) 1 and 2 can be differentiated but 3 and 4 can't be differentiated from each other
    (B) 1 and 3 can be differentiated but 2 and 4 can't be differentiated from each other
    (C) 1, 2 and 3 can't be differentiated but 4 can be differentiated from each other
    (D) 1,2,3,4 can be differentiated from each other
2. Which of the following statements is false regarding Follicular Thyroid carcinoma?
    (A) It's a disease of older population compared to Papillary Thyroid carcinoma
    (B) FTC typically spreads via hematogenous route
    (C) Most commonly osteoblastic bone and lung seconadries are encountered in metastatic FTC
    (D) It has a less favorable prognosis compared to Papillary Thyroid carcinoma

3. Which of the following is not routinely used as adjuvant treatment of non metastatic FTC without extra thyroidal extension?
   (A) Whole body Radioactive Iodine scan and therapy
   (B) Suppressive doses of Thyroxine
   (C) Periodical follow up with Serum Tg and Anti Tg
   (D) External beam radiotherapy to neck

Answers:
1.   C.
   The differentiation between Follicular adenoma and carcinoma is made on basis of capsular invasion. Hurthle cell carcinoma is a variant of FTC
2.   C
   Osteolytic lesions are commonly encountered in FTC
3.   D

References:
1.   ZH Krukowski. The Thyroid and Parathyroid glands. In: Williams NS, Bulstrode CJK, O'Connell PR (Eds). Bailey and Love's Short Practice of Surgery. 26th ed. CRC Press: Boca Raton 2013. pp 765-768
2.   Philip W. Smith, Leslie J. Salomone, and John B. Hanks. In: Thyroid Townsend CM, Beuchamp RD, Evers BM, Mattox KL(Eds). Sabiston Textbook of Surgery: The Biological Basis of Modern Surgical Practice. 19th ed. Elsevier: Philadelphia 2012. pp 909-12

WOUND HEALING
Dr. Anurag Rai, Assistant Professor, Department of Surgery

A healthy 20 year old boy presents to emergency room in evening with a 3-cm contaminated laceration on his right arm that he received in the morning .The wound is deep extending to deep fascia.

1. Which of the following cell types are the first infiltrating cells to enter the wound site, peaking at 24 to 48 hours?
   (A) Macrophages
   (B) Neutrophills
   (C) Fibroblasts
   (D) Lymphocyte
2. Which of the following solutions should be used to irrigate this wound ?
   (A) Sterile water
   (B)Normal saline
   (C) Dilute iodine solution
   (D) Dakin solution
3. Which of the following is the most appropriate management of the wound?
   (A) Closure of the skin only and administration of oral antibiotics for 5 days
   (B) Local wound care without wound closure or antibiotics
   (C) Closure of skin and subcutaneous tissue and administration of oral antibiotics
   (D) A single dose of intravenous antibiotics and closure of skin only

Answers:
1.   B
   PMN are the first infiltrating cells to enter the wound site, peaking at 24-48 hrs. Macrophages achieve significant numbers in the wound 48-96 hrs post injury and remain until wound healing is complete.
2.   B
   Irrigation to visualize all areas of the wound and remove foreign material is best accomplished with normal saline(without additives). Iodine, hydrogen peroxide and organically based antibacterial preparation have been shown to impair wounded healing due to injury to wound neutrophils and macrophages,and they should not be used.
3.   B

Reference:
1.   Barbul A, Efron DT, Kavalukas SL. Wound Healing. In: Brunicardi FC, Andersen DK, Billiar TR, Dunn DL, Hunter JG, Matthews JB, Pollock RE (Eds) Schwartz's Principles of Surgery, 10th Edition. McGraw Hill Educations: New York 2015, pp 241-272.

SHOCK

Dr. Anurag Rai, Assistant Professor, Department of Surgery

38-year-old 70 kgs woman sustains blunt abdominal trauma following a motor vehicle crash. Her BP is 90/50mm Hg, HR >120 beats/min,RR 35 beats /min. She is confused with urine output 12ml/h.

1. The initiating event in shock is?
   (A) Hypotension
   (B) Decreased cardiac output
   (C) Decreased oxygen delivery
   (D) Cellular energy deficit

2. Which of the following can initiate afferent impulses to the CNS which triggers the neuroendocrine response of shock?
   (A) Severe alkalosis
   (B) Hypothermia
   (C) Hyperthermia
   (D) Hyperglycaemia

3. Which of the following cytokines is released immediately after major injury?
   (A) IL-10
   (B) IL-2
   (C) TNF-alpha
   (D) TNF-beta

4. Expected amount of blood loss in this patient would be?
   (A) 750-1500 ml
   (B) <750 ml
   (C) >2000 ml
   (D) 1500-2000 ml

Answers:

1. A.

   Regardless of the etiology,the initial physiological responses in shock are driven by tissue hypo perfusion and the developing cellular energy deficit.

2. B.

   Afferent impulses transmitted from the periphery are processed with in the central nervous system and activate the reflexive effector responses. These effector responses are designed to expand plasma volume, maintain peripheral perfusion and tissue O2 delivery and homeostasis.The initial inciting event usually is loss of circulating blood volume. Other stimuli that produce the neuroendocrine response are pain,hypoxemia,hypercarbia,acidosis,and change in temperature or hypoglycaemia.

3. C.

   TNF-alpha level peak within 90 minutes of stimulus and return frequently to baseline within 4hrs.Its release is triggered by bacteria or endotoxins, hemorrhage and ischemia.

4. D

   Blood volume in a adult can roughly calculated as 70 ml per kg. So this patient would have volume of 4900 ml.15% loss of circulating volume(700-750ml) may produce little in terms of symptoms, while loss of 30% circulating volume (1.5L) may result in tachycardia,tachypnea and anxiety.Hypotension, marked tachycardia (>110-120bpm) and confusion may not be evident until more than 30% of blood volume has been lost; loss of 40% volume is immediately life threatening.

Reference:

1. Zuckerbraun BB, Peitzman AB, Billiar TR. Shock. In: Brunicardi FC, Andersen DK, Billiar TR, Dunn DL, Hunter JG, Matthews JB, Pollock RE (Eds) Schwartz's Principles of Surgery, 10th Edition. McGraw Hill Educations: New York 2015, pp 109-134.

LIVER TRAUMA

Dr. Anurag Rai, Asssitant Professor, Department of Surgery

32-year-old man sustains blunt abdominal trauma following a motor vehicle crash. His HR is 110 beats /min ,RR is 25 beats/min, mildly anxious with only minimal tenderness in her right upper quadrant. FAST is positive with fluid in hepato-renal pouch and pelvis. He remains hemodynamically stable and abdominal computed tomography (CT) scan is remarkable for liver laceration.

1. What percentage of blood volume do you estimate he has lost ?

(A) <15%
(B) 15%-30%
(C) 30%-40%
(D) >40%
2. Which of the following is the next best step in his management?
(A) Observation only
(B) CECT abdomen
(C) Laparoscopy
(D) Exploratory laparotomy
3. After CT scan , she is shown to have a laceration of 3 cm into right lobe with a 10 cm subcapsular hematoma. What is grade of liver injury does he have ?
(A) Grade I
(B) Grade II
(C) Grade III
(D) Grade IV
4. Which of the following is the next step in management?
(A) Observation only
(B) Laparoscopy
(C) Exploratory laparotomy
(D) None of the above
5. The best criteria that would indicate failure with the non operative management would be ?
(A) Grade III laceration or greater
(B) Greater than 150 ml of intraperitoneal blood.
(C) Transfusion of >2 units during the first 12 hours.
(D) CT intravenous contrast extravasation.

Answers:
1. B.
   He has class II hemorrhagic shock(based on vital signs) with loss of between 15% and 30% of his blood volume.
2. B.
   Patient with fluid on FAST examination, considered a 'positive FAST', who do not have immediate indications for laparotomy and are hemodynamically stable undergo CT scan to quantify their injuries. Because of the risk of a solid organ injury, observation is not indicated. If he has an isolated liver or spleen injury, the correct treatment is most like likely observation; therefore, both laparoscopy and laparotomy would not be indicated.
3. C.
   Injury grading using the American Association for the surgery of trauma grading scale is a key component of non operative management of solid organ injuries. Because he has a laceration of 3cm,she had Gd III Injury.
4. A.
   Patient with fluid on FAST examination,considered a 'positive FAST', who do not have immediate indications for laparotomy and are hemodynamically stable undergo CT scan to quantify their injuries.Because of the risk of a solid organ injury, observation is not indicated. If he has an isolated liver or spleen injury,the correct treatment is most like likely observation; therefore, both laparoscopy and laparotomy would not be indicated.
5. D.
   Currently as many as 80%to 90% of low grade lesions (I,II,III) and as many as 50% of more severe lesions Grade IV and V are being managed non operatively.The extravasation of contrast material is a universally agreed-on indication of active bleeding and most consider this a criterion not to pursue non-operative management. Role of angiography in these circumstances is being evaluated but is not a routine until its role is defined. Operative management of patients with CT contrast extravasation should be followed.

Reference:
1. Burlew CC, Moore EE. Trauma. In: Brunicardi FC, Andersen DK, Billiar TR, Dunn DL, Hunter JG, Matthews JB, Pollock RE (Eds) Schwartz's Principles of Surgery, 10th Edition. McGraw Hill Educations: New York 2015, pp 161-226.

GERD (GASTROESOPHAGEAL REFLUX DISEASE)

Dr. Faraz Ahmad, Assistant Professor, Department of Surgery

A healthy 45-year-old woman is seen with a 6-month history of worsening heartburn, regurgitation, and dysphagia. Over the-counter antacids have resulted in mild improvement in her symptoms.

1. Which of the following is least likely to contribute to her symptoms?
    (A) Presence of a hiatal hernia
    (B) Cigarette smoking and alcohol consumption
    (C) High-protein diet
    (D) Obesity
2. The procedure of choice for above mentioned patient is
    (A) Nissen fundoplication
    (B) Toupet's fundoplication
    (C) Hills procedure
    (D) Belsey work IV operation
3. Which of the following is the least importantwhen performing a laparoscopic Nissen fundoplication for reflux disease?
    (A) Use of pledgets to prevent suture tears
    (B) Lengthening the intra-abdominal esophagus
    (C) Division of the short gastric vessels
    (D) Hiatal dissection and closure
4. Seven years after her initial ARS, a patient undergoes a reoperation for recurrence of symptoms. During the reoperation,what is the most likely finding?
    (A) Disrupted wrap
    (B) Loose wrap
    (C) Herniated wrap
    (D) Slipped wrap

Answers:

1. C

   Gastroesophageal reflux disease (GERD) is an imbalance of this normal physiology because of a defect in either the antireflux mechanism or esophageal protection.

2. A
3. A

   The principles of antireflux surgery (ARS) that have been studied and accepted are hiatal dissection and closure, lengthening of the intra-abdominal esophagus, division of the short gastric vessels, creation of a short (2 cm) and floppy fundoplication, and the use of a bougie.

4. C

   The most common operative finding on repeated fundoplication is a herniated fundoplication (33%) above the diaphragm, followed by a disrupted wrap (18%), a tight wrap (13%), and a slipped wrap (10%) on to the body of the stomach.

Reference:

1. Peterson RP, Pellegrini CA, Oelschlager BK. Hiatal hernia & GERD. In: Townsend CM, Beauchamp RD, Evers BM, Mattox KL(Eds). Sabiston Textbook of surgery; The Biological Basis of Modern Surgical Practice. 19th ed. Elsevier: Philadelphia 2012. pp 1068-1086

CARCINOMA ESOPHAGUS

Dr . Faraz Ahmad, Assistant Professor, Department of Surgery

A 75-year-old white man with a history of alcohol abuse,40-pack-year tobacco use, and long-standing GERD controlled by antacids is evaluated for dysphagia and weight loss. Esophagography shows an apple core lesion at the distal end of theesophagus.

1. Which of the following is true regarding further work-up?
   (A) Endoscopic biopsy should be avoided because of the riskfor perforation.
   (B) Computed tomography (CT) is excellent for tumor staging.
   (C) Positron emission tomography (PET) is an excellent toolfor staging and can be used as a single diagnosticmodality.
   (D) EUS is more sensitive than CT for evaluating the celiaclymph nodes.
2. The patient above underwent EUS that showed a T2lesion. The biopsy specimen is positive for adenocarcinomaof the esophagus. His chance of having a positive lymphnode is:
   (A) 20%
   (B) 40%
   (C) 60%
   (D) 80%
3. The patient above undergoes neoadjuvant chemo-radiation. Which of the following is true regarding multimodality therapy?
   (A) A complete histologic response occurs in approximately25% of patients.
   (B) Squamous cell carcinoma and adenocarcinoma cell typeshave similar response rates to radiation therapy.
   (C) Survival beyond 5 years has not been reported in patientswith stage IV disease.
   (D) Cisplatin-based combination therapy is no longer usedbecause of the high rate of neuropathy.
4. The patient above undergoes transhiatal esophagectomy.Which of the following is true of the procedure?
   (A) Three incisions are required: cervical, thoracic, andabdominal.
   (B) A gastric conduit is preferred, and the blood supply is basedon the right gastroepiploic artery.
   (C) More lymph nodes can be harvested than with en blocesophagectomy.
   (D) A substernal route of the replacement conduit is preferredbecause of the shorter route and improved function.

Answers:
1. D
   Endoscopic ultrasound is the most important diagnostic tool in esophageal cancer staging. Tissue samples can be obtained from lymph nodes, as well as from the primary lesion. EUS is more sensitive and specific than CT in evaluating the celiac lymph nodes.
2. C
   The incidence of positive lymph nodes is 18% for T1a intramucosa, 55% for T1b submucosa, 60% for T2 not beyond the muscularis propria, 80% for T3 with involvement of paraesophageal tissue but not adjacent structures, and 100% for T4 with involvement of adjacent structures.
3. A
   Squamous cell carcinoma is much more radioresponsive than adenocarcinoma, although with the latter, a complete histologicresponse is seen in approximately 25% of patients undergoing neoadjuvant chemoradiation therapy.
4. B
   A gastric pull-up procedure, based on the right gastroepiploic artery, in the posterior mediastinal position has the best functional result.

Reference:
1. Maish M S. Esophagus.In:Townsend CM, Beuchamp RD, Evers BM, Mattox KL(Eds). Sabiston Textbook of surgery; The Biological Basis of Modern Surgical Practice. 19th ed. Elsevier: Philadelphia 2012. pp 1013-1067.

DUODENAL ULCER PERFORATION
Dr.Faraz Ahmad, Assistant Professor, Department of Surgery

A 75-year-old man taking NSAIDs for arthritis has an acuteabdomen and pneumoperitoneum. His symptoms are 6 hoursold and his vital signs are stable after the infusion of 1 L ofnormal saline solution.

1. What should be the next step in themanagement of this patient?
   (A) Computed tomography of the abdomen
   (B) Esophagogastroduodenoscopy (EGD)
   (C) Antisecretory drugs, antibiotics for *H. pylori*, and surgeryif he fails to improve in 6 hours
   (D) Surgery
2. The patient above is found to have a perforated duodenalulcer. Which of the following best describes the requiredoperation?
   (A) Suture closure of the perforation
   (B) Omental patch of the perforation
   (C) Repair of the perforation and highly selective vagotomy
   (D) Repair of the perforation and truncal vagotomy

Answers:
1. D
   Treatment of a perforated duodenal ulcer is resuscitation and prompt surgery.
2. B
   Operative management requires closure of the perforation, which is generally best accomplished with an omental (Graham) patch.

Reference:
1. Mahvi DM, Krantz SB. Stomach. In: Townsend CM, Beuchamp RD, Evers BM, Mattox KL(Eds) Sabiston Textbook of surgery; The Biological Basis of Modern Surgical Practice. 19th ed. Elsevier: Philadelphia 2012. pp 1182-1226.

MEN SYNDROME
Dr. Gitika Nanda Singh, Assistant Professor, Department of Surgery

A 24-year-old male has an anterior neck swelling, which has not been investigated. He presents to a surgeon with right inguinal hernia, for which he was planned for surgery under GA. On table he had high BP; 200/140 at the time of induction and the course of surgery was marked by rapid BP fluctuations due to which surgery was deferred and patient was referred for further workup. Detailed evaluation found him hypertensive with marfanoid habitus. His mother had thyroid swelling and HTN and died of thyroid cancer.

1. What is the most probable diagnosis?
   (A) Hyperaldosteronism
   (B) Essential hypertension
   (C) Pheochromocytoma
   (D) Thyrotoxicosis
2. What is the possible syndrome associated?
   (A) MEN 1
   (B) MEN 2
   (C) NF1
   (D) VHL
3. How would you work up this patient?
   (A) 24 hour urine metanephrines
   (B) Urinary VMA
   (C) ACTH
   (D) S. PRA/Aldosterone ratio
4. What is the most common gene involved?
   (A) RET/PTC
   (B) PTEN
   (C) P53
   (D) Rb

Answers:

1. C

   Hypertension in a young patient which is uncontrolled by multiple drugs with intraoperative fluctuations, should raise the suspicion of pheochromocytoma.

2. B

   MEN 2 is characterized by pheochromocytoma, medullary carcinoma and hyperparathyroidism. Patient can have marfanoid habitus and multiple neuromas. It is characterized by RET/PTC gene mutation, AD mode of inheritance. Patient can have marfanoid habitus and multiple neuromas.

3. A

   Serum metanephrines and 24 hour urine metanephrines is the most sensitive investigation for the work up of pheochromocytoma.

4. A

Reference:

1. Martucci VL, Pacak K. Pheochromocytoma and paraganglioma: diagnosis, genetics, management and treatment. Curr Probl Cancer. 2014 Jan-Feb;38(1):7-41.

ADRENO CORTICAL CARCINOMA

Dr. Gitika Nanda Singh, Assistant Professor, Department of Surgery

A 57-year-old lady presented with the features of vague right upper abdominal pain with dragging sensation and loss of appetite. She also gave a recent history of hirsutism, deepening of voice, loss of frontal hair. She underwent a USG for the same, which showed a right hetero-echoic 4x3.8 cm right suprarenal mass.

1. What is the probable diagnosis?
   - (A) PCOD
   - (B) Adrenogenital syndrome
   - (C) Virilising adrenal tumor
   - (D) Cushing syndrome
2. What is the next investigation required?
   - (A) Diagnostic laproscopy
   - (B) CECT Abdomen
   - (C) MRI abdomen
   - (D) PET Scan
3. How do you treat this patient?
   - (A) Ketoconazole
   - (B) Mitotane
   - (C) Surgery
   - (D) Chemo-embolisation
4. What is the approved adjuvant treatment?
   - (A) RT
   - (B) Mitotane
   - (C) Streptozocin
   - (D) IGF 1 Inhibitors

Answers:

1. C

   ACC is a slow growing tumor and clinical presentation is characterized by dull pain in lumbar region along with decreased appetite. It can be functional or non functional. Though cushing syndrome is the most common manifestation of ACC, androgenic features can be seen in patients with androgen secreting tumors, which is second most common.

2. B

   CECT abdomen should be done in ACC for anatomic delineation of tumor, relation to neighboring organs, to assess resectability and to r/o metastasis. PET scan is also recommended now to rule out a metastasis.

3. C

   Surgery is the treatment of choice in all-resectable tumors. Ketoconazole can be used to palliate Cushing's syndrome, chemo-embolisation can be done for palliation of pain and role of RT is uncertain in ACC

4. B

Mitotane is FDA approved drug for ACC with streptozocin and IGF inhibitors, in trial phases.

Reference:

1. Golden SH et al. Clinical review: Prevalence and incidence of endocrine and metabolic disorders in the United States: a comprehensive review. J Clin Endocrinol Metab. 2009 Jun; 94(6):1853-78.

DIABETIC FOOT

Dr. Gitika Nanda Singh, Assistant Professor, Department of Surgery

A 40-year-old male presents with an ulcer on dorsum of right foot following trivial trauma. O/E he has a 4x3 cm superficial ulcer on dorsum of right foot with underlying tendons exposed. He has absent DPA and PTA pulsations and diminishes sensations below knee bilaterally. He gives a family history of diabetes. His Hb 8.1, RBS is 270 mg/dl and HbA1c is 10.4, TLC: 4800; N55L44E1,S. Creat 1.9, S. Sodium 131, potassium 2.8.

1. What is the probable diagnosis?
    (A) Atherosclerotic foot ulcer
    (B) Buerger's disease
    (C) Diabetic foot ulcer
    (D) Acute embolic ulcer
2. What do his blood tests indicate?
    (A) Chronic kidney disease
    (B) Stress induced hyperglycemia
    (C) Chronic uncontrolled sugars with MRD
    (D) Sepsis
3. How would you manage this patient?
    (A) Extensive debridement
    (B) Foot off loading and daily normal saline wash
    (C) Thorough cleaning of ulcer by betadine, chlorine and peroxide
    (D) Amputation

Answers:

1.C

Foot ulcer in a non smoker, middle aged patient following a trivial trauma is suggestive of diabetic ulcer.

2.A

His blood investigations are suggestive of uncontrolled sugars with acute rise in blood sugars and deranged creatinine suggestive of Medical renal disease.

3.B

Foot off loading and daily dressing is recommended for treatment of diabetic foot. However betadine, free radicals should be avoided in already flow compromised limb.

Reference:

1. Yazdanpanah Let al. Literature reviews on the management of diabetic foot ulcer. World J Diabetes. 2015 Feb 15;6(1):37-53.

CARCINOMA PENIS

Dr. Ajay Kumar Pal, Lecturer, Department of Surgery

A 50 year old male presents with 4 × 2 cm growth over glans penis and multiple small palpable and fixed lymph nodes in left inguinal region.

1. Which of the following can preclude curative surgical resection?
    (A) No more than 2 positive lymph nodes.
    (B) Positive pelvic lymph nodes.
    (C) Unilateral metastasis.
    (D) Single metastasis of only 6 cm.
2. If left sided adenopathy comes out to be positive unilateral metastasis then all of the following are true about surgical considerations except:

(A) Ipsilateral ilioinguinal lymphadenectomy should be done

(B) Contralateral staging is not indicated

(C) Both a superficial and deep ipsilateral dissection are performed

(D) Ipsilateral pelvic dissection provides useful prognostic information.

3. Adjuvant or neoadjuvant chemotherapy should be considered in addition of surgery for all of following except:

(A) Single pelvic nodal metastasis

(B) Extranodal extension of cancer

(C) Fixed inguinal masses

(D) Two unilateral inguinal lymph nodes with focal metastasis.

Answers:

1.   B.

Radical ilioinguinal lymphadenectomy is indicated in patients with resectable metastatic adenopathy and may be curative when the disease is limited to the inguinal nodes.

2.   D.

In patients at risk for the development of inguinal metastaticdisease and with no palpable adenopathy, modified inguinal lymphadenectomy provides excellent assessmentof the regional nodes and may be converted to a full lymphadenectomy if metastatic disease is detected.

3.   D.

References:

1.   Curtis A. Pettaway, Raymond S. Lance, John W. Davis. Tumors of the Penis In: Alan J. Wein et al (Eds) Campbell-Walsh Urology. 10th ed. Saunders Elsevier; Philadelphia 2012. pp 930-947.

2.   Eardley Ian. Penis and Urethra In: Williams NS, Bulstrode CJK, O'Connell PR (Eds). Bailey and Love's Short Practice of Surgery, 26th edition. CRC Press: Boca Raton 2013: pp1375.

INFECTED PANCREATIC NECROSIS
Dr. Ajay Kumar Pal, Lecturer, Department of Surgery

An alcoholic patient has acute pancreatitis with 5 points on Ranson criteria. He gradually improves on 14 day hospitalization but then a Pulse of 120 beats per minute, a temperature of 39˙ and abdominal distension develop

1. Which is next best investigation?

(A) MRI abdomen.

(B) Contrast enhanced CT.

(C) USG abdomen.

(D) Dynamic pancreatography.

2. Which is next appropriate therapy if patient is having infected pancreatic necrosis?

(A) Antibiotics

(B) Pecutaneous catheter drainage

(C) Peritoneal lavage

(D) Operative drainage

3. For the above patient which of the following antibiotics does not achieve adequate levels in pancreas?

(A) Imipenem

(B) Metronidazole

(C)Aminoglycoside

(D) Flouroquinolones

Answers:

1.   B.

Necrotic areas can be identified by an absence of contrast enhancement on CT. These are sterile to begin with, but can become subsequently infected, probably due to translocation of gut bacteria.

2.   B.

A CT scan should be performed and a needle passed into the area under CT guidance, choosing a path that does not traverse hollow viscera. This may be done under ultrasonographic guidance as well. If the aspirate is purulent, percutaneous drainage of the infected fluid should be carried out. The tube drain inserted should have the widest bore possible. The aspirate should be sent for microbiological assessment, and appropriate antibiotic therapy should be commenced as per the sensitivity report.

3.   C.

Because of their penetration into the pancreas and spectrum coverage, carbapenems are the first option of treatment. Alternative therapy includes quinolones, metronidazole, third-generation cephalosporins, and piperacillin.

References:
1. Bhattacharya S. The pancreas In: Williams NS, Bulstrode CJK, O'Connell PR (Eds). Bailey and Love's Short Practice of Surgery, 26th edition. CRC Press: Boca Raton 2013: pp 1129.
2. Eric H. Jensen, Daniel Borja-Cacho, Waddah B. Al-Refaie, and Selwyn M. Vickers. The Exocrine Pancreas In: Townsend CM, Beauchamp RD, Evers BM, Mattox KL(Eds). Sabiston Textbook of Surgery. The Biological Basis of Modern Surgical Practice. 19th ed. Elsevier; Philadelphia 2012: pp 1539-1542.

CARCINOMA HEAD OF PANCREAS
Dr. Ajay Kumar Pal, Lecturer, Department of Surgery

A jaundiced otherwise healthy patient is noted to have a 3 cm mass in head of pancreas on CT. EUS(endoscopic ultrasound) guided FNA shows cancer. The mass abuts the portal vein but there is no clear evidence of vessel involvement or metastatic disease .

1. Which of the following is most appropriate next step?
   (A) MRCP to better assess vascular involvement.
   (B) Operative exploration and potential resection.
   (C) Endoscopic placement of biliary stent.
   (D) Chemotherapy and radiation therapy.
2. In which of the following situations is resection of ductal carcinoma of pancreas contraindicated?
   (A) Age $\geq$ 80 years
   (B) Tumor located in body of pancreas
   (C) Tumor invading portal vein
   (D) Presence of small peritoneal metastasis.
2. Which of the following could be appropriate for above patient?
   (A) Pancreaticoduodenectomy with preservation of stomach and pylorus
   (B) Duodenum sparing pancreatectomy
   (C) Total pancreaticoduodenectomy
   (D) All are potentially appropriate.

Answers:
1. B
   Staging laparoscopy has been advocated by several authors as a means to reduce the frequency of nontherapeutic laparotomy for patients with unsuspected metastatic or locally advanced unresectable disease identified at the time of surgery
2. D
   Unresectable tumors are those that exhibit metastasis, including lymph node metastasis outside the field of resection, ascites, or vascular involvement
3. A

References:
1. Bhattacharya Satyajit. The pancreas In: Williams NS, Bulstrode CJK, O'Connell PR (Eds). Bailey and Love's Short Practice of Surgery, 26th edition. CRC Press: Boca Raton 2013: pp 1138.
2. Eric H. Jensen, Daniel Borja-Cacho, Waddah B. Al-Refaie, and Selwyn M. Vickers. The Exocrine Pancreas In: Townsend CM, Beauchamp RD, Evers BM, Mattox KL(Eds). Sabiston Textbook of Surgery. The Biological Basis of Modern Surgical Practice. 19th ed. Elsevier; Philadelphia 2012: pp 1539-1542.

PAROTID TUMOR (PLEOMORPHIC ADENOMA)
Dr. Akshay Anand, Lecturer, Department of Surgery

A 40 yrs. old woman comes to surgical OPD with complaints of a left swelling anterior to ear, which is progressively increasing for past 7 months. The swelling is non-tender, firm in consistency; smooth surface and non-adhered to overlying skin. There are no signs of facial nerve involvement.
FNAC of the lesion is suggestive of pleomorphic adenoma of the parotid gland.

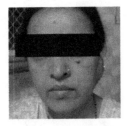

1. How should a benign tumor involving tail of parotid be managed?
   (A) Enucleation
   (B) Superficial parotidectomy
   (C) Total parotidectomy
   (D) Radiotherapy
2. Which of the following landmarks is used to locate the facial nerve trunks?
   (A) Insertion of sternocleidomastoid muscle
   (B) Greater horn of hyoid
   (C) Conley's pointer - the superior most portion of cartilaginous ear canal.
   (D) Upper border of posterior belly of digastric muscle.
3. After parotidectomy, what does Frey's syndrome refer to?
   (A) Gustatory sweating
   (B) Dry mouth due to reduction in salivary flow.
   (C) Permanent numbness of the ear lobe associated with great auricular nerve transection
   (D) Development of sialocele over the parotid bed

Answers:
1. B.
   All tumors of the superficial lobe of the parotid gland should be managed by superficial parotidectomy. There is no role for enucleation even if a benign lesion is suspected. The aim of superficial parotidectomy is to remove the tumor with a cuff of normal surrounding tissue.
2. D.
   Landmarks commonly used to aid identification of the trunk of the facial nerve are:
   The inferior portion of the cartilaginous canal. This is termed Conley's pointer and indicates the position of the facial nerve, which lies 1 cm deep and inferior to its tip.
   The upper border of the posterior belly of the digastric muscle. Identification of this muscle not only mobilizes the parotid gland, but also exposes an area immediately superior, in which the facial nerve is usually located.
3. A.
   Frey's syndrome (gustatory sweating) is now considered an inevitable consequence of parotidectomy, unless preventative measures are taken. It results from damage to the autonomic innervation of the salivary gland with inappropriate regeneration of parasympathetic nerve fibres that stimulate the sweat glands of the overlying skin.

Reference:
1. Smith WP. Disorders of the salivary glands. In: Williams NS, Bulstrode CJK, O'Connell PR (Eds) Bailey and Love's Short Practice of Surgery, 26th edition. CRC Press: Boca Raton 2013,pp 729-735.

PANCREATITIS WITH ITS COMPLICATIONS
Dr. Akshay Anand, Lecturer, Department of Surgery

A 30 years old man presents to surgical emergency with history of severe pain in abdomen, nausea and vomiting. Patient is non-alcoholic and non-smoker with past history of similar episode 6 months back.

On history pain was experienced first in the epigastrium but now is felt diffusely throughout the abdomen. On examination patient has generalized abdominal tenderness with guarding. Pain is radiating to back. Icterus is absent and patient is afebrile. PR – 120 beats/min, RR – 28/min, BP - 90/60 mm Hg; GCS -15/15.

USG abdomen is s/o cholelithiasis (multiple stones) with dilated common bile duct. Pancreas could not be commented upon due to excessive bowel gases. CECT abdomen reveals following picture:

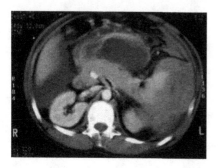

Lab reports: Hb- 10.2 gm%, TLC - 12500, DLC – P79L20E1M0, S. urea - 78, S. creat - 1.3, S. Na -138, S K – 3.8, S.Ca – 3.6, S Amylase - 3310 IU/l, S. Lipase – 1890 IU/L,
AST – 60 IU/L, ALT – 80 IU/L, SALP – 1240 IU/L, T. Bil – 1.4 mg%, Direct Bil -1.0 mg%, S LDH – 383 IU/L.

1. Which of the following is not a parameter to assess the severity of acute pancreatitis in either Ranson or Glasgow Score?
   (A) Age
   (B) Serum amylase
   (C) Serum calcium
   (D) Blood urea
2. Which of the following statement is TRUE in relation to pancreatic pseudocyst?
   (A) Pseudocyst may occur within the first week of onset of acute pancreatitis.
   (B) Pseudocyst rarely communicates with the main pancreatic duct.
   (C) GI bleeding is not a complication of a pseudocyst.
   (D) Pseudocyst can even arise after blunt trauma to upper abdomen.
3. Which of the following statements is FALSE regarding to complications in acute pancreatitis?
   (A) Patients with severe acute pancreatitis require a CECT scan to detect pancreatic necrosis.
   (B) Pseudocyst rarely resolves spontaneously.
   (C) Majority of patients with peri-pancreatic sepsis can be treated conservatively.
   (D) Pleural effusion is seen in 10-20% of patients.

Answers:
1. B

Ranson score	Glasgow scale
On admission	**On admission**
Age >55 years	Age >55 years
White blood cell count >16 × 10⁹/L	White blood cell count >15 × 10⁹/L
Blood glucose >10 mmol/L	Blood glucose >10 mmol/L (no history of diabetes)
LDH >700 units/L	Serum urea >16 mmol/L (no response to intravenous fluids)
AST >250 Sigma Frankel units per cent	Arterial oxygen saturation (PaO₂) <8 kPa (60 mmHg)
Within 48 hours	**Within 48 hours**
Blood urea nitrogen rise >5 mg per cent	Serum calcium <2.0 mmol/L
Arterial oxygen saturation (PaO₂) <8 kPa (60 mmHg)	Serum albumin <32 g/L
Serum calcium <2.0 mmol/L	LDH >600 units/L
Base deficit >4 mmol/L	AST/ALT >600 units/L
Fluid sequestration >6 litres	

ALT, alanine aminotransferase; AST, aspartate aminotransferase; LDH, lactate dehydrogenase; PaO₂, arterial oxygen tension.

2. D

   Pseudocyst typically arises following an attack of acute pancreatitis, but can develop in chronic pancreatitis or after pancreatic trauma.
3. B

   Pseudocysts will resolve spontaneously in most instances, but complications can develop. Pseudocysts that are thick-walled or large (over 6 cm in diameter), have lasted for a long time (over 12 weeks) or have arisen in the context of chronic pancreatitis are less likely to resolve spontaneously, but these factors are not specific indications for intervention.

Reference:

1. Bhattacharya S. The pancreas. In: Williams NS, Bulstrode CJK, O'Connell PR (Eds) Bailey and Love's Short Practice of Surgery, 26th edition. CRC Press: Boca Raton 2013,pp 1127-1133.

HYDATID DISEASE OF LIVER

Dr. Akshay Anand, Lecturer, Department of Surgery, KGMU, Lucknow

A 56 yrs. old female presents to surgical OPD with c/o right hypochondrial pain. There is no h/o fever, jaundice and altered bowel movements. On per abdomen examination only hepatomegaly is present.

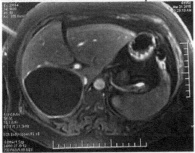

On USG abdomen a well-circumscribed cystic lesion is present in the segment V, VI, VII with budding sign on cyst membrane. MRI abdomen is as follows:

1. Which of the following statement is TRUE regarding hydatid cyst disease?
   (A) Dogs are definite host of E. Granulosus.
   (B) Human is definite host of E. Granulosus.
   (C) Human is intermediate host of E. Granulosus.
   (D) Sheep is definite host of E. Granulosus.
2. Which of the following statement is TRUE regarding hydatid cyst?
   (A) The cyst wall three layered – pericyst, ectocyst and endocyst.
   (B) The cyst wall is two layered - ectocyst and endocyst.
   (C) Calcified cyst denotes a dead cyst
   (D) Hydatid cyst is more common in left lobe of liver.
3. Regarding management of hydatid cyst, all are true except?
   (A) Small, asymptomatic densely calcified cyst in elderly can be managed conservatively.
   (B) During preoperative preparation, steroids have been recommended.
   (C) Bile duct communication diagnosed at operation needs to taken care of either by suture repair or post op ERCP.
   (D) Cyst disappear with medical therapy is more common and should be tried first hand.

Answers:

1. A.
   Dogs are the definitive host of E. granulosus; the adult tapeworm is attached to the villi of the ileum. Up to thousands of ova are passed daily and deposited in the dog's feces. Sheep are the usual intermediate host, but humans are an accidental intermediate host. Humans are an end stage to the parasite.
2. B.
   Three weeks after infection, a visible hydatid cyst develops, which then slowly grows in a spherical manner. A pericyst or fibrous capsule derived from host tissues develops around the hydatid cyst. The cyst wall itself has two layers, an outer gelatinous membrane (ectocyst) and an inner germinal membrane (endocyst).
3. D.
   Treatment of echinococcosis with albendazole or mebendazole is effective at shrinking cysts in many patients with E. granulosus, but cyst disappearance occurs in well under 50% of patients. Medical therapy without definitive resection or drainage should only be considered for widely disseminated disease or poor surgical candidates.

Reference:
Sicklick JK, D'Angelica M, Fong Y. The Liver. In: Townsend CM JR, Beauchamp RD, Evers BM, Mattox KL (Eds). Sabiston Textbook of Surgery: the biological basis of modern practice. 19 edition. Elsevier: Saunders, Philadelphia 2012, pp 1447 – 1449.

CARCINOMA OVARY
Dr. Saumya Singh, Lecturer, Department of Surgery

A 25 years young female, married nullipara, a school teacher, undergoes laparoscopic cystectomy for ovarian cyst lt. ovary, which on HPE revealed serous cystadenocarcinoma. Her LFT,RFT and CXR is within normal limits and presently she is asymptomatic.

1. What should be done next?
   (A) Hysterectomy and B/L salpingoopherectomy
   (B) Hysterectomy and radiotherapy
   (C) Radiotherapy
   (D) Serial CA-125 measurement and follow up
2. Chemotherapeutic drug of choice in this type of tumours is
   (A) Gemcitabine
   (B) Carboplatin
   (C) Methotrexate
   (D) Cyclophosphamid
3. Histological characteristic of serous epithelial tumour is
   (A) Reinke's Crystal
   (B) Schiller dual bodies
   (C) Signet ring cell
   (D) Psammoma bodies

Answers:
   1. D
       Doing an oopherectomy will suffice, as the pt. is young and nullipara.
       Next step is to follow the patient with regular CA-125.
   2. B
       Treatment with carboplatin and Paclitaxel is desirable in younger pts.
   3. B
       Histological charecteristics of epithelial tumours is psammoma bodies.

Reference:
   1. Berek JS et. al. Ovarian and Fallopian Tube Cancer. In: Berek JS, Jonathan S (Eds). Berek & Novak's Gynecology. 15th ed. Lippincott Williams & Wilkins 2012. pp 1317 -1371.

ENDOMETRIAL CARCINOMA
Dr. Saumya Singh, Lecturer, Department of Surgery

A 43 years married female, presented with well differentiated adenocarcinoma of uterus has more than half of myometrial invasion, vaginal metastasis and inguinal lymph node metastasis .LFT and CXR is within normal limits.

1. Her AJCC staging is?
   (A) III b
   (B) IV a
   (C) III c
   (D) IVb
2. All of the following are risk factors for Endometrial Carcinoma except
   (A) Hypertension
   (B) Multiparity
   (C) Diabetes mellitus
   (D) Obesity
3. All of the following are prognostic factors in Endometrial Cancer, except
   (A) Lymph node metastasis

(B) Stage of disease

(C) CA-125

(D) Histologic type

Answers:
1. C

    As per FIGO,vaginal and /or parametrial involvement is stage III b.
2. B

    Nulliparity and not multiparity is a risk factor.
3. C

    CA -125 is prognostic marker of Ca ovary and not Ca endometrium.

Reference:
1. Lurain JR et. al. Uterine Cancer. In: Berek JS, Jonathan S (Eds). Berek & Novak's Gynecology. 15th ed. Lippincott Williams & Wilkins 2012. pp 1317 -1371.

CARCINOMA LUNG
Dr. Saumya Singh, Lecturer, Department of Surgery

A 56 years male, chronic smoker, presented with hoarseness of voice and hemoptysis. There is H/O fever off and on, decreased appetite and weight loss. On examination patient is anemic with a single large painless lymph node felt in left supraclavicular region.

1. Next appropriate Investigation to be done is?

    (A) CT chest

    (B) Sputum examination for AFB

    (C) Laryngoscopy and CXR

    (D) Excision biopsy of node
2. Most common tumor to produce metastasis to supraclavicular lymph node is?

    (A) Glottic Ca

    (B) Ca lip

    (C) Nasopharyngeal Ca

    (D) Ca base of tounge
3. Biopsy report of above mentioned patient states Squamous cell carcinoma. What is the most probable diagnosis?

    (A) Ca Stomach

    (B) Ca Lip

    (C) Ca Lung

    (D) Ca Pancreas

Answers:
1. D

    In cases of lymphadenopathy, if the patient's history and physical findings are suggestive of malignancy, then a prompt LN biopsy should be done. FNAC is not of much use.
2. C

    Nasopharyngeal carcinoma is most common tumor to produce cervical LN metastasis.
3. C

    SCC is a variant of lung cancer, which is coherent with the clinical features of this pt.

Reference:
1. Ramaswamy Govindan. Devita, Hellman & Rosenberg's Cancer: Principles & Practice of Oncology. Lippincott Williams & Wilkins; New Delhi 2012. pp 396-397.

CARDIAC TAMPONADE
Dr. Suresh Kumar, Professor, Department of Surgery

A 30 year male car driver presented in casualty department with history steering wheel injury to the anterior chest wall with complaints of chest pain and breathlessness. On examination pulse rate 120/min, low volume, B.P 86/50 mmHg, , respiratory rate 28/mins,neck veins distended. On auscultation bilateral normal vesicular breath sounds with muffled heart sounds were present.

1. What is the clinical diagnosis?
    (A) Fail chest
    (B) Cardiac tamponade
    (C) Massive haemothorax
    (D) Tension pneumothorax
2. What is FAST?
    (A) Focussed assessment sonography in trauma
    (B) Focussed assessment study in trauma
    (C) Focussed assessment sonography in thorax
    (D) Fast assessment sonography in trauma
3. What is Becks triad?
    (A) Raised JVP,muffled heart sounds, hypertension
    (B) Raised JVP,muffled heart sounds, hypotension
    (C) Raised JVP,muffled heart sounds, normal B.P
    (D) Raised JVP, normal heart sounds, hypotension

Answers
    1.   B
    2.   A
    3.   B

Reference:
    1.   Advanced Trauma Life Support (ATLS) 8TH ed., American college of Surgeons ,Chicago , Pg 91

CHYLOTHORAX
Dr. Suresh Kumar, Professor, Department of Surgery

A 45 years male operated for carcinoma oesophagus presented with complains of chest pain, breathlessness and malaise. On local examination right side chest movements were restricted. On auscultation air entry was decreased on right side, trachea was shifted to left side. On percussion dull note was present on right side. X-ray was s/o massive pleural effusion on right side. On pleural tap the fluid was grossly milky.
1. What is the clinical diagnosis?
    (A) Malignant pleural effusion
    (B) Chylothorax
    (C) Empyema thoracis
    (D) Haemothorax
2. What should be the treatment of the above condition?
    (A)ICD, low fat diet, aggressive fluid, electrolytes correction and nutritional support.
    (B) ICD, high fat diet, fluid restriction, electrolytes correction and nutritional support.
    (C) ICD, fluid therapy, electrolytes correction and nill orally till ICD drainage stops.
    (D) Wait and watch, fluids and nutritional support.
3. Expected fluid loss per day via inercostal drainage tube ?
    (A) >1liter
    (B) >2liters
    (C) >3liters
    (D) >4liters
4. For how long conservative management for the above condition can be continued?
    (A) 1 –2 weeks
    (B) 2 -4 weeks
    (C) 4 -6 weeks
    (D) 6 -8 weeks
5. If conservative management fails, what surgical intervention can be taken?
    (A) Ligation of the cysterna chyli.
    (B) Ligation of thoracic duct at the diaphragmatic hiatus through right thoracotomy.
    (C) Ligation of thoracic duct at the site of insertion.
    (D) Ligation of the cysterna chyliand thoracic duct at the level of insertion.

Answers:
    1.   B
    2.   A
    3.   C

4.   A
5.   B
Reference:
1.   In: Townsend CM, Beuchamp RD, Evers BM, Mattox KL (Eds). Sabiston Textbook of Surgery. The Biological Basis of Modern Surgical Practice. 19th Ed. Elsevier: Philadephia 2012: pp 1598-99.

TENSION PNEUMOTHORAX

Dr. Suresh Kumar, Professor, Department of Surgery

A young male presented in emergency department after sustaining RTA with complains of chest pain, air hunger and respiratory distress. Pulse rate was 120/min, B.P 90/60 mmHg,respiratory rate 35/mins with cyanosis. Local examination revealed restricted right side chest movements,distended neck veins, tracheal shift to left side. On percussion right side chest was hyper- resonant. On auscultation air entry was decreased on right side.

1. What is the clinical diagnosis?
   (A) Cardiac tamponade
   (B) Tension pneumothorax
   (C) Massive haemothorax
   (D) Traumatic diaphragmatic hernia
2. What is the initial management of the above condition?
   (A) Urgent insertion of large calibre needle into second intercostal space in mid-clavicular line.
   (B)Urgent insertion of pigtail catheter in second intercostal space in midclavicular line on the affected side.
   (C) Emergency thoracotomy.
   (D) Immediately shift the patient on ventilator,start I.V. fluids, sodabicarbonate and antibiotics.
3. What is the ideal site for chest tube insertion in haemothorax?
   (A) 2nd intercostals space in midclavicular line
   (B)5th intercostals space in anterior axillary line
   (C) 5th intercostals space posterior axillary line
   (D) 5th intercostals space in just anterior to the mid axillary line

Answers:
   1.   B
   2.   A
   3.   D

Reference:
1.   Advanced Trauma Life Support (ATLS) 8TH ed., American college of Surgeons, Chicago, Pg 87.

Chapter-28

Surgery Gastroenterology

POST LAPAROSCOPIC CHOLECYSTECTOMY BILE DUCT INJURY

Dr. Abhijit Chandra, Professor and Head, Dr. Vishal Gupta, Associate Professor &
Dr. Rahul, Senior Resident, Department of Surgical Gastroenterology

30 year female underwent laparoscopic cholecystectomy for symptomatic gall stone disease. Surgery was uneventful. She was not feeling well on POD 1. She was discharged on POD 2 on pain killers after reassurance. The patient returned on POD 5 with complains of respiratory distress, abdominal distension, pedal edema, jaundice. The patient remained afebrile. On examination, vitals were stable. Pulse – 92/minute. Blood pressure – 112/70 mmHg. Abdomen was distended but soft. There was no obvious lump palpable. Shifting dullness was positive. Abdominal sounds were decreased.

1. What is the most likely diagnosis?
    (A) Biliary ascitis/bilioma following biliary injury
    (B) Decompensated liver cirrhosis
    (C) Acute intestinal obstruction
    (D) Biliary peritonitis following biliary injury
2. Most appropriate next step?
    (A) Ultrasound abdomen
    (B) Contrast enhanced CT scan
    (C) X ray abdomen
    (D) Ultrasound abdomen with paracentesis
3. What should be the initial management?
    (A) Resuscitation, pig tail drainage and antibiotics
    (B) Resuscitation, pig tail drainage and ERCP with stenting
    (C) Resuscitation, paracentesis, biliary refeeding and monitoring
    (D) Resuscitation and immediate exploration with an attempt to repair the injury
4. External biliary fistula was established (500mL/day for last 7 days). Which investigation will give the correct diagnosis?
    (A) Magnetic resonance cholangiography (MRCP)
    (B) Endoscopic retrograde cholangiography(ERC)
    (C) Percutaneous transhepatic cholangiography (PTC)
    (D) Fistulography
5. Surgical reconstruction should be done at:
    (A) 6 weeks after index surgery
    (B) 8 weeks after the closure of the fistula
    (C) 8 weeks after the establishment of controlled external biliary fistula
    (D) 6 months after the establishment of external biliary fistula

Answers:

1. A

    The patient did not have fever and abdomen was soft on examination. This rules out peritonitis. Jaundice cannot be explained by intestinal obstruction. Liver decompensation without previous history of liver disease and without major liver resection is unlikely. So, the patient most likely has biliary ascitis/bilioma

2. D

    Most appropriate step will be ultrasound and guided paracentesis to establish the diagnosis of bilioma

3. A

    Best initial management of bilioma is control of sepsis. This can be easily achieved by resuscitation, pig tail drainage and antibiotics. ERCP as the first step is not a good option. Biliary refeeding in a case of bilioma is not indicated. Exploration and repair is not indicated after 72 hours of injury and undrained collection.

4. D

    Fistulography is the cheapest and most informative initial investigation. Magnetic resonance cholangiography will not be useful in collapsed system. ERC and PTC are invasive & not warranted.

5. C

    Optimum time of repair – 6 to 8 weeks of establishment of controlled external biliary fistula.

References:

1. Blumgart LH. Blumgart. Surgery of the Liver, Biliary Tract and Pancreas. Chapter 42a, Benign biliary strictures. 5th ed. Philadelphia: Saunders Elsevier; 2012. p 615-643.

Blumgart LH. Blumgart. Surgery of the Liver, Biliary Tract and Pancreas. 5th ed. Philadelphia: Saunders Elsevier; 2012. Chapter 42b. Biliary fistulae. P. 644-669.

ACUTE DIVERTICULITIS WITH COLOVESICAL FISTULA

Dr. Abhijit Chandra, Professor and Head, Dr. Vishal Gupta, Associate Professor, Dr. Rahul, Senior Resident, Department of Surgical Gastroenterology

50 years male, otherwise asymptomatic before, presented with history of constipation and recurrent lower abdominal pain (left sided) for 7 days, developed hematuria and fever for last 2 days. The patient also complains of pneumaturia for the last 3-4 hours. Patient is vitally stable and has tenderness in left lower abdomen.

1. Most likely cause which can explain the above features?
   (A) Carcinoma colon with colovesical fistula
   (B) Acute diverticulitis with colovesical fistula
   (C) Crohns disease with enterovesical fistula
   (D) Severe cystitis
2. What is the most appropriate diagnostic investigation?
   (A) Intravenous pyelogram
   (B) Cystoscopy
   (C) CECT abdomen + pelvis
   (D) Colonoscopy
3. What is the opt treatment in colovesical fistula?
   (A) Diversion and allow the fistula to heal
   (B) Single stage operation after possible bowel preparation
   (C) 3 stage procedure – colostomy followed by closure of fistula and then reversal of the colostomy as the final step
   (D) Cystoscopic glue injection

Answers:
   1. B
       Short history of seven days with fever and age of 50 years correlates best with option
   2. C
       Best investigation for colovesical fistula is CECT abdomen with pelvis. Colonoscopy is not advised in acute diverticulitis and may not be able to locate colovesical fistula. Cystoscopy may establish the diagnosis of enterovesical fistula but is not accurate to locate the site of fistula and will not give any clue regarding the colonic pathology.
   3. B
       Single stage procedure is feasible if the patient is in good condition which shall include dismantling of fistula and resection anastomosis of the colon.

Reference:
   1. Charles JY. Shackelford's Surgery of the Alimentary Tract. Diverticular disease. 7th ed. Philadelphia: Elsevier Saunders; 2013. p. 1879-95.

POST TRANSHIATAL ESOPHAGECTOMY CERVICAL ANASTOMOSIS LEAK

Dr. Abhijit Chandra, Professor and Head; Dr. Vishal Gupta, Associate Professor; Dr. Rahul, Senior Resident, Department of Surgical Gastroenterology

Patient underwent Transhiatal Esophagectomy (THE) for lower one third of carcinoma Esophagus. On POD 5, he suddenly developed respiratory distress. On chest auscultation, bilateral air entry was normal. There was no limb edema. Patient was febrile with a pulse rate of 104/minute and blood pressure of 108/64 mm Hg. On per abdomen examination, abdomen was soft, non tender.

1. What is the most likely diagnosis?
   (A)Pulmonary embolism.
   (B)Mucus plug
   (C)Cervical anastomotic leak
   (D)Bronchopneumonia

2. What is the immediate treatment?
   (A)Cardiopulmonary consultation and anticoagulation
   (B)Cervical wound exploration
   (C)Mucolytics and antibiotics
   (D)Compression stockings and limb elevation
3. After development of cervical fistula, what is the management?
   (A)NPO with adequate drainage and jejunostomy feeds
   (B)Ryle's tube insertion with antibiotics
   (C)Immediate endoscopy to assess the leak and clipping
   (D)Re-exploration and suture reinforcement
4. Most common reason for cervical anastomotic leak?
   (A)Poor vascular supply of cervical esophagus
   (B)Arterial ischemia of the gastric conduit
   (C)Venous ischemia of gastric conduit
   (D)Compression from the trachea
5. True about cervical and intrathoracic esophagogastric anastomoses
   (A)Cervical anastomotic leak is more common than intrathoracic anastomoses
   (B)Stapled anastomosis has higher leak rate than hand sewn
   (C)Substernal route is the best route
   (D)Cervical anastomotic leak is difficult to manage than intrathoracic anastomosis

Answers:

1. C

   Post THE, the patient's condition can be best explained by cervical anastomotic leak. There is no evidence of DVT, so chances of pulmonary embolism as the cause is less likely. Musus plug does not correlate with bilateral normal air entry. Patient with bronchopneumonia will have complains of cough with or without expectoration and the onset is likely to be gradual.

2. B

   Immediate treatment for cervical anastomosis leak is drainage of the wound.

3. A

   Subsequently, the patient is maintained on feeding jejunostomy and is kept nil per orally. Adequate drainage is assured.

4. C

   Most common cause of the cervical anastomosis leak is venous ischemia of the gastric conduit.

5. A

   Cervical anastomosis leaks more often than intrathoracic, but are easier to manage. They usually heal by conservative management but inthoracic leaks result in high morbidity and mortality. Leak rate is not affected much by the technique of anastomosis and the native posterior mediastinal route of esophagus is the best route for the conduit.

References:

1. Charles JY. Shackelford's Surgery of the Alimentary Tract. 7th ed. Philadelphia: Elsevier Saunders; 2013. Chapter 43, Techniques of esophageal reconstruction.p. 518-36.
2. Charles JY. Shackelford's Surgery of the Alimentary Tract. 7th ed. Philadelphia: Elsevier Saunders; 2013. Chapter 44, Complications of esophagectomy. p 537-46.

PSEUDOCYST OF THE PANCREAS

Dr. Abhijit Chandra, Professor and Head, Dr. Vishal Gupta, Associate Professor,
Dr. Rahul, Senior Resident, Department of Surgical Gastroenterology

A patient with a history of alcoholic acute pancreatitis 2 month back managed conservatively presented with a gradually increasing swelling in epigastrium with the history of early satiety and vomiting. CECT abdomen as

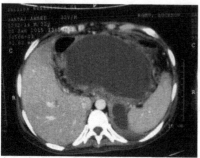

shown in the picture below.

1. What is the most probable diagnosis?
   - (A)Gastric Outlet Obstruction
   - (B)Pseudocyst pancreas
   - (C)Cystic neoplasm of pancreas
   - (D)Mesenteric cyst
2. Best management modality for the patient.
   - (A)Cystoenteric bypass
   - (B)Exploration and cyst deroofing
   - (C)Percutaneous drainage
   - (D)Total pancreatectomy + cyst excision
3. After admission, the patient developed acute onset abdominal pain with small amount of hematemesis without hemodynamic instability and no major fall in Hb levels. Most likely cause of UGI bleed?
   - (A)Gastritis.
   - (B)Stress Ulcers
   - (C)Pseudoaneurysm
   - (D)Esophageal varices
4. What is the most appropriate management?
   - (A)Monitor Hb levels, wait and watch
   - (B)Stop NSAIDS and start on sucralfate
   - (C)Immediate exploration
   - (D)CT angiography

Answers:

1. B

   With the history of acute pancreatitis and appearance of the cyst in the CECT, the most probable diagnosis appears to be pseudocyst pancreas. Pressure symptoms can explain early satiety and vomiting.

2. A

   Best treatment is cystoenteric bypass for symptomatic cysts – endoscopic or laparoscopic. This can also be done after laparotomy. In this case, endoscopic intervention in the form of endoscopic cystogastrostomy appears most appropriate.

3. C

   Acute onset pain associated with hematemesis in a patient with acute pseudocyst pancreas usually points towards sentinel bleed due to pseudoaneurysm. Gastritis and stress ulcers donot usually cause hematemsis. Esophageal Variceal bleed is usually painless.

4. D

   In a stable patient with sentinel bleed and suspected pseudoaneurysm, an early evaluation with CT angiography is very informative. Endoscopy can be done to rule out other causes of UGI bleed and to look for ongoing bleed.

Reference:
1. Charles JY. Shackelford's. Surgery of the Alimentary Tract. Chapter 90. Pseudocysts and other complications of pancrfeatitis. 7th ed. Philadelphia: Elsevier Saunders; 2013. p. 1144-67.

PERIAMPULLARY CARCINOMA

Dr. Abhijit Chandra, Professor and Head, Dr. Vishal Gupta, Associate Professor,
Dr. Rahul, Senior Resident, Department of Surgical Gastroenterology

A 50 yr male patient presented with painless progressive jaundice with intense itching for last one month. On examination, icterus was present. Per abdomen examination revealed palpable cystic gall bladder. DRE normal. No ascites present. CECT abdomen of the patient revealed the following picture.

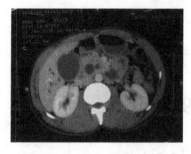

1. What is the most likely diagnosis?
   (A) Gall bladder carcinoma
   (B) Periampullary carcinoma
   (C) Benign biliary stricture
   (D)Choledocholithiasis
2. Definitive treatment for the patient?
   (A) Radical cholecystectomy
   (B) Roux en Y Hepaticojejunostomy
   (C) Whipple's procedure
   (D) ERCP stenting
3. The same patient is planned for definitive surgery. On the morning of surgery, the patient develops high grade fever. What should be done next?
   (A) Go for the definitive procedure as per plan
   (B) ERCP stenting and plan for surgery within 48 hours
   (C) Drainage procedure by surgery and definitive procedure to be done later
   (D) ERCP stenting and wait for the patient to stabilize

Answers:
1. B
   CECT abdomen shows double duct sign which is classical in periampullary carcinoma
2. C
   Definite treatment for periampullary carcinoma will be Whipple's pancreaticoduodenectomy if resectable.
3. D
   The patient appears to develop cholangitis on the day of surgery. Best option will be ERCP stenting, treat the patient with antibiotics and wait for the fever to subside before taking for surgery.

Reference:
1. Charles JY. Shackelford's. Surgery of the Alimentary Tract. Chapter 93, pancreatic and periampullary cancer. 7th ed. Philadelphia: Elsevier Saunders; 2013. p. 1187-1205.

Chapter-29

Surgical Oncology

CARCINOMA HEAD OF PANCREAS

Dr. Vijay Kumar, Associate Professor, Dr. Naseem Akhtar, Assistant Professor,
Department of Surgical Oncology

A 45 yr old lady presented with painless progressively increasing jaundice since last 15 days. It was associated with itching all over body and clay coloured stools with dark yellow urine. On examination, patient was having deep icterus and a non- tender globular lump was palpable in right hypochondrium, moving with respiration.

1. What is the most probable site of origin of lump?
(A) Pancreas
(B) Kidney
(C) Bile duct
(D) Gall bladder

2. What is the least probable diagnosis?
(A) Carcinoma head of pancreas
(B) Carcinoma bile duct
(C) Carcinoma gallbladder fundus
(D) Carcinoma ampulla

3. What is the initial investigation of choice?
(A) CT scan
(B) Magnetic Resonance Imaging
(C) Positron Emission Tomography
(D) USG

4. Which is the best investigation to assess biliary anatomy?
(A) Contrast enhanced CT scan
(B) Magnetic Resonance CholangioPancreatography
(C) USG
(D) HIDA scan

5. The investigation shows periampullary carcinoma with multiple liver metastases. What is the most appropriate next step?
(A) Whipple's procedure
(B) Radiation
(C) Explore and put T-tube in Common Bile Duct
(D) ERCP and stenting

Answers:

1. D
   Globular lump in right hypochondrium is highly suggestive of gallbladder lump.
2. C
   Carcinoma gallbladder fundus is away from biliary tree hence would not present with such scenario commonly.
3. D
   USG is initial investigation of choice as it is cheap, easily available and reproducible.
4. B
   Magnetic resonance cholangiopancreatography is best diagnostic modality for biliary anatomy.
5. D
   In case of multiple metastasis, palliation of jaundice is the main goal which is best done by ERCP guided stenting.

Reference:

1. Richard E. Royal, Robert A. Wolff, and Christofer H. Crane. Cancer of the Pancreas. In: Vincent T. DeVita Jr., Theodore S. Lawrence, and Steven A. Rosenberg. Principles and Practice of Oncology.10th ed. Philadelphia. Wolters Kluwer health / Lippincott Williams and Wilkins; 2015; pp 961-86.

PAROTID CARCINOMA

Dr. Vijay Kumar, Associate Professor, Department of Surgical Oncology

A 28 yr old man presented with swelling at right cheek behind the angle of mandible since last one year, which is progressively increasing in size and is painless. On examination, a 4x3 cm swelling is present below and behind right ear and has lifted up the ear lobule. Swelling is having restricted mobility and is non-tender. Tonsils are not pushed medially.

1. Which is the most probable diagnosis?
(A)   Temporal lobe tumor
(B)   Mandibular bone tumor
(C)   Carotid body tumor
(D)   Parotid gland tumor

2. Which is the most common tumor of parotid gland?
(A)   Mucoepidermoid tumor
(B)   Adenoid cystic
(C)   Pleomorphic adenoma
(D)   Acinic cell tumor

3. FNAC from lesion is suggestive of pleomorphic adenoma. What is the best treatment further?
(A)   Total parotidectomy
(B)   Radiotherapy
(C)   Superficial parotidectomy
(D)   Cryotherapy

4. Which type of incision is given for parotid surgery?
(A)   Lazy L incision
(B)   Lazy M incision
(C)   Lazy S incision
(D)   Lazy P incision

5.   Which nerve is most likely to get damaged during surgery?
(A)   Hypoglossal nerve
(B)   Glossopharyngeal nerve
(C)   Auditory nerve
(D)   Facial nerve

Answers:

1.   D
        Swelling behind ear lifting ear lobule is typical of parotid gland tumor.
2.   C
        Pleomorphic adenoma is overall the most common tumor of salivary gland .
3.   C
        Pleomorphic adenoma limited to superficial lobe is best treated by superficial parotidectomy.
4.   C
        Lazy S incision is given in front of tragus extending along lower border of mandible.
5.   D
        Facial nerve passes through the parotid gland and is thus more at risk during surgery.

Reference:

1.   William M. Mendenhall, John W. Werning, David J. Pfister. Treatment Of Head And Neck Cancer. In:Vincent T. DeVita Jr., Theodore S. Lawrence, and Steven A. Rosenberg. Principles and Practice of Oncology.10th ed. Philadelphia. Wolters Kluwer health / Lippincott Williams and Wilkins; 2015; pp 774-80.

CARCINOMA BREAST

Dr. Vijay Kumar, Associate Professor, Department of Surgical Oncology

A 50 yr old female patient, presented with lump involving left breast. It was insidious in onset and gradually increasing in size and not associated with pain. She was married at the age of 20 and has given birth to 3 children. All the children were breast fed for approximately six months. She attained menopause one year back. On examination 6 x 4 cm hard lump was palpable in left lower and outer quadrant involving nipple areola complex with no peau'd orange overlying the lump. The nipple is found retracted. The lump has restricted mobility in the breast tissue. On examining the left axilla, two palpable lymph nodes were found. They are soft and mobile. There are no supraclavicular lymphnodes. Opposite breast and axilla are normal.

1. What is the most likely diagnosis?
   (A) Fibro adenoma
   (B) Carcinoma breast
   (C) Tubercular breast lump
   (D) Mastitis

2. The clinical staging of above lesion is
   (A) T1 N1
   (B) T2 N1
   (C) T3 N1
   (D) T3 N2

3. In patients with breast cancer chest wall involvement means involvement of any of the following except
   (A) Serratus anterior
   (B) Pectoralis muscle
   (C) Intercostal muscles
   (D) Ribs

4. Commonest type of breast cancer is
   (A) Papillary carcinoma
   (B) Paget's disease
   (C) Fibro sarcoma
   (D) Infiltrating ductal carcinoma

5. Carcinoma breast which is multi-centric and bilateral:
   (A) Ductal
   (B) Lobular
   (C) Mucoid
   (D) Colloid

Answers:
1. B
   Carcinoma breast.
2. C
   T3 is > 5cm and clinical N1 is mobile axillary lymph nodes.
3. B
   Involvement of Pectoralis major and minor will not come under chest wall involvement.
4. D
   Infiltrating ductal carcinoma is the most common type of cancer.
5. D
   Lobular carcinoma is usually bilateral and multicentric.

Reference:
1. Harold J. Burstein, Jay R. Harris, and Monica Morrow. Malignant Tumors of the Breast. In: Vincent T. DeVita Jr., Theodore S. Lawrence, and Steven A. Rosenberg. Principles and Practice of Oncology.10th ed. Philadelphia. Wolters Kluwer health / Lippincott Williams and Wilkins; 2015; pp 1401-39.

CARCINOMA THYROID
Dr. Vijay Kumar, Associate Professor, Department of Surgical Oncology

A 50 years female patient presented with a swelling in the front and sides of the neck for last 6 months. It was increasing in size over this span. She complains dull aching pain over the swelling for 15 days. She also complains of slight hoarseness of voice for one month. On examination, 6x5 cm swelling in front of neck towards right side of midline, which moves on deglutition. Serum TSH was normal. Right vocal cord was not moving on indirect laryngoscopy.

1. What is the most likely diagnosis
   (A) Carcinoma larynx
   (B) Carcinoma parotid
   (C) Carcinoma thyroid
   (D) Carcinoma submandibular gland

2. Most common form of differentiated thyroid carcinoma is :
    (A) Papillary carcinoma
    (B) Follicular carcinoma
    (C) Medullary carcinoma
    (D) Anaplastic carcinoma
3. Tubercle of zuckerkandl is in relation to :
    (A) Adrenal gland
    (B) Thyroid gland
    (C) Parotid gland
    (D) Submandibular gland
4. Retrosternal goiter true is :
    (A) Extends into posterior mediastinum
    (B) Anterior to subclavian and innominate vein in the anterior mediastinum
    (C) Almost always needs sternotomy
    (D) None of the above
5. Sistrunk's operation is done :
    (A) Bronchial cyst
    (B) Thyroglossal cyst
    (C) Sebaceous cyst
    (D) None of the above

Answers:

1.   C
    Female patient with swelling in anterior neck for 6 months and gradually progressive
    and examination finding revealed mobility of swelling with deglutition and right vocal cord fixed
    indicates towards carcinoma thyroid as probable diagnosis.
2.   A
    Papillary carcinoma thyroid is most common form of differentiated thyroid cancer.
3.   B
    Tubercle of zuckerkandl is in related to thyroid gland.
4.   B
    Retrosternalgoiter lies anterior to subclavian and innominate vein in the anterior mediastinum
    and seldom requires sternotomy for excision.
5.   B
    Sistrunk's operation is performed for thyroglossal cyst excision.

References:

1.   Carlson HE. Endocrine neoplasms. In: Casciato DA, Territo MC (Eds). Manual of clinical oncology.7th edition.Wolter Kluwer (India); 2012; pp 408-32.
2.   Carling T, Udelsman R. Thyroid tumors. In: Vincent T. DeVita Jr., Theodore S. Lawrence, and Steven A. Rosenberg. Principles and Practice of Oncology.10th ed. Philadelphia. Wolters Kluwer health / Lippincott Williams and Wilkins; 2015; pp1457-72.

CARCINOMA COLON

Dr. Vijay Kumar, Associate Professor, Department of Surgical Oncology

A 50 yr old male patient presented with fresh bleeding per rectum which was painless, not associated with abdominal cramps. On general examination, pallor was present. Abdominal examination was unrevealing. On per-rectal examination, no growth was palpable, however finger was stained with blood.Proctoscopic examination was done which did not reveal any source of bleeding . Colonoscopy was performed which revealed growth in sigmoid colon from which biopsy was taken which later revealed malignancy.

1. What is the next best step?
    (A) Magnetic Resonance Imaging
    (B) Barium enema
    (C) Positron Emission Tomography
    (D) CECT abdomen
2. Appropriate tumor marker for carcinoma colon is
    (A) CA 125
    (B) Carcino-Embryonic Antigen

(C) CA15.3

(D) Prostate Specific Antigen

3. Radiological investigations suggest single liver metastasis in left lobe with rest of metastatic workup normal. Next best step is

    (A) Palliative chemotherapy as disease is already metastatic

    (B) Colon resection with chemotherapy for liver metastasis

    (C) Colon resection with cryotherapy

    (D) Colon resection with left lobectomy

4. Which type of cancer is most common in colon?

    (A) Adenocarcinoma

    (B) Squamous cell carcinoma

    (C) Adenosquamous carcinoma

    (D) Neuroendocrine tumor

5. What is most commonly involved in carcinoma colon?

    (A) Caecum

    (B) Rectosigmoid

    (C) Transverse colon

    (D) Ascending colon

Answers:

1.   D

Contrast enhanced CT abdomen is best next step to assess staging

2.   B

Carcinoembryogenic antigen is tumor marker for carcinoma colon

3.   D

Resectable isolated liver metastasis in carcinoma colon can be resected along with primary resection

4.   A

Adenocarcinoma is most common cancer of colon

5.   B

Rectosigmoid is most common site of cancer colon

Reference:

1.   Steven K. Libutti, Leonard B. Saltz, and Christofer G. Willett. Cancer of the Colon. In: Vincent T. DeVita Jr., Theodore S. Lawrence, and Steven A. Rosenberg. Principles and Practice of Oncology.10th ed. Philadelphia. Wolters Kluwer health / Lippincott Williams and Wilkins; 2015; pp 1084-1126.

SOFT TISSUE SARCOMA

Dr. Vijay Kumar, Associate Professor, Department of Surgical Oncology

A 28 years old male, shopkeeper, presented with gradually progressive swelling over middle of thigh after fall from cycle four months back associated with pain. On physical examination 12X8 cms swellingis present over left mid thigh which is hard, tender and multiple tortuous veins present over it. X-ray of thigh shows soft tissue involvement and extra osseous calcification.

1. All are etiological factor for soft tissue sarcoma except

    (A) Lymphedema

    (B) Chemical

    (C) Hormonal

    (D) Genetic

2. Most common site of origin of soft tissue sarcoma is

    (A) Retroperitoneal

    (B) Head and Neck

    (C) Visceral

    (D) Lower extremity

3. Most common radiation induced sarcoma is

    (A) Malignant Peripheral Sheath Tumour

    (B) Pleomorphic Malignant Fibrous Histiocytoma

    (C) Myxofibrosarcoma

    (D) Angiosarcoma

4. Characteristic genetic abnormality associated with synovial sarcoma is

    (A) T(12:16)

    (B) T(X:18)

(C) T(12:22)

(D) Giant chromosome

5.Stewart-Treves syndrome is

    (A) Lymphangiosarcoma of post mastectomy irradiated arm of women

    (B) A variant of Dermato fibroma Sarcoma Protuberans with melanin pigmentation

    (C) Malignant Peripheral Nerve Sheath Tumour with rhabdomyosarcomatous element

    (D) Multiple intramuscular myxoma associated with Fibrous dysplasia

Answers:

    1.   C

        Hormone imbalance is not a etiological factor for soft tissue sarcoma

    2.   D

        Lower extremity is most common site of origin of soft tissue sarcoma

    3.   B

        Pleomorphic Malignant Fibrous Histiocytomais the most common soft tissue sarcoma associated with radiation

    4.   B

        T(X:18) is hallmark for synovial sarcoma

    5.   A

        Lymphangiosarcoma of post mastectomy irradiated arm of women

References:

    1.   Samuel Singer, Robert G. Maki, and Brian O' Sullivan. Soft Tissue Sarcoma. In: Vincent T. DeVita Jr., Theodore S. Lawrence, and Steven A. Rosenberg. Principles and Practice of Oncology.10th ed. Philadelphia. Wolters Kluwer health / Lippincott Williams and Wilkins; 2015; pp 1533-77

ENDOMETRIAL CARCINOMA

Dr. Vijay Kumar, Associate Professor, Department of Surgical Oncology

A 60 year old obese hypertensive female with BMI 40 presented with post-menopausal bleeding since 3 months. The abdominal examination is within normal limits. USG Abdomen revealed thickened endometrium wall. Fractional curettage was done and biopsy showed adenocarcinoma.

1.What is best way to stage carcinoma endometrium?

    (A) Contract Enhanced CT Whole Abdomen

    (B) Magnetic Resonance Imaging Abdomen

    (C) Positron Emission Tomography Scan

    (D) Surgery

2.What is predominant route of metastasis of carcinoma endometrium?

    (A) Direct

    (B) Lymphatic

    (C) Haematogenous

    (D) Peritoneal transplants

3.What is the most common pathology of Endometrial carcinoma?

    (A) Adenocarcinomas

    (B) Papillary carcinoma

    (C) Squamous cell carcinoma

    (D) Clear cell carcinoma

4.Most common malignancy associated with carcinoma endometrium

    (A) Carcinoma Ovary

    (B) Carcinoma Cervix

    (C) Carcinoma Colon

    (D) Carcinoma Lung

Answers:

    1.   D

        Unless contraindicated, laparotomy is required for staging of patients withcarcinomaendometrium.

    2.   A

        Endometrial Cancer metastasizes to inguinal lymph node primarily by direct extensions to adjacent structures.

    3.   B

Ninety percent of all endometrial cancers are adenocarcinomas.

4. A

Upto 20% of the patients havesynchronous or metastatic ovarian carcinoma.

Reference:
1. Pedro T. Ramirez, Arno J Mundt, Franco Muggia.Cancer of Uterine BodyIn: Vincent T. DeVita Jr., Theodore S. Lawrence, and Steven A. Rosenberg. Principles and Practice of Oncology.9th ed. Philadelphia. Wolters Kluwer health / Lippincott Williams and Wilkins; 2011;pp 1345.

CARCINOMA CERVIX

Dr. Vijay Kumar, Associate Professor, Department of Surgical Oncology

A 45 year old multiparous woman presented with complains of whitish discharge per vaginum since 2 months accompanied with post coital bleeding. There is no other complains. PV examinations reveal ulcerative growth on anterior lip of cervix with obliteration of left fornix. Punch Biopsy is done which reveals squamous cell carcinoma.

1. Which is most useful in staging of carcinoma Cervix?
   (A) Clinical examination
   (B) Contract Enhanced CT Abdomen
   (C) Magnetic Resonance Imaging Abdomen
   (D) Surgery
2. What is most common histology of carcinoma Cervix?
   (A) Squamous cell carcinoma
   (B) Adenocarcinoma
   (C) Transitional cell Carcinoma
   (D) Mixed
3. Which virus is most commonly associated with carcinoma Cervix?
   (A) HPV 16
   (B) HPV 18
   (C) HPV 31
   (D) HPV 33
4. What is management of patient in this case?
   (A) Surgery
   (B) Radiotherapy
   (C) Chemotherapy
   (D) Neo Adjuvant Chemotherapy followed by surgery

Answers:
1. A
   Cervical cancer is staged by the results of clinical examination.
2. A
   85% of all cervical cancers is squamous cell carcinomas.
3. A
   HPV 16 is most common virus implicated in carcinomaCervix.
4. B
   Radiotherapy as the lesion appears to be involving the left side parametrium.

References:
1. Patricia J Eifel , Jonathan S Berek and Maurie A Marksman.Cancer of Cervix, Vagina and Vulva.In: Vincent T. DeVita Jr., Theodore S. Lawrence, and Steven A. Rosenberg. Principles and Practice of Oncology.9th ed. Philadelphia. Wolters Kluwer health / Lippincott Williams and Wilkins; 2011;pp 1311

CARCINOMA VULVA

Dr. Vijay Kumar, Associate Professor, Department of Surgical Oncology

A 60 year old woman presented with a nodule on labia since 3 months which was accompanied by itching on the lesions. There was no other complaint. On local examination there was 2x1cm ulcerative proliferative growth located in left labia majora which bleeds on touch. There were no inguinal nodes. Per-abdomen examination was within normal limits. Punch biopsy of the lesion was done which was positive for malignancy.

1.Which is most common histology of carcinoma Vulva?
  (A) Squamous cell carcinoma
  (B) Adenocarcinoma
  (C) Malignant melanoma
  (D) Basal cell Carcinoma

2.Most common site for carcinoma vulva
  (A) Labia Majora
  (B) Labia Minora
  (C) Pre clitorial area
  (D) Perineum

3.Surgical dissection of Inguinal nodes is mandatory when tumor thickness is greater than
  (A) 10mm
  (B) 5mm
  (C) 2mm
  (D) 1mm

4.Most common virus associated with carcinomavulva
  (A) HPV
  (B) EBV
  (C) HIV
  (D) HSV

Answers:
  1.   A
        85% of vulvar malignancies are squamous cell carcinomas.
  2.   A
        Lesions in vulva arise from labia majora (40%) labia minora (20%), preclitorial area (15%), and perineum (15%).
  3.   D
        Groin dissection is mandatory if depth of lesion is greater than 1 mm.
  4.   A
        HPV is most commonly associated with carcinoma Vulva although the association is not as strong ascarcinomaCervix.

Reference:
  1.   Patricia J Eifel , Jonathan S Berek and Maurie A Marksman.Cancer of Cervix, Vagina and Vulva.In: Vincent T. DeVita Jr., Theodore S. Lawrence, and Steven A. Rosenberg. Principles and Practice of Oncology.9th ed. Philadelphia. Wolters Kluwer health / Lippincott Williams and Wilkins; 2011; pp 1335

EWINGS SARCOMA
Dr. Vijay Kumar, Associate Professor, Department of Surgical Oncology

A 12 years old male child, resident of Gorakhpur, presented with 20 X15 cms swelling over left lower end of femur associated with pain and difficulty in walking . On X ray of knee joint there is lytic as well sclerotic lesion with extensive soft tissue involvement.

1.Most probable diagnosis is
  (A) Osteosarcoma
  (B) Ewings sarcoma
  (C) Pleomorphic sarcoma
  (D) Osteomyelitis

2.Most common site of origin of Ewings sarcoma is
  (A) Thigh
  (B) Arm
  (C) Pelvis
  (D) Trunk

3.Most common translocation associated with Ewing's Sarcoma is
  (A) T(11:22)
  (B) T(21:22)
  (C) T(7:22)

(D) T(17:22)

4.All are small round blue cell tumor except

    (A) Ewings sarcoma

    (B) Neuroblastoma

    (C) Rhabdomyosarcoma

    (D) Wilms tumor

5.All are regimen used for management of Ewing's Sarcoma except

    (A) IE+VAC

    (B) VACD

    (C) M-VAC

    (D) VAID

Answers

    1.   B

         Most probable diagnosis is Ewings sarcoma.

    2.   A

         Most common site of origin is thigh.

    3.   A

         Translocation between chromosome 11 & 22 is most common.

    4.   D

         Wilms tumor.

    5.   C

         M-VAC is not used in treatment of ES.

Reference:

    1.   Martin M Malawer, Lee J Hellman ,BrianO'Sullivan.Sarcoma of BoneIn: Vincent T. DeVita Jr., Theodore S. Lawrence, and Steven A. Rosenberg. Principles and Practice of Oncology.9th ed. Philadelphia. Wolters Kluwer health / Lippincott Williams and Wilkins; 2011; pp1578

CARCINOID TUMOURS

Dr. Vijay Kumar, Associate Professor, Department of Surgical Oncology

60 yr old male patient presented with pain in abdomen accompanied by episodes of intermittent vomiting. Patient also describes intermittent episodes of diarrhea which are accompanied by flushing and respiratory distress. There was no history of dysphagia , weight loss, constipation.On examination,Pulse 80 per minute; blood pressure 124/80 mm of Hg

Abdomen is soft on palpation.All Blood investigations were within normal limits

1.What is most likely diagnosis?

    (A) Pheochromocytoma

    (B) Carcinoid Tumour

    (C) Celiac Disease

    (D) Small Bowel adenocarcinoma

2.What is most common site of GI Carcinoid tumor?

    (A) Rectum

    (B) Small Bowel

    (C) Stomach

    (D) Appendix

3.Which markers are used for diagnosis of carcinoid syndrome ?

    (A) Urinary VMA

    (B) Urinary Catecholamines

    (C)) Urine 5-HIAA

    (D) Urinary b-HCG

4.Which is most sensitive diagnostic test for diagnosis for detection of Carcinoid Tumour?

    (A) CECT

    (B) Barium meal follow thru

    (C) Octreotide Scan

    (D) MRI with contrast

Answers:

1. B.
   Carcinoid syndrome represents a constellation of symptoms including flushing, diarrhea and bronchospasm
2. B.
   Majority of GI Carcinoids occur in small intestine (41.8%)
3. C
   Biochemically urinary 5-HIAA have been used as tumor markers of midgut carcinoids
4. C
   Octreotide scans are diagnostic in 90% of the cases

Reference:

1. Amer H Zureikat, MattewT.Heller& Herbert J Zeh. Neuroendocrine tumors and the Carcinoid SyndromeIn: Vincent T. DeVita Jr., Theodore S. Lawrence, and Steven A. Rosenberg. Principles and Practice of Oncology.9th ed. Philadelphia. Wolters Kluwer health / Lippincott Williams and Wilkins; 2011; pp 1578.

CARCINOMA PENIS

Dr. Vijay Kumar, Associate Professor, Department of Surgical Oncology

A 50 yr old male patient, farmer by occupation resident of Unnao, presented with ulcerinvolving penis since 8 months. The ulcer was insidious in onset and gradually increasing in size and not associated with pain. On examination a 4 x 4 cm ulcero-proliferative growth involving distal shaft and glans of the penis 4 cm from the base of penis. The ulcer is irregular in shape; surface covered with necrotic material and hasfoul smelling discharge. Margins are everted. The inguinal region has sub centimeter lymphnodes palpable on both sides. They are mobile and soft in consistency. Biopsy of the lesion is done. Ultrasound scan of the bilateral inguinal and iliac region is done to evaluate regional lymph nodes and it showed sub-centimetrelymph nodes in both the inguinal region and there are no iliac lymph nodes.

1. What is the most likely diagnosis?
   (A) Balanitis xerotica obliterans
   (B) Carcinoma penis
   (C) Syphilitic ulcer
   (D) Tubercular ulcer
2. Not true about carcinoma penis
   (A) Erythroplasia ofQueret is a precancerous condition
   (B) Smoking is a etiological factor
   (C) Circumcision if done any time before puberty provides 100% protection against carcinoma penis
   (D) More than 50% pts have inguinal lymph nodes enlarged when they present
3. Cause of death in carcinoma penis
   (A) Pulmonary metastasis
   (B) Liver metastasis
   (C) Erosion of femoral vessels
   (D) Urinary obstruction
4. Circumcision is included in management of carcinoma penis present at
   (A) Glans
   (B) Prepuce
   (C) Glandulo-prepucial
   (D) Shaft of penis
5. What is true about carcinoma penis?
   (A) Metastasis is rare
   (B) Occurs more commonly in circumcised males
   (C) Pain is frequent
   (D) Grade of the tumor is important in management of the groin.

Answers:

1. B
   Carcinoma Penis.
2. C
   Circumcision that is done soon after birth in infancy offers 100% protection.
3. C
   The most common cause of death in ca penis is due to erosion of femoral vessels by lymph nodal metastasis.
4. B

Circumcision is done at prepuce.
5. D
Grade of the tumor is important in management. Depending on the grade of the tumor in early penile cancer inguinal lymph node dissection is done. In T1 high grade lesions groin alsoinguinal lymph node dissection is done.

Reference:

1. Edouard JT, Leonard GG. Cancer of Urethra and Penis.In: Vincent T. DeVita Jr., Theodore S. Lawrence, and Steven A. Rosenberg. Principles and Practice of Oncology.9th ed. Philadelphia. Wolters Kluwer health / Lippincott Williams and Wilkins; 2011; pp 1274

BASAL CELL CARCINOMA NOSE

Dr. Vijay Kumar, Associate Professor, Department of Surgical Oncology

A 60 yr old male patient, labourer by occupation, resident of Lucknow presented with ulcer over nose since 6 months. The ulcer was insidious in onset, initially of peanut size, gradually increasing and not associated with pain. He had the history of chronic exposure to sunlight due to his occupation. On examination a black colored ulcer of size 2 x 2 cms is seen on the upper part of the dorsum of the nose just below the glabella. Nearly round in shape, edges everted. No parotid or cervical lymphadenopathy was seen. Biopsy of the lesion is done.

1.What is the most likely diagnosis?
   (A) Basal cell carcinoma
   (B) Marjolin's ulcer
   (C) Soft tissue sarcoma
   (D) None of the above
2. An ulcer over the cheek skin which is pearly white with central necrosis and telangiectasia
   (A) Basal cell carcinoma
   (B) Squamous cell carcinoma
   (C) Amelanotic melanoma
   (D) Kaposis' sarcoma
3.Commonest site of rodent ulcer?
   (A) Limbs
   (B) Face
   (C) Abdomen
   (D) Trunk
4.One of the following malignancies does not spread through the lymphatics
   (A) Squamous cell carcinoma
   (B) Basal cell carcinoma
   (C) Melanoma
   (D) Kaposis' sarcoma
5.Diagnostic procedure for basal cell carcinoma
   (A) Wedge biopsy
   (B) Incisional biopsy
   (C) Shave
   (D) Punch biopsy

Answers:

1. A
   Basal cell carcinoma. Malignantmelanoma sometimes mimics basal cell carcinoma but amelanotic melanoma does not look like basal cell carcinoma.
2. A
   Basal cell carcinoma, it has central necrosis with pearly white and is telangiectatic.
3. B
   The most common site of basal cell carcinomais face.
4. B
   Basal cell carcinoma is locally aggressive and it does not spread to lymphatic.
5. A
   The diagnostic procedure of choice is wedge biopsy.

Reference:

1. Anetta R, Sumaira ZA, Lynn DW, David JL. Cancert of Skin In: Vincent T. DeVita Jr., Theodore S. Lawrence, and Steven A. Rosenberg. Principles and Practice of Oncology.9th ed. Philadelphia. Wolters Kluwer health / Lippincott Williams and Wilkins; 2011;pp 1616

PRIMARY PERITONEAL CARCINOMATOSIS

Dr. Vijay Kumar, Associate Professor, Department of Surgical Oncology

A 68 yr-old female presented to the emergency department of with complaints of shortness of breath and abdominal distension. Her past medical history was significant for Type II diabetes mellitus and hypertension. Abdominal ascites and a mild right pleural effusion were present. Ultrasound imaging (US) of the abdomen and pelvis was normal except for the known ascites. Computed tomography (CT) of the abdomen and pelvis demonstrated moderate ascites, a right pleural effusion and omental thickening. US and CT imaging failed to demonstrate any masses. Magnetic resonance imaging of the abdomen and pelvis revealed pelvic peritoneal masses suspicious for metastatic implants. Paracentesis was performed and the ascitic fluid obtained was positive for malignant cells consistent with metastatic adenocarcinoma. Immunohistochemical staining of the malignant ascitic cells was positive for CA 125, WT-1 and CK7 but negative for CK20, TTF-1. Her CA-125 was found to be 544 IU/L.

1. What is the most likely diagnosis?
   (A) Primary serous ovarian carcinoma
   (B) Primary peritoneal cyst adenocarcinoma
   (C) Mucinous carcinoma appendix
   (D) Mucinous carcinoma of ovary
2. Peritoneal Carcinomatosis may arise from tumors of which of the following structures?
   (A) The peritoneal lining
   (B) Intra-abdominal viscera
   (C) Extra abdominal organs.
   (D) All of the above.
3. Which is the most common type of cancer presenting with isolated peritoneal carcinomatosis?
   (A) Ovarian
   (B) Appendiceal
   (C) Colon
   (D) Both A & B
4. What imaging modality is best tool to detect peritoneal recurrence?
   (A) Magnetic Resonance Imaging
   (B) CT Scan
   (C) USG
   (D) Positron Emission Tomography

5. What is the most important prognostic factor associated with pseudomyxomaperitonei ?
   (A) Presence of malignancy
   (B) Amount of mucin
   (C) Abdominal distention
   (D) Abdominal pain

Answers:

1.   B
     Primary peritoneal cystadenocarcinoma is the most likely diagnosis as primary ovarian disease without any radiological diagnosis is rare.
2.   D
     Primary peritoneal carcinoma can arise from tumors of all these structures with or without concurrent systemic metastases.
3.   D
     Intra abdominal viscera, including ovary and appendix are most common source of tumors presenting with isolated peritoneal carcinomatosis.
4.   B
     MRI has been found to be superior to helical CT in assessment of bowel and mesenteric thickening.
5.   A

Presence of tumor cells in peritoneal washings obtained at time of surgical resection correlates with increased recurrence and decreased survival, even in the absence of nodal or systemic metastases.

Reference:
1. Stephen AC, David MG, Abram R. Ovarian Cancer, Fallopian Tube Carcinoma, and Peritoneal Carcinoma, In: Vincent T. DeVita Jr., Theodore S. Lawrence, and Steven A. Rosenberg. Principles and Practice of Oncology.9th ed. Philadelphia. Wolters Kluwer health / Lippincott Williams and Wilkins; 2011;pp 1389

CARCINOMA TESTIS

Dr. Vijay Kumar, Associate Professor, Department of Surgical Oncology

A 22 year old male patient presents in OPD with c/o testicular lump since 20 days which he incidentally noticed during self-examination. It is painless, not associated with fever or any significant past history of trauma. On examination, his left testis is enlarged, non-tender and hard. Spermatic cord and rest of the clinical examination were normal. HRUSG scrotum was suggestive of a hypo echoic intra-testicular mass. Contrast enhanced CT abdomen corroborated USG findings along with presence of multiple retroperitoneal lymph nodes. Blood examination revealed significantly raised levels of levels of serum B-HCG and LDH but normal levels of AFP.

1. What is the most likely diagnosis?
   (A) Testicular tumor
   (B) Hematocele
   (C) Hydrocele
   (D) Epididymo-orchitis
2. Which germ cell tumor is associated with widespread haematogenous metastasis and high levels of HCG?
   (A) Pure chorio-carcinoma
   (B) Yolk sac tumor
   (C) Embryonal carcinoma
   (D) Seminoma
3. Which IHC markers are commonly expressed in patients with seminoma?
   (A) CD 117
   (B) Placental alkaline phosphatase
   (C) None of the above
   (D) A & B
4. Which of the following characterizes a pathological stage T3 testicular GCT?
   (A) Invasion of tunica vaginalis
   (B) Invasion of tunica albuginea
   (C) Invasion of spermatic cord
   (D) None of the above
5. Which of the following defines seminoma with poor prognosis?
   (A) Mediastinal primary site
   (B) Brain metastasis
   (C) A & B
   (D) None of the above.

Answers:
1. A
   Testicular mass in young adult with characteristic raised markers is highly suggestive of Testicular GCT.
2. A
   Metastases from testicular cancer usually follow the lymphatic drainage, reaching retroperitoneal nodes in a predictable way. This is the case for seminoma and most non seminomas except pure chorio-carcinoma, which are associated with haematogenous metastases.
3. D
   Virtually all seminoma express CD 117 (c-kit) and Placental alkaline phosphatase
4. C
   According to 7[th]ed AJCC, T3 is defined as invasion of spermatic cord.
5. D
   Poor risk category is not applicable in Seminoma.

Reference:
1. George JB, Darren RF, Dean FB, Joel S, Robert JM, Victor ER, Marisa AK, Raju SKC.Cancer of Testes. In: Vincent T. DeVita Jr., Theodore S. Lawrence, and Steven A. Rosenberg. Principles and Practice of Oncology.9th ed. Philadelphia. Wolters Kluwer health / Lippincott Williams and Wilkins; 2011;pp 1280-98

HEPATOCELLULAR CARCINOMA
Dr. Vijay Kumar, Associate Professor, Department of Surgical Oncology

A 70 year old male presents in OPD with complains of lump in right upper abdomen associated with loss of appetite and dull aching pain since 2 months. There is no history of jaundice or fever .Clinical examination is suggestive of hepatomegaly which is hard and non tender. Blood examination revealed abnormal liver function and an elevated serum AFP > 1000 IU/L. USG abdomen suggested a 4 cm hypo echoic lesion in left hepatic lobe, and a Contrast enhanced CT Scan revealed no evidence of metastatic disease.

1. What is the most likely diagnosis?
   (A) Hepatocellular carcinoma
   (B) Focal nodular hyperplasia
   (C) Hydatid cyst of liver
   (D) Hemangioma of liver
2. All of these are risk factors for development of Hepatocellular Carcinoma except
   (A) Wilson disease
   (B) Hemochromatosis
   (C) Alpha 1- antitrypsin deficiency
   (D) Primary biliary cirrhosis
3. Which biochemical abnormality is both a paraneoplastic syndrome associated with Hepatocellular Carcinoma, and may also be caused by end stage liver failure?
   (A) Hypoglycaemia
   (B) Erythrocytosis
   (C) Hypercalcemia
   (D) Hypercholesterolemia
4. Which of the following statements regarding fibro-lamellar Hepatocellular Carcinoma is incorrect?
   (A) It occurs in equal frequency in male and females
   (B) Uncommonly associated with prior cirrhosis
   (C) Commonly presents with lymph node metastasis
   (D) Most patients are diagnosed in third decade of life
5. Which one of these is not included in Milan Criteria for selection of patients appropriate for liver transplantation?
   (A) Solitary tumor less than or equal to 5 cm
   (B) Multifocal disease with less than or equal to 3 tumors
   (C) Child Pugh B & C
   (D) Child Pugh A

Answers:
1. A
   Hepatocellular carcinoma is the most common primary liver tumor in elderly males.
2. D
   Primary biliary cirrhosis is associated with an increased risk of cholangio- carcinoma.
3. A
   Hypoglycemia may be seen in Hepatocellular Carcinoma due to both.
4. D
   Presence of arterial hypervascularity, rapid enhancement during arterial phase of contrast and wash out during the later portal venous and delayed phase are characteristic finding in four phase CT scan.
5. D
   All others are included in Milan Criteria

Reference:
1. David LB, Adrian MD, Laura AD. Cancer of Liver.In: Vincent T. DeVita Jr., Theodore S. Lawrence, and Steven A. Rosenberg. Principles and Practice of Oncology.9th ed. Philadelphia. Wolters Kluwer health / Lippincott Williams and Wilkins; 2011; pp 997-1008

NON HODGKIN'S LYMPHOMA

Dr. Vijay Kumar, Associate Professor, Department of Surgical Oncology

A 56 years old male, farmer, presented with fever of unknown origin for 2 months, bilateral multiple neck swelling and loss of weight and appetite. On examination bilateral multiple non matted neck node, right axillary lymph node enlargement and hepato-spleenomegaly present.

1. What is the most probable diagnosis of this patient?
    (A) Tuberculosis
    (B) Kala azar
    (C) Non Hodgkin's Lymphoma
    (D) Hodgkin's lymphoma
2. Most common variant of NHL is
    (A) Mantle cell
    (B) Diffuse Large B-cell Lymphoma(DLBCL)
    (C) Follicular
    (D) T-cell
3. All are EBV associated lympho-proliferative disorder except
    (A) Burkitt's Lymphoma
    (B) Mantle cell
    (C) Post transplant lympho-proliferative disorder
    (D) HIV associated lympho-proliferative disorder
4. All are used for staging of NHL except
    (A) CT/Magnetic Resonance Imaging
    (B) Bone marrow ex.
    (C) Serum LDH
    (D) Positron Emission Tomography Scan
5. All regimen used in management of NHL except
    (A) ABVD
    (B) CHOP
    (C) R-CHOP
    (D) ACVBP

Answers:
1. C
    Most probable diagnosis is NHL.
2. B
    Most common NHL variant is DLBCL.
3. B
    Mantle cell lymphoma not associated with EBV.
4. D
    PET scan is not recommended for NHL staging.
5. A
    ABVD used in Hodgkin's lymphoma.

Reference:
1. Jonathan WF, Peter MM, Lisa R, Richard IF. In: Vincent T. DeVita Jr., Theodore S. Lawrence, and Steven A. Rosenberg. Principles and Practice of Oncology.9th ed. Philadelphia. Wolters Kluwer health / Lippincott Williams and Wilkins; 2011; pp 1869

CARCINOMA ESOPHAGUS

Dr. Vijay Kumar, Associate Professor, Department of Surgical Oncology

A 55 yrs female presented with c/o of dysphagia initially to solids and now to liquids since 3 months a/w with loss of appetite and loss of weight.On examination patient is dehydrated and cachexic.UGIE was done showing ulceroproliferative lesion at 30 cm from incisors with biopsy showing Sq cell scan.CT SCAN was done showing lesion starting just below carina for 7cm in length with GE junction free without lymphadenopathy and with no evidence of metastatic disease.

1.All are the risk factors for development of scc of esophagus except

(A) Plummer-vinson syndrome
(B) Gastroesophageal reflux disease
(C) Achalasia
(D) Tylosis

2.Most common site of scc in esophagus is
(A) Upper 1/3rd
(B) Middle 1/3rd
(C) Lower 1/3rd
(D) GE junction

3. Definitive investigation of choice for diagnosis of carcinoma esophagus is
(A) CECT thorax
(B) UGIE endoscopy and biopsy
(C) Barium swallow
(D) PET scan

4.Metastatic disease in carcinoma esophagus include all except
(A) Pleural effusion
(B) Pericardium involvement
(C) Ascites
(D) Supraclavicular lymphnode

5.Toc in scc of middle 1/3rd esophagus
(A) Surgery
(B) Definitive chemoradiation
(C) A and B
(D) Chemotherapy

Answers:

1. B
   GE reflux is associated with adenocarcinoma of lower 1/3 rd of esophagus.
2. B
   Middle 1/3rd is the mc site of scc 50% ,while adenocarcinoma is more common in lower 1/3rd esophagus.
3. B
   Upper gi endoscopy and biopsy is the definitive investigation of choice.
4. B
   Pericardium involvement is T4a locally advanced but resectable.
5. C
   Surgery and definitive ctrt are both the treatment options recommended for middle 1/3rd scc esophagus.

Reference:

1. Mitchell C.Posner, Bruce D. Minsky, and David H. Ilson. Cancer of the Esophagus. In: Vincent T. DeVita Jr., Theodore S. Lawrence, and Steven A. Rosenberg. Principles and Practice of Oncology.9th ed. Philadelphia. Wolters Kluwer health / Lippincott Williams and Wilkins; 2011; pp 887-923

CARCINOMA STOMACH

Dr. Vijay Kumar, Associate Professor, Department of Surgical Oncology

A 45 yrs old male patient presented with c/o sensation of fullness after meals and intermittent vomitings for the last 5 months.He has complaint of loss of appetite and loss of weight with occasional h/o melena.On physical examination pt is dehydrated without evidence of supraclavicular lymphadenopathy.On local examination of abdomen there is visible peristalsis in upper abdomen from left to right hypochondrium.A firm globular intraabdominal lump is palpable in epigastrium ,irregular surface with well defined margins, moving cephalo caudally with respiration.No others lump was felt with no evidence of free fluid in the abdomen.

1.What is the probable diagnosis?
(A) Acute peptic ulcer with edema
(B) GOO from peptic stricture
(C) External compression from ca head of pancreas
(D) GOO due to carcinoma stomach

2. Clinical features of carcinoma stomach include
(A) Melena

(B) Satiety

(C) Vommiting

(D) Diarrhea

3. MC metabolic abnormality in carcinoma stomach with GOO

(A) Metabolic alkalosis

(B) Hyperchloremic metabolic acidosis

(C) Respiratory alkalosis

(D) Hypochloremic hypokalemic metabolic alkalosis with paradoxical aciduria

4. Workup of carcinoma stomach include a/e

(A) CECT whole abdomen

(B) UGIE and biopsy

(C) Chest x-ray

(D) Urease breath test

5. TOC for non metastatic carcinoma stomach include

(A) Surgery

(B) Chemotherapy

(C) Radiotherapy

(D) Surgery with perioperative chemotherapy

Answers:

1. D

Mass in epigasrium with features of goo with fullness and vomitings and mass moving cephalo caudally is carcinoma stomach.

2. D

Diarrhoea is not a feature of ca stomach and satiety in carcinoma stomach is due to linitis plastic.

3. D

Vomittings due to GOO causes loss of h+,cl-and k+ which causes hypochloremic hypokalemic met alkalosis and if vomittings increase body conserves na+ by excreting h+in urine which leads to paradoxical aciduria.

4. D

Urease breath test is done to detect peptic ulcer disease due to h pylori.

5. D

Perioperative chemotherapy with surgery is toc in non metastatic carcinoma stomach.

Reference:

1. Itzhak Avital, Peter W. T. Pisters, David P. Kelsen, and Christofer G. Willett. Cancer of the Stomach. In: Vincent T. DeVita Jr., Theodore S. Lawrence, and Steven A. Rosenberg. Principles and Practice of Oncology.9th ed. Philadelphia. Wolters Kluwer health / Lippincott Williams and Wilkins; 2011;pp 924-54

BRONCHOGENIC CARCINOMA

Dr. Vijay Kumar, Associate Professor, Department of Surgical Oncology

A 55 yr old man with a 30 pack-year history of smoking,presents to the opd with shortness of breath.Chest radiograph demonstrates a right upper lobe opacity. CECT reveals a 3.5cm spiculated mass in the peripheral right upper lobe without any hilar and mediastinal lymphadenopathy. USG abdomen was done and was normal.

1. What is the probable diagnosis?

(A) Carcinoma lung

(B) Hamartoma

(C) Lung mets

(D) Fibrosis due to tuberculosis

2. What is the next best step in management?

(A) Bronchoscopy and biopsy of the mass

(B) CT guided biopsy of the mass

(C) Brain MRI

(D) Refer to thoracic surgeon for resection

3. Pancoast syndrome includes all except

(A) Shoulder and arm pain

(B) Horner syndrome

(C) Weakness or atrophy of the hand muscles

(D) Upper limb edema

4. Workup of NSCLC(non small cell lung carcinoma) include all except
   (A) CT thorax and upper abdomen
   (B) Bone marrow biopsy
   (C) Mediastinoscopy
   (D) Pulmonary assessment(fev1,dlco,vo2max)
5 Treatment options in NSCLC of lung include
   (A) Surgery
   (B) Radiotherapy
   (C) CT RT followed by surgery
   (D) All of the above

Answers:

1. A
   H/O smoking with large large single peripheral sol is ca lung ,lungmets are also peripherall located but multiple and non spiculated.
2. B
   As lesion is peripherally located , CT guided biopsy is the modality of choice.
3. D
   Rt apical lobe lesion causes pancoast tumor and symptoms are due to compression of sympathetic chain and brachial plexus and not axillary vessels.
4. B
   Bone marrow biopsy,bone scan and mri brain are done in small cell carcinoma of lung not in nsclc.
5. D
   Surgery for early stage disease,radiotherapy for early lesion with poor performance status and chemoradiotherapy followed by surgery in few stage 3A lesions.

Reference:

1. David S. Schrump, Darryl Carter, Christofer R. Kelsey, Lawrence B. Marks, and Giuseppe Giaccone. Non- Small Cell Lung Carcinoma In: Vincent T. DeVita Jr., Theodore S. Lawrence, and Steven A. Rosenberg. Principles and Practice of Oncology.9th ed. Philadelphia. Wolters Kluwer health / Lippincott Williams and Wilkins; 2011; pp 79

CARCINOMA OVARY

Dr. Vijay Kumar, Associate Professor, Department of Surgical Oncology

A 50yrs old postmenopausal women with 2 children is c/o vague abdominal symptoms followed by distension of abdomen since the last 4 months.On local examination of the abdomen there is free fluid in the abdomen and palpable intra-abdominal lump in the lower abdomen freely mobile side to side.CXR was done which was wnl and CECT whole abdomen was done showing b/l adnexal masses with omental deposits with free fluid in abdomen.

1. What is the probable diagnosis?
   (A) Carcinoma ovary
   (B) Krukenbergstumour
   (C) Simple ovarian cysts
   (D) Uterine sarcoma
2. Serum markers that can be elevated in carcinoma ovary
   (A) CA-125
   (B) CA 19-9
   (C) Activin -A
   (D) All of the above
3. Risk factor for developing ovarian cancer include
   (A) Usage of ocp pills for >5yrs
   (B) Nulliparity
   (C) Breast feeding
   (D) Tubal ligation
4. Ascites and omental deposits in carcinoma ovary is
   (A) Stage 1
   (B) Stage 2
   (C) Stage 3

(D) Stage 4
5. Treatment options in carcinoma ovary
   (A) NACT followed by surgery
   (B) Surgery followed by adjuvant chemotherapy
   (C) Surgery
   (D) All of the above

Answers:
1. A
   Krukenbergs tumors occur in premenopausal women, b/l adnexal masses with ascites is carcinoma ovary.
2. D
   CA 125 is commonly used serum tumor marker in carcinoma ovary but ca 19-9 and ca 15-3 are elevated in mucinous carcinoma of ovary.
3. B
   OCP pills,multiparity .breast feeding decrease ovulation so reduce risk of ca ovary. Fewstudies have shown tubal ligation also decreases the risk.
4. C
   Ascites and omental deposits in GI malignancies is stage 4 (metastatic) but in carcinoma ovary it is stage 3.
5. D
   Early stage disease surgery is the option and in advanced disease NACT(neo adjuvant chemotherapy) followed by surgery followed by adjuvant treatment is the option.

Reference:
1. Stephen A. Cannistra, David M. Gershenson, Abram Recht. Ovarian cancer, Fallopian Tube Carcinoma, and Peritoneal Carcinoma In: Vincent T. DeVita Jr., Theodore S. Lawrence, and Steven A. Rosenberg. Principles and Practice of Oncology.9th ed. Philadelphia. Wolters Kluwer health / Lippincott Williams and Wilkins; 2011; pp 1368-1391

OSTEOSARCOMA
Dr. Vijay Kumar, Associate Professor, Department of Surgical Oncology

A 17 years old male, presented with gradually progressive swelling over lower end of thigh after fall from cycle four months back associated with pain which worsens at night. On physical examination , a 20x15 cm swelling is present over left lower thigh which is hard, tender and multiple tortuous veins arecpresent over it. X-ray of knee joint shows new bone formation.

1.What is the most probable diagnosis?
   (A) Ewing's Sarcoma
   (B) Osteosarcoma
   (C) Chondrosarcoma
   (D) Osteoclastoma
2.All are the radiological features of osteosarcoma except
   (A) Sun-ray appearance
   (B) Codman's triangle
   (C) Periosteal reaction
   (D) Soap bubble appearance
3.Investigation not required for diagnosis
   (A) MRI femur
   (B) Bone marrow examination
   (C) CT chest
   (D) Bone scan
4.Which variant of osteosarcoma has best prognosis?
   (A) Classical
   (B) Periosteal
   (C) Parosteal
   (D) Paget's sarcoma
5.All are contraindication of limb sparing surgery except
   (A) Major neurovascular involvement
   (B) Pathological fracture

(C) Inappropriate biopsy site

(D) Adjacent joint involvement

Answers:

1. B

Most probable diagnosis is osteosarcoma.

2. D

Soap bubble appearance is not seen in osteosarcoma.

3. B

Bone marrow examination is not required for diagnosis of OS.

4. C

Parosteal variant has best prognosis.

5. D

Adjacent bone involvement is not a contraindication of limb sparing surgery.

Reference:

1. Martin A. Malawer, Lee J. Helman, and Brian O' Sullivan. Sarcomas of Bone. In: Vincent T. DeVita Jr., Theodore S. Lawrence, and Steven A. Rosenberg. Principles and Practice of Oncology.9th ed. Philadelphia. Wolters Kluwer health / Lippincott Williams and Wilkins; 2011;pp 1578-1609.

GASTRO INTESTINAL STROMAL TUMOUR

Dr. Vijay Kumar, Associate Professor, Department of Surgical Oncology

A 23 years old housewife presented with generalized weakness, severe anaemia, pedal edema, loss of appetite and melena. In USG abdomen there is outward growth involving lesser curvature of stomach near pylorus and on endoscopic biopsy both spindle cell &epithelioid cells are present.

1.What is the most probable diagnosis of this patient?

(A) Stomach cancer

(B) Gastro Intestinal Stromal Tumour(GIST)

(C) Lymphoma

(D) Amyloidosis

2.Which is the cell of origin of GIST?

(A) Interstitial cell of Cajal

(B) Argyrophillic cell

(C) Kulchitsky cell

(D) Totipotent cell

3.Hallmark Immunohistochemistry for GIST is

(A) KIT(CD117)

(B) KIT+DOG 1

(C) NF related GIST

(D) SDH deficient GIST

4.Treatment of choice of localized GIST of stomach is

(A) Surgery

(B) Imatinib

(C) Radiotherapy

(D) Sunitinib

5.All agent are used in GIST except

(A) Imatinib

(B) Sunitinib

(C) Pazopinib

(D) Regorafinib

Answers:

1. B

Most probable diagnosis is Gatrointestinal stromal tumor.

2. A

Interstitial cell of Cajal are cells of origin of GIST,which are pacemakers of gastrointestinal motility.

3. B

KIT(CD117)+DOG 1 are hallmark IHC for diagnosis of GIST.

4. A

Surgery is the treatment of choice for localized disease.

5. C

Pazopanib is not used in the treatment of GIST.

Reference:

1. Paolo G.Casali,Angelo Paolo Dei Tos, and Alessandro Gronchi. Gastrointestinal Stromal Tumor. In: Vincent T. DeVita Jr., Theodore S. Lawrence, and Steven A. Rosenberg. Principles and Practice of Oncology.9th ed. Philadelphia. Wolters Kluwer health / Lippincott Williams and Wilkins; 2011;pp 745-56.

CARCINOMA LARYNX

Dr. Vijay Kumar, Associate Professor, Dr. Naseem Akhtar, Assistant Professor Department of Surgical Oncology

A 60 years male patient presented with hoarseness of voice for two months and a small swelling in left side neck for one month. Patient had history of bidi smoking for 30 years. He did not have other complaints like cough, dyspnea or haemoptysis. On examination, a 2x1.5 cm mobile, hard lymph node at left level II was found.

1.What is the most likely diagnosis?

(A) Carcinoma larynx

(B) Carcinoma lung

(C) Carcinoma tongue

(D) Carcinoma esophagus

2.What investigation would your perform to confirm the diagnosis?

(A) Upper Gastro Intestinal Endoscopy

(B) Video-laryngoscopy and biopsy

(C) X Ray Neck

(D) Orthopantomogram

3.Most common site of carcinoma larynx is ?

(A) Supra glottis

(B) Glottis

(C) Sub-glottis

(D) None of the above

4.Glottis cancers involving both vocal cords but cords are mobile. What is the stage of disease

(A) T1a

(B) T1b

(C) T2

(D) T3

5.Supraglottic cancer limited to larynx with vocal cord fixation without thyroid cartilage invasion is

(A) T1

(B) T2

(C) T3

(D) T4a

Answers:

1. A

In a 60 years male chronic smoker and history of hoarseness of voice with neck nodes probable diagnosis is carcinoma larynx.

2. B

Videolaryngoscopy and biopsy confirm the diagnosis and mucosal extent of the disease.

3. B

Most common site of carcinoma larynx is glottis. Supraglottic cancers are 2nd most common laryngeal cancers.

4. B

Tumor invading both vocal cords but in mobile cords disease is termed as T1b.

5. C

In a case of supraglottic cancer, tumour limited to larynx with cord fixation is included in T3 in TNM staging.

References:

1. Lee SP, John MAS, Wong SG, Casciato DA. Head and neck cancers. In: Casciato DA, Territo MC (Eds). Manual of clinical oncology.7th edition WolterKluwer (India) 2012, pp 170-04.
2. Mendenhall WM, Werning JW, PfisteDG.Treatment of head and neck cancerIn: Vincent T. DeVita Jr., Theodore S. Lawrence, and Steven A. Rosenberg. Principles and Practice of Oncology.9th ed. Philadelphia. Wolters Kluwer health / Lippincott Williams and Wilkins; 2011; pp 729-88.

CARCINOMA LIP

Dr. Vijay Kumar, Associate Professor,Dr. Naseem Akhtar, Assistant Professor Department of Surgical Oncology

A 45 years female patient presented with history of a painless ulcer over midline lower lip for 3 months. There was no history of bleeding from ulcer. Patient was addicted for tobacco chewing for 15 years. On examination, 3x2 cm ulcero-proliferative growth over midline lower lip and lower gingiva labial sulcus was not involved. Neck examination revealed a 1x1 cm hard palpable, mobile lymph node at level IA. Other findings were unremarkable.

1. The most likely diagnosis is :
    (A) Carcinoma tongue
    (B) Carcinoma skin
    (C) Carcinoma lip
    (D) Apthous ulcer
2. What investigation would be needed to confirm the diagnosis ?
    (A) CT scan
    (B) Orthopantomogram
    (C) Punch biopsy
    (D) Magnetic Resonance Imaging
3. Most common site of carcinoma on lip is ?
    (A) Upper lip
    (B) Lower lip
    (C) Commissure
    (D) None of the above
4. Which one of the following is not correct regarding T4a in oral cavity according to AJCC 2010 TNM staging?
    (A) Invasion through cortical bone
    (B) Skin infiltration
    (C) Maxillary sinus invasion
    (D) Carotid artery invasion
5. Which one of the following is not correct regarding T4b in oral cavity according to AJCC 2010TNM staging?
    (A) Invasion into masticator space
    (B) Pterygoid plate infiltration
    (C) Skull base infiltration
    (D) Invasion into floor of mouth

Answers:

1. C
    Painless progressive increasing in size ulceroproliferative growth over lower lip in a middle aged woman is likely carcinoma lip.
2. C
    Punch or incisional biopsy will be required for histopathological examination, which will confirm the diagnosis.
3. B
    Lower lip constitutes 90% of all cancers on lip, while remaining occurs on upper lip.
4. D
    According to 7th edition of AJCC TNM staging for oral cavity, carotid artery invasion is considered in T4b (very advanced).

5. D

   Invasion into floor of mouth is not included in T4b according to 7th edition of AJCC TNM staging for oral cavity.

References:

1. Lee SP, John MAS, Wong SG, Casciato DA. Head and neck cancers. In: Casciato DA, Territo MC (Eds). Manual of clinical oncology. 7th edition Wolter Kluwer (India) 2012, pp 170-204.
2. Mendenhall WM, Werning JW, PfisteDG.Treatment of head and neck cancer. In: Vincent T. DeVita Jr., Theodore S. Lawrence, and Steven A. Rosenberg. Principles and Practice of Oncology.9th ed. Philadelphia. Wolters Kluwer health / Lippincott Williams and Wilkins; 2011; pp 729-88.

CARCINOMA TONGUE

Dr. Vijay Kumar, Associate Professor, Dr. Naseem Akhtar, Assistant Professor
Department of Surgical Oncology

A 60 years female patient presented with ulcer over right lateral border tongue for 3 months associated with difficulty in eating. She had history of tobacco chewing for 18 years. On examination, revealed an ulceroproliferative growth 3.5x2 cm on right lateral border tongue, involving floor of mouth and ankyloglossia. The lesion was not crossing midline and base of tongue was not involved on palpation.

1.What is the most probable diagnosis?
   (A) Apthous ulcer
   (B) Carcinoma tongue
   (C) Carcinoma buccal mucosa
   (D) Lingual thyroid
2.What is the probable stage of this patient?
   (A) T1
   (B) T2
   (C) T3
   (D) T4a
3.Early carcinoma of tongue can be treated by
   (A) Surgery only
   (B) Radiotherapy only
   (C) Both of above
   (D) Chemotherapy only
4.Carcinoma of base of tongue, treatment of choice is
   (A) Surgery
   (B) Chemotherapy
   (C) Radiotherapy
   (D) Laser therapy
5.Carcinoma of tongue mainly spread through
   (A) Haematogenous
   (B) Lymphatics
   (C) None of the above
   (D) Peritoneal

Answers:

1. B

   In an elderly female patient ulcerative growth over tongue progressive increasing in size with addiction of tobacco chewing indicates towards the carcinoma tongue.

2. D

   Ankyloglossia occurs due to tumor invasion into deep extrinsic muscles of tongue, which is included in T4a in TNM staging.

3. C

   Early carcinoma of tongue can be treated with either surgery or radiotherapy both.

4. C

   Base of tongue cancer included in the oropharynx and oropharyngeal cancers are treated primarily by radiotherapy.

5. B

Oral cavity cancers primarily spread through lymphatics to the neck nodes.

References:
1. Lee SP, John MAS, Wong SG, Casciato DA. Head and neck cancers. In: Casciato DA, Territo MC (Eds). Manual of clinical oncology. 7th edition Wolter Kluwer (India) 2012, pp 170-204.
2. Mendenhall WM, Werning JW, PfisteDG.Treatment of head and neck cancer. In: Vincent T. DeVita Jr., Theodore S. Lawrence, and Steven A. Rosenberg. Principles and Practice of Oncology.9th ed. Philadelphia. Wolters Kluwer health / Lippincott Williams and Wilkins; 2011; pp 729-88.

CARCINOMA THYROID

Dr. Vijay Kumar, Associate Professor, Department of Surgical Oncology

A 50 years female patient presented with a swelling in the front and sides of the neck for last 6 months. It was increasing in size over this span. She complains dull aching pain over the swelling for 15 days. She also complains of slight hoarseness of voice for one month. On examination, 6x5 cm swelling is present on right side probably right lobe of thyroid, which moves on deglutition. Serum TSH was normal. Right vocal cord was not moving on indirect laryngoscopy.

1.What is the most likely diagnosis ?
   (A) Carcinoma larynx
   (B) Carcinoma parotid
   (C) Carcinoma thyroid
   (D) Carcinoma submandibular gland

2.Most common form of differentiated thyroid carcinoma is
   (A) Papillary carcinoma
   (B) Follicular carcinoma
   (C) Medullary carcinoma
   (D) Anaplastic carcinoma

3.Tubercle ofZukerkendle is in relation to
   (A) Adrenal gland
   (B) Thyroid gland
   (C) Parotid gland
   (D) Submandibular gland

4.Retrosternal goiter true is
   (A) Extends into posterior mediastinum
   (B) Anterior to subclavian and innominate vein in the anterior mediastinum
   (C) Almost always needs sternotomy
   (D) None of the above

5.Sistrunk's operation is done
   (A) Bronchial cyst
   (B) Thyroglossal cyst
   (C) Sebacous cyst
   (D) None of the above

Answers:
1. C
   Female patient with swelling in anterior neck for 6 months and gradually progressive and examination finding revealed mobility of swelling with deglutition and right vocal cord fixed indicates towards carcinoma thyroid as probable diagnosis.
2. A
   Papillary carcinoma thyroid is most common form of differentiated thyroid cancer.
3. B
   Tubercle of Zuekerkendle is in related to thyroid gland.
4. B
   Retro sternalgoiter lies anterior to subclavian and innominate vein in the anterior mediastinum and seldom requires sternotomy for excision.
5. B
   Sistrunk's operation is performed for thyroglossal cyst excision.

References:

1   Carlson HE. Endocrine neoplasms. In: Cas.ciato DA, Territo MC (Eds). Manual of clinical oncology.7th edition Wolter Kluwer (India) 2012, pp 408-32.
2.   Carling T, Udelsman R. Thyroid tumors. In: Devia, Hellman, and Rosenberg (Eds). Cancer Principles and practice of oncology 9th edition Lippincott Williams &wilkins USA 2011, pp 1457-72.

CARCINOMA URINARY BLADDER

Dr. Vijay Kumar, Associate Professor, Department of Surgical Oncology

A 50 years male patient working in rubber factory for 30 years presented with haematuria for one month. Patient had no history of pain, burning micturition, fever or chills etc. Clinical examination was unremarkable. Urine examination for cytology revealed malignant cells. Cystoscopy showed a large ulcerated growth arising from right lateral and posterior wall of bladder.

1.   Most likely diagnosis of this patient is
     (A) carcinoma kidney
     (B) carcinoma urinary bladder
     (C) carcinoma prostate
     (D) carcinoma of testis
2.   Schistosomiumhaematobium infection of the bladder is associated with which type of bladder cancer in (A) endemic regions
     (A) Transitional cell carcinoma
     (B) Adenocarcinoma
     (C) Squamous cell carcinoma
     (D) None of the above
3.   Which statement is correct?
     (A) Low grade superficial carcinoma have better prognosis than CIS
     (B) CIS in not multifocal
     (C) It does not spread by lymphatics
     (D) Sessile cancers are often low grade
4.Most common presenting feature of carcinoma of urinary bladder
     (A) Burning Micturition
     (B) Haematuria
     (C) Pain
     (D) Edema Of Lower Extremities
5. Tumor invasion into prostatic stroma in carcinoma of urinary bladder is
     (A) T2
     (B) T3
     (C) T4a
     (D) T4b

Answers:

1.   B
     An elderly male patient having haematuria and chronic exposure of rubber industry, along with urinary cytology positive for malignant cells is a classical example of transitional cell carcinoma urinary bladder.
2.   C
     Schistosomiumhaematobium infection of the bladder is associated with squamous cell carcinoma.
3.   A
     Low grade superficial carcinoma of bladder have better prognosis than CIS. CIS is usually multifocal.
4.   B
     Most common presenting feature of carcinoma of urinary bladder is haematuria.
5.   C
     Tumor invasion into prostatic stroma, seminal vesicle uterus or vagina is included in T4a according to 7th AJCC TNM staging system.

References:

1.   Pal SK, Kim HL, Figlin RA. Urinary tract cancers. In: Casciato DA, Territo MC (Eds). Manual of clinical oncology 7th edition Wolter Kluwer (India) 2012, pp 365-94.

2. McDoughal WS, Shipley WU, Kaufman DS, Dahl DM, Michaelson MD, Zietman AL. Cancer of the bladder, ureter and renal pelvisIn: Vincent T. DeVita Jr., Theodore S. Lawrence, and Steven A. Rosenberg. Principles and Practice of Oncology.9th ed. Philadelphia. Wolters Kluwer health / Lippincott Williams and Wilkins; 2011; pp 1192-1211.

RENAL CELL CARCINOMA

Dr. Vijay Kumar, Associate Professor, Department of Surgical Oncology

A 55 years male, chronic smoker, shopkeeper, presented with hematuria, left flank pain and left testicular swelling for two and half months. On physical examination there is 10 x 8 cms lump present in left lumbar region with varicocele of left testis.

1.What is the most probable diagnosis of this patient ?
  (A) Retroperitoneal sarcoma
  (B) Renal cell carcinoma
  (C) Prostate cancer
  (D) Left Testicular carcinoma
2.All are paraneoplastic syndromes associated with RCC except
  (A) Polycythemia
  (B) Hypertension
  (C) Stauffer syndrome
  (D) Hypocalcemia
3.All are hereditary syndrome associated with RCC except
  (A) Li-Fraumani syndrome
  (B) Von Hippel Lindau
  (C) HPRC
  (D) Birt-Hogg –Dube
4.Targeted therapy used in metastatic RCC except
  (A) Pazopanib
  (B) Bevacizumab
  (C) Trastuzumab
  (D) Sunitinib
5.Which is not a variant of RCC ?
  (A) Clear cell
  (B) Papillary
  (C) Small cell
  (D) Chromophobe

Answers:

  1. B
      Most probable diagnosis in this elderly patient with hematuria, lump in left lumber region and varicocele is renal cell carcinoma
  2. D
      Hypercalcaemia is seen in renal cell carcinoma not hypocalcaemia.
  3. A
      Li Fraumani syndrome is not associated with renal cell carcinoma. Rest of the all mentioned in options are associated with renal cell carcinoma.
  4. C
      Trastuzumab is not used in the management of renal cell carcinoma
  5. C
      Small cell is not a variant of renal cell carcinoma.

Reference:

  1. Marston Linehan W, Rini BI, Yang JC. Cancer of the kidneyIn: Vincent T. DeVita Jr., Theodore S. Lawrence, and Steven A. Rosenberg. Principles and Practice of Oncology.9th ed. Philadelphia. Wolters Kluwer health / Lippincott Williams and Wilkins; 2011; pp 1161-82.

Chapter-30

Transfusion Medicine

DELAYED HEMOLYTIC TRANSFUSION REACTION

Dr. Tulika Chandra, Professor & Head, Department of Transfusion Medicine

A 40 year old man was admitted to hospital with GIT bleeding. Patient gave a history of recurrent epigastric pain with vomiting and a previous episode of gastric bleeding 5 months back. He was a diagnosed case of peptic ulcer. Hemoglobin on admission was 7.0 gm%. He was transfused 4 units of PRBC's after compatibility testing. Four days post transfusion patient developed mild jaundice and low grade fever. CBC showed haemoglobin of 6gm% and a low hematocrit. PBS showed spherocytes. Two more PRBC's were ordered for transfusion but they were found to be incompatible. Antibody screen was positive. Pretransfusion DAT result was negative. Repeat crossmatch tests with pre and post transfusion patients specimens with donor units revealed no incompatibility

1. The first mode of action in relation to transfusion which should be done should be
   (A) Check for clerical errors in blood transfusion chain
   (B) Review the diagnosis of the patient
   (C) Repeat haemoglobin and CBC
   (D) Assess the fluids transfused

2. In a transfusion reaction what is expected in this case
   (A) Pretransfusion DAT result negative and post transfusion DAT result negative
   (B) Pretransfusion DAT result positive and post transfusion DAT result negative
   (C) Pretransfusion DAT result negative and post transfusion DAT result positive
   (D) Pretransfusion DAT result positive and post transfusion DAT result positive

3. If patients and donor unit blood culture was negative are there chances that patients serum and eluate will reveal antibody
   (A) Yes
   (B) No
   (C) Antigen will be present
   (D) None of the above

4. What type of transfusion reaction has occurred in the above patient
   (A) Transfusion associated graft versus host diseases
   (B) Delayed non haemolytic transfusion reaction
   (C) Transfusion related acute lung injury
   (D) Delayed haemolytic transfusion reaction

5. The antibody type expected to be present is
   (A) IgM
   (B) IgG
   (C) IgD
   (D) IgA

Answers :

1. A
   First step in case for transfusion reaction is to check for clerical errors which is one of the most commonest cause for a reaction
2. C
   Post transfusion DAT result positive due to IgG sensitization
3. A
   Patients serum and eluate will reveal antibody as it will cause Hemolytic reaction which is depicted by above clinical picture
4. D
   Delayed haemolytic transfusion reaction
5. B
   IgG as it develops due to sensitization

References:

1. Salama. A and Mueller Eckhardt,C : Delayed haemolytic transfusion reactions. Transfusion 24-188.1984
2. Denise M Harmening : Modern Blood Banking and Transfusion Practices. Fifth Edition

FEBRILE NON-HEMOLYTIC REACTION

Dr. Tulika Chandra, Professor & Head, Department of Transfusion Medicine

A 21 year old female living was admitted for a discharge from the nose, fever, lethargy, neck stiffness and pain. The patient was underweight and with poor nutritional status. Diagnosis of meningitis was made. Patient was treated with standard protocols, he responded and was afebrile. After a week the patients hemoglobin was dropping quickly and the physician decided to transfuse 2 units of packed red blood cells (PRBC).

BLOOD TEST RESULTS

Hemoglobin 6.0 gm%

Hematocrit 20 l/L

Platelets 5.9×10^6 cells / cmm

PAST MEDICAL HISTORY

Pt had ben given chemotherapy for rhabdomyosarcoma 10 years back.

TRANSFUSION SERVICE LABORATORY

The patients blood sample was given along with requisition form , 2 units of PRBC were crossmatched and sent to patients ward for transfusion.

TRANSFUSION - PRBC #1

The first unit was started at 10:55 am. Vital signs were recorded:

Blood pressure: 128/70

Oxygen saturation: 94%

Temperature: 36.7°C

Pulse: 110/min.

As the nurse was unable to get an infusion rate faster than 1 drop/10sec., she flushed the port-o-cath with 350 U of heparin. The rate did not increase and she replaced the needle with no success. Finding a new IV access was unlikely because patient had poor vein access and would have required a new port-o-cath insertion or a central venous access, not considered possible as the patient was already unstable.

The nurse followed the order and ran the transfusion over a little more than 8 hours. No further vital signs were taken.

TRANSFUSION - PRBC #2

The second unit was started by the same nurse (who was working a 12-hour shift) at 20:15 h. Vital signs were taken with no untoward results. No further vital signs were taken until 21:30 h. when the patient started shaking and stiffness was noted. The transfusion was stopped, the physician was contacted, and the nurse followed standard procedures in the nursing manual.

Vital signs were

Temperature: 41.0 °C (axillary)

Pulse: 230/min.

Blood pressure: 160/100

Oxygen saturation: 97% on rebreather

The patient presented with but loss of consciousness. The patient was then transferred to an intensive care unit. The patient was finally intubated and put into artificial coma. Blood culture was done and blood bag returned to blood bank for investigation.

LABORATORY SERVICES

Upon detecting the suspected transfusion reaction, the transfusion service was contacted and they performed a transfusion reaction investigation, eliminating a hemolytic transfusion reaction as the cause.

Because a bacteriogenic reaction was suspected due to fever subsequent to a prolonged transfusion time (8 hrs.+), the hospital microbiology laboratory performed gram stains and cultures of both PRBC contents, as well as recipient blood cultures. All were negative.

1. What types of transfusion reactions are possible in this scenario of fever following transfusion?
   (A)Febrile haemolytic transfusion reaction
   (B)Febrile non haemolytic transfusion reaction
   (C) Bacterial transfusion reaction
   (D)All of the above
2. What is the maximum time limit for transfusion to complete.
   (A)8 hours
   (B)4 hours
   (C)16 hors
   (D)10 hours
3. What patient consequences could happen if nurses do not properly chart a transfusion and take vital signs for the entire transfusion and a blood component culture is found to be positive?
   (A)No effect on patient

(B)Monitoring of vital records only in the initial phase is essential , hence patient will have no changes during transfusion

(C)Patient will always have a reaction if monitoring for the entire transfusion process does not take place

(D) Patient may have a reaction if monitoring for the entire transfusion process does not take place

4. What is the key learning point from the above case

(A)Proper education and training of the paramedical and medical staff is essential to perform a safe transfusion.

(B)Blood unit should always be warmed before transfusion

(C)Infusion by heparin should be done in case of blockage

(D)Monitoring should be done during transfusion only in serious cases

Answers:

1. D

   All the above three reactions can occur in the above case

2. B

   Maximum time limit for transfusion to complete is 4 hours

3. D

   Patient may have a reaction if monitoring for the entire transfusion process does not take place.

4. A

   Proper education and training of the paramedical and medical staff is essential to perform a safe transfusion

References:

1. Carroll JS, Quijada MA. Redirecting traditional professional values to support safety: changing organisational culture in health care. Qual Saf Health Care 2004 Dec;13 Suppl 2:ii16?21.

2. Mancini ME. Performance improvement in transfusion medicine. What do nurses need and want? Arch Pathol Lab Med 1999;123(6):496?502.

Chapter-31
Urology

CARCINOMA PENIS

Dr. Bimalesh Purkait, SR, Dr. Madhusudan Patodia, SR, Dr. Bhupendra Pal Singh, Professor, Dr. Divakar Dalela, Professor, Dr. Apul Goel, Professor, Dept. of Urology

A 47-year old gentleman, presented with penile growth for last 7 months. He also had pain, itching and foul smelling discharge from growth. Further enquiry revealed that the growth has increased rapidly in last 2 months. Local examination revealed a 2 x 3 cm fungating, ulcerated growth involving glans and distal penis with no palpable inguinal lymphadenopathy. Proximally about 4 cm of penile shaft is free from tumour margin. Abdominal and chest examination were unremarkable. All the blood investigations were normal.

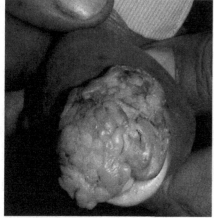

1. What is the most likely diagnosis?
   (A) Penile wart
   (B) Carcinoma penis
   (C) Vascular malformation
   (D) Lymphogranuloma
2. All of the following are preventive strategies to decrease the incidence of penile cancer EXCEPT:
   (A) Circumcision after 21 years of age
   (B) Daily genital hygiene
   (C) Avoiding cigarette smoke
   (D) Circumcision before puberty
3. What is the most important predisposing factor for carcinoma penis?
   (A) Alcohol
   (B) Gonorrhoea
   (C) Phimosis
   (D) Urinary tract infection
4. What is the best test for confirming the diagnosis?
   (A) Biopsy
   (B) High resolution ultrasonography of penis
   (C) CT Scan lower abdomen
   (D) PET scan
5. What is the most common histological variety?
   (A) Squamous cell carcinoma
   (B) Adenocarcinoma
   (C) Transitional Cell Carcinoma
   (D) Basal Cell Carcinoma
6. What is the strongest prognostic factor for survival in penile cancer?
   (A) The extent of lymph node metastasis
   (B) The grade of the primary tumour
   (C) The stage of the primary tumour
   (D) Vascular invasion presence in the primary tumour
7. A watchful waiting strategy toward the management of the inguinal region in this patient (no palpable adenopathy) is recommended for all of the following situations EXCEPT:
   (A) Primary tumour stage Ta.

(B)Primary tumour stage T1, grade I.

(C)Primary tumour stage T1, grade II.

(D)Noncompliant patients.

8. Adjuvant or neo-adjuvant chemotherapy should be considered in addition to surgery for all of the Following EXCEPT:

(A)Single pelvic nodal metastasis.

(B)Extra nodal extension of cancer.

(C)Fixed inguinal masses.

(D)Two unilateral inguinal nodes with focal metastases.

9. Patient underwent surgery and histopathology shows T1G2 with no vascular invasion and ifthe right Inguinal Lymph node (LN) is palpable, and then what will be the next management for the LN

(A)Observation

(B)Fine needle aspiration cytology

(C)Ipsi-lateral superficial and deep inguinal lymph node dissection

(D)Four weeks of antibiotics and then reassess

Answers:

1. B

    Carcinoma Penis.

    In view of rapidly growing fungating lesion with foul odour, clinical diagnosis of Ca penis is correct.

2. A

    Circumcision after 21 years of age

3. C

    Phimosis

    Phimosis allows accumulation of smegma and this allows stagnation of viral and other carcinogenic factors in preputial sac.

4. A

    Biopsy

    HPE is the only sure way of diagnosing carcinoma penis.

5. A

    Squamous cell carcinoma

    The most common histological type of penile carcinoma is sqamous cell carcinoma.

6. A

    The extent of lymph node metastasis

    The presence and extent of metastasis to the inguinal region are the most important prognostic factors for survival in patients withsquamous penile cancer.

7. D

    Noncompliant patients.

8. D

    Two unilateral inguinal nodes with focal metastases.

    For patients requiring ilioinguinal lymphadenectomy because of the presence of metastases,adjuvant chemotherapy should be considered for those exhibiting more than two positive lymph nodes, extranodal extension of cancer, or pelvic nodal metastasis. Reports from one center further confirmed the value of adjuvant chemotherapy.

9. B

    FNAC

References:

1. Currtis A. Pettaway, Raymond S. Lance, John W. Davis. Tumors of the Penis. In: Alan J. Wein, Louis R. Kavoussi, Andrew C. Novick, Alan W. Partin, Craig A. Peters, editors. Campbell-Walsh Urology, 10[th]International edition. Philadelphia. Saunders, Elsevier. 2012. Ch 34, Page-901-933.

2. Currtis A. Pettaway, Raymond S. Lance. John W. Davis. Tumors of the Penis. In: Alan J. Wein, Louis R. Kavoussi, Andrew C. Novick, Alan W. Partin, Craig A. Peters,editors. Campbell-Walsh Urology, 10[th]International edition. Philadelphia. Saunders, Elsevier;2012. Ch 34, Page-901-933.

3. Maden C, Sherman KJ, Beckman AM, et al. History of circumcision, medical conditions, and sexual activity and risk of penile cancer. J Natl Cancer Inst 1993;85:19–24

4. Misra S, Chaturvedi A, Misra NC. Penile carcinoma: a challenge for the developing world. Lancet Oncol 2004; 5:240–7.

5. Currtis A. Pettaway, Raymond S. Lance, John W. Davis. Tumors of the Penis. In: Alan J. Wein, Louis R. Kavoussi, Andrew C. Novick, Alan W. Partin, Craig A. Peters, editors. Campbell-Walsh Urology, 10th International edition. Philadelphia. Saunders, Elsevier; 2012. Ch 34, Page-901-933.
6. Buechner SA. Common skin disorders of the penis. BJU Int 2002; 90: 498–506.
7. Currtis A. Pettaway, Raymond S. Lance, John W. Davis. Tumors of the Penis. In: Alan J. Wein, Louis R. Kavoussi, Andrew C. Novick, Alan W. Partin, Craig A. Peters, editors. Campbell-Walsh Urology, 10th International edition. Philadelphia. Saunders, Elsevier; 2012. Ch 34, Page-901-933.

CARCINOMA URINARY BLADDER

Dr. Bimalesh Purkait, SR, Dr. Madhusudan Patodia, SR, Dr. Bhupendra Pal Singh, Professor, Dr. Divakar Dalela, Professor, Dr. Apul Goel, Professor, Dept. of Urology

A 56 years old man, chronic smoker with painless haematuria with irregular clots on and off for last 2 months. He did not have fever, voiding or storage lower urinary tract symptoms (LUTS), urinary retention or any systemic illness. General examination revealed anaemia with poor nutrition. Chest and abdominal examination did not reveal any abnormality. Urine microscopy showed plenty of red blood cells. Urine cytology was positive for malignant cells. Ultrasonography of bladder shows the following:

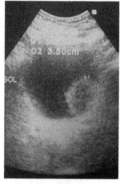

1. What is the most likely clinical diagnosis?
   (A)Blood clots
   (B)Bladder calculus
   (C)Bladder carcinoma
   (D)Foreign body
2. What is the most important risk factor for this condition?
   (A)Smoking
   (B)Alcohol
   (C)Trauma
   (D)Infection
3. What is best way to confirm the diagnosis?
   (A)Cystoscopic Biopsy
   (B)PET scan
   (C)Uitrasonography guided needle biopsy
   (D)Magnetic resonance imaging
4. What is the initial ideal treatment?
   (A)Immunotherapy
   (B)Transurethral resection
   (C)Chemotherapy
   (D)Radiotherapy
5. What is the most common histological cell type?
   (A)Squamous.
   (B)Adeno.
   (C)Urothelial.
   (D)Small cell.
6. General anaesthesia is most important when resecting a bladder tumour in which setting?
   (A)Large, mobile papillary tumour

(B)Tumour in a posterior wall diverticulum

(C)Lateral location, at about 4 or 8 o'clock

(D)Extensive carcinoma in situ (CIS)

7. Cystoscopy shows 3-cm bladder tumor in a posterior wall bladder diverticulum. After tumour resection histopathology demonstrates a pT1G3 bladder tumor with associated areas of carcinoma in situ (CIS). Muscularis mucosa is involved, but there is no definite muscularis propria in the specimen. Optimal management includes:

(A)Repeat resection to stage the cancer.

(B)Intravesical BCG therapy.

(C)Partial cystectomy with excision of the diverticulum.

(D)Radical cystectomy and urinary diversion.

8. Restaging transurethral resection of bladder tumour (TURBT) is indicated in which of the following situations?

(A)pT1, G2 tumor with no muscularis propria identified

(B)pTa, G1 tumor that is multifocal ($n = 5$) with complete resection,

(C)pT1, G3 tumor with muscularis propria identified and negative

(D)Both a and c

Answers:

1. C

Bladder Carcinoma

In view of positive urinary cytology and a mass lesion attached to wall of urinary bladder, carcinoma of bladder is the most tenable diagnosis.

2. A

Smoking

Long duration of regular smoking leads to carcinogenic changes in transitional epithelium of urinary bladder.

3. A

Cystoscopic Biopsy

By cystoscopy one can see the appearance of lesion and also obtain tissue for histopathological confirmation.

4. B

Transurethral resection

TURBT as the initial step of treatment, it not only removes all endoscopically visiable tumour but also allows for pathological staging by detecting the degree of muscle invasion.

5. C

Urothelial

6. C

Lateral location, at about 4 or 8 o'clock

7. E

radical cystectomy and urinary diversion.

8. D

a and c

References:

1. J Stephen Jones, William A. Larchian. Non Muscle Invasive Bladder Cancer (Ta, T1, and CIS). In: Alan J. Wein, Louis R. Kavoussi, Andrew C. Novick, Alan W. Partin, Craig A. Peters, editors. Campbell-Walsh Urology, 10th International edition. Philadelphia.Saunders, Elsevier; 2012. Ch 81, Page 2335-2345.

2. Thompson I, Fair W: Occupational and environmental factors in bladder cancer. In: Chisolm GD, Fair WR (editors): *Scientific Foundationsof Urology*, 2nd ed. Heinemann Medical Books, 1990.

3. Jemal A, Siegel R, Ward E, et al. Cancer statistics, 2008. CA Cancer J Clin 2008;58(2):71–96

4. J Stephen Jones, William A. Larchian. Non Muscle Invasive Bladder Cancer (Ta, T1, and CIS). In: Alan J. Wein, Louis R. Kavoussi, Andrew C. Novick, Alan W. Partin, Craig A. Peters, editors. Campbell-Walsh Urology, 10th International edition. Philadelphia.Saunders, Elsevier; 2012. Ch 81, Page 2335-2345.

5. J Stephen Jones, William A. Larchian. Non Muscle Invasive Bladder Cancer (Ta, T1, and CIS). In: Alan J. Wein, Louis R. Kavoussi, Andrew C. Novick, Alan W. Partin, Craig A. Peters, editors. Campbell-Walsh Urology, 10th International edition. Philadelphia.Saunders, Elsevier; 2012. Ch 81, Page 2335-2345.

CARCINOMA TESTS

Dr. Bimalesh Purkait, SR, Dr. Madhusudan Patodia, SR, Dr. Bhupendra Pal Singh, Professor, Dr. Divakar Dalela, Professor, Dr. Apul Goel, Professor, Dept. of Urology

A 42 years young man presented with painless progressively increasing swelling in the right scrotum for last 4 months. He had hydrocele surgery for the same somewhere but the swelling gradually increased in size. He had no fever, vomiting, burning micturition. Local examination revealed an enlarged and hard right testis with normal left testis. There was no inguinal lymphadenopathy. Ultrasonography of scrotum showed the following findings –

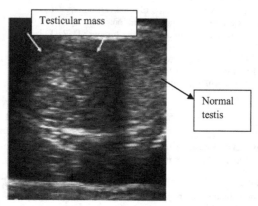

1. What is the most likely diagnosis?
   (A) Carcinoma testis
   (B) Lipoma of cord
   (C) Organised Pyocele
   (D) Haematocele
2. What blood tests will you recommend for prognostication of this condition?
   (A) Serum protein, albumin and bilirubin
   (B) Serum LDH, AFP and beta HCG
   (C) Hb, Serum creatinine and blood urea
   (D) Serum LDH, serum calcium and serum protein
3. What is the initial treatment?
   (A) Chemotherapy
   (B) Radiotherapy
   (C) Scrotal orchidectomy
   (D) High inguinal orchidectomy
4. What are the main histological types of testicular tumour?
   (A) Seminoma and non seminoma
   (B) Leukaemia and lymphoma
   (C) Squamous cell and adeno carcinoma
   (D) Leydig cell and Sertoli cell tumour
5. Which of the following is TRUE regarding testicular anatomy?
   (A) The right testicular vein drains to the right renal vein.
   (B) The left testicular artery arises from the left renal artery.
   (C) The left testicular lymphatic drainage is to the interaortocaval and paracaval nodes.
   (D) The right testicular lymphatic drainage is to paracaval, interaortocaval, and para-aortic nodes.
6. In testicular cancer, staging done according to TNM S. What does 'S' stand for?
   (A) Staging
   (B) Serum tumour marker
   (C) Society
   (D) Serum testosterone,
7. What is most common type of testicular tumour in prepubertal children?
   (A) Seminoma.
   (B) Yolk sac tumours.
   (C) Embryonal carcinoma.
   (D) Teratoma.

8. Which of the following is an acceptable indication for testis-sparing surgery?
   (A)1.3-cm solid intratesticular mass with a normal contra lateral testis
   (B)Suspected benign testicular lesion
   (C)2.4-cm solid mass in a solitary testis
   (D)Hypogonadal male with 1.2-cm solid intratesticular mass in a solitary testis
9. Patient underwent high inguinal orchidectomy with cytopathology shows seminoma testis. On CT scan a 10 cm mass was seen in the retro peritoneum. His tumour markers are normal both before and after chemotherapy. After treatment his mass is 5 cm. What will be the next treatment?
   (A)Complete resection of the mass
   (B)PET scan
   (C)Percutaneous biopsy is accurate.
   (D)Radiotherapy
10. The most common site for recurrence after retroperitoneal lymph node dissection (RPLND) is the:
   (A)Interaortocaval region.
   (B)Paracaval region.
   (C)Para-aortic region.
   (D)Interiliac region.

Answers:

1. A
   Carcinoma testis
   In view of the rapidly increasing testicular swelling, which is hard on clinical examination, and echogenic on ultrasound examination, carcinoma of the testis is the most logical clinical diagnosis.
2. B
   Serum LDH, AFP and beta HCG
   The elevation of these biochemical parameters help to differentiate between seminoma and non seminoma and thus are useful in prognosticating the outcome.
3. D
   High inguinal orchidectomy
   High inguinal orchiectomy allows removal of substantial length of spermatic cord along with testis, both of which are later submitted for HPE and diagnostic confirmation.
4. A
   Seminoma and non seminoma
   Seminoma and non- seminoma are two major types of germ cell tumors of testis, rest are very uncommon.
5. B
   Serum tumour marker
   5d. the right testicular lymphatic drainage is to paracaval, interaortocaval, and para-aortic nodes.
6. B
   Yolk sac tumours.
   7b. PET scan
7. C
   Para-aortic region.
8. B
   Suspected benign testicular lesion
9. B
   PET scan
10. C
   Para-aortic region.

References:

1. Vogelzang NJ, Scardino PT, Shipley WU, Coffey DS, editors. Genitourinary oncology. Philadelphia: Lippincott Williams & Wilkins; 1999.

2. Sobin LH, Wittekind CH. UICC: TNM classification of malignant tumors. 6th ed. New 2. York: Wiley-Liss; 2002.

3. Anderw J.Stephenson, Timothy D.Gilligan. Neoplasms of the Testis. In: Alan J. Wein, Louis R. Kavoussi, Andrew C. Novick, Alan W. Partin, Craig A. Peters, editors. Campbell-Walsh Urology, 10th International edition. Philadelphia. Saunders, Elsevier; 2012. Ch 31, Page-837-870.

4. International Germ Cell Consensus Classification: a prognostic factor-based staging system for metastatic germ cell cancers. International Germ Cell Cancer Collaborative Group. J Clin Oncol 1997; 15:594–603.

5. Anderw J.Stephenson, Timothy D.Gilligan. Neoplasms of the Testis. In: Alan J. Wein, Louis R. Kavoussi, Andrew C. Novick, Alan W. Partin, Craig A. Peters, editors . Campbell-Walsh Urology, 10th International edition. Philadelphia. Saunders, Elsevier; 2012. Ch 31, Page-837-870.

BENIGN PROSTATIC HYPERPLASIA (BPH)

Dr. Bimalesh Purkait, SR, Dr. Madhusudan Patodia, SR, Dr. Bhupendra Pal Singh, Professor, Dr. Divakar Dalela, Professor, Dr. Apul Goel, Professor, Dept. of Urology

A 64 years old gentle man complains of of voiding and storage lower urinary tracts symptoms (LUTS) for last 1 year. He had no fever, hematuria or pain during micturition. There was no previous urinary tract intervention. On digital rectal examination, he was found to have smooth, non tender enlarged prostate. Urine test showed no abnormality. The serum PSA was 3.5 ng/ml, Ultrasonography of bladder region shows following findings

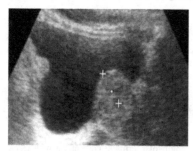

1.What is most likely diagnosis?
   (A)Benign prostatic hyperplasia with median lobe enlargement
   (B)Carcinoma urinary bladder
   (C)Rectal mass protruding into bladder
   (D)Cystitis Cystic

2.Which drug may be suitable for this patient?
   (A)Tamsulosin
   (B)Buscopan
   (C)Magnamycin
   (D)Tetracycline

3.Which one is not a treatment option for this case?
   (A)Tamsulosin
   (B)Trans urethral resection of prostate (TURP)
   (C)Holmium enucleation of prostate (HOLEP)
   (D)Watchful waiting

4.Benign prostatic hyperplasia (BPH) is more common in which region of prostate?
   (A)Periurethral and peripheral zone
   (B)Periurethral and transitional zone
   (C)Peripheral zone
   (D)Anterior stroma

5. The tension of prostate smooth muscle is mediated by the:
   (A)$\alpha 1$ receptor.
   (B)$\alpha 2$ receptor.
   (C)$\beta 2$ receptor.
   (D)Androgen receptor

6. Imaging of the upper tract in benign prostatic hyperplasia patient is indicated if:
   (A)Prostate glands weighing more than 50 gm.
   (B)Urinalysis demonstrating hematuria.
   (C)Bladder trabeculation.
   (D)Severe lower urinary tract symptoms.

7. Dutasteride:
   (A)Is a dual inhibitor of type 1 and type 2 5α-reductase?
   (B)Is more effective than finasteride.
   (C)Results in a 95% reduction in prostate specific antigen (PSA) after 6 months of therapy.
   (D)Improves erectile function.
8. The most common complication after TURP surgery is:
   (A)Failure to void.
   (B)Hemorrhage requiring transfusion.
   (C)Clot retention.
   (D)Urinary tract infection.

Answers:

1. A
   BPH with median lobe enlargement .
   As per the classical symptoms, no haematuria and the USG picture showing bulge of median lobe, the likely clinical diagnosis should be BPH with median lobe enlargement.

2. A
   Tamsulosin
   Since the patient is symptomatic, he needs medical therapy and tamsulosin is current drug of choice.

3. D
   Watchful waiting
   In view of multiple symptoms – both of storage and voiding phase, watchful waiting is not justified.

4. B
   Periurethral and transitional zone
   The classical BPH occurs in periurethral and transitions zone of prostate and cancer occurs in peripheral zone.

5. A
   α1 receptor.

6. B
   urinalysis demonstrating hematuria.

7. A
   is a dual inhibitor of type 1 and type 2 5α-reductase.

8. A
   failure to void.

References:

1. American Urological Association Practice Guidelines Committee. AUA guideline on management of benign prostatic hyperplasia. Chapter 1: Diagnosis and treatment recommendations. J Urol 2003;170 (2 Pt. 1):530–47.
2. Barry MJ, Cockett AT, Holtgrewe HL, et al. Relationship of symptoms of prostatism to commonly used physiological and anatomical measures of the severity of benign prostatic hyperplasia. J Urol 1993; 150:351–8.
3. Thomas Anthony McNicholas, Roger Sinclair Kirby, Herbert Lepor. In: Alan J. Wein, Louis R. Kavoussi, Andrew C. Novick, Alan W. Partin, Craig A. Peters, editors. Campbell-Walsh Urology, 10th International edition. Philadelphia. Saunders, Elsevier; 2012. Ch 92, Page-2611-2654.
4. Thomas Anthony McNicholas, Roger Sinclair Kirby, Herbert Lepor. In: Alan J. Wein, Louis R. Kavoussi, Andrew C. Novick, Alan W. Partin, Craig A. Peters, editors. Campbell-Walsh Urology, 10th International edition. Philadelphia. Saunders, Elsevier; 2012. Ch 92, Page-2611-2654.
5. Thomas Anthony McNicholas, Roger Sinclair Kirby, Herbert Lepor. In: Alan J. Wein, Louis R. Kavoussi, Andrew C. Novick, Alan W. Partin, Craig A. Peters, editors. Campbell-Walsh Urology, 10th International edition. Philadelphia. Saunders, Elsevier; 2012. Ch 92, Page-2611-2654.

CARCINOMA PROSTATE

Dr. Bimalesh Purkait, SR, Dr. Madhusudan Patodia, SR, Dr. Bhupendra Pal Singh, Professor, Dr. Divakar Dalela, Professor, Dr. Apul Goel, Professor, Dept. of Urology

Eighty two years old gentle man had complains of voiding lower urinary tract symptoms (LUTS) for last 7 months. He had no fever, vomiting, cough or bony pain. On digital rectal examination, prostate was enlarged with one discrete hard nodule palpable on right side. Urine gross and microscopic analysis showed 10-12 RBCs /hpf. Serum PSA was 8.0 ng/dl. Trans rectal ultrasound evaluation shows following findings.

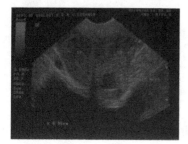

1. What is the most likely diagnosis in this patient?
   (A)Carcinoma prostate, early stage
   (B)Benign prostatic hyperplasia
   (C)Prostatitis
   (D)Carcinoma prostate, late stage
2. A hypoechoic lesion of the prostate can be caused by all of the following EXCEPT:
   (A)Hematologic malignancies.
   (B)Prostate cancer.
   (C)Transition zone, benign prostatic hyperplasia nodules.
   (D)Normal urethra.
3. What is the most important risk factor for this condition?
   (A)Smoking
   (B)Positive family history
   (C)Lead exposure
   (D)Aromatic amine exposure
4. What is the most useful first-line test for the diagnosis of prostate cancer?
   (A)Digital rectal examination (DRE)
   (B)Prostate-specific antigen (PSA) assay
   (C)Transrectal ultrasonography (TRUS)
   (D)Combination of DRE and PSA
5. Which one is not a treatment options for this condition?
   (A)Radiation therapy
   (B)Observation
   (C)Surgery
   (D)Transurethral Microwave Thermotherapy (TUMT)
6. For describing the pathological features of the lesion, which grading system is followed?
   (A)Minnesota
   (B)MSKCC
   (C)Atlanta
   (D)Gleason
7. What outcome do the Partin tables predict?
   (A)Clinical stage
   (B)Gleason score
   (C)Pathologic stage
   (D)Cancer-specific survival probability
8. Watchful waiting is appropriate for men who:
   (A)Are 70 years of age or older.
   (B)Have impalpable cancer not visible on imaging studies.
   (C)Have a serum prostate-specific antigen (PSA) level less than 10 ng/mL.
   (D)Have a life expectancy approximately 10 years or less and well to moderately differentiated cancer.
9. Two years after definitive radiotherapy for prostate cancer, what should the serum PSA level be?
   (A)Undetectable
   (B)Less than 0.5ng/mL
   (C)Stable and not rising

(D)Normal

Answers:

1. A

   Carcinoma prostate, early stage. In a symptomatic elderly male, a discrete hard nodule palpable on DRE along with elevated PSA of 8.0 mg/dl and demonstrable localized nodule on TRUS, a diagnosis of localized carcinoma prostate is most tenable.

2. A

   hematologic malignancies.

3. B

   Positive family history. In most countries, a positive family history is the most major risk factors observed.

4. D

   Combination of DRE and PSA

5. D

   TUMT. TUMT is an option for treatment of small sized BPH, not cancer prostate.

6. D

   Gleason. Gleason grading is the only system of pathological grading for cancer prostate.

7. C

   Pathologic stage

8. D

   Have a life expectancy approximately 10 years or less and well- to moderately-differentiated cancer.

9. C

   Stable and not rising

References:

1. Andriole GL, Grubb 3rd RL, Buys SS, et al. Mortality results from a randomized prostate-cancer screening trial. N Engl J Med 2009; 360 (13):1310–19.
2. Stacy Loeb, Herbert Ballentine Carter. Early Detection, Diagnosis, and Staging of Prostate Cancer.In: Alan J. Wein, Louis R. Kavoussi, Andrew C. Novick, Alan W. Partin, Craig A. Peters, editors. Campbell-Walsh Urology, 10th International edition. Philadelphia. Saunders, Elsevier;2012, Ch 99, page-2763-2771.
3. Witte JS. Prostate cancer genomics: towards a new understanding. Nat Rev Genet 2009; 10:77–82.
4. Stacy Loeb, Herbert Ballentine Carter. Early Detection, Diagnosis, and Staging of Prostate Cancer.In: Alan J. Wein, Louis R. Kavoussi, Andrew C. Novick, Alan W. Partin, Craig A. Peters, editors. Campbell-Walsh Urology, 10th International edition. Philadelphia. Saunders, Elsevier;2012, Ch 99, page-2763-2771.
5. Michael O. Koch. High-Intensity Focused Ultrasound for the Treatment of Prostate Cancer.In: Alan J. Wein, Louis R. Kavoussi, Andrew C. Novick, Alan W. Partin, CraigA. Peters, editors. Campbell-Walsh Urology, 10th International edition. Philadelphia. Saunders, Elsevier;2012, Ch 106, page- 2897-2902.
6. Eble JN, Sauter G, Epstein JI, Sesterhenn IA. Pathology and genetics: tumours of the urinary system and male genital organs. Lyon (France): IARC Press; 2004.Partin AW, Yoo J, Carter HB, et al. The use of prostate specific antigen, clinical stage and Gleason score to predict pathological stage in men with localized prostate cancer. J Urol 1993; 150 (1) : 110 –14.
7. James A. Eastham, Peter T. Scardino. Expectant Management of Prostate Cancer. In: Alan J. Wein, Louis R. Kavoussi, Andrew C. Novick, Alan W. Partin, Craig A. Peters, editors. Campbell-Walsh Urology, 10 th International edition. Philadelphia. Saunders, Elsevier;2012. Ch 101. Page-2789-2800.
8. Anthony V. D'Amico, Juanita M. Crook, Clair J. Beard, Theodore L. DeWeese, Mark Hurwitz, Irving D. Kaplan. Radiation Therapy for Prostate Cancer.In: Alan J. Wein, Louis R. Kavoussi, Andrew C. Novick, Alan W. Partin, Craig A. Peters, editors. Campbell-Walsh Urology, 10th International edition. Philadelphia. Saunders, Elsevier; 2012. Ch 104. Page-2850-2872.

Metastatic Carcinoma Prostate

Dr. Bimalesh Purkait, SR, Dr. Madhusudan Patodia, SR, Dr. Bhupendra Pal Singh, Professor, Dr. Divakar Dalela, Professor, Dr. Apul Goel, Professor, Dept. of Urology

A 78-years old man known case of adeno carcinoma prostate (Gleason grade 5 + 4) on hormonal therapy for last 1 year presented with complain of severe low back pain for last 1 month. Serum prostate specific antigen (PSA) was 35 ng/dl. No history fever, Tuberculosis, cough, haemoptysis or any localized neurological deficit. On general examination, he was found to have pallor, cachexia and tenderness over spine. Abdominal and Chest examination-No abnormality detected. Bone scan is depicted below.

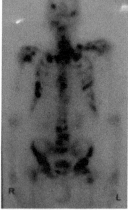

1.What is the most likely diagnosis?
   (A)Early prostate carcinoma
   (B)Prostate carcinoma with bone metastasis
   (C)Prostate carcinoma with osteoporosis
   (D)Multiple Myeloma
2.What are the findings in the bone scan?
   (A)Osteoporosis
   (B)Post radiation changes
   (C)Multiple fractures
   (D)Multiple metastases
3.Best test to estimate prostate volume?
   (A)Digital rectal examination
   (B)Prostate specific antigen level
   (C)PET scan
   (D)Transrectal ultrasonography
4.What could be the next management option for this condition?
   (A)Docetaxel
   (B)Defcortisone
   (C)Denosumab
   (D)Octreotide
5.If patient develops severe back pain and the PSA level is stable. The next step is:
   (A)Give analgesics as needed and consider a workup when the PSA value rises.
   (B)Add zoledronate to management.
   (C)Consider radiation therapy.
   (D)Order magnetic resonance imaging (MRI) of the spine to rule out cord compression.

Answers:
   1. B
      Prostate carcinoma with bone metastasis
      An elderly male with H/o carcinoma prostate now having markedly elevated S. PSA with multiple metastasis seen on bone scan, the most likely diagnosis is metastatic carcinoma prostate.
   2. D
      Multiple metastases

The bone scan picture is showing multiple localized hot spots which in this clinical background will high S. PSA, indicate multiple metastases.

3. D
TRUS
TRUS is a reliable method for accurately estimating the prostatic volume.

4. A
Docetaxel
Once patient develops hormone refractory disease, the most useful option is Docetaxel.

5. D
order magnetic resonance imaging (MRI) of the spine to rule out cord compression

References:

1. Maxwell V.Meng, Peter R.Carroll. Treatment of Locally Advanced Prostate Cancer.In: Alan J. Wein, Louis R. Kavoussi, Andrew C. Novick, Alan W. Partin, Craig A. Peters, editors. Campbell-Walsh Urology, 10th International edition. Philadelphia. Saunders, Elsevier; 2012. Ch 107, Page-2903-2920.

2. Antonarakis ES, Carducci MA, Eisenberger MA. Novel targeted therapeutics for metastatic castration-resistant prostate cancer. Cancer Lett 2010; 291:1–13.

3. Petrylak DP, Tangen CM, Hussain MH, et al. Docetaxel and estramustine compared with mitoxantrone and prednisone for advanced refractory prostate cancer. N Engl J Med 2004; 351:1513–20.

4. Maxwell V.Meng, Peter R.Carroll. Treatment of Locally Advanced Prostate Cancer. In: Alan J. Wein, Louis R. Kavoussi, Andrew C. Novick, Alan W. Partin, Craig A. Peters, editors. Campbell-Walsh Urology, 10th International edition. Philadelphia. Saunders, Elsevier;2012. Ch 107, Page-2903-2920.

5. Emmanuel S. Antonarakis, Michael A. Carducci, Mario A. Eisenberger.Treatment of Castration-Resistant Prostate Cancer. In: Alan J. Wein, Louis R. Kavoussi, Andrew C. Novick, Alan W. Partin, Craig A. Peters, editors. Campbell-Walsh Urology, 10th International edition.Philadelphia. Saunders, Elsevier;2012. Ch 110, page- 2954-2971.

EMPHYSEMATOUS PYELONEPHRITIS

Dr. Durgesh Kumar Saini, SR, Dr. Gaurav Prakash, SR, Dr. Vishwajeet Singh, Professor, Dr. Apul Goel, Professor, Dr. Divakar Dalela, Professor, Dept. of Urology

A 50-year old diabetic woman presented with high-grade fever with rigors, vomiting and severe right flank pain for last 6 days. On examination, she appeared toxic with pulse rate of 120/min, BP 90/60 mm Hg. Abdominal examination revealed a tender right renal lump. On investigations her total leukocyte count was 22,000/mm^3, platelet 60,000/mm^3, urinalysis showed >100 pus cells/hpf. Ultrasonography showed renal enlargement with multiple echoes and fluid accumulation. Her contrast-enhanced CT scan showed the following picture:

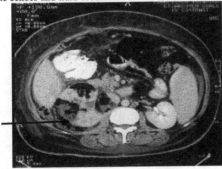

1.What is the diagnosis
(A)Right-sided multifocal bacterial nephritis
(B)Right-sided emphysematous pyelonephritis
(C)Right-sided renal abscess
(D)Right-sided pyonephrosis

2. Emphysematous pyelonephritis is usually seen in patients suffering from
    (A)Hypertension
    (B)Clostridium infection
    (C)Diabetes
    (D)All
3. Gas produced in emphysematous pyelonephritis is
    (A)NO_2
    (B)N_2O
    (C)CO
    (D)CO_2
4. Most common organism identified in emphysematous pyelonephritis is
    (A)Proteus
    (B)Klebsiella
    (C)Clostridium
    (D)E. coli
5. In the picture given above, arrow indicates
    (A)Bowel loop
    (B)Gas in kidney parenchyma
    (C)Hydronephrosis
    (D)Extrarenal collection

Answers:

1. B

The typical clinical picture in a diabetic lady with CECT showing multiple air pocketsinrenal parenchyma suggest emphysematous pyelonephritis.

2. C

Diabetics are most prone to develop this type of infection.

3. D

CO_2 is the gas produced following bacterial action.

4. D

E. coli is the commonest organism responsible for this disease.

5. B

Gas in kidney parenchyma

RENAL ABSCESS

Dr. Durgesh Kumar Saini, SR, Dr. Gaurav Prakash, SR, Dr. Vishwajeet Singh, Professor, Dr. Apul Goel, Professor, Dr. Divakar Dalela, Professor, Dept. of Urology

A 50-year old man presented with fever with rigors, left flank pain, weight loss and malaise of 1 month duration. General exam revealed tachycardia and normal blood pressure. On abdominal examination there was tenderness in left renal angle. Blood report showed marked leukocytosis and uncontrolled diabetes. Ultrasonography showed fluid collection adjacent to posterior surface of left kidney. CT showed the following picture.

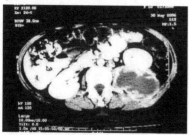

1. What is the diagnosis?
    (A)Emphysematous pyelonephritis
    (B)Renal abscess
    (C)Hydronephrosis
    (D)Tuberculosis
2. Patient with renal abscess typically shows

(A)Bacteriuria
(B)Positive urine culture
(C)Leucocytosis
(D)All
3. What is the diagnostic investigation of choice for renal abscess?
(A)CT scan
(B)MRI
(C)Ultrasonography
(D)DMSA Renal Scan
4. If size of abscess is 10 cm then treatment of choice for renal abscess in this patient?
(A)Antibiotics alone
(B)Percutaneous drainage with antibiotics
(C)Nephrectomy
(D)Surgical drainage

Answers:

1. B
   Since it is a solitory fluid containing lesion coming out of renal parenchyma, producing a toxic clinical picture, it is a case of renal abscess.
2. C
   Patient typically has marked leucocytosis. Blood cultures but not the urine cultures are usually positive. Unless the abcess communicates with collecting system pyuria or bacteriuria may not be evident.
3. A
   CT Scan is the most useful test
4. D
   Treatment of choice according to size of renal abscess
   <3 cm and early in course-> intravenous antimicrobials
   3-5 cm-> percutaneous drainage
   >5 cm-> surgical drainage

INFECTED HYDRONEPHROSIS

Dr. Durgesh Kumar Saini, SR, Dr. Gaurav Prakash, SR, Dr. Vishwajeet Singh, Professor, Dr. Apul Goel, Professor, Dr. Divakar Dalela, Professor, Dept. of Urology

A 50-year old man presented with high-grade fever with chills and right flank pain of 10 days duration. There was previous history of urinary tract calculi. On examination, patient was toxic, febrile with pulse rate 130/min, BP 100/70 mm Hg. His abdominal exam showed tender right renal lump which felt firm and immobile. On ultrasonography there was markedly dilated pelvicaliceal system, focal areas of decreased echogenicity with sludge in collecting system. X-ray KUB showed a 15-mm stone in the midureter. CT showed following picture

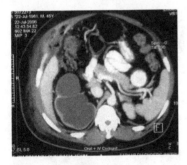

1. What is the likely diagnosis?
(A)Pyonephrosis
(B)Perinephric abscess
(C)Pyelonephritis
(D)Bacterial nephritis
2. Pyonephrosis is defined as:
(A)Collection of purulent material in renal parenchyma
(B)Collection of pus in hydronephrotic kidney

(C)Infected hydronephrosis with suppurative destruction of renal parenchyma

(D)Acute necrotising parenchyma and perirenal infection

3. In pyonephrosis, USG shows which of the following features:

(A)Acoustic shadow

(B)Internal echoes in collecting system

(A)Hyperechoic mass with fluid echoes in pelvicaliceal system

(D)None

4. Emergency best measure to control sepsis in this patient would be:

(A)Parenteral antibiotics alone

(B)Percutaneous drainage with antibiotics

(C)Emergency Nephrectomy

(D)Ureteral stenting

5. What is the usual method of treatment

(A)Immediate ureterolithomy with antibiotics

(B)Ureteroscopic stone removal with antibiotics

(C)Immediate decompression with nephrostomy and antibiotics; later removal of ureteric stone

(D)Nephrectomy

Answers:

1. A

Patient is toxic and ultrasonography shows sludge in kidney, suggestive of pyonephrosis.

2. C

3. B

4. B

Since general condition of patient is unstable, definitive treatment is deferred and sepsis is controlled with percutaneous drainage

5. C

PERINEPHRIC ABSCESS WITH INFECTED HYDRONEPHROSIS

Dr. Durgesh Kumar Saini, SR, Dr. Gaurav Prakash, SR, Dr. Vishwajeet Singh, Professor, Dr. Apul Goel, Professor, Dr. Divakar Dalela, Professor, Dept. of Urology

A 35-year old woman presented with insidious onset of fever, right flank pain and dysuria of 20 days duration. On examination, there was subcutanous edema with buldging in right flank. A flank mass was felt. Lab investigations showed leucocytosis, elevated levels of serum creatinine (1.8mg%) and pyuria. The patient was given parenteral antibiotics but fever persisted even after 3 days of antibiotic therapy. CECT showed right hydronephrotic kidney with normal right ureter with collection (following picture; see arrow). Percutaneous drains were placed in collecting system of the kidney and outside the kidey, which drained pus and patient respoded well. Lab investigations settled down with serum creatinine 1 mg%.

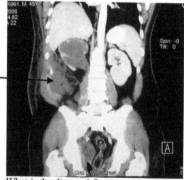

1. What is the diagnosis?

(A)Right renal abscess in hydronephrotic kidney

(B)Right perinephric abscess with hydronephrotic kidney

(C)Pyelonephritis in right kidney

(D)Renal Cell Carcinoma of right kidney

2. What is the investigation of choice for perinephric abscess

(A)X-ray
(B)USG
(C)MRI
(D)CT scan

3. Perinephric abscess is collection of suppurative material
    (A)Within Gerota fascia
    (B)Outside Gerota fascia
    (C)Irrespective of Gerota's fascia, but goes in subcutaneous plane
    (D)All of above

4. Organism mostly responsible for perinephric abscess
    (A)Clostridium
    (B)Streptococci
    (C)E. coli
    (D)Salmonella

5. What is the likely cause of hydronephrosis in this patient?
    (A)Uretero-pelvic junction obstruction
    (B)Stone in ureter
    (C)Compression from the peri-nephric collection
    (D)Residual hydronephrosis from a recently passed stone

Answers:

1. B

    The classical clinical picture and CT showing fluid accumulation in perinephric space with reactive pockets of edema in subcutaneous plane and cephalad displacement of liver, suggest a diagnosis of perinephric abscess with HN kidney.

2. D

    CT, as shown in this case too, gives most appreciable imaging.

3. A

    Classically, perinephric space is limited within Gerota's fascia and so should be the PN abscess.

4. C

    E-coli is the commonest pathogen.

5. A

    Perinephric abscess is formed as a consequence of rupture of infected hydronephrosis in perinephric space.

CHYLURIA

Dr. Durgesh Kumar Saini, SR, Dr. Gaurav Prakash, SR, Dr. Vishwajeet Singh, Professor, Dr. Apul Goel, Professor, Dr. Divakar Dalela, Professor, Dept. of Urology

A 18-year old lady from Bihar presented with passage of milky white urine for last 3 months associated with passage of white clots. Her ultrasonography of bladder and retrograde pyelography picture are given below.

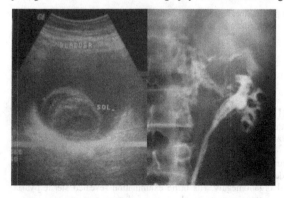

1. What is the likely diagnosis
    (A)Genitourinary TB
    (B)Chyluria
    (C)Chronic UTI

(D)Calculi in kidney with infection
2. What is the most common cause of chyluria in India
    (A)Schistosomiasis
    (B)Trauma
    (C)Strongyloidiasis
    (D)Filariasis
3. Most common cause of lymphatic filariasis is
    (A)Wuchereria bancrofti
    (B)Brugia malayi
    (C)Brugia timori
    (D)Onchocerca volvulus
4. Surgical procedure done for refractory chyluria is known as
    (A)Lymphatico-pelvic dissconnection (Nephrolysis)
    (B)Mainz procedure
    (C)Nephrostomy
    (D)Pyeloplasty
5. What are typical findings on urine examination:
    (A)lymphocyturia
    (B)presence of glucose
    (C)presence of acetone
    (D)presence of casts
6. What is the diagnostic finding on urine examination:
    (A)presence of protein
    (B)presence of trigycerides
    (C)presence of sugar
    (D)presence of Tamm-Horsfall protein
7. What is the dietary advice for patient with chyluria
    (A)high fat low carbohydrate diet
    (B)high fat protein rich diet
    (C)low fat diet with medium chain triglycerides
    (D)fat free diet

Answers:
    1.   B
          The passage of milky urine, demonstration of hetrogenous clot in bladder and classical pyelolymphatic fistulous communications on retrograde pyelography indicate the diagnosis of chyluria.
    2.   D
          The clyluria in India is considered to be felarial in origin until proved otherwise.
    3.   A
          Wacheresia barcrofti is the most common cause.
    4.   A
          Dissonnection of fistulae between pelvicaliceal system and retroperitoneal lymphatics, either done by open surgery or by laparoscopic method, is the main surgical procedure.
    5.   A
    6.   B
    7.   C
          Medium chain triglycerides are absorbed directly into blood stream thereby lymphatic absorption is bypassed.

GENITOURINARY TUBERCULOSIS

Dr. Durgesh Kumar Saini, SR, Dr. Gaurav Prakash, SR, Dr. Vishwajeet Singh, Professor, Dr. Apul Goel, Professor, Dr. Divakar Dalela, Professor, Dept. of Urology

A 30-ycar man presented with intractable urinary frequency for 2 years which was refractory to antibiotics. He was not febrile. 4 months ago, he had an episode of mild self-limiting haematuria. On examination, he appeared thin and abdominal examination did not reveal organomegaly. His urine examination revealed sterile pyuria. Plain x-ray KUB did not show any stone while the intravenous urography shows following picture.

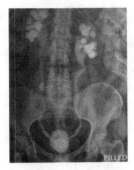

1. What is the likely diagnosis
   (A)Overactive bladder
   (B)Chyluria
   (C)Bladder Calculus
   (D)Genitourinary tuberculosis
2. What is the diagnostic test to document urinary tuberculosis-
   (A)Urine for acid fast bacilli
   (B)Contrast-enhanced CT KUB
   (C)Montoux test
   (D)Intravenous urography
3. The most common primary site of hematogenous spread of TB in the urinary tract is
   (A)Kidney
   (B)Ureter
   (C)Bladder
   (D)Prostate
4. Sample mostly preferred for urinalysis and culture in genitourinary TB is
   (A)24 hr sample
   (B)Single early morning sample
   (C)3-5 early morning samples
   (D)Any of the above
5. What is treatment of thimble bladder
   (A)Antitubercular drugs
   (B)Bladder augmentation with bowel segment
   (C)Hydrodistension of bladder
   (D)Ureteric reimplantation

Answers:
1. D
   The clinical history of intractable frequency with mild haematuria, urine showing sterile pyuria and IVU demonstrated B/l hydro ureteronephrosis and thimble bladder – all indicate towards genito-urinary tuberculosis.
2. A
3. A
   The kidney, on account of its rich vascularity is the most common site for haematogenous seeding.
4. C
   Multiple early morning samples are mostly needed because the bacilluria is an intermittent phenomenon.
5. B
   Since bladder is small in capacity, augmentation of bladder would be required to increase capacity and compliance.

Reference:
1. Schaeffer AJ, Schaeffer EM. Infection of the Urinary Tract. Wein AJ, Kavoussi LR, Novick AC, Partin AW, Peters CA (eds). Campbell-Walsh Urology, 10th ed. Philadelphia: Elsevier, 2012. P. 257-326

VARICOCELE

Dr. Ashok Kumar Gupta, SR, Dr. Siddarth Singh, SR, Dr. S.N. Sankhwar, Professor,
Dr. Diwakar Dalela, Professor, Dr. Apul Goel, Professor, Dept. of Urology

A 35-year old male presented with infertility. He was married for 4 years. On examination of genitalia in lying position, there was visible swelling on left side of scrotum above upper pole of left testis with bag of worm feeling on palpation. Semen analysis showed reduced motility with sperm count 20 million/ml with alkaline reaction.

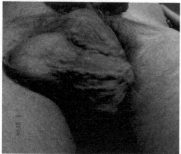

1. What is possible clinical diagnosis
   (A) Left varicocele
   (B) Left hydrocele
   (C) Left inguino-scrotal hernia
   (D) Left spermatocele
2. Left gonadal vein drains into:
   (A) Left renal vein
   (B) Inferior Vena Cava
   (C) Left Iliac Vein
   (D) Left Lumbar vein
3. The mechanism of varicocele-induced impaired spermatogenesis is thought to be because of:
   (A) Heat injury from excess pooling of blood in dilated spermatic veins.
   (B) Turbulent flow through dilated veins that causes a pressure injury to the testis.
   (C) Reflux of splenic metabolites, which is directly gonadotoxic.
   (D) All of the above.
4. Indications for varicocelectomy include all of the following EXCEPT:
   (A) A clinical varicocele in a male with known infertility.
   (B) Dull ipsilateral scrotal pain.
   (C) A subclinical varicocele in a patient with abnormal semen parameters.
   (D) Adolescent males with ipsilateral testis size reduction of 20% compared with the   contralateral testis.
5. Which parameter usually improves after varicocelectomy?
   (A) Motility
   (B) Counts
   (C) Viability
   (D) All of the above
6. Most popular method for varicocelectomy is:
   (A) Microscopic subinguinal varicocelectomy
   (B) Open inguinal varicocelectomy
   (C) Laparoscopic varicocelectomy
   (D) Open suprainguinal approach

Answers:
1.   A
2.   A
3.   A
4.   C
5.   A
6.   A

Reference:

1. Goldstein M. Surgical management of Male infertility. Wein AJ, Kavoussi LR, Novick AC, Partin AW, Peters CA (eds). Campbell-Walsh Urology, 10th ed. Philadelphia: Elsevier, 2012; C.2012 .p.648-687

TORSION TESTIS (SPERMATIC CORD TORSION)

Dr. Ashok Kumar Gupta, SR, Dr. Siddarth Singh, SR, Dr. S.N. Sankhwar, Professor,
Dr. Diwakar Dalela, Professor, Dr. Apul Goel, Professor, Dept. of Urology

10-year old child presented after 8 hours of sudden severe scrotal pain during sleep. He had history of previous episodes of scrotal pain lasting for 30 minutes, usually on the same side which resolved conservatively. Urine examination revealed 5-6 pus cells/hpf.

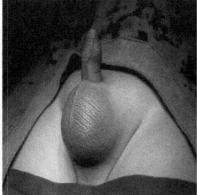

Fig 1.Erythematous left hemiscrotum   Fig 2. Necrosed testis with twisted cord

1. What is the probable diagnosis?
   (A)Spermatic cord torsion
   (B)Epididymo orchitis
   (C)UTI
   (D)Varicocele

2. Which of the following is most specific in diagnosing spermatic cord torsion?
   (A)High-riding testis
   (B)Absence of the cremasteric reflex
   (C)Transverse lie of the testis
   (D)Spermatic cord twist on high-resolution Doppler ultrasonography

3. After manual de-torsion of the spermatic cord, which of the following is appropriate management?
   (A)Color Doppler ultrasonography
   (B)Radionuclide scan
   (C)Doppler examination of the testis and spermatic cord
   (D)Immediate scrotal exploration

4. Irreversible ischemic injury of the testicular parenchyma may begin as early as how many hours after torsion of the spermatic cord?
   (A)1
   (B)2
   (C)4
   (D)6

5. What treatment should be offered to this patient
   (A)Detorsion of spermatic cord
   (B)Left orchidopexy
   (C)Left orchidectomy
   (D)Conservative management should have been extended

Answers:
1. A
2. D
3. D

4. C
5. C

Reference:
1. Barthold JS.Abnormalities of the Testis and Scrotum and Their Surgical Management. . Wein AJ, Kavoussi LR, Novick AC, Partin AW, Peters CA (eds). Campbell-Walsh Urology, 10th ed. Philadelphia: Elsevier, 2012.p.3557-3596

TRAUMATIC URETHRAL STRICTURE

Dr. Ashok Kumar Gupta, SR, Dr. Siddarth Singh, SR, Dr. S.N. Sankhwar, Professor,
Dr. Diwakar Dalela, Professor, Dr. Apul Goel, Professor, Dept. of Urology

A 22 year old boy sustained injury over perineum while falling over a manhole. He noticed blood at urinary meatus and inability to void. On examination he was found to have bruising at perineum and palpable bladder lump. His micturating cystourethrogram (MCU) and retrograde urethrogram (RGU) is shown below.

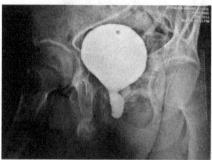 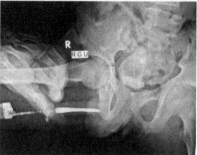

Fig A. MCU   Fig B. RGU

1. What is possible diagnosis?
    (A)Bulbar urethral injury
    (B)Prostatic urethral injury
    (C)Membranous urethral injury
    (D)Penile urethral injury
2. Emergency RGU shows extravasation of contrast in perineum, with no contrast reaching the bladder. What is the ideal treatment?
    (A)Perineal exploration and repair of urethra
    (B)Cystoscopy to bypass the injury
    (C)Suprapubic catherization
    (D)Immediate urethroplasty
3. What is the first-line investigation in urethral injury?
    (A)Endoscopy of urethra
    (B)RGU
    (C)MRI Pelvis
    (D)High resolution ultrasonography of perineum
4. What is the desired time period after pelvic fracture to proceed for reconstruction of urethral injury?
    (A)1-2 months
    (B)3-4 months
    (C)4-6 months
    (D)6- 8 months
5. Which of the following statements concerning pelvic fracture urethral distraction defects is TRUE?
    (A)It involves the tissues of the epithelium as well as the underlying erectile tissues of the corpora cavernosa.
    (B)It involves the tissues of the epithelium as well as the underlying erectile tissue of the corpus spongiosum.
    (C)It is not a true stricture but rather fibrosis that results in distraction of the urethra.
    (D)The stricture process can often be occult because of the unpredictable involvement of the urethral tissues.

Answers:
    1. A
    2. C

3. B
4. C
5. C

Reference:
1. Jordan GH. Surgery of the Penis and Urethra. . Wein AJ, Kavoussi LR, Novick AC, Partin AW, Peters CA (eds). Campbell-Walsh Urology, 10th ed. Philadelphia: Elsevier, 2012 .p.956-1000

BULBOUS URETHRAL STRICTURE

Dr. Ashok Kumar Gupta, SR, Dr. Siddarth Singh, SR, Dr. S.N. Sankhwar, Professor,
Dr. Diwakar Dalela, Professor, Dr. Apul Goel, Professor, Dept. of Urology

A 65-year old man presented with poor urinary stream with dysuria with history of urethral catheterization 6 years back for inguinal hernia surgery. Ultrasound KUB showed normal prostate volume, while his urine examination showed 7-8 pus cell/hpf, culture being sterile. The retrograde urethrogram film is shown below:

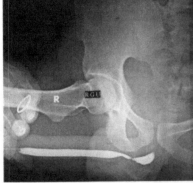

1. In determining the anatomy of the stricture, all of the following provide useful information EXCEPT:
    (A)MRI.
    (B)High-resolution ultrasonography.
    (C)Contrast studies.
    (D)Urethroscopy
2. What is the site of stricture in the urethra?
    (A)Bulbar
    (B)Membranous
    (C)Penile
    (D)Penobulbar
3. Which organism does not cause urethral stricture
    (A)Neisseria
    (B)Chlamydia
    (C)LGV
    (D)Mycoplasma
4. What is the most likely cause of stricture in above mentioned case?
    (A)Infection
    (B)Catheter induced
    (C)Idiopathic
    (D)Previous trivial trauma

Answers:
    1. A
    2. B
    3. D
    4. B

Reference:
1. Jordan GH. Surgery of the Penis and Urethra. Wein AJ, Kavoussi LR, Novick AC, Partin AW, Peters CA (eds). Campbell-Walsh Urology, 10th ed. Philadelphia: Elsevier, 2012.p.956-1000

ELEPHANTIASIS OF PENIS

Dr. Ashok Kumar Gupta, SR, Dr. Siddarth Singh, SR, Dr. S.N. Sankhwar, Professor,
Dr. Diwakar Dalela, Professor, Dr. Apul Goel, Professor, Dept. of Urology

A 40-year old male from Bihar presented with gross enlargement of penis with thickened rough and dry skin with recurrent history of fever with chills and left lower limb swelling

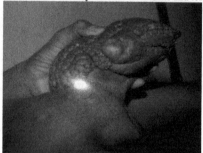

1. What is best method to diagnose penile elephantiasis?
   (A)History and physical examination
   (B)Blood for parasitemia
   (C)Penile ultrasound
   (D)Penile skin biopsy
2. Filarial disease is characterized by all of the following EXCEPT:
   (A)Elephantiasis of the limbs, chyluria, fever, localized lymphangitis, and hydrocele.
   (B)Biopsy and removal of involved lymph nodes are often necessary.
   (C)Obstructive lymphatic disease occurs in patients who are repeatedly infected.
   (D)The female mosquito *(Culex pipiens)* is the vector
3. The vector for filariasis is
   (A)Culex fatigans
   (B)Anopheles
   (C)Culex pipiens
   (D)Tsy Tsy fly
4. What is the ideal treatment for above shown condition?
   (A)DEC
   (B)Penectomy
   (C)Excision of thickened skin and flap/graft to cover raw area
   (D)all of the above

Answers:
    1. A
    2. B
    3. C
    4. C

Reference:

1. Ghoneim IA. Tuberculosis and Other Opportunistic Infections of the Genitourinary System. Wein AJ, Kavoussi LR, Novick AC, Partin AW, Peters CA (eds). Campbell-Walsh Urology, 10th ed. Philadelphia: Elsevier, 2012.p.468-494

SCROTAL CANCER

Dr. Ashok Kumar Gupta, SR, Dr. Siddarth Singh, SR, Dr. S.N. Sankhwar, Professor,
Dr. Diwakar Dalela, Professor, Dr. Apul Goel, Professor, Dept. of Urology

A 60-year old male presented with non healing ulcer over his scrotum for last 6 months. On examination an ulceroproliferative , nontender ,indurated lesion was found on scrotum with few enlarged hard inguinal nodes.

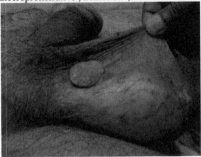

1. What is clinical diagnosis?
   - (A)Squamous Cell carcinoma of scrotum
   - (B)Basal Cell Carcinoma of scrotum
   - (C)Syphilis
   - (D)Chancroid
2. Commonest site of metastasis is:
   - (A)Inguinal nodes
   - (B)Pelvic nodes
   - (C)Liver
   - (D)Lungs
3. Gold standard for diagnosis
   - (A)Incisional Biopsy
   - (B)FNAC
   - (C)USG
   - (D)MRI
4. Treatment of choice
   - (A)Wide Local excision
   - (B)EBRT
   - (C)Chemotherapy
   - (D)Observation

Answers:
1. A
2. B
3. A
4. A

Reference:
1. EdwardR. Cutaneous Diseases of the External Genitalia. Wein AJ, Kavoussi LR, Novick AC, Partin AW, Peters CA (eds). Campbell-Walsh Urology, 10th ed. Philadelphia: Elsevier, 2012.p.436-467

FRACTURE PENIS

Dr. Ashok Kumar Gupta, SR, Dr. Siddarth Singh, SR, Dr. S.N. Sankhwar, Professor,
Dr. Diwakar Dalela, Professor, Dr. Apul Goel, Professor, Dept. of Urology

A 30-year male presented to emergency department with pain, swelling and rapid detumescence of penis during coital act following a snap sound. On examination ecchymosis was limited to penis resulting in typical "egg plant" deformity.

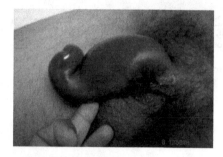

1. Best way to diagnose is:
   (A)History & physical examination
   (B)Ultrasound of penis
   (C)Contrast-enhanced CT scan penis
   (D)MRI penis
2. Penile fracture result due to tear in:
   (A)Buck's fascia
   (B)Tunica Albuginea
   (C)Dartos fascia
   (D)Carpora spongiosa
3. Which of the following statements regarding penile fracture is FALSE?
   (A)Most injuries occur ventro-laterally.
   (B)Rupture of a superficial vein can sometimes mimic the presentation of a corporeal tear.
   (C)Retrograde urethrography should be uniformly performed to assess for urethral injury.
   (D)Physical examination is usually sufficient in making the diagnosis or for deciding on surgical exploration.
4. Treatment of choice is:
   (A)Immediate surgical exploration
   (B)Angio-embolisation
   (C)Observation
   (D)Delayed exploration

Answers:
   1.   A
   2.   B,
   3.   C
   4.   A

Reference:
   1.   Morey AF. Genital and Lower Urinary Tract Trauma In: Dugi DD . Wein AJ,   Kavoussi LR, Novick AC, Partin AW, Peters CA (eds). Campbell-Walsh Urology,   10th ed. Philadelphia: Elsevier, 2012.p.436-467

BLADDER DIVERTICULUM
Dr. Ashok Sokhal, SR, Dr. Ankur Jhanwar, SR, Dr. Manoj Kumar, Assist. Professor, Dr. D. Dalela, Professor, Dr. S.N. Sankhwar, Professor, Dept. of Urology

30-years old man presented with slow urinary stream for last 6-months. Ultrasonography revealed a large bladder diverticulum with thickened bladder wall and normal upper tracts. Cystoscopy under anesthesia revealed a large wide-mouth bladder diverticulum near left ureteric orifice. The urodynamic study revealed high pressure, low flow pattern. The voiding cystourethrogram picture showed the following:

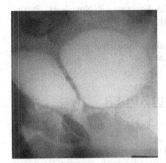

1. Voiding cystourethrogram evaluation should include-
   (A)Static antero-posterior and lateral film
   (B)Voiding antero-posterior and lateral film
   (C)Static as well as voiding antero-posterior and lateral film
   (D)Oblique film only
2. Cysto-pan-endoscopy evaluation for bladder diverticulum should include-
   (A)Anterior and posterior urethra for obstruction
   (B)Bladder for presence of other diverticula
   (C)Diverticula position in relation to ureteric orifices
   (D)All of above
3. The gold standard investigation for the diagnosis of bladder diverticulum is-
   (A)Intravenous urography
   (B)Ultrasonography
   (C)Voiding cystourethrogram (VCUG)
   (D)MR urography
4. Hutch diverticulum is-
   (A)Herniation of bladder mucosa through hiatus above the ureter.
   (B)A space created below fibro-muscular sheath extending longitudinally over the ureter.
   (C)A diverticulum formed due to enlargement of prostatic utricle.
   (D)Herniation of bladder mucosa through hiatus at trigone.
5. In acquired bladder diverticulum, first thing to be done is-
   (A)Conservative management
   (B)Infra-vesical obstruction elimination
   (C)2-week antibiotic course
   (D)Supra pubic cystostomy

Answers:

1. C
   Static as well as Voiding antero-posterior and lateral film
2. D
   All of above
   (Cysto-pan-endoscopy evaluation for bladder diverticulum should include anterior and posterior urethra for obstruction, bladder for presence of other diverticula and diverticula position in relation to ureteric orifices)
3. C
   VCUG -The voiding cystourethrogram (VCUG) remains the gold standard study in diagnosing bladder diverticula because it defines the anatomy and gross function of the bladder, bladder neck, and urethra and reveal possible accompanying VUR.
4. A
   Chronic increases in intravesical pressure resulting from bladder outlet obstruction can cause herniation of the bladder mucosa through the weakest point of the hiatus above the ureter and produces a "Hutch diverticulum"
5. B
   In acquired bladder diverticulum, the infravesical obstruction has to be eliminated first

References:

1.   Rovner ES. Bladder and Female Urethral Diverticula. Wein AJ, Kavoussi LR, Novick AC, Partin AW, Peters CA (eds). Campbell-Walsh Urology, 10th ed. Philadelphia: Elsevier, 2012. P. 2262-2289.
2.   Berrocal T, Lopez-Pereira P, Arjonilla A, Gutierrez J. Anomalies of the distal ureter, bladder and urethra in children: embryologic, radiologic and pathologic features.

SPINAL DYSRAPHISM/NEUROGENIC BLADDER

Dr. Ashok Sokhal, SR, Dr. Ankur Jhanwar, SR, Dr. Manoj Kumar, Assist. Professor, Dr. D. Dalela, Professor, Dr. S.N. Sankhwar, Professor, Dept. of Urology

A 14-years old girl presented with urinary incontinence since birth. Physical examination revealed a dimple with tuft of hair on the back in the sacral region. Digital rectal examination revealed lax anal sphincter. Her blood reports showed hemoglobin of 8.5 g%, TLC- 7200/mm³, blood urea-23 mg%, serum creatinine 0.7 mg%. Ultrasonography revealed bilateral hydroureteronephrosis (R>L) with thickened bladder with post void residual urine of 250 ml. X-ray KUB region and voiding cystourethrography images are shown below. Urodynamic study showed low compliance with stable bladder. She underwent cystoscopy under GA and was found to have normal urethra with trabeculated bladder wall.

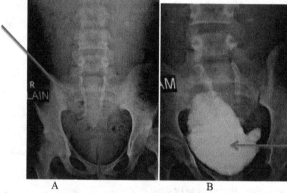

| A | B |

1. Which vitamin plays a major role in the prevention of neural tube defects?
   (A)Niacin
   (B)Riboflavin
   (C)Folic acid
   (D)B12
2. All of the following may be an external physical sign of an occult spinal dysraphism EXCEPT:
   (A)A subcutaneous mass overlying the thoracic spine.
   (B)An asymmetrical gluteal cleft.
   (C)A draining pilonidal dimple.
   (D)One leg slightly longer than the other.
3. In figure A arrow shows-
   (A)Normal sacrum
   (B)Sacral bifid spines
   (C)Lumbo-sacral disc prolapse
   (D)Sacral agenesis
4. In figure B arrow shows appearance of bladder in neurogenic conditions-
   (A)Fir tree appearance
   (B)Umbrella appearance
   (C)Cobra head appearance
   (D)Drooping lily appearance
5. What type of incontinence this patient is having-
   (A)Stress urinary incontinence
   (B)Overflow urinary incontinence
   (C)Incontinence due to abnormal communication
   (D)Incontinence due to detrusor overactivity
6. What would be the appropriate definitive treatment for this girl if she presents with gradually increasing

serum creatinine (present value 1.5 mg%) with bilateral hydroureteronephrosis-

(A)Clean intermittent self catheterization (CISC) with anti-cholinergic medications

(B)CISC with antibiotics

(C)Bladder augmentation

(D)Anti-cholinergic

Answers:

1. C

   Folic acid.

   Folic acid has been shown to reduce the incidence of neural tube defects in several large populations

2. A

   A subcutaneous mass overlying the thoracic spine

   In more than 90% of children with an occult spinal dysraphism there is a cutaneous abnormality overlying the lower spine in the lower lumbar or upper sacral areas.

3. B

   Sacral bifid spines

4. A

   Fir tree appearance

5. B

   Overflow urinary incontinence

6. C

   Bladder augmentation

References:

1. Canning DA, Lambert SM. Evaluation of the Pediatric Urology Patient. Wein AJ, Kavoussi LR, Novick AC, Partin AW, Peters CA (eds). Campbell-Walsh Urology, 10th ed. Philadelphia: Elsevier, 2012. P. 3067-3084.

2. Lapides J, Diokno AC, Silber SJ, Lowe BS. Clean intermittent self- catheterization in the treatment of urinary tract disease. J Urol 1972;107:458.

3. Palmer LS, Richards I, Kaplan WE. Age related bladder capacity and bladder capacity growth in children with myelomeningocele. J Urol 1997;158: 1261–4.

POSTERIOR URETHRAL VALVE

Dr. Ashok Sokhal, SR, Dr. Ankur Jhanwar, SR, Dr. Manoj Kumar, Assist. Professor, Dr. D. Dalela, Professor, Dr. S.N. Sankhwar, Professor, Dept. of Urology

A 3-years boy presented with weak urinary stream, crying during micturition and intermittent fever since birth. His investigations showed hemoglobin of 12.5g/dl, TLC- 10400 mm³, blood urea 30 mg% and serum creatinine 1.0mg%. Ultrasonography revealed hydroureteronephrosis with thickened trabeculated bladder with post void residue of 114 ml. The voiding cystourethrography image is shown below –

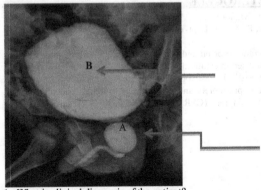

1. What is clinical diagnosis of the patient?

   (A) Anterior urethral valve

   (B) Posterior urethral valve

   (C) Phimosis

   (D) Urethral stricture

2. Name structures pointed by arrow in correct sequence-

(A)Dilated posterior urethra, B- Bladder diverticulum
(B)Bladder diverticulum, B- Dilated posterior urethra
(C)Hypertrophied bladder neck, B- Bladder diverticulum
(D)Hypertrophied bladder neck, B- Dilated posterior urethra
3. If this boy presents with azotemia and sepsis, management would be-
   (A)Temporary bladder drainage
   (B)Transurethral fulguration of the valves
   (C)Intravenous antibiotics only
   (D)Temporary bladder drainage and Intravenous antibiotics
4. Investigation of choice for diagnosis of posterior urethral valve-
   (A)Ultrasonography abdomen
   (B)Intravenous urography
   (C)Voiding cystourethrography
   (D)MAG-3 renal scan
5. Commonest site of posterior urethral valve fulguration is-
   (A) 7 O'clock
   (B) 5 O'clock
   (C) 12 O'clock
   (D) Can be fulgurated at any site

Answers:
1. B
   Posterior urethral valve
2. A
   Dilated posterior urethra, B- Bladder diverticulum
3. D
   Temporary bladder drainage and Intravenous antibiotics
4. C
   Voiding cystourethrography
5. C
   12 O'clock

References:
1. Casale AJ. Posterior Urethral Valves. Wein AJ, Kavoussi LR, Novick AC, Partin AW, Peters CA (eds). Campbell-Walsh Urology, 10th ed. Philadelphia: Elsevier, 2012. P. 3389-3410.
2. Young HH, Frontz WA, Baldwin JC. Congenital obstruction of the posterior urethra. J Urol 1919;3:289.
3. Hassan JM, Pope JC, Brock JW, et al. Vesicoureteral reflux in patients with posterior urethral valves. J Urol 2003;170:1677.

URETEROCELE

Dr. Ashok Sokhal, SR, Dr. Ankur Jhanwar, SR, Dr. Manoj Kumar, Assist. Professor, Dr. D. Dalela, Professor, Dr. S.N. Sankhwar, Professor, Dept. of Urology

6-years old girl presented with dysuria with low-grade fever on and off for last 2 years. Blood investigations showed hemoglobin of 12.7 g%, TLC 6300/mm³ and serum creatinine 0.9 mg%. Urine analysis showed 5-6 pus cells/hpf. Urine culture grew E. coli (colony count >10^5). Ultrasonography and intravenous urography revealed left duplex collecting system with hydronephrotic upper moiety and dilated ureters. Renal scan revealed left kidney contributing 40% to total glomerular filtration rate (GFR). Ultrasonography (A) and intravenous urography (B) films are shown below-

A   B

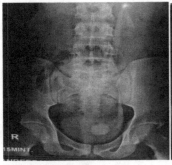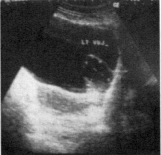

1. The diagnosis of this case is-
   (A)Bladder diverticulum
   (B)Bladder cancer
   (C)Ureterocele
   (D)Cystic rhabdo-myo-sarcoma bladder
2. In male patients it can present as all EXCEPT-
   (A)Incontinence
   (B)Urinary tract infection
   (C)Incidental detection
   (D)Pain in flank

3. During transurethral incision of ureterocele, the type incision given is-
   (A)Vertical
   (B)Transverse
   (C)Sigmoid
   (D)Any of above
4.In a case of ureterocele the classic IVU finding is-
   (A)Cobra head appearance
   (B)Drooping lilly appearance
   (C)Soap bubble appearance
   (D)Spider leg appearance

Answers:
   1. C
      ureterocele
      Ureteroceles may be seen to represent a version of the ectopic ureter with a cystic dilation of the distal aspect of the ureter that is located either within the bladder or spanning the bladder neck and urethra.
   2. A
      Incontinence
      Urinary incontinence may be due to an ectopic ureter in a girl but not in a boy. In boys ureterocele/ectopic ureters remain confined to above the external sphincter.
   3. B
      Transverse
      A transverse incision through the full thickness of the ureterocele wall using the cutting current and making the incision as distally on the ureterocele and as close to the bladder floor as possible lessens the chance of postoperative reflux into the ureterocele.
   4. A
      Cobra head appearance

References:
   1. Peters CA, Schlussel RN, Mendelsohn C. Ectopic Ureter, Ureterocele,and Ureteral Anomalies. Wein AJ, Kavoussi LR, Novick AC, Partin AW, Peters CA (eds). Campbell-Walsh Urology, 10th ed. Philadelphia: Elsevier, 2012. P. 3236-3266.
   2. Byun E, Merguerian PA. A meta-analysis of surgical practice patterns in the endoscopic management of ureteroceles. J Urol 2006;176:1871-7; discussion 1877.
   3. Stephens D. Caecoureterocele and concepts on the embryology and aetiology of ureteroceles. Aust N Z J Surg 1971;40:239-48.
   4. Lewis JM, Cheng EY, Campbell JB, et al. Complete excision or marsupialization of ureteroceles: does choice of surgical approach affect outcome? J Urol 2008;180:1819-22; discussion 1822-3.

VESICOURETERAL REFLUX

Dr. Ashok Sokhal, SR, Dr. Ankur Jhanwar, SR, Dr. Manoj Kumar, Assist. Professor, Dr. D. Dalela, Professor, Dr. S.N. Sankhwar, Professor, Dept. of Urology

A 6-years boy presented with dysuria and intermittent fever for last 10 months. His blood investigations showed hemoglobin 12 gm%, total leukocyte count of 7500/mm³, serum creatinine of 0.7 mg%. Urine culture grew >10^5 colony counts of E. coli. Ultrasonography revealed right kidney 7X3X3 cm with thickened bladder. Voiding cystourethrogram revealed bilateral reflux. Renal scan showed hydronephrotic right kidney contributing 16% to total glomerular filtration rate (GFR). His voiding cystourethrogram film is depicted below -

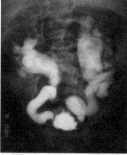

1. What is the ratio of tunnel length to ureteral diameter found in normal children without reflux?
   (A) 5:1
   (B) 4:1
   (C) 3:1
   (D) 2:1

2. Which of the following statements is TRUE regarding secondary vesico-ureteric reflux?
   (A) The most common cause of anatomic bladder outlet obstruction in the pediatric population is posterior urethral valves, and vesico-ureteral reflux is present in a great majority of these children.
   (B) Anatomic obstruction of the bladder outlet is a common cause of secondary vesico-ureteral reflux in female patients.
   (C) Patients with neuro-functional etiology for secondary vesico-ureteral reflux benefit from immediate surgical intervention to try to correct vesico-ureteral reflux.
   (D) A sacral dimple or hairy patch on the lower back is not a significant finding in regard to evaluation and treatment of vesico-ureteral reflux.

3. What is the grade of reflux seen is this voiding cystourethrogram?
   (A) I
   (B) II
   (C) III
   (D) IV to V

4 In a case of vesico-ureteral reflux, what is the best study for the detection of pyelonephritis and cortical renal scarring?
   (A) Di-ethylene tri-amine penta acetic acid (DTPA) renal scan
   (B) DMSA renal scan
   (C) Mercaptoacetyltriglycine (MAG3) renal scan
   (D) Renal ultrasonographic scan

5. Surgical management is indicated in this case if-
   (A) Grade 4 or 5 VUR
   (B) Low pressure VUR and significant hydroureter
   (C) Multiple breakthrough infections
   (D) All of above

6. If voiding cystourethrogram shows contrast in ureter   and   renal pelvis without dilatation VUR grade would be-
   (A) Grade I
   (B) Grade II
   (C) Grade III
   (D) Grade IV

Answers:
1. A
   5:1
   In Paquin's novel study, a 5:1 tunnel length:ureteral diameter ratio was found in normal children without reflux.
2. A
   The most common cause of anatomic bladder outlet obstruction in the pediatric population is posterior urethral valves, and vesicoureteral reflux is present in a great majority of these children. Between 48% and 70% of patients with posterior urethral valves have vesicoureteralreflux. The most common structural obstruction in female patients is the presence of a ureterocele that prolapses and obstructs the bladder neck.
3. D
   IV to V, both the ureters are severely dilated and tortuous.
4. B
   DMSA renal scan.
   Renal scintigraphy with technetium 99m-labeled DMSA is the best study for detection of pyelonephritis and the cortical renal scarring.
5. D
6. B
   Grade II

References:
1. Khoury AE, Bägli DJ. Vesicoureteral Reflux. Wein AJ, Kavoussi LR, Novick AC, Partin AW, Peters CA (eds). Campbell-Walsh Urology, 10th ed. Philadelphia: Elsevier, 2012. P. 3267-3309.
2. Arant Jr BS. Medical management of mild and moderate vesicoureteral reflux: follow-up studies of infants and young children. A preliminary report of the Southwest Pediatric Nephrology Study Group. J Urol 1992;148:1683–7.
3. Hodson CJ, Maling TM, McManamon PJ, et al. The pathogenesis of reflux nephropathy (chronic atrophic pyelonephritis). Br J Radiol 1975;(Suppl. 13):1–26.
4. Tamminen-Mobius T, Brunier E, Ebel KD, et al. Cessation of vesicoureteral reflux for 5 years in infants and children allocated to medical treatment.The International Reflux Study in Children. J Urol 1992;148:1662–6.

RENAL CALCULI

Dr. Ved Bhaskar, SR, Dr. Ankur Bansal, SR, Dr Rahul J Sinha, Assoc. Professor,Dr Apul Goel, Professor, Dr. Diwakar Dalela, Professor, Dept. of Urology

A 40 year old woman presented with intermittent pain in right flank since last 6 months. It was associated with vomiting and fever. There was no hematuria or dysuria. The urine examination showed 20 RBC/hpf and many leucocytes. Urine culture was sterile. X-ray KUB is shown below.

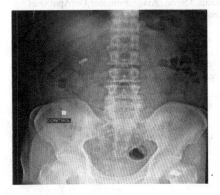

1. What is the probable diagnosis?
   (A)Right renal stone
   (B)Gall stones

(C)Calcified lymph node

(D)Normal

2. This condition can present in all of the following manners except

(A)Asymptomatic

(B)Hematuria

(C)Dysuria

(D)Suprapubic pain

3. What is investigation of choice to confirm the diagnosis -

(A)PET Scan

(B)Non contrast CT KUB

(C)Ultrasonography KUB

(D)MRI

4. What is the most common treatment option preferred for this pt

(A)Open nephrolithotomy

(B)Percutaneous nephrolithotomy (PCNL)

(C)Extracorporeal shock wave lithotripsy (ESWL)

(D)Exploratory laparotomy

Answers:

1. A

    Renal Calculus

    In a patient who presents with typical flank pain, shows microscopic haematuria, this radio-opaque shadow is likely to be renal calculus.

2. D

    Suprapubic pain

    Renal Calculus will not cause suprapubic pain if kidney is located in normal location.

3. B

    NCCT KUB

    This is regarded as investigation of choice because of high sensitivity and specificity.

4. B

    PCNL

    This stone, as is apparent by its shape, is most probably located in inferior calyx. Hence, out of all, PCNL will be most preferred option.

Reference:

1. FerrandinoMN, Wein AJ, Kavoussi LR, Novick AC, Partin AW, Peters CA (eds) Evaluation and Medical Management of Urinary Lithiasis. Campbell-Walsh Urology, 10th ed. Philadelphia: Elsevier, 2012; p1287-1323

STAGHORN CALCULUS

Dr. Ved Bhaskar, SR, Dr. Ankur Bansal, SR, Dr Rahul J Sinha, Assoc. Professor,Dr. Apul Goel, Professor, Dr. Diwakar Dalela, Professor, Dept. of Urology

A 45-year old diabetic woman presented with intermittent pain in right flank radiating from loin to groin for last 7 years sometimes accompanied with fever. There was no hematuria or dysuria. Urine analysis showed RBCs and WBCs. Urine culture grew *Proteus mirabilis*. Her serum creatinine was 3.4 mg% and serum uric acid level was 6.8 mg%. On radiological evaluation, she was found to have the following picture

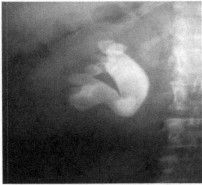

1. What is the investigation shown here?
   (A)CT scan
   (B)Plain X ray KUB
   (C)Intravenous urogram
   (D)Ultrasonogram
2. What may by the likely composition of this staghorn calculus
   (A)Calcium oxalate monohydrate
   (B)Calcium oxalate dehydrate
   (C)Calcium-Magnisium-Ammonium phosphate
   (D)Calcium Phosphate
3. What other investigations you may like to do
   (A)Contrast-enhanced CT KUB
   (B)DTPA Renal scan
   (C)Intravenous pyelography
   (D)MRI KUB
4. What are the most common treatment options available for this patient?
   (A)One-stage PCNL
   (B)Open extended pyelolithotomy
   (C)ESWL
   (D)Retrograde Intra-renal surgery (RIRS)
5. All these can be the problem if the condition is not treated timely EXCEPT
   (A)Non-functioning kidney
   (B)Hydronephrosis
   (C)Pyonephrosis
   (D)Adenocarcinoma kidney

Answers:

1. B

   Plain X ray KUB

   The radio opacity of the calculus in same as that of vertebral bodies. Hence the picture is that of plain x-ray KUB

2. C

   Calcium –Mag. – Ammonium Phosphate

   In a diabetic female, who has been having history of febrile UTI and urine culture grows Proteus bacteriastruvite (Ca-Mag.Ammo. Phos.) in the most likely composition.

3. C

   MRI

   Because the patient is having renal failure, only test that may be done is MRI.

4. B

   Open extended pyelolithotomy

   In presence of history of fever and positive urine C/s in a diabetic lady, it may not be prudent to do once stage PCNL or ESWL or RIRS. Open extended pyelolithotomy, shall be better.

5. D

   Adenocarcinoma Kidney

   Renal adenocarcinoma is not known to develop on account of renal stone.

Reference:
1. FerrandinoMN.Evaluation andMedical Management of Urinary Lithiasis. Wein AJ, Kavoussi LR, Novick AC, Partin AW, Peters CA (eds). Campbell-Walsh Urology, 10th ed. Philadelphia: Elsevier, 2012; p1287-1323

URETERIC CALCULUS

Dr. Ved Bhaskar, SR, Dr. Ankur Bansal, SR, Dr Rahul J Sinha, Assoc. Professor, Dr ApulGoel, Professor, Dr. Diwakar Dalela, Professor, Dept. of Urology

A 35-year old man presented with intermittent severe colicky pain in left lumbar and iliac region for 3 months. It was associated with 2 episodes of hematuria. His urinalysis showed plenty of RBCs and WBCs. His serum creatinine is 0.9 mg%, serum uric acid is 7.0 mg% and serum calcium is 8.7 mg%. USG KUB showed normal right kidney and mild hydroureteronephrosis on left side. X ray KUB image is shown below

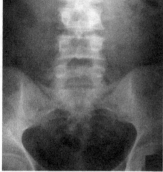

1. What is the probable diagnosis?
   (A)Fecolith
   (B)Ureteric calculus (Left)
   (C)Calcified lymph node
   (D)Bladder calculus
2. Investigations done in such patients may be all of the following **except**
   (A)Intravenous pyelography
   (B)CT Urography
   (C)DTPA Renal scan
   (D)PET scan
3. What may be the treatment options available for this patient?
   (A)Open ureterolithotomy
   (B)Ureteroscopic removal
   (C)Medical Expulsive Therapy
   (D)All the above
4. Medicines used to manage these stones conservatively may be all of the following except -
   (A)Calcium channel blockers
   (B)B.Tamsulosin
   (C)Deflazacort
   (D)Hydrocortisone
5. All of the following may be the problems if the condition is not treated timely, **Except**
   (A)Progressive Hydroureterohephrosis
   (B)Pyonephrosis
   (C)Non-functioning kidney
   (D)Metabolic acidosis

Answers:
1. B
    Ureteric calculus (left),
    In view of typical symptoms, microscopic haematuria & pyuria, most probable diagnosis will be ureteric calculus, the radio opaque shadow of which is seen on x-ray KUB.
2. D

PET Scan

PET scan is usually done for malignancies.

3. D

All the above,

Lower ureteric calculus may be managed by any of these methods depending upon availability and technical experience of surgeons.

4. D

Hydrocortisone,

Hydrocortisone is not needed, rest all have been used as part of medical expulsive therapy.

5. D

Metabolic acidosis

Metabolic acidosis occurs only when there is acute renal failure. This is unlikely due to normal opposite kidney an evident by her USG KUB.

Reference:

1. FerrandinoMN.Evaluation andMedical Management of Urinary Lithiasis. Wein AJ, Kavoussi LR, Novick AC, Partin AW, Peters CA (eds). Campbell-Walsh Urology, 10th ed. Philadelphia: Elsevier, 2012; p1287-1323

VESICAL CALCULUS

Dr. Ved Bhaskar, SR, Dr. Ankur Bansal, SR, Dr Rahul J Sinha, Assoc. Professor,Dr Apul Goel, Professor, Dr. Diwakar Dalela, Professor, Dept. of Urology

A 65-year old man presented with intermittent suprapubic pain and terminal hematuria for last 6 months. He has been having obstructed urinary stream with increased frequency and nocturia for last 6 years. His urinalysis showed plenty of RBCs and WBCs. The urine culture showed *E. coli.*On evaluation with X ray KUB he was found to have the following picture.

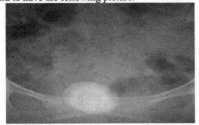

1. What is can be the probable diagnosis?
   (A)Fecolith
   (B)Bladder calculus
   (C)Calcified Prostate
   (D)Osteoma of Pubis
2. What are the treatment options available for this patient?
   (A)Transurethral Pneumatic Cystolitholapaxy
   (B)Percutaneous cystolitholapaxy
   (C)Open cystolithotomy
   (D)All the above
3. What can be the problems if the condition is not treated timely?
   (A)Recurrent UTI
   (B)Hydroureteronephrosis
   (C)Urinary retention
   (D)All the above
4. What is the composition of Jackstone calculus?
   (A)Calcium oxalate dihydrate
   (B)Calcium oxalate monohydrate
   (C)Uric acid
   (D)Cystine

Answers:

1. B

Bladder calculus

In view of history of suprapubic pain, haematuria, positive culture and x-ray showing laminated radio-opaque shadow, calculus in bladder in most probable diagnosis.

2. D

All of above

As per the availability of facility and technical expertise any of the method may be used for removal of this bladder calculus.

3. D

All the above

All the problems can occur either singly or in various combinations.

4. A

Calcium**oxalate dihydrate**

Jackstone is a very hard, dark brown stone developing in bladder. Commonly this is made of calcium oxalate monohydrate.

Reference:

1. Benway BM.Lower Urinary Tract Calculi. Wein AJ, Kavoussi LR, Novick AC, Partin AW, Peters CA (eds). Campbell-Walsh Urology, 10th ed. Philadelphia: Elsevier, 2012; p2581-2532

POST ESWL STEINSTRASSE

Dr. Ved Bhaskar, SR, Dr. Ankur Bansal, SR, Dr Rahul J Sinha, Assoc. Professor,Dr Apul Goel, Professor, Dr. Diwakar Dalela, Professor, Dept. of Urology

A 36-year old man presented with right flank pain since 3 months. On evaluation with X-ray KUB and intravenous pyelography he was found to have right superior calyceal calculus. He underwent Extracorporeal Shock Wave Lithotripsy (ESWL) for the same. 15 days post-ESWL his plain X ray is shown below

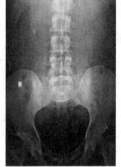

1. What does this picture show?
   (A)Renal calculus
   (B)Lower ureteric calculus
   (C)Steinstrasse
   (D)All are true
2. This condition is common after which procedure
   (A)Percutaneous Nephrolithotomy
   (A)Extracorporeal Shockwave Lithotripsy
   (C)Open pyelolithotomy
   (D)All of above
3. What is the treatment option available for this patient?
   (A)Conservative
   (B)Double J stent placement
   (C)Ureteroscopic removal
   (D)All the above
4. What should be the treatment at this stage?
   (A)Continue with another session of ESWL for the remaining renal stone fragment
   (B)Treat lower ureteric calculi first
   (C)Wait & watch
   (D)Parenteral antibiotics

5. The word "Steinstrasse" means
   (A)House of stones
   (B)Street of stones
   (C)Pack of stones
   (D)Fragmented Stones

Answers:
   1. D
      All are true
      This x-ray KUB is showing all of these.
   2. B
      ESWL
      In ESWL, the intact calculus is broken into many small fragments which themselves pass down. In that process, sometimes many small particles pile up behind a leading fragment.
   3. D
      All the above
      Either of method may be utilized for treating this case, depending upon availability technology and proper expertise.
   4. B
      Treat for lower ureteric calculi first
      If the lead fragment is removed somehow, rest of the fragments may themselves pass out.
   5. B
      Street of stones
      "Steinstrasse" word in German language means, a street of stones.

Reference:
   1. Wolf JS. Percutaneous Approaches to the Upper Urinary Tract Collecting System. Wein AJ, Kavoussi LR, Novick AC, Partin AW, Peters CA (eds). Campbell-Walsh Urology, 10th ed. Philadelphia: Elsevier, 2012; C.2012 .p.1324-1356

RENAL CELL CARCINOMA

Dr Kawaljeet Singh, SR, Dr Gautam Kanodia, SR, Dr Manmeet Singh, Assist. Professor, Dr Apul Goel, Professor, Dr. D. Dalela, Professor, Dept. of Urology

A 35-years man with left cervical lymphadenopathy of 2-months duration underwent FNAC that revealed clear cell pathology that prompted further evaluation. Clinical examination revealed pallor and left cervical lymph node enlargement. His BP was 170/85mm Hg and laboratory examination showed polycythemia and serum calcium 13.1mg/dl. Ultrasonography showed left renal mass (7X6cm) in lower pole and contrast-enhanced CT scan revealed a well-defined solid-cystic lesion with areas of hemorrhage and calcification measuring 7.8X6.9X7.0 cm involving the lower pole of left kidney, abutting adjacent bowel loops, left ureter and left renal vessels with few well-defined lesions seen in both lobes of liver (suspicious metastasis) and multiple lymph nodes in para-aortic region

1. What is the most probable diagnosis?
   (A)Renal cell cancer
   (B)Transitional Cell Carcinoma
   (C)Renal Sarcoma

(D)Renal Tuberculosis
2. Identify the structure shown by the arrow in the above shown CT scan film.
 (A)Right Kidney
 (B)Left Kidney
 (C)Liver
 (D)Retroperitoneum mass
3. What is the best initial management in this patient?
 (A)Left Radical Nephrectomy.
 (B)Chemotherapy.
 (C)Radiotherapy.
 (D)Targeted therapy.
4. What is the cause of hypertension in this patient?
 (A)Increased production of rennin directly by the tumor
 (B)Compression of the renal artery leading to renal artery stenosis
 (C)Arteriovenous fistula within the tumor
 (D)All of the above
5. What is the cause of hypercalcemia in RCC?
 (A)Paraneoplastic phenomenon
 (B)Osteolytic metastatic involvement
 (C)Both of the above
 (D)None of the above

Answers:
1. A
2. A
3. A
4. D
5. C

Reference:
1. Campbell SC, Lane BR. Malignant Renal Tumours. Wein AJ, Kavoussi LR, Novick AC, Partin AW, Peters CA (eds). Campbell-Walsh Urology, 10th ed. Philadelphia: Elsevier, 2012;1413-73.

PELVIC – URETERIC JUNCTION OBSTRUCTION (PUJO)
Dr Kawaljeet Singh, SR, Dr Gautam Kanodia, SR, Dr Manmeet Singh, Assist. Professor, Dr Apul Goel, Professor, Dr. D. Dalela, Professor, Dept. of Urology

A 15 years old girl presented with right flank pain associated with nausea for last 2 months with no fever or haematuria. Clinical examination showed pallor with hypertension (B.P.= 145/92mm of Hg). Urine analysis showed 0-2 pus cells, 12 RBCs/hpf and urine culture was sterile. Ultrasonography abdomen showed moderate hydronephrosis of right side with normal left kidney. CT film is depicted below:

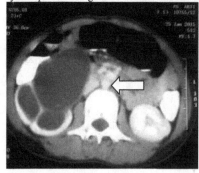

1. What is the probable diagnosis:
 (A)Right renal cyst
 (B)Right polycystic Kidney
 (C)Multicystic dysplastic kidney

(D)Right pelvi-ureteral junction obstruction
2. What is the next best step after contrast-enhanced CT scan to assess the functional status of kidney in this patient?
   (A)Contrast-enhanced CT scan is adequate and gives information of renal function
   (B)MRI
   (C)Diuretic DTPA/EC Nuclear Renal Scan
   (D)Doppler of renal arteries
3. What are the acquired causes of PUJO?
   (A)Vesicoureteral reflux in children
   (B)Fibroepithelial polyps
   (C)Urothelial malignancy
   (D)All of the above
4. What is the structure shown by arrow in the above shown contrast enhanced CT scan film?
   (A)Aorta
   (B)Inferior Vena Cava
   (C)Superior Mesenteric Artery
   (D)Artery of Drummond
5. What are the indications of intervention in this patient?
   (A)Presence of symptoms associated with the obstruction
   (B)Impairment of overall renal function
   (C)Stones or infection
   (D)All of the above

Answers:
   1. D
   2. C
   3. D
   4. A
   5. D

Reference:

1. Campbell SC, Lane BR. Malignant Renal Tumours. Wein AJ, Kavoussi LR, Novick AC, Partin AW, Peters CA (eds). Campbell-Walsh Urology, 10th ed. Philadelphia: Elsevier, 2012;1413-73.

ADULT POLYCYSTIC KIDNEY DISEASE

Dr Kawaljeet Singh, SR, Dr Gautam Kanodia, SR, Dr Manmeet Singh, Assist. Professor, Dr Apul Goel, Professor, Dr. D. Dalela, Professor, Dept. of Urology

A 50-year old chronic smoker presented with hematuria and flank pain of 6-months duration. He lost 11 kg weight in past 6 months and clinical examination showed pallor. There was no jaundice, thyroid enlargement or lymphadenopathy. Urine culture was sterile and urine for malignant cells only showed epithelial cells. His serum creatinine was 1.2 mg%. Ultrasound abdomen revealed multiple space occupying lesions of variable sizes in bilateral kidneys with a suspicious lesion (0.5 X 1cm) in liver. Contrast enhanced CT scan film is shown below:

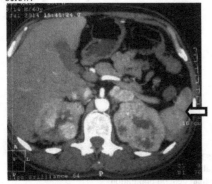

1. What is the most probable diagnosis?
   (A)Adult Polycystic Kidney Disease
   (B)Bilateral Renal Cell Carcinoma
   (C)Angiomyolipoma
   (D)Lymphoma
2. What is the most common familial syndrome associated with bilateral renal   tumours?
   (A)Von Hippel-Lindau syndrome
   (B)Hereditary papillary RCC
   (C)Familial leiomyomatosis and RCC
   (D)Birt-Hogg-Dubé syndrome
3. What is the structure shown in the above CT scan picture?
   (A)Spleen
   (B)Stomach
   (C)Left colon
   (D)Hepatic flexure.

Answers:
   1. B
   2. A
   3. A

Reference:
   1. Pope JC. Renal Dysgenesis and Cystic Disease of the Kidney. Wein AJ, Kavoussi LR, Novick AC, Partin AW, Peters CA (eds). Campbell-Walsh Urology, 10th ed. Philadelphia: Elsevier, 2012; 3161-96.

RENAL CELL CARCINOMA IN HORSE SHOE KIDNEY

Dr Kawaljeet Singh, SR, Dr Gautam Kanodia, SR, Dr Manmeet Singh, Assist. Professor, Dr Apul Goel, Professor, Dr. D. Dalela, Professor, Dept. of Urology

A 60 years old man presented with hematuria for last 1 month. Few days back he had an episode of acute urinary retention for which foley catheter (16) Fr was placed at a primary health center and patient was referred to higher center for further management. Patient was urgently taken for cystoscopic clot evacuation and no bladder growth was found on cystoscopy. Urine analysis revealed epithelial cells with abundant RBCs. Ultrasound abdomen revealed horseshoe kidney with a space occupying lesion (5 X 7cm in size) present in its right moiety. On further evaluation with CECT, the following picture was obtained:

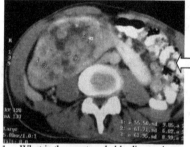

1.   What is the most probable diagnosis
     (A)Renal cell carcinoma
     (B)Renal Pelvic Tumour
     (C)Renal lymphoma
     (D)Renal carcinoids
2.   What is the most common fusion anomaly of kidney?
     (A)Horseshoe kidney
     (B)Pelvic kidney
     (C)Thoracic Kidney
     (D)Pancake kidney
3.   Which of the following is true?
     (A)Incidence of renal pelvis tumours in horseshoe kidney is more than general population
     (B)Incidence of RCC in horseshoe kidney is same as general population
     (C)Incidence of wilms tumour in horseshoe kidney is more than general population
     (D)All of the above.

4. What is the structure shown by the arrow in above shown CT scan film?
   (A)Isthmus of horseshoe kidney
   (B)Right kidney mass
   (C)Retroperitoneal fibrosis
   (D)Left kidney mass
5. What is the ideal management plan of the above mentioned patient?
   (A)Right Radical Nephrectomy with preservation of normal moiety
   (B)Right Partial nephrectomy
   (C)Preoperative sunitinib
   (D)Radiotherapy and chemotherapy.

Answers:
   1. A
   2. A
   3. D
   4. A
   5. A

Reference:
   1. Shapiro E. Anomalies of the Upper Urinary Tract. Wein AJ, Kavoussi LR, Novick AC, Partin AW, Peters CA (eds). Campbell-Walsh Urology, 10th ed. Philadelphia: Elsevier, 2012; 3123-60.

ADULT POLYCYSTIC KIDNEY DISEASE
Dr Kawaljeet Singh, SR, Dr Gautam Kanodia, SR, Dr Manmeet Singh, Assist. Professor, Dr Apul Goel, Professor, Dr. D. Dalela, Professor, Dept. of Urology

A 35 year lady presented with pain right flank region for last 2 months. There was history of her mother dying of renal failure at the age of 52 years. Her B.P. was 150/88mm of Hg. Abdomen examination revealed that the liver was palpable up to 3 fingers below the right costal margin.
Biochemistry showed Hb 12.5mg/dl and urine examination consists of plenty of RBCs. Evaluation with ultrasonography showed multiple cysts (of variable sizes) in both kidneys and liver. Further evaluation with CT showed the following picture:

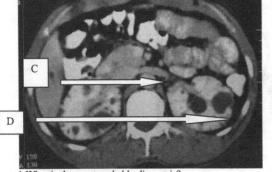
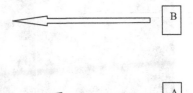

1.What is the most probable diagnosis?
   (A)Autosomal dominant polycystic kidney disease
   (B)Juvenile nephronophthisis
   (C)Simple cysts of kidney
   (D)Renal Cell Carcinoma.
2.In the above shown contrast enhanced CT scan film, liver is shown by:
   (A)A
   (B)B
   (C)C
   (D)D
3.What is true about hypertension in this patient?
   (A)50% patients with normal renal function are hypertensive.
   (B)Hypertension is renin mediated

(C)Early treatment of hypertension is essential to slow the progression to renal failure.
(D)All of the above

4.What is the incidence risk of RCC in this patient?
    (A)More than general population
    (B)less than general population
    (C)Equal to general population
    (D)None

5.Which is true regarding screening of this patient for renal cell carcinoma?
    (A)Routinely done
    (B)Screening not done routinely
    (C)Screening only done in patients with cerebral involvement
    (D)Screening done only in patients presenting with renal failure.

Answers:
    1. A
    2. C
    3. D
    4. C
    5. B

Reference:
1. Pope JC. Renal Dysgenesis and Cystic Disease of the Kidney. Wein AJ, Kavoussi LR, Novick AC, Partin AW, Peters CA (eds). Campbell-Walsh Urology, 10th ed. Philadelphia: Elsevier, 2012; 3161-96.

TRANSITIONAL CELL CARCINOMA OF RENAL PELVIC

Dr Kawaljeet Singh, SR, Dr Gautam Kanodia, SR, Dr Manmeet Singh, Assist. Professor, Dr Apul Goel, Professor, Dr. D. Dalela, Professor, Dept. of Urology

A 50 year old labourer working in a tyre manufacturing company, presented with gross haematuria for last 2 months with 5 kg weight loss in last 6 months. There was no family history of malignancy. He was a chronic smoker for last 25 years. His B.P was 138/78mm of Hg and pallor was present. Urine examination for malignant cells showed two out of three samples positive for malignant cells. Ultrasonography revealed a space occupying lesion (2X2cm) in left renal sinus. Intravenous pyelogram (A) and CT scan (B) films are shown below:

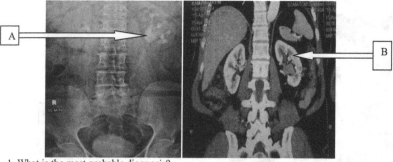

1. What is the most probable diagnosis?
    (A)Renal cell carcinoma
    (B)Transitional cell carcinoma of left renal pelvis
    (C)Clots in left renal pelvis
    (D)Renal staghorn calculus

2.What is the most important risk factor causally associated with this disease?
    (A)Smoking
    (B)Alcohol consumption
    (C)Family history
    (D)Arsenic

3.What is the most common sign shown on intravenous pyelogram (A) to depict this disease?
    (A)Filling defect
    (B)Cullen sign
    (C)Grey Turner sign
    (D)Hour glass sign

4.What is the incidence of bladder cancer in this patient in near future?
   (A)15% – 75% over 5 years
   (B)10% -20% over 5 years
   (C)5% – 10% over 5 years
   (D)>90% over 5 years
5.What is the structure shown as (B) in the above contrast enhanced CT scan picture?
   (A)Left renal pelvis with growth
   (B)Left renal vein with clot
   (C)Left renal artery
   (D)Left kidney lower pole tumour

Answers:
   1.   B
   2.   A
   3.   A
   4.   A
   5.   A

Reference:
   1.   Sagalowsky AI. Urothelial Tumors of the Upper Urinary Tract and Ureter. Wein AJ, Kavoussi LR, Novick AC, Partin AW, Peters CA (eds). Campbell-Walsh Urology, 10th ed. Philadelphia: Elsevier, 2012; 1516-53.

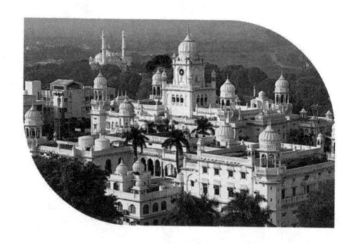

Printed in the United States
By Bookmasters